D1369435

Evidence-Based Geriatric Nursing Protocols for Best Practice

Marie Boltz, PhD, RN, APRN-BC, is an assistant professor at New York University (NYU) where she has directed the undergraduate course in Nursing Care of Adults and Elders. Dr. Boltz is also practice director of the NICHE (Nurses Improving Care for Healthsystem Elders) program, which is the only national nursing program designed to improve care of the older adult patient. Her areas of research are the geriatric care environment including measures of quality, the geriatric nurse practice environment, and the prevention of functional decline in hospitalized older adults. She has presented nationally and internationally and authored and coauthored numerous journal publications, organizational tools, and book chapters in these areas. Dr. Boltz is a John A. Hartford Foundation Claire M. Fagin fellow and the 2009–2010 American Nurses Credentialing Center (ANCC) Margretta Madden Styles Credentialing scholar.

Elizabeth Capezuti, PhD, RN, FAAN, is the Dr. John W. Rowe Professor in Successful Aging at the College of Nursing at NYU. She also serves as codirector for the Hartford Institute for Geriatric Nursing where she directs the research center. She is an internationally recognized geriatric nurse researcher, known for her work in improving the care of older adults by interventions and models that positively influence a health care provider's knowledge and work environment. Her current studies focus primarily on translating effective interventions into actual practice, specifically, testing of new technologies for promoting independence and system change approaches to transform provider behavior. A recipient of more than $8 million in research and training grants, she has disseminated the findings of 35 funded projects in four coedited books and more than a hundred peer reviewed articles and book chapters. Dr. Capezuti received her doctoral degree in nursing from the University of Pennsylvania in 1995. She joined the NYU faculty in 2003 and was promoted to professor in 2008. She has also been on the faculty of the University of Pennsylvania School of Nursing from 1984 to 2000 where she received the 1995 Provost's Award for Distinguished Teaching. From 2000 to 2003, she held the Independence Foundation—Wesley Woods Chair in Gerontologic Nursing at Emory University. She is a fellow of the American Academy of Nursing, the Gerontological Society of America, the American Association of Nurse Practitioners, and the New York Academy of Medicine.

Terry Fulmer, PhD, RN, FAAN, is the dean of the Bouvé College of Health Sciences at Northeastern University. She received her bachelor's degree from Skidmore College, her master's and doctoral degrees from Boston College, and her Geriatric Nurse Practitioner Post-Master's Certificate from NYU. Dr. Fulmer's program of research focuses on acute care of the elderly and, specifically, elder abuse and neglect. She has received the status of fellow in the American Academy of Nursing, the Gerontological Society of America, and the New York Academy of Medicine. She completed a Brookdale National Fellowship and is a distinguished practitioner of the National Academies of Practice. Dr. Fulmer was the first nurse to be elected to the board of the American Geriatrics Society and the first nurse to serve as the president of the Gerontological Society of America.

DeAnne Zwicker, DrNP, APRN, BC is an ANCC certified adult nurse practitioner and is currently working as independent geriatric consultant. She completed her doctor of nursing practice (DrNP) in 2010 with a primary focus as a clinical scientist and secondary in education at Drexel University in Philadelphia. Her dissertation was entitled *Preparedness, Appraisal of Behaviors, and Role Strain in Dementia Family Caregivers and the Caregiver Perspective of Preparedness* and was a mixed-method study. She was a coeditor and chapter author for the fourth edition of *Evidence-based Geriatric Nursing Protocols* (in press) as well as the third edition (2008), and managing editor for the second edition (2003). She has served as the content editor of www.ConsultGeriRN.org since its inception. She recently instituted the NICHE program at Washington Hospital Center, which was awarded national NICHE designation. Ms. Zwicker has been a registered nurse for 32 years, with clinical practice experience as a geriatric nurse practitioner since 1992 in primary care, subacute care, long-term care, and clinical expert consultant in geriatrics. She has also taught nursing at the graduate level at NYU and Drexel University. Her areas of interest in geriatrics include proactive interventions in older adults, including prevention of adverse drug events and iatrogenesis in persons with dementia and prevention and/or early recognition of delirium.

Ardis O'Meara, MA manages *Geriatric Nursing, Heart and Lung: The Journal of Acute and Critical Care,* and other geriatric nursing books. Her experience includes cardiology and research.

Evidence-Based Geriatric Nursing Protocols for Best Practice

4th Edition

Marie Boltz, PhD, RN, APRN-BC
Elizabeth Capezuti, PhD, RN, FAAN
Terry Fulmer, PhD, RN, FAAN
DeAnne Zwicker, DrNP, APRN, BC
EDITORS

Ardis O'Meara, MA
MANAGING EDITOR

SPRINGER PUBLISHING COMPANY
NEW YORK

Copyright © 2012 Springer Publishing Company, LLC

All rights reserved.

No part of this publication may be reproduced, stored in a retrieval system, or transmitted in any form or by any means, electronic, mechanical, photocopying, recording, or otherwise, without the prior permission of Springer Publishing Company, LLC, or authorization through payment of the appropriate fees to the Copyright Clearance Center, Inc., 222 Rosewood Drive, Danvers, MA 01923, 978-750-8400, fax 978-646-8600, info@copyright.com or on the web at www.copyright.com.

Springer Publishing Company, LLC
11 West 42nd Street
New York, NY 10036
www.springerpub.com

Acquisitions Editor: Margaret Zuccarini
Composition: Absolute Service, Inc.

ISBN 978-0-8261-7128-3
E-book ISBN: 978-0-8261-7129-0
11 12 13 / 5 4 3 2 1

The author and the publisher of this work have made every effort to use sources believed to be reliable to provide information that is accurate and compatible with the standards generally accepted at the time of publication. The author and the publisher shall not be liable for any special, consequential, or exemplary damages resulting, in whole or in part, from the readers' use of, or reliance on, the information contained in this book. The publisher has no responsibility for the persistence or accuracy of URLs for external or third party Internet websites referred to in this publication and does not guarantee that any content on such websites is, or will remain, accurate or appropriate.

Library of Congress Cataloging-in-Publication Data

Evidence-based geriatric nursing protocols for best practice / [edited by] Marie Boltz ... [et al.]. — 4th ed.
    p. ; cm.
  Includes bibliographical references and index.
  ISBN 978-0-8261-7128-3 — ISBN 978-0-8261-7129-0 (e-book)
  I. Boltz, Marie.
  [DNLM: 1. Geriatric Nursing—methods. 2. Nursing Care. 3. Aged. 4. Evidence-Based Nursing. 5. Nursing Assessment. WY 152]

  618.97'0231—dc23
                            2011038613

Special discounts on bulk quantities of our books are available to corporations, professional associations, pharmaceutical companies, health care organizations, and other qualifying groups.

If you are interested in a custom book, including chapters from more than one of our titles, we can provide that service as well.

For details, please contact:
Special Sales Department, Springer Publishing Company, LLC
11 West 42nd Street, 15th Floor, New York, NY 10036-8002
Phone: 877-687-7476 or 212-431-4370
Fax: 212-941-7842
Email: sales@springerpub.com

Printed in the United States of America by Bang Printing

Contents

v

Contributors

Elaine J. Amella, PhD, RN, FAAN Professor, Medical University of South Carolina, Mt. Pleasant, SC

Melissa B. Aselage, MSN, RN-BC, FNP-BC Lecturer, University of North Carolina, Wilmington, NC

Elizabeth Ann Ayello, PhD, RN, APRN, BC, CWOCN, FAPWCA, FAAN President, Ayello, Harris & Associates, Inc., Clinical Associate Editor, Advances in Skin & Wound Care, Faculty, Excelsior College, School of Nursing, Executive Editor, Journal of World Council of Enterostomal Therapists

Michele C. Balas, PhD, RN, APRN-NP, CCRN Assistant Professor, University of Nebraska Medical Center (UNMC), Omaha, NE

Marie Boltz, PhD, RN, APRN-BC Assistant Professor, New York University, New York, NY

Cheryl M. Bradas, RN, MSN, GCNS-BC, CHPN Geriatric Clinical Nurse Specialist, MetroHealth Medical Center, Cleveland, OH

Christine Bradway, PhD, RN, CRNP Assistant Professor, University of Pennsylvania, Philadelphia, PA

Tom Braes, RN, MSN Managing Director, Nursing Home Zoniën, OCMW Tervuren, Belgium

Pamela Z. Cacchione, PhD, RN, GNP-BC Associate Professor, University of Pennsylvania, Philadelphia, PA

Elizabeth Capezuti, PhD, RN, FAAN Dr. John W. Rowe Professor in Successful Aging at the College of Nursing, New York University, New York, NY

Billy A. Caceres, RN, BSN, BA Research Assistant, New York University, New York, NY

Colleen M. Casey, PhD, MS, RN, CCRN, CNS Nurse Practitioner, Internal Medicine and Geriatrics Oregon Health Sciences University Healthcare

Eileen R. Chasens, DSN Assistant Professor, University of Pittsburgh, Pittsburgh, PA

Deborah A. Chyun, MSN, PhD, RN Associate Professor, Yale University, New Haven, CT

Valerie T. Cotter, DrNP, CRNP, FAANP Advanced Senior Lecturer, University of Pennsylvania School of Nursing, Philadelphia, PA

Jessica Coviello, MSN, APRN Associate Professor, Yale University, New Haven, CT

Rose Ann DiMaria-Ghalili, PhD, RN, CNSN Associate Professor, Drexel University, Philadelphia, PA

Annemarie Dowling-Castronovo, MA, RN, GNP Assistant Professor, Wagner College, Staten Island, NY

Regina M. Fink, RN, PhD, FAAN, AOCN Research Nurse Scientist, University of Colorado Hospital, Aurora, CO

Kathleen Fletcher, RN, MSN, APRN-BC, GNP, FAAN Administrator of Senior Services, University of Virginia Health System, Charlottesville, Virginia.

Marquis D. Foreman, PhD, RN, FAAN Professor and Chairperson, Rush University, Chicago, IL

Janice Foust, PhD, RN Assistant Professor, University of Massachusetts, Boston, MA

Deborah C. Francis, RN, MSN, GCNS-BC Geriatric Clinical Nurse Specialist, Kaiser Permanente Medical Center, South Sacramento, CA

Terry Fulmer, PhD, RN, FAAN Dean of the Bouvé College of Health Sciences, Northeastern University, Boston, MA

Elizabeth Galik, PhD, CRNP Assistant Professor, University of Maryland, Baltimore, MD

Mindy Grall, PhD, APRN, BC Advanced Registered Nurse Practitioner, Baptist Medical Center, Jacksonville, FL

Deanna Gray-Miceli, PhD, GNP-BC, FAANP Assistant Professor, Rutgers University, New Brunswick, NJ

Mary Beth Happ, PhD, RN, FAAN Professor, University of Pittsburgh, Pittsburgh, PA

Theresa A. Harvath, PhD, RN, CNS, FAAN Professor, Oregon Health & Science University, Portland, OR

Ann L. Horgas, PhD, RN, FGSA, FAAN Associate Professor, University of Florida, Gainesville, FL

Susan Kaplan Jacobs, MLS, MA, RN, AHIP Health Sciences Librarian/Associate Curator, Elmer Holmes Bobst Library, New York University, New York, NY

Meredith Wallace Kazer, PhD, APRN, A/GNP-BC Associate Professor, Fairfield University, Fairfield, CT

Denise M. Kresevic, RN, PhD, GNP-BC, GCNS-BC Nurse Researcher, Louis Stokes Cleveland VAMC, University Hospitals Case Medical Center, Case Western Reserve University, Cleveland, OH

Jeanne M. Lahaie, RN, MS, GCNS-BC Elder Life Nurse Specialist, Hospital Elder Life Program (HELP), California Pacific Medical Center, San Francisco, CA

Rona F. Levin, PhD, RN Professor, Pace University and Visiting Faculty, Visiting Nurse Service of New York, New York, NY

Fidelindo Lim, RN, MA Clinical Instructor, New York University, New York, NY

Glenise L. McKenzie, RN, MN, PhD Assistant Professor, Oregon Health & Science University, Ashland, OR

Mary Beth Flynn Makic, RN, PhD, CNS, CCNS, CCRN   Research Nurse Scientist, University of Colorado Hospital and Assistant Professor, Adjoint, University of Colorado, Aurora, CO

Janet C. Mentes, PhD, APRN, BC, FGSA   Associate Professor, University of California, Los Angeles, Los Angeles, CA

Deborah C. Messecar, PhD, MPH, GCNS-BC, RN   Associate Professor, Oregon Health & Science University, School of Nursing, Portland, OR

Koen Milisen, PhD, RN   Professor, Katholieke Universiteit, Leuven, Belgium

Lorraine C. Mion, PhD, RN, FAAN   Independence Foundation Professor of Nursing, Vanderbilt University, Nashville, TN

Ethel L. Mitty, EdD, RN   Adjunct Clinical Professor, New York University, New York, NY

Madeline Naegle, APRN, BC, PhD, FAAN   Professor, New York University, New York, NY

Cynthia J. Nigolian, RN, GCNS, BC   NICHE Clinical Administrator, New York, NY

Linda J. O'Connor, MSN, RNC, GCNS-BC, CLNC   Assistant Administrator for Nursing and Hospital Affairs, Mount Sinai Hospital, New York, NY

Kathleen S. Oman, RN, MS, PhD   Research Nurse Scientist, Assistant Professor (Adjoint), University of Colorado Hospital, Aurora, CO

Janine Overcash, PhD, GNP   Assistant Professor, University of South Florida, Tampa, FL

Lenard L. Parisi, RN, MA, CPHQ, FNAHQ   Vice President, Quality Management/ Performance Improvement, Metropolitan Jewish Health System, Brooklyn, NY

Linda Farber Post, JD, MA, BSN   Director, Bioethics, Hackensack University Medical Center, Hackensack, NJ

Patricia A. Quigley, PhD, MPH, APRN, CRRN, FAAN, FAANP   Associate Chief, Nursing Service for Research, Health Service and Rehabilitation Research Center of Excellence: Maximizing Rehabilitation Outcomes and Associate Director, VISN 8 Patient Safety Center, James A. Haley VA Hospital, Tampa, FL

Barbara Resnick, PhD, CRNP, FAAN, FAANP   Professor and Sonya Ziporkin Gershowitz Chair in Gerontology, University of Maryland, Baltimore, MD

Satinderpal K. Sandhu, MD   Assistant Professor, MetroHealth Medical Center and Case Western Reserve University School of Medicine, Cleveland, OH

Judith E. Schipper, MS, NP-C, CLS, FNLA, FPCNA   Clinical Coordinator, Heart Failure Program, New York University Langone Medical Center, New York, NY

R. Gary Sibbald, MD, FRCPC, ABIM, DABD, Med   Director, Wound Healing Clinic, The New Women's College Hospital and Professor, Public Health Sciences and Medicine, University of Toronto, Toronto, CA

Constance M. Smith, PhD, RN   Wilmington, DE

Dorothy F. Tullmann, PhD, RN   Assistant Professor, University of Virginia, School of Nursing, Charlottesville, VA

Mary Grace Umlauf, RN, PhD, FAAN   Professor, The University of Alabama, Tuscaloosa, AL

Janet Van Cleave, MBA, MSN, PhD   Post-Doctoral Research Fellow, University of Pennsylvania, Philadelphia, PA

Heidi L. Wald, MD, MSPH   Assistant Professor, University of Colorado, Denver, CO

Saunjoo L. Yoon, PhD, RN   Assistant Professor, University of Florida, College of Nursing, Gainesville, FL

DeAnne Zwicker, DrNP, APRN, BC   ANCC certified adult nurse practitioner and is currently working as independent geriatric consultant.

Foreword

The first book I reached for in 2001 when I began my serious inquiry of best nursing practices for older adults was the initial edition of this very text. In fact, I had both a home version and an office version. It was never far from my reach, and I used it daily when developing a series of teaching plans to educate nurses on the care of hospitalized elders. Because each protocol was and remains research or evidence based, it represented the state of the science on care problems faced by staff nurses caring for older adults.

So, you might imagine how thrilled I was to be asked to write the foreword for the fourth edition of *Evidence-Based Geriatric Nursing Protocols for Best Practice*. Initially only 15 chapters, the fourth edition now has 34 chapters—testimony to the growing body of geriatric nursing knowledge. New chapters include function-focused care, catheter-associated urinary tract infection prevention, mistreatment detection, acute care models, and transitional care. There is a heightened sense of urgency to deploy these protocols in practice and education because of recent reports and policy changes that are spotlighted by the debate and discussion surrounding the passage of the 2010 Affordable Care Act. Whereas the final outcome of the law remains to be seen, Americans agree that there is an urgent resolve for action. The public is waking up to the fact that "It's tomorrow already," as discussed in a recent AARP Bulletin—speaking to the multitude of complex national issues, not the least of which is health care reform (Toedtman, 2011). The message to nurses is that we must embrace this reality and work to fully use and promote these geriatric nursing protocols and motivate others to do the same.

Proposed changes to the Centers for Medicare and Medicaid Services (CMS) measurements of quality and cost in health care delivery include the introduction of accountable care organizations (ACO) and value-based purchasing (VBP; CMS, 2011; Welton, 2010). Delivery model innovation mandates that health care must break away from traditional models and practices and move toward more efficient and safer care—a clinical transformation calling for the use of clinical protocols and improved coordination and collaboration (Health Care Advisory Board, 2010). Although the new language may seem daunting, geriatric nurses have used this paradigm for years. A recent Wall Street Journal report on health care summarized it best by saying, "Sometimes innovation means getting back to basics" (Landro, 2011). In truth, it is exactly why geriatric nursing protocols may be better received and, most importantly, implemented in the years ahead. These protocols address basic gerontological tenets: access and quality of care, especially for vulnerable populations; prevention of iatrogenic conditions; the institutionalization of best practices; and the application of innovative and interdisciplinary models of care.

These are uncertain times in health care, with new payment systems and models of care being developed; however, the overriding theme is urgency and delivering results. Therefore, take these protocols and adopt them as your unit based standards. Talk to your patients and families about how nurses have developed methods to improve their care and reduce the risk of complications. Create teaching plans that supplement the protocols with actual patient situations, develop documentation templates to integrate the protocols into your charting system, and develop quality improvement initiatives to measure the degree to which you are currently using these protocols and set goals to improve their use.

The 2011 Institute of Medicine (IOM) report, *The Future of Nursing: Leading Change, Advancing Health*, makes our directive clear and powerful. The IOM was founded on the following premise: *"Knowing is not enough; we must apply. Willing is not enough, we must do"* (von Goethe).

Now, more than ever, nurses are called upon to lead efforts to embed evidence-based practice in daily operations. As the IOM report states, "nurses have key roles to play as team members and leaders for a reformed and better-integrated, patient-centered health care system" (p. xii). The process of implementing sweeping change in health care will likely take years; however, nurses must start pragmatically and focus on these critically important protocols that have demonstrated improved outcomes for older adults. Simply stated, "Pick this book up and use it."

Susan L. Carlson, MSN, APRN, ACNS-BC, GNP-BC, FNGNA
President
National Gerontological Nursing Association

REFERENCES

Centers for Medicare & Medicaid Services. (2011). *Special open door forum: Hospital inpatient value-based purchasing program. Fiscal year 2013. Proposed rule overview.* Baltimore, MD.

Health Care Advisory Board. (2010). *Health care's accountability moment: 15 imperatives for success under risk-based reimbursement.* Washington, DC: The Advisory Board Company.

Institute of Medicine. (2011). *The future of nursing: Leading change, advancing health.* Washington, DC: National Academies Press.

Landro, L. (2011, March 28). The time to innovate is now. *The Wall Street Journal,* R1.

Toedtman, J. (2011, March 3). It's tomorrow already. *AARP Bulletin.*2.Centers for Medicare & Medicaid Services (CMS). *Special Open Door Forum: Hospital Value-Based Purchasing Proposed Rule Overview for Facilities, Providers, and Suppliers.* Baltimore, MD; 2011.

Welton, J. M. (2010). Value-based nursing care. *Journal of Nursing Administration, 40*(10), 399–401.

Acknowledgments

We would like to thank the following for their involvement, support, and leadership during the production of this book:

- All of the expert contributors for this fourth edition
- Those nursing experts who participated in the Nurse Competence in Aging project and contributed protocols to www.HartfordIGN.org, many of which were the impetus for new topics added to this edition
- The institutions that supported faculty and geriatric clinicians participating as contributors of the evidence-based protocols
- Those who provided a valuable contribution in the first and second editions and their ongoing geriatric research
- Faculty and clinicians involved in the project of the American Association of Colleges of Nursing to develop geriatric content for upper-division baccalaureate nursing programs
- Springer Publishing Company for its ongoing support of quality geriatric nursing publications
- Nurses Improving Care for HealthSystem Elders (NICHE) hospitals that bring many of these protocols to the bedside and are leaders in ensuring geriatric nursing best practices

Introduction

Older adults are overwhelmingly the majority of hospitalized patients and are, by far, the most complicated patients to care for in the acute care setting. They suffer from multiple complex medical problems, take multiple medications, are the most vulnerable to iatrogenic events, experience prolonged hospital stays, and are the more likely to die in the hospital (versus community or other setting). Acute care nurses have an enormous responsibility when providing care to older adults in this rapidly changing healthcare environment with increasing regulatory requirements and short staffing. Even though older persons are our fastest growing segment in the United States, most nursing programs, like medical programs, are just now incorporating geriatrics into the curriculum. Many unfamiliar with geriatrics might ask: What's so different about older people? Don't they have the same diagnoses as younger adults, like diabetes, hypertension, and heart disease? The answer to that is yes, they do have the same diseases; however, physiological changes that occur with aging, multiple coexisting medical problems, and multiple medications place older adults at significantly higher risk for complications, including death, while hospitalized. The nurse armed with information on the unique ways in which older adults present with subtle signs and symptoms may actually avert complications. Additionally, the nurse equipped with knowledge about and implementation of proactive assessment and interventions may actually prevent these complications in the first place.

As in the previous, second edition (honored as *American Journal of Nursing*, Geriatric Book of the Year, 2003), we will present assessment and interventions for common geriatric syndromes. Geriatric syndromes are increasingly recognized as being related to preventable iatrogenic complications, or those that occur as a direct result of medical and nursing care, causing serious adverse outcomes in older patients (See Iatrogenesis chapter). We are also very happy to present five new topics and several new expert contributors in this edition. Many of these topics have been updated from the protocols that appear on the website of the Hartford Institute for Geriatric Nursing at NYU (www.HartfordIGN.org). The new topics in this edition are:

- Interventions to Prevent Functional Decline in the Acute Care Setting
- Catheter-Associated Urinary Tract Infection Prevention
- Mistreatment Detection
- Acute Care Models
- Transitional Care

In this fourth edition of *Evidence-Based Geriatric Nursing Protocols for Best Practice*, we provide guidelines that are developed by experts on the topics of each chapter and are based on best available evidence. A systematic method, the AGREE appraisal process (AGREE Next Steps Consortium, 2009; Levin & Vetter, 2007; Singleton & Levin, 2008), was used to evaluate the protocols in the second edition and identify a process to help us improve validity of the book's content. Thus, a systematic process, described in Chapter 1, was developed to retrieve and evaluate the level of evidence of key references related to specific assessment and management strategies in each chapter. The purpose in determining the best available evidence was to answer the clinical questions posed. The chapter authors rated the levels of evidence based on the work of Stetler and colleagues (1998) and Melnyk and Fineout-Overholt (2011). The first chapter in this book, "Developing and Evaluating Clinical Practice Guidelines: A Systematic Approach," details the process of how the clinical practice guidelines were developed and how they complied with the AGREE items for rigour of development (AGREE Next Steps Consortium, 2009). Chapter 1, written by leaders in the field of evidence-based practice in the United States, will most likely be the most important chapter reference for understanding the rating of the levels of evidence. Most of the protocols reflect assessment and intervention strategies for acute care recommended by expert authors who have reviewed the evidence using this process; the evidence provided may come from all levels of care and may not have been specifically tested in the hospital setting.

How to Best Use This Book

The standard nursing approach was used as a guideline for the outline of each topic as deemed appropriate by the chapter author(s) providing: overview and background information on the topic, evidence-based assessment and intervention strategies, and a topic-specific case study with discussion. The text of the chapter provides the context and detailed evidence for the protocol; the tabular protocol is not intended to be used in isolation of the text. We recommend the reader to take the following into consideration when reviewing the chapters:

- Review the objectives to ascertain what is to be achieved by reviewing the chapter.
- Review the text, noting the level of evidence presented in the reference section— Level I, being the highest (e.g., systematic review/meta-analysis) and Level VI, the lowest (e.g., expert opinion). Refer back to Chapter 1, Figure 1.2 for definitions of level of evidence to understand the quantitative evidence that supports each of the recommendations. Keep in mind that it is virtually impossible to have evidence for all assessments and interventions, which *does not* mean it is not going to be used as an intervention. Many interventions that have been successfully used for years have not been quantitatively researched but are well known to be effective to experts in the field of geriatrics.
- Review the protocols, and keep in mind they reflect assessment and intervention strategies for acute care, recommended by experts who have reviewed the evidence. This evidence is from all levels of care (e.g., community, primary care, long-term care) and not necessarily the hospital setting and should be applied to the unique needs of the individual patient.
- The focus should always be patient centered, which takes into consideration many other factors specific to the individual.
- Review the case study and discussion in each topic, which provides a more real life, practical manner in which the protocol may be applied in clinical practice.
- Resources in each chapter to provide easy access to tools discussed in the chapter and to link readers with organizations that provide on-going, up-to-date information and resources on the topic.
- An Appendix provides additional geriatric-specific resources for the reader that can be applied to all topics.

Although this book is entitled *Evidence-Based Geriatric Nursing: Protocols for Best Practice*, the text may be utilized by educators for geriatric nursing courses and advance practice nurses and by many other disciplines including interdisciplinary team members, nursing home and other staff educators, social workers, dieticians, advance practice nurses, physician assistants, and physicians. Many interventions that are proactively identified and implemented by nurses can make a significant difference in improving outcomes, but nurses cannot provide for the complex needs of older adults in isolation. Research has shown that interdisciplinary teams have dramatically improved geriatric patient care and outcomes. We know that communication and collaboration are essential to improve care coordination and prevent iatrogenic complications (IOM, 2001). Caring for the older adult, as the baby boom population continues to "age in," will be an ultimate challenge in healthcare. Each of us must work together and be committed to provide a culture of safety that vulnerable older adults need in order to receive the safest, evidence-based clinical care with optimum outcomes.

Marie Boltz
Elizabeth Capezuti
Terry Fulmer
DeAnne Zwicker

REFERENCES

AGREE Next Steps Consortium. (2009). *Appraisal of guidelines for research & evaluation II*. Retrieved from http://www.agreetrust.org/?o=1397

Institute of Medicine. (2001). *Crossing the quality chasm: A new health system for the 21st century*. Washington, DC: National Academy Press.

Levin, R. F., & Vetter, M. (2007). Evidence-based practice: A guide to negotiate the clinical practice guideline maze. *Research and Theory for Nursing Practice, 21*(1), 5–9.

Melnyk, B. M., & Fineout-Overholt, E. (2011). *Evidence-based practice in nursing & healthcare: A guide to best practice* (2nd ed.). Philadelphia, PA: Lippincott Williams & Wilkins.

Singleton, J. K., & Levin, R. F. (2008). Strategies for learning evidence-based practice: Critically appraising clinical practice guidelines. *Journal of Nursing Education, 47*(8), 380–383.

Stetler, C. B., Morsi, D., Rucki, S., Broughton, S., Corrigan, B., Fitzgerald, J., . . . Sheridan, E. A. (1998). Utilization-focused integrative reviews in a nursing service. *Applied Nursing Research, 11*(4), 195–206.

Evidence-Based Geriatric Nursing
Protocols for Best Practice

Developing and Evaluating Clinical Practice Guidelines: A Systematic Approach

1

Rona F. Levin and Susan Kaplan Jacobs

Clinical decision making that is grounded in the best available evidence is essential to promote patient safety and quality health care outcomes. With the knowledge base for geriatric nursing rapidly expanding, assessing geriatric clinical practice guidelines (CPGs) for their validity and incorporation of the best available evidence is critical to the safety and outcomes of care. In the second edition of this book, Lucas and Fulmer (2003) challenged geriatric nurses to take the lead in the assessment of geriatric clinical practice guidelines (CPGs), recognizing that in the absence of best evidence, guidelines and protocols have little value for clinical decision making. In the third edition of this book, Levin, Singleton, and Jacobs (2008) proposed a method for ensuring that the protocols included in the book were based on a systematic review of the literature and synthesis of best evidence.

The purpose of this chapter is to describe the process that was used to create the fourth edition of *Evidence-Based Geriatric Nursing Protocols for Best Practice*. Prior to the third edition of this book, each chapter author individually gathered and synthesized evidence on a particular topic and then developed a "nursing standard of practice protocol" based on that evidence. There was no standard process or specific criteria for protocol development nor was there any indication of the "level of evidence" of each source cited in the chapter (i.e., the evidence base for the protocol). In the third edition and this fourth edition, the process previously used to develop the geriatric nursing protocols has been enhanced. This chapter is a guide to understanding how the geriatric nursing protocols in these third and fourth editions were developed and describes how to use the process to guide the assessment and/or development and updating of practice protocols in any area of nursing practice.

DEFINITION OF TERMS

Evidence-based practice (EBP) is a framework for clinical practice that integrates the best available scientific evidence with the expertise of the clinician and with patients' preferences and values to make decisions about health care (Levin & Feldman, 2006; Straus, Richardson, Glasziou, & Haynes, 2005). Health care professionals often use the terms *recommendations*, *guidelines*, and *protocols* interchangeably, but they are not synonymous.

A recommendation is a suggestion for practice, not necessarily sanctioned by a formal, expert group. A clinical practice guideline is an "official recommendation" or suggested approach to diagnose and manage a broad health condition (e.g., heart failure, smoking

1

cessation, or pain management). A protocol is a more detailed guide for approaching a clinical problem or health condition and is tailored to a specific practice situation. For example, guidelines for falls prevention recommend developing a protocol for toileting elderly, sedated, or confused patients (Rich & Newland, 2006). The specific practices or protocol each agency implements, however, is agency specific. The validity of any of these practice guides can vary depending on the type and the level of evidence on which they are based. Using standard criteria to develop or refine CPGs or protocols assures reliability of their content. Standardization gives both nurses, who use the guideline/protocol, and patients, who receive care based on the guideline/protocol, assurance that the geriatric content and practice recommendations are based on the best evidence.

In contrast to these practice guides, "standards of practice" are not specific or necessarily evidence based; rather, they are a generally accepted, formal, published framework for practice. As an example, the American Nurses Association document, *Nursing: Scope and Standards of Practice* (American Nurses Association, 2010), contains a standard regarding nurses' accountability for making an assessment of a patient's health status. The standard is a general statement. A protocol, on the other hand, may specify the assessment tool(s) to use in that assessment—for example, an instrument to predict pressure-ulcer risk.

THE AGREE INSTRUMENT

The AGREE (*Appraisal of Guidelines for Research & Evaluation*) instrument (http://www.agreecollaboration.org/), created and evaluated by international guideline developers and researchers for use by the National Health Services (AGREE Collaboration, 2001), was initially supported by the UK National Health Services Management Executive and later by the European Union (Cluzeau, Littlejohns, Grimshaw, Feder, & Moran, 1999).

Released in 2001 in its initial form, the purpose of the AGREE instrument is to provide standard criteria with which to appraise CPGs. This appraisal includes evaluation of the methods used to develop the CPG, assessment of the validity of the recommendations made in the guideline, and consideration of factors related to the use of the CPG in practice. Although the AGREE instrument was created to critically appraise CPGs, the process and criteria can also be applied to the development and evaluation of clinical practice protocols. Thus, the AGREE instrument has been expanded for that purpose: to standardize the creation and revision of the geriatric nursing practice protocols in this book.

The initial AGREE instrument and the one used for clinical guideline/protocol development in the third edition of this book has six quality domains: (a) *scope and purpose*, (b) *stakeholder involvement*, (c) *rigour of development*, (d) *clarity and presentation*, (e) *application*, and (f) *editorial independence*. A total of 23 items divided among the domains were rated on a 4-point Likert-type scale from *strongly disagree* to *strongly agree*. Appraisers evaluate how well the guideline they are assessing meets the criteria (i.e., items) of the six quality domains. For example, when evaluating the rigour of development, appraisers rated seven items. The reliability of the AGREE instrument is increased when each guideline is appraised by more than one appraiser. Each of the six domains receives an individual domain score and, based on these scores, the appraiser subjectively assesses the overall quality of a guideline.

Important to note, however, is that the original AGREE instrument was revised in 2009 (http://www.agreetrust.org/), is now called AGREE II, and is the version that we used for this fourth edition (AGREE Next Steps Consortium, 2009). The revision added one new item to the rigour of development domain. This is the current Item 9, which underscores the importance of evaluating the evidence that is applied to practice. Item 9

TABLE 1.1

Sample domain and items from the AGREE II instrument for critical appraisal of clinical practice guidelines with rating scale.

Domain 3: Rigour of Development

7. Systematic methods were used to search for evidence.

8. The criteria for selecting the evidence are clearly described.

9. The strengths and limitations of the body of evidence are clearly described

10. The methods for formulating the recommendations are clearly described.

11. The health benefits, side effects, and risks have been considered in formulating the recommendations.

12. There is an explicit link between the recommendations and the supporting evidence.

13. The guideline has been externally reviewed by experts prior to its publication.

14. A procedure for updating the guideline is provided.

Source: The AGREE Research Trust. (2009). *Appraisal of Guidelines for Research and Evaluation, AGREE II Instrument.* Retrieved from http://www.agreetrust.org/index.aspx?o=1397

---

reads: "The strengths and limitations of the body of evidence are clearly described." The remainder of the changes included a revision of the Likert-type scale used to evaluate each item in the AGREE II, a reordering of the number assigned to each item based on the addition of the new Item 9 and minor editing of items for clarity. No other substantive changes were made. Table 1.1 includes the items that are in the rigour of development domain and were used for evaluation of evidence in the current edition of this book.

The rigour of development section of the AGREE instrument provides standards for literature-searching and documenting the databases and terms searched. Adhering to these criteria to find and use the best available evidence on a clinical question is critical to the validity of geriatric nursing protocols and, ultimately, to patient safety and outcomes of care.

Published guidelines can be appraised using the AGREE instrument as discussed previously. In the process of guideline development, however, the clinician is faced with the added responsibility of appraising all available evidence for its quality and relevance. In other words, how well does the available evidence support recommended clinical practices? The clinician needs to be able to support or defend the inclusion of each recommendation in the protocol based on its level of evidence. To do so, the guideline must reflect a systematic, structured approach to find and assess the available evidence.

The Search for Evidence Process

Models of EBP describe the evidence-based process in five steps:

1. Develop an answerable question.
2. Locate the best evidence.
3. Critically appraise the evidence.
4. Integrate the evidence into practice using clinical expertise with attention to patient's values and perspectives.
5. Evaluate outcome(s).
   (Flemming, 1998; McKibbon, Wilczynski, Eady, & Marks, 2009; Melnyk & Fineout-Overholt, 2011)

Locating evidence to support development of protocols, guidelines, and reviews requires a comprehensive and systematic review of the published literature, following Steps 1 and 2. A search begins with Step 1, developing an answerable question, which may be in the form of a specific "foreground" question (one that is focused on a particular clinical issue), or it may be a broad question (one that asks for overview information about a disease, condition, or aspect of healthcare) (Flemming, 1998; Melnyk & Fineout-Overholt, 2011; Straus et al., 2005) to gain an overview of the practice problem and interventions and gain insight into its significance. This step is critical to identifying appropriate search terms, possible synonyms, construction of a search strategy, and retrieving relevant results. One example of an answerable foreground question asked in this book is "What is the effectiveness of restraints in reducing the occurrence of falls in patients 65 years of age and older?" Foreground questions are best answered by individual primary studies or syntheses of studies, such as systematic reviews or meta-analyses. PICO templates work best to gather the evidence for focused clinical questions (Glasziou, Del Mar, & Salisbury, 2003). PICO is an acronym for *population, intervention* (or occurrence or risk factor), *comparison* (or control), and *outcome*. In the preceding question, the population is patients at risk of falling, 65 years of age and older; the intervention is use of restraints; the implied comparison or control is no restraints; and the desired outcome is decreased incidence of falls. An initial database search would consider the problem (falls) and the intervention (restraints) to begin to cast a wide net to gather evidence. A broader research query, related to a larger category of disease or problem and encompassing multiple interventions, might be "What is the best available evidence regarding the use of restraints in residential facilities?" (Griggs, 2009)

General or overview/background questions may be answered in textbooks, review articles, and "point-of-care" tools that aggregate overviews of best evidence, for example, online encyclopedias, systematic reviews, and synthesis tools (BMJ Publishing Group Limited; The Cochrane Collaboration; Joanna Briggs Institute; UpToDate; Wolters Kluwer Health). This may be helpful in the initial steps of gathering external evidence to support the significance of the problem you believe exists prior to developing your PICO question and investing a great deal of time in a narrow question for which there might be limited evidence.

Step 2, locating the evidence, requires a literature search based on the elements identified in the clinical question. Gathering the evidence for the protocols in this book presented the challenge to conduct literature reviews, encompassing *both* the breadth of overview information as well as the depth of specificity represented in high-level systematic reviews and clinical trials to answer specific clinical questions.

Not every nurse, whether he or she is a clinical practitioner, educator, or administrator, has developed proficient database search skills to conduct a literature review to locate evidence. Beyond a basic knowledge of Boolean logic, truncation, and applying categorical limits to filter results, competency in "information literacy" (Association of College & Research Libraries, 2000) requires experience with the idiosyncrasies of databases, selection of terms, and ease with controlled vocabularies and database functionality. Many nurses report that limited access to resources, gaps in information literacy skills, and, most of all, a lack of time are barriers to "readiness" for EBP (Pravikoff, Tanner, & Pierce, 2005).

For both the third and current edition of this book, the authors enlisted the assistance of a team of New York University health sciences librarians to assure a standard and efficient approach to collecting evidence on clinical topics. Librarians as intermediaries have been called "an essential part of the health care team by allowing knowledge consumers to focus on the wise interpretation and use of knowledge for critical decision making, rather than spending unproductive time on its access and retrieval" (Homan, 2010, p. 51). The *Cochrane Handbook for Systematic Reviews of Interventions* points out the complexity of conducting a systematic literature review and highly recommends enlisting the help of a healthcare librarian when searching for studies to support locating studies for systematic reviews (Section 6.3.1; Higgins & Green, 2008). The team of librarian/searchers were given the topics, keywords, and suggested synonyms, as well as the evidence pyramid we agreed upon, and they were asked to locate the best available evidence for each broad area addressed in the following chapters.

Search Strategies for Broad Topics

The literature search begins with database selection and translation of search terms into the controlled vocabulary of the database if possible. The major databases for finding the best primary evidence for most clinical nursing questions are CINAHL (Cumulative Index to Nursing and Allied Health Literature) and MEDLINE. The PubMed interface to MEDLINE was used, as it includes added "unprocessed" records to provide access to the most recently published citations. For most topics, the PsycINFO database was searched to ensure capturing relevant evidence in the literature of psychology and behavioral sciences. The Cochrane Database of Systematic Reviews and the Joanna Briggs Institute's evidence summaries (The Cochrane Collaboration; Joanna Briggs Institute) were also searched to provide authors with another synthesized source of evidence for broad topic areas.

The AGREE II instrument was used as a standard against which we could evaluate the process for evidence searching and use in chapter and protocol development (AGREE Next Steps Consortium, 2009). Domain 3, rigour of development, Item 7, states: "The search strategy should be as comprehensive as possible and executed in a manner free from potential biases and sufficiently detailed to be replicated." Taking a tip from the *Cochrane Handbook*, a literature search should capture both the subject terms and the methodological aspects of studies when gathering relevant records (Higgins & Green, 2008). Both of these directions were used to develop search strategies and deliver results to chapter authors using the following guidelines:

- ■ To facilitate replication and update of searches in all databases, search results sent to authors were accompanied by a *search strategy*: listing the keywords/ descriptors and search string used in each database searched (e.g., MEDLINE, PsycINFO, CINAHL).
- ■ The time period searched was specified (e.g, 2006–2010).
- ■ Categorical limits or methodological filters were specified. (Some examples are the article type: "meta-analysis" or the "systematic review subset" in Pubmed; the "methodology" limit in PsycINFO for meta-analysis OR clinical trial; the "research" limit in CINAHL.)
- ■ To facilitate replication and update of MEDLINE/PubMed searches, searches were saved and chapter authors were supplied with a login and password for a *My NCBI* account (National Center for Biotechnology Information, U.S. National Library of Medicine), linking to Saved Searches to be rerun at later dates.

The librarian then aggregated evidence in a RefWorks database and sent this output to all chapter authors to enhance their knowledge base and provide a foundation for further exploration of the literature.

Limits, Hedges, and Publication Types

Most bibliographic databases have the functionality to exploit the architecture of the individual citations to *limit* to articles tagged with publication types (such as "meta-analysis" or "randomized controlled trial" in MEDLINE). In CINAHL, methodological filters or "hedges" (Haynes, Wilczynski, McKibbon, Walker, & Sinclair, 1994) for publication types "systematic review," "clinical trials," or "research" articles are available. The commonly used PubMed "Clinical Queries" feature (http://www.nlm.nih.gov/pubs/techbull/mj10/mj10_clin_query.html) is designed for *specific* clinical questions such as the example mentioned previously. Gathering evidence to support broader topics, such as the protocols in this book, presents the searcher with a larger challenge. Limiting searches by methodology can unwittingly eliminate the best evidence for study designs that do not lend themselves to these methods. For example, a cross-sectional retrospective design may provide the highest level of evidence for a study that examines "nurses' perception" of the practice environment (Boltz et al., 2008). Methodological filters have other limitations, such as retrieving citations tagged "randomized controlled trials as topic" or abstracts that state a "systematic review of the literature" was conducted (which is not the same as retrieving a study that is actually a systematic review). Chapter authors were cautioned that the CINAHL database assigns publication type "systematic review" to numerous citations that upon review, we judged to be "Level V" review articles (narrative reviews or literature reviews), not necessarily the high level of evidence we would call "Level I," (which according to our scheme are studies that do a rigorous synthesis and pooling or analysis of research results). It may not be easily discernible from an article title and abstract whether the study is a systematic review with evidence synthesis or a narrative literature review (Lindbloom, Brandt, Hough, & Meadows, 2007). These pitfalls of computerized retrieval are justification for the review by the searcher to weed false hits from the retrieved list of articles.

Precision and Recall

An additional challenge to an intermediary searcher is the need to balance the comprehensiveness of recall (or "sensitivity") with precision ("specificity") to retrieve a "useful" number of references. The *Cochrane Handbook* states: "Searches should seek high sensitivity, which may result in relatively low precision" (Section 6.3; Higgins & Green, 2008). Thus, retrieving a large set of articles may include many irrelevant hits. Conversely, putting too many restrictions on a search may exclude relevant studies. The goal of retrieving the relevant studies for broad topic areas required "sacrificing precision" and deferring to the chapter authors to filter false or irrelevant hits (Jenkins, 2004; Matthews et al., 1999). The iterative nature of a literature search requires that an initial set of relevant references for both broad or specific research questions serves to *point* authors toward best evidence as an adjunct to their own knowledge, their own pursuit of "chains of citation" (McLellan, 2001) and related records, and their clinical expertise. Thus, a list of core references on physical restraints, supplied to a chapter author, might lead to exploring citations related to wandering, psychogeriatric care, or elder abuse (Fulmer, 2002).

LEVELS OF EVIDENCE

Step 3, critical appraisal of the evidence, begins with identifying the methodology used in a study (often evident from reviewing the article abstract) followed by a critical reading and evaluation of the research methodology and results. The coding scheme described in the subsequent text provides the first step in filtering retrieved studies based on research methods.

Levels of evidence offer a schema that, once known, helps the reader to understand the value of the information presented to the clinical topic or question under review. There are many schemas that are used to identify the level of evidence sources. Although multiple schemas exist, they have commonalities in their hierarchical structure, often represented by a pyramid or "publishing wedge" (DiCenso, Bayley, & Haynes, 2009; McKibbon et al., 2009). The highest level of evidence is seen at the top of a pyramid, characterized by increased relevance to the clinical setting in a smaller number of studies. The schema used by the authors in this book for rating the level of evidence comes from the work of Stetler et al. (1998) and Melnyk and Fineout-Overholt (2005; See Figure 1.1).

A Level I evidence rating is given to evidence from synthesized sources (systematic reviews), which can either be meta-analyses or structured integrative reviews of evidence, and CPG's based on Level I evidence. Evidence rated as Level II comes from a randomized controlled trial. A quasi-experimental study such as a nonrandomized controlled single

---

FIGURE 1.1

Levels of quantitative evidence.

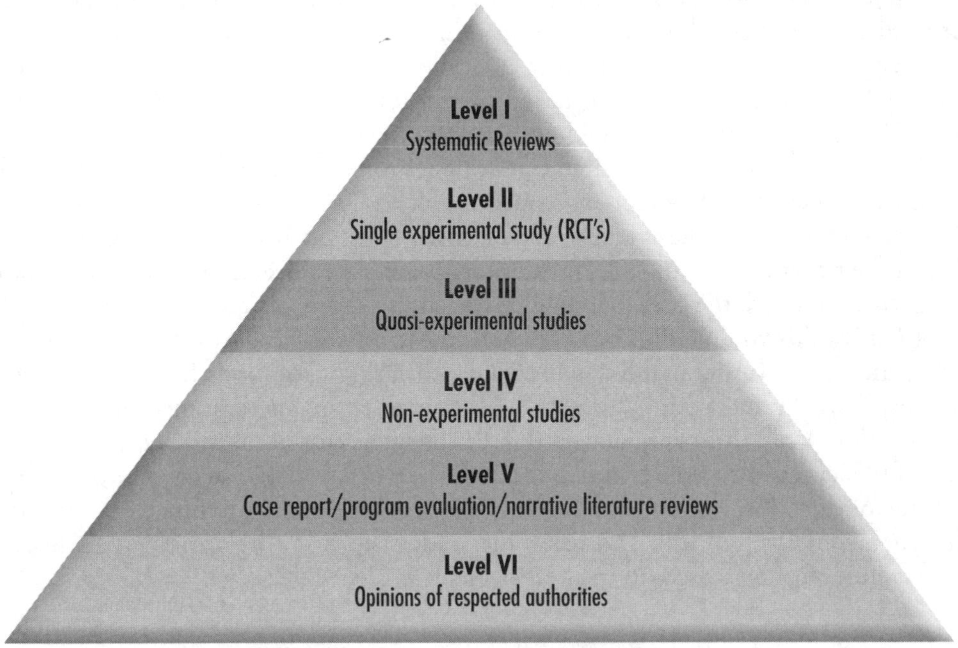

Level I
Systematic Reviews

Level II
Single experimental study (RCT's)

Level III
Quasi-experimental studies

Level IV
Non-experimental studies

Level V
Case report/program evaluation/narrative literature reviews

Level VI
Opinions of respected authorities

Systematic Reviews (Integrative/Meta-analyses/CPG's based on systematic reviews) Adapted from Stetler, C. B., Morsi, D., Rucki, S., Broughton, S., Corrigan, B., Fitzgerald, J., . . . Sheridan, E. A. (1998). Utilization-focused integrative reviews in a nursing service. *Applied Nursing Research, 11*(4), 195–206; Melnyk, B. M., & Fineout-Overholt, E. (2005). *Evidence-based practice in nursing & healthcare: A guide to best practice* (p. 608). Philadelphia, PA: Lippincott Williams & Wilkins.

EXHIBIT 1.1

An example of a coded literature citation supplied to protocol author.

REF ID: 22449 Level IV

Boltz, M., Capezuti, E., Bowar-Ferres, S., Norman, R., Secic, M., Kim, H. et al. (2008). Hospital nurses' perception of the geriatric nurse practice environment. *Journal of Nursing Scholarship,* *40*(3), 282-289.
Purpose: To test the relationship between nurses' perceptions of the geriatric nurse practice environment (GNPE) and perceptions of geriatric-care delivery, and geriatric nursing knowledge. Design: A secondary analysis of data collected by the New York University Hartford Institute Benchmarking Service staff using a retrospective, cross-sectional, design. Methods: Responses of 9,802 direct-care registered nurses from 75 acute-care hospitals in the US that administered the GIAP (Geriatric Institutional Assessment Profile) from January 1997 to December 2005 were analyzed using linear mixed effects modeling to explore associations between variables while controlling for potential covariates. Findings: Controlling for hospital and nurse characteristics, a positive geriatric nurse practice environment was associated with positive geriatric care delivery ($F=4,686$, $p<.0001$) but not geriatric nursing knowledge. The independent contribution of all three dimensions of the geriatric nurse practice environment (resource availability, institutional values, and capacity for collaboration) influences care delivery for hospitalized older-adult patients. Conclusions: Organizational support for geriatric nursing is an important influence upon quality of geriatric care. Clinical Relevance: Hospitals that utilize an organizational approach addressing the multifaceted nature of the GNPE are more likely to improve the hospital experience of older adults.

---

group pretest and posttest time series or matched case-controlled study is considered Level III evidence. Level IV evidence comes from a nonexperimental study, such as correlational descriptive research and qualitative or case-control studies. A narrative literature review, a case report systematically obtained and of verifiable quality, or program evaluation data are rated as Level V. Level VI evidence is identified as the opinion of respected authorities (e.g., nationally known) based on their clinical experience or the opinions of an expert committee, including their interpretation of non-research-based information. This level also includes regulatory or legal opinions. Level I evidence is considered the strongest.

For all topics, the results of literature searches were organized in a searchable, web-based RefWorks "shared" folder and coded for level of evidence. The authors were then charged with reviewing the evidence and deciding on its quality and relevance for inclusion in their chapter or protocol. The critical appraisal of research uses specialized tools designed to evaluate the methodology of the study. Examples are the AGREE instrument (which this volume of protocols conforms to) (AGREE Next Steps Consortium, 2009), the Critical Appraisal Skills Programme (CASP) (Solutions for Public Health), and the PRISMA Statement (PRISMA: Transparent reporting) among others.

An additional feature implemented in the previous edition of this book is the inclusion of the level and type of evidence for each reference, which leads to a recommendation for practice (See Exhibit 1.1). Using this type of standard approach ensures that this book contains protocols and recommendations for use with geriatric patients and their families that are based on the best available evidence.

SUMMARY

The protocols contained in this edition, therefore, have been refined, revised, and/or developed by the authors using the best available research evidence as a foundation, with the ultimate goal of improving patient safety and outcomes. The systematic process we used for finding, retrieving, and disseminating the best evidence for the fourth edition of *Geriatric Nursing Protocols for Best Practice* provides a model for the use of research evidence in nursing education and in clinical practice. Translating nursing research into practice requires competency in information literacy, knowledge of the evidence-based process, and the ability to discern the context of a research study as ranked hierarchically. The following chapters and protocols present both overview and foreground information in readiness for taking the next steps in the EBP process: Step 4, integrate the evidence with clinical expertise and patient's values and perspective, and Step 5, evaluate outcome.

REFERENCES

American Nurses Association. (2010). *Nursing: Scope and standards of practice.* Silver Spring, MD: Authors.

AGREE Collaboration. (2001). Appraisal of Guidelines Research and Evaluation. Retrieved from http://www.agreecollaboration.org/

AGREE Next Steps Consortium. (2009). Appraisal of guidelines for research & evaluation II. Retrieved from http://www.agreetrust.org/?o=1397

Association of College & Research Libraries. (2000). Information literacy competency standards for higher education. Retrieved from http://www.ala.org/ala/mgrps/divs/acrl/standards/informationliteracycompetency.cfm

Boltz, M., Capezuti, E., Bowar-Ferres, S., Norman, R., Secic, M., Kim, H., . . . Fulmer, T. (2008). Hospital nurses' perception of the geriatric nurse practice environment. *Journal of Nursing Scholarship, 40*(3), 282–289.

BMJ Publishing Group Limited. (2011). BMJ Clinical Evidence. Available at http://clinicalevidence.bmj.com/ceweb/index.jsp

Cluzeau, F. A., Littlejohns, P., Grimshaw, J. M., Feder, G., & Moran, S. E. (1999). Development and application of a generic methodology to assess the quality of clinical guidelines. *International Journal for Quality in Health Care, 11*(1), 21–28.

The Cochrane Collaboration. (2010). Cochrane Reviews. Available at http://www2.cochrane.org/reviews/

DiCenso, A., Bayley, L., & Haynes, R. B. (2009). Accessing pre-appraised evidence: Fine-tuning the 5S model into a 6S model. *Evidence-based Nursing, 12*(4), 99–101.

Flemming, K. (1998). Asking answerable questions. *Evidence-Based Nursing, 1*(2), 36–37.

Fulmer, T. (2002). Elder mistreatment. *Annual Review of Nursing Research, 20*, 369–395.

Glasziou, P., Del Mar, C., & Salisbury, J. (2003). *Evidence-based medicine workbook: Finding and applying the best research evidence to improve patient care.* London, United Kingdom: BMJ Publishing.

Griggs, K. (2009). Restraint: Physical. *Evidence Summaries - Joanna Briggs Institute.*

Haynes, R. B., Wilczynski, N., McKibbon, K. A., Walker, C. J., & Sinclair, J. C. (1994). Developing optimal search strategies for detecting clinically sound studies in MEDLINE. *Journal of the American Medical Informatics Association, 1*(6), 447–458.

Higgins, J. P., & Green, S. (2008). Planning the search process. In *Cochrane handbook for systematic reviews of interventions.* West Sussex, United Kingdom: John Wiley & Sons. Retrieved from http://www.cochrane-handbook.org/

Homan, J. M. (2010). Eyes on the prize: reflections on the impact of the evolving digital ecology on the librarian as expert intermediary and knowledge coach, 1969–2009. *Journal of Medical Library Association, 98*(1), 49–56.

Jenkins, M. (2004). Evaluation of methodological search filters—a review. *Health Information and Libraries Journal, 21*(3), 148–163.

Joanna Briggs Institute. (n.d.). Clinical online network of evidence for care & therapeutics: JBI COnNECT. Available at http://connect.jbiconnectplus.org/Search.aspx

Levin, R. F., & Feldman, H. R. (2006). *Teaching evidence-based practice in nursing: A guide for academic and clinical settings.* New York, NY: Springer Publishing.

Levin, R. F., Singleton, J. K., & Jacobs, S. K. (2008). Developing and evaluating clinical practice guidelines: A systematic approach. In E. Capezuti, D. Zwicker, M. Mezey, T. Fulmer, D. Gray-Miceli, & M. Kluger (Eds.), *Evidence-based geriatric nursing protocols for best practice* (3rd ed.). New York, NY: Springer Publishing.

Lindbloom, E. J., Brandt, J., Hough, L. D., & Meadows, S. E. (2007). Elder mistreatment in the nursing home: A systematic review. *Journal of the American Medical Directors Association, 8*(9), 610–616.

Lucas, J. A., & Fulmer, T. (2003). Evaluating clinical practice guidelines: A best practice. In M. D. Mezey, T. Fulmer, & I. Abraham (Eds.), *Geriatric nursing protocols for best practice* (2nd ed.). New York, NY: Springer Publishing.

Matthews, E. J., Edwards, A. G., Barker, J., Bloom, M., Covey, J., Hood, K., . . . Wilkinson, C. (1999). Efficient literature searching in diffuse topics: Lessons from a systematic review of research on communicating risk to patients in primary care. *Health Libraries Review, 16*(2), 112–120.

McKibbon, A., Wilczynski, N., Eady, A., & Marks, S. (2009). *PDQ evidence-based principles and practice.* (2nd ed.). Shelton, CT: People's Medical Publishing House.

McLellan, F. (2001). 1966 and all that—when is a literature search done? *Lancet, 358*(9282), 646.

Melnyk, B. M., & Fineout-Overholt, E. (2005). *Evidence-based practice in nursing & healthcare: A guide to best practice* (p. 608). Philadelphia, PA: Lippincott Williams & Wilkins.

Melnyk, B. M., & Fineout-Overholt, E. (2011). *Evidence-based practice in nursing & healthcare: A guide to best practice* (2nd ed.). Philadelphia, PA: Lippincott Williams & Wilkins.

National Center for Biotechnology Information, U.S. National Library of Medicine. (2009). My NCBI. Available at http://www.ncbi.nlm.nih.gov/sites/myncbi/

Pravikoff, D. S., Tanner, A. B., & Pierce, S. T. (2005). Readiness of U.S. nurses for evidence-based practice. *American Journal of Nursing, 105*(9), 40–52.

PRISMA: Transparent reporting of systematic reviews and meta-analyses. (n.d.). Available at http://www.prisma-statement.org/

Rich, E. R., & Newland, J. A. (2006). Creating clinical protocols with an Apgar of 10. In R. F. Levin & H. Feldman (Eds.), *Teaching evidence-based practice in nursing: A guide for academic and clinical settings.* New York, NY: Springer Publishing.

Solutions for Public Health. (2010). Critical Appraisal Skills Programme. Available at http://www.sph.nhs.uk/what-we-do/public-health-workforce/resources/critical-appraisals-skills-programme

Stetler, C. B., Morsi, D., Rucki, S., Broughton, S., Corrigan, B., Fitzgerald, J., . . . Sheridan, E. A. (1998). Utilization-focused integrative reviews in a nursing service. *Applied Nursing Research, 11*(4), 195–206.

Straus, S. E., Richardson, W. S., Glasziou, P., & Haynes, R. B. (2005). *Evidence-based medicine: How to practice and teach EBM* (3rd ed.). Edinburgh, United Kingdom: Churchill Livingstone.

UpToDate. (2011). Available at http://www.uptodate.com/

Wolters Kluwer Health. (2011). Clin-eguide. Available at http://www.clineguide.com/index.aspx

Measuring Performance, Improving Quality

2

Lenard L. Parisi

EDUCATIONAL OBJECTIVES

After completion of this chapter, the reader will be able to:

1. discuss key components of the definition of quality as outlined by the Institute of Medicine (IOM)
2. describe three challenges of measuring quality of care
3. delineate three strategies for addressing the challenges of measuring quality
4. list three characteristics of a good performance measure

Nadzam and Abraham (2003) state that, "The main objective of implementing best practice protocols for geriatric nursing is to stimulate nurses to practice with greater knowledge and skill, and thus improve the quality of care to older adults" (p. 11). Although improved patient care and safety certainly is a goal, providers also need to be focused on the implementation of evidence-based practice and on improving outcomes of care. The implementation of evidenced-based nursing practice as a means to providing safe, quality patient care, and positive outcomes is well supported in the literature. However, in order to ensure that protocols are implemented correctly, as is true with the delivery of all nursing care, it is essential to evaluate the care provided. Outcomes of care are gaining increased attention and will be of particular interest to providers as the health care industry continues to move toward a "pay-for-performance (P4P)/value-based purchasing (VBP)" reimbursement model.

BACKGROUND AND STATEMENT OF PROBLEM

The improvement of care and clinical outcomes—or, as it is commonly known as Performance Improvement—requires a defined, organized approach. Improvement efforts are typically guided by the organization's Quality Assessment (measurement) and Performance Improvement (process improvement) model. Some well-known models or approaches for improving care and processes include Plan-Do-Study-Act (PDSA; Institute for Health Care Improvement, see http://www.ihi.org/IHI/Topics/Improvement/ImprovementMethods/Tools/Plan-Do-Study-Act%20(PDSA)%20Worksheet) and Six

Sigma (see http://asq.org/learn-about-quality/six-sigma/overview/overview.html). These methodologies are simply an organized approach to defining improvement priorities, collecting data, analyzing the data, making sound recommendations for process improvement, implementing identified changes, and then reevaluating the measures. Through Performance Improvement, standards of care (e.g., Nurses Improving Care for Health-system Elders [NICHE] protocols, in this case) are identified, evaluated, analyzed for variances, and improved. The goal is to standardize and improve patient care and outcomes. Restructuring, redesigning, and innovative processes aid in improving the quality of patient care. However, nursing professionals must be supported by a structure of continuous improvement that empowers nurses to make changes and delivers reliable outcomes (Johnson, Hallsey, Meredith, & Warden, 2006).

From the very beginning of the NICHE project in the early 1990s (Fulmer et al., 2002), the NICHE team has struggled with the following questions: How can we measure whether the combination of models of care, staff education and development, and organizational change leads to improvements in patient care? How can we provide hospitals and health systems that are committed to improving their nursing care to older adults with guidance and frameworks, let alone tools for measuring the quality of geriatric care? In turn, these questions generated many other questions: Is it possible to measure quality? Can we identify direct indicators of quality? Or do we have to rely on indirect indicators (e.g., if 30-day readmissions of patients older than the age of 65 drop, can we reasonably state that this reflects an improvement in the quality of care)? What factors may influence our desired quality outcomes, whether these are unrelated factors (e.g., the pressure to reduce length of stay) or related factors (e.g., the severity of illness)? How can we design evaluation programs that enable us to measure quality without adding more burden (of data collection, of taking time away from direct nursing care)? No doubt, the results from evaluation programs should be useful at the "local" level. Would it be helpful, though, to have results that are comparable across clinical settings (within the same hospital or health system) and across institutions (e.g., as quality benchmarking tools)? Many of these questions remain unanswered today, although the focus on defining practice through an evidence-based approach is becoming the standard, for it is against a standard of care that we monitor and evaluate expected care. Defining outcomes for internal and external reporting is expected, as is the improvement of processes required to deliver safe, affordable, and quality patient care.

This chapter provides guidance in the selection, development, and use of performance measures to monitor quality of care as a springboard to Performance Improvement initiatives. Following a definition of quality of care, the chapter identifies several challenges in the measurement of quality. The concept of performance measures as the evaluation link between care delivery and quality improvement is introduced. Next, the chapter offers practical advice on what and how to measure (Fulmer et al., 2002). It also describes external comparative databases sponsored by Centers for Medicare & Medicaid Services (CMS) and other quality improvement organizations. It concludes with a description of the challenge to selecting performance measures.

It is important to reaffirm two key principles for the purposes of evaluating nursing care in this context. First, at the management level, it is indispensable to measure the quality of geriatric nursing care; however, doing so must help those who actually provide care (nurses) and must impact on those who receive care (older adult patients). Second, measuring quality of care is not the end goal; rather, it is done to enable the continuous use of quality-of-care information to improve patient care.

ASSESSMENT OF THE PROBLEM

Quality Health Care Defined

It is not uncommon to begin a discussion of quality-related topics without reflecting on one's own values and beliefs surrounding quality health care. Many have tried to define the concept; but like the old cliché "beauty is in the eye of the beholder," so is our own perception of quality. Health care consumers and providers alike are often asked, "What does quality mean to you?" The response typically varies and includes statements such as "a safe health care experience," "receiving correct medications," "receiving medications in a timely manner," "a pain-free procedure or postoperative experience," "compliance with regulation," "accessibility to services," "effectiveness of treatments and medications," "efficiency of services," "good communication among providers," "information sharing," and "a caring environment." These are important attributes to remember when discussing the provision of care with clients and patients.

The IOM defines *quality of care* as "the degree to which health services for individuals and populations increase[s] the likelihood of desired health outcomes and are consistent with current professional knowledge" (Kohn, Corrigan, & Donaldson, 2000, p. 211). Note that this definition does not tell us what quality is, but what quality should achieve. This definition also does not say that quality exists if certain conditions are met (e.g., a ratio of x falls to y older orthopedic surgery patients, a 30-day readmission rate of z). Instead, it emphasizes that the likelihood of achieving desired levels of care is what matters. In other words, quality is not a matter of reaching something but, rather, the challenge, over and over, of improving the odds of reaching the desired level of outcomes. Thus, the definition implies the cyclical and longitudinal nature of quality: What we achieve today must guide us as to what to do tomorrow—better and better, over and over. The focus being on improving processes while demonstrating sustained improvement.

The IOM definition stresses the framework within which to conceptualize quality: knowledge. The best knowledge to have is research evidence—preferably from randomized clinical trials (experimental studies)—yet without ignoring the relevance of less rigorous studies (nonrandomized studies, epidemiological investigations, descriptive studies, even case studies). Realistically, in nursing, we have limited evidence to guide the care of older adults. Therefore, professional consensus among clinical and research experts is a critical factor in determining quality. Furthermore, knowledge is needed at three levels: To achieve quality, we need to know what to do (knowledge about best practice), we need to know how to do it (knowledge about behavioral skills), and we need to know what outcomes to achieve (knowledge about best outcomes).

The IOM definition of quality of care contains several other important elements. "Health services" focuses the definition on the care itself. Granted, the quality of care provided is determined by such factors as knowledgeable professionals, good technology, and efficient organizations; however, these are not the focus of quality measurement. Rather, the definition implies a challenge to health care organizations: The system should be organized in such a way that knowledge-based care is provided and that its effects can be measured. This brings us to the "desired health outcomes" element of the definition. Quality is not an attribute (as in "My hospital is in the top 100 hospitals in the United States as ranked by *U.S. News & World Report*"), but an ability (as in "Only $x\%$ of our older adult surgical patients go into acute confusion; of those who do, $y\%$ return to normal cognitive function within z hours after onset").

In the IOM definition, *degree* implies that quality occurs on a continuum from unacceptable to excellent. The clinical consequences are on a continuum as well. If the care is of unacceptable quality, the likelihood that we will achieve the desired outcomes is nil. In fact, we probably will achieve outcomes that are the opposite of what are desired. As the care moves up the scale toward excellent, the more likely the desired outcomes will be achieved. Degree also implies quantification. Although it helps to be able to talk to colleagues about, say, unacceptable, poor, average, good, or excellent care, these terms should be anchored by a measurement system. Such systems enable us to interpret what, for instance, poor care is by providing us with a range of numbers that correspond to *poor*. In turn, these numbers can provide us with a reference point for improving care to the level of average: We measure care again, looking at whether the numbers have improved, then checking whether these numbers fall in the range defined as *average*. Likewise, if we see a worsening of scores, we will be able to conclude whether we have gone from, say, good to average. *Individuals* and *populations* underscores that quality of care is reflected in the outcomes of one patient and in the outcomes of a set of patients. It focuses our attention on providing quality care to individuals while aiming to raise the level of care provided to populations of patients.

In summary, the IOM definition of quality of care forces us to think about quality in relative and dynamic rather than in absolute and static terms. Quality of care is not a state of being but a process of becoming. Quality is and should be measurable, using performance measures—"a quantitative tool that provides an indication of an organization's performance in relation to a specified process or outcome" (Schyve & Nadzam, 1998, p. 222).

Quality improvement is a process of attaining ever better levels of care in parallel with advances in knowledge and technology. It strives toward increasing the likelihood that certain outcomes will be achieved. This is the professional responsibility of those who are charged with providing care (clinicians, managers, and their organizations). On the other hand, consumers of health care (not only patients but also purchasers, payors, regulators, and accreditors) are much less concerned with the processes in place, as with the results of those processes.

Clinical Outcomes and Publicly Reported Quality Measures

Although it is important to evaluate clinical practices and processes, it is equally important to evaluate and improve outcomes of care. Clinical outcome indicators are receiving unprecedented attention within the health care industry from providers, payors, and consumers alike. Regulatory and accrediting bodies review outcome indicators to evaluate the care provided by the organization prior to and during regulatory and accrediting surveys, and to evaluate clinical and related processes. Organizations are expected to use outcome data to identify and prioritize the processes that support clinical care and demonstrate an attempt to improve performance. Providers may use outcomes data to support best practices by benchmarking their results with similar organizations. The benchmarking process is supported through publicly reported outcomes data at the national and state levels. National reporting occurs on the CMS website, where consumers and providers alike may access information and compare hospitals, home-care agencies, nursing homes, and managed care plans. For example, the websites http://www.hospitalcompare.hhs.gov, http://www.medicare.gov/nhcompare/, and http://www.medicare.gov/HomeHealthCompare

list outcome indicators relative to the specific service or delivery model. Consumers may use those websites to select organizations and compare outcomes, one against another, to aid in their selection of a facility or service. These websites also serve as a resource for providers to benchmark their outcomes against those of another organization. Outcomes data also become increasingly important to providers as the industry shifts toward a P4P/ VBP model.

In a P4P/VBP model, practitioners are reimbursed for achieved quality-of-care outcomes. Currently, the CMS has several P4P initiatives and demonstration projects (see http://www.cms.gov/DemoProjectsEvalRpts/ for details). The *Hospital Quality Initiative* (see http://www.cms.gov/HospitalQualityInits/ and http://www.cms.gov/HospitalQualityInits/Downloads/Hospital_VBP_102610.pdf for a detailed overview) is part of the U.S. Department of Health and Human Services' broader national quality initiative that focuses on an initial set of 10 quality measures by linking reporting of those measures to the payments the hospitals receive for each discharge. The purpose of the Premier Hospital Quality Incentive Demonstration (see http://www.cms.gov/HospitalQualityInits/35_HospitalPremier.asp for more details and outcomes) was to have improved the quality of inpatient care for Medicare beneficiaries by giving financial incentives to almost 300 hospitals for high quality. The Physician Group Practice Demonstration, mandated by the Medicare, Medicaid, and State Children's Health Insurance Program (SCHIP) Benefits Improvement and Protection Act of 2000 (BIPA), is the first P4P initiative for physicians under the Medicare program. The Medicare Care Management Performance Demonstration (Medicare Modernization Act [MMA] section 649), modeled on the "bridges to excellence" program, is a 3-year P4P demonstration with physicians to promote the adoption and use of health information technology to improve the quality of patient care for chronically ill Medicare patients. The Medicare Health Care Quality Demonstration, mandated by section 646 of the MMA, is a 5-year demonstration program under which projects enhance quality by improving patient safety, reducing variations in utilization by appropriate use of evidence-based care and best practice guidelines, encouraging shared decision making, and using culturally and ethnically appropriate care.

INTERVENTIONS AND CARE STRATEGIES

Measuring Quality of Care

Schyve and Nadzam (1998) identified several challenges to measuring quality. First, the suggestion that quality of care is in the eye of the beholder points to the different interests of multiple users. This issue encompasses both measurement and communication challenges. Measurement and analysis methods must generate information about the quality of care that meets the needs of different stakeholders. In addition, the results must be communicated in ways that meet these different needs. Second, we must have good and generally accepted tools for measuring quality. Thus, user groups must come together in their conceptualization of quality care so that relevant health care measures can be identified and standardized. A common language of measurement must be developed, grounded in a shared perspective on quality that is cohesive across, yet meets the needs of various user groups. Third, once the measurement systems are in place, data must be collected. This translates into resource demands and logistic issues as to who is to report, record, collect, and manage data. Fourth, data must be analyzed in statistically appropriate ways. This is not just a matter of using the right statistical methods. More important, user groups must agree on a framework for analyzing quality data to interpret the results. Fifth, health care environments are complex and dynamic in nature. There are differences across health care environments, between types of provider organizations, and within organizations. Furthermore, changes in health care occur frequently, such as the movement of care from one setting to another and the introduction of new technology. Finding common denominators is a major challenge.

Addressing the Challenges

These challenges are not insurmountable. However, making a commitment to quality care entails a commitment to putting the processes and systems in place to measure quality through performance measures and to report quality-of-care results. This commitment applies as much to a quality-improvement initiative on a nursing unit as it does to a corporate commitment by a large health care system. In other words, once an organization decides to pursue excellence (i.e., quality), it must accept the need to overcome the various challenges to measurement and reporting. Let us examine how this could be done in a clinical setting.

McGlynn and Asch (1998) offer several strategies for addressing the challenges to measuring quality. First, the various user groups must identify and balance competing perspectives. This is a process of giving and taking: not only proposing highly clinical measures (e.g., prevalence pressure ulcers) but also providing more general data (e.g., use of restraints). It is a process of asking and responding: not only asking management for monthly statistics on medication errors but also agreeing to provide management with the necessary documentation of the reasons stated for restraint use. Second, there must be an accountability framework. Committing to quality care implies that nurses assume several responsibilities and are willing to be held accountable for each of them: (a) providing the best possible care to older patients, (b) examining their own geriatric nursing knowledge and practice, (c) seeking ways to improve it, (d) agreeing to evaluation of their practice, and (e) responding to needs for improvement. Third, there must be objectivity in the evaluation of quality. This requires setting and adopting explicit criteria for judging performance, then building the evaluation process on these criteria. Nurses, their colleagues, and their managers need to reach consensus on how performance will be measured and what will be considered excellent (and good, average, etc.) performance. Fourth, once these indicators have been identified, nurses need to select a subset of indicators for routine reporting. Indicators should give a reliable snapshot of the team's care to older patients. Fifth, it is critical to separate as much as possible the use of indicators for evaluating patient care and the use of these indicators for financial or nonfinancial incentives. Should the team be cost conscious? Yes, but cost should not influence any clinical judgment as to what is best for patients. Finally, nurses in the clinical setting must plan how to collect the data. At the institutional level, this may be facilitated by information systems that allow performance measurement and reporting. Ideally, point-of-care documentation will also provide the data necessary for a systematic and goal-directed quality-improvement program, thus, eliminating separate data abstraction and collection activities.

The success of a quality-improvement program in geriatric nursing care (and the ability to overcome many of the challenges) hinges on the decision as to what to measure.

We know that good performance measures must be objective, that data collection must be easy and as burdenless as possible, that statistical analysis must be guided by principles and placed within a framework, and that communication of results must be targeted toward different user groups. Conceivably, we could try to measure every possible aspect of care; realistically, however, the planning for this will never reach the implementation stage. Instead, nurses need to establish priorities by asking these questions: Based on our clinical expertise, what is critical for us to know? What aspects of our care to older patients are high risk or high volume? What parts of our elder care are problem-prone, either because we have experienced difficulties in the past or because we can anticipate problems caused by the lack of knowledge or resources? What clinical indicators would be of interest to other user groups: patients, the general public, management, payors, accreditors, and practitioners? Throughout this prioritization process, nurses should keep asking themselves: What questions are we trying to answer, and for whom?

Measuring Performance—Selecting Quality Indicators

The correct selection of performance measures or quality indicators is a crucial step in evaluating nursing care and is based on two important factors: frequency and volume. Clearly, high-volume practices or frequent processes require focused attention—to ensure that the care is being delivered according to protocol or processes are functioning as designed. Problem-prone or high-risk processes would also warrant a review because these are processes with inherent risk to patients or variances in implementing the process. The selection of indicators must also be consistent with organizational goals for improvement. This provides buy-in from practitioners as well as administration when reporting and identifying opportunities for improvement. Performance measures (indicators) must be based on either a standard of care, policy, procedure, or protocol. These documents, or standards of care, define practice and expectations in the clinical setting and, therefore, determine the criteria for the monitoring tool. The measurement of these standards simply reflects adherence to or implementation of these standards. Once it is decided what to measure, nurses in the clinical geriatric practice setting face the task of deciding how to measure performance. There are two possibilities: either the appropriate measure (indicator) already exists or a new performance measure must be developed. Either way, there are a number of requirements of a good performance measure that will need to be applied.

Although indicators used to monitor patient care and performance do not need to be subject to the rigors of research, it is imperative that they reflect some of the attributes necessary to make relevant statements about the care. The measure and its output need to focus on improvement, not merely the description of something. It is not helpful to have a very accurate measure that just tells the status of a given dimension of practice. Instead, the measure needs to inform us about current quality levels and relate them to previous and future quality levels. It needs to be able to compute improvements or declines in quality over time so that we can plan for the future. For example, to have a measure that only tells the number of medication errors in the past month would not be helpful. Instead, a measure that tells what types of medication errors were made, perhaps even with a severity rating indicated, compares this to medication errors made during the previous months, and shows in numbers and graphs the changes over time that will enable us to do the necessary root-cause analysis to prevent more medication errors in the future.

Performance measures need to be clearly defined, including the terms used, the data elements collected, and the calculation steps employed. Establishing the definition prior to implementing the monitoring activity allows for precise data collection. It also facilitates benchmarking with other organizations when the data elements are similarly defined and the data collection methodologies are consistent. Imagine that we want to monitor falls on the unit. The initial questions would be as follows: What is considered a fall? Does the patient have to be on the floor? Does a patient slumping against the wall or onto a table while trying to prevent himself or herself from falling to the floor constitute a fall? Is a fall due to physical weakness or orthostatic hypotension treated the same as a fall caused by tripping over an obstacle? The next question would be the following: Over what time are falls measured: a week, a fortnight, a month, a quarter, a year? The time frame is not a matter of convenience but of accuracy. To be able to monitor falls accurately, we need to identify a time frame that will capture enough events to be meaningful and interpretable from a quality improvement point of view. External indicator definitions, such as those defined for use in the National Database of Nursing Quality Indicators, provide guidance for both the indicator definition as well as the data collection methodology for *nursing-sensitive indicators*. The nursing-sensitive indicators reflect the structure, process, and outcomes of nursing care. The *structure* of nursing care is indicated by the supply of nursing staff, the skill level of the nursing staff, and the education/certification of nursing staff. *Process* indicators measure aspects of nursing care such as assessment, intervention, and registered nurse (RN) job satisfaction. Patient *outcomes* that are determined to be nursing sensitive are those that improve if there is a greater quantity or quality of nursing care (e.g., pressure ulcers, falls, intravenous [IV] infiltrations) and are not considered "nursing-sensitive" (e.g., frequency of primary C-sections, cardiac failure; see http://www.nursingquality .org/FAQPage.aspx#1 for details). Several nursing organizations across the country participate in data collection and submission, which allows for a robust database and excellent benchmarking opportunities.

Additional indicator attributes include validity, sensitivity, and specificity. *Validity* refers to whether the measure "actually measures what it purports to measure" (Wilson, 1989). *Sensitivity* and *specificity* refer to the ability of the measure to capture all true cases of the event being measured, and only true cases. We want to make sure that a performance measure identifies true cases as true, and false cases as false, and does not identify a true case as false or a false case as true. Sensitivity of a performance measure is the likelihood of a positive test when a condition is present. Lack of sensitivity is expressed as false positives: The indicator calculates a condition as present when in fact it is not. Specificity refers to the likelihood of a negative test when a condition is not present. False-negatives reflect lack of specificity: The indicators calculate that a condition is not present when in fact it is. Consider the case of depression and the recommendation in Chapter 9, Depression in Older Adults, to use the Geriatric Depression Scale, in which a score of 11 or greater is indicative of depression. How robust is this cutoff score of 11? What is the likelihood that someone with a score of 9 or 10 (i.e., negative for depression) might actually be depressed (false-negative)? Similarly, what is the likelihood that a patient with a score of 13 would not be depressed (false positive)?

Reliability means that results are reproducible; the indicator measures the same attribute consistently across the same patients and across time. Reliability begins with a precise definition and specification, as described earlier. A measure is reliable if different people calculate the same rate for the same patient sample. The core issue of reliability is measurement error, or the difference between the actual phenomenon and its measurement: The greater the difference, the less reliable the performance measure. For example, suppose that we want to focus on pain management in older adults with end-stage cancer. One way of measuring pain would be to ask patients to rate their pain as none, a little, some, quite a bit, or a lot. An alternative approach would be to administer a visual analog scale, a 10-point line on which patients indicate their pain levels. Yet another approach would be to ask the pharmacy to produce monthly reports of analgesic use by type and dose. Generally speaking, the more subjective the scoring or measurement, the less reliable it will be. If all these measures were of equal reliability, they would yield the same result. Concept of reliability, particularly inter-rate reliability, becomes increasingly important to consider in those situations where data collection is assigned to several staff members. It is important to review the data collection methodology and the instrument in detail to avoid different approaches by the various people collecting the data.

Several of the examples given earlier imply the criterion of interpretability. A performance measure must be interpretable; that is, it must convey a result that can be linked to the quality of clinical care. First, the quantitative output of a performance measure must be scaled in such a way that users can interpret it. For example, a scale that starts with 0 as the lowest possible level and ends with 100 is a lot easier to interpret than a scale that starts with 13.325 and has no upper boundary except infinity. Second, we should be able to place the number within a context. Suppose we are working in a hemodialysis center that serves quite a large proportion of patients with end-stage renal disease (ESRD) and are older than the age of 60—the group least likely to be fit for a kidney transplant yet with several years of life expectancy remaining. We know that virtually all patients with ESRD develop anemia (hemoglobin [Hb] level less than 11 g/dL), which in turn impacts on their activities of daily living (ADL) and independent activities of daily living (IADL) performance. In collaboration with the nephrologists, we initiate a systematic program of anemia monitoring and management, relying in part on published best practice guidelines. We want to achieve the best practice guideline of 85% of all patients having Hb levels equal to or greater than 11 g/dL. We should be able to succeed because the central laboratory provides us with Hb levels, which allows us to calculate the percentage of patients at Hb of 11 g/dL or greater.

The concept of risk-adjusted performance measures or outcome indicators is an important one. Some patients are more sick than others, some have more comorbidities, and some are older and frailer. No doubt, we could come up with many more risk variables that influence how patients respond to nursing care. Good performance measures take this differential risk into consideration. They create a "level playing field" by adjusting quality indicators on the basis of the (risk for) severity of illness of the patients. It would not be fair to the health care team if the patients on the unit are a lot sicker than those on the unit a floor above. The team is at greater risk for having lower quality outcomes, not because they provide inferior care, but because the patients are a lot more sick and are at greater risk for a compromised response to the care provided. The more sick patients are more demanding in terms of care and ultimately are less likely to achieve the same outcomes as less ill patients. Performance measures must be easy to collect. The many examples cited earlier also refer to the importance of using performance measures for which data are readily available, can be retrieved from existing sources or can be collected with little burden. The goal is to gather good data quickly without running the risk of having "quick and dirty" data.

We begin the process of deciding how to measure by reviewing existing measures. There is no need to reinvent the wheel, especially if good measures are out there. Nurses should review the literature, check with national organizations, and consult with colleagues. Yet, we should not adopt existing measures blindly. Instead, we need to subject them to a thorough review using the characteristics identified previously. Also, health care organizations that have adopted these measures can offer their experience.

It may be that after an exhaustive search, we cannot find measures that meet the various requirements outlined previously. We decide instead to develop our own in-house measure. The following are some important guidelines:

1. *Zero in on the population to be measured.* If we are measuring an undesirable event, we must determine the group at risk for experiencing that event, then limit the denominator population to that group. If we are measuring a desirable event or process, we must identify the group that should experience the event or receive the process. Where do problems tend to occur? What variables of this problem are within our control? If some are not within our control, how can we zero in even more on the target population? In other words, we exclude patients from the population when good reason exists to do so (e.g., those allergic to the medication being measured).
2. *Define terms.* This is a painstaking but essential effort. It is better to measure 80% of an issue with 100% accuracy than 100% of an issue with 80% accuracy.
3. *Identify and define the data elements and allowable values required to calculate the measure.* This is another painstaking but essential effort. The 80/100 rule applies here, as well.
4. *Test the data collection process.* Once we have a prototype of a measure ready, we must examine how easy or difficult it is to get all the required data.

IMPLEMENTING THE QUALITY ASSESSMENT AND PERFORMANCE IMPROVEMENT PROGRAM

Successful Performance Improvement programs require an organizational commitment to implementation of the Performance Improvement processes and principles outlined in this chapter. Consequently, this commitment requires a defined, organized approach that most organizations embrace and define in the form of a written plan. The plan outlines the approach the organization uses to improve care and safety for its patients. There are several important elements that must be addressed in order to implement the Performance Improvement program effectively. The scope of service, which addresses the types of patients and care that is rendered, provides direction on the selection of performance measures. An authority and responsibility statement in the document defines who is able to implement the quality program and make decisions that will affect its implementation. Finally, it is important to define the committee structure used to effectively analyze and communicate improvement efforts to the organization.

The success of the Performance Improvement program is highly dependent on a well-defined structure and appropriate selection of performance measures. The following is a list of issues that, if not addressed, may negatively impact the success of the quality program:

1. *Lack of focus*: a measure that tries to track too many criteria at the same time or is too complicated to administer, interpret, or use for quality monitoring and improvement
2. *Wrong type of measure*: a measure that calculates indicators the wrong way (e.g., uses rates when ratios are more appropriate; uses a continuous scale rather than a discrete scale; measures a process when the outcome is measurable and of greater interest)
3. *Unclear definitions*: a measure that is too broad or too vague in its scope and definitions (e.g., population is too heterogeneous, no risk adjustment, unclear data elements, poorly defined values)

4. *Too much work*: a measure that requires too much clinician time to generate the data or too much manual chart abstraction
5. *Reinventing the wheel*: a measure that is a reinvention rather than an improvement of a performance measure
6. *Events not under control*: measure focuses on a process or outcome that is out of the organization (or the unit's) control to improve
7. *Trying to do research rather than quality improvement*: data collection and analysis are done for the sake of research rather than for improvement of nursing care and the health and well-being of the patients
8 *Poor communication of results*: the format of communication does not target and enable change
9. *Uninterpretable and underused*: uninterpretable results are of little relevance to improving geriatric nursing care

In summary, the success of the Quality Assessment Performance Improvement Program's ability to measure, evaluate, and improve the quality of nursing care to health system elders is in the planning. First, it is important to define the scope of services provided and those to be monitored and improved. Second, identify performance measures that are reflective of the care provided. Indicators may be developed internally or may be obtained from external sources of outcomes and data collection methodologies. Third, it is important to analyze the data, pulling together the right people to evaluate processes, make recommendations, and improve care. Finally, it is important to communicate findings across the organization and celebrate success.

RESOURCES

Hospital Compare
http://www.hospitalcompare.hhs.gov/

Nursing Home Compare
http://www.medicare.gov/nhcompare/

Home Health Compare
http://www.medicare.gov/HomeHealthCompare

Centers for Medicare and Medicaid Services Hospital Quality Initiatives
http://www.cms.gov/HospitalQualityInits/

Centers for Medicare and Medicaid Services Hospital Quality Initiatives Press Release, dated 9/17/09
http://www.cms.gov/HospitalQualityInits/downloads/HospitalPremierPressReleases20090817.pdf

Centers for Medicare and Medicaid Services Demonstration Projects and Evaluation Reports
http://www.cms.gov/DemoProjectsEvalRpts/MD/list.asp?intNumPerPage=all

REFERENCES

Fulmer, T., Mezey, M., Bottrell, M., Abraham, I., Sazant, J., Grossman, S., & Grisham, E. (2002). Nurses Improving Care for Health System Elders (NICHE): Using outcomes and benchmarks for evidence-based practice. *Geriatric Nursing, 23*(3), 121–127.

Johnson, K., Hallsey, D., Meredith, R. L., & Warden, E. (2006). A nurse-driven system for improving patient quality outcomes. *Journal of Nursing Care Quality, 21*(2), 168–175.

Kohn, L. T., Corrigan, J. M., & Donaldson, M. S. (Eds.). (2000). *To err is human: Building a safer health system* (p. 222). Washington, DC: National Academy Press.

McGlynn, E. A., & Asch, S. M. (1998). Developing a clinical performance measure. *American Journal of Preventive Medicine, 14*(3 Suppl.), 14–21.

Nadzam, D. M., & Abraham, I. L. (2003). Measuring performance, improving quality. In M. D. Mezey, T. Fulmer, & I. Abraham (Eds.), *Geriatric nursing protocols for best practice* (2nd ed., pp. 15–30). New York, NY: Springer Publishing Company.

Schyve, P. M., & Nadzam, D. M. (1998). Performance measurement in healthcare. *Journal of Strategic Performance Measurement, 2*(4), 34–42.

State Children's Health Insurance Program (SCHIP). (2010). The National Center for Public Policy Research. Accessed August 23, 2011, from http://www.schip-info.org

Wilson, H. S. (1989). *Research in nursing* (2nd ed., p. 355). Reading, MA: Addison-Wesley.

ADDITIONAL READINGS

Albanese, M. P., Evans, D. A., Schantz, C. A., Bowen, M., Disbot, M., Moffa, J. S., . . . Polomano, R. C. (2010). Engaging clinical nurses in quality and performance improvement activities. *Nursing Administration Quarterly, 34*(3), 226–245.

Bowling, A. (2001). *Measuring disease: A review of disease-specific quality of life measurement scales* (2nd ed.). Philadelphia, PA: Open University Press.

Bryant, L. L., Floersch, N., Richard, A. A., & Schlenker, R. E. (2004). Measuring healthcare outcomes to improve quality of care across post-acute care provider settings. *Journal of Nursing Care Quality, 19*(4), 368–376.

Coopey, M., Nix, M. P., & Clancy, C. M. (2006). Translating research into evdience-based nursing practice and evaluating effectiveness. *Journal of Nursing Care Quality, 21*(3), 195–202.

Hart, S., Bergquist, S., Gajewski, B., & Dunton, N. (2006). Reliability testing of the National Database of Nursing Quality Indicators pressure ulcer indicator. *Journal of Nursing Care Quality, 21*(3), 256–265.

Hoo, W. E., & Parisi, L. L. (2005). Nursing informatics approach to analyzing staffing effectiveness indicators. *Journal of Nursing Care Quality, 20*(3), 215–219.

Kliger, J., Lacey, S. R., Olney, A., Cox, K. S., & O'Neil, E. (2010). Nurse-driven programs to improve patient outcomes: Transforming care at the bedside, integrated nurse leadership program, and the clinical scene investigator academy. *The Journal of Nursing Administration, 40*(3), 109–114.

Kovner, C. T., Brewer, C. S., Yingrengreung, S., & Fairchild, S. (2010). New nurses' views of quality improvement education. *Joint Commission Journal on Quality and Patient Safety/Joint Commission Resources, 36*(1), 29–35.

Lageson, C. (2004). Quality focus of the first line nurse manager and relationship to unit outcomes. *Journal of Nursing Care Quality, 19*(4), 336–342.

Age-Related Changes in Health

3

Constance M. Smith and Valerie T. Cotter

EDUCATIONAL OBJECTIVES

On completion of this chapter, the reader should be able to:

1. describe the structural and functional changes in multiple body systems that occur during the normal aging process
2. understand the clinical significance of these age-related changes regarding the health and disease risks of the older adult
3. discuss the components of a nursing assessment for the older adult in light of the manifestations of normal aging
4. identify care strategies to promote successful aging in older adults, with consderation of age-related changes

The process of normal aging, independent of disease, is accompanied by a myriad of changes in body systems. As evidenced by longitudinal studies such as the Baltimore Longitudinal Study of Aging (2010), modifications occur in both structure and function of organs and are most pronounced in advanced age of 85 years or older (Hall, 2002). Many of these alterations are characterized by a decline in physiological reserve, so that, although baseline function is preserved, organ systems become progressively less capable of maintaining homeostasis in the face of stresses imposed by the environment, disease, or medical therapies (Miller, 2009). Age-related changes are strongly impacted by genetics, as well as by long-term lifestyle factors, including physical activity, diet, alcohol consumption, and tobacco use (Kitzman & Taffet, 2009). Furthermore, great heterogeneity occurs among older adults; clinical manifestations of aging can range from stability to significant decline in function of specific organ systems (Beck, 1998).

The clinical implications of these age-related alterations are important in nursing assessment and care of the older adult for several reasons. First, changes associated with normal aging must be differentiated from pathological processes in order to develop appropriate interventions (Gallagher, O'Mahony, & Quigley, 2008). Manifestations of aging can also adversely impact the health and functional capability of older adults and

For description of Evidence Levels cited in this chapter, see Chapter 1, Developing and Evaluating Clinical Practice Guidelines: A Systematic Approach, page 7.

require therapeutic strategies to correct (Matsumura & Ambrose, 2006). Age-associated changes predispose older persons to selected diseases (Kitzman & Taffet, 2009). Thus, nurses' understanding of these risks can serve to develop more effective approaches to assessment and care. Finally, aging and illness may interact reciprocally, resulting in altered presentation of illness, response to treatment, and outcomes (Hall, 2002).

This chapter describes age-dependent changes for several body systems. Clinical implications of these alterations, including associated disease risks, are then discussed followed by nursing assessment and care strategies related to these changes.

CARDIOVASCULAR SYSTEM

Cardiac reserve declines in normal aging. This alteration does not affect cardiac function at rest and resting heart rate, ejection fraction, and cardiac output remain virtually unchanged with age. However, under physiological stress, the ability of the older adult's heart to increase both rate and cardiac output, in response to increased cardiac demand, such as physical activity or infection, is compromised (Lakatta, 2000). Such diminished functional reserve results in reduced exercise tolerance, fatigue, shortness of breath, slow recovery from tachycardia (Watters, 2002), and intolerance of volume depletion (Mick & Ackerman, 2004). Furthermore, because of the decreased maximal attainable heart rate with aging, a heart rate of greater than 90 beats per minute (bpm) in an older adult indicates significant physiological stress (Kitzman & Taffet, 2009).

Age-dependent changes in both the vasculature and the heart contribute to the impairment in cardiac reserve. An increase in the wall thickness and stiffness of the aorta and carotid arteries results in diminished vessel compliance and greater systemic vascular resistance (Thomas & Rich, 2007). Elevated systolic blood pressure (BP) with constant diastolic pressure follows, increasing the risk of isolated systolic hypertension and widened pulse pressure (Joint National Committee [JNC], 2004). Strong arterial pulses, diminished peripheral pulses, and increased potential for inflamed varicosities occur commonly with age. Reductions in capillary density restrict blood flow in the extremities, producing cool skin (Mick & Ackerman, 2004).

As an adaptive measure to increased workload against noncompliant arteries, the left ventricle and atrium hypertrophy become rigid. The ensuing impairment in relaxation of the left ventricle during diastole places greater dependence on atrial contractions to achieve left ventricular filling (Lakatta, 2000). In addition, sympathetic response in the heart is blunted because of diminished β-adrenergic sensitivity, resulting in decreased myocardial contractility (Thomas & Rich, 2007).

Additional age-related changes include sclerosis of atrial and mitral valves, which impairs their tight closure and increases the risk of dysfunction. The ensuing leaky heart valves may result in aortic regurgitation or mitral stenosis, presenting on exam as heart murmurs (Kitzman & Taffet, 2009). Loss of pacemaker and conduction cells contributes to changes in the resting electrocardiogram (ECG) of older adults. Isolated premature atrial and ventricular complexes are common arrhythmias, and the risk of atrial fibrillation is increased (Thomas & Rich, 2007). Because of atrial contractions in diastole, S_4 frequently develops as an extra heart sound (Lakatta, 2000).

Baroreceptor function, which regulates BP, is impaired with age, particularly with change in position. Postural hypotension with orthostatic symptoms may follow, especially after prolonged bed rest, dehydration, or cardiovascular drug use, and can cause dizziness and potential for falls (Mukai & Lipsitz, 2002).

Cardiac assessment of an older adult includes performing an ECG and monitoring heart rate (40–100 bpm within normal limits), rhythm (noting whether it is regular or irregular), heart sounds (S_1, S_2, or extra heart sounds S_3 in heart disease or S_4 as a common finding), and murmurs (noting location where loudest). The apical impulse is displaced laterally. In palpation of the carotid arteries, asymmetric volumes and decreased pulsations may indicate aortic stenosis and impaired left cardiac output, respectively. Auscultation of a bruit potentially suggests occlusive arterial disease. Peripheral pulses should be assessed bilaterally at a minimum of one pulse point in each extremity. Assessment may reveal asymmetry in pulse volume suggesting insufficiency in arterial circulation (Docherty, 2002). The nurse should examine lower extremities for varicose veins and note dilation or swelling. In addition, dyspnea with exertion and exercise intolerance are critical to note (Mahler, Fierro-Carrion, & Baird, 2003).

BP should be measured at least twice (Kestel, 2005) on the older adult and performed in a comfortably seated position with back supported and feet flat on the floor. The BP should then be repeated after 5 minutes of rest. Measurements in both supine and standing positions evaluate postural hypotension (Mukai & Lipsitz, 2002).

Nursing care strategies include referrals for older adults who have irregularities of heart rhythm and decreased or asymmetric peripheral pulses. The risk of postural hypotension emphasizes the need for safety precautions (Mukai & Lipsitz, 2002) to prevent falls. These include avoiding prolonged recumbency or motionless standing and encouraging the older adult to rise slowly from lying or sitting positions and wait for 1 to 2 minutes after a position change to stand or transfer. Overt signs of hypotension such as a change in sensorium or mental status, dizziness, or orthostasis should be monitored, and fall-prevention strategies should be instituted. Sufficient fluid intake is advised to ensure adequate hydration and prevent hypovolemia for optimal cardiac functioning (Docherty, 2002; Watters, 2002).

Older adults should be encouraged to adopt lifestyle practices for cardiovascular fitness with the aim of a healthy body weight (body mass index [BMI] 18.5–24.9 kg/m²; American Heart Association Nutrition Committee et al., 2006) and normal BP (JNC, 2004). These practices involve a healthful diet (Knoops et al., 2004), physical activity appropriate for age and health status (Netz, Wu, Becker, & Tenenbaum, 2005), and elimination of the use of and exposure to tobacco products (U.S. Department of Health and Human Services [USDHHS], 2004a).

PULMONARY SYSTEM

Respiratory function slowly and progressively deteriorates with age. This decline in ventilatory capacity seldom affects breathing during rest or customary limited physical activity in healthy older adults (Zeleznik, 2003); however, with greater than usual exertional demands, pulmonary reserve against hypoxia is readily exhausted and dyspnea occurs (Imperato & Sanchez, 2006).

Several age-dependent anatomic and physiologic changes combine to impair the functional reserve of the pulmonary system. Respiratory muscle strength and endurance deteriorate to restrict maximal ventilatory capacity (Buchman et al., 2008). Secondary to calcification of rib cage cartilage, the chest wall becomes rigid (Imperato & Sanchez, 2006), limiting thoracic compliance. Loss of elastic fibers reduces recoil of small airways, which can collapse and cause air trapping, particularly in dependent portions of the lung. Decreases in alveolar surface area, vascularization, and surfactant production adversely affect gaseous exchange (Zeleznik, 2003).

Additional clinical consequences of aging include an increased anteroposterior chest diameter caused by skeletal changes. An elevated respiratory rate of 12–24 breaths per minute accompanies reduced tidal volume for rapid, shallow breathing. Limited diaphragmatic excursion and chest/lung expansion can result in less effective inspiration and expiration (Buchman et al., 2008; Mick & Ackerman, 2004). Because of decreased cough reflex effectiveness and deep breathing capacity, mucus and foreign matter clearance is restricted, predisposing to aspiration, infection, and bronchospasm (Watters, 2002). Further, elevating the risk of infection is a decline in ciliary and macrophage activities and drying of the mucosal membranes with more difficult mucous excretion (Htwe, Mushtaq, Robinson, Rosher, & Khardori, 2007). With the loss of elastic recoil comes the potential for atelectasis. Because of reduced respiratory center sensitivity, ventilatory responses to hypoxia and hypercapnia are blunted (Imperato & Sanchez, 2006), putting the older adult at risk for development of respiratory distress with illness or administration of narcotics (Zeleznik, 2003).

The modifications in ventilatory capacity with age are reflected in changes in pulmonary function tests measuring lung volumes, flow rates, diffusing capacity, and gas exchange. Whereas total lung capacity remains constant, vital capacity is reduced and residual volume is increased. Reductions in all measures of expiratory flow (forced expiratory volume in 1 second [FEV_1], forced vital capacity [FVC], FEV_1/FVC, peak expiratory flow rate [PEFR]) quantify a decline in useful air movement (Imperato & Sanchez, 2006). Because of impaired alveolar function, diffusing capacity of the lung for carbon monoxide (DLCO) declines as does pulmonary arterial oxygen tension (PaO_2), indicating impaired oxygen exchange; however, arterial pH and partial pressure of arterial carbon dioxide ($PaCO_2$) remain constant (Enright, 2009). Reductions in arterial oxygen saturation and cardiac output restrict the amount of oxygen available for use by tissues, particularly in the supine position, although arterial blood gas seldom limits exercise in healthy subjects (Zeleznik, 2003).

Respiratory assessment includes determination of breathing rate, rhythm, regularity, volume (hyperventilation/hypoventilation), depth (shallow, deep; Docherty, 2002), and effort (dyspnea; Mahler et al., 2003). Auscultation of breath sounds throughout the lung fields may reveal decreased air exchange at the lung bases (Mick & Ackerman, 2004). Thorax and symmetry of chest expansion should be inspected. A history of respiratory disease (tuberculosis, asthma), tobacco use (expressed as pack years), and extended exposure to environmental irritants through work or avocation is contributory (Imperato & Sanchez, 2006).

Subjective assessment of cough includes questions on quality (productive/nonproductive), sputum characteristics (note hemoptysis; purulence indicating possible infection), and frequency (during eating or drinking, suggesting dysphagia and aspiration; Smith & Connolly, 2003).

Secretions and decreased breathing rate during sedation can reduce ventilation and oxygenation (Watters, 2002). Oxygen saturation can be followed through arterial blood gases and pulse oximetry (Zeleznik, 2003) while breathing rate (greater than 24 respirations per minute), accessory muscle use, and skin color (cyanosis, pallor) should also be monitored (Docherty, 2002). The inability to expectorate secretions, the appearance of dyspnea, and decreased saturation of oxygen (SaO_2) levels suggest the need for suctioning to clear airways (Smith & Connolly, 2003). Optimal positioning to facilitate respiration should be regularly monitored with use of upright positions (Fowler's or orthopneic position) recommended (Docherty, 2002). Pain assessment may be necessary to allow ambulation and deep breathing (Mick & Ackerman, 2004). See Atypical Presentation of Disease section for assessment of pneumonia, tuberculosis, and influenza.

Nursing care strategies useful in facilitating respiration and maintaining patent airways in the older adult include positioning to allow maximum chest expansion through the use of semi- or high-Fowler's or orthopneic position (Docherty, 2002). Additionally, frequent repositioning in bed or encouraging ambulation, if mobility permits, is advised (Watters, 2002). Analgesics may be necessary for ambulation and deep breathing (Mick & Ackerman, 2004).

Hydration is maintained through fluid intake (6–8 oz per day) and air humidification, which prevent desiccation of mucous membranes and loosen secretions to facilitate expectoration (Suhayda & Walton, 2002). Suctioning may be necessary to clear airways of secretions (Smith & Connolly, 2003) while oxygen should be provided as needed (Docherty, 2002). Incentive spirometry, with use of sustained maximal inspiration devices (SMIs), can improve pulmonary ventilation, mainly inhalation, as well as loosen respiratory secretions, particularly in older adults who are unable to ambulate or are declining in function (Dunn, 2004).

Deep breathing exercises, such as abdominal (diaphragmatic) and pursed-lip breathing, in addition to controlled and huff coughing, can further facilitate respiratory function. Techniques for healthy breathing, including sitting and standing erect, nose breathing (Dunn, 2004), and regular exercise (Netz et al., 2005) should be promoted. Education on eliminating the use of and exposure to tobacco problems should be emphasized (USDHHS, 2004a).

RENAL AND GENITOURINARY SYSTEMS

In normal aging, the mass of the kidney declines with a loss of functional glomeruli and tubules in addition to a reduction in blood flow. Concomitantly, changes occur in the activity of the regulatory hormones, vasopressin (antidiuretic hormone), atrial natriuretic hormone, and renin-angiotensin-aldosterone system (Miller, 2009). These alterations combine to result in diminished glomerular filtration rate (GFR), with a 10% decrement per decade starting at age 30, as well as impaired electrolyte and water management (Beck, 1998).

Despite these changes, the older adult maintains the ability to regulate fluid balance under baseline conditions; however, with age, the renal system is more limited in its capacity to respond to externally imposed stresses. This reduced functional reserve increases vulnerability to disturbances in fluid homeostasis as well as to renal complications and failure (Lerma, 2009), particularly from fluid/electrolyte overload and deficit, medications, or illness (Miller, 2009).

The decline in functional nephrons emphasizes the risk from nephrotoxic agents including nonsteroidal anti-inflammatory drugs (NSAIDs), β-lactam antibiotics, and radiocontrast dyes. Reduced GFR impairs the older adult's ability to excrete renally cleared medications such as aminoglycoside antibiotics (e.g., gentamicin) and digoxin, increasing the risk of adverse drug reactions (Beyth & Shorr, 2002). Dosages should be based on GFR estimated by the Cockcroft-Gault equation for creatinine clearance (Péquignot et al., 2009) or the modification of diet in renal disease (MDRD) rather than by serum creatinine concentration (Miller, 2009; National Kidney Disease Education Program, 2009). Values of serum creatinine remain unchanged despite an age-associated decline in GFR because of the parallel decrease in both older adults' skeletal muscle mass, which produces creatinine and GFR for creatinine elimination. Thus, serum creatinine levels overestimate GFR to result in potential drug overdose (Beck, 1998).

Increased risk of electrolyte imbalances can result from an age-dependent impairment in the excretion of excessive sodium loads, particularly in heart failure and with NSAID use, leading to intravascular volume overload. Clinical indicators include weight gain (greater than 2%); intake is greater than output; edema; change in mental status; tachycardia; bounding pulse; pulmonary congestion with dyspnea, rales; increased BP and central venous pressure (CVP); and distended neck/peripheral veins (Beck, 1998).

Conversely, sodium wasting or excess sodium excretion when maximal sodium conservation is needed, can occur with diarrhea. Hypovolemia and dehydration may ensue (Stern, 2006), manifesting as acute change in mental status (may be the initial symptom), weight loss (greater than 2%), decreased tissue turgor, dry oral mucosa, tachycardia, decreased BP, postural hypotension, flat neck veins, poor capillary refill, oliguria (less than 30 mL/hr), increased hematocrit and specific gravity of urine, blood urea nitrogen (BUN): plasma creatinine ratio greater than 20:1, and serum osmolality greater than 300 mOsm/kg (Mentes, 2006).

Impaired potassium excretion puts the older adult at risk for hyperkalemia, particularly in heart failure and with use of potassium supplements, potassium-sparing diuretics, NSAIDs, and angiotensin-converting enzyme (ACE) inhibitors (Mick & Ackerman, 2004). Clinical indicators include diarrhea, change in mental status, cardiac dysrhythmias or arrest, muscle weakness and areflexia, paresthesias and numbness in extremities, ECG abnormalities, and serum potassium greater than 5.0 mEq/L (Beck, 1998).

Limited acid excretion capability can cause metabolic acidosis during acute illness in the older adult. This condition presents as Kussmaul's respirations, change in mental status, nausea, vomiting, arterial blood pH less than 7.35, serum bicarbonate less than 22 mEq/L, and $PaCO_2$ less than 38 mm Hg with respiratory compensation (Beck, 1998).

Causes of abnormal water metabolism with age include diminution in maximal urinary concentrating ability, which, in concert with blunted thirst sensation and total body water, can result in hypertonic dehydration and hypernatremia (Mentes, 2006). Often associated with insensible fluid loss from fever (Miller, 2009), hypernatremia presents with thirst; dry oral mucosa; dry, furrowed tongue; postural hypotension; weakness; lethargy; serum sodium less than 150 mEq/L; and serum osmolality less than 290 mOsm/kg. Disorientation, seizures, and coma occur in severe hypernatremia (Suhayda & Walton, 2002).

Impaired excretion of a water load, exacerbated by ACE inhibitors, thiazide diuretics (Miller, 2009), and selective serotonin reuptake inhibitors (SSRIs; Mentes, 2006), predisposes the older adult to water intoxication and hyponatremia (Beck, 1998). Clinical indicators involve lethargy, nausea, muscle weakness and cramps, serum sodium less than 135 mEq/L, and serum osmolality less than 290 mOsm/kg. Confusion, coma, and seizures are seen in severe hyponatremia (Suhayda & Walton, 2002).

Changes in the lower urinary tract with age include reduced bladder elasticity and innervation, which contribute to decreases in urine flow rate, voided volume, and bladder capacity, as well as increases in postvoid residual and involuntary bladder contractions. A delayed or decreased perception of the signal from the bladder to void translates into urinary urgency (Kevorkian, 2004). Increased nocturnal urine flow, which results from altered regulatory hormone production, impaired ability to concentrate urine, and bladder–muscle instability, can lead to nocturnal polyuria (Miller, 2009). In older men, benign prostatic hyperplasia (BPH) can result in urinary urgency, hesitancy, and frequency. All these changes combine to increase the risk of urinary incontinence in the older adult. Further, urgency and nocturia increase the risk of falls. Changes with age in the physiology of the urinary tract such as increased vaginal pH and decreased antibacterial activity of urine in addition to the functional changes of the bladder contribute to the development of bacteriuria, with potential for urinary tract infection (UTI; Htwe et al., 2007; Stern, 2006).

Renal assessment includes monitoring for renal function (GFR) based on creatinine clearance, particularly in acute and chronic illness (Lerma, 2009; Miller, 2009; Péquignot et al., 2009). The choice, dose, need, and alternatives for nephrotoxic and renally excreted agents should be considered (Beyth & Shorr, 2002).

Dehydration, volume overload, and electrolyte status are assessed first by screening for risk of fluid/electrolyte imbalances based on the older adult's age, medical and nutritional history, medications, cognitive and functional abilities, psychosocial status, and bowel and bladder patterns. Data on fluid intake and output; daily weights; and vital signs, including orthostatic BP measurements, are needed. Heart rate is a less reliable indicator for dehydration in older adults because of the effects of medications and heart disease (Suhayda & Walton, 2002).

Physical assessment for fluid/electrolyte status focuses on skin for edema and turgor. Note that turgor in older adults is a less reliable indicator for dehydration because of poor skin elasticity, and assessment over the sternum or inner thigh is recommended. Additional assessment involves the oral mucosa for dryness as well as cardiovascular, respiratory, and neurologic systems. Acute changes in mental status, reasoning, memory, or attention may be initial symptoms of dehydration (Suhayda & Walton, 2002). Pertinent laboratory tests include serum electrolytes, serum osmolality, complete blood count (CBC), urine pH and specific gravity, BUN, hematocrit (Mentes, 2006), and arterial blood gases (Beck, 1998).

Evaluations of urinary incontinence, UTI, and nocturnal polyuria using a 72-hour voiding diary are recommended. See Atypical Presentation of Diseases section for UTI. Voiding history and rectal exam are required to diagnose BPH (see Chapter 18, Urinary Incontinence). Fall risk should be addressed when nocturnal or urgent voiding is present (see Chapter 15, Fall Prevention: Assessment, Diagnoses, and Intervention Strategies).

Ongoing care involves monitoring for renal function (Lerma, 2009; Miller, 2009; Péquignot et al., 2009) and for levels of nephrotoxic and renally cleared drugs (Beyth & Shorr, 2002). Maintenance of fluid/electrolyte balance is paramount (Beck, 1998). To prevent dehydration, older adults weighing between 50 and 80 kg are advised to have a minimum fluid intake of 1,500–2,500 mL/day (unless contraindicated by medical condition; Suhayda & Walton, 2002) from both fluids and food sources including fruits, vegetables, soups, and gelatin with avoidance of high salt and caffeine (Mentes, 2006; Ney, Weiss, Kind, & Robbins, 2009).

Incontinence care and exercise can contribute to management of voiding problems, including reduced incontinence, of nursing home residents (Schnelle et al., 2002). Behavioral interventions recommended for nocturnal polyuria include limited fluid intake in the evening, avoidance of caffeine and alcohol, and prompted voiding schedule (Miller, 2009). Institution of safety precautions and fall prevention strategies are needed in nocturnal or urgent voiding (see Chapter 15, Fall Prevention: Assessment, Diagnoses, and Intervention Strategies).

OROPHARYNGEAL AND GASTROINTESTINAL SYSTEMS

Age-specific alterations in the oral cavity can adversely affect the older adult's nutritional status. Deterioration in the strength of muscles of mastication as well as potential for tooth loss and xerostomia because of dehydration or medications may reduce food intake (Hall, 2009). Contributing to poor appetite are an altered taste perception and a diminished sense of smell (see Chapter 20, Oral Health Care; Ney et al., 2009; Visvanathan & Chapman, 2009).

Changes in the esophagus with age include delayed emptying in addition to decreases in upper and lower esophageal sphincter pressures, sphincter relaxation, and peristaltic contractions. Although these alterations rarely impair esophageal function and swallowing sufficiently to cause dysphagia or aspiration in normal aging, such conditions can develop in conjunction with disease or medication side effects in older adults (Gregersen, Pedersen, & Drewes, 2008; Ney et al., 2009). Diminished gastric motility with delayed emptying contributes to altered oral drug passage time and absorption in the stomach; elevated risk of gastroesophageal reflux disease (GERD; Hall, 2009); and decreased postprandial hunger, leading to diminished food intake and possible malnutrition (Visvanathan & Chapman, 2009). Reduced mucin secretion impairs the protective function of the gastric mucosal barrier and increases the incidence of NSAID-induced gastric ulcerations (Newton, 2005). Although the motility and most absorptive functions of the small intestine are preserved with age, absorption of vitamin B_{12}, folic acid, and carbohydrates declines (Hall, 2009). In addition, malabsorption of calcium and vitamin D contributes to the risk of osteoporosis. Supplementation with calcium and vitamins D and B_{12} is now recommended for older adults (USDHHS, 2005; Visvanathan & Chapman, 2009).

Age-dependent weakening of the large intestine wall predisposes older adults to diverticulosis and may lead to diverticulitis (Hall, 2009). Because motility of the colon appears to be preserved with age, increased self-reports of constipation in older adults may be attributed instead to altered dietary intake, medications, inactivity, or illness. Diminished rectal elasticity, internal anal sphincter thickening, and impaired sensation to defecate contribute to the risk of fecal incontinence in older adults (Gallagher et al., 2008), although this condition is primarily found in combination with previous bowel surgery or disease and not in normal aging (Hall, 2009).

Pancreatic exocrine output of digestive enzymes is preserved to allow normal digestive capacity with aging (Hall, 2009). Regarding endocrine function, aging changes in carbohydrate metabolism allow a genetic predisposition for diabetes to become manifest (Meneilly, 2010). An age-related decrease in gallbladder function increases the risk of gallstone formation. Although liver size and blood flow decline with age, reserve capacity maintains adequate hepatic function, and values of liver function tests remain stable; however, the liver is more susceptible to damage by stressors including alcohol and tobacco. Associated with changes in the hepatic and intestinal cytochrome P450 system (Hall, 2009), clearance of a range of medications, including many benzodiazepines, declines to result in increased potential for dose-dependent adverse reactions to these drugs (Beyth & Shorr, 2002).

Reductions in antimicrobial activity of saliva and immune response of the gastrointestinal tract with age contribute to a high risk for infectious and inflammatory diseases of this system (Htwe et al., 2007). Further, impaired enteric neuronal function may blunt the older adult's reaction to infection and inflammation and result in atypical presentation of disease (see Atypical Presentation of Disease section; Hall, 2002).

In the gastrointestinal evaluation, the abdomen and bowel sounds are assessed. Liver size, as well as reports of pain, anorexia, nausea, vomiting, and altered bowel habits should be noted (Visvanathan & Chapman, 2009). Assessment of the oral cavity includes dentition and chewing capacity (Chapman, 2007; see Chapter 20, Oral Health Care).

Weight is monitored with calculation of BMI and compared to recommended values (American Hearth Association Nutrition Committee et al., 2006; Visvanathan & Chapman, 2009). Deficiencies in diet can be identified through comparisons of dietary intake, using a 24- to 72-hour food intake record, with nutritional guidelines (Chapman, 2007; Roberts & Dallal, 2005; USDHHS, 2005). In addition, laboratory values of serum albumin, prealbumin, and transferrin are useful nutritional indicators. Low albumin concentration can also affect efficacy and potential for toxicity of selected drugs, including digoxin and warfarin (Beyth & Shorr, 2002). Several instruments for screening the nutritional status, eating habits, and appetite of older adults are available (see Resources section and Chapter 22, Nutrition; Ney et al., 2009).

Signs of dysphagia such as coughing or choking with solid or liquid food intake should be reported for further evaluation. If aspiration from dysphagia is suspected, the lungs must be assessed for the presence of infection, typically indicated by unilateral or bilateral basilar crackles in the lungs, dyspnea, tachypnea, and cough (Imperato & Sanchez, 2006). A decline in function or change in mental status may signal atypical presentation of respiratory infection from aspiration (Ney et al., 2009). Evaluation of GERD is based on typical and atypical symptoms (see Atypical Presentation of Disease section; Hall, 2009).

To assess constipation or fecal incontinence, a careful history with a 2-week bowel log noting laxative use is needed. Fecal impaction is assessed by digital examination of the rectum as a hardened mass of feces, which can be palpated. The impaction may also be palpated through the abdomen (Gallagher et al., 2008).

For continuing care, referrals should be provided to a registered dietician for poor food intake, unhealthy BMI (healthy BMI: 18.5–24.9 kg/m²; overweight: 25–29.9 kg/m²; obesity: 30 kg/m² or greater; American Hearth Association Nutrition Committee et al., 2006), and unintentional weight loss of 10% or greater in 6 months (Chapman, 2007; Ney et al., 2009). Drug levels and liver function tests are monitored if drugs are metabolized hepatically (Beyth & Shorr, 2002). Explanation of normal bowel frequency, the importance of diet and exercise, and recommended types of laxatives addresses constipation problems (Gallagher et al., 2008). Mobility should be encouraged to prevent constipation, and prophylactic laxatives should be provided if constipating medications such as opiates are prescribed (Stern, 2006). Community-based food and nutrition programs (Visvanathan & Chapman, 2009) and education on healthful diets using the food pyramid for older adults may be useful in improving dietary intake (see Chapter 22, Nutrition; JNC, 2004; USDHHS, 2005).

MUSCULOSKELETAL SYSTEM

Musculoskeletal tissues undergo age-associated changes that can negatively impact function in the older adult. In sarcopenia or the loss of muscle mass and strength, a decline in the size, number, and quality of skeletal muscle fibers occurs with aging. Lean body mass is replaced by fat and fibrous tissue (Loeser & Delbono, 2009) so that by age 75, only 15% of the total body mass is muscle compared to 30% in a young, healthy adult (Matsumura & Ambrose, 2006). These alterations result in diminished contractile muscle force with increased weakness and fatigue plus poor exercise tolerance. Age-specific physiological alterations contributing to sarcopenia include reductions in muscle innervation, insulin activity, and sex steroid (estrogen, testosterone) and growth hormone levels. Additionally, individual factors such as weight loss, protein deficiency, and physical inactivity can accelerate development of this condition to progress to a clinically significant problem (Jones et al., 2009). Sarcopenia has been documented to affect function adversely in older adults by increasing the risk of disability, falls, unstable gait, and need for assistive devices. Physical activity, particularly strength training, and adequate intake of energy and protein can prevent or reverse sarcopenia (Narici, Maffulli, & Maganaris, 2008).

Age-dependent bone loss occurs in both sexes and at all sites in the skeleton. Whereas bone mass peaks between ages 30 and 35, density decreases thereafter at a rate of 0.5% per year. This decrement, caused by reduced osteoblast activity in the deposition of new bone, is accompanied by deterioration in bone architecture and strength. Further, from 5–7 years following menopause during estrogen decline, bone loss in women accelerates to a 3%–5% annual rate (USDHHS, 2004b). This loss, resulting from osteoclast activation with elevated bone breakdown or resorption, occurs mainly in cancellous or trabecular bone such as the vertebral body and may develop into Type I osteoporosis in women aged 51–75 years who risk vertebral fractures. Following this postmenopausal period, bone loss slows again in women and involves cortical bone in the long bones of the extremities. With aging, both women and men may develop Type II osteoporosis and are susceptible to hip fractures and kyphosis from vertebral compression fractures in later life (Simon, 2005).

An age-associated decline in the strength of ligaments and tendons, which are integral to normal joint function, predisposes to increased ligament and tendon injury, more limited joint range of motion (ROM), and reduced joint stability, leading to osteoarthritis (Narici et al., 2008). Degeneration of intervertebral discs caused by dehydration and poor nutrient influx elevates the risk of spinal osteoarthritis, spondylosis, and stenosis with aging (Loeser & Delbono, 2009).

Age-related changes in articular cartilage, which covers the bone endings in joints to allow smooth movement, involve increased dehydration, stiffening, crystal formation, calcification, and roughening of the cartilage surface. Although these alterations have a minor effect on joint function under baseline conditions, the aging joint is less capable of withstanding mechanical stress, such as the stress caused by obesity or excess physical activity, and is also more susceptible to disease including osteoarthritis (Loeser, 2010).

Age-dependent changes in stature include dorsal kyphosis, reduction in height, flexion of the hips and knees, and a backward tilt of the head to compensate for the thoracic curvature. A shorter stride, reduced velocity, and broader base of support with feet more widely spaced characterize modifications in gait with age (Harris et al., 2008).

The musculoskeletal assessment includes inspection of posture, gait, balance, symmetry of body parts, and alignment of extremities. Kyphosis, bony enlargements, or other abnormalities should be noted. The clinician should palpate bones, joints, and surrounding muscles, evaluating muscle strength on a scale of 0/5, and noting symmetry and signs of atrophy of major upper and lower extremity muscle groups. Active and passive ROM for major joints is evaluated, noting pain, limitation of ROM, and joint laxity. Joint stabilization and slow movements in ROM examinations are advised to prevent injury. Functionality, mobility, fine and gross motor skills, balance, and fall risk should be assessed (see Chapter 6, Assessment of Physical Function and Chapter 15, Fall Prevention: Assessment, Diagnoses, and Intervention Strategies; Harris et al., 2008).

For continuing care, referrals to physical or occupational therapy may be appropriate. Increased physical activity, including exercises for ROM (Netz et al., 2005) and muscle strengthening and power (Narici et al., 2008) are recommended to maintain maximal function. Interventions to promote such behavior in older adults involve health education, goal setting, and self-monitoring (Conn, Minor, Burks, Rantz, & Pomeroy, 2003). Pain medication may be needed to enhance functionality (see Chapter 14, Pain Management; McCleane, 2008). Strategies to prevent falls (see Chapter 15, Falls Prevention: Assessment, Diagnoses, and Intervention Strategies) and avoid physical restraints (see Chapter 13, Physical Restraints and Side Rails in Acute and Critical Care Settings) are appropriate.

To prevent and treat osteoporosis, adequate daily intake of calcium (1,200 mg for women aged 50 years and older) and vitamin D (400 IU for women aged 50–70 years and 600 IU for women aged 71 years and older), physical exercise, and smoking cessation are recommended (USDHHS, 2004b). In addition, routine bone mineral density screening for osteoporosis is advised for women aged 65 years and older, as well as for women aged 60–64 years at increased risk for osteoporotic fractures (Agency for Healthcare Research and Quality, 2010).

NERVOUS SYSTEM AND COGNITION

Age-related alterations in the nervous system can affect function and cognition in older adults. Changes include a reduced number of cerebral and peripheral neurons (Hall, 2002), modifications in dendrites and glial support cells in the brain, and loss and remodeling of synapses. Decreased levels of neurotransmitters, particularly dopamine, as well as deficits in systems that relay signals between neurons and regulate neuronal plasticity also occur with aging (Mattson, 2009).

Combined, these neurological changes contribute to decrements in general muscle strength; deep tendon reflexes; sensation of touch, pain, and vibration; and nerve conduction velocity (Hall, 2002), which result in slowed coordinated movements and increased response time to stimuli (Matsumura & Ambrose, 2006). These clinical consequences, although relatively mild in normal aging, cause an overall slowing of motor skills with potential deficits in balance, gait, coordination, reaction time, and agility (Harris et al., 2008; Narici et al., 2008). Such decline in function can adversely affect an older adult's daily activities, notably ambulation and driving, and predispose to falls and injury (Craft, Cholerton, & Reger, 2009).

Neurological changes, along with thinning of the skin, compromise thermoregulation in the older adult. These result in decreased sensitivity to ambient temperature as well as impaired heat conservation, production, and dissipation with predisposition to hypothermia and hyperthermia (Kuchel, 2009). Febrile responses to infection may be blunted or absent (see Atypical Presentation of Disease section; High, 2009; Htwe et al., 2007; Watters, 2002).

With age, the speed of cognitive processing slows (Bashore & Ridderinkhof, 2002) and some degree of cognitive decline is common (Park, O'Connell, & Thomson, 2003) but not universal in the older adult population (Stewart, 2004). Older adults demonstrate significant heterogeneity in cognitive performance, which may be positively impacted by education, good health, and physical activity (Christensen, 2001; Colcombe & Kramer, 2003).

Specific cognitive abilities exhibit differing levels of stability or decline with age. For example, crystallized intelligence, or the information and skills acquired from experience, remains largely intact, whereas fluid intelligence, or creative reasoning and problem solving, declines (Christensen, 2001). Sustained attention is unaffected by aging, although divided attention, or the ability to concentrate on multiple tasks concurrently, deteriorates. The mild decline in executive function, which includes the capability of directing behavior and completing multistep tasks, usually has minimal impact on an older adult's ability to manage daily activities. Although language abilities and comprehension appear stable, spontaneous word finding may deteriorate and is often a complaint of older adults. Remote memory, or recalling events in the distant past, and procedural memory, or remembering ways to perform tasks, remain intact but declarative memory, or learning new information, is slowed (Craft et al., 2009). However, despite some deficits, memory functions are adequate for normal life in successful aging (Henry, MacLeod, Phillips, & Crawford, 2004).

Changes in the nervous system increase the risk of sleep disorders (Espiritu, 2008) and delirium in the older adult, especially in acute care (see Chapter 11, Delirium). Neural changes affect the perception, tolerance, and response to treatment of pain (McCleane, 2008). In addition, age-specific alterations predispose neurons to degeneration, contributing to Alzheimer's disease (Charter & Alekoumbides, 2004), Parkinson's disease, and Huntington's disease (Mattson, 2009).

Assessment, with periodic reassessment, of baseline functional status (see Chapter 6, Assessment of Physical Function) should include evaluation of fall risk, gait, and balance (see Chapter 15, Falls Prevention: Assessment, Diagnoses, and Intervention Strategies) as well as basic, instrumental, and advanced activities of daily living (ADLs). During acute illness, functional status, pain (see Chapter 14, Pain Management), and symptoms of delirium (see Chapter 11, Delirium) should be monitored. Evaluation of baseline cognition with periodic reassessment (see Chapter 8, Assessing Cognitive Function) and sleep disorders (Espiritu, 2008) is warranted. The impact of physical and cognitive changes of aging on an older adult's level of safety and attentiveness in daily tasks should be determined (Bashore & Ridderinkhof, 2002; Craft et al., 2009; Henry et al., 2004; Park et al., 2003). Temperature indicating hypothermia (less than 95 °F or less than 35 °C) or hyperthermia (greater than 105 °F or greater than 40.6 °C) must be closely watched (Kuchel, 2009; Lu, Leasure, & Dai, 2010).

For care of the older adult, fall prevention strategies should be implemented (see Chapter 15, Fall Prevention: Assessment, Diagnoses, and Intervention Strategies). If delirium is identified, nursing interventions for its treatment are needed (see Chapter 11, Delirium). Particularly during surgery, procedures such as the use of warmed intravenous fluids and humidified gases should be instituted to maintain normal temperatures and prevent hypothermia in the older patient (Watters, 2002). Lifestyle modifications recommended to improve cognitive function include regular physical exercise (Colcombe & Kramer, 2003), intellectual stimulation (Mattson, 2009), and a healthful diet (JNC, 2004; USDHHS, 2005). Behavioral interventions for sleep disorders may be warranted (Irwin, Cole, & Nicassio, 2006).

IMMUNE SYSTEM AND VACCINATION

Immunosenescence, or the age-related dysfunction in immune response, is characterized by reduced cell-mediated immune function and humoral immune responses (Weiskopf, Weinberger, & Grubeck-Loebenstein, 2009), as well as increased inflammatory response (High, 2009; Hunt, Walsh, Voegeli, & Roberts, 2010). In older adults, it is responsible, in part, for the increased susceptibility to and severity of infectious diseases (Htwe et al., 2007), the lower efficacy of vaccination (Weiskopf et al., 2009), and the chronic inflammatory state, which may contribute to chronic disease with age (Hunt et al., 2010).

Infectious diseases are a critical threat to older adults, especially since vaccination efficacy declines with age. Mortality rates for infectious diseases are highest for adults older than 85 years (Htwe et al., 2007), whereas reactivation of viruses, particularly varicella zoster leading to herpes zoster, occurs significantly more frequently in older adults (High, 2009). Immunosenescence, by dampening the induction of adaptive immune responses, results in reduced response rates to vaccination. For example, influenza vaccination has a protection rate of only 56% in older persons. Further, antibody titers following booster vaccinations, such as against tetanus, are lower and decline faster with diminished antibody function in older adults compared to younger individuals (Weiskopf et al., 2009).

Current immunization recommendations for older adults are available from the Centers for Disease Control and Prevention (CDC, 2010). Vaccination with pneumococcal polysaccharide for pneumococcal infections is recommended for individuals 65 years of age and older, with one-time revaccination indicated if the patient was vaccinated 5 or more years previously and was aged younger than 65 years at the time of primary vaccination. For seasonal influenza, all individuals 50 years of age and older should be vaccinated with the inactivated vaccine just prior to influenza season each year. A single dose of zoster vaccine is recommended for all adults 60 years of age and older regardless of prior zoster history. A complete tetanus vaccine series is indicated for individuals having an uncertain history of tetanus immunization or having received fewer than three doses. Boosters should be given at 10-year intervals or more frequently with high-risk injuries. Hepatitis vaccines should also be considered for older adults depending on circumstances such as potential exposure and travel (CDC, 2010; High, 2009).

ATYPICAL PRESENTATION OF DISEASE

Diseases, particularly infections, often manifest with atypical features in older adults. Signs and symptoms are frequently subtle in the very old. These may initially involve nonspecific declines in functional or mental status, anorexia with reduced oral intake, incontinence, falls (Htwe et al., 2007), fatigue (Hall, 2002), or exacerbation of chronic illness such as heart failure or diabetes (High, 2009).

As a presenting sign of infection, fever is often blunted or absent, particularly in the very old (High, 2009), frail, or malnourished (Watters, 2002) adults. Compared to young adults with a normal mean baseline body temperature of 98.6 °F (37 °C), frail older adults have a lower mean oral baseline temperature of 97.4 °F (36.3 °C; Lu et al., 2010). A blunted response to inflammatory stimuli in combination with lower basal temperature can result in a lack of measurable febrile response. Increasing age is a predisposing factor for the absence of fever (Htwe et al., 2007).

Assessment of the older patient should note any changes from baseline (including those that are subtle and nonspecific) in functioning, mental status and behavior (e.g., increased/new onset confusion), appetite, or exacerbation of chronic illness (High, 2009; Watters, 2002). This is especially important in individuals with cognitive impairment who are unable to describe symptoms.

To detect fever, normal temperature should be established for the older adult and monitored for changes of 2–2.4 °F (1.1–1.3 °C) above baseline (Htwe et al., 2007). Oral temperatures of 99 °F (37.2 °C) or greater on repeated measurements also can be used to signify fever. The difficulty of diagnosing infection based on signs and symptoms may result in greater reliance on laboratory and radiologic evaluations (High, 2009).

In the assessment of disease, both typical and atypical symptoms must be considered. Evaluation for pneumococcal pneumonia includes monitoring for typical symptoms such as productive cough, fever, chills, and dyspnea as well as insidious, atypical symptoms including tachypnea, lethargy (Bartlett et al., 2000), weakness, falls, decline in functional status, delirium, or increased/new-onset confusion with absent high fever. Decreased appetite and dehydration may be the only initial symptoms in the older adult (Imperato & Sanchez, 2006). Although chest radiograph is basic to diagnosis, the older adult who is dehydrated may not show infiltrate or consolidation, and these findings may appear only after hydration (Htwe et al., 2007).

Clinical features of tuberculosis in the older person are often atypical and nonspecific. Presenting symptoms may include dizziness, nonspecific pain, or impaired cognition rather than the typical manifestations of fever, night sweats, cough, or hemoptysis (High, 2009). Typical influenza symptoms of cough, fever, and chills may be combined with altered mental status in older adults (Htwe et al., 2007).

UTI in older adults may present with classical symptoms of dysuria, flank or suprapubic discomfort, hematuria, and urinary frequency and urgency, or atypical symptoms of new-onset/worsening incontinence, anorexia, confusion, nocturia, or enuresis (Htwe et al., 2007).

For peritonitis, atypical symptoms such as confusion and fatigue may be manifest rather than the typical symptoms of rigidity (Hall, 2002). Evaluation of GERD is based on typical presenting symptoms of heartburn (pyrosis) and acid regurgitation, as well as atypical symptoms in the older adult of dysphagia, chest pain, hoarseness, vomiting, chronic cough, or recurrent aspiration pneumonia (Hall, 2009).

CASE STUDY

Ms. M is an 89-year-old woman presenting with productive cough, dyspnea, fatigue, and increased confusion over the past week. Her vital signs are pulse, 96 bpm; temperature, 98.6 °F; respiration, 31 bpm; and BP, 110/55. A chest radiograph shows multilobe infiltrates with a diagnosis of pneumonia. How severe is her pneumonia?

Ms. M's symptoms of a respiratory rate greater than 30 respirations per minute, multilobe infiltrates on a chest radiograph, and diastolic BP of less than 60 mm Hg characterize her pneumonia as severe (Bartlett et al., 2000), and she is likely to require admission to an intensive care unit. However, several age-related changes affect her symptoms of pneumonia. Pneumonia may present in the older adult with typical symptoms of productive cough, fever, and dyspnea or with more insidious, atypical symptoms of tachypnea, lethargy (Bartlett et al., 2000), weakness, falls, decline in functional status, or increased/new-onset confusion. Decreased appetite and dehydration may be the only initial symptoms (Imperato & Sanchez, 2006).

Because of reduced sympathetic innervation of the heart with age, the heart rate of an older adult does not increase in response to stress comparable to that of a younger individual (Kitzman & Taffet, 2009). Thus, 96 bpm in an 89-year-old person is tachycardic and indicates a severe stress reaction. Furthermore, because of a blunted febrile response to infection particularly in a very old, frail, or malnourished adult, a fever may not be manifest even with severe infection (High, 2009; Htwe, 2007; Lu et al., 2010; Watters, 2002).

SUMMARY

Changes that occur with age strongly impact the health and functional status of older adults. Thus, recognition of and attention to these alterations are critically important in nursing assessment and care. Armed with knowledge of age-related changes and using the clinical protocol described in this chapter, nurses can play a vital role in improving geriatric standards of practice. Designing interventions that take age-related changes into consideration, educating patients and family caregivers on these alterations, and sharing information with professional colleagues will all serve to ensure optimal care of older adults.

NURSING STANDARD OF PRACTICE

Protocol 3.1: Age-Related Changes in Health

I. GOAL: To identify anatomical and physiological changes, which are attributed to the normal aging process.

II. OVERVIEW: Age-associated changes are most pronounced in advanced age of 85 years or older, may alter the older person's response to illness, show great variability among individuals, are often impacted by genetic and long-term lifestyle factors, and commonly involve a decline in functional reserve with reduced response to stressors.

III. STATEMENT OF PROBLEM: Gerontological changes are important in nursing assessment and care because they can adversely affect health and functionality and require therapeutic strategies; must be differentiated from pathological processes to allow development of appropriate interventions; predispose to disease, thus emphasizing the need for risk evaluation of the older adult; and can interact reciprocally with illness, resulting in altered disease presentation, response to treatment, and outcomes.

IV. AGE-ASSOCIATED CARDIOVASCULAR CHANGES
   A. Definition(s)
     Isolated systolic hypertension: systolic BP >140 mm Hg and diastolic BP <90 mm Hg.
   B. Etiology
     1. Arterial wall thickening and stiffening, decreased compliance.
     2. Left ventricular and atrial hypertrophy. Sclerosis of atrial and mitral valves.
     3. Strong arterial pulses, diminished peripheral pulses, cool extremities.
   C. Implications
     1. Decreased cardiac reserve.
       a. At rest: No change in heart rate, cardiac output.
       b. Under physiological stress and exercise: Decreased maximal heart rate and cardiac output, resulting in fatigue, shortness of breath, slow recovery from tachycardia.

(continued)

Protocol 3.1: Age-Related Changes in Health *(cont.)*

    c. Risk of isolated systolic hypertension; inflamed varicosities.
    d. Risk of arrhythmias, postural, and diuretic-induced hypotension. May cause syncope.
  D. Parameters of Cardiovascular Assessment
    1. Cardiac assessment: ECG; heart rate, rhythm, murmurs, heart sounds (S_4 common, S3 in disease). Palpate carotid artery and peripheral pulses for symmetry (Docherty, 2002).
    2. Assess BP (lying, sitting, standing) and pulse pressure (Mukai & Lipsitz, 2002).

V. AGE-ASSOCIATED CHANGES IN THE PULMONARY SYSTEM
  A. Etiology
    1. Decreased respiratory muscle strength; stiffer chest wall with reduced compliance.
    2. Diminished ciliary and macrophage activity, drier mucus membranes. Decreased cough reflex.
    3. Decreased response to hypoxia and hypercapnia.
  B. Implications
    1. Reduced pulmonary functional reserve.
      a. At rest: No change.
      b. With exertion: Dyspnea, decreased exercise tolerance.
    2. Decreased respiratory excursion and chest/lung expansion with less effective exhalation. Respiratory rate of 12–24 breaths per minute.
    3. Decreased cough and mucus/foreign matter clearance.
    4. Increased risk of infection and bronchospasm with airway obstruction.
  C. Parameters of Pulmonary Assessment
    1. Assess respiration rate, rhythm, regularity, volume, depth (Docherty, 2002), and exercise capacity (Mahler et al., 2003). Ascultate breath sounds throughout lung fields (Mick & Ackerman, 2004).
    2. Inspect thorax appearance, symmetry of chest expansion. Obtain smoking history.
    3. Monitor secretions, breathing rate during sedation, positioning (Watters, 2002; Docherty, 2002), arterial blood gases, pulse oximetry (Zeleznik, 2003).
    4. Assess cough, need for suctioning (Smith & Connolly, 2003).
  D. Nursing Care Strategies
    1. Maintain patent airways through upright positioning/repositioning (Docherty, 2002), suctioning (Smith & Connolly, 2003).
    2. Provide oxygen as needed (Docherty, 2002); maintain hydration and mobility (Watters, 2002).
    3. Incentive spirometry as indicated, particularly if immobile or declining in function (Dunn, 2004).
    4. Education on cough enhancement (Dunn, 2004), smoking cessation (USDHHS, 2004a).

(continued)

Protocol 3.1: Age-Related Changes in Health *(cont.)*

VI. AGE-ASSOCIATED CHANGES IN THE RENAL AND GENITOURINARY SYSTEMS

A. Definition(s)

To determine renal function (GFR):

Cockcroft-Gault equation: Calculation of creatinine clearance in older adults (Péquignot et al., 2009).

For Men

$$\text{Creatinine clearance (mL/min)} = \frac{(140 - \text{age in years}) \times (\text{body weight in kg})}{72 \times (\text{serum creatinine, mg/dL})}$$

For women, the calculated value is multiplied by 85% (0.85).

MDRD: see National Kidney Disease Education Program calculator (National Kidney Disease Education Program, 2009).

B. Etiology
1. Decreases in kidney mass, blood flow, GFR (10% decrement/decade after age 30). Decreased drug clearance.
2. Reduced bladder elasticity, muscle tone, capacity.
3. Increased postvoid residual, nocturnal urine production.
4. In males, prostate enlargement with risk of BPH.

C. Implications
1. Reduced renal functional reserve; risk of renal complications in illness.
2. Risk of nephrotoxic injury and adverse reactions from drugs.
3. Risk of volume overload (in heart failure), dehydration, hyponatremia (with thiazide diuretics), hypernatremia (associated with fever), hyperkalemia (with potassium-sparing diuretics). Reduced excretion of acid load.
4. Increased risk of urinary urgency, incontinence (not a normal finding), urinary tract infection, nocturnal polyuria. Potential for falls.

D. Parameters of Renal and Genitourinary Assessment
1. Assess renal function (GFR through creatinine clearance; Lerma, 2009; Miller, 2009; National Kidney Disease Education Program, 2009; Péquignot et al., 2009).
2. Assess choice/need/dose of nephrotoxic agents and renally cleared drugs (Beyth & Shorr, 2002; see Chapter 17, Reducing Adverse Drug Events.
3. Assess for fluid/electrolyte and acid/base imbalances (Suhayda & Walton, 2002).
4. Evaluate nocturnal polyuria, urinary incontinence, BPH (Miller, 2009). Assess UTI symptoms (see Atypical Presentation of Disease section; Htwe et al., 2007).
5. Assess fall risk if nocturnal or urgent voiding (see Chapter 15, Fall Prevention: Assessment, Diagnoses, and Intervention Strategies)

E. Nursing Care Strategies
1. Monitor nephrotoxic and renally cleared drug levels (Beyth & Shorr, 2002).
2. Maintain fluid/electrolyte balance. Minimum 1,500–2,500 mL/day from fluids and foods for 50- to 80-kg adults to prevent dehydration (Suhayda & Walton, 2002).
3. For nocturnal polyuria: limit fluids in evening, avoid caffeine, use prompted voiding schedule (Miller, 2009).

(continued)

Protocol 3.1: Age-Related Changes in Health *(cont.)*

4. Fall prevention for nocturnal or urgent voiding (see Chapter 15, Fall Prevention: Assessment, Diagnoses, and Intervention Strategies).

VII. AGE-ASSOCIATED CHANGES IN THE OROPHARYNGEAL AND GASTROINTESTINAL SYSTEMS

A. Definition(s)

BMI: Healthy, 18.5–24.9 kg/m^2; overweight, 25–29.9 kg/m^2; obesity, 30 kg/m^2 or greater.

B. Etiology
  1. Decreases in strength of muscles of mastication, taste, and thirst perception.
  2. Decreased gastric motility with delayed emptying.
  3. Atrophy of protective mucosa.
  4. Malabsorption of carbohydrates, vitamins B$_{12}$ and D, folic acid, calcium.
  5. Impaired sensation to defecate.
  6. Reduced hepatic reserve. Decreased metabolism of drugs.

C. Implications
  1. Risk of chewing impairment, fluid/electrolyte imbalances, poor nutrition.
  2. Gastric changes: altered drug absorption, increased risk of GERD, maldigestion, NSAID-induced ulcers.
  3. Constipation not a normal finding. Risk of fecal incontinence with disease (not in healthy aging).
  4. Stable liver function tests. Risk of adverse drug reactions.

D. Parameters of Oropharyngeal and Gastrointestinal Assessment
  1. Assess abdomen, bowel sounds.
  2. Assess oral cavity (see Chapter 20, Oral Health Care); chewing and swallowing capacity, dysphagia (coughing, choking with food/fluid intake; Ney et al., 2009). If aspiration, assess lungs (rales) for infection and typical/atypical symptoms (Bartlett et al., 2000; High, 2009; see Atypical Presentation of Disease section).
  3. Monitor weight, calculate BMI, compare to standards (American Hearth Association Nutrition Committee et al., 2006). Determine dietary intake, compare to nutritional guidelines (Chapman, 2007; USDHHS, 2005; Visvanathan & Chapman, 2009; see Chapter 22, Nutrition).
  4. Assess for GERD; constipation and fecal incontinence; fecal impaction by digital examination of rectum or palpation of abdomen.

E. Nursing Care Strategies
  1. Monitor drug levels and liver function tests if on medications metabolized by liver. Assess nutritional indicators (Chapman, 2007; USDHHS, 2005; Visvanathan & Chapman, 2009).
  2. Educate on lifestyle modifications and over-the-counter (OTC) medications for GERD.
  3. Educate on normal bowel frequency, diet, exercise, recommended laxatives. Encourage mobility, provide laxatives if on constipating medications (Stern, 2006).
  4. Encourage participation in community-based nutrition programs (Visvanathan & Chapman, 2009); educate on healthful diets (USDHHS, 2005).

(continued)

Protocol 3.1: Age-Related Changes in Health *(cont.)*

VIII. AGE-ASSOCIATED CHANGES IN THE MUSCULOSKELETAL SYSTEM

A. Definition(s)

Sarcopenia: Decline in muscle mass and strength associated with aging.

B. Etiology

1. Sarcopenia evokes increased weakness and poor exercise tolerance.
2. Lean body mass replaced by fat with redistribution of fat.
3. Bone loss in women and men after peak mass at age 30 to 35 years.
4. Decreased ligament and tendon strength. Intervertebral disc degeneration. Articular cartilage erosion. Changes in stature with kyphosis, height reduction.

C. Implications

1. Sarcopenia: increased risk of disability, falls, unstable gait.
2. Risk of osteopenia and osteoporosis.
3. Limited ROM, joint instability, risk of osteoarthritis.

D. Nursing Care Strategies

1. Encourage physical activity through health education and goal setting (Conn, 2003) to maintain function (Netz et al., 2005).
2. Pain medication to enhance functionality (see Chapter 14, Pain Management). Implement strategies to prevent falls (see Chapter 15, Fall Prevention: Assessment, Diagnoses, and Intervention Strategies and Chapter 13, Physical Restraints and Side Rails in Acute and Critical Care Settings).
3. Prevent osteoporosis by adequate daily intake of calcium and vitamin D, physical exercise, smoking cessation (USDHHS, 2004b). Advise routine bone mineral density screening (Agency for Healthcare Research and Quality, 2010).

IX. AGE-ASSOCIATED CHANGES IN THE NERVOUS SYSTEM AND COGNITION

A. Etiology

1. Decrease in neurons and neurotransmitters.
2. Modifications in cerebral dendrites, glial support cells, synapses.
3. Compromised thermoregulation.

B. Implications

1. Impairments in general muscle strength; deep tendon reflexes; nerve conduction velocity. Slowed motor skills and potential deficits in balance and coordination.
2. Decreased temperature sensitivity. Blunted or absent fever response.
3. Slowed speed of cognitive processing. Some cognitive decline is common but not universal. Most memory functions are adequate for normal life.
4. Increased risk of sleep disorders, delirium, neurodegenerative diseases.

C. Parameters of Nervous System and Cognition Assessments

1. Assess, with periodic reassessment, baseline functional status (Craft et al., 2009; see Chapter 6, Assessment of Physical Function and Chapter 15, Fall Prevention: Assessment, Diagnoses, and Intervention Strategies). During acute illness, monitor functional status and delirium (see Chapter 11, Delirium).
2. Evaluate, with periodic reassessment, baseline cognition (see Chapter 8, Assessing Cognitive Function) and sleep disorders (Espiritu, 2008).

(continued)

Protocol 3.1: Age-Related Changes in Health *(cont.)*

    3. Assess impact of age-related changes on level of safely and attentiveness in daily tasks (Park et al., 2003; Henry et al., 2004).
    4. Assess temperature during illness or surgery (Kuchel, 2009).
  D. Nursing Care Strategies
    1. Institute fall preventions strategies (see Chapter 15, Fall Prevention: Assessment, Diagnoses, and Intervention Strategies).
    2. To maintain cognitive function, encourage lifestyle practices of regular physical exercise (Colcombe & Kramer, 2003), intellectual stimulation (Mattson, 2009), healthful diet (JNC, 2004).
    3. Recommend behavioral interventions for sleep disorders.

X. AGE-ASSOCIATED CHANGES IN THE IMMUNE SYSTEM
  A. Etiology
    1. Immune response dysfunction (Kuchel, 2009) with increased susceptibility to infection, reduced efficacy of vaccination (Htwe et al., 2007), chronic inflammatory state (Hunt et al., 2010).
  B. Nursing Care Strategies
    1. Follow CDC immunization recommendations for pneumococcal infections, seasonal influenza, zoster, tetanus, and hepatitis for the older adult (CDC, 2010; High, 2009).

XI. ATYPICAL PRESENTATION OF DISEASE
  A. Etiology
    1. Diseases, especially infections, may manifest with atypical symptoms in older adults.
    2. Symptoms/signs often subtle include nonspecific declines in function or mental status, decreased appetite, incontinence, falls (Htwe et al., 2007), fatigue (Hall, 2002), exacerbation of chronic illness (High, 2009).
    3. Fever blunted or absent in very old (High, 2009), frail, or malnourished (Watters, 2002) adults. Baseline oral temperature in older adults is 97.4 °F (36.3 °C) versus 98.6 °F (37 °C) in younger adults (Lu et al., 2010).
  B. Parameters of Disease Assessment
    1. Note any change from baseline in function, mental status, behavior, appetite, chronic illness (High, 2009).
    2. Assess fever. Determine baseline and monitor for changes 2–2.4 °F (1.1–1.3 °C) above baseline (Htwe et al., 2007). Oral temperatures above 99 °F (37.2 °C) or greater also indicate fever (High, 2009).
    3. Note typical and atypical symptoms of pneumococcal pneumonia (Bartlett et al., 2000; Htwe et al., 2007; Imperato & Sanchez, 2006), tuberculosis (Kuchel, 2009), influenza (Htwe et al., 2007), UTI (Htwe et al., 2007), peritonitis (Hall, 2002), and GERD (Hall, 2009).

XII. EVALUATION/EXPECTED OUTCOMES (FOR ALL SYSTEMS)
  A. Older adult will experience successful aging through appropriate lifestyle practices and health care.

(continued)

Protocol 3.1: Age-Related Changes in Health *(cont.)*

  B. Health care provider will
     1. Identify normative changes in aging and differentiate these from pathological processes.
     2. Develop interventions to correct for adverse effects associated with aging.
  C. Institution will
     1. Develop programs to promote successful aging.
  D. Will provide staff education on age-related changes in health.

XIII. FOLLOW-UP MONITORING OF CONDITION
  A. Continue to reassess effectiveness of interventions.
  B. Incorporate continuous quality improvement criteria into existing programs.

RESOURCES

Government Informational Agencies

Agency for Healthcare Research and Quality
http://www.ahrq.gov

Administration on Aging
http://www.aoa.gov

National Institute on Aging
http://www.nia.nih.gov

Non-Profit Organizations

Health and Age Foundation
http://www.healthandage.org

American Federation of Aging Research
http://www.afar.org

Alliance for Aging Research
http://www.agingresearch.org

National Council on Aging
http://www.ncoa.org

Smith-Kettlewell Eye Research Institute
http://www.ski.org

CRONOS
http://www.unu.edu/unupress/food/V183e/begin.htm

Professional Societies

The National Gerontological Nursing Association
http://www.ngna.org

The National Conference of Gerontological Nurse Practitioners
http://www.ncgnp.org/

The American Geriatrics Society
http://www.americangeriatrics.org/

REFERENCES

Agency for Healthcare Research and Quality. (2010). *Guide to clinical preventive services, 2010–2011: Recommendations of the U.S. preventive services task force.* AHRQ Publication No. 10-05145. Rockville, MD. Retrieved from http://www.ahrq.gov/clinic/pocketgd1011/

American Heart Association Nutrition Committee, Lichtenstein, A. H., Appel, L. J., Brands, M., Carnethon, M., Daniels, S., . . . Wylie-Rosett, J. (2006). Diet and lifestyle recommendations revision 2006: A scientific statement from the American Heart Association Nutrition Committee. *Circulation, 114*(1), 82–96. Evidence Level I.

Baltimore Longitudinal Study of Aging. (2010). Retrieved from http://www.grc.nia.nih.gov/branches/blsa/blsa.htm/. Evidence Level I.

Bartlett, J. G., Dowell, S. F., Mandell, L. A., File, T. M., Jr., Musher, D. M., & Fine, M. J. (2000). Practice guidelines for the management of community-acquired pneumonia in adults. Infectious Diseases Society of America. *Clinical Infectious Diseases, 31*(2), 347–382. Evidence Level I.

Bashore, T. R., & Ridderinkhof, K. R. (2002). Older age, traumatic brain injury, and cognitive slowing: Some convergent and divergent findings. *Psychological Bulletin, 128*(1), 151–198. Evidence Level I.

Beck, L. H. (1998). Changes in renal function with aging. *Clinics in Geriatric Medicine, 14*(2), 199–209. Evidence Level V.

Beyth, R. J., & Shorr, R. I. (2002). Principles of drug therapy in older patients: Rational drug prescribing. *Clinics in Geriatric Medicine, 18*(3), 577–592. Evidence Level V.

Buchman, A. S., Boyle, P. A,, Wilson, R. S., Gu, L., Bienias, J. L., & Bennett, D. A. (2008). Pulmonary function, muscle strength and mortality in old age. *Mechanisms of Ageing and Development, 129*(11), 625–631. Evidence Level V.

Centers for Disease Control and Prevention. (2010). *Recommendations and guidelines: Adult immunization schedule.* Retrieved from www.cdc.gov/vaccines/recs/schedules/adult-schedule.htm#hcp/. Evidence Level I.

Chapman, I. M. (2007). The anorexia of aging. *Clinics in Geriatric Medicine, 23*(4), 735–756. Evidence Level V.

Charter, R. A., & Alekoumbides, A. (2004). Evidence for aging as the cause of Alzheimer's disease. *Psychological Reports,* 95(3 Pt. 1), 935–945. Evidence Level I.

Christensen, H. (2001). What cognitive changes can be expected with normal ageing? *Australian and New Zealand Journal of Psychiatry, 35*(6), 768–775. Evidence Level I.

Colcombe, S., & Kramer, A. F. (2003). Fitness effects on the cognitive function of older adults: A meta-analytic study. *Psychological Science, 14*(2), 125–130. Evidence Level I.

Conn, V. S., Minor, M. A., Burks, K. J., Rantz, M. J., & Pomeroy, S. H. (2003). Integrative review of physical activity intervention research with aging adults. *Journal of the American Geriatrics Society, 51*(8), 1159–1168. Evidence Level I.

Craft, S., Cholerton, B., & Reger, M. (2009). Cognitive changes with normal and pathological aging. In J. B. Halter, J. G. Ouslander, M. E. Tinetti, S. Studenski, K. P. High, & S. Asthana (Eds.), *Hazzard's geriatric medicine and gerontology* (6th ed., pp. 751–765). New York, NY: McGraw-Hill. Evidence Level V.

Docherty, B. (2002). Cardiorespiratory physical assessment for the acutely ill: 1. *British Journal of Nursing, 11*(11), 750–758. Evidence Level I.

Dunn, D. (2004). Preventing perioperative complications in an older adult. *Nursing, 34*(11), 36–41. Evidence Level V.

Enright, P. L. (2009). Aging of the respiratory system. In J. B. Halter, J. G. Ouslander, M. E. Tinetti, S. Studenski, K. P. High, & S. Asthana (Eds.), *Hazzard's geriatric medicine and gerontology* (6th ed., pp. 983–986). New York, NY: McGraw-Hill. Evidence Level V.

Espiritu, J. R. (2008). Aging-related sleep changes. *Clinics in Geriatric Medicine, 24*(1), 1–14. Evidence Level V.

Gallagher, P. F., O'Mahony, D., & Quigley, E. M. (2008). Management of chronic constipation in the elderly. *Drugs & Aging, 25*(10), 807–821. Evidence Level V.

Gregersen, H., Pedersen, J., & Drewes, A. M. (2008). Deterioration of muscle function in the human esophagus with age. *Digestive Diseases and Sciences, 53*(12), 3065–3070. Evidence Level II.

Hall, K. E. (2002). Aging and neural control of the GI tract. II. Neural control of the aging gut: Can an old dog learn new tricks? *American Journal of Physiology. Gastrointestinal and Liver Physiology, 283*(4), G827–G832. Evidence Level V.

Hall, K. E. (2009). Effect of aging on gastrointestinal function. In J. B. Halter, J. G. Ouslander, M. E. Tinetti, S. Studenski, K. P. High, & S. Asthana (Eds.), *Hazzard's geriatric medicine and gerontology* (6th ed., pp. 1059–1064). New York, NY: McGraw-Hill. Evidence Level V.

Harris, M. H., Holden, M. K., Cahalin, L. P., Fitzpatrick, D., Lowe, S., & Canavan, P. K. (2008). Gait in older adults: A review of the literature with an emphasis toward achieving favorable clinical outcomes, Part I. *Clinical Geriatrics, 16*(7), 33–42. Evidence Level I.

Henry, J. D., MacLeod, M. S., Phillips, L. H., & Crawford, J. R. (2004). A meta-analytic review of prospective memory and aging. *Psychology and Aging, 19*(1), 27–39. Evidence Level I.

High, K. P. (2009). Infection in the elderly. In J. B. Halter, J. G. Ouslander, M. E. Tinetti, S. Studenski, K. P. High, & S. Asthana (Eds.), *Hazzard's geriatric medicine and gerontology* (6th ed., pp. 1507–1515). New York, NY: McGraw-Hill. Evidence Level V.

Htwe, T. H., Mushtaq, A., Robinson, S. B., Rosher, R. B., & Khardori, N. (2007). Infection in the elderly. *Infectious Disease Clinics of North America, 21*(3), 711–743. Evidence Level V.

Hunt, K. J., Walsh, B. M., Voegeli, D., & Roberts, H. C. (2010). Inflammation in aging part I: Physiology and immunological mechanisms. *Biological Research for Nursing, 11*(3), 245–252. Evidence Level V.

Imperato, J., & Sanchez, L. D. (2006). Pulmonary emergencies in the elderly. *Emergency Medicine Clinics of North America, 24*(2), 317–338. Evidence Level V.

Irwin, M. R., Cole, J. C., & Nicassio, P. M. (2006). Comparative meta-analysis of behavioral interventions for insomnia and their efficacy in middle-aged adults and in older adults 55+ years of age. *Health Psychology, 25*(1), 3–14. Evidence Level I.

Joint National Committee. (2004). *The seventh report of the Joint National Committee on prevention, detection, evaluation, and treatment of high blood pressure.* Retrieved from http://www.nhlbi.nih.gov/guidelines/hypertension/jnc7full.htm/. Evidence Level I.

Jones, T. E., Stephenson, K. W., King, J. G., Knight, K. R., Marshall, T. L., & Scott, W. B. (2009). Sarcopenia—Mechanisms and treatments. *Journal of Geriatric Physical Therapy, 32*(2), 83–89. Evidence Level II.

Kestel, F. (2005). The best BP. *Advance for Nurses, 12*, 33–34. Evidence Level V.

Kevorkian, R. (2004). Physiology of incontinence. *Clinics in Geriatric Medicine, 20*(3), 409–425. Evidence Level V.

Kitzman, D., & Taffet, G. (2009). Effects of aging on cardiovascular structure and function. In J. B. Halter, J. G. Ouslander, M. E. Tinetti, S. Studenski, K. P. High, & S. Asthana (Eds.), *Hazzard's geriatric medicine and gerontology* (6th ed., pp. 883–895). New York, NY: McGraw-Hill. Evidence Level V.

Knoops, K. T., de Groot, L. C., Kromhout, D., Perrin, A. E., Moreiras-Varela, O., Menotti, A., & van Staveren, W. A. (2004). Mediterranean diet, lifestyle factors, and 10-year mortality in elderly European men and women: The HALE project. *Journal of the American Medical Association, 292*(12), 1433–1439. Evidence Level II.

Kuchel, G. A. (2009). Aging and homeostatic regulation. In J. B. Halter, J. G. Ouslander, M. E. Tinetti, S. Studenski, K. P. High, & S. Asthana (Eds.), *Hazzard's geriatric medicine and gerontology* (6th ed., pp. 621–629). New York, NY: McGraw-Hill. Evidence Level V.

Lakatta, E. G. (2000). Cardiovascular aging in health. *Clinics in Geriatric Medicine, 16*(3), 419–444. Evidence Level V.

Lerma, E. V. (2009). Anatomic and physiologic changes of the aging kidney. *Clinics in Geriatric Medicine, 25*(3), 325–329. Evidence Level V.

Loeser, R. F. (2010). Age-related changes in the musculoskeletal system and the development of osteoarthritis. *Clinics in Geriatric Medicine, 26*(3), 371–386. Evidence Level V.

Loeser, R. F., Jr., & Delbono, O. (2009). Aging of the muscles and joints. In J. B. Halter, J. G. Ouslander, M. E. Tinetti, S. Studenski, K. P. High, & S. Asthana (Eds.), *Hazzard's geriatric medicine and gerontology* (6th ed., pp. 1355–1368). New York, NY: McGraw-Hill. Evidence Level V.

Lu, S. H., Leasure, A. R., & Dai, Y. T. (2010). A systematic review of body temperature variations in older people. *Journal of Clinical Nursing, 19*(1–2), 4–16. Evidence Level I.

Mahler, D. A., Fierro-Carrion, G., & Baird, J. C. (2003). Evaluation of dyspnea in the elderly. *Clinics in Geriatric Medicine, 19*(1), 19–33. Evidence Level V.

Matsumura, B. A., & Ambrose, A. F. (2006). Balance in the elderly. *Clinics in Geriatric Medicine, 22*(2), 395–412. Evidence Level V.

Mattson, M. (2009). Cellular and neurochemical aspects of the aging human brain. In J. B. Halter, J. G. Ouslander, M. E. Tinetti, S. Studenski, K. P. High, & S. Asthana (Eds.), *Hazzard's geriatric medicine and gerontology* (6th ed., pp. 739–750). New York, NY: McGraw-Hill. Evidence Level V.

McCleane, G. (2008). Pain perception in the elderly patient. *Clinics in Geriatric Medicine, 24*(2), 203–211. Evidence Level V.

Meneilly, G. S. (2010). Pathophysiology of diabetes in the elderly. *Clinical Geriatrics, 18*, 25–28. Evidence Level V.

Mentes, J. (2006). Oral hydration on older adults: Greater awareness is needed in preventing, recognizing, and treating dehydration. *American Journal of Nursing, 106*(6), 40–49. Evidence Level V.

Mick, D. J., & Ackerman, M. H. (2004). Critical care nursing for older adults: Pathophysiological and functional considerations. *Nursing Clinics of North America, 39*(3), 473–493. Evidence Level V.

Miller, M. (2009). Disorders of fluid balance. In J. B. Halter, J. G. Ouslander, M. E. Tinetti, S. Studenski, K. P. High, & S. Asthana (Eds.), *Hazzard's geriatric medicine and gerontology* (6th ed., pp. 1047–1058). New York, NY: McGraw-Hill. Evidence Level V.

Mukai, S., & Lipsitz, L. A. (2002). Orthostatic hypotension. *Clinics in Geriatric Medicine, 18*(2), 253–268.

Narici, M. V., Maffulli, N., & Maganaris, C. N. (2008). Ageing of human muscles and tendons. *Disability and Rehabilitation, 30*(20–22), 1548–1554. Evidence Level V.

National Kidney Disease Education Program. (2009). *Health professionals: GFR MDRD calculators for adults (conventional units)*. Retrieved from http://www.nkdep.nih.gov/professionals/gfr_calculators/orig_con.html/. Evidence Level I.

Netz, Y., Wu, M. J., Becker, B. J., & Tenenbaum, G. (2005). Physical activity and psychological well-being in advanced age: A meta-analysis of intervention studies. *Psychology & Aging, 20*(2), 272–284. Evidence Level I.

Newton, J. L. (2005). Effect of age-related changes in gastric physiology on tolerability of medications for older people. *Drugs & Aging, 22*(8), 655–661. Evidence Level V.

Ney, D. M., Weiss, J. M., Kind, A. J., & Robbins, J. (2009). Senescent swallowing: Impact, strategies, and interventions. *Nutrition in Clinical Practice, 24*(3), 395–413. Evidence Level V.

Park, H. L., O'Connell, J. E., & Thomson, R. G. (2003). A systematic review of cognitive decline in the general elderly population. *International Journal of Geriatric Psychiatry, 18*(12), 1121–1134. Evidence Level I.

Péquignot, R., Belmin, J., Chauvelier, S., Gaubert, J. Y., Konrat, C., Duron, E., & Hanon, O. (2009). Renal function in older hospital patients is more accurately estimated using the Cockcroft-Gault formula than the modification diet in renal disease formula. *Journal of the American Geriatrics Society, 57*(9), 1638–1643. Evidence Level II.

Roberts, S. B., & Dallal, G. E. (2005). Energy requirements and aging. *Public Health Nutrition*, *8*(7A), 1028–1036. Evidence Level I.

Schnelle, J. F., Alessi, C. A., Simmons, S. F., Al-Samarrai, N. R., Beck, J. C., & Ouslander, J. G. (2002). Translating clinical research into practice: A randomized controlled trial of exercise and incontinence care with nursing home residents. *Journal of the American Geriatrics Society*, *50*(9), 1476–1483. Evidence Level II.

Simon, L. S. (2005). Osteoporosis. *Clinics in Geriatric Medicine*, *21*(3), 603–629. Evidence Level V.

Smith, H. A., & Connolly, M. J. (2003). Evaluation and treatment of dysphagia following stroke. *Topics in Geriatric Rehabilitation*, *19*(1), 43–59. Evidence Level V.

Stern, M. (2006). Neurogenic bowel and bladder in the older adult. *Clinics in Geriatric Medicine*, *22*(2), 311–330. Evidence Level V.

Stewart, R. (2004). Review: In older people, decline of cognitive function is more likely than improvement, but rate of change is very variable. *Evidence-Based Mental Health*, *7*(3), 92. Evidence Level I.

Suhayda, R., & Walton, J. C. (2002). Preventing and managing dehydration. *Medsurg Nursing*, *11*(6), 267–278. Evidence Level V.

Thomas, S., & Rich, M. W. (2007). Epidemiology, pathophysiology, and prognosis of heart failure in the elderly. *Clinics in Geriatric Medicine*, *23*(1), 1–10. Evidence Level V.

U.S. Department of Health and Human Services. (2004a). *The health consequences of smoking: A report of the Surgeon General.* Retrieved from http://www.cdc.gov/tobacco/data_statistics/sgr/2004/index.htm/. Evidence Level I.

U.S. Department of Health and Human Services. (2004b). *Bone health and osteoporosis: A report of the Surgeon General.* Retrieved from http://www.surgeongeneral.gov/library/bonehealth/. Evidence Level I.

U.S. Department of Health and Human Services. (2005). *Dietary guidelines for Americans.* Retrieved from http://www.healthierus.gov/dietaryguidelines/. Evidence Level I.

Visvanathan, R., & Chapman, I. M. (2009). Undernutrition and anorexia in the older person. *Gastroenterology Clinics of North America*, *38*(3), 393–409. Evidence Level V.

Watters, J. M. (2002). Surgery in the elderly. *Canadian Journal of Surgery*, *45*(2), 104–108. Evidence Level V.

Weiskopf, D., Weinberger, B., & Grubeck-Loebenstein, B. (2009). The aging of the immune system. *Transplant International*, *22*(11), 1041–1050. Evidence Level V.

Zeleznik, J. (2003). Normative aging of the respiratory system. *Clinics in Geriatric Medicine*, *19*(1), 1–18. Evidence Level V.

Sensory Changes

4

Pamela Z. Cacchione

EDUCATIONAL OBJECTIVES

On completion of this chapter, the reader should be able to:

1. describe the normal changes of aging that affect the senses in the older adult
2. identify common disorders that impact the senses in the older adult
3. determine how best to assess sensory status in the older adult
4. identify nursing strategies to manage sensory impairment in the older adult
5. collaborate with interprofessional team members who can assist the older adults with sensory impairment

BACKGROUND AND STATEMENT OF PROBLEM

Individuals experience and interact with their environments through their senses. Vision, hearing, smell, taste, and peripheral sensation allow us to safely experience and enjoy the world around us. As people age, they often experience changes in their sensory function (vision, hearing, smell, taste, and peripheral sensation). These sensory changes can negatively impact the older adults' ability to interact with their environment, decreasing their quality of life. For example, changes in hearing can impact an older person's communication skills; changes in vision can impact their health literacy limiting their ability to take medications safely. *Healthy People 2020* emphasizes the importance of healthy senses, including vision, hearing, balance, smell, and taste. Vision and hearing abilities are essential to language, whether spoken, signed, or read (U.S. Department of Health and Human Services [USDHHS], 2010). Decreases in sense of smell can interfere with an older adult's ability to smell smoke in a fire or recognize spoiled food. Many adults report a decrease in taste that impacts their desire to eat. Decreased peripheral sensation sets up an individual for falls.

Understanding how to assess the senses as well as manage sensory deficits is essential to holistic nursing. A goal of *Healthy People 2020* is to decrease the prevalence and

For description of Evidence Levels cited in this chapter, see Chapter 1, Developing and Evaluating Clinical Practice Guidelines: A Systematic Approach, page 7.

severity of disorders of vision, hearing, balance, smell, and taste, as well as voice, speech, and language (USDHHS, 2010). This chapter on sensory changes addresses common age-related changes associated with the senses as well as disease states and injuries to the senses that occur more commonly with aging. Nursing care related to the *Healthy People 2020* goals regarding sensory changes will also be addressed.

Normal Changes of Aging Senses

The senses—vision, hearing, taste, smell, balance, and peripheral sensation—change with aging, usually presenting primarily with a slowing of function. A summary table is presented describing the changes that occur and the functional outcomes for each sense (Table 4.1).

Vision

There are several changes that occur with vision as people age. The eyelids start to lag, potentially obscuring vision; the pupil takes longer to dilate and contract, slowing accommodation; and presbyopia is widespread.

Presbyopia

A loss of elasticity in the lens and stiffening of the muscle fibers of the lens of the eye leads to a decrease in the eyes' ability to change the shape of the lens to focus on near objects, such as fine print, and decreases ability to adapt to light (National Eye Institute [NEI], 2004a; Whiteside, Wallhagen, & Pettengill, 2006).

Hearing

Normal changes of aging impacting hearing include the decrease in function of the hair fibers in the ear canal that normally aid in the natural removal of cerumen and the protection of the ear canal from external elements.

Presbycusis

Presbycusis is the most common form of hearing loss in the United States (Bagai, Thavendiranathan, & Detsky, 2006). This high-frequency sensorineural hearing loss is a multifactorial process that varies in severity and is associated with aging (Gates & Mills, 2005). Presbycusis usually has a bilateral progressive onset and is caused by gradual loss of hair cells and fibrous changes in the small blood vessels that supply the cochlea. Risk factors include heredity, environmental exposure, free radical, and mitochondrial deoxyribonucleic acid (DNA) damage (Huang & Tang, 2010). Presenting clinical symptoms of this irreversible condition includes high-frequency hearing loss and difficulty hearing high-pitched sounds such as /t/, /p/, /k/, /s/, /z/, /sh/, and /ch/ (Huang & Tang, 2010; Wallhagen, Strawbridge, Shema, & Kaplan, 2004). Background noise further aggravates this hearing deficit.

Smell

Changes in smell are common as we age, but are not considered a normal part of aging. Frequently, older adults complain of distortions of smell. Factors associated with loss of sense of smell include age and sex with older males being more prone to smell loss (Hoffman, Cruickshanks, & Davis, 2009). The environment, trauma, diseases, or illness can diminish

TABLE 4.1

Normal Changes of Aging

Sense	Change of Aging	Functional Outcome
Vision	■ Decreased dark adaptation ■ Decreased upward gaze ■ Eyes become drier and produce less tears ■ Cornea becomes less sensitive ■ Pupils decrease in size ■ Visual fields become smaller	■ Increased safety risk in changing environmental light ■ Decreased field of vision ■ Dry irritated eyes ■ Slow to recognize injury to the cornea ■ Inability to adjust to glare and change in lighting conditions ■ Safety risk for driving and maneuvering in the environment
Hearing	■ Ear drum thickens ■ Loss of high-frequency hearing acuity ■ Decreased ability to process sounds after age 50 ■ Increased cerumen impactions	■ Thickened ear drum decreases sound moving across the ear canal ■ Decreased ability to hear sounds, such as /p/, /w/, /f/, /sh/, and women's and children's voices ■ Requires more time to process and respond to auditory stimuli ■ Decreased hearing because of blockage of sound
Smell	■ Decreased ability to identify odors ■ Impacts ability to taste	■ Inability to identify spoiled food or smoke ■ Limits enjoyment in eating
Taste	■ Decreased number of taste buds ■ Limited decrease in taste supported by studies ■ Less saliva production	■ Decreased sensitivity to flavors ■ Dry mouth affecting ability to swallow
Sensation	■ Decreased vibratory sense ■ Decreased two-point discrimination ■ Decreased temperature sensitivity ■ Decreased balance ■ Decreased proprioception ■ Changed pain sensation	■ Increases risk for injury ■ Decreased ability to sense pressure ■ Decreased protective response to withdraw from hot objects ■ Risk of falls ■ Risk of falls ■ Decreased protective mechanism

Note. Adapted from: Bromley, S. M. (2000). Smell and taste disorders: A primary care approach. *American Family Physician, 61*(2), 427–436, 438. Evidence Level VI. Linton, A. D. (2007). Age-related changes in the special senses. In A. D. Linton & H. W. Lach (Eds.), *Matteson & McConnell's gerontological nursing, concepts and practice* (3rd ed., pp. 600–630). St. Louis, MO: Saunders Elsevier. Evidence Level V. Murphy, C., Schubert, C. R., Cruickshanks, K. J., Klein, B. E., Klein, R., & Nondahl, D. M. (2002). Prevalence of olfactory impairment in older adults. *Journal of the American Medical Association, 288*(18), 2307–2312. Evidence Level III. Schiffman, S. S. (1997). Taste and smell losses in normal aging and disease. *Journal of the American Medical Association, 278*(16), 1357–1362. Evidence Level V. Seiberling, K. A., & Conley, D. B. (2004). Aging and olfactory and taste function. *Otolaryngologic Clinics of North America, 37*(6), 1209–1228. Evidence Level V. Wallhagen, M. I., Pettengill, E., & Whiteside, M. (2006). Sensory impairment in older adults: Part 1: Hearing loss. *The American Journal of Nursing, 106*(10), 40–48. Evidence Level VI. Whiteside, M. M., Wallhagen, M. I., & Pettengill E. (2006). Sensory impairment in older adults: Part 2: Vision loss. *The American Journal of Nursing, 106*(11), 52–61. Evidence Level V.

the sense of smell (Hoffman et al., 2009). Changes in the sense of smell have also been found to correlate with neurological conditions such as Parkinson's disease and Alzheimer's disease (Albers, Tabert, & Devanand, 2006; Wilson, Arnold, Schneider, Tang, & Bennett, 2007).

Taste

Common changes in taste include a decreased ability to detect the intensity of taste but not somatic sensations such as touch and burning pain in the tongue when compared to younger adults (Fukunaga, Uematsu, & Sugimoto, 2005). However, complete loss of taste is rare and changes in taste are more often related to dental concerns; diseases or illness such as rhinitis, allergies, or infections; and medications or cancer treatments to the head and neck (Fukunaga et al., 2005; Hoffman et al., 2009).

Peripheral Sensation

Peripheral nerve function that controls the sense of touch declines slightly with age. Two-point discrimination and vibratory sense both decrease with age. The ability to perceive painful stimuli is preserved in aging. However, there may be a slowed reaction time for pulling away from painful stimuli with aging (Linton, 2007).

ASSESSMENT OF THE PROBLEM

Vision

The prevalence of visual impairment increases with age and the settings in which older adults live. Data from the National Health and Nutrition Examination Survey (NHANES; Dillon, Gu, Hoffman, & Ko, 2010) in older adults aged 70 years and older identified, 15.4% were found to be visually impaired but this varied by race and ethnicity with non-Hispanic Whites (13.8%), non-Hispanic Blacks (21.1%), and Mexican Americans (24%). In adults aged 80 years and older, 24.6% were found to be visually impaired (Dillon et al., 2010). In another study, adults aged 80 years and older are 7.7% of one study but accounted 69% of the cases of blindness (Congdon et al., 2004). This is worrisome because this is the fastest growing segment of our population.

Studies evaluating older adults in long-term care settings demonstrate prevalence rates from 27% to 54% of older adults with visual impairment (Bron & Caird, 1997; Cacchione, Culp, Dyck, & Laing, 2003). Uncorrected refractive error was also found to be common in visually impaired older adults. In one study, of the 8.8% of the older adults found to be visually impaired, 59% of those were impaired because of an uncorrected refractive error (Vitale, Cotch, & Sperduto, 2006). Leading causes of blindness by race and ethnicity was found to be macular degeneration in Whites, cataracts and open-angle glaucoma in Blacks, and open-angle glaucoma in Hispanic persons (Congdon et al., 2004). Cataracts, one of the leading causes of blindness, are unilateral or bilateral clouding of the crystalline lens that presents as painless, progressive loss of vision (NEI, 2004a).

The definition of visual impairment varies by different groups and by country (Agency for Healthcare Research and Quality [AHRQ], 2004). The United States defines low vision as best corrected visual acuity:

- Normal vision: visual acuity of 20/20 or better
- Mild vision impairment: 20/25 to 20/50
- Moderate visual impairment: 20/60 to 20/160
- Severe visual impairment (legally blind): 20/200 to 20/400
- Profound vision impairment: 20/400 to 20/1,000
- Near-total vision loss: less than or equal to 20/1,250
- Total blindness: no light perception

Low vision can also be defined based on visual field limitations. *Severe visual impairment* is defined as best corrected field less than or equal to 20 degrees (legal blindness). *Profound visual impairment* is defined as visual field less than or equal to 10 degrees (AHRQ, 2004).

Nursing Assessment of Vision

The health history is an essential part of vision assessment. Several health conditions predispose older adults to visual impairment. Diabetes is a common cause of disease-related blindness related to diabetic retinopathy, with 6% of diabetics older than the age of 65 years developing diabetic retinopathy (Baker, 2003; NEI, 2004b). Hypertension carries with it the risk of hypertensive retinopathy. Ascertaining a thorough baseline health history with yearly reviews and updates is essential in maintaining visual health. Health questions related to visual health include the questions shown in Table 4.2 (Cacchione, 2007; Wallhagen, Pettengill, & Whiteside, 2006).

Examination of the Eye

The external structures can cause decreased vision if the lids lag because of laxity of the skin of the upper eyelid. Lid lag can interfere with visual acuity and fields, which may require surgery. A decreased level of tear function can negatively impact visual acuity. Cataracts in severe cases can be visible with the naked eye and appear as a whitish gray pupil instead of black. Cloudiness of the whole cornea of the eye is indicative of a corneal problem, not a cataract. If the person has had cataract surgery, the lens implant may be visible on close inspection.

Fundus Exam. Using an ophthalmoscope, a nurse can visualize the red reflex and, with experience and practice, the fundus of the eye. This is often difficult with small pupils. Darkening the room may help with dilating the pupils. Optometrists and ophthalmologists

---

TABLE 4.2
Vision History Questions

- When was your last eye exam?
- How would you describe your eyesight?
- Any change in your eyesight?
- When did you notice this change?
- Are you experiencing any blurred vision?
- Are you having any double vision?
- Are you bothered by glare?
- Are you experiencing any eye pain?
- Are you using any eye drops for any reason?
- Any history of trauma or injury to your eyes?
- Have you had any eye surgeries?
- Do you have cataracts?
- Any family history of eye problems?

Note. Adapted from: Cacchione, P. Z. (2007). Nursing care of older adults with age-related vision loss. In S. Crocker-Houde (Ed.), *Vision loss in older adults: Nursing assessment and care management* (pp. 131–148). New York, NY: Springer Publishing. Evidence Level VI. Whiteside, M. M., Wallhagen, M. I., & Pettengill E. (2006). Sensory impairment in older adults: Part 2. Vision loss. *The American Journal of Nursing, 106*(11), 52–61. Evidence Level V.

dilate the pupils to allow for a better view of the fundus. Cataracts will appear as a dark shadow in the anterior portion of the lens in front of the retina.

Vision Testing. Vision testing should be completed before the eyes are dilated and completed with both uncorrected and corrected (with glasses) vision.

Distance Vision. The "gold standard" in eye charts, the Snellen chart, is one of the most commonly used to assess distance vision. Visual acuity is tested at 20 ft. The individual is asked to read the letters on the chart until he or she miss more than two on a line of acuity. Acuity equals the line above the line with more than two errors. Acuity measures range from 20/10 to 20/800 on the Snellen chart.

Early Treatment Diabetic Retinopathy Study. The Early Treatment Diabetic Retinopathy Study (ETDRS; Ferris, Kassoff, Bresnick, & Bailey, 1982) eye chart is also used frequently and can be used at a distance of 4 m. At this distance, the greatest visual acuity measured is 20/200—the equivalent of legal blindness.

Pin-Hole Test. With best vision, with or without glasses, a card with a small pin hole or a multiple pin-hole occluder can be placed in front of the eye, and the vision is tested again at the last line the individual was able to read. This test identifies refractive error of the peripheral cornea of the lens of the eye by allowing only perpendicular light to the lens (Kalinowski, 2008). If the individual can read farther down the chart with the pin hole, his or her vision may be improved with better refraction of his or her eyeglasses or, if he or she do not have glasses, with eyeglasses.

Near Vision. Near vision is important for health literacy, especially regarding reading food or medication labels. There are several ways to assess near vision. Two commonly used tools are the Rosenbaum Pocket Eye Screener and the Lighthouse for the Blind Near Vision Screener. The Rosenbaum Pocket Eye Screener is a non-copyrighted tool based on the Snellen chart that can be useful in assessing near vision in the acute care and primary care settings. The Rosenbaum is true to scale when compared with the Snellen chart at the 20/200, 20/400, and 20/800 acuity levels. However, the other levels are slightly too large, causing an overestimation of visual acuity (Horton & Jones, 1997).

Lighthouse for the Blind Near Vision Screener (Lighthouse for the Blind). This handheld vision screener has a cord that can be used at 40 and 20 cm to measure the proper distance for testing near vision. This near vision screener mimics the ETDRS eye chart in a smaller version but is not pocket size. It does not, however, have the concern over the scale matching of the ETDRS distance acuity level. For research purposes, it has the added feature of the cord for measuring a consistent distance.

Contrast Sensitivity. Contrast sensitivity is often compromised by aging and diseases or conditions of the eye. Decreases in contrast sensitivity occur with cataracts, glaucoma, and retinopathies (Mäntyjärvi & Laitinen, 2001; Wilensky & Hawkins, 2001). Contrast sensitivity provides information on how well an individual may perform in real-life conditions. Decline in contrast sensitivity impacts one's ability to distinguish when one step ends and another begins, identify light switches on the wall, read materials not made in high-contrast font, or identify the buttons on the remote. Intact contrast sensitivity is important for day-to-day safety and function within the environment.

The Pelli–Robson Contrast Sensitivity Chart (Pelli, Robson, & Wilkins, 1988) is read at the 1- or 3-m distance. All letters are presented at the 20/200 acuity level but in decreasing shades of black to gray. The Pelli–Robson Contrast Sensitivity Chart is widely used in practice and works well for older adults who are experienced in recognizing letters (Hirvelä & Laatikainen, 1995; Morse & Rosenthal, 1997). The Vistech Contrast Sensitivity Test, another contrast sensitivity measure, has four patches of gray circles with lines in different directions (Kennedy & Dunlap, 1990). The person being examined points to the direction the lines within the circle are pointed (Morse & Rosenthal, 1997).

Visual Fields. Fields of vision refers to the area of peripheral vision visible when the individual is focusing straight ahead (Cassin & Rubin, 2001). The vision in visual fields can be affected by many eye conditions, as well as neurological disorders that inhibit eye movement or affect the blood supply to the optic nerve. Intact visual fields are important to function safely in one's environment. In assessing visual fields by confrontation, a gross clinical measure of visual fields, the examiner faces the patient and determines if the patient can identify the examiner's moving fingers as they are moving into their field of view (Seidel, Dains, Ball, & Benedict, 2003). Although subjective and dependent on the examiner having normal fields of vision, the confrontation test is useful in quickly identifying large losses in visual fields.

The Humphrey Visual Field Test is completed by an ophthalmologist and assesses visual fields using a static type of perimetry (Gianutsos & Suchoff, 1997). This measure provides a more reliable measure of functional visual fields. The Goldman VI4e kinetic perimetry visual field testing, on the other hand, assesses kinetic type of functional visual fields (Gillmore, 2002). Kinetic perimetry entails the introduction of a moving stimulus moving from a nonvisible area toward the fixed point of view. The Goldman VI4e kinetic perimetry visual field testing is hard to standardize because it is operator dependent (Gillmore, 2002). Because these automated methods are more widely used, the location of the visual field deficit may clue the examiner about the type of eye condition. For example, unilateral visual field deficits may be related to a cerebral vascular accident, glaucoma will affect the peripheral fields, and macular degeneration has associated central field of vision loss.

Stereopsis. Stereopsis is the process where humans have the ability to use the different viewpoints provided by their eyes to produce a vivid perception of depth and three-dimensional shapes (Norman et al., 2008; Read, Phillipson, Serrano-Pedraza, Milner, & Parker, 2010). There are multiple methods of measuring stereopsis and it is not thought to be affected by aging but may be negatively impacted by distance acuity and eye diseases (Norman et al., 2008).

Visual Function Questionnaire-25

The NEI Visual Function Questionnaire (VFQ) is a 25-item survey that assesses the functional impact visual impairment. It provides a subjective report on 12 functional subscales: General Vision, Near Vision, Distance Vision, Driving, Peripheral Vision, Color Vision, Ocular Pain, General Health, Vision Specific Role Difficulties, Dependency, Social Function, and Mental Health (Revicki, Rentz, Harnam, Thomas, & Lanzetta, 2010). The NEI VFQ-25 has sound psychometric properties in cognitively intact older adults (Mangione et al., 2001).

Conditions of the Eye

Diseases That Alter Vision Seen More Frequently as People Age

Cataracts. Clouding of the crystalline lens that presents either unilaterally or bilaterally as painless, progressive loss of vision (NEI, 2009). Cataracts are usually age related but they can be secondary to glaucoma, diabetes, Alzheimer's disease; congenital; injury related; or related to medications or radiation (NEI, 2009). The management of cataracts includes early identification and monitoring followed by surgical extraction and lens implantation once vision is affected.

Macular Degeneration. Involves the development of drusen deposits in the retinal pigmented epithelium and is the leading cause of central vision loss and legal blindness in older adults (Revicki et al., 2010). Macular degeneration is more common in fair-haired, blue-eyed individuals. Other risk factors include smoking and excessive sunlight exposure. There are wet and dry forms of macular degeneration. The wet form of macular degeneration is more easily treated than the dry form. Newer treatments of expensive injectable medications are available to slow the progression of dry macular degeneration.

Glaucoma. Glaucoma is a progressive, serious form of eye disease that can damage the optic nerve and result in vision loss and blindness (NEI, 2009). Primary open-angle glaucoma is the most common form of glaucoma in older adults (Linton, 2007). Increased intraocular pressure causes atrophy and cupping of the optic nerve head that leads to visual field deficits that can progress to blindness. Vision changes include loss of peripheral vision, intolerance to glare, decreased perception of contrast, and decreased ability to adapt to the dark.

Diabetic Retinopathy. This results from end-organ damage from diabetes causing retinopathy and spotty vision. Risk can be reduced by tight blood sugar control. Almost 6% of diabetics aged 65–74 years old develop diabetic retinopathy (NEI, 2004a). Diabetic retinopathy starts as mild nonproliferative retinopathy with microaneurysms on the retina and progresses as moderate-to-severe nonproliferative retinopathy where blood vessels in the retina are blocked, depriving the retina with adequate blood supply, then progressing to proliferative retinopathy where the growth of new abnormal blood vessels that leak can cause blindness (NEI, 2009).

Hypertensive Retinopathy. This is caused by end-organ damage from poorly controlled hypertension causing background and eventual proliferative retinopathy. Hypertensive retinopathy is usually treated with laser photocoagulation and tight blood pressure control.

Temporal Arteritis. This is an autoimmune disorder that causes inflammation of the temporal artery, also known as *giant cell arteritis*. It presents as malaise, scalp tenderness, unilateral temporal headache, jaw claudication, and sudden vision loss (usually unilateral). This vision loss is a medical emergency but is potentially reversible if identified immediately. The client should see an ophthalmologist or go to the emergency room immediately if symptoms develop.

Detached Retina. This is a condition that can occur in patients with cataracts or recent cataract surgery, trauma, or occur spontaneously. A detached retina presents as a curtain coming down across a patient's line of vision. An individual experiencing this should see an ophthalmologist or proceed to the closest emergency room immediately. See Table 4.3 for the implications of vision changes on an older adult's function.

TABLE 4.3

Implications of Vision Changes in Older Adults

Impact on safety
  Inability to read medication labels
  Difficulty navigating stairs of curbs
  Difficulty driving
  Difficulty crossing streets

Impact on quality of life
  Reduces ability to remain independent
  Difficulty or unable to read
  Falls

INTERVENTIONS AND CARE STRATEGIES

Vision

The nurse should obtain a past medical history to avoid disruption in the management of chronic eye conditions, assuring continuation of ongoing regimens such as eye drops for glaucoma. Without the continuation of the individual's eye drops, eye pressures could precipitously increase causing an acute exacerbation of their glaucoma, potentially dramatically limiting their vision. If an acute change in an individual's vision occurs, the primary care provider should be notified immediately. Depending on the signs and symptoms present, the individual may need to see an ophthalmologist or go to the emergency room to receive treatment to restore the vision or limit the deterioration.

Lighting is important in an individual's environment. Too little light can limit an individual's vision. Too much light depending on the individual's eye condition, such as cataracts or macular degeneration, may cause eye pain and glare. It is important to ascertain whether an individual is sensitive to light. If he or she is sensitive to light, indirect light and night lights may be helpful to provide a safe environment. The majority of older adults benefit from improved lighting. To avoid glare, directing incandescent lamps directly on a task such as sewing or reading often improves visual acuity and is well tolerated. Glare occurs when a light shines directly into the eye or reflects off a shiny surface. Low vision specialists recommend trying different positions and wattage of lighting to find what works best for each individual (Community Services for the Blind and Partially Sighted, 2004).

Encourage the use of the person's eyeglasses. Older adults' eyeglasses should be labeled with the person's name so they can be reconnected to their owner if they are set down and left behind. Even with eyeglasses, magnification may be helpful. Have family provide lighted magnification if needed (large lighted magnifiers are available at low vision centers). A low vision optometrist or specialist can assist in recommending appropriate levels of magnifiers.

Contrast sensitivity is a problem with several eye conditions including cataracts, glaucoma, and macular degeneration. Adding contrast to the edge of each step, fixtures in the home, light switches that blend into the wall, or faucets that blend into the sink can create a safer and more functional environment.

Annual mass screening is not recommended in the older adult (Chou, Dana, & Bougatsos, 2009). However, nurses should encourage an annual dilated eye exam either with an optometrist or ophthalmologist. This is crucial in people who have a diagnosis of diabetes or hypertension (NEI, 2009). Nurses are members of the interprofessional team responsible for preventing unnecessary disability. Therefore, nurses should make sure that there is a mechanism in place to trigger these visits on an annual basis.

Hearing Impairment

Surveys to identify older adults with hearing impairment often suffer from underreporting on self-report instruments. The latest version of the NHANES included audiometric testing in older adults and found a prevalence rate of 26.3% in those older than age 70 years and 45.4% in those older than age 80 years (Dillon et al., 2010). Hearing loss has been found to be greater in men and progresses more quickly than in women (Chao & Chen, 2009; National Institute on Deafness and Other Communication Disorders [NIDCD], 2007). This dramatic increase in prevalence rates is magnified in the nursing home population. Prevalence rates of hearing impairment in the nursing home are similar to rates of visual impairment, approximately 24% (Warnat & Tabloski, 2006). When hearing is tested through audiometry, the prevalence rates increase to 42%–90% (Bagai et al., 2006; Cacchione et al., 2003; Tolson, Swan, & Knussen, 2002). The American Academy of Audiology defines hearing loss based on decibels or loudness and the hertz or the pitch of sound. Normal speech is in the 0- to 25-dB level, mild hearing loss is defined as hearing in the 25- to 40-dB level. Hearing between 40 and 70 dB is considered moderate hearing loss. Severe hearing loss is between 70 and 90 dB. Greater than 90 dB is considered profound hearing loss (Mehr, 2007). Aging impairs the processing of sound through the ear canal as well as the central nervous system processing of sounds, making it more difficult to hear the higher frequencies including women's and children's voices (Huang & Tang, 2010).

Assessment of Hearing

Often, it is easy to determine when an older adult is hard of hearing just by having a conversation with them. The older adult may lean closer in an attempt to hear better, turn their head to their "good ear," or cup their hand behind their ear. Older adults may have to ask for things to be repeated; they may report having trouble hearing their grandchildren's or other's high-pitched voices. Older adults often complain that people are mumbling. Any or all of these signs may be present. Regardless of whether any of these signs are present, all older adults should have their hearing screened annually at their primary care visit (Bagai et al., 2006). Primary care providers play an important role in screening for hearing loss and making appropriate referrals for older adults (Johnson, Danhauer, Bennett, & Harrison, 2009). Methods of screening are described herein.

Hearing Handicap Inventory for the Elderly-Screen

The Hearing Handicap Inventory for the Elderly-Screen (HHIE-S; Ventry & Weinstein, 1983) is a 10-item scale to determine how hearing is impacting an older adult's daily life and to assist in identifying who might benefit from a hearing aid and an audiology referral. The scale takes approximately 5 minutes to complete and is targeted for community-dwelling older adults. This scale is available online through the Hartford Foundation Institute for Geriatric Nursing "Try This Best Practices in Care for Older Adults" (Demers, 2001). The HHIE-S has reported excellent sensitivity and specificity for severe hearing loss, but the sensitivity and specificity decreases as the level of hearing impairment lessens (Adams-Wendling, Pimple, Adams, & Titler, 2008).

Whisper Test

The whisper test involves covering or rubbing one ear canal, and from a distance of 2 ft, whispering a three-syllable word on an exhale that the patient either correctly or incorrectly repeats back. An incorrect response triggers a repeat attempt to see if the older adult can identify a different three-syllable word. The consistency of the level of the whispered word makes this test difficult to compare from examiner to examiner. However, despite this difficulty, it has been found to be a valid and reliable test to screen for hearing loss (Bagai et al., 2006).

Handheld Audioscope

The handheld audioscope is a device developed to specifically screen for hearing impairment. It has a test tone that is presented at the 60-dB level. The decibel levels that may be tested include the 20-, 25-, and 40-dB levels at the 500-, 1,000-, 2,000-, and 4,000-Hz levels (Yueh et al., 2007). The audioscope has an otoscope that allows for the direct inspection of the tympanic membrane or cerumen impactions that can result in conductive hearing loss present in up to 30% of older adults (Lewis-Cullinan & Janken, 1990; Yueh, Shapiro, MacLean, & Shekelle, 2003). Testing using the audioscope should be performed in a quiet setting and may not be as useful in the long-term care environment with high noise levels.

Pure Tone Audiometry

This is the gold standard of hearing tests, particularly if completed in a sound-proof booth with 92% sensitivity and 94% specificity in detecting sensorineural hearing loss (Frank & Petersen, 1987). Pure tone audiometry allows for testing of a wide range of decibels and hertz levels, or loudness and pitch or frequencies, allowing for testing at the 5- to 120-dB level and 250–4,000 Hz. Portable pure tone audiometers with noise-reduction earphones are available and can be used in the community, outpatient, and long-term care settings when access to an audiologist is limited. This wide range of tones allows for a better understanding of the individual's functional hearing. Pure tone audiometry by an audiologist is the next step after screening has identified a hearing deficit (Yueh et al., 2003).

Tuning Fork Tests

Two tuning fork tests have been used in hearing screenings, although a recent systematic review discouraged their use because they were found to be unreliable with limited accuracy (Bagai et al., 2006). The tuning fork should be either 256 or 512 Hz (M. I. Wallhagen, personal communication, 2006). The Rinne test is meant to differentiate whether an older adult hears better by bone or air conduction and can help determine if an individual had sensorineural or conductive hearing loss. The Weber test is used to help identify unilateral hearing loss.

Hearing Changes Common in Older Adults

Conductive hearing loss usually involves abnormalities of the middle or external ear, including the ear canal, tympanic membrane, and ossicular chain of bones in the middle ear (Marcincuk & Roland, 2002; Yueh et al., 2003). Causes of conductive hearing impairment include cerumen impactions or foreign bodies, ruptured eardrum, otitis media, and otosclerosis (Wallhagen et al., 2006; Yueh et al., 2003).

Sensorineural hearing loss is the most common form of hearing loss in older adults (Linton, 2007) that involves damage to the inner ear, the cochlea, or the fibers of the eighth cranial nerve. Sensorineural hearing loss is usually a bilateral progressive onset and is caused by gradual loss of hair cells, and fibrous changes in the small blood vessels that supply the cochlea. Risk factors include heredity, environmental exposure, free radical, and mitochondrial DNA damage (Huang & Tang, 2010). Additional causes of sensorineural hearing loss include viral or bacterial infections, trauma, tumors, noise exposure, cardiovascular conditions, ototoxic drugs, and Ménière's disease (Wallhagen et al., 2006).

Central auditory processing disorder is an uncommon disorder that includes an inability to process incoming signals and is often found in patients with stroke and older adults with neurological conditions such as Alzheimer's disease and Parkinson's disease (Pekkonen et al., 1999). The person's hearing is intact but his or her ability to process the sound is impaired.

Tinnitus, otherwise known as *ringing in the ear*, is of two types: subjective and objective. Subjective tinnitus is a condition where there is perceived sound in the absence of acoustic stimulus (Ahmad & Seidman, 2004; Lockwood, Salvi, & Burkard, 2002). Objective tinnitus is considered rare and presents as ringing in the ear that is audible by the individual and others. It is thought to have a vascular or neurological condition or Eustachian tube dysfunction (Crummer & Hassan, 2004). Subjective ringing in the ears may fluctuate and can be caused by damage to the hair receptors of the cochlear nerve and age-related changes in the organs of hearing and balance. Patients with tinnitus should be referred to an ear, nose, and throat (ENT) specialist.

Ménière's disease is characterized by fluctuating hearing loss, dizziness, vertigo, tinnitus, and a sensation of pressure in the affected ear (NIDCD, 2001). Unfortunately, the fluctuating hearing loss can become permanent hearing loss over time. Possible causes of Ménière's disease include hypothyroidism, diabetes, and neurosyphilis.

Implications of Hearing Changes

Older adults who have hearing impairment experience a decreased quality of communication, social isolation, low self-esteem, and generally lower quality of life. Decreased hearing impacts an individual's word recognition, decreasing the ability to communicate. This in turn can lead to significant safety issues. For example, if patient education about medication administration is provided only verbally, key information can be misheard and misinterpreted. Difficulty understanding the spoken word can lead to fatigue and speech paucity of friends and loved ones.

Speech paucity is described as decreased attempts to have meaningful conversations because of the difficulty in getting the message through to a hearing-impaired loved one. Speech paucity (Wallhagen et al., 2006) leads to social isolation of the hearing impaired because only the necessary information is transferred and no everyday social information is shared (Wallhagen et al., 2004). This can lead to depression and low self-esteem in the hearing-impaired individual and the partner. Other factors that lead to social isolation in hearing-impaired older adults include the inability to hear the phone or the doorbell ringing or knocking at the door.

Ideally, an older adult who develops hearing loss will see an audiologist and obtain unilateral or bilateral hearing aids to improve their ability to communicate with the people around them. Unfortunately, the stigma, cost, and delay in pursuing hearing aids are barriers to their success. Hearing aids should be pursued early in the course of hearing impairment. For example, hearing aids can be very helpful when hearing is impaired to the point that background noise interferes with understanding the spoken word. Success in using hearing aids at this level of hearing improves the chance that older adults will continue with hearing aids. Once an individual is offered a hearing aid, hearing rehabilitation should accompany the hearing aid dispensing; this will increase the use of the hearing aid and positively impact their independent living and quality of life (Yueh & Shekelle, 2007). Once older adults become used to the silence, it is hard to adapt to the increased ambient noise heard with hearing aids. Often, older adults require extensive coaching from an audiologist to get through the transition phase of wearing hearing aids. Technology has improved to the point of analog hearing aids that can be finely tuned to the individual's needs (Wallhagen et al., 2006). In one intervention group of older adults fitted with hearing aids, 98% experienced benefit and their caregivers perceived significant benefit as well (Tolson et al., 2002). University settings are often the most cost-effective locations to pursue hearing aids. The cost of hearing aids is an important factor because most insurance plans including Medicare do not cover hearing aids.

Cochlear implants are another technological advancement that has demonstrated positive outcomes in older adults in the areas of speech recognition. A cochlear implant works by bypassing the damaged parts of the ear and stimulating the auditory nerve. These impulses are sent to the brain through the auditory nerve and the brain recognizes them as sound (NIDCD, 2001). Severe hearing impairment must be present unilaterally or bilaterally prior to this surgical intervention will be considered. Cochlear implants were found in one study to improve word recognition and health-related quality of life (Francis, Chee, Yeagle, Cheng, & Niparko, 2002). At this time, there is only evidence for unilateral cochlear implants in profoundly deaf adults rather than bilateral cochlear implants because of cost and limited functional gain (Bond et al., 2009). Despite these improvements, relatively few adults have received this new technology. According to the U.S. Food and Drug Administration, nearly 22,000 adults have received cochlear implants (NIDCD, 2001). Technological advances will continue to improve our options for hearing-impaired older adults.

Smell and Taste

Smell and taste are two senses that are difficult to separate because they overlap, particularly, when food is involved. Both these senses are dependent on chemosensation, the ability of the nose, mouth, and throat to identify tastes and smells based on chemical reactions that occur when odors or tastes are present in the environment (American Academy of Otolaryngology-Head and Neck Surgery, 2001). The sense of smell and ability to identify odors decreases because of normal changes in aging. Up to 50% of octogenarians have smell disorders (Murphy et al., 2002). This can be problematic for safety reasons. An inability to smell smoke for instance could put an older adult at risk. Studies have also linked the loss of smell to Alzheimer's disease and Parkinson's disease (Mesholam, Moberg, Mahr, & Doty, 1998; Müller, Reichmann, Livermore, & Hummel, 2002). Taste problems are rare, ranging in those aged 65 years and older (0.72%) to those aged 85 years and older (1.7%; Hoffman et al., 2009).

CHANGES IN SMELL AND TASTE COMMON TO OLDER ADULTS

There are four medical terms used when describing olfactory disorders: (a) *hyposmia* is the reduction of the sense of smell; (b) *parosmia* is the distortion in the sense of smelling the presence of an odor; (c) *anosmia* is no sense of smell; and (d) *phantosmia* is the perception of an odor when no odor source is present (Albers et al., 2006). Olfactory disorders impact quality of life in older adults. Common complaints from people with olfactory disorders include difficulty with cooking, decreased appetite, eating spoiled food, too little perception of body odor, and inability to detect gas leaks or smoke (Albers et al., 2006; Murphy et al., 2002).

Because of the impact on quality of life, it is important to take a complete history and physical with older adults. A thorough cranial nerve exam and head and neck examination should be included. If an olfactory disorder is identified, the individual should be referred to an otorhinolaryngologist (ENT; Miwa et al., 2001).

Most changes in taste are thought to occur because of an oral condition, xerostomia (dry mouth), decreased sense of smell, medications, diseases, and tobacco use (Seiberling & Conley, 2004). Dysgeusias or taste disorders may resolve spontaneously. The taste sensory system has the capacity to recover function after being damaged (Hoffman et al., 2009). However, because of the poor outcomes for older adults with taste disorders, referral for treatment is indicated either to an otolaryngologist, neurologist, or a subspecialist at a smell and taste center (Bromley, 2000; Hoffman et al., 2009).

As with olfactory disorders, disorders of taste are often identified on history not by physical exam. There are very few tests to assess for taste disorders. Therefore, the history is essential. Substance abuse including tobacco, alcohol, and cocaine should be reviewed. The individual's dietary habits should be reviewed. Questions regarding recent dental work or procedures should also be asked. Ascertaining whether the individual has a history of gastric reflux could surface manageable conditions impacting taste. A thorough review of their medications is fundamental in the evaluation of a taste disorder (Bromley, 2000).

Diseases That Alter Taste Seen More Frequently as People Age

Burning Mouth Syndrome

This is a sensation that one's tongue is tingling or burning. There may be several contributing factors: vitamin B deficiencies, local trauma, gastrointestinal disorders causing reflux, allergies, salivary dysfunction, and diabetes.

Xerostomia

Dry mouth is common with many medications used to treat disorders common to older adults, including anticholinergic medications, antidepressants, antihistamines, angiotensin-converting enzyme (ACE)-inhibitors, lipid-lowering agents, antiparkinsonian medications, and anticonvulsants to name a few (Bromley, 2000; Seiberling & Conley, 2004).

Implications of Taste and Smell Changes

Inability to smell limits some of the pleasures of everyday life. The smell of a spring rain, smell of a Christmas tree, flowers, or coffee brewing may not be detectable. Taste is diminished because of inability to smell. Of significant concern in older adults who have smell and taste disorders is malnutrition. Appetite is detrimentally affected because of inability to smell and taste the food. Inability to smell is a safety hazard because of the inability to smell smoke in a fire or a gas leak. Decreased sense of taste may also result in inability to recognize spoiled food resulting in nausea, vomiting, or infectious diarrhea.

Peripheral Sensation

Two percent to 7% of all patients presenting with symptoms of neuropathy in a general medical practice will have peripheral neuropathy (Smith & Singleton, 2004). In older adults in the NHANES study older than the age of 70 years, 27% reported the loss of feeling in their feet, this grew to 34% in adults older than 80 years (Dillon et al., 2010). A prospective study evaluating older adults for peripheral sensory neuropathy found prevalence rates of 26% for those 65–74 years old and 54% for those 85 years and older (Mold, Vesely, Keyl, Schenk, & Roberts, 2004). Common disorders that increase the risk of peripheral neuropathy include diabetes, alcoholism, osteoporosis with compression fractures, peripheral vascular disease, infections, nutritional deficiencies particularly vitamins (e.g., thiamine and B_{12}), and malignancies (Mold et al., 2004). Because of the multitude of risk factors for peripheral neuropathy and neurology, consultation is recommended for complicated presentations of peripheral neuropathy to help tease out the best evaluation and management of the condition.

Changes in Peripheral Sensation Common to Older Adults

Conditions that alter peripheral sensation are seen more frequently as people age and include peripheral neuropathy, diabetic neuropathy, phantom limb pain, and acute sensory loss.

Peripheral Neuropathy. This is nerve pain in the distal extremities related to nerve damage from circulatory problems or vitamin deficiencies. Common vitamin deficiencies that impact peripheral nerves include thiamine and B_{12}.

Diabetic Neuropathy. This is end-organ damage to the peripheral nerves from microvascular changes that occur with diabetes. It often leads to loss of sensation in the feet of diabetics, contributing to undetected trauma to the extremities and subsequent refractory infections because of poor vascular supply to the extremity. It is extremely important to teach diabetics and patients with peripheral neuropathy to provide special care to their feet.

Phantom Limb Pain. This is the experience of pain that can range from dull ache to crushing pain where an amputated limb once was. The sensory cortex of the brain has influence in this mechanism. This pain is often chronic and requires special interventions to control and manage the pain, including electronic prosthetics, analgesics, and psychosocial support.

Acute Sensory Loss. Acute sensory loss may be caused by a stroke, acute nerve entrapment in the spine, or compartment syndrome because of trauma to a limb and presents with acute onset of numbness, tingling, or lack of sensation and function in the affected extremity.

Implications of Peripheral Sensation Changes

Inability to recognize position sense, pressure, or to ascertain where feet are on the floor can lead to falls, burns, lacerations, calluses, and pressure ulcers. Intact peripheral sensation is essential for keeping ourselves safe in our environment.

Nursing Assessment and Care Strategies of Peripheral Sensation

Nurses should take appropriate health histories to ascertain the presence of decreased sensation or pain in limbs. Physical exams should always include a thorough inspection and physical examination of the individual's legs and feet (Hellman, 2002). Diabetics and people known to have peripheral neuropathy should have thorough neurological exams including vibratory sense with a tuning fork over bony prominences and Semmes–Weinstein monofilament testing of the feet and proprioception (Boike & Hall, 2002).

Semmes–Weinstein Monofilament Test

This inexpensive simple procedure is used to screen for decreased sensation in several plantar sites on the foot. The monofilament is placed against the sole of the foot in eight different areas on the foot. The individual is asked to report any sensations (Boike & Hall, 2002). The Semmes–Weinstein nylon monofilament 5.04 gauge buckles at a pressure of 10 g. Loss of sensation at this level of pressure indicates a risk for ulcer development. Identification of this risk is important for improving the vigilance of foot care (Armstrong & Lavery, 1998).

Vibratory Sense

This is assessed by using a 128-Hz vibrating tuning fork on a lower extremity bony prominence and asking the individual if they feel any vibration (Boike & Hall, 2002). Older adults should be able to feel the vibration.

Proprioception

This is the ability for an individual to determine where they are in space. To assess for deficits in proprioception in the feet that may set the older adult up for falls and local trauma, have the individual close his or her eyes then hold the large toe on the sides and move the foot up or down and ask the individual to identify which direction the toe was moved. Inability to correctly identify the direction is an indication of decreased proprioception.

Individualized Sensory Enhancement of the Elderly

The Individualized Sensory Enhancement of the Elderly (I-SEE) program was developed to tailor nursing interventions to the type and level of sensory impairment experienced by the older adult (Wilensky & Hawkins, 2001). Originally developed to address hearing and visually impaired older adults, the I-SEE can logically be extended to address sensory impairment in smell, taste, and peripheral sensation. There are three levels to the I-SEE program: nursing assessments, nursing actions, and nursing referrals.

NURSING SENSORY ASSESSMENTS

History

- Ask questions about changes in hearing, vision, sense of smell, and taste as well as any numbness and tingling in extremities.
- Review medications that may be exacerbating the sensory problem, such as anticholinergic medications, antibiotics, aminoglycosides, and high-dose aspirin.

- Determine if symptoms occurred suddenly or gradually.
- Clarify if symptoms are unilateral or bilateral.
- Inquire whether the individual has had any prior treatment for sensory conditions.
- Ascertain if sensory conditions interfere with daily function.
- Ask about ability to drive, both daytime and nighttime driving can be impacted by visual impairment as well as hearing and the peripheral nervous system.
- Determine interest in receiving treatment for these conditions.

For each positive symptom reported, gather more information by asking about the Character, Associated symptoms, Radiation, Location, Intensity, and Duration, as well as what makes it Better, what Medications the individual has tried for these symptoms, and what makes it Worse. These questions can be easily remembered by using the acronym CAR LID BMW. These questions provide a better understanding of the individual's concerns.

Physical Exam for All Systems

- Inspect the external structures of the eyes and ears; examine ear canal for cerumen using otoscope.
- Check visual acuity with a near vision screener and distance acuity measure and contrast sensitivity.
- Perform whisper test to assess rough hearing. If available in your setting, use a handheld audioscope to assess up to 40-dB hearing. If a greater range of hearing testing is needed, use a portable audiometer with noise reduction earphones—a referral to audiology may be indicated.
- Assess the nares, determine if they are patent using the otoscope.
- Inspect the mouth and tongue for any obvious lesions or deviations from normal.
- Perform a neurosensory exam of the extremities including a monofilament test.
- Complete a monofilament test on all diabetics. This test quantifies the level of sensory impairment in the feet of patients with diabetes.
- Assess vibratory sense of the extremities with a 128-Hz tuning fork and proprioception.

Nursing Actions and Referrals

Vision

- Avoid disruption in the management of chronic eye conditions by obtaining past history and assuring continuation of ongoing regimens such as eye drops for glaucoma.
- Notify the primary care provider of any acute change in vision.
- Encourage the use of good lighting in patient rooms. Avoid glare whenever possible.
- Encourage the use of the patient's eyeglasses. Have family provide lighted magnification if needed. (These are the large magnifiers with a light attached. Available for purchase on a sliding scale at low vision centers.)
- Add contrast to the fixtures and electronics in the room if light switches blend into the wall or faucets blend into the sink. Other low contrast items in the environment include remote controls, television sets, and radios.
- Encourage annual eye exams either with an optometrist or ophthalmologist.

- Schedule an annual dilated exam for patients with diabetes and hypertension by ophthalmologist.
- Written materials should be provided in 14–16 high contrasting fonts with generous white space to improve visual tracking.
- Encourage use of adaptive equipment.

Hearing

- Assess for cerumen impactions. Request cerumen softening drops followed by cerumen removal or ENT consultation.
- Get the person's attention and face them before speaking to assist the individual with lip reading, if female consider wearing red lipstick to increase the contrast of your lips, a common compensatory mechanism for older adults.
- Have at least one pocket amplifier on the nursing unit to use with hard of hearing individuals.
- Do not shout at people with hearing impairments, but rather use lower tones of your voice.
- Provide written instructions (use large black marker if person is also visually impaired).
- Assure appropriate care for hearing aids: remove batteries out at night; use brush provided to gently clean the tubes to reduce wax accumulation. Before sending bed linens or clothing to the laundry, determine if the patient has hearing aid in his or her ear or in their designated location (bedside table or medication cart).
- Notify the primary care provider of any sudden change in hearing.
- Referral to audiologist and/or ENT as indicated (i.e., complicated cerumen impactions, new onset tinnitus, or vertigo).
- Encourage use of adaptive equipment.

Taste and Smell

- Take all complaints of inability or decreased ability to smell or taste seriously. Do not pass them off to medications or poor dentition.
- Notify primary care provider of an abrupt change in taste or smell.
- ENT referral for evaluation for change in smell or taste.
- Patient teaching should focus on safety issues with odors of gas and spoiled food.
- Educate seniors to have smoke and carbon monoxide detectors in their home and to date all food at time refrigerator, evaluate food with other methods other than sense of smell and taste.

Peripheral Sensation

- The individual should be taught to examine his or her feet daily, as well as look inside his or her shoes daily prior to putting them on each day.
- The individual should be taught to always wear shoes or protective slippers when he or she is ambulating to avoid unintentional injury to his or her feet.
- The individual should be instructed to inform his or her primary provider of any lesions, calluses, or red areas.
- Extremities should be kept clean and thoroughly dry prior to applying lotion.
- Encourage the individual to bring in footwear for evaluation by the advanced practice nurse if he or she has concerns about the safety. Most medical supply

companies carry diabetic healing shoes that have wide toe boxes and Velcro straps that can be purchased for less than $50.

■ Refer diabetics to facilities with certified diabetes educator and foot care specialist.

■ Implement fall precautions and initiate referral to physical therapy for all diabetics with peripheral neuropathy.

■ Refer all older adults with decreased sensation or circulation to a podiatrist of foot care specialist for ongoing foot care.

■ Encourage a diet rich in thiamine and B_{12}.

Expected Outcomes

■ Baseline visual acuity and hearing acuity for all older patients will be performed prior to discharge from the hospital, and on admission to home care or nursing home.

■ Fall precautions should be in place for all older patients with sensory impairments. Older adults should avoid falls and injuries to extremities if they have decreased sensation of lower extremities.

■ Accidental exposure to toxins either in the air or in food because of decreased sense of smell or taste should be avoided.

Follow-up Monitoring

■ Annual vision assessment—Medicaid in most states will pay for a new pair of eyeglasses every 2 years.

■ When vision is worse than 20/125, individuals should be referred to a low vision specialist to provide training in the use of visual assistive devices.

■ Given that hearing can change significantly over time, an audiological evaluation for hearing impaired older adults every 2 years is important. Some states will pay through Medicaid for one hearing aid under limited conditions. Hearing aids have been shown to be better accepted if older adults receive them when they start having difficulty with word finding with background noise. Encouragement and hearing rehabilitation is needed to improve the consistent use of hearing aid. Audiologists can help train older adults and their families in the use of hearing aids that may be necessary.

■ When abrupt changes in smell or taste are reported, a referral to a dentist or ENT is indicated.

■ Long-term adjustments must be made in the home when smell and taste are affected. First, food should be dated and discarded after 48 hours to avoid accidentally eating spoiled food. Smoke and carbon monoxide detectors must be present.

■ When xerostomia (severe dry mouth) is found, a referral to a dentist is indicated.

■ Older adults with decreased peripheral sensation should be followed regularly by a podiatrist or foot care specialist.

Interprofessional Care of Sensory Changes

Care of the aging senses is an interdisciplinary endeavor. Nurses who frequently have the most contact with clients can take the lead in assessing and screening older adults for decreased sensory function. Once these deficits are identified, it is important to take the appropriate steps and identify the resources available to the older adult. Occupational therapists, low vision specialists, audiologists, nutritionists, otolaryngologists, and neurologists are just some of the interprofessionals who may be part of the team caring for the sensory-impaired older adult. Good communication among disciplines is essential to assist the older adult benefit from each specialist.

CASE STUDY

MR. SWEETS

Mr. Sweets is a 75-year-old African American male living by himself in the community. He lives in a senior apartment building where he receives housekeeping services and can participate in a meal plan if he would like. He arrives on the Acute Care of the Elderly (ACE) Unit in your hospital with a diagnosis of hyperglycemia and a urinary tract infection. He also has a history of hypertension, hyperlipidemia, and osteoarthritis of the left hip. He is widowed and has three children: two live in the area, the other lives out of state. He is a retired aeronautical engineer. His medications include Amaryl 6 mg that was recently increased from 4 mg; Zocor, 40 mg p.o. daily; lisinopril, 20 mg daily; hydrochlorothiazide (HCTZ), 25 mg daily; and Tylenol ES, 1,000 mg three times a day for his hip discomfort.

Upon your admission assessment, you discover that he remembers receiving verbal instructions to cut his diabetic pills in half. Thus, since that appointment, he has only been taking 2 mg of Amaryl instead of 6 mg. His primary care provider had instructed him to take one and one half tablets of his Amaryl not just one half tablet. You were not sure if it was just a misunderstanding or if Mr. Sweets was having difficulty hearing. You are also concerned that his vision may be a problem as well because of his 5-year history of known diabetes.

After you complete taking your history, you gather your supplies to complete your physical exam. Your supplies include an audioscope, Lighthouse for the Blind Near Vision Screener, three plastic bags—one full of coffee, baby powder, and peppermint candies—128-Hz tuning fork, and a Semmes–Weinstein monofilament test. The audioscope reveals that Mr. Sweets' ear canals are completely occluded with cerumen and he can only hear the test tone that is delivered at the 60-dB level. On the near vision screener, he scored 20/125 in both eyes with his dirty glasses. Unfortunately, because his blood sugar is and has been elevated, it is unclear how much of the decreased vision is caused by his elevated blood sugar and how much is related to possible refractive error or diabetic retinopathy. Mr. Sweets was able to correctly identify each scent in the plastic bags. When you examine his feet, you identify that he has significant sensation loss on the bottom of his feet. He has intact vibratory sense in the ankle but his vibratory sense is decreased in both toes. His feet are currently free of any calluses, deformities, or open wounds. He does have some thickened toe nails.

These assessments impact the care plan for Mr. Sweets. His sensory deficits most likely precipitated his hospital admission. Written instructions may have helped prevent this, but his near vision may have interfered with the understanding of the written directions as well. He should have written instructions in large font, ideally because

(continued)

CASE STUDY *(continued)*

of his vision in 24-point font. Because of bilateral cerumen impactions, he will need cerumen softening drops started and the cerumen removed with a cerumen spoon after a few days. If this is not successful, he may need to be seen by an otolaryngologist (ENT) to have the cerumen removed. If his hearing is still impaired after the cerumen is removed, Mr. Sweets should see an audiologist.

If his vision does not improve with blood sugar control, he should be seen by an ophthalmologist to determine if any treatments for his diabetic retinopathy are necessary. He should also see an ophthalmologist if he has not been to one in a year. He would qualify for low vision services if his acuity remained at 20/125. He would also benefit from increased contrast. Older adults with diabetic retinopathy often need enhanced contrast. This can be achieved by adding red or white to light fixtures, remote controls, and other electrical devices that are usually solid colors with limited contrast. A low vision specialist could be very helpful here to make his home environment more safe and user friendly.

Mr. Sweets should be evaluated by a diabetic foot nurse and a podiatrist to have his nails trimmed and to learn more about foot care. He will need to learn how to complete daily foot inspections as well as assistance learning of what type of foot wear is appropriate for his feet. His hip may cause him some difficulty reaching his feet. It will be important for him to use mirrors and palpation to assist him in his self-care. A diabetic nurse educator can assist him with further information on the management of the disease and empower him to ask more questions and clarify when information does not appear compatible with what his symptoms are.

Mr. Sweets was discharged from the hospital after 4 days. His Amaryl was increased to 6 mg; he is afebrile and discharged on oral antibiotics for his urinary tract infection. He had his ears cleaned out over those 4 days so his hearing has improved to where he can hear at the 40-dB level. He has an appointment to see the audiologist. An appointment was also made for ophthalmology. Follow-up appointments have also been made with endocrine, with the diabetic nurse educator and diabetic foot nurse on the same visit. These appointments were written out on a 4- 3 6-in, index card with a black marker that he could read with his glasses.

Sensory impairment is an interprofessional health care problem. Good communication between disciplines is essential in maintaining Mr. Sweets' functional status and ability to stay in the community. Nurses are best prepared to help Mr. Sweets navigate and coordinate visits to the other disciplines. Screening completed by nurses either in the community, acute care, or long-term care settings can identify problems that have often been passed off by the older adult as they are just getting older.

RESOURCES

Related Professional Organizations and Informational Sites

Administration on Aging
http://www.aoa.gov

American Speech-Language-Hearing Association
http://www.asha.org

Assisted Listening Devices: Summary of available assisted listening devices
http://www.asha.org/public/hearing/treatment/assist_tech.htm

Cochlear Implants
General information including video on cochlear implants.
http://www.fda.gov/cdrh/cochlear

Hear Now
Will accept donated hearing aids to refit for the underserved.
http://www.starkeyhearingfoundation.org/hear-now.php

The Lighthouse for the Blind
Consumer and health professional information on visual impairment and dual impairment. Will
    accept donated hearing aids to refit for the underserved.
http://www.lighthouse.org

Lighting Research Center
Consumer, Builders, and Health Professional information on lighting.
http://www.lrc.rpi.edu/programs/lightHealth/AARP/index.asp

The National Eye Institute
Contains health information for consumers and health professionals. Also have images of eye diseases
    and eye charts.
http://www.nei.nih.gov

National Institute on Aging Information Center
http://www.nia.nih.gov

National Institute on Deafness and Other Communication Disorders
Contains information for health care providers and consumers.
http://www.nidcd.nih.gov

Talking Tapes
Access to talking books for visually impaired older adult.
http://www.talkingtapes.org

For Patients and Families

Aging in the Know
Your gateway to health and aging resources on the web. Created by the American Geriatrics Society
    Foundation for Health in Aging (FHA).
http://www.healthinaging.org/agingintheknow/

League for Hard of Hearing
http://www.lhh.org/

Prentiss Care Networks Project
Care networks for formal and informal caregivers of older adults.
http://caregiving.case.edu

REFERENCES

Adams-Wendling, L., Pimple, C., Adams, S., & Titler, M. G. (2008). Nursing management of hear-
    ing impairment in nursing facility residents. *Journal of Gerontological Nursing, 34*(11), 9–17.
    Evidence Level V.
Agency for Healthcare Research and Quality. (2004). *Technology assessment: Vision rehabilitation for
    elderly individuals with low vision and blindness.* Rockville, MD: Author. Evidence Level VI.

Ahmad, N., & Seidman, M. (2004). Tinnitus in the older adult: Epidemiology, pathophysiology and treatment options. *Drugs & Aging, 21*(5), 297–305. Evidence Level VI.

Albers, M. W., Tabert, M. H., & Devanand, D. P. (2006). Olfactory dysfunction as a predictor of neuro-degenerative disease. *Current Neurology and Neuroscience Reports, 6*(5), 379–386. Evidence Level I.

American Academy of Otolaryngology-Head and Neck Surgery. (2001). *Smell and taste*. Retrieved from http://www.entnet.org/HealthInformation/smellTaste.cfm. Evidence Level VI.

Armstrong, D. G., & Lavery, L. A. (1998). Diabetic foot ulcers: Prevention, diagnosis and classification. *American Family Physician, 57*(6), 1325–1332, 1337–1338. Evidence Level VI.

Bagai, A., Thavendiranathan, P., & Detsky, A. S. (2006). Does this patient have hearing impairment? *Journal of the American Medical Association, 295*(4), 416–428. Evidence Level I.

Baker, R. S. (2003). Diabetic retinopathy in African Americans: Vision impairment, prevalence, incidence, and risk factors. *International Ophthalmology Clinics, 43*(4), 105–122. Evidence Level I.

Boike, A. M., & Hall, J. O. (2002). A practical guide for examining and treating the diabetic foot. *Cleveland Clinic Journal of Medicine, 69*(4), 342–348. Evidence Level VI.

Bond, M., Mealing, S., Anderson, R., Elston, J., Weiner, G., Taylor, R. S., . . . Stein, K. (2009). The effectiveness and cost-effectiveness of cochlear implants for severe to profound deafness in children and adults: A systematic review and economic model. *Health Technology Assessment, 13*(44), 1–330. Evidence Level I.

Bromley, S. M. (2000). Smell and taste disorders: A primary care approach. *American Family Physician, 61*(2), 427–436, 438. Evidence Level VI.

Bron, A. J., & Caird, F. I. (1997). Loss of vision in the ageing eye. Research into Ageing Workshop, London, 10 May 1995. *Age and Ageing, 26*(2), 159–162. Evidence Level VI.

Cacchione, P. Z. (2007). Nursing care of older adults with age-related vision loss. In S. Crocker-Houde (Ed.), *Vision loss in older adults: Nursing assessment and care management* (pp. 131–148). New York, NY: Springer Publishing. Evidence Level VI.

Cacchione, P. Z., Culp, K., Dyck, M. J., & Laing, J. (2003). Risk for acute confusion in sensory-impaired, rural, long-term-care elders. *Clinical Nursing Research, 12*(4), 340–355. Evidence Level III.

Cassin, B., & Rubin, M. L. (2001). *Dictionary of eye terminology* (4th ed.). Gainesville, FL: Triad Publishing. Retrieved from http://www.eyeglossary.net. Evidence Level IV.

Chao, T. K., & Chen, T. H. (2009). Predictive model for progression of hearing loss: Meta-analysis of multi-state outcome. *Journal of Evaluation in Clinical Practice, 15*(1), 32–40. Evidence Level I.

Chou, R., Dana, T., & Bougatsos, C. (2009). Screening older adults for impaired visual acuity: A review of the evidence for the U.S. Preventive Services Task Force. *Annals of Internal Medicine, 151*(1), 44–58. Evidence Level I.

Community Services for the Blind and Partially Sighted. (2004). *Enhancing low vision: Lighting*. Retrieved from http://www.independentliving.org/donet/217_community_services_for_the_blind_and_partially_sighted.html. Evidence Level VI.

Congdon, N., O'Colmain, B., Klaver, C. C., Klein, R., Muñoz, B., Friedman, D. S., . . . Eye Diseases Prevalence Research Group. (2004). Causes and prevalence of visual impairment among adults in the United States. *Archives of Ophthalmology, 122*(4), 477–485. Evidence Level I.

Crummer, R. W., & Hassan, G. A. (2004). Diagnostic approach to tinnitus. *American Family Physician, 69*(1), 120–126. Evidence Level V.

Demers, K. (2001). *Hearing screening. Try This: Best Practices in Nursing care for older adults*. Hartford Institute for Geriatric Nursing 12. Evidence Level V.

Dillon, C. F., Gu, Q., Hoffman, H. J., & Ko, C. W. (2010, April). *Vision, hearing, balance and sensory impairments in Americans aged 70 years and older: United States, 1999–2006* (NCHS Data Brief No. 31). Hyattsville, MD: National Center for Health Statistics. Evidence Level II.

Ferris, F. L., III, Kassoff, A., Bresnick, G. H., & Bailey, I. (1982). New visual acuity charts for clinical research. *American Journal of Ophthalmology, 94*(1), 91–96. Evidence Level III.

Francis, H. W., Chee, N., Yeagle, J., Cheng, A., & Niparko, J. K. (2002). Impact of cochlear implants on the functional health status of older adults. *Laryngoscope, 112*(8 Pt. 1), 1482–1488. Evidence Level III.

Frank, T., & Petersen, D. R. (1987). Accuracy of a 40 dB HL Audioscope and audiometer screening for adults. *Ear and Hearing, 8*(3), 180–183. Evidence Level II.

Fukunaga, A., Uematsu, H., & Sugimoto, K. (2005). Influences of aging on taste perception and oral somatic sensation. *The Journals of Gerontology. Series A, Biological Sciences and Medical Sciences, 60*(1), 109–113. Evidence Level II.

Gates, G. A., & Mills, J. H. (2005). Presbycusis. *Lancet, 366*(9491), 1111–1120. Evidence Level V.

Gianutsos, R., & Suchoff, I. B. (1997). Visual fields after brain injury: Management issues for the occupational therapist. In M. Scheiman (Ed.), *Understanding and managing vision deficits: A guide for occupational therapists* (pp. 333–358). Thorogare, NJ: SLACK. Evidence Level VI.

Gillmore, G. (2002). *Modules 12: Visual field testing. Glaucoma I, Continuing education module.* Retrieved from http://www.eyetec.net/group3/M12Start.htm. Evidence Level VI.

Hellman, C. (2002). Nurse practitioner management of the patient with diabetic foot ulcers. *Clinical Excellence for Nurse Practitioners, 5*(5), 11–15. Evidence Level VI.

Hirvelä, H., & Laatikainen, L. (1995). Visual acuity in a population aged 70 years or older; prevalence and causes of visual impairment. *Acta Ophtalmologica Scandinavica, 73*(2), 99–104. Evidence Level III.

Hoffman, H. J., Cruickshanks, K. J., & Davis, B. (2009). Perspectives on population-based epidemiological studies of olfactory and taste impairment. *Annals of the New York Academy of Sciences, 1170*, 514–530. Evidence Level I.

Horton, J. C., & Jones, M. R. (1997). Warning on inaccurate Rosenbaum cards for testing near vision. *Survey of Ophthalmology, 42*(2), 169–174. Evidence Level VI.

Huang, Q., & Tang, J. (2010). Age-related hearing loss or presbycusis. *European Archives of Otorhinolaryngology, 267*(8), 1179–1191. Evidence Level I.

Johnson, C. E., Danhauer, J. L., Bennett, M., & Harrison, J. (2009). Systematic review of physicians' knowledge of, participation in, and attitudes toward hearing and balance screening in the elderly population. *Seminars in Hearing, 30*(3), 193–206. Evidence Level I.

Kalinowski, M. A. (2008). "Eye" dentifying vision impairment in the geriatric patient. *Geriatric Nursing, 29*(2), 125–132. Evidence Level V.

Kennedy, R. S., & Dunlap, W. P. (1990). Assessment of the Vistech contrast sensitivity test for repeated-measures applications. *Optometry and Vision Science, 67*(4), 248–251. Evidence Level II.

Lewis-Cullinan, C., & Janken, J. K. (1990). Effect of cerumen removal on the hearing ability of geriatric patients. *Journal of Advanced Nursing, 15*(5), 594–600. Evidence Level II.

Linton, A. D. (2007). Age-related changes in the special senses. In A. D. Linton & H. W. Lach (Eds.), *Matteson and McConnell's gerontological nursing, concepts and practice* (3rd ed., pp. 600–627). St. Louis, MO: Saunders Elsevier. Evidence Level V.

Lockwood, A. H., Salvi, R. J., & Burkard, R. F. (2002). Tinnitus. *New England Journal of Medicine, 347*(12), 904–910. Evidence Level V.

Mangione, C. M., Lee, P. P., Gutierrez, P. R., Spritzer, K., Berry, S., Hays, R. D., & National Eye Institute Visual Function Questionnaire Field Test Investigators. (2001). Development of the 25-item National Eye Institute Visual Function Questionnaire. *Archives of Ophthalmology, 119*(7), 1050–1058. Evidence Level II.

Mäntyjärvi, M., & Laitinen, T. (2001). Normal values for the Pelli-Robson contrast sensitivity test. *Journal of Cataract and Refractive Surgery, 27*(2), 261–266. Evidence Level III.

Marcincuk, M. C., & Roland, P. S. (2002). Geriatric hearing loss. Understanding the causes and providing appropriate treatment. *Geriatrics, 57*(4), 44, 48–50. Evidence Level VI.

Mehr, A. S. (2007). *Understanding your audiogram.* Retrieved from American Association of Audiology website: http://www.aurorahealthcare.org/yourhealth/healthgate/getcontent.asp?URLhealthgate=%22100920.html%22. Evidence Level IV.

Mesholam, R. I., Moberg, P. J., Mahr, R. N., & Doty, R. L. (1998). Olfaction in neurodegenerative disease: A meta-analysis of olfactory functioning in Alzheimer's and Parkinson's diseases. *Archives of Neurology, 55*(1), 84–90. Evidence Level I.

Miwa, T., Furukawa, M., Tsukatani, T., Costanzo, R. M., DiNardo, L. J., & Reiter, E. R. (2001). Impact of olfactory impairment on quality of life and disability. *Archives of Otolaryngology— Head & Neck Surgery, 127*(5), 497–503. Evidence Level II.

Mold, J. W., Vesely, S. K., Keyl, B. A., Schenk, J. B., & Roberts, M. (2004). The prevalence, predictors, and consequences of peripheral sensory neuropathy in older patients. *The Journal of the American Board of Family Practice, 17*(5), 309–318. Evidence Level II.

Morse, A. R., & Rosenthal, B. P. (1997). Vision and vision assessment. In J. A. Teresi, M. P. Lawton, D. Holmes, & M. Ory (Eds.), *Measurement in elderly chronic care populations* (pp. 45–60). New York, NY: Springer Publishing. Evidence Level VI.

Müller, A., Reichmann, H., Livermore, A., & Hummel, T. (2002). Olfactory function in idiopathic Parkinson's disease (IPD): Results from cross-sectional studies in IPD patients and long-term follow-up of de-novo IPD patients. *Journal of Neural Transmission, 109*(5–6), 805–811. Evidence Level II.

Murphy, C., Schubert, C. R., Cruickshanks, K. J., Klein, B. E., Klein, R., & Nondahl, D. M. (2002). Prevalence of olfactory impairment in older adults. *The Journal of the American Medical Association, 288*(18), 2307–2312. Evidence Level III.

National Eye Institute. (2004). *Age-related eye diseases study—results*. Retrieved from http://www.nei.nih.gov/amd/background.asp. Evidence Level VI.

National Eye Institute. (2004). *Statistics and data: Prevalence of blindness data*. Retrieved from http://www.nei.nih.gov/eyedata/pbd_tables.asp. Evidence Level VI.

National Eye Institute. (2009). *Diabetic retinopathy*. Retrieved from http://www.nei.nih.gov/health/. Evidence Level VI.

National Institute on Deafness and Other Communication Disorders. (2001). *Ménière's Disease*. Retrieved from http://www.nidcd.nih.gov/health/balance/meniere.asp. Evidence Level VI.

National Institute on Deafness and Other Communication Disorders. (2007). *Statistics about hearing, balance, ear infections, and deafness*. Retrieved from http://www.nidcd.nih.gov/health/statistics/hearing.asp. Evidence Level VI.

Norman, J. F., Norman, H. F., Craft, A. E., Walton, C. L., Bartholomew, A. N., Burton, C. L., . . . Crabtree, C. E. (2008). Stereopsis and aging. *Vision Research, 48*(23–24), 2456–2465. Evidence Level II.

Pekkonen, E., Jääskeläinen, I. P., Hietanen, M., Huotilainen, M., Näätänen, R., Ilmoniemi, R. J. & Erkinjuntti, T. (1999). Impaired preconscious auditory processing and cognitive functions in Alzheimer's disease. *Clinical Neurophysiology, 110*(11), 1942–1947. Evidence Level II.

Pelli, D. G., Robson, J. G., & Wilkins, A. J. (1988). The design of a new letter chart for measuring contrast sensitivity. *Clinical Vision Science, 2*(3), 187–199. Evidence Level III.

Read, J. C., Phillipson, G. P., Serrano-Pedraza, I., Milner, A. D., & Parker, A. J. (2010). Stereoscopic vision in the absence of lateral occipital cortex. *PLoS One, 5*(9), 1–14. Evidence Level I.

Revicki, D. A., Rentz, A. M., Harnam, N., Thomas, V. S., & Lanzetta, P. (2010). Reliability and validity of the National Eye Institute Visual Function Questionnaire-25 in patients with age-related macular degeneration. *Investigative Ophthalmology & Visual Science, 51*(2), 712–717. Evidence Level II.

Seiberling, K. A., & Conley, D. B. (2004). Aging and olfactory and taste function. *Otolaryngologic Clinics of North America, 37*(6), 1209–1228. Evidence Level V.

Seidel, H. M., Dains, J. E., Ball, J. W., & Benedict, G. W. (2003). *Mosby's guide to physical examination* (5th ed., pp. 278–312). St. Louis, MO: Mosby. Evidence Level VI.

Smith, A. G., & Singleton, J. R. (2004). The diagnostic yield of a standardized approach to idiopathic sensory-predominant neuropathy. *Archives of Internal Medicine, 164*(9), 1021–1025. Evidence Level III.

Tolson, D., Swan, I., & Knussen, C. (2002). Hearing disability: A source of distress for older people and carers. *British Journal of Nursing, 11*(15), 1021–1025. Evidence Level II.

U.S. Department of Health and Human Services. (2010). *Healthy People 2020*. Retrieved from http://www.healthypeople.gov/2020/topicsobjectives2020/default.aspx. Evidence Level VI.

Ventry, I. M., & Weinstein, B. E. (1983). Identification of elderly people with hearing problems. *American Speech and Hearing Association, 25*(7), 37–42. Evidence Level III.

Vitale, S., Cotch, M. F., & Sperduto, R. D. (2006). Prevalence of visual impairment in the United States. *Journal of the American Medical Association, 295*(18), 2158–2163. Evidence Level III.

Wallhagen, M. I., Pettengill, E., & Whiteside, M. (2006). Sensory impairment in older adults: Part 1. Hearing Loss. *The American Journal of Nursing, 106*(10), 40–48. Evidence Level VI.

Wallhagen, M. I., Strawbridge, W. J., Shema, S. J., & Kaplan, G. A. (2004). Impact of self-assessed hearing loss on a spouse: A longitudinal analysis of couples. *The Journals of Gerontology. Series B, Psychological Sciences and Social Sciences, 59*(3), S190–S196. Evidence Level III.

Warnat, B. M., & Tabloski, P. (2006). Sensation: Hearing, vision, taste, touch, and smell. In P. A. Tabloski (Ed.), *Gerontological nursing* (Vol. 1, pp. 384–420). Upper Saddle River, NJ: Pearson Education. Evidence Level VI.

Whiteside, M. M., Wallhagen, M. I., & Pettengill E. (2006). Sensory impairment in older adults: Part 2. Vision loss. *The American Journal of Nursing, 106*(11), 52–61. Evidence Level V.

Wilensky, J. T., & Hawkins, A. (2001). Comparison of contrast sensitivity, visual acuity, and Humphrey visual field testing in patients with glaucoma. *Transactions of the American Ophthalmological Society, 99*, 213–217. Evidence Level III.

Wilson, R. S., Arnold, S. E., Schneider, J. A., Tang, Y., & Bennett, D. A. (2007). The relationship between cerebral Alzheimer's disease pathology and odour identification in old age. *Journal of Neurology, Neurosurgery, and Psychiatry, 78*(1), 30–35. Evidence Level II.

Yueh, B., Collins, M. P., Souza, P. E., Heagerty, P. J., Liu, C. F., Boyko, E. J., . . . Hedrick, S. C. (2007). Screening for Auditory Impairment—Which Hearing Assessment Test (SAI-WHAT): RCT design and baseline characteristics. *Contemporary Clinical Trials, 28*(3), 303–315. Evidence Level II.

Yueh, B., Shapiro, N., MacLean, C. H., & Shekelle, P. G. (2003). Screening and management of adult hearing loss in primary care: Scientific review. *Journal of the American Medical Association, 289*(15), 1976–1985. Evidence Level I.

Yueh, B., & Shekelle, P. (2007). Quality indicators for the care of hearing loss in vulnerable elders. *Journal of the American Geriatrics Society, 55*(Suppl. 2), S335–S339. Evidence Level II.

Excessive Sleepiness

5

Eileen R. Chasens and Mary Grace Umlauf

EDUCATIONAL OBJECTIVES

On completion of this chapter, the reader should be able to:

1. identify the signs and symptoms of excessive sleepiness and quantify them using a standardized scale
2. describe the signs, symptoms, and usual treatments for the most primary sleep disorders causing excessive sleepiness in older adults: obstructive sleep apnea, restless leg syndrome, insomnia, and short sleep duration
3. discuss the implications of chronic illness, medications, and acute hospitalization on sleep
4. provide nursing care that incorporates sleep hygiene measures and provide consistent ongoing treatment for existing sleep disorders
5. educate patients and families about sleep disorders and sleep hygiene measures

OVERVIEW

Excessive sleepiness, sometimes called *excessive daytime sleepiness,* is common in older adults. Fatigue manifests as difficulty in sustaining a high level of physical performance; *excessive sleepiness* refers to the inability to maintain alertness or vigilance because of hypersomnolence. Many factors can affect nighttime sleep and result in daytime sleepiness in older adults. These include psychological disorders, symptoms of chronic illnesses (e.g., pain), medication side effects, environmental factors, and lifestyle preferences. Increases in sleepiness can result from age-related changes in chronobiology and sleep disorders. In older adults, the most common primary sleep disorders are obstructive sleep apnea (OSA), restless leg syndrome, and insomnia. The extent to which changes in sleep patterns experienced by older adults are caused by normal physiological alterations, pathological events, sleep disorders, or poor sleep hygiene remains unclear. Hospitalization and institutionalization can also interfere with sleep quality or quantity. There are many effective treatments for sleep disorders, but the first step is to identify the cause of excessive daytime

For description of Evidence Levels cited in this chapter, see Chapter 1, Developing and Evaluating Clinical Practice Guidelines: A Systematic Approach, page 7.

sleepiness and then to quantify and aggressively treat this condition in the older adult. This chapter outlines an overview of sleep disorders common in older adults, describes how to assess sleep, and provides interventions to improve sleep in older adults.

BACKGROUND AND STATEMENT OF PROBLEM

The Institute of Medicine (Colten & Altevogt, 2006) reports that 50–70 million Americans are affected by chronic disorders of sleep and wakefulness. Recent data from the Behavioral Risk Factor Surveillance System (BRFSS) conducted by the Centers for Disease Control and Prevention (CDC) found that among community dwelling persons older than age 65 years ($n = 23,167$), nearly a quarter (24.5%) reported sleeping, on average, less than 7 hours in a 24-hour period and more than half (50.5%) of these older adults reported snoring (CDC, 2011b). Data from the 2005–2008 National Health and Nutrition Examination Survey (NHANES) show that 32% of persons older than age 60 years ($n = 3,716$) slept less than 7 hours per night on weekdays or workdays (CDC, 2011a). Likewise, the Cardiovascular Health Study documented excessive sleepiness in 20% among subjects older than age 65 years ($n = 4,578$; Whitney et al., 1998). Further, some sleep disorders are more common in patients in acute and chronic care settings. Ancoli-Israel and colleagues (1991) and Ancoli-Israel, Kripke, and Mason (1987) studied only persons older than age 65 years and found undiagnosed sleep apnea in 24% of those living independently in the community, in 33% of those in acute care settings, and in 42% of older adults in nursing home settings.

CONSEQUENCES OF EXCESSIVE SLEEPINESS

The primary consequences of sleepiness are decreased alertness, delayed reaction time, and reduced cognitive performance (Ohayon & Vecchierini, 2002). The BRFSS found that nearly half (44%) of subjects in this telephone survey reported that they unintentionally fell asleep during the day at least once in the preceding month and that one out of 50 older adults had fallen asleep while driving in the preceding month (CDC, 2011a). The 2005–2008 NHANES data also show that older adults reported difficulty concentrating (18%) and remembering (14.7%) because of sleep-related problems (CDC, 2011a). Recent studies show that daytime sleepiness is significantly associated with declining cognitive function (Cohen-Zion et al., 2001), falls (Brassington, King, & Bliwise, 2000), and cardiovascular events (Whitney et al., 1998). In the Cardiovascular Health Study, daytime sleepiness was the only sleep symptom associated with mortality, incident cardiovascular disease morbidity and mortality, myocardial infarction, and congestive heart failure, particularly among women (Newman et al., 2000). This linkage between sleep and medical conditions is consistent with the 2005–2008 NHANES results that demonstrated a greater rate of sleep-related problems with concentration, memory, and activities of daily living among women (CDC, 2011a).

PHYSIOLOGICAL CHANGES IN SLEEP THAT ACCOMPANY AGING

Normal changes in sleep that occur as part of human development and lifestyle choices must be differentiated from pathological sleep conditions that are common among older adults. Although older adults require as much sleep as younger adults, older adults may divide their sleep between nighttime slumber and daytime naps, rather than a single consolidated period. The endogenous circadian pacemaker, located in the suprachiasmatic nucleus, along with exogenous environmental cues and a homeostatic need for sleep, mediate the normal wake and sleep pattern. With aging, the circadian pattern for sleep-wake decreases in amplitude, possibly in association with less robust changes in core body temperature (Richardson, Carskadon, Orav, & Dement, 1982). Compared with younger adults, healthy older adults have a more pronounced biphasic pattern of sleepiness during the afternoon hours (about 2–6 p.m.) and a phase advancement of nighttime sleepiness earlier in the evening (Roehrs, Turner, & Roth, 2000).

Changes in sleep architecture associated with normal aging include increased difficulty in falling asleep, poorer sleep quality with decreased sleep efficiency, more time awake after sleep onset, increased "light" sleep (Stages 1 and 2 sleep), and decreased quantity and amplitude of restorative "deep" slow-wave sleep (Stages 3 and 4). Although older women report more sleep disturbances than older men, studies indicate that their sleep is less disturbed than that of men (Rediehs, Reis, & Creason, 1990).

PRIMARY CAUSES OF EXCESSIVE DAYTIME SLEEPINESS

Obstructive Sleep Apnea

OSA is a condition in which intermittent pharyngeal obstruction causes cessation of respiratory airflow (apneas) or reductions of airflow (hypopneas) that lasts for at least 10 seconds. This results in a microarousal that restores upper airway patency, permitting breathing and airflow to resume. According to the American Academy of Sleep Medicine (AASM, 2005) Task Force, OSA is diagnosed when these events occur at a rate of greater than five per hour of sleep and is accompanied by daytime sleepiness and impaired daytime functioning. It is common for patients with severe symptoms to experience multiple arousals during the night. These multiple arousals severely fragment sleep, preventing the deep sleep (Stages 3 and 4) and rapid eye movement (REM) sleep necessary for healthy mental and physical functioning.

OSA is both an age-related and an age-dependent condition, with an overlap in both distributions in the 60- to 70-year-old age range (Bliwise, King, & Harris, 1994). Age-related risk factors for OSA in older adults include an increased prevalence of overweight and obesity. Conversely, age-dependent risk factors include increased collapsibility of the upper airway, decreased lung capacity, altered ventilatory control, decreased muscular endurance, and altered sleep architecture (Brassington et al., 2000).

Treatments for OSA depend on the contributing pathology and patient preference and include nocturnal positive airway pressure, surgical procedures designed to increase the posterior pharyngeal area, oral appliances, and weight reduction when obesity is a contributing factor. Nasal continuous positive airway pressure (CPAP) therapy, which is highly effective when individually titrated to eliminate apneas and hypopneas, is currently the gold standard for treating OSA (Morgenthaler et al., 2006). Older adults tolerate CPAP therapy, with patterns of compliance similar to that of middle-aged adults (Weaver & Chasens, 2007). Although oral appliances offer a low-tech treatment option, they require a stable dentition that may be problematic for persons with extensive tooth loss or dentures.

Insomnia

Insomnia can be defined as delayed sleep onset, difficulty in maintaining sleep, premature waking, and/or very early arousals that result in insufficient sleep (Ancoli-Israel & Martin, 2006). Insomnia can be transient or chronic, and the perception of sleep loss may not correspond to objective assessment. The frequent awakenings suggestive of insomnia may be a conditioned arousal response because of environmental (e.g., noise or extremes of temperature) or behavioral cues. Anxiety associated with emotional conflict, stress, recent loss, feeling insecure at night, or significant changes in living arrangements can also produce insomnia (Ancoli-Israel & Martin, 2006). Chronic insomnia can result in a conditioned response of anxiety and arousal at bedtime in anticipation of difficulty falling asleep; this may prompt use of hypnotic medications, over-the-counter (OTC) drugs, or alcohol. Although the use of hypnotics may produce short-term relief, they also affect sleep architecture and consequently lead to deterioration of sleep quality. The cycle of dependency and substance abuse is a potential problem in this age group (see Chapter 17, Reducing Adverse Drug Events). At this time, the general recommendation is, when hypnotics are indicated, the most short-acting drug should be selected and, optimally, used in conjunction with an appropriate behavioral intervention (Ancoli-Israel, 2000).

Both the cause and duration of insomnia should inform the choice of treatment. For example, insomnia associated with a psychological origin, such as depression or anxiety, is best treated from that perspective. If pain is affecting sleep, pain management should be addressed first and strategies to promote sleep onset should be added secondarily. Short-term pharmacotherapy may be appropriate if insomnia is situational and of recent onset. When insomnia has been "learned" and the behavior becomes chronic, behavioral interventions are most appropriate. Behavioral treatments for insomnia include stimulus control, progressive muscle relaxation, paradoxical intention, sleep restriction, biofeedback, and multifaceted cognitive behavior therapy (Morin et al., 1999). Data show that 70%–80% of patients benefit from behavioral therapies and that improvement in sleep are often sustained for a minimum of 6 months after treatment.

Restless Legs Syndrome

Restless legs syndrome (RLS) is a neurological condition that is characterized by the irresistible urge to move the legs. It is usually associated with disagreeable leg sensations that become worse during inactivity and often interferes with initiating and maintaining sleep. As a secondary condition, this movement disorder can be caused by iron deficiency anemia, uremia, neurological lesions, diabetes, Parkinson's disease, rheumatoid arthritis, or it can be a side effect of certain drugs (e.g., tricyclic antidepressants, serotonin reuptake inhibitors, lithium, dopamine blockers, xanthines). Periodic leg movement disorder (PLMD) is a similar condition also known as *nocturnal myoclonus*. However, PLMD is characterized by involuntary flexion of the leg and foot that produces microarousals or full arousals from sleep that interfere with achieving and maintaining restorative slow-wave sleep (Stages 3 and 4). Although the etiology and associated mechanism of this specific movement disorder are not well defined, this condition has been linked to metabolic, vascular, and neurologic causes. Dopaminergic drugs are the most effective agents for treating RLS and PLMD as well as opioids, benzodiazepines, anticonvulsants, adrenergics, and iron supplements. However, their efficacy for long-term treatment in older adults has not been sufficiently evaluated (Ancoli-Israel & Martin, 2006; Gamaldo & Earley, 2006).

SECONDARY CAUSES OF EXCESSIVE DAYTIME SLEEPINESS

Medical and psychiatric illness can interfere with sleep quality and disturb sleep. For example, depression or anxiety appears to have a bidirectional relationship with insomnia (Buysse, 2004). Painful chronic conditions, such as arthritis, reduce sleep efficiency, or simply changing body position, may be painful enough to cause awakenings. Because older adults frequently have multiple medical conditions, they are also more likely to take OTC and prescription medications for symptom relief. However, many medications and nonprescription drugs (e.g., pseudoephedrine, alcohol, caffeine, and nicotine) interfere with sleep. Thus, health care providers must be acutely aware of which OTC medications and beverages can cause sleep problems. Symptom management must be balanced against preventing polypharmacy in older adults to maintain sleep quality (Ancoli-Israel, 2005).

Sleep Disturbance During Hospitalization

Studies have shown that as many as 22%–61% of hospitalized patients experience impaired sleep (Redeker, 2000). Many older adults have primary sleep disorders (OSA, insomnia, restless leg syndrome) and these conditions can become more pronounced or acute during acute illness and hospitalization. Sleep disorders may go unrecognized in acute care settings, thus patients may experience acute sleep deprivation concurrently with a medical crisis or surgical intervention.

Protecting sleep and monitoring sleep quality should be routine elements of care in hospital settings (Young, Bourgeois, Hilty, & Hardin, 2008). There are three common causes for sleep disruption in hospitals that are often overlooked by nursing staff: noise, light, and patient-care activities (Redeker, 2000). Further, anesthesia, cardiopulmonary disorders, and pain medications can reduce the respiratory drive and lead to hypopnea and apnea. Medications typically administered postoperatively can affect alertness by causing excessive sedation, changes in sleep architecture, decreased REM sleep, nightmares, or insomnia. Pain and anxiety may also cause older patients to have insomnia. Inadequate sleep impedes healing and recovery and may be associated with acute mental confusion in older adults (Young, Bourgeois, Hilty, & Hardin, 2009). In summary, older adults in acute care settings are exposed to many conditions that can negatively affect sleep and result in excessive daytime sleepiness.

The sleep environment and the quality of patients' sleep can be improved in hospital settings if caregivers recognize the essential importance of sleep in illness and health. As a standard practice, nurses should include a thorough sleep history (Table 5.1) during admission to determine usual sleep patterns and/or symptoms of sleep disorders. Patients with OSA who use CPAP at home should be instructed to bring their machines with them to the hospital. Sleep hygiene measures should be incorporated into nursing care routines during evening and night hours and also incorporated into care plans on every nursing unit. This includes simple practices such as reducing light intensity, maintaining a quiet environment, and efficient delivery of patient care to minimize sleep disruption among patients. Anticipatory and preventive pain management is also an important element of care to promote adequate sleep in the hospital setting (Young et al., 2009).

ASSESSMENT OF THE PROBLEM

There are several valid and reliable measures to screen for sleepiness. One of the most commonly used instruments is the Epworth Sleepiness Scale (ESS; Johns, 1991). Although OSA can only be diagnosed with a sleep study, the risk of OSA can be determined using

TABLE 5.1

Sleep History

Basic Sleep History Questions	Follow-Up Questions	Sleep Disorders to Consider
■ Do you have any difficulty falling asleep? ■ Are you having any difficulty sleeping until morning? ■ Are you having difficulty sleeping throughout the night? ■ Have you or anyone else ever noticed that you snore loudly or stop breathing in your sleep? ■ Do you find yourself falling asleep during the day when you do not want to?	■ What time do you usually go to bed? ■ Fall asleep? ■ What prevents you from falling asleep? ■ Review intake of alcohol, nicotine, caffeine, all medications. ■ Review of depressive symptoms: weight loss, sadness, or recent losses. ■ How often do you waken? ■ How long are you awake? ■ Do you have any pain, discomfort, or shortness of breath during the night? ■ What prevents you from falling back to sleep? ■ Are you sleepy or tired during the day? ■ Review risk factors (e.g., obesity, arthritis, poorly controlled illnesses). ■ Do your legs kick or jump around while you sleep? ■ Do you stay outdoors in natural daylight on most days?	■ Shift work/sleep schedule disorders ■ Psychophysiologic insomnia ■ Restless leg syndrome ■ Psychiatric disorders ■ Substance/medications related disorders ■ Depression ■ Insomnia ■ Medical causes of sleep disturbance ■ Obstructive sleep apnea ■ Obstructive sleep apnea ■ Functional impairment resulting from sleep disorder ■ Periodic leg movement disorders

Note. Adapted from Avidan, A. Y. (2005). Sleep in the geriatric patient population. *Seminars in Neurology, 25*(1), 52–63. Evidence Level I. Bloom, H. G., Ahmed, I., Alessi, C. A., Ancoli-Israel, S., Buysse, D. J., Kryger, M. H., . . . Zee, P. C. (2009). Evidence-based recommendations for the assessment and management of sleep disorders in older persons. *Journal of the American Geriatrics Society, 57*(5), 761–789. Evidence Level I.

the Multivariable Apnea Prediction Index (Maislin et al., 1995), the Berlin Questionnaire (Netzer, Stoohs, Netzer, Clark, & Strohl, 1999), or the STOP-Bang Questionnaire (Chung et al., 2008). The STOP-Bang questionnaire (Table 5.2), first developed to screen for OSA in persons scheduled for anesthesia, consists of eight questions and has sensitivity from 76% to 96%. The Functional Outcomes of Sleep Questionnaire (Weaver et al., 1997b) is used to evaluate the impact of sleepiness on functional status; the Pittsburgh Sleep Quality Index (PSQI) (Buysse, Reynolds, Monk, Berman, & Kupfer, 1989) quantifies sleep quality over the past month (see Sleep topic at http://www.hartfordign.org). Many sleep clinicians use the ESS to screen for sleepiness and track symptoms over the previous week during common activities such as sitting and reading, watching TV, or riding in a car. It is easy to administer and includes a scoring parameter to indicate the need for a medical evaluation. A brief sleep history can be obtained by using the questionnaire in Table 5.1. In a sleep laboratory setting, a completed evaluation of sleep is conducted using polysomnography that includes electroencephalography (EEG), electromyogram (EMG), electro-oculogram (EOG), respiratory effort,

---

TABLE 5.2

STOP-Bang (OSA Risk Questionnaire)

1. Snoring
   Do you snore loudly (louder than talking or loud enough to be heard through closed doors)? Yes or No
2. Tired
   Do you often feel tired, fatigued, or sleepy during daytime? Yes or No
3. Observed
   Has anyone observed you stop breathing during your sleep? Yes or No
4. Blood pressure
   Do you have or are you being treated for high blood pressure? Yes or No
5. BMI
   BMI more than 35 kg/m^2? Yes or No
6. Age
   Age over 50 years old? Yes or No
7. Neck circumference
   Neck circumference greater than 40 cm? Yes or No
8. Gender
   Gender male? Yes or No

Scoring
High risk of OSA: answering yes to three or more items
Low risk of OSA: answering yes to less than three items

Note. OSA = obstructive sleep apnea. Adapted from Chung, F., Yegneswaran, B., Liao, P., Chung, S. A., Vairavanathan, S., Islam, S., . . . Shapiro, C. M. (2008). STOP questionnaire: A tool to screen patients for obstructive sleep apnea. *Anesthesiology*, *108*(5), 812–821.

---

oxygen saturation, and electrophysiological cardiac aspects of sleep. Additional electrophysiological tests, such as the Multiple Sleep Latency Test, are also used to quantify daytime sleepiness. Most important in the assessment of sleepiness is an evaluation of the patient's knowledge and application of sleep hygiene measures (Table 5.3) that are also effective behavioral strategies to maximize, promote, and protect sleep.

TABLE 5.3

Sleep Hygiene Measures

- Use the bed only for sleeping or sex.
- Develop consistent and rest-promoting bedtime routines.
- Maintain the same bedtime and waking time every day.
- Exposure to bright sunlight is desirable upon awakening.
- Upon awakening, get out of bed slowly, no matter what time it is to prevent postural hypotension.
- If awakened during the night, avoid looking at the clock; frequent time checks may heighten anxiety and hinder sleep onset.
- Avoid naps if they negatively affect nighttime sleep. Limit naps to 15–30 minutes' duration.
- Sleep in a cool, quiet environment.
- If you cannot fall asleep after 15 or 20 minutes in bed, get up and go into another room, read, or do a quiet activity, using dim lighting, until you are sleepy again.
- Before bedtime, avoid the following:
  - caffeine and nicotine after noon
  - alcohol intake (more than three drinks)
  - large meals or exercise 3–4 hours before bedtime
  - emotional upset or emotionally charged activities including television programs that are troubling

INTERVENTIONS AND CARE STRATEGIES

The first line of defense against excessive sleepiness is a lifestyle that promotes and ensures adequate sleep and rest. Although humans have a natural drive to sleep, environment and habituation play an important behavioral role in sleep. Sleep hygiene, those practices that permit and promote sleep onset and sleep maintenance, has many aspects and requires regular reinforcement. Regardless of health status, sleep hygiene practices and routines are as important for older adults as they are for children, adolescents, and other adults.

CASE STUDY

Scenario

Mrs. M. complained to her friends that she sleeps poorly because her husband snores "loud enough to wake the dead" and "he even stops breathing on and off all night." She relates that they "don't have sex very often," he had difficulty with "doing it." In addition, they are both too tired to be "in the mood" so she has started sleeping in the guest room. Her friends have urged her to talk to their primary care physician about his symptoms and her concerns.

History

Mr. M. is a 62-year-old man who is obese (height, 6′2″; weight, 260 lbs; body mass index [BMI], 33.4). He is hypertensive (sitting blood pressure, 154/98 mm Hg) and takes several medications to control his blood pressure (i.e., amlodipine, digoxin, hydrochlorothiazide, lisinopril, pravastatin, enteric-coated aspirin). He was diagnosed with Type II diabetes almost 10 years ago (HbA1c, 8.2%) and is on metformin 1,000 mg BID and glimepiride 2 mg daily. He has a history of snoring (more than 20 years) and was a smoker until 12 years ago.

Symptoms

Mr. M. says, "I have no energy. I can sleep anytime and anywhere, but I am tired all the time. I went to the Diabetic Educator and learned what I need to do with exercise and diet. Usually, I am so tired I just grab some fast food on the way home and then do nothing when I get home." He reports that he wakes unrefreshed, has morning headaches, and that his sleep is disturbed by nocturia four times per night. He reports that he has heartburn at night and his legs jerk during sleep. He has difficulty driving any distance on the highway because of extreme sleepiness, and cannot attend church or movies without falling asleep. Although he takes frequent naps, he consumes more than six cups of coffee per day. Mr. M. has one or two alcoholic beverage in the evenings before bedtime.

Assessment

The patient has severe daytime sleepiness and symptoms of OSA. His sleep hygiene habits are poor and he self-medicates with caffeine as a daytime stimulant and uses

(continued)

CASE STUDY *(continued)*

alcohol as a hypnotic. With a BMI greater than 30, he has a high risk for both OSA and poorly controlled Type II diabetes. Clearly, Mr. M. is a high-risk driver, even during daylight hours. Although depression can cause sleep disruption, this patient's medical history and symptoms are compelling indicators of excessive sleepiness and warrant a referral to a sleep specialist for evaluation and treatment.

Interventions

The immediate intervention was referral to sleep specialist who ordered an overnight polysomnography to evaluate for OSA and begin treatment. The results of the overnight polysomnography are as follows:

TABLE 5.4

Results of Overnight Polysomnography

Total recording time	368 min	REM sleep	0
Total sleep time	256 min	Stage 1 sleep	92%
Sleep efficiency	70%	Stage 2 sleep	8%
Lowest O_2 saturation	65%	Stages 3 & 4 sleep	0
Apnea/Hypopnea index	56/hr of sleep	Longest apnea	39 s

Note. REM = rapid eye movement.

Intermediate interventions include a referral to the dietician for assistance in managing his diabetic diet and achieving weight loss. He requires instruction on sleep hygiene measures, avoidance of sedating OTC drugs (i.e., alcohol), which can exacerbate OSA symptoms, and avoidance of driving long distances alone or at night until treatment of OSA has begun. With CPAP treatment adherence, Mr. M. is more likely to be successful with weight loss involving increased activity, which can improve hypertension and glucose control. In addition, effective treatment of OSA often improves nocturia as well as reduced libido.

Diagnosis

Severe obstructive sleep apnea.

Treatment

Because of the obstructive character of the patient's sleep-related breathing disorder, CPAP at 14 cm water pressure.

Six-Month Follow-Up

Since starting CPAP, Mr. M. has lost 30 lbs, and his CPAP pressures and antihypertensive medications have already been titrated downward. His blood pressure has dropped to 132/88 mm Hg, his HbA1c has improved (7.6%), and he seldom has

(continued)

CASE STUDY *(continued)*

nocturia or takes naps. The patient reduced his caffeine intake to one or two cups of coffee per day and stopped using OTC products or alcohol as a sleeping aid. He no longer feels tired and has driven his car on several car trips without feeling sleepy. Mr. M. also states that he has started taking 30-minute walks with his wife at least four times a week. He reports, "I did not know how tired I was until I started on this breathing machine at night. I will admit, a few nights I haven't used it. But, the next day, I always know that I made a mistake by skipping the night before."

SUMMARY

Nurses must be able to identify, screen, and refer patients with excessive daytime sleepiness and symptoms of sleep disorders. No other group of health care providers watch more people sleep than nurses, and sleep disorders can affect all aspects of health and illness. Sleep medicine is a relatively new specialty, and many health care providers have had no preparation in the science of sleep. Nurses also must incorporate sleep hygiene measures and actively address existing sleep disorders in care plans of older adults to ensure adequate sleep in all settings: acute care, primary care, and at home. Failing to identify, diagnose, or treat excessive sleepiness and its underlying cause(s) can adversely affect the health and longevity of older adults.

NURSING STANDARD OF PRACTICE

Protocol 5.1: Excessive Sleepiness

I. GOAL: Older adults will maintain an optimal state of alertness while awake and optimal quality and quantity of sleep during their preferred sleep interval.

II. OVERVIEW: Although normal aging is accompanied by decreased "deep sleep," sleep efficiency, and increased time awake after sleep onset, these changes should not result in excessive daytime sleepiness. Daytime sleepiness is not only a symptom of sleep disorders but also results in decreased health and functional outcomes in the older adult.

III. BACKGROUND
  A. Definition
     Excessive sleepiness: somnolence, hypersomnia, excessive daytime sleepiness, subjective sleepiness. Sleepiness is an ubiquitous phenomenon, experienced not only as a symptom in a number of medical, psychiatric, and primary sleep disorders, but also as a normal physiological state by most individuals over any

(continued)

Protocol 5.1: Excessive Sleepiness *(cont.)*

given 24-hour period. Sleepiness can be considered abnormal when it occurs at inappropriate times, or does not occur when desired (Shen, Barbera, & Shapiro, 2006).

B. Etiology and Epidemiology
 1. Excessive sleepiness may be caused by difficulty initiating sleep, impaired sleep maintenance, waking prematurely, sleep disorders, or sleep fragmentation.
 2. There are many types of sleep diagnoses and the most common disorders reported by older adults are obstructive sleep apnea (OSA), insomnia, and restless leg syndrome.
 3. Many sleep disorders share excessive sleepiness as a common symptom, but this symptom is often not evaluated or treated because health care providers are uninformed about the nature of sleep disorders, the symptoms of these disorders, and the many effective treatments available for these conditions.

IV. PARAMETERS OF ASSESSMENT
 A. A sleep history (see Table 5.1) should include information from both the patient and family members. People who share living and sleeping spaces can provide important information about sleep behavior that the patient may not be able to convey.
 B. The Epworth Sleepiness Scale (Johns, 1991) is a brief instrument to screen for severity of daytime sleepiness in the community setting. It can also be found under "Resources" at http://consultgerirn.org/resources
 C. The Pittsburgh Sleep Quality Index (PSQI; Buysse et al., 1989) is useful to screen for sleep problems in the home environment and to monitor changes in sleep quality. This instrument can be found under "Resources" at http://consultgerirn.org/resources

V. NURSING CARE STRATEGIES
 A. Vigilance by nursing staff in observing patients for snoring, apneas during sleep, excessive leg movements during sleep, and difficulty staying awake during normal daytime activities (Ancoli-Israel & Martin, 2006; Avidan, 2005).
 B. Management of medical conditions, psychological disorders, and symptoms that interfere with sleep, such as depression, pain, hot flashes, anemia, or uremia (Ancoli-Israel & Martin, 2006; Avidan, 2005).
 C. For patients with a current diagnosis of a sleep disorder, ongoing treatments such as continuous positive airway pressure (CPAP) should be documented, maintained, and reinforced through patient and family education (Avidan, 2005). Nursing staff should reinforce patient instruction in cleaning and maintaining positive airway pressure equipment and masks.
 D. Instruction for patients and families regarding sleep hygiene techniques to protect and promote sleep among all family members (see Table 5.3; Avidan, 2005).
 E. Review and, if necessary, adjustment of medications that interact with one another or whose side effects include drowsiness or sleep impairment (Ancoli-Israel & Martin, 2006).

(continued)

Protocol 5.1: Excessive Sleepiness *(cont.)*

F. Referral to a sleep specialist for moderate or severe sleepiness or a clinical profile consistent with major sleep disorders such as OSA or restless leg syndrome (Avidan, 2005).

G. Aggressive planning, monitoring, and management of patients with OSA when sedative medications or anesthesia are given (Avidan, 2005).

H. Ongoing assessment of adherence to prescriptions for sleep hygiene, medications, and devices to support respiration during sleep (Avidan, 2005).

VI. EVALUATION AND EXPECTED OUTCOMES

A. Quality Assurance Actions
   1. Provide staff education on the major causes of excessive sleepiness (i.e., OSA, insomnia, restless leg syndrome).
   2. Provide staff with in-services on how to use and monitor CPAP equipment.
   3. Have individual nursing units conduct environmental surveys regarding noise level during the night hours and then develop strategies to reduce sleep disruption caused by noise and care patterns.
   4. Add sleep as a parameter of the admission assessment for patients and provide written instructions for patients using CPAP at home to always bring the equipment with them to the hospital.
      Include sleep quality (e.g., see PSQI tool; http://www.hartfordign.org).
   5. Utilize posthospital surveys of patient satisfaction with their sleep while in the hospital and provide feedback for nursing staff (see http://www.hartfordign.org, Sleep topic).

B. Quality Outcomes
   Improved quality and/or quantity of sleep during normal sleep intervals as reported by patients and staffs.

VII. FOLLOW-UP MONITORING

A. Depending on the diagnosis, follow-up may include long-term reinforcement of the original interventions along with support for adhering to treatments prescribed by a sleep specialist. For example, patient compliance with CPAP therapy for OSA is critical to its efficacy and should be assessed during the first week of treatment (Weaver et al., 1997a). All patients benefit from positive reinforcement while trying to acclimate to nightly use of a positive airway pressure device.

B. CPAP masks may require minor adjustments or refitting to find the most comfortable fit. Most such changes are needed during the acclimation period, but patients should be encouraged to seek assistance if mask problems develop (Weaver et al., 1997a). In the acute care setting, respiratory care technicians are valuable in-house resources when staff from a sleep center are not readily available.

C. During the initial treatment phase of insomnia, sleep deprivation may cause rebound sleepiness, which should subside over time. Follow-up should include ongoing assessment of napping habits and sleepiness to track treatment effectiveness (Avidan, 2005).

(continued)

Protocol 5.1: Excessive Sleepiness *(cont.)*

D. If obesity has been a complicating health factor, weight loss is a desirable long-term goal. With reduction in daytime sleepiness, the timing is ripe for increasing the activity level. Treatment of sleep disorders should include planning for strategic changes in lifestyle that include regular exercise, which is also consistent with cardiovascular health and long-term diabetes control (Ancoli-Israel & Ayalon, 2006).

RESOURCES

American Academy of Sleep Medicine (AASM)
This organization for sleep professionals is also a great source of information for the public and for practice guidelines for professionals.
http://www.aasmnet.org/

Basics of Sleep Guide
This Sleep Research Society publication is designed for students, sleep researchers, and nonsleep professionals interested in studying sleep across the life cycle, sleep deprivation or restriction, and sleep physiology. Information about this publication and how to order it can be found on the *Sleep Research Society* website.
http://www.sleepresearchsociety.org/Products.aspx

National Institutes of Health, National Center on Sleep Disorders Research
This site includes brochures that may be downloaded or printed for distribution to patients or for the education of other health care providers.
For patients and the general public: http://www.nhlbi.nih.gov/health/public/sleep/index.htm
For health care professionals: http://www.nhlbi.nih.gov/health/prof/sleep/index.htm

New Abstracts and Papers in Sleep
This free online subscription service is an excellent resource for professionals to find the most recent research on sleep disorders and their treatments on a regular basis. Services include weekly personalized e-mail alerts of new citations, author abstracts, a compilation of the current week's literature in sleep, and an archive of the current year's literature in sleep.
http://www.websciences.org/bibliosleep/naps/

Restless Leg Syndrome Foundation
This organization is dedicated to improving the lives of the men, women, and children who live with this often devastating disease. The organization's goals are to increase awareness of RLS, to improve treatments, and, through research, to find a cure.
http://www.rls.org

Sleep Research Society
This professional organization fosters scientific investigation, professional education, and career development in sleep research and academic sleep medicine. It is an excellent resource for nurses who are interested in studying issues of sleep and circadian processes.
http://www.sleepresearchsociety.org/

REFERENCES

American Academy of Sleep Medicine. (2005). *International classification of sleep disorders: Diagnostic and Coding Manual* (2nd ed.). Westchester, MN: Author.

Ancoli-Israel, S. (2000). Insomnia in the elderly: A review for the primary care practitioner. *Sleep*, *23*(Suppl. 1), S23–S30; discussion S36–S38. Evidence Level I.

Ancoli-Israel, S. (2005). Sleep and aging: Prevalence of disturbed sleep and treatment considerations in older adults. *The Journal of Clinical Psychiatry*, *66*(Suppl. 9), 24–30; quiz 42–43. Evidence Level I.

Ancoli-Israel, S., & Ayalon, L. (2006). Diagnosis and treatment of sleep disorders in older adults. *The American Journal of Geriatric Psychiatry*, *14*(2), 95–103. Evidence Level I.

Ancoli-Israel, S., Kripke, D. F., Klauber, M. R., Mason, W. J., Fell, R., & Kaplan, O. (1991). Sleep-disordered breathing in community-dwelling elderly. *Sleep*, *14*(6), 486–495. Evidence Level IV.

Ancoli-Israel, S., Kripke, D. F., & Mason, W. (1987). Characteristics of obstructive and central sleep apnea in the elderly: An interim report. *Biological Psychiatry*, *22*(6), 741–750. Evidence Level IV.

Ancoli-Israel, S., & Martin, J. L. (2006). Insomnia and daytime napping in older adults. *Journal of Clinical Sleep Medicine*, *2*(3), 333–342. Evidence Level VI.

Avidan, A. Y. (2005). Sleep in the geriatric patient population. *Seminars in Neurology*, *25*(1), 52–63. Evidence Level I.

Bliwise, D. L., King, A. C., & Harris, R. B. (1994). Habitual sleep durations and health in a 50–65 year old population. *Journal of Clinical Epidemiology*, *47*(1), 35–41.

Bloom, H. G., Ahmed, I., Alessi, C. A., Ancoli-Israel, S., Buysse, D. J., Kryger, M. H., . . . Zee, P. C. (2009). Evidence-based recommendations for the assessment and management of sleep disorders in older persons. *Journal of the American Geriatrics Society*, *57*(5), 761–789. Evidence Level I.

Brassington, G. S., King, A. C., & Bliwise, D. L. (2000). Sleep problems as a risk factor for falls in a sample of community-dwelling adults aged 64–99 years. *Journal of the American Geriatrics Society*, *48*(10), 1234–1240. Evidence Level III.

Buysse, D. J. (2004). Insomnia, depression and aging. Assessing sleep and mood interactions in older adults. *Geriatrics*, *59*(2), 47–51. Evidence Level VI.

Buysse, D. J., Reynolds, C. F., III, Monk, T. H., Berman, S. R., & Kupfer, D. J. (1989). The Pittsburgh Sleep Quality Index: A new instrument for psychiatric practice and research. *Psychiatry Research*, *28*(2), 193–213.

Centers for Disease Control and Prevention. (2011a). Effect of short sleep duration on daily activities—United States, 2005–2008. *Morbidity and Mortality Weekly Report*, *60*(8), 239–242. Evidence Level IV.

Centers for Disease Control and Prevention (2011b). Unhealthy sleep-related behaviors—12 States, 2009. *Morbidity and Mortality Weekly Report*, *60*(8), 233–238. Evidence Level IV.

Chung, F., Yegneswaran, B., Liao, P., Chung, S. A., Vairavanathan, S., Islam, S., . . . Shapiro, C. M. (2008). STOP questionnaire: A tool to screen patients for obstructive sleep apnea. *Anesthesiology*, *108*(5), 812–821.

Cohen-Zion, M., Stepnowsky, C., Marler, Shochat, T., Kripke, D. F., & Ancoli-Israel, S. (2001). Changes in cognitive function associated with sleep disordered breathing in older people. *Journal of the American Geriatrics Society*, *49*(12), 1622–1627. Evidence Level III.

Colten, H. R., & Altevogt, B. M. (Eds.). (2006). *Sleep disorders and sleep deprivation: An unmet public health problem*. Washington, DC: The National Academies Press. Evidence Level I.

Gamaldo, C. E., & Earley, C. J. (2006). Restless legs syndrome: A clinical update. *Chest*, *130*(5), 1596–1604. Evidence Level I.

Johns, M. W. (1991). A new method for measuring daytime sleepiness: The Epworth sleepiness scale. *Sleep*, *14*(6), 540–545.

Maislin, G., Pack, A. I., Kribbs, N. B., Smith, P. L., Schwartz, A. R., Kline, L. R., . . . Dinges, D. F. (1995). A survey screen for prediction of apnea. *Sleep*, *18*(3), 158–166.

Morgenthaler, T. I., Kapen, S., Lee-Chiong, T., Alessi, C., Boehlecke, B., Brown, T., . . . Swick, T. (2006). Practice parameters for the medical therapy of obstructive sleep apnea. *Sleep, 29*(8), 1031–1035. Evidence Level I.

Morin, C. M., Hauri, P. J., Espie, C. A., Spielman, A. J., Buysse, D. J., & Bootzin, R. R. (1999). Nonpharmacologic treatment of chronic insomnia. An American Academy of Sleep Medicine review. *Sleep, 22*(8), 1134–1156. Evidence Level I.

Netzer, N. C., Stoohs, R. A., Netzer, C. M., Clark, K., & Strohl, K. P. (1999). Using the Berlin Questionnaire to identify patients at risk for the sleep apnea syndrome. *Annals of Internal Medicine, 131*(7), 485–491.

Newman, A. B., Spiekerman, C. F., Enright, P., Lefkowitz, D., Manolio, T., Reynolds, C. F., & Robbins, J. (2000). Daytime sleepiness predicts mortality and cardiovascular disease in older adults. The Cardiovascular Health Study Research Group. *Journal of the American Geriatrics Society, 48*(2), 115–123. Evidence Level III.

Ohayon, M. M., & Vecchierini, M. F. (2002). Daytime sleepiness and cognitive impairment in the elderly population. *Archives of Internal Medicine, 162*(2), 201–208. Evidence Level IV.

Redeker, N. S. (2000). Sleep in acute care settings: An integrative review. *Journal of Nursing Scholarship, 32*(1), 31–38. Evidence Level I.

Rediehs, M. H., Reis, J. S., & Creason, N. S. (1990). Sleep in old age: Focus on gender differences. *Sleep, 13*(5), 410–424. Evidence Level I.

Richardson, G. S., Carskadon, M. A., Orav, E. J., & Dement, W. C. (1982). Circadian variation of sleep tendency in elderly and young adult subjects. *Sleep, 5*(Suppl. 2), S82–S94.

Roehrs, T., Turner, L., & Roth, T. (2000). Effects of sleep loss on waking actigraphy. *Sleep, 23*(6), 793–797. Evidence Level IV.

Shen, J., Barbera, J., & Shapiro, C. M. (2006). Distinguishing sleepiness and fatigue: Focus on definition and measurement. *Sleep Medicine Reviews, 10*(1), 63–76. Evidence Level VI.

Weaver, T. E., & Chasens, E. R. (2007). Continuous positive airway pressure treatment for sleep sleep apnea in older adults. *Sleep Medicine Reviews, 11*(2), 99–111. Evidence Level I.

Weaver, T. E., Kribbs, N. B., Pack, A. I., Kline, L. R., Chugh, D. K., Maislin, G., . . . Dinges, D. F. (1997a). Night-to-night variability in CPAP use over the first three months of treatment. *Sleep, 20*(4), 278–283. Evidence Level II.

Weaver, T. E., Laizner, A. M., Evans, L. K., Maislin, G., Chugh, D. K., Lyon, K., . . . Dinges, D. F. (1997b). An instrument to measure functional status outcomes for disorders of excessive sleepiness. *Sleep, 20*(10), 835–843.

Whitney, C. W., Enright, P. L., Newman, A. B., Bonekat, W., Foley, D., & Quan, S. F. (1998). Correlates of daytime sleepiness in 4578 elderly persons: The Cardiovascular Health Study. *Sleep, 21*(1), 27–36. Evidence Level III.

Young, J. S., Bourgeois, J. A., Hilty, D. M., & Hardin, K. A. (2008). Sleep in hospitalized medical patients, part 1: Factors affecting sleep. *Journal of Hospital Medicine, 3*(6), 473–482. Evidence Level VI.

Young, J. S., Bourgeois, J. A., Hilty, D. M., & Hardin, K. A. (2009). Sleep in hospitalized medical patients, part 2: Behavioral and pharmacological management of sleep disturbances. *Journal of Hospital Medicine, 4*(1), 50–59. Evidence Level VI.

Assessment of Physical Function

6

Denise M. Kresevic

EDUCATIONAL OBJECTIVES

On completion of this chapter, the reader should be able to:

1. describe common components of standardized functional assessment instruments for acute care
2. identify unique challenges to gathering information from older adults regarding functional assessments
3. describe common nursing care strategies to restore, maintain, and promote functional health in older adults in acute care settings

OVERVIEW

Physical functioning is a dynamic process of interaction between individuals and their environments. The process is influenced by motivation, physical capacity, illness, cognitive ability, and the external environment including social supports. Management of these day-to-day activities (e.g., eating, bathing, ambulating, managing money) serves as the foundation for safe, independent functioning of all adults. Functional assessment instruments provide a common language of health for patients, family members, and health care providers across settings, especially for care of older adults.

The consequences of not assessing for change in status are significant. Acute changes in functional ability often signal an acute illness and an increased need for assistance to maintain safety. These changes have important implications for nursing care across settings, but especially during hospitalization. The ability to assess functional status is critical in accurately identifying normal aging changes, illness, and disability, and in developing an individualized plan for continuity of care across settings. The failure to assess function can lead to increased decline (e.g., malnutrition, falls), decreased quality of life, and the need for institutional care.

For description of Evidence Levels cited in this chapter, see Chapter 1, Developing and Evaluating Clinical Practice Guidelines: A Systematic Approach, page 7.

BACKGROUND AND STATEMENT OF PROBLEM

The ability to manage day-to-day functioning (e.g., bathing, dressing, managing medications), rather than the absence of disease, is the cornerstone of health for older adults. As individuals age or become ill, they may require assistance to accomplish these activities independently. Hospitalization can also contribute to functional decline, with decline experienced by an estimated 20%–40% of hospitalized older adults (Landefeld, Palmer, Kresevic, Fortinsky, & Kowal, 1995). Although the exact cause of the decline is often a combination of factors including acute illness, it can in part be caused by environmental factors of hospitalization that could be prevented or ameliorated by skilled nursing care (McCusker, Kakuma, & Abrahamowicz, 2002). In fact, hospitalization provides a unique opportunity to assess function, plan for services, and promote "successful aging."

Common risk factors for functional decline include falls, injuries, acute illness, medication side effects, depression, malnutrition, baseline functional impairment, and decreased mobility associated with iatrogenic complications such as incontinence, falls, and pressure sores (Creditor, 1993). In one randomized clinical trial of hospitalized older adults, the daily nursing assessment of ability to perform bathing, dressing, grooming, toileting, transferring, and ambulation during routine nursing care yielded information necessary for maintenance of function in self-care activities (Landefeld et al., 1995).

This chapter addresses the need for and goals of functional assessment of older adults in acute care, and it provides a clinical practice protocol to guide nurses in this assessment (Protocol 6.1).

ASSESSMENT OF THE PROBLEM

Assessment of function includes an ongoing systematic process of identifying the older person's physical abilities and need for help. Functional assessment also provides the opportunity to identify individual strengths and measures of "successful aging." This information is especially important for nurses in planning for discharge and evaluating continuity of care. Nurses are in a pivotal position in all care settings, but particularly during hospitalization, to assess the functional status of older adults by direct observation during routine care and through information gathered from the individual patient, the patient's family, and any other long-term caregivers.

Including critical components of functional assessments into routine assessments in the acute care setting can provide (a) baseline functional capacity and recent changes in level of independence indicative of possible illness, especially infections; (b) baseline information to benchmark patients' response to treatment as they move along the continuum from acute care to rehabilitation or from acute to subacute care (e.g., following a new stroke or hip replacement surgery); (c) information regarding care needs and eligibility for services, including safety, physical therapy, and posthospitalization needs; and (d) information on quality of care. The ongoing use of a standardized functional assessment instrument promotes systematic communication of the patient's health status between care settings. It also allows units to compare their level of care with other units in the facility, measure outcomes, and plan for continuity of care (see Table 6.1; Campbell, Seymour, Primrose, & ACMEPLUS Project, 2004).

Although gathering information about functional status is a critical indicator of quality care in geriatrics, it requires significant time, skill, and knowledge. Older persons often present to the care setting with multiple medical conditions resulting in fatigue and pain. Acute illnesses may be superimposed upon multiple interrelated medical comorbidities.

TABLE 6.1

Functional Assessment of Older Adults

Dimension	Assessment Parameter	Standardized Instrument	Nursing Strategy
ADLs Bathing Dressing Eating Toileting Hygiene Transferring	Self-report of patient Surrogate report Observation during hospitalization	Katz ADL index (Katz et al., 1963)	Orient to environment Encourage active participation in ADLs Range of motion exercises Encourage to be out of bed Promote continence Consult PT/OT for strengthening exercises
Mobility Balance sitting and standing Gait steadiness Turns	Self-report Surrogate report Observation	"Get Up and Go" test (Mathias et al., 1986)	Ambulate PT/OT consult Mobility aids Community referrals
IADLs Housework Finances Driving Shopping Meal preparation Reading Medication adherence Aware of current events Hobbies Employment Volunteer work	Self-report (include normal daily routine) Surrogate report (able to balance check book, traffic violations)	Lawton IADL scale Lawton & Brody, 1969; Gurland et al., 1994) DAFA–for patients with dementia (Karagiozis et al., 1998)	Assess ability to: ■ Find hospital room ■ Read newspaper ■ Read pill bottles ■ Order hospital meals from menu Facilitate as needed: ■ Community referrals for transportation and/or Meals on Wheels ■ OT consult to assess home management skills (cooking, laundry, etc.) ■ Home care referral including medication management, follow-up medical care, rehabilitation, home safety management, and ADL support

Note. ADLs = activities of daily living; IADLs = instrumental activities of daily living; PT/OT = physical therapist/occupational therapist

In addition, sensory aging changes, particularly vision and hearing, can threaten the accuracy of responses. Ideally, information regarding functional status should be elicited as part of the routine history of older adults and incorporated into daily care routines of all caregivers. In addition, comprehensive assessment of function provides an opportunity to teach patients and families about normal aging as well as indicators of pathology.

Assessment Instruments

Collecting systematic information regarding tasks of daily living (e.g., bathing, dressing, ambulating, using a phone, taking medications, managing finances) can be accomplished by the use of standardized instruments. The use of standardized instruments serves to ensure inclusive assessments, the ability to communicate in a common language, and the ability to benchmark information over time. Several instruments have been developed over the years to measure function. Although all measure components of function, the decision of which instrument to use depends on the primary purpose of the assessment and the institutional preferences and resources (Kane & Kane, 2000). No single instrument will meet the needs of all care settings.

Many performance-based measures and observational instruments can be incorporated into routine care practices without significantly burdening caregivers. Incorporating electronic medical record templates into routine documentation can function as a prompt for providers, decreasing the time and increasing the communication of the results of these assessments.

The Katz Index of Independence in Activities of Daily Living (commonly referred to as *Katz ADL index*) assesses activities of daily living (ADL) including bathing, dressing, transferring, toileting, continence, and feeding (Katz, Ford, Moskowitz, Jackson, & Jaffe, 1963). This scale is used widely to assess function of older adults in all settings including during hospitalization (Mezey, Rauckhorst, & Stokes, 1993). Originally, the Katz ADL index was proposed as an observation tool with scores ranging from 1 to 3, indicating *independent ability, limited assistance,* and *extensive assistance* for each activity. Over time, the instrument has evolved into a dichotomized tool with independent versus dependent ability of each task (Kane & Kane, 2000). With established reliability (0.94–0.97), it is easy to use either as an observational or self-reported measure of level of independence (Kane & Kane, 2000). The Katz ADL index is easily incorporated into history and physical assessment flowsheets and takes little time to complete. Many other tools exist to assess ADLs, including the Barthel index for physical functioning and the Older Americans Resources and Services ADL scale (Burton, Damon, Dillinger, Erickson, & Peterson, 1978; Mahoney & Barthel, 1965; Mezey et al., 1993).

In addition to ADL tools, instruments to measure more complex physical function called *instrumental activities of daily living* (IADLs) have been proposed to be included in a comprehensive assessment of function in older adults. The majority of these instruments assess the individual's function in relation to the environment. Common IADL skills identified include using a phone, shopping, meal preparation, housekeeping, laundry, medication administration, transportation, and money management (Kane & Kane, 2000). Although assessment of ADLs provides useful information for nursing care needs both during and after hospitalization, IADL information helps target critical posthospital care needs. Although direct observation of the patient's IADLs may not occur during an acute hospitalization, it is important for the nurse to assess this information to plan for the patient's discharge. Common instruments used to measure IADLs include the Lawton IADL scale, the Older Americans Resource and Services IADL (OARS-IADL) scale, and the Direct Assessment of Functional Abilities (DAFA) scale.

Perhaps the most widely used IADL instrument for hospitalized older adults is the Lawton IADL scale. This scale assesses eight items with each scored from 0 (*dependence*) to 8 (*independent self-care*). Reliability coefficients have been reported to be 0.96 for men and 0.93 for women (Kane & Kane, 2000).

Assessment of function in individuals with dementia presents a unique challenge. A recently developed instrument, the DAFA, is a 10-item observational measure of IADLs useful in assessing function in the presence of dementia (Karagiozis, Gray, Sacco, Shapiro, & Kawas, 1998; see http://www.consultgerirn.org/resources and the Resources section of this chapter for assessment instruments).

Regardless of the instrument used, basic ADL and IADL function should be assessed for each patient, including capacity for dressing, eating, transferring, toileting, hygiene, ambulation, and medication adherence (see Chapter 17, Reducing Adverse Drug Events). Appropriate assessment instruments should be readily available on the acute care unit for reference and/or incorporated into routine documentation instruments for history, daily assessment, and discharge planning. To adequately assess function, sensory and cognitive capacity should be established and environmental adaptations, such as magnifying glasses or hearing amplifiers, may be necessary and should be accessible to nursing staff.

Direct Assessment of Patient

Although nurses often rely on reports of physical functioning and capacity for ADL and IADL from patients and family members, direct observation provides strong evidence for current capacity versus past ability.

Functional assessments are constantly conducted by nurses every time they notice that a patient can no longer pick up a fork or has difficulty walking. A comprehensive functional assessment leads to more than simply noticing a change in activity or ability, however. In a systematic manner, nurses need to assess the ability of a patient to perform ADLs in the context of the patient's baseline functional and hospitalization status.

While assessing functional status, the patient should be made as comfortable as possible, with frequent rest periods allowed. Adaptive aids, such as glasses and hearing aids, should be applied. Often, family members accompany the older person and can assist in answering questions regarding function. It is important for patients and family members to understand that baseline functional levels as well as any recent changes in function need to be reported. Many older adults may be reluctant to report decline in function, fearing that such reports will threaten their autonomy and independent living.

Occasionally, the history and physical exam may reveal clues to further identify functional status. Muscle weakness and atrophy of legs may indicate lack of ability to safely ambulate independently. Temporal muscle wasting may indicate moderate-to-severe malnutrition resulting from inability to shop, prepare meals, or adequately consume sufficient calories. Hand contractures present with arthritis or cerebral vascular accidents alert the nurse to pay particular attention to performance versus self-report of ability to open pill bottles, dial a phone, or write checks. General appearance (e.g., hair, teeth, fingernails) and condition of clothing (e.g., clean and dry versus urine-soaked undergarments) may give rise to information on bathing, dressing, continence, and ability to do laundry.

Specific Functional Assessments

Ambulation

Inherent in both ADLs and IADLs is ambulation, a critical parameter for functional assessment. Early nursing assessment of the hospitalized patient's ability to walk is very important in order to ensure safety and prevent falls and injuries (see Chapter 15, Fall Prevention: Assessment, Diagnoses, and Intervention Strategies). The ability to safely ambulate is contingent on the ability to transfer, propel forward, and pivot with sufficient strength and balance. Ambulation is necessary for self-care both in the hospital and posthospital discharge. It is also a very sensitive indicator of acute health changes. Therefore, the ability to ambulate should be assessed by both self- or proxy report and by direct observation.

Some instruments used to assess ambulation, balance, and gait are sensitive measures of mobility (Applegate, Blass, & Franklin, 1990); however, they are also complex and time consuming to use. Therefore, direct observation of an individual's ability to get out of bed, sit in a chair, assume a standing position, and steadily walk a short distance—with or without assistive devices—is much simpler to do yet important to ensure safety (Applegate et al., 1990; Cress et al., 1995).

An efficient performance-based measure of ambulation, balance, and gait that can be observed during routine care of the hospitalized patient is the "Get Up and Go" test (Cress et al., 1995). To do a Get Up and Go test, patients are observed sitting in a chair, standing, walking, and pivoting. Direct observation of the patient should include an assessment of speed of performance, hesitancy, stumbling, swaying, grabbing for support, or unsafe maneuvers such as sitting too close to the edge of a chair or dizziness while pivoting (Tinetti & Ginter, 1998). Performance is scored from 1 (*normal balance and steady gait*) to 5 (*severely abnormal balance and gait*) which is clear evidence of falls risk (Kane & Kane, 2000). Assessment of unsafe transfers or ambulation indicates the need to begin immediate restorative therapies to prevent falls and injuries. These can include attention to environmental designs such walking paths free of clutter, hand rails, and rest areas to encourage daily ambulation as opposed to bed rest and immobility (Creditor, 1993). Although the Get Up and Go test is easy to do, it is relatively subjective. Objectivity may be enhanced by timing the tasks (Kane & Kane, 2000).

Sensory Capacity

Evaluation of the potential impact of sensory changes on the performance of ADLs is often underestimated. Impaired vision is especially important in medication adherence and safety. A simple test for functional vision is to have older adults read from a newspaper. A moderate impairment can be noted if only the headline can be read (Tinetti & Ginter, 1998). Another way to assess vision is to have older persons read prescription bottles. Functional assessment of safe medication administration includes the ability to read pill bottles and repeat directions for use, potential side effects, and instructions of when to contact a health care provider. Glasses should be available with clean lenses. Inability to read raises questions of literacy, undiagnosed vision difficulties, and safety for medication administration. Often overlooked is the number of older people who may not be able to read but are too embarrassed to reveal that information. As part of routine care, older adults should be encouraged to actively participate each day in learning about medications. In addition, at the time of discharge, nurses need to verify patient and family knowledge and skills regarding medications. This may include discussing medications as well as directly observing older adults opening pill bottles and identifying the correct pills.

Hearing ability is also essential for functioning and cognition. Individuals with decreased hearing may be inaccurately labeled as *cognitively impaired*. Hearing aids may not have been sent to the hospital with the older patient and should be obtained by the family. Hearing acuity may be validated by asking patients to identify the sound of a ticking watch. The "whisper test" may also be used. This is performed by whispering 10 words while standing 6 in. away from the individual. Inability to repeat 5 of the 10 words indicates a need for further assessment of hearing acuity. Occlusion of the external ear canal by cerumen, an easily treatable cause of decreased hearing acuity, may be evident with visualization (Mathias, Nayak, & Isaacs, 1986). Individuals with hearing deficits detected as part of bedside assessment should be referred for additional assessment and treatment. Amplifier devices may be useful and are an inexpensive item to stock on hospital nursing units.

Cognitive Capacity

Cognitive function is a major factor in a person's functional capacity, and baseline data regarding cognitive function should be gathered. However, such assessments most often initially rely on information provided by family members because acute illness may manifest as acute confusional states and not reflect baseline cognitive function (Kruianski & Gurland, 1976; see Chapter 8, Assessing Cognitive Function). Fluctuating attention may indicate an acute, reversible impairment (delirium) or temporary reactions to hospitalization. An acute change in cognition should be evaluated immediately for the presence of a potentially life-threatening, reversible medical condition (see Chapter 11, Delirium).

Cause of Functional Decline

All instances of functional decline should be assessed for an underlying reversible cause such as acute illness. With the resolution of acute illness (e.g., urinary tract infection [UTI], pneumonia, postoperative recovery), impaired ADLs are expected to return to baseline with appropriate care and rehabilitation. Comprehensive musculoskeletal or neurologic examination, laboratory tests, or referral for a therapeutic trial of physical or occupational therapy may be needed to boost recovery.

INTERVENTIONS AND CARE STRATEGIES

Functional ability is a sensitive indicator of health in older adults. The need for assistance with ADLs is an important nursing assessment that aids in care planning during and after a hospital stay. Sudden loss of function, including the ability to ambulate, is the hallmark of acute illness in older adults. Although recovery from illness may be associated with improvements in function, early nursing interventions to address care needs, refer to therapy, and modify environments of care help to ensure safety and decrease further loss of function. Therefore, all nurses must be skilled at incorporating a comprehensive functional assessment into all patient care assessments. Nurses need to be knowledgeable and skilled in assessment of function, implementing supportive environments, and providing geriatric-sensitive care to prevent functional decline. Geriatric-sensitive care incorporates strategies to prevent bed rest, encourage exercise and ambulation, ensure adequate nutrition, and encourage ongoing communication among all team members. Such care is essential in maximizing safe, independent functioning of hospitalized older adults (see Chapter 7, Interventions to Prevent Funtional Decline in the Acute Care Setting).

Use of Assessment Information

Knowledge of ADL and IADL abilities, including shopping, housework, finances, food preparation, medication administration, and transportation, is an important part of providing individual nursing care for comprehensive discharge planning (Woolf, 1990). In summary, for older people, the evaluation of function represents the cornerstone of good nursing care and affords a sound baseline by which to provide information essential to plan for continued care across settings.

CASE STUDY

Mrs. Hope, a 74-year-old retired night nurse and recent widow, is admitted to the hospital from her physician's office. Her admitting diagnosis is pneumonia, dehydration, and weakness. She is accompanied by her daughter. Her past medical history is significant for hypertension, congestive heart failure (CHF), and chronic obstructive pulmonary disease (COPD). She is extremely hard of hearing, but has refused to wear her hearing aid. She smokes approximately 10 cigarettes a day, which she has done for more than 50 years. Her daughter admits that lately, Mrs. Hope has not been taking most of her pills, although she has been taking aspirin for pain. She has also been losing weight and has poor appetite and intake. Laboratory values indicate anemia with a very low hematocrit and a UTI.

While on the unit, Mrs. Hope prefers to sleep in the recliner, saying she is most comfortable there and prefers to nap during the day. Despite intravenous fluids, blood transfusions, diuresis for fluid overload, oxygen therapy, occupational therapy for energy conservation, and round-the-clock acetaminophen for "aches and pains," Mrs. Hope continues to be weak and need assistance with daily bathing and ambulation. She is able to communicate well using an amplifier, after her ears are cleaned from wax. She is assessed by the multidisciplinary care team over the next several days. After the team meeting consultations are obtained for physical therapy, nutrition services, pharmacy, geriatric clinical nurse specialist, and social work. Her fatigue improves. Referrals for home care are made for nursing and therapy as well as for telehealth to monitor her CHF. Mrs. Hope's medication regimen is adjusted, substituting acetaminophen rather than aspirin for her pain. She and her daughter are instructed on a high-calorie diet and are provided with information on senior care and smoking cessation programs. She is given vaccines for influenza and pneumonia. A future outpatient appointment for a comprehensive geriatric evaluation is made to do an anemia workup and more accurately assess her cognitive status once her acute conditions resolve.

Mrs. Hope is discharged home with her daughter after medications, diet, and exercises are reviewed. The numbers for the home care agency and directions to the outpatient appointment are printed out for her at the time of discharge.

Case Study Review

This case study indicates the need to assess baseline function, changes in function, and trajectory of function following acute care. Assessment in this case used components from several standardized functional assessment instruments and incorporated them into existing care routines. Care was enhanced by collaboration between multiple disciplines and across settings. Opportunities for assessment and resolution of impairment rely on institutional preferences and resources, as well as the functional level of the patient. Despite impaired function of Mrs. Hope, hospital staff worked to enhance her physical functioning as much as possible within the current care setting and a context of safety.

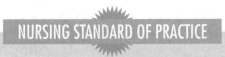

Protocol 6.1: Assessment of Physical Function

I. GOAL: The following nursing care protocol has been designed to help bedside nurses to monitor function in older adults, prevent decline, and maintain the function of older adults during acute hospitalization.

II. OBJECTIVE: To maximize physical functioning, prevent or minimize decline in activity of daily living (ADL) function, and plan for transitions of care.

III. BACKGROUND

A. Functional status of individuals describes the capacity and performance of safe ADLs and instrumental activities of daily living (IADLs; Applegate et al., 1990; Kane & Kane, 2000; Katz et al., 1963; Lawton & Brody, 1969); and is a sensitive indicator of health or illness in older adults. It is therefore a critical nursing assessment (Byles, 2000; Campbell et al., 2004; Kresevic et al., 1998; Mezey et al., 1993).

B. Some functional decline may be prevented or ameliorated with prompt and aggressive nursing intervention (e.g., ambulation, toileting schedules, enhanced communication, adaptive equipment, and attention to medications and dosages [Bates-Jensen et al., 2004; Counsell et al., 2000; Landefeld et al., 1995; Palmer, Counsell, & Landefeld, 1998]).

C. Some functional decline may occur progressively and is not reversible. This decline often accompanies chronic and terminal disease states such as degenerative joint disease, Parkinson's disease, dementia, heart failure, and cancer (Hirsch, Sommers, Olsen, Mullen, & Winograd, 1990).

D. Functional status is influenced by physiological aging changes, acute and chronic illness, and adaptation to the physical environment. Functional decline is often the initial symptom of acute illness such as infections (e.g., pneumonia and urinary tract infection). These declines are usually reversible and require medical evaluation (Applegate et al., 1990; Sager & Rudberg, 1998). Functional status is contingent on motivation, cognition, and sensory capacity, including vision and hearing (Pearson, 2000).

E. Risk factors for functional decline include injuries, acute illness, medication side effects, pain, depression, malnutrition, decreased mobility, prolonged bed rest (including the use of physical restraints), prolonged use of Foley catheters, and changes in environment or routines (Counsell et al., 2000; Landefeld et al., 1995; McCusker et al., 2002).

F. Additional complications of functional decline include loss of independence, falls, incontinence, malnutrition, decreased socialization, and increased risk for long-term institutionalization and depression (Covinsky et al., 1998; Creditor, 1993; Landefeld et al., 1995). (See related chapters.)

G. Recovery of function can also be a measure of return to health, such as for those individuals recovering from exacerbations of cardiovascular or respiratory diseases and acute infections, recovering from joint replacement surgery, or new strokes (Katz et al., 1963).

(continued)

Protocol 6.1: Assessment of Physical Function *(cont.)*

H. Functional status evaluation assists in planning future care needs posthospital-
    ization, such as short-term skilled care, home care, and need for community
    services (Graf, 2006; Landefeld et al., 1995).
I. Physical environments of care with attention to the special needs of older adults
    serve to maintain and enhance function (i.e., chairs with arms, elevated toilet
    seat, levers versus door knobs, enhanced lighting; Kresevic et al., 1998; Lande-
    feld et al., 1995).

IV. ASSESSMENT PARAMETERS

A. Comprehensive functional assessment of older adults includes independent
    performance of basic ADLs, social activities, or IADLs, the assistance needed
    to accomplish these tasks, and sensory ability, cognition, and capacity to ambu-
    late (Campbell et al., 2004; Doran et al., 2006; Freedman, Martin, & Schoeni,
    2002; Kane & Kane, 2000; Katz et al., 1963; Lawton & Brody, 1969; Light-
    body & Baldwin, 2002; McCusker et al., 2002; Tinetti & Ginter, 1998).
    1. Basic ADLs (bathing, dressing, grooming, eating, continence, transferring)
    2. IADLs (meal preparation, shopping, medication administration, house-
        work, transportation, accounting)
    3. Mobility (ambulation, pivoting)
B. Older adults may view their health in terms of how well they can function
    rather than in terms of disease alone. Strengths should be emphasized as well as
    needs for assistance (Depp & Jeste, 2006; Pearson, 2000).
C. The clinician should document baseline functional status and recent or pro-
    gressive decline in function (Graf, 2006).
D. Function should be assessed over time to validate capacity, decline, or progress
    (Applegate et al., 1990; Callahan, Thomas, Goldhirsh, & Leipzig, 2002; Kane
    & Kane, 2000).
E. Standard instruments selected to assess function should be efficient to adminis-
    ter and easy to interpret. They should provide useful practical information for
    clinicians and be incorporated into routine history taking and daily assessments
    (Kane & Kane, 2000; Kresevic et al., 1998). (see "Function" topic at http://
    www.consultgerirn.org for tools.)
F. Interdisciplinary communication regarding functional status, changes, and
    expected trajectory should be part of all care settings and should include the
    patient and family whenever possible (Counsell et al., 2000; Covinsky et al.,
    1998; Kresevic et al., 1998; Landefeld et al., 1995).

V. CARE STRATEGIES

A. Strategies to maximize functional status and to prevent decline
    1. Maintain individual's daily routine. Help to maintain physical, cognitive,
        and social function through physical activity and socialization. Encourage
        ambulation, allow flexible visitation, including pets, and encourage reading
        the newspaper (Kresevic & Holder, 1998; Landefeld et al., 1995).
    2. Educate older adults, family, and formal caregivers on the value of indepen-
        dent functioning and the consequences of functional decline (Graf, 2006;
        Kresevic & Holder, 1998; Vass, Avlund, Lauridsen, & Hendriksen, 2005).
        a. Physiological and psychological value of independent functioning

(continued)

Protocol 6.1: Assessment of Physical Function *(cont.)*

  b. Reversible functional decline associated with acute illness (Hirsch et al., 1990; Sager & Rudberg, 1998)

  c. Strategies to prevent functional decline: exercise, nutrition, pain management, and socialization (Kresevic & Holder, 1998; Landefeld et al., 1995; Siegler, Glick, & Lee, 2002; Tucker, Molsberger, & Clark, 2004)

  d. Sources of assistance to manage decline

 3. Encourage activity, including routine exercise, range of motion, and ambulation to maintain activity, flexibility, and function (Counsell et al., 2000; Landefeld et al., 1995; Pedersen & Saltin, 2006).

 4. Minimize bed rest (Bates-Jensen et al., 2004; Covinsky et al., 1998; Kresevic & Holder, 1998; Landefeld et al., 1995).

 5. Explore alternatives to physical restraint use (Covinsky et al., 1998; Kresevic & Holder, 1998; see Chapter 13, Physical Retraints and Side Rails and Critical Care Settings).

 6. Judiciously use medications, especially psychoactive medications, in geriatric dosages (Inouye, Rushing, Foreman, Palmer, & Pompei, 1998; see Chapter 17, Reducing Adverse Drug Events).

 7. Assess and treat for pain (Covinsky et al., 1998).

 8. Design environments with handrails, wide doorways, raised toilet seats, shower seats, enhanced lighting, low beds, and chairs of various types and height (Cunningham & Michael, 2004; Kresevic et al., 1998).

 9. Help individuals regain baseline function after acute illnesses by using exercise, physical or occupational therapy consultation, nutrition, and coaching (Conn, Minor, Burks, Rantz, & Pomeroy, 2003; Covinsky et al., 1998; Engberg, Sereika, McDowell, Weber, & Brodak, 2002; Forbes, 2005; Hodgkinson, Evans, & Wood, 2003; Kresevic et al., 1998).

B. Strategies to help older individuals cope with functional decline

 1. Help older adults and family members determine realistic functional capacity with interdisciplinary consultation (Kresevic & Holder, 1998).

 2. Provide caregiver education and support for families of individuals when decline cannot be ameliorated in spite of nursing and rehabilitative efforts (Graf, 2006).

 3. Carefully document all intervention strategies and patient response (Graf, 2006).

 4. Provide information to caregivers on causes of functional decline related to acute and chronic conditions (Covinsky et al., 1998).

 5. Provide education to address safety care needs for falls, injuries, and common complications. Short-term skilled care for physical therapy may be needed; long-term care settings may be required to ensure safety (Covinsky et al., 1998).

 6. Provide sufficient protein and caloric intake to ensure adequate intake and prevent further decline. Liberalize diet to include personal preferences (Edington et al., 2004; Landefeld et al., 1995).

 7. Provide caregiver support and community services, such as home care, nursing, and physical and occupational therapy services to manage functional decline (Covinsky et al., 1998; Graf, 2006).

(continued)

Protocol 6.1: Assessment of Physical Function *(cont.)*

VI. EXPECTED OUTCOMES
A. Patients can
1. Maintain safe level of ADL and ambulation.
2. Make necessary adaptations to maintain safety and independence, including assistive devices and environmental adaptations.
3. Strive to attain highest quality of life despite functional level.
B. Providers can demonstrate
1. Increased assessment, identification, and management of patients susceptible to or experiencing functional decline. Routine assessment of functional capacity despite level of care.
2. Ongoing documentation and communication of capacity, interventions, goals, and outcomes.
3. Competence in preventive and restorative strategies for function.
4. Competence in assessing safe environments of care that foster safe independent function.
C. Institution will experience
1. System-wide incorporation of functional assessment into routine assessments.
2. A reduction in incidence and prevalence of functional decline.
3. A decrease in morbidity and mortality rates associated with functional decline.
4. Reduction in the use of physical restraints, prolonged bed rest, and Foley catheters.
5. Decreased incidence of delirium.
6. An increase in prevalence of patients who leave hospital with baseline or improved functional status.
7. Decreased readmission rate.
8. Increased early utilization of rehabilitative services (occupational and physical therapy).
9. Evidence of geriatric sensitive physical care environments that facilitate safe, independent function, such as caregiver educational efforts and walking programs.
10. Evidence of continued interdisciplinary assessments, care planning, and evaluation of care related to function.

VII. RELEVENT PRACTICE GUIDELINES
Several resources are now available to guide adoption of evidenced based nursing interventions to enhance function in older adults.
A. Agency for Healthcare Research and Quality & National Guideline Clearinghouse; http://www.guideline.gov/
B. McGill University Health Centre Research & Clinical Resources for Evidence Based Nursing; http://www.muhc-ebn.mcgill.ca/
C. National Quality Forum; http://www.qualityforum.org/Home.aspx
D. Registered Nurses Association of Ontario. (2005). *Clinical practice guidelines.* Retrieved from http://www.rnao.org/Page.asp?PageID=861&SiteNodeID=270&BL_ExpandID
E. University of Iowa Hartford Center of Geriatric Nursing Excellence. *Evidence-based practice guidelines.* Retrieved from http://www.nursing.uiowa.edu/hartford/nurse/ebp.htm

RESOURCES

Agency for Healthcare Research and Quality & National Guideline Clearinghouse
http://www.guideline.gov/

McGill University Health Centre Research & Research and Clinical Resources for Evidence Based Nursing
http://www.muhc-ebn.mcgill.ca/

National Quality Forum
http://www.qualityforum.org/Home.aspx

Registered Nurses Association of Ontario. *Clinical practice guidelines.*
http://www.rnao.org/Page.asp?PageID=861&SiteNodeID=270&BL_ExpandID

University of Iowa Hartford Center of Geriatric Nursing Excellence. *Evidence-based practice guidelines.*
http://www.nursing.uiowa.edu/hartford/nurse/ebp.htm

REFERENCES

Applegate, W. B., Blass, J., & Franklin, T. F. (1990). Instruments for the functional assessment of older patients. *New England Journal of Medicine, 322*(17), 1207–1214. Evidence Level IV.

Bates-Jensen, B. M., Alessi, C. A., Cadogan, M., Levy-Storms, L., Jorge, J., Yoshii, J., . . . Schnelle, J. F. (2004). The minimum data set bedfast quality indicators: Differences in nursing homes. *Nursing Research, 53*(4), 260–272. Evidence Level V.

Burton, R. M., Damon, W. W., Dillinger, D. C., Erickson, D. J., & Peterson, D. W. (1978). Nursing home rest and care: An investigation of alternatives. In E. Pfeiffer (Ed.), *Multidimensional functional assessment: The DARS methodology.* Durham, NC: Duke Center for Study of Aging Human Development. Evidence Level III.

Byles, J. E. (2000). A thorough going over: Evidence for health assessments for older persons. *Austrialian and New Zealand Journal of Public Health, 24*(2), 117–123. Evidence Level I.

Callahan, E. H., Thomas, D. C., Goldhirsh, S. L., & Leipzig, R. M. (2002). Geriatric hospital medicine. *Medical Clinics of North America, 86*(4), 707–729. Evidence Level VI.

Campbell, S. E., Seymour, D. G., Primrose, W. R., & ACMEPLUS Project. (2004). A systematic literature review of factors affecting outcome in older medical patients admitted to hospital. *Age and Ageing, 33*(2), 110–115. Evidence Level I.

Conn, V. S., Minor, M. A., Burks, K. J., Rantz, M. J., & Pomeroy, S. H. (2003). Integrative review of physical activity intervention research with aging adults. *Journal of the American Geriatrics Society, 51*(8), 1159–1168. Evidence Level I.

Counsell, S. R., Holder, C. M., Liebenauer, L. L., Palmer, R. M., Fortinsky, R. H., Kresevic, D. M., . . . Landefeld, C. S. (2000). Effects of a multicomponent intervention on functional outcomes and process of care of hospitalized older patients: A randomized controlled tiral of Acute Care for Elders (ACE) in a community hospital. *Journal of the American Geriatric Society, 48*(12), 1572–1581. Evidence Level II.

Covinsky, K. E., Palmer, R. M., Kresevic, D. M., Kahana, E., Counsell, S. R., Fortinsky, R. H., & Landefeld, C. S. (1998). Improving functional outcomes in older patients: Lessons from an acute care for elders unit. *The Joint Commission Journal on Quality Improvement, 24*(2), 63–76. Evidence Level II.

Creditor, M. C. (1993). Hazards of hospitalization of the elderly. *Annals of Internal Medicine, 118*(3), 219–223. Evidence Level VI.

Cress, M. E., Schechtman, K. B., Mulrow, C. D., Fiatarone, M. A., Gerety, M. B., & Buchner, D. M. (1995). Relationship between physical performance and self-perceived physical function. *Journal of the American Geriatrics Society, 43*(2), 93–101. Evidence Level IV.

Cunningham, G. O., & Michael, Y. L. (2004). Concepts guiding the study of the impact of the built environment on physical activity for older adults: A review of the literature. *American Journal of Health Promotion, 18*(6), 435–443. Evidence Level I.

Depp, C. A., & Jeste, D. V. (2006). Definitions and predictors of successful aging: A comprehensive review of larger quantitative studies. *American Journal of Geriatric Psychiatry, 14*(1), 6–20. Evidence Level I.

Doran, D. M., Harrison, M. B., Laschinger, H. S., Hirdes, J. P., Rukholm, E., Sidani, S., . . . Tourangeau, A. E. (2006). Nursing-sensitive outcomes data collection in acute care and long-term-care settings. *Nursing Research, 55*(Suppl. 2), S75–S81. Evidence Level VI.

Edington, J., Barnes, R., Bryan, F., Dupree, E., Frost, G., Hickson, M., . . . Coles, S. J. (2004). A prospective randomised controlled trial of nutritional supplementation in malnourished elderly in the community: Clinical and health economic outcomes. *Clinical Nutrition, 23*(2), 195–204. Evidence Level II.

Engberg, S., Sereika, S. M., McDowell, B. J., Weber, E., & Brodak, I. (2002). Effectiveness of prompted voiding in treating urinary incontinence in cognitively impaired homebound older adults. *Journal of Wound, Ostomy, and Continence Nursing, 29*(5), 252–265. Evidence Level II.

Forbes, D. A. (2005). An educational programme for primary healthcare providers improved functional abiltiy in older people living in the community. *Evidence-Based Nursing, 8*(4), 122. Evidence Level VI.

Freedman, V. A., Martin, L. G., & Schoeni R. F. (2002). Recent trends in disability and functioning among older adults in the United States: A systematic review. *Journal of the American Medical Association, 288*(24), 3137–3146. Evidence Level I.

Graf, C. (2006). Functional decline in hospitalized older adults. *American Journal of Nursing, 106*(1), 58–67. Evidence Level V.

Gurland, B. J., Cross, P., Chen, J., Wilder, D. E., Pine, Z. M., Lantigua, R. A., & Fulmer, T. (1994). A new performance test of adaptive cognitive functioning: The Medication Management (MM) test. *International Journal of Geriatric Psychiatry, 9*(11), 875–885. Evidence Level VI.

Hirsch, C. H., Sommers, L., Olsen, A., Mullen, L., & Winograd, C. H. (1990). The natural history of functional morbidity in hospitalized older patients. *Journal of the American Geriatrics Society, 38*(12), 1296–1303. Evidence Level IV.

Hodgkinson, B., Evans, D., & Wood, J. (2003). Maintaining oral hydration in older adults: A systematic review. *International Journal of Nursing Practice, 9*(3), S19–S28. Evidence Level I.

Inouye, S. K., Rushing, J. T., Foreman, M. D., Palmer, R. M., & Pompei. P. (1998). Does delirium contribute to poor hospital outcomes? A three-site epidemiologic study. *Journal of General Internal Medicine, 13*(4), 234–242. Evidence Level III.

Kane, R. A., & Kane, R. L. (Eds.). (2000). *Assessing older persons: Measures, meaning, and practical applications.* New York, NY: Oxford University Press. Evidence Level VI.

Karagiozis, H., Gray, S., Sacco, J., Shapiro, M., & Kawas C. (1998). The Direct Assessment of Functional Abilities (DAFA): A comparison to an indirect measure of instrumental activities of daily living living. *Gerontologist, 38*(1), 113–121. Evidence Level III.

Katz, S., Ford, A. B., Moskowitz, R. W., Jackson, B. A., & Jaffe, M. W. (1963). Studies of illness and the aged. The index of ADL: A standardized measure of biological and psychosocial function. *Journal of the American Medical Association, 185*, 914–919. Evidence Level I.

Kresevic, D. M., Counsell, S. R., Covinsky, K., Palmer, R., Landefeld, C. S., Holder, C., & Beeler, J. (1998). A patient-centered model of acute care for elders. *Nursing Clinics of North America, 33*(3), 515–527. Evidence Level VI.

Kresevic, D., & Holder, C. (1998). Interdisciplinary care. *Clinics in Geriatric Medicine, 14*(4), 787–798. Evidence Level VI.

Kruianski, J., & Gurland, B. (1976). The performance test of activities of daily living. *International Journal of Aging & Human Development, 7*(4), 343–352. Evidence Level VI.

Landefeld, C. S., Palmer, R. M., Kresevic, D. M., Fortinsky, R. H., & Kowal, J. (1995). A random-ized trial of care in a hospital medical unit especially designed to improve the functional out-comes of acutely ill older patients. *The New England Journal of Medicine, 332*(20), 1338–1344. Evidence Level II.

Lawton, M. P., & Brody, E. M. (1969). Assessment of older people: Self-maintaining and instrumen-tal activities of daily living. *Gerontologist, 9*(3), 179–186. Evidence Level IV.

Lightbody, E., & Baldwin, R. (2002). Inpatient geriatric evaluation and management did not reduce mortality but reduced functional decline. *Evidence-Based Mental Health, 5*(4), 109. Evidence Level VI.

Mahoney, F. I., & Barthel, D. W. (1965). Functional evaluation: The Barthel index. *Maryland State Medical Journal, 14*, 61–65. Evidence Level III.

Mathias, S., Nayak, U. S., & Isaacs, B. (1986). Balance in elderly patients: The "get-up and go" test. *Archives of Physical Medicine and Rehabilitation, 67*(6), 387–389. Evidence Level VI.

McCusker, J., Kakuma, R., & Abrahamowicz, M. (2002). Predictors of functional hospitalized elderly patients: A systematic review. *Journals of Geronotology. Series A, Biological Sciences and Medical Sciences, 57*(9), M569–M577. Evidence Level I.

Mezey, M. D., Rauckhorst, L. H., & Stokes, S. A. (1993). *Health assessment of the older individual.* New York, NY: Springer Publishing. Evidence Level VI.

Palmer, R. M., Counsell, S., & Landefeld, C. S. (1998). Clinical interventions trials: The ACE unit. *Clinics in Geriatric Medicine, 14*(4), 831–849. Evidence Level I.

Pearson, V. I. (2000). Assessment of function in older adults. In R. I. Kane & R. A. Kane (Eds.), *Assessing older persons: Measures, meanings and practical applications* (pp. 17–34). New York, NY: Oxford University Press. Evidence Level VI.

Pedersen, B. K., & Saltin, B. (2006). Evidence for prescribing exercise as therapy in chronic disease. *Scandinavian Journal of Medicine & Science in Sports, 16*(Suppl. 1), 3–63. Evidence Level I.

Sager, M. A., & Rudberg, M. A. (1998). Functional decline associated with hospitalization for acute illness. *Clinics in Geriatric Medicine, 14*(4), 669–679. Evidence Level II.

Siegler, E. L., Glick, D., & Lee, J. (2002). Optimal staffing for Acute Care of the Elderly (ACE) units. *Geriatric Nursing, 23*(3), 152–155. Evidence Level VI.

Tinetti, M. E., & Ginter, S. F. (1998). Identifying mobility dysfunctions in elderly patients. Standard neuromuscular examination or direct assessment? *Journal of the American Medical Association, 259*(8), 1190–1193. Evidence Level I.

Tucker, D., Molsberger, S. C., & Clark, A. (2004). Walking for wellness: A collaborative program to maintain mobility in hospitalized older adults. *Geriatric Nursing, 25*(4), 242–245. Evidence Level VI.

Vass, M., Avlund, K., Lauridsen, J., & Hendriksen, C. (2005). Feasible model for prevention of functional decline in older people: Municipality-randomized, controlled trial. *Journal of the American Geriatrics Society, 53*(4), 563–568. Evidence Level II.

Woolf, S. H. (1990). Screening for hearing impairment. In R. B. Goldbloom & R. S. Lawrence (Eds.), *Preventing disease: Beyond the rhetoric* (pp. 331–346). New York, NY: Springer-Verlag. Evidence Level VI.

7

Interventions to Prevent Functional Decline in the Acute Care Setting

Marie Boltz, Barbara Resnick, and Elizabeth Galik

EDUCATIONAL OBJECTIVES

On completion of this chapter, the reader should be able to:

1. discuss the functional trajectory of the hospitalized older adult
2. identify risk factors for functional decline
3. describe the influence of the care environment upon physical function
4. discuss interventions to optimize physical function of hospitalized older adults

OVERVIEW

As described in Chapter 6, Assessment of Function, functional decline is a common complication in hospitalized older adults, even in those with good baseline function (Gill, Allore, Gahbauer, & Murphy, 2010). Loss of physical function is associated with poor long-term outcomes, including increased likelihood of being discharged to a nursing home setting (Fortinsky, Covinsky, Palmer, & Landefeld, 1999), increased morbidity and mortality (Boyd, Xue, Guralnik, & Fried, 2005; Rozzini et al., 2005), increased rehabilitation costs, and decreased functional recovery (Boyd et al., 2008; Boyd et al., 2005; Gill, Allore, Holford, & Guo, 2004; Volpato et al., 2007). The immobility associated with functional decline results in infections, pressure ulcers, falls, a persistent decline in function and physical activity and nonelective rehospitalizations (Gill et al., 2004).

The promotion of function is a basic gerontological tenet, and functional status is a key determinant of quality of life for older adults (Boltz, Capezuti, Shabbat, & Hall, 2010). Although the acute care setting, with its focus on correcting the admitting medical problem, typically prioritizes nursing tasks such as medication administration, coordination of care, and documentation over the promotion of function as a clinical outcome, there is growing awareness of the need to attend to the functional status of the hospitalized older adult (Nolan & Thomas, 2008). Older adults themselves expect that an acute care

For description of Evidence Levels cited in this chapter, see Chapter 1, Developing and Evaluating Clinical Practice Guidelines: A Systematic Approach, page 7.

stay will not result in functional decline but instead lead to the resumption of normal roles and activities posthospitalization (Boltz, Capezuti, Shabbat, & Hall, 2010). This chapter addresses the trajectory of change in physical function during the acute care stay, the factors associated with functional decline, and function-promoting interventions that can potentially modify these factors. Finally, a clinical practice protocol to guide a unit-level approach to function-focused care (Protocol 7.1: Protocol for FFC) is provided.

BACKGROUND AND STATEMENT OF PROBLEM

Physical Function as a Clinical Measure

Functional decline may result from the acute illness and can begin preadmission (Fortinsky et al., 1999) and continue after discharge (Sager et al., 1996). In a large prospective observational study, Covinsky and colleagues (2003) evaluated the changes in performance of activities of daily living (ADL) function prior to and posthospitalizations of older adults with medical illness. Over one third declined in ADL function between baseline (2 weeks before admission) and discharge. This included the 23% of patients who declined between baseline and admission and failed to recover to baseline function between admission and discharge, and the 12% of patients who did not decline between baseline and admission but declined between hospital admission and discharge. Older adults age 85 and older comprised the age cohort demonstrating the most functional loss, with rates exceeding 50%.

In their examination of the functional trajectory of hospitalized older adults, Wakefield and Holman (2007) also assessed function at baseline, as well as upon admission and Day 4. The largest change in functional status was a decline in ADL from baseline to the time of admission; ADL did not return to baseline during the first 4 days in the hospital. The older adults whose ADL scores declined during hospitalization (regardless of baseline status) were more likely than others to die within 3 months of discharge.

The results of these studies demonstrate that ADL status is unstable in large percentage of older adults. Consequently, Covinsky et al. (2003) suggest that an older adult's functional trajectory is a critical "vital sign," an important prognostic marker, and an indicator to guide care delivery and transitional care. Baseline function may serve as a useful benchmark when developing discharge goals. Older adults who have sustained loss of ADL function prior to admission would ideally have rehabilitation as a goal of their hospital care. For those patients who have acquired ADL disability from admission to discharge, aggressive post-acute rehabilitation plans could be mobilized with the goal of preventing disability.

Patient Risk Factors for Functional Decline

Intrinsic vulnerabilities to functional decline include prehospitalization functional status, the presence of two or more comorbidities, taking five or more prescription medications, and having had a hospitalization or emergency room visit in the previous 12 months (McCusker, Kakuma, & Abrahamowicz, 2002). Depression scores are associated with ADL decline before admission (Covinsky, Fortinsky, Palmer, Kresevic, & Landefeld, 1997). Symptoms of depression during hospitalization have also been associated with dependence in basic ADL at discharge and 30 and 90 days after discharge (Covinsky et al., 1997).

The association between functional status and cognitive status must also be considered (Inouye, Schlesinger, & Lydon, 1999). Cognitive impairment, including delirium, increases the risk of functional decline in the older adults during and after hospitalization

(McCusker et al., 2002). A study of 2,557 patients from two teaching hospitals examined the association between performance on a cognitive status screen and maintenance and recovery of functioning from admission to discharge (Narain et al., 1988). Among patients who needed help performing one or more ADLs at the time of admission, 23% had moderate-to-severe cognitive impairment, 49% had mild impairment, and 67% had little or no impairment in cognitive performance recovered the ability to independently execute an additional ADL by discharge ($p < 0.001$; Narain et al., 1988).

Pain (Reid, Williams, & Gill, 2005), nutritional problems, and adverse medication effects also contribute to functional decline (Graf, 2006). Fear of falling (Boltz, Capezuti, & Shabbat, 2010; Boltz, Capezuti, Shabbat, & Hall, 2010), self-efficacy, and outcome expectations (McAuley et al., 2006; Resnick, 2002), attitudes towards functional independence, and views on hospitalization (Boltz, Capezuti, & Shabbat, 2010; Boltz, Capezuti, Shabbat, & Hall, 2010; Brown, Williams, Woodby, Davis, & Allman, 2007) influence the level of engagement in physical activity and mobility in older adults in general and thus may influence acute care functional outcomes.

ASSESSMENT OF THE PROBLEM

A social ecological perspective assumes that the physical, social, and organizational environment contribute to patient outcomes (Moos, 1979; Stokols, 1992), including functional measures (Galik, 2010). The hospital environment, with its emphasis on biomedical interventions for acute medical and surgical problems is challenged to "fit" the complex physical, social, and psychological circumstances, which predisposes the hospitalized older adult to functional decline. Parke and Chappell (2010) recommend that the older adult hospital environment fit be viewed through four dimensions: care systems and processes, social climate, policy and procedure, and physical design.

Hospital Care Systems and Processes

Hospitalization is associated with significantly greater loss of total, lean, and fat mass and strength in older persons. These effects appear particularly important in persons hospitalized for 8 or more days per year (Alley et al., 2010). Hospitalization itself may also pose risks for functional decline due to the deleterious effects of bed rest and restricted activity (Gill, Allore, & Guo, 2004). Bed rest results in loss of muscle strength and lean muscle mass (Kortebein, Ferrando, Lombeida, Wolfe, & Evans, 2007; Kortebein et al., 2008), decreased aerobic capacity (Kortebein et al., 2008), diminished pulmonary ventilation, altered sensory awareness, reduced appetite and thirst, and decreased plasma volume (Creditor, 1993; Harper & Lyles, 1988; Hoenig & Rubenstein, 1991). Brown, Redden, Flood, and Allman (2009) describe bed rest and low mobility as an "underrecognized epidemic." In their study of hospitalized older veterans, they used accelerometers to measure activity level. Despite the fact that most were able to walk independently (78%), 83% of the measured hospital stay was spent lying in bed (Brown et al., 2009).

Another study (Brown, Friedkin, & Inouye, 2004) that evaluated the outcomes associated with mobility level found that 66 (83%) were on complete bed rest for at least 24 hours during hospitalization. Almost 60% of the observations had no documented medical reason for the bed rest. Physician's orders for bed rest were present on the date of bed rest for only 92 (52%) of the 176 observations. Low mobility (defined as having an average mobility level of bed rest or bed to chair for the entire hospitalization) was compared with high mobility (ambulation two or more times with partial or no assistance, on average). The low mobility group had a statistically significant higher rate of ADL decline, new institutionalization, and death. Similarly, Zisberg and colleagues (2011) found that low versus high in-hospital mobility was associated with worse functional status at discharge and at 1-month follow-up, even in older adults who were functionally stable prior to admission.

Also indicative of the low priority placed upon mobility promotion is the common process of restricting the patients' ability to walk to tests and procedures within the hospital. Other care processes associated with immobility include physical restraints and "tethering devices" such as catheters, intravenous (IV) lines, and medications that contribute to delirium and/or cause sedation (Boltz, Capezuti, & Shabbat, 2010; Graf, 2006; King, 2006). Additionally, there is a tendency for staff to perform ADLs for patients that could participate or do it for themselves, placing older adults at risk for loss of self-care ability (Boltz, Capezuti, & Shabbat, 2010). This "doing for," as opposed to promoting functional independence, is often associated with a lack of understanding of the patient's underlying capability. Interdisciplinary rounds support a functional approach, with the goal of preventing functional decline and discharging the older adult to the least restrictive setting (McVey, Becker, Saltz, Feussner, & Cohen, 1989). Key elements to be addressed include functional assessment (baseline, admission, and current ADL status, as well as physical capability), alternatives to the use of potentially restrictive devices and agents, and a plan for progressive mobility and engagement in ADL (McVey et al., 1989).

Social Climate

Leadership commitment to rehabilitative values is essential to support a social climate conducive to the promotion of function (Boltz, Capezuti, & Shabbat, 2010; Resnick, 2004). Older adults have identified that respectful, encouraging communication and engagement in decision making as important to facilitating independence (Boltz, Capezuti, Shabbat, & Hall, 2010; Jacelon, 2004). Staff education that addresses the physiology, manifestations, and prevention of hospital-acquired deconditioning; assessment of physical capability; rehabilitative techniques and use of adaptive equipment; interdisciplinary collaboration; and communication that motivates are associated with a function-promoting philosophy (Boltz, Capezuti, & Shabbat, 2010; Jacelon, 2004; Gillis, MacDonald, & MacIsaac, 2008; Weitzel & Robinson, 2004). Nursing staff have also described the need for well-defined roles, including areas of accountability for follow-through for function-promoting activities (Jacelon, 2004; Resnick, et al., 2011). Clear communication of patient needs among staff and dissemination of data (e.g., compliance with treatment plans and functional outcomes) also support these activities (Boltz, Capezuti, & Shabbat, 2010).

Policy and Procedure

Policies that clearly define staff roles in assessing physical function and cognition and implementing interventions are foundational to implement function-promoting care (Boltz, Capezuti, & Shabbat, 2010). Additionally, protocols that minimize adverse effects of selected procedures (e.g., urinary catheterization) and medications (e.g., sedative-hypnotic agents) contribute to positive functional outcomes (Kleinpell, 2007). Other supporting policies address identification and storage of sensory devices (e.g., glasses, hearing aids/amplifiers) and mobility and other assistive devices (St. Pierre, 1998).

Physical Design

Acute care environments directly impact patient function and physical activity. The bed is often the only accessible furniture in the room and the height of toilets, beds, and available chairs does not always fall within the range in which transfers and function are optimized (Capezuti et al., 2008). Accessible functional seating and safe walking areas with relevant destination areas promote functional mobility. Adequate lighting, nonglare flooring, door levers, and hand rails (including in the patient room) are basic requirements to promote safe mobility (Gulwadi & Calkins, 2008; Ulrich et al., 2008). Environmental enhancements to promote orientation include large-print calendars and clocks (Kleinpell, 2007) and control of ambient noise levels, especially in critical care units (Gabor et al., 2003).

In addition to the environment in general, it is important to consider person–environment (P–E) fit. P–E Fit can be measured using the Housing Enabler instrument (Iwarsson, 1999), which includes an assessment of the patient's functional limitations, dependence on mobility devices, and a detailed assessment of environmental barriers to engaging in functional activities. Assessments include a focus on the outdoor environment, entrances, indoor environment, and communication features (e.g., signage) of a community. For each environmental barrier item, the instrument comprises predefined severity ratings and is scored from 1 (*potential accessibility problem*) to 4 (*very severe accessibility problem*). The assessment of the individuals' limitations is matched with the environment and a score calculated using Housing Enabler software. Higher scores are indicative of a less desirable P–E fit. Areas of concern can then be altered to improve the fit between the individual and the environment to optimize function (Iwarsson, 1999).

INTERVENTIONS AND CARE STRATEGIES

Support for Cognition

Cognition and physical function are closely linked in older adults. The ability to engage in ADL and physical activity requires varying types and degrees of cognitive capability, including memory, executive function, and visuospatial ability. Therefore, an appraisal of the older adult's cognition (baseline, admission, and ongoing) is an essential activity associated with promoting physical function (see Chapter 8, Assessing Cognitive Function) in order to develop, implement, and evaluate a plan to promote maximum physical functioning (Coelho, Santos-Galduroz, Gobbi, & Stella, 2009; Yu, Kolanowski, Strumpf, & Eslinger, 2006).

Interventions to prevent, detect, and manage delirium are associated with improved cognition and, thus, are integral components of a plan to prevent functional decline (Foreman, Wakefield, Culp, & Milisen, 2001). Liberal visiting hours and familiar items brought in from home (e.g., photos, blanket) provide meaningful sensory input and along with control of excessive noise and attention to sleep hygiene enhance function-promoting interventions (Galik et al., 2008; Landefeld, Palmer, Kresevic, Fortinsky, & Kowal, 1995). Diversional activities such as TV, movies, and word games are associated with "keeping the mind active" and engagement in self-care and physical activity (Boltz, Capezuti, Shabbat, & Hall, 2010). For patients with cognitive challenges, including dementia, activity kits that include tactile, auditory, and visual items enhance cognitive integration, perceptual processing, and neuromuscular strength as well as provide solace and an opportunity for emotional expression and relief of boredom (Kresevic & Holder, 1998). Activity kits can include a wide range of items such as audiotapes and nontoxic art supplies. In addition, items such as pieces of textured fabric, cloth to fold, tools, and key and lock boards, are included for the person with more advanced dementia (Conedera & Mitchell, 2010; Glantz & Richman, 2007). For more information, see Chapter 11, Delirium.

Older adults with cognitive impairment can benefit from function-promoting interventions with demonstrated improvements in mood and behavior (Galik et al., 2008). Galik, Resnick, and Pretzer-Aboff (2009), in their work with nursing assistants, identified critical factors associated with successfully engaging persons with cognitive impairment in restorative care activities. An understanding of the person's values, past experiences, and relationships supports meaningful communication to motivate them, along with the use of humor and verbal cues. In addition, teamwork with other nursing staff, rehabilitative staff, medical providers, and families was considered a key component in facilitating self-care and physical activity (Galik et al., 2009).

In addition, adapted communication techniques are necessary to accommodate receptive difficulties associated with cognitive impairment, including dementia. The ability to participate in ADLs is often more preserved than clinicians believe because activities like washing face, brushing teeth, and walking rely on psychomotor memory that is preserved even in those with moderate to severe cognitive impairment. Communicating with short simple verbal requests and visual cues and modeling the activity can be helpful in promoting independence in ADLs. (For example, assist the person to the sink, set them up to brush teeth, hand them tooth brush, and model the behavior; Galik et al., 2008; Galik et al., 2009.)

Physical Therapy and Exercise

Interventions such as implementation of physical therapy and individualized, targeted exercise programs as soon as possible postadmission have all been tested as ways in which to increase physical activity and prevent deconditioning and functional decline in hospitalized older adults. A single-blinded randomized controlled trial was conducted in a tertiary metropolitan hospital involving 180 acute general medical patients aged 65 years and older(Jones, Lowe, MacGregor, & Brand, 2006). In addition to usual physiotherapy care, the intervention group performed an exercise program for 30 minutes twice daily, with supervision and assistance provided by an allied health assistant (AHA). In older adults with low admission ADL scores (modified Barthel Index score lower than 48), there was improvement in function among individuals exposed to the exercise interventions versus those who were not (Jones et al., 2006). Similarly, an individually tailored exercise program to maintain functional mobility, prescribed and progressed by a physical therapist and supervised by an AHA, provided in addition to usual physiotherapy care was associated with reduced likelihood of referral for nursing home admissions (Nolan & Thomas, 2008). Despite the known benefit of staying engaged in function and physical activity when hospitalized a 2007 Cochrane review (de Morton, Keating, & Jeffs, 2007) concluded that, in general, patient participation in these programs has been poor. Challenges to feasibility and implementation of these interventions included competing care demands (e.g., test schedules), illness severity, short hospital stays, a general unwillingness of patients to consent to or actively participate in exercise interventions, and a persistent belief among patients that bed rest will assure recovery (Brown, Peel, Bamman, & Allman, 2006; de Morton, Keating, Berlowitz, Jackson, & Lim, 2007; de Morton et al., 2007).

Functional Mobility Programs

One of the most common forms of physical activity encouraged in acute care settings are functional mobility programs. Mobility is conceptualized as a continuum progressing from bedbound to independent walking (Callen, Mahoney, Wells, Enloe, & Hughes, 2004). The benefits of interventions aimed at promoting functional mobility have recently received growing attention. Tucker, Molsberger, and Clark (2004) demonstrated the feasibility of a "Walking for Wellness" program comprised of a patient education program, a screening process to identify patients who would benefit from physical therapy daily walking assistance from cross-trained transportation staff. Walking opportunities included "walking trails" marked inside the hospital, with markers placed every 10 ft at the baseboard of the hallways provided a measure of walking distance as well as a visual incentive for patients walking in the halls. Unless otherwise indicated by the medical provider, the goal for participants was to walk in the hallways two to three times a day with trained escorts, nursing staff, family, or friends. Weitzel and Robinson (2004) developed an educational program for nursing assistants on a medical unit that emphasized promoting the functional status of hospitalized older adults. Content included therapeutic communication, promotion of functional mobility, skin care, and eating/feeding problems. Discharge destination (home or nursing home) and length of stay were compared for patients preimplementation and postimplementation. There was a significant reduction on length of stay (2.4 days) and increase in the percentage of patients discharged to the home setting (Weitzel & Robinson, 2004).

The positive association between mobility and shorter length of stay was also supported on the Acute Care for Elderly (ACE) unit, where ambulation was measured by a step monitor (Fisher et al., 2011). Patients on the ACE unit who had shorter stays tended to ambulate more on the first complete day of hospitalization and had a markedly greater increase in mobility on the second day than patients with longer length of stay. There were no significant differences in mean daily steps according to illness severity or reason for admission.

To address motivational issues, Mudge and colleagues (2008) evaluated a functional mobility program enhanced with cognitive interventions. This research team used an individualized, graduated exercise, and mobility program with an activity diary, progressive encouragement of functional independence by nursing staff and other members of the multidisciplinary team, and cognitive stimulation sessions in older adults age 70 and older on a medical unit. The intervention group had greater improvement in functional status than the control group, with a median modified Barthel Index improvement of 8.5 versus 3.5 points ($p = .03$). In the intervention group, there was a reduction in delirium (19.4% vs. 35.5%, $p = .04$) and a trend to reduced falls (4.8% vs. 11.3%, $p = .19$).

In patients recovering from hip surgery, functional mobility programs are enhanced with measures to prevent postoperative complications. Siu, Penrod, et al. (2006) and Siu, Boockvar, et al. (2006) found that positive processes related to mobilization (including time from admission to surgery, mobilization to and beyond the chair, use of anticoagulants and prophylactic antibiotics, pain control, physical therapy, catheter and restraint use, and active clinical issues) were associated with improved locomotion and self-care at 2 months postdischarge. Patients who experienced no hospital complications and no readmissions retained benefits in locomotion at 6 months. Olsson, Karlsson, and Ekman (2007) demonstrated that interventions focused on skin care, pain control, and progressive ambulation yielded improved functional discharge outcomes.

Critical Care Initiatives to Prevent Functional Decline

The geriatric imperative to support physical function has also been recognized in critical care, and studies are emerging that examine mobility promotion in the critically ill patient, including older adults. A study conducted in a respiratory intensive care unit (RICU) examined the feasibility of early mobility as well as its safety in six activity-related adverse events: fall to knees, tube removal, systolic blood pressure higher than 200 mm Hg, systolic blood pressure lower than 90 mm Hg, oxygen desaturation less than 80%, and extubation. There were less than 1% activity-related adverse events; most survivors (69%) were able to ambulate farther than 100 ft at RICU discharges (Bailey et al., 2007).

Similarly, a mobility team (critical care nurse, nursing assistant, and physical therapist) in a medical intensive care unit (ICU) initiated a mobility protocol for patients with acute respiratory failure. The protocol consisted of progressive mobility interventions ranging from passive range of motion for unconscious patients, to active assistive and active range of motion exercise, to functional activities such as transfer to edge of bed; safe transfers to and from bed, chair, or commode; seated balance activities; pregait standing activities (forward and lateral weight shifting, marching in place); and ambulation. As compared to usual care (passive range of motion only), protocol patients were out of bed earlier (5 vs. 11 days, $p \leq .001$), had therapy initiated more frequently in the ICU (91% vs. 13%, $p \leq .001$), and had similar low complication rates. For protocol patients, ICU length of stay was 5.5 vs. 6.9 days for usual care ($p = .025$); hospital length of stay for protocol patients was 11.2 versus 14.5 days for usual care ($p = .006$). (The ICU/hospital length of stay adjusted for body mass index, Acute Physiology, and Chronic Health Evaluation II, and use of a vasopressor.) There were no adverse events during an ICU mobility session and no cost difference between the protocol and usual care costs (Morris et al., 2008).

Function-Focused Care: A Multimodal Intervention

Function-focused care (FFC) is a comprehensive, system–level approach that prioritizes the preservation and restoration of functional capability. It is predicated on the philosophy that physical function is as important a treatment goal as correcting the acute admitting problem and recognizing the multifactorial nature of functional decline (Jacelon, 2004). FFC, previously referred to as *restorative care* from its use in long-term care (Resnick, Gruber-Baldini, et al., 2009; Resnick & Simpson, 2003; Resnick, Rogers, Galik, & Gruber-Baldini, 2007), uses a philosophy of care in which nurses acknowledge older adults' physical and cognitive capabilities with regard to function and integrate functional and physical activities into all care interactions. The components of FFC are

- assessment of Environment and Policy/Procedures for Function and Physical Activity;
- education of nursing staff and other members of the interdisciplinary team (e.g., social work, physical therapy) on rehabilitative techniques (Resnick, Cayo, Galik, & Pretzer-Aboff, 2009);
- education of patients and families regarding FFC;
- establishing FFC goals, including discharge goals based on capability assessments, communication with other members of the team (e.g., medicine, physical therapy), and input from patients;
- addressing risk factors that impact goal achievement (e. g., cognitive status, anemia, nutritional status, pain, fear of falling, fatigue, medications and drug side

effects such as somnolence) by the interdisciplinary team to optimize patient participation in functional and physical activity; and

■ mentoring and motivating provided by a nurse change agent (e.g., geriatric resource nurse) using theoretically based interventions for monitoring and motivating the nursing staff to provide FFC and thereby help the nurses to motivate patients to engage in functional and physical activity.

When implemented in long-term care settings, FFC interventions increased nursing knowledge of beliefs in and observed performance of FFC and resulted in improvements in function (ambulation, gait, and balance) and physical activity in nursing home and assisted-living residents and decreased transfers from nursing homes to acute care settings (Resnick, Gruber-Baldini, et al., 2009; Resnick & Simpson, 2003; Resnick et al., 2007). Additionally, Resnick and colleagues (2011) demonstrated that nurses were willing to be engaged in a FFC educational intervention on medical–surgical units and showed improvements in knowledge and outcome expectations associated with FFC. FFC interactions between patient and nurses have also demonstrated an association with a decrease in the overall loss of ADL function from baseline to discharge (Boyd, Capezuti, & Shabbat, in press).

CASE STUDY

TS is an 80-year-old man who was admitted from an assisted living to the Emergency Department after he was found on the floor. His workup is negative for fractures and head trauma. His admitting diagnoses include pneumonia, anemia, and dehydration. His past medical history, per his daughter's report, is remarkable for mild hypertension, treated with hydrochlorothiazide (HCTZ) and captopril, and dementia. Upon admission to the floor, TS was somnolent but able to respond to his name. He is receiving IV antibiotics and hydration. The IV site is "camouflaged" with kling and covered with his sweater so as to not cue him to remove it.

The admitting nurse learns from TS's daughter and the staff at the assisted-living facility that TS's normal or baseline function is that he is independent in ambulation, continent, (although at times has trouble wayfinding), and needs verbal cues ("prompting") to get dressed and bathe. After hydration, TS becomes more alert. He is able to respond to one-step commands and is moving all extremities, with good range of motion. The interdisciplinary team makes rounds that afternoon and develops the following plan:

■ Monitor confusion assessment method (CAM) and mental status when able to respond

■ Daughter to bring in familiar robe, shoes, and family photo; she also plans to complete social profile "all about me" to be shared with hospital staff.

■ Glasses were labeled with his name and placed on TS.

■ No restraints; adjustable height low bed, in low position, then adjusted to lower leg length to promote safe transfers.

■ Switch to oral antibiotics; cap IV when able to take sufficient fluids by mouth.

■ Assist out of bed for meals, starting that evening.

■ In AM, attempt to ambulate to bathroom; not to be left unattended. Ambulate as tolerated in room, progress to hallway ambulation three times a day.

(continued)

CASE STUDY *(continued)*

- Pressure reducing mattress.
- Assist, cue, and redirect as needed during meal; monitor for aspiration.
- Encourage self-care during bathing; cue as needed.
- Anemia workup.
- Plan to discharge back to assisted living at baseline level of function; estimated discharge in 48–72 hours.

Discussion

The case study demonstrates decision making that recognizes the potential of TS to return to his baseline physical function. The interdisciplinary team implements measures to correct his delirium and prevent avoidable complications (falls and pressure ulcers) that could negatively impact his function. The plan to promote physical activity and independence in ADL is adapted to his cognitive impairment. His daughter is engaged in his care and the nurse leverages this support to benefit TS.

SUMMARY

Hospitalization poses many challenges to the functional health of older adults. However, functional decline is not inevitable. Interventions formerly perceived to be relevant only for the rehabilitation setting are slowly being recognized as integral to the care and treatment of the older adult in the acute setting. Function-focused care employs nursing care practices that acknowledge the older person's capabilities and potential while positively modifying the care environment to prevent avoidable functional decline.

NURSING STANDARD OF PRACTICE

Protocol 7.1: Function-Focused Care (FFC) Interventions

I. GOAL: The following protocol has been designed to help nurses collaborate with the interdisciplinary team to implement interventions that maximize the older adult's functional abilities and performance. This protocol can be used in combination with Chapter 6, Assessment of Physical Function.

II. OBJECTIVE: As stated in Chapter 3, to restore or maximize physical functioning, prevent or minimize decline in ADL function, and plan for transitions of care.

III. BACKGROUND
  A. Functional decline is a common complication in hospitalized older adults, even in those with good baseline function (Gill et al., 2010).

(continued)

Protocol 7.1: Function-Focused Care (FFC) Interventions *(cont.)*

B. Loss of physical function is associated with poor long-term outcomes, including increased likelihood of being discharged to a nursing home setting (Fortinsky et al., 1999), increased mortality (Boyd et al., 2005; Rozzini et al, 2005), increased rehabilitation costs, and decreased functional recovery (Boyd et al., 2008; Boyd et al., 2005; Gill et al., 2004; Volpato et al., 2007). The immobility associated with functional decline results in infections, pressure ulcers, falls, a persistent decline in function and physical activity, and nonelective rehospitalizations (Gill et al., 2004).

C. Functional decline may result from the acute illness and can begin preadmission (Fortinsky et al., 1999) and continue after discharge (Sager et al., 1996). Baseline function serves as a useful benchmark when developing discharge goals (Covinsky et al., 2003; Fortinsky et al., 1999; Sager et al., 1996; Wakefield & Holman, 2007).

D. Patient risk factors for functional decline include prehospitalization functional loss; the presence of two or more comorbidities; taking five or more prescription medications; having had a hospitalization or emergency room visit in the previous 12 months (McCusker et al., 2002); depression (Covinsky et al., 1997); impaired cognition, including delirium (Inouye et al., 1999; Narain et al., 1988); pain (Reid et al., 2005); nutritional problems; adverse medication effects (Graf, 2006); fear of falling (Boltz, Capezuti, & Shabbat, 2010); low self-efficacy and outcome expectations (McAuley et al., 2006; Resnick, 2002); and attitudes toward functional independence and views on hospitalization (Boyd, Capezuti, & Shabbat, 2010; Boltz, Capezuti, Shabbat, & Hall, 2010; Brown et al., 2007).

E. Bed rest results in loss of muscle strength and lean muscle mass (Kortebein et al., 2007; Kortebein et al., 2008), decreased aerobic capacity (Kortebein et al., 2008), diminished pulmonary ventilation, altered sensory awareness, reduced appetite and thirst, and decreased plasma volume (Creditor, 1993; Harper et al., 1988; Hoenig & Rubenstein, 1991). Care processes that curtail mobility such as the use of restraints and tethering devices (Boltz, Capezuti, & Shabbat, 2010; Graf, 2006; King, 2006) are associated with low mobility, higher rate of ADL decline (Brown et al, 2004; Zisberg et al., 2011), new institutionalization, and death (Brown et al., 2004).

F. Interdisciplinary rounds support promotion of function by addressing functional assessment (baseline and current), evaluate potentially restrictive devices and agents, and yield a plan for progressive mobility (McVey et al., 1989).

G. Leadership commitment to rehabilitative values is essential to support a social climate conducive to the promotion of function (Boltz, Capezuti, & Shabbat, 2010; Resnick, 2004).

H. FFC educational intervention on medical–surgical units have shown improvements in knowledge and outcome expectations associated with function-promoting care (Resnick et al., 2011).

IV. FUNCTION-FOCUSED CARE INTERVENTIONS
A. Hospital care systems and processes
  1. Evaluation of leadership commitment to rehabilitative values (Boltz, Capezuti, & Shabbat, 2010; Resnick, 2004).

(continued)

Protocol 7.1: Function-Focused Care (FFC) Interventions *(cont.)*

2. Interdisciplinary rounds that address functional assessment (baseline and current), evaluate potentially restrictive devices and agents, and yield a plan for progressive mobility (McVey et al., 1989).
3. Well-defined roles, including areas of accountability for assessment and follow-through for function-promoting activities (Jacelon, 2004; Resnick et al., 2011).
4. Method of evaluating communication of patient needs among staff (Boyd, Capezuti, & Shabbat, 2010).
5. Process of disseminating data (e.g., compliance with treatment plans and functional outcomes; Boyd, Capezuti, & Shabbat, 2010).

B. Policy and procedures to support function promotion
1. Protocols that minimize adverse effects of selected procedures (e.g., urinary catheterization) and medications (e.g., sedative-hypnotic agents) contribute to positive functional outcomes (Kleinpell, 2007).
2. Supporting policies: identification and storage of sensory (e.g., glasses, hearing aids/amplifiers) and mobility devices and other assistive devices (Boyd, Capezuti, & Shabbat, 2010; St. Pierre, 1998).
3. Discharge policies that address the continuous plan for function promotion (Boyd, Capezuti, & Shabbat, 2010; Boyd, Capezuti, Shabbat, & Hall, 2010)

C. Physical design
1. Toilets, beds, and chairs at appropriate height to promote safe transfers and function (Capezuti et al., 2008).
2. Functional and accessible furniture and safe walking areas with relevant/interesting destination areas (Gulwadi & Calkins, 2008; Ulrich et al., 2008) and with distance markers (Callen et al., 2004).
3. Adequate lighting, nonglare flooring, door levers, and hand rails (including in the patient room; Gulwadi & Calkins, 2008; Ulrich et al., 2008).
4. Large-print calendars and clocks to promote orientation (Kleinpell, 2007).
5. Control of ambient noise levels (Gabor et al., 2003).

D. Education of nursing staff, and other members of the interdisciplinary team (e.g., social work, physical therapy), regarding
1. the physiology, manifestations, and prevention of hospital-acquired deconditioning (Boyd, Capezuti, & Shabbat, 2010; Gillis et al., 2008; Resnick et al., 2011; Weitzel & Robinson, 2004);
2. assessment of physical capability (Resnick, Cayo et al., 2009; Resnick et al., 2011);
3. rehabilitative techniques and use of adaptive equipment (Weitzel & Robinson, 2004; Resnick et al., 2011; Resnick, Cayo et al., 2009);
4. interdisciplinary collaboration (Resnick et al., 2011; Resnick, Cayo et al., 2009);
5. engagement in decision making (Boltz, Capezuti, & Shabbat, 2010; Boltz, Capezuti, Shabbat, & Hall, 2010; Jacelon, 2004); and
6. communication that motivates are associated with a function-promoting philosophy (Boltz, Capezuti, & Shabbat, 2010; Gillis et al., 2008; Jacelon, 2004; Weitzel & Robinson, 2004).

(continued)

Protocol 7.1: Function-Focused Care (FFC) Interventions *(cont.)*

E. Education of patients and families regarding FFC (Resnick, Cayo, et al., 2009), including the benefits of FFC, the safe use of equipment, and self-advocacy (Boltz, Capezuti, Shabbat & Hall, 2010)

F. Clinical Assessment and interventions
   1. Assessment of physical function and capability (baseline, at admission and daily) and cognition (at a minimum daily; Boltz, Capezuti, & Shabbat, 2010; Covinsky et al., 2003; Fortinsky et al., 1999; Sager et al., 1996; Wakefield & Holman, 2007).
   2. Establishing functional goals based on assessments and communication with other members of the team and input from patients (Resnick, Cayo, et al., 2009; Resnick et al., 2011; Resnick, Gruber-Baldini, et al., 2009; Resnick et al., 2007; Resnick & Simpson, 2003).
   3. Social assessment: history, roles, values, living situation, and methods of coping (Boltz, Capezuti, & Shabbat, 2010; Boltz, Capezuti, Shabbat, & Hall, 2010).
   4. Addressing risk factors that impact goal achievement (e. g., cognitive status, anemia, nutritional status, pain, fear of falling, fatigue, medications and drug side effects such as somnolence) by the interdisciplinary team to optimize patient participation in functional and physical activity (Boltz et al., in press; Resnick, Cayo, et al., 2009; Resnick et al., 2011; Resnick, Gruber-Baldini, et al., 2009; Resnick et al., 2007; Resnick & Simpson, 2003).
   5. Development of discharge plans that include carryover of functional interventions, and addressing the unique preferences and needs of the patient (Nolan & Thomas, 2008).

V. EXPECTED OUTCOMES
   A. Patients will
      1. Be discharged, functioning at their maximum level.
   B. Providers can demonstrate
      1. Competence in assessing physical function and devloping an individualized plan to promote function, in collaboration with the patient and interdisciplinary team.
      2. Physical and social environments that enable optimal physical function for older adults.
      3. Individualized discharge plans.
   C. Institution will experience
      1. A reduction in incidence and prevalence of functional decline.
      2. Reduction in the use of physical restraints, prolonged bed rest, Foley catheters.
      3. Decreased incidence of delirium and other advserse events (pressure ulcers and falls).
      4. An increase in prevalence of patients who leave hospital at their baseline or with improved functional status.
      5. Physical environments that are safe and enabling.
      6. Increased patient satisfaction.
      7. Enhanced staff satisfaction and teamwork.

(continued)

> **Protocol 7.1: Function-Focused Care (FFC) Interventions** *(cont.)*
>
> ## VI. RELEVANT PRACTICE GUIDELINES
> Several resources are now available to guide adoption of evidence-based nursing interventions to enhance function in older adults.
>   1. Agency for Healthcare Research and Quality, National Guideline Clearinghouse; http://www.guideline.gov/
>   2. McGill University Health Centre. Research & Clinical Resources for Evidence Based Nursing (EBN); http://www.muhc-ebn.mcgill.ca/
>   3. National Quality Forum; http://www.qualityforum.org/Home.aspx
>   4. Registered Nurses Association of Ontario. Clinical Practice Guidelines Program; http://www.rnao.org/Page.asp?PageID=861&SiteNodeID=270&BL _ExpandID
>   5. University of Iowa Hartford Center of Geriatric Nursing Excellence (HCGNE). Evidence-Based Practice Guidelines; http://www.nursing.uiowa.edu/hartford/ nurse/ebp.htm

REFERENCES

Alley, D. E., Koster, A., Mackey, D., Cawthon, P., Ferrucci, L., Simonsick, E. M., . . . Harris, T. (2010). Hospitalization and change in body composition and strength in a population-based cohort of older persons. *Journal of the American Geriatrics Society, 58*(11), 2085–2091. doi:10.1111/j.1532-5415.2010.03144.x. Evidence Level IV.

Bailey, P., Thomsen, G. E., Spuhler, V. J., Blair, R., Jewkes, J., Bezdjian, L., . . . Hopkins, R. O. (2007). Early activity is feasible and safe in respiratory failure patients. *Critical Care Medicine, 35*(1), 139–145. Evidence Level IV.

Gulwadi, G. B., & Calkins, M. P., (2008). *The impact of healthcare environmental design on patient falls.* Concord, CA: Center for Healthcare Design. Evidence Level V.

Boltz, M., Capezuti, E., & Shabbat, N. (2010). Nursing staff perceptions of physical function in hospitalized older adults. *Applied Nursing Research.* Retrieved from http://www.appliednursingresearch.org/ article/S0897-1897(10)00002-9/abstract. Evidence Level IV.

Boltz, M., Capezuti, E., & Shabbat, N. (in press). Function-focused care and changes in physical function in Chinese American and non-Chinese American hospitalized older adults. *Rehabilitation Nursing.* Evidence Level IV.

Boltz, M., Capezuti, E., Shabbat, N., & Hall, K. (2010). Going home better not worse: Older adults' views on physical function during hospitalization. *International Journal of Nursing Practice, 16*(4), 381–388. Evidence Level IV.

Boyd, C. M., Landefeld, C. S., Counsell, S. R., Palmer, R. M., Fortinsky, R. H., Kresevic, D., . . . Covinsky, K. E. (2008). Recovery of activities of daily living in older adults after hospitalization for acute medical illness. *Journal of the American Geriatrics Society, 56*(12), 2171–2179. Evidence Level IV.

Boyd, C. M., Xue, Q. L., Guralnik J. M., & Fried, L. P. (2005). Hospitalization and development of dependence in activities of daily living in a cohort of disabled older women: The Women's Health and Aging Study. *The Journals of Gerontology. Series A, Biological Sciences and Medical Sciences, 60*(7), 888–893. Evidence Level IV.

Brown, C. J., Friedkin, R. J., & Inouye, S. K. (2004). Prevalence and outcomes of low mobility in hospitalized older patients. *Journal of the American Geriatrics Society, 52*(8), 1263–1270. Evidence Level IV.

Brown, C. J., Peel, C., Bamman, M. M., & Allman, R. (2006). Exercise program implementation proves not feasible during acute care hospitalization. *Journal of Rehabilitation Research and Development, 43*(7), 939–946. Evidence Level III.

Brown, C. J., Redden, D. T., Flood, K. L., & Allman, R. M. (2009). The underrecognized epidemic of low mobility during hospitalization of older adults. *Journal of the American Geriatrics Society, 57*(9), 1660–1665. Evidence Level IV.

Brown, C. J., Williams, B. R., Woodby, L. L., Davis, L. L., Allman, R. M. (2007). Barriers to mobility during hospitalization from the perspective of older patients, their nurses and physicians. *Journal of Hospital Medicine, 2*(5), 305–313. Evidence Level IV.

Callen, B., L., Mahoney, J. E., Wells, T. J., Enloe, M., & Hughes, S. (2004). Admission and discharge mobility of frail hospitalized older adults. *Medsurg Nursing: Official Journal of the Academy of Medical-Surgical Nurses. 13*(3), 156–164. Evidence Level III.

Capezuti, E., Wagner, L., Brush, B. L., Boltz, M., Renz, S., & Secic, M. (2008). Bed and toilet heights as potential environmental risk factors. *Clinical Nursing Research, 17*(1), 50–66. Evidence Level IV.

Coelho, F. G., Santos-Galduroz, R. F., Gobbi, S., & Stella, F. (2009). Systematized physical activity and cognitive performance in elderly with Alzheimer's dementia: A systematic review. *Revista Brasileira de Psiquiatria, 31*(2), 163–170. Evidence Level I.

Conedera, F., & Mitchell, L. (2010). Try this: Therapeutic activity kits. Retrieved from http://consultgerirn.org/uploads/File/trythis/theraAct.pdf. Evidence Level VI.

Covinsky, K. E., Fortinsky, R. H., Palmer, R. M., Kresevic, D. M., & Landefeld, C. S. (1997). Relation between symptoms of depression and health status outcomes in acutely ill hospitalized older persons. *Annals of Internal Medicine, 126*(6), 417–425. Evidence Level IV.

Covinsky, K. E., Palmer, R. M., Fortinsky, R. H., Counsell, S. R., Stewart, A. L., Kresevic, D., . . . Landefeld, C. S. (2003). Loss of independence in activities of daily living in older adults hospitalized with medical illness: Increased vulnerability with age. *Journal of the American Geriatrics Society, 51*(4), 451–458. Evidence Level IV.

Creditor, M. C. (1993). Hazards of hospitalization of the elderly. *Annals of Internal Medicine, 118*(3), 219–223. Evidence Level VI.

de Morton, N. A., Keating, J. L., Berlowitz, D. J., Jackson, B., & Lim, W. K. (2007). Additional exercise does not change hospital or patient outcomes in older medical patients: A controlled clinical trial. *The Australian Journal of Physiotherapy, 53*(2), 105–111. Evidence Level III.

de Morton, N. A., Keating, J. L., & Jeffs, K. (2007). The effect of exercise on outcomes for older acute medical inpatients compared with control or alternative treatments: A systematic review of randomized controlled trials. *Clinical Rehabilitation, 21*(1), 3–16. Evidence Level I.

Fisher, S. R., Goodwin, J. S., Protas, E. J., Kuo, Y. F., Graham, J. E., Ottenbacher, K. J., & Ostir, G. V. (2011). Ambulatory activity of older adults hospitalized with acute medical illness. *Journal of the American Geriatrics Society, 59*(1), 91–95. doi:10.1111/j.1532-5415.2010.03202.x. Evidence Level IV.

Foreman, M. D., Wakefield, B., Culp, K., & Milisen, K. (2001). Delirium in elderly patients: An overview of the state of the science. *Journal of Gerontological Nursing, 27*(4), 12–20. Evidence Level V.

Fortinsky, R. H., Covinsky, K. E., Palmer R. M., & Landefeld, C. S. (1999). Effects of functional status changes before and during hospitalization on nursing home admission of older adults. *The Journals of Gerontology. Series A, Biological Sciences and Medical Sciences, 54*(10), M521–M526. Evidence Level IV.

Gabor, J. Y., Cooper, A. B., Crombach, S. A., Lee, B., Kadikar, N., Bettger, H. E., & Hanly, P. J. (2003). Contribution of the intensive care unit environment to sleep disruption in mechanically ventilated patients and healthy subjects. *American Journal of Respiratory and Critical Care Medicine, 167*(5), 708–715. Evidence Level III.

Galik, E. (2010). Function-focused care for long-term care residents with moderate to severe cognitive impairment: A social ecological approach. *Annals of Long-Term Care: Clinical Care and Aging, 18*(6), 27–32. Evidence Level V.

Galik, E. M., Resnick, B., Gruber-Baldini, A., Nahm, E. S., Pearson, K., & Pretzer-Aboff, I. (2008). Pilot testing of the restorative care intervention for the cognitively impaired. *Journal of the American Medical Directors Association, 9*(7), 516–522. Evidence Level III.

Galik, E. M., Resnick, B., & Pretzer-Aboff, I. (2009). "Knowing what makes them tick": Motivating cognitively impaired older adults to participate in restorative care. *International Journal of Nursing Practice, 15*(1), 48–55. Evidence Level IV.

Gill, T. M., Allore, H. G., Gahbauer, E. A., & Murphy, T. E. (2010). Change in disability after hospitalization or restricted activity in older persons. *The Journal of the American Medical Association, 304*(17), 1919–1928. Evidence Level IV.

Gill, T. M., Allore, H., & Guo, Z. (2004). The deleterious effects of bed rest among community-living older persons. *The Journals of Gerontology. Series A, Biological Sciences and Medical Sciences, 59*(7), 755–761. Evidence Level IV.

Gill, T. M., Allore, H. G., Holford, T. R., & Guo, Z. (2004). Hospitalization, restricted activity, and the development of disability among older persons. *The Journal of the American Medical Association, 292*(17), 2115–2124. Evidence Level IV.

Gillis, A., MacDonald, B., & MacIsaac, A. (2008). Nurses' knowledge, attitudes, and confidence regarding preventing and treating deconditioning in older adults. *Journal of Continuing Education in Nursing, 39*(12), 547–554. Evidence Level IV.

Glantz, C., & Richman, N. (2007). Occupation-based, ability-centered care for people with dementia. *Occupational Therapy Practice, 12*(2), 10–16. Evidence Level VI.

Graf, C. (2006). Functional decline in hospitalized older adults. *The American Journal of Nursing, 106*(1), 58–67. Evidence Level V.

Harper, C. M., & Lyles, Y. M. (1988). Physiology and complications of bed rest. *Journal of the American Geriatrics Society, 36*(11), 1047–1054. Evidence Level VI.

Hoenig, H. M., & Rubenstein, L. Z. (1991). Hospital-associated deconditioning and dysfunction. *Journal of the American Geriatrics Society, 39*(2), 220–222. Evidence Level IV.

Inouye, S. K., Schlesinger, M. J., & Lydon, T. J. (1999). Delirium: A symptom of how hospital care is failing older persons and a window to improve quality of hospital care. *The American Journal of Medicine, 106*(5), 565–573. Evidence Level VI.

Iwarsson, S. (1999). The housing enabler: An objective tool for assessing accessibility. *The British Journal of Occupational Therapy, 62*(11), 491–497. Evidence Level V.

Jacelon, C. S. (2004). Managing personal integrity: The process of hospitalization for elders. *Journal of Advanced Nursing, 46*(5), 549–557. Evidence Level IV.

Jones, C. T., Lowe, A. J., MacGregor, L., Brand, C. A. (2006). A randomised controlled trial of an exercise intervention to reduce functional decline and health service utilisation in the hospitalised elderly. *Australasian Journal on Ageing, 25*(3), 126–133. Evidence Level II.

King, B. D. (2006). Functional decline in hospitalized elders. *MedSurg Nursing: Official Journal of the Academy of the Medical-Surgical Nurses, 15*(5), 265–271.Evidence Level V.

Kleinpell, R. (2007). Supporting independence in hospitalized elders in acute care. *Critical Care Nursing Clinics of North America, 19*(3), 247–252. Evidence Level V.

Kortebein, P., Ferrando, A., Lombeida, J., Wolfe, R., & Evans, W. J. (2007). Effect of 10 days of bed rest on skeletal muscle in healthy older adults. *The Journal of the American Medical Association, 297*(16), 1772–1774. Evidence Level III.

Kortebein, P., Symons, T. S., Ferrando, A., Paddon-Jones, D., Ronsen, O., Protas, E., . . . Evans, W. J. (2008). Functional impact of 10 days of bed rest in healthy older adults. *The Journals of Gerontology. Series A, Biological Sciences and Medical Sciences, 63*(10), 1076–1081. Evidence Level III.

Kresevic, D., & Holder, C. (1998). Interdisciplinary care. *Clinics in Geriatric Medicine, 14*(4), 787–798. Evidence Level VI.

Landefeld, C. S., Palmer, R. M., Kresevic, D. M., Fortinsky, R. H., & Kowal, J. (1995). A randomized trial of care in a hospital medical unit especially designed to improve the functional outcomes of acutely ill older patients. *The New England Journal of Medicine, 332*(20), 1338–1344. Evidence Level II.

McAuley, E., Konopack, J. F., Motl, R. W., Morris, K. S., Doerksen, S. E., & Rosengren, K. R. (2006). Physical activity and quality of life in older adults: Influence of health status and self-efficacy. *Annals of Behavioral Medicine, 31*(1), 99–103. Evidence Level IV.

McCusker, J., Kakuma, R., & Abrahamowicz, M. (2002). Predictors of functional decline in hospitalized elderly patients: A systematic review. *The Journal of Gerontology. Series A, Biological Sciences and Medical Sciences, 57*(9), M569–M577. Evidence Level I.

McVey, L., J., Becker, P. M., Saltz, C. C., Feussner, J. R., & Cohen, H. J. (1989). Effect of geriatric consultation team on functional status of elderly hospitalized patients. A randomized, controlled clinical trial. *Annals of Internal Medicine, 110*(1), 79–84. Evidence Level II.

Moos, R. H. (1979). Social-ecological perspectives on health. In G. C. Stone, F. Cohen, N. E. Alder, (eds.), *Health psychology—a handbook: Theories, applications, and challenges of a psychological approach to the health care system* (pp. 523–547). San Francisco, CA: Jossey Bass. Evidence Level VI.

Morris, P. E., Goad, A., Thompson, C., Taylor, K., Harry, B., Passmore, L., . . . Haponik, E. (2008). Early intensive care unit mobility therapy in the treatment of acute respiratory failure. *Critical Care Medicine, 36*(8), 2238–2243. Evidence Level III.

Mudge, A. M., Giebel, A. J., & Cutler, A. J. (2008). Exercising body and mind: An integrated approach to functional independence in hospitalized older people. *Journal of the American Geriatrics Society, 56*(4), 630–651. Evidence Level III.

Narain, P., Rubenstein, L. Z., Wieland, G. D., Rosbrook, B., Strome, L. S., Pietruszka, F., & Morley, J. E. (1988). Predictors of immediate and 6-month outcomes in hospitalized elderly patients. The importance of functional status. *Journal of the American Geriatrics Society, 36*(9), 775–783. Evidence Level IV.

Nolan, J., & Thomas, S. (2008). Targeted individual exercise programmes for older medical patients are feasible, and may change hospital and patient outcomes: A service improvement project. *BMC Health Services Research, 8*, 250. Evidence Level III.

Olsson, L. E., Karlsson, J., Ekman, I. (2007). Effects of nursing interventions within an integrated care pathway with hip fracture. *Journal of Advanced Nursing, 58*(2), 116–125. Evidence Level III.

Parke, B., & Chappell, N. L. (2010). Transactions between older people and the hospital environment: A social ecological analysis. *Journal of Aging Studies, 24*, 115–124. Evidence Level IV.

Reid, M., Williams, C. S., & Gill, T. M. (2005). Back pain and decline in lower extremity physical function among community-dwelling older persons. *The Journals of Gerontology. Series A, Biological Sciences and Medical Sciences, 60*(6), 793–797. Evidence Level IV.

Resnick, B. (2002). Geriatric Rehabilitation: The influence of efficacy beliefs and motivation. *Rehabilitation Nursing: The Official Journal of the Association of Rehabilitation Nurses, 27*(4), 152–159. Evidence Level IV.

Resnick, B. (2004). *Restorative care nursing for older adults: A guide for all care settings.* New York, NY: Springer Publishing. Evidence Level VI.

Resnick, B., Cayo, C., Galik, E., Pretzer-Aboff, I. (2009). Implementation of the 6-week educational component in the Res-Care intervention: Process and outcomes. *Journal of Continuing Education in Nursing, 40*(8), 353–360. doi:10.3928/00220124-20090723-04.Evidence Level III: Quasi Experimental Study.

Resnick, B., Galik, E., Enders, H., Sobol, K., Hammersla, M., Dustin, I., . . . Trotman, S. (2011). Pilot testing of function-focused care for acute care intervention. *Journal of Nursing Care Quality, 26*(2), 169–177. Evidence Level III.

Resnick, B., Gruber-Baldini, A. L., Galik, E., Pretzer-Aboff, I., Russ, K., Hebel, J. R., & Zimmerman, S. (2009). Changing the philosophy of care in long-term care: Testing of the restorative care intervention. *Gerontologist, 49*(2), 175–184. Evidence Level III.

Resnick, B., Rogers, V., Galik E., & Gruber-Baldini, A. L. (2007). Measuring restorative care provided by nursing assistants: Reliability and validity of the Restorative Care Behavior Checklist. *Nursing Research, 56*(6), 387–398. Evidence Level III.

Resnick, B., & Simpson, M. (2003). Restorative care nursing activities: Pilot testing self-efficacy and outcome expectation measures. *Geriatric Nursing, 24*(2), 82–89. Evidence Level III.

Rozzini R, Sabatini T, Cassinadri A, Boffelli, S., Ferri, M., Barbisoni, P., . . . Trabucchi, M. (2005). Relationship between functional loss before hospital admission and mortality in elderly persons with medical illness. *The Journals of Gerontology. Series A, Biological Sciences and Medical Sciences, 60*(9), 1180–1183. Evidence Level IV.

Sager, M. A., Franke, T., Inouye, S. K., Landefeld, C., S., Morgan, T. M., Rudberg, M. A., . . . Winograd, C. H. (1996). Functional outcomes of acute medical illness and hospitalization in older persons. *Archives of Internal Medicine, 156*(6), 645–652. Evidence Level IV.

Siu, A. L., Boockvar, K. S., Penrod, J. D., Morrison, R. S., Halm, E. A., Litke, A., . . . Magaziner, J. (2006). Effect of inpatient quality of care on functional outcomes in patients with hip fracture. *Medical Care, 44*(9), 862–869. Evidence Level IV.

Siu, A. L., Penrod, J. D., Boockvar, K. S., Koval, K., Strauss, E., & Morrison, R. S. (2006). Early ambulation after hip fracture: Effects on function & mortality. *Archives of Internal Medicine, 166*(7), 766–771. Evidence Level IV.

St. Pierre, J. (1998). Functional decline in hospitalized elders: Preventive nursing measures. *AACN Clinical Issues, 9*(1), 109–118. Evidence Level V.

Stokols, D. (1992). Establishing and maintaining healthy environments: Toward a social ecology of health promotion. *American Psychologist, 47*(1), 6–22. Evidence Level VI.

Tucker, D., Molsberger, S. C., & Clark, A. (2004). Walking for wellness: A collaborative program to maintain mobility in hospitalized older adults. *Geriatric Nursing, 25*(4), 242–245. Evidence Level V.

Ulrich, R., Zimring, C., Barch, X. Z., Dubose, J., Seo, H. B., Choi, Y. S., . . . Joseph, A. (2008). A review of the research literature on evidence-based healthcare design. *Health Environments Research & Design Journal, 1*(3), 61–125. Evidence Level V.

Volpato, S., Onder, G., Cavalieri, M., Guerra, G., Sioulis, F., Maraldi, C., . . . Italian Group of Pharmacoepidemiology in the Elderly Study. (2007). Characteristics of nondisabled older patients developing new disability associated with medical illnesses and hospitalization. *Journal of General Internal Medicine, 22*(5), 668–674. Evidence Level IV.

Wakefield, B. J., & Holman, J. E. (2007). Functional trajectories associated with hospitalization in older adults. *Western Journal of Nursing Research, 29*(2), 161–177. Evidence Level IV.

Weitzel, T., & Robinson, S. B. (2004). A model of nurse assistant care to promote functional status in hospitalized elders. *Journal for Nurses in Staff Development, 20* (4), 181–186. Evidence Level V.

Yu, F., Kolanowski, A. M., Strumpf, N. E., & Eslinger, P. (2006). Improving cognition and function through exercise intervention in Alzheimer's Disease. *Journal of Nursing Scholarship, 38*(4), 358–365. Evidence Level I.

Zisberg, A., Shadmi, E., Sinoff, G., Gur-Yaish, N., Srulovici, E., & Admi, H. (2011). Low mobility during hospitalization and functional decline in older adults. *Journal of the American Geriatrics Society, 59*(2), 266-273. doi:10.1111/j.1532-5415.2010.03276.x. Evidence Level IV.

Assessing Cognitive Function

8

Koen Milisen, Tom Braes, and Marquis D. Foreman

EDUCATIONAL OBJECTIVES

On completion of this chapter, the reader should be able to:

1. discuss the importance of assessing cognitive function
2. describe the goals of assessing cognitive function
3. compare and contrast the clinical features of delirium, dementia, and depression
4. incorporate the assessment of cognitive function into daily practice

OVERVIEW

Cognitive functioning comprises perception, memory, and thinking—the processes by which a person perceives, recognizes, registers, stores, and uses information (Foreman & Vermeersch, 2004). Cognitive functioning can be affected, positively and negatively, by illness and its treatment. Consequently, assessing an individual's cognitive functioning is paramount for identifying the presence of specific pathological conditions, such as dementia and delirium, for monitoring the effectiveness of various health interventions, and for determining an individual's readiness to learn and ability to make decisions (Foreman & Vermeersch, 2004). Despite the importance of assessing cognitive functioning, physicians and nurses routinely fail to assess an individual's cognitive functioning (Foreman & Milisen, 2004). This failure to assess cognitive functioning has profoundly serious consequences that include the failure to detect a potentially correctable condition of cognitive impairment and death (Inouye, Foreman, Mion, Katz, & Cooney, 2001) and outcomes that could be prevented or minimized by early recognition of their existence afforded by the routine assessment of cognitive functioning (Foreman & Milisen, 2004).

For description of Evidence Levels cited in this chapter, see Chapter 1, Developing and Evaluating Clinical Practice Guidelines: A Systematic Approach, page 7.

BACKGROUND AND STATEMENT OF PROBLEM

Declines in cognitive functioning are a hallmark of aging (McEvoy, 2001); however, most declines in cognition with aging are not pathological. Examples of nonpathological changes include a diminished ability to learn complex information, a delayed response time, and minor loss of recent memory; declines are especially evident with complex tasks or with those requiring multiple steps for completion (McEvoy, 2001).

Pathological conditions of cognitive impairment that are prevalent with aging include delirium, dementia, and depression (please see Table 8.1 for a comparison of the clinical features and also refer to the respective chapters, Chapter 9, Depression, Chapter 10, Dementia, and Chapter 11, Delirium). There are protocols to prevent and treat delirium, and protocols to slow the progression of decline with dementia (Protocol 8.1; however, these opportunities exist only when and if these conditions are detected early, and the possibility of early detection exists only when cognitive function is assessed systematically (Chow & MacLean, 2001; Registered Nurse Association of Ontario, 2003). Without systematic assessment, these pathological conditions go unchecked, and the individuals with these conditions face much greater accelerated and long-term cognitive and functional decline and death (Fick, Agostini, & Inouye, 2002; Fick & Foreman, 2000; Hopkins & Jackson, 2006; Lang et al., 2006).

Despite these profoundly negative consequences, nurses and physicians fail to access cognitive function (Ely et al., 2004; Foreman & Milisen, 2004; Inouye et al., 2001). Yet, it is clear that the assessment of cognitive function is the first and most crucial step in a cascade of strategies to prevent, reverse, halt, or minimize cognitive decline (Chow & MacLean, 2001; Registered Nurse Association of Ontario, 2003).

ASSESSMENT OF THE PROBLEM

Reasons for Assessing Cognitive Functioning

There are several reasons for assessing an individual's cognitive functioning:

Screening is conducted to determine the presence or absence of impairment. Bedside screening methods, however, are not useful in and of themselves for diagnosing specific pathological conditions of impairment such as delirium or dementia. Screening is also an important element in determining an individual's readiness to learn, and capacity to consent (Shekelle, MacLean, Morton, & Wenger, 2001). As a result, screening activities enable the early detection of impairment that affords the opportunity to determine the nature of the impairment. That is, is the impairment delirium, dementia, or depression, or possibly one superimposed upon another? Only through early detection can treatment be initiated promptly and accurately to either reverse, halt, or slow the progression of impairment (Chow & MacLean, 2001; Registered Nurse Association of Ontario, 2003).

Monitoring is conducted to track cognitive function over time as a means for following the progression or regression of impairment especially in response to treatment (Registered Nurse Association of Ontario, 2003; Shekelle et al., 2001).

How to Assess Cognitive Functioning

For assessing cognitive functioning, Folstein's Mini-Mental State Examination (MMSE; Folstein, Folstein, & McHugh, 1975) is the most frequently recommended instrument (British Geriatrics Society Clinical Guidelines, 2005; Fletcher, 2007; Registered Nurse Association of Ontario, 2003). The MMSE is a brief instrument, consisting of 11 items

TABLE 8.1

A Comparison of the Clinical Features of Delirium, Dementia, and Depression

Clinical Feature	Delirium	Dementia	Depression
Onset	Sudden/abrupt; depends on cause; often at twilight	Insidious/slow and often unrecognized; depends on cause	Coincides with major life changes; often abrupt, but can be gradual
Course	Short; diurnal fluctuations in symptoms; worse at night, in darkness, and on awakening	Long, no diurnal effects, symptoms progressive yet relatively stable over time, may see deficits with increased stress	Diurnal effects, typically worse in the morning; situational fluctuations in symptoms, but less than with delirium
Progression	Abrupt	Slow but uneven	Variable; rapid or slow but generally even
Duration	Hours to less than 1 month; longer if unrecognized and untreated	Months to years	At least 6 weeks, can be several months to years
Consciousness	Disturbed	Clear	Clear
Alertness	Fluctuates from stuporous to hypervigilant	Generally normal	Normal
Attention	Inattentive, easily distractible and may have difficulty shifting attention from one focus to another	Generally normal	Minimal impairment, but is distractible
Orientation	Generally impaired; disoriented to time and place, should not be disoriented to person	Generally normal	Selective disorientation
Memory	Recent and immediate impaired; unable to recall events of hospitalization and current illness, forgetful, unable to recall instructions	Recent and remote impaired	Selective or "patchy" impairment, "islands" of intact memory, evaluation often difficult due to low motivation
Thinking	Disorganized; rambling, irrelevant and incoherent conversation; unclear or illogical flow of ideas	Difficulty with abstraction, thoughts impoverished; judgment impaired; words difficult to find	Intact but with themes of hopelessness, helplessness, or self-deprecation
Perception	Perceptual disturbances such as illusions and visual and auditory hallucinations; misperceptions of common people and objects common	Misperceptions usually absent	Intact; delusions and hallucinations absent except in severe cases
Psychomotor behavior	Variable; hypoactive, hyperactive, and mixed	Normal, may have apraxia	Variable; psychomotor retardation or agitation
Associated features	Variable affective changes; symptoms of autonomic hypo-hyperarousal	Affect tends to be superficial, inappropriate, and labile; attempts to conceal deficits in intellect; personality changes, aphasia, agnosia may be present; lacks insight	Affect depressed; dysphoric mood, exaggerated and detailed complaints; preoccupied with personal thoughts; insight present; verbal elaboration; somatic complaints, poor hygiene, and neglect of self
Assessment	Distracted from task; fails to remember instructions, frequent errors without notice	Failings highlighted by family, frequent "near miss" answers, struggles with test, great effort to find an appropriate reply, frequent requests for feedback on performance	Failings highlighted by individual; frequent "don't know" answers, little effort; frequently gives up; indifferent toward test: does not care or attempt to find answer

and taking about 7–10 minutes to complete. It is composed of items assessing orientation, attention, memory, concentration, language, and constructional ability (Tombaugh & McIntyre, 1992). Each question is scored as either correct or incorrect; the total score ranges from 0 to 30 and reflects the number of correct responses. A score less than 24 is considered evidence of impaired cognition (Tombaugh & McIntyre, 1992).

Although considered the best available method for screening for impairment, the performance on the MMSE is significantly influenced by education (individuals with less than an 8th grade education commit more errors), language (individuals for whom English is not their primary language commit more errors) and verbal ability (the MMSE can only be used with individuals who can respond verbally to questioning), and age (older people do less well; Tombaugh & McIntyre, 1992). Others contend that the MMSE takes too long to administer in hectic, fast-paced health care environments (e.g., more than 10 minutes; Borson, Scanlan, Watanabe, Tu, & Lessiq, 2005).

To minimize the limitations of the MMSE while maximizing practical aspects of assessing cognitive function, the Mini-Cog was developed (Borson, Scanlan, Brush, Vitaliano, & Dokmak, 2000). The aim was to have a brief screening test that required no equipment and little training to use while not being negatively influenced by age, education, or language (Borson, Scanlan, Brush, et al., 2000; Borson, Scanlan, Watanabe, et al., 2005). The Mini-Cog is a four-item screening test consisting of three-item recall similar to the MMSE, and a clock-drawing item (e.g., draw the face of a clock, number the clock face, and place the hands on the clock face to indicate a specific time such as 11:10).

Since its initial development in 2000, the Mini-Cog has been used with various samples of people from different cultural, educational, age, and language backgrounds. In a recent systematic review, it was reported that the Mini-Cog was suitable for the routine screening for cognitive impairment (Brodaty, Low, Gibson, & Burns, 2006) and, even more recently, was found to predict the development of in-hospital delirium (Alagiakrishnan et al., 2007).

Another brief cognitive assessment tool (The Sweet 16) has recently been developed to address the aforementioned limitations of the MMSE. It is reported to be an easy-to-use instrument that can be completed in 2–3 minutes. In contrast to MMSE and Mini-Cog, it requires no pen, paper, or props to administer. It may be, therefore, more appropriate in frail older patients admitted to an acute hospital setting in which ability to write and manipulate props may be limited for reasons other than cognitive impairment (IV tubing, positioning in bed, etc.). Initial validation of the Sweet 16 indicates its performance to be equivalent or superior to that of the MMSE; however, much more research is needed to further validate the Sweet 16 (Fong et al., 2010).

With respect to MMSE, Mini-Cog, and Sweet 16, they are classified as simple bedside cognitive screens. This means that they are all qualified for determining the presence or absence of cognitive impairment; however, none are capable of determining if the impairment is delirium, dementia, or depression. If the results of this cognitive assessment or screening indicate the individuals to be impaired, further in-depth evaluation is necessary to confirm a diagnosis of dementia, depression, delirium, or some other health problem (see Chapter 10, Dementia, and Chapter 11, Delirium).

INTERVENTIONS AND CARE STRATEGIES

When to Assess Cognitive Functioning

When and how frequently to assess cognitive functioning, either using the MMSE, Mini-Cog, or Sweet 16, is in part a function of the purpose for the assessment, the condition of the patient, and the results of prior or current testing. Recommendations for the systematic assessment of cognition using standardized and validated tools include on admission to and discharge from an institutional care setting (British Geriatrics Society Clinical Guidelines, 2005; Shekelle et al., 2001); upon transfer from one care setting to another (Shekelle et al., 2001); during hospitalization, every 8–12 hours throughout hospitalization (http://www.mc.vanderbilt.edu/icudelirium/); as follow-up to hospital care, within 6 weeks of discharge (Shekelle et al., 2001); before making important health care decisions as an adjunct to determining an individual's capacity to consent; on the first visit to a new care provider; following major changes in pharmacotherapy (Shekelle et al., 2001); and with behavior that is unusual for the individual and/or inappropriate to the situation (Foreman & Vermeersch, 2004).

It is also recommended that formal cognitive testing be supplemented with information from close intimate others (Cole et al., 2002; Registered Nurse Association of Ontario, 2003) and from naturally occurring observations and conversations (Foreman, Fletcher, Mion, & Trygslad, 2003). One method for obtaining information from intimate others (Cole et al., 2002) is through the use of the Informant Questionnaire on Cognitive Decline in the Elderly (IQCDE; Jorm, 1994). Obtaining information from intimate others about an individual's cognitive functioning assists in determining the duration of impairment necessary for determining whether the impairment is delirium or dementia (see Chapter 10, Dementia, and Chapter 11, Delirium). Whereas naturally occurring observations and conversations during everyday nursing care activities in which it becomes apparent that the individual is inattentive, and responding unusually or inappropriately to conversation or questioning may be the first indication of the need to formally assess the individual's cognitive functioning by using one of the aforementioned instruments. However, formal assessment is not always possible (e.g., patient is too sick for formal testing). In contrast with formal testing, naturally occurring observations are based on daily and routine contacts with the patient (e.g., during bathing, feeding, transferring the patient) in a natural setting (e.g., not in a formal test setting). One criticism of naturally occurring observations (Persoon, 2010) is that they lack standardization. Since well-validated observation scales are scarce and cognitive functioning is often assessed in a limited way by these instruments, Persoon and colleagues recently developed and validated the new Nurses' Observation Scale for Cognitive Abilities (NOSCA; Persoon, 2010). By using this instrument, nurses can easily—and in a nonthreatening way—evaluate the patients' cognitive functioning in a comprehensive way (e.g., consciousness, attention, perception, orientation, memory, thoughts, higher cognitive functioning, language, and praxis).

Cautions for Assessing Cognitive Functioning

Various characteristics of the physical environment should be considered to ensure that the results of the cognitive assessment accurately reflect the individual's abilities and not extraneous factors. Overall, the ideal assessment environment should maximize the comfort and privacy of both the assessor and the individual. The environment should enhance performance by maximizing the individual's ability to participate in the assessment process (Dellasega, 1998). To accomplish this, the room should be well lit and of comfortable ambient temperature. Lighting must be balanced to be sufficient for the individual to see adequately the examination materials, while not being so bright that it creates glare. Additionally, the environment should be free from distractions that can result from extraneous noise, scattered assessment materials, or brightly colored and/or patterned clothing and flashy jewelry on the assessor (Lezak, Howieson, & Loring, 2004).

It will be vital to prepare the individual for the assessment, explaining what will take place and how long it will take, this way reducing anxiety and creating an emotionally nonthreatening environment and a safe individual–assessor relationship (Engberg & McDowell, 2000). Performing the assessment in the presence of others should be avoided when possible because the other individual may be distracting. If the other is a significant intimate relative, additional problems may arise. For example, when the individual fails to respond or responds in error, significant others have been known to provide the answer, or to say such things as "Now, you know the answer to that," or "Now, you know that's wrong." In most instances, the presence of another only heightens anxiety. Rarely does the presence of another facilitate the performance of an individual on cognitive assessment. Older adults are especially sensitive to any insinuation that they may have some "memory problem"; therefore, the dilemma for the assessor is to stress the importance of the assessment while taking care not to increase the individual's anxiety. Further, it can be counterproductive to describe the assessment as consisting of "simple," "silly," or "stupid" questions. Such explanations tend to diminish motivation to perform and only heighten anxiety when errors are committed.

The assessment can be perceived by the individual as intrusive, intimidating, fatiguing, and offensive—characteristics that can seriously and negatively affect performance. Consequently, Lezak et al., 2004 recommends an initial period to establish rapport with the individual. This period also allows a determination of the individual's capacity for assessment. For example, do conditions exist that could alter the performance of the individual or interpretation of results such as sensory decrements? As a consequence, the assessor can alter the testing environment through simple methods (e.g., by taking a position across from the individual or a little to the side). In this position, the individual can readily use the assessor's nonverbal communication as well as read the assessor's lips. Positioning also is important relative to lighting and glare.

Finally, avoid assessment periods immediately upon awakening from sleep (wait at least 30 minutes); immediately before and after meals, medical diagnostic, or therapeutic procedures; and when the individual is in pain or is uncomfortable (Foreman et al., 2003).

CASE STUDY

Mrs. O is a 79-year-old retired nurse who lives at home with her husband who is physically frail. Mrs. O was diagnosed with probable Alzheimer's disease approximately 3 years ago. In addition, she has Type II diabetes that is generally well controlled on Actoplus (pioglitazone hydrochloride and metformin hydrochloride). She and her husband are able to remain living in their own home with help from their children, neighbors, friends, and a monthly visit from a home health nurse. Mrs. O. is quite mobile but recently has begun to wander at times. Her husband reports that she seems more confused in the past few days and has fallen twice since yesterday. There is evidence of minor physical injury, which Mrs. O insists is "nothing." Her husband is also concerned that she has not been taking her Actoplus as prescribed; although she has been eating okay, but she has not been drinking enough. Because of these concerns,

(continued)

CASE STUDY *(continued)*

he calls the home health nurse to come and evaluate the situation. Mr. O's concerns are real and the call to the home health nurse is appropriate.

When the nurse arrives, she assesses Mrs. O, including her cognitive functioning. The results of her assessment indicate that Mrs. O's cognitive functioning has deteriorated significantly in the past. Mrs. O is more disoriented to time and place, more easily distracted, her conversation is disorganized, and she has greater difficulty following commands and remembering simple objects. In talking with the husband, the nurse learns that these changes occurred in the past 2 days. The nurse suspects delirium as evidenced by the sudden and dramatic decline in Mrs. O's cognitive abilities. The nurse thinks that Mrs. O may be severely dehydrated because her diabetes is no longer controlled, and is concerned about impending hyperosmolar, nonketotic coma. The nurse seeks an emergency admission to the local hospital for further diagnostic workup to determine the cause for her suspected delirium; is she hyperglycemic and dehydrated? (The nurse's suspected diagnosis is certainly a health emergency warranting further diagnostic workup to confirm a diagnosis of delirium and the identification of the underlying causes.)

Mrs. O is admitted with a diagnosis of mental status changes, and is described by the hospital nurse as "cooperative, lying quietly in bed, but being slow to respond"— changes the nurse attributes to merely a worsening of her dementia and nothing new. The hospital nurse moves on to more "important" patient care concerns. A couple of hours later, the nurse goes back to check on Mrs. O only to find her obtunded, unresponsive to physical stimuli, hypotensive, and tachycardic. The nurse calls a code, but Mrs. O fails to respond and dies. (What went wrong here? It is likely that the assessment performed by the home health nurse was not transmitted to the nurse in the hospital. Thus, vital information was missing, and the nurse in the hospital was working at a disadvantage.) In addition, it is not uncommon for health care providers to assume because an older person is "confused," that this confusion is either a result of their age or an exacerbation of their underlying dementia or both (Fick & Foreman, 2000). However, this is an erroneous assumption, and in this case dangerous as the undetected worsening of Mrs. O's cognitive impairment resulted in lack of treatment of the underlying hyperglycemia and severe dehydration leading to her eventual death. The cascade of mortal events could have been prevented with detection of the impairment, diagnosis of delirium, and prompt treatment of the underlying cause.

SUMMARY

The determination of an individual's cognitive status is critical in the process and outcomes of illness and its treatment. Being competent in the assessment of cognitive functioning requires (a) knowledge and skill as they relate to the performance of the assessment of cognitive functioning, (b) sensitivity to the issues that can negatively bias the results and interpretation of this assessment, (c) accurate and comprehensive documentation of the assessment, and (d) the incorporation of the results of the assessment in the development of the individual's plan of care.

Protocol 8.1: Assessing Cognitive Functioning

I. GOAL: The goals of cognitive assessment include:
A. To determine an individual's cognitive abilities.
B. To recognize early the presence of an impairment in cognitive functioning.
C. To monitor an individual's cognitive response to various treatments.

II. OVERVIEW
A. Undetected impairment in cognition is associated with greater morbidity and mortality (Inouye et al., 2001).
B. Assessing cognitive function is the foundation for early detection and prompt treatment of impairment (Shekelle et al., 2001).

III. BACKGROUND AND STATEMENT OF PROBLEM
A. Definition of cognitive functioning includes the processes by which an individual perceives, registers, sores, retrieves, and uses information.
B. Conditions in which cognitive functioning is impaired:
   1. *Dementia* (e.g., Alzheimer's or vascular) is a syndrome of cognitive deterioration that involves memory impairment and a disturbance in at least one other cognitive function (e.g., aphasia, apraxia, or agnosia that result in changes in function and behavior; American Psychiatric Association, 2000).
   2. *Delirium* is a disturbance of consciousness with impaired attention and disorganized thinking that develops rapidly. Evidence of an underlying physiologic or medical condition is generally present (American Psychiatric Association, 2000).
   3. *Depression* is a syndrome of either depressed mood or loss of interest or pleasure in most activities of the day; these symptoms represent a change from usual functioning for the individual and have been present for at least 2 weeks (American Psychiatric Association, 2000).

IV. ASSESSMENT OF COGNITIVE FUNCTION
A. Reasons/Purposes of Assessment
   1. Screening: to determine the absence or presence of impairment (Foreman et al., 2003).
   2. Monitoring: to track cognitive status over time, especially response to treatment (Foreman et al., 2003).
B. How to Assess Cognitive Function
   1. Mini-Mental State Examination (MMSE; Folstein, Folstein, & McHugh, 1975) can be used to screen for or monitor cognitive function instrument; however, performance on the MMSE is adversely influenced by education, age, language, and verbal ability. The MMSE is also criticized for taking too long to administer and score.
   2. Mini-Cog (Borson, Scanlan, Watanabe, et al., 2005) or Sweet-16 (Fong et al., 2010) can also be used to screen and monitor cognitive function; is not

(continued)

Protocol 8.1: Assessing Cognitive Functioning *(cont.)*

adversely influenced by age, language, and education; and takes about half as much time to administer and score as the MMSE.

3. Informant Questionnaire on Cognitive Decline in the Elderly (IQCDE) is useful to supplement testing with the MMSE or Mini-Cog as it is useful to determining onset, duration and functional impact of the cognitive impairment. Information from intimate others can be obtained by using the IQCDE (Jorm, 1994).

4. Naturally occurring interactions: Observations and conversations during naturally occurring care interactions can be the impetus for additional screening/monitoring of cognitive function with the MMSE or Mini-Cog (Foreman et al., 2003). Furthermore, observations should be standardized by using a formal observation instrument such as the Nurses' Observation Scale for Cognitive Abilities (NOSCA; Persoon, 2010).

C. When to Assess Cognitive Function

1. On admission to and discharge from an institutional care setting (British Geriatrics Society Clinical Guidelines, 2005; Shekelle et al., 2001)

2. Upon transfer from one care setting to another (Shekelle et al., 2001)

3. During hospitalization, every 8–12 hours throughout hospitalization (http://www.mc.vanderbilt.edu/icudelirium/)

4. As follow-up to hospital care, within 6 weeks of discharge (Shekelle et al., 2001)

5. Before making important health care decisions as an adjunct to determining an individual's capacity to consent (Shekelle et al., 2001)

6. On the first visit to a new care provider (Shekelle et al., 2001).

7. Following major changes in pharmacotherapy (Shekelle et al., 2001)

8. With behavior that is unusual for the individual and/or inappropriate to the situation (Foreman & Vermeersch, 2004)

D. Cautions for Assessing Cognitive Function

1. Physical environment (Dellasega, 1998)
   a. Comfortable ambient temperature
   b. Adequate lighting (not glaring)
   c. Free of distractions (e.g., should be conducted in the absence of others and other activities)
   d. Position self to maximize individual's sensory abilities

2. Interpersonal environment (Engberg & McDowell, 2000)
   a. Prepare individual for assessment
   b. Initiate assessment within nonthreatening conversation
   c. Let individual set pace of assessment
   d. Be emotionally nonthreatening

3. Timing of assessment (Foreman et al., 2003)
   a. Select time of assessment to reflect actual cognitive abilities of the individual.
   b. Avoid the following times.
      i. Immediately upon awakening from sleep, wait at least 30 minutes
      ii. Immediately before and after meals

(continued)

Protocol 8.1: Assessing Cognitive Functioning *(cont.)*

     iii. Immediately before and after medical diagnostic or therapeutic procedures

     iv. In the presence of pain or discomfort

V. EVALUATION/EXPECTED OUTCOMES
  A. Patient
    1. Is assessed at recommended time points
    2. Any impairment detected early
    3. Care tailored to appropriately address cognitive status/impairment
    4. Satisfaction with care improved
  B. Health Care Provider
    1. Competent to assess cognitive function
    2. Able to differentiate among delirium, dementia, and depression
    3. Uses standardized cognitive assessment protocol
    4. Satisfaction with care improved
  C. Institution
    1. Improved documentation of cognitive assessments
    2. Impairments in cognitive function identified promptly and accurately
    3. Improved referral to appropriate advanced providers (e.g., geriatricians, geriatric nurse practitioners) for additional assessment and treatment recommendations
    4. Decreased overall costs of care

VI. FOLLOW-UP MONITORING
  A. Provider competence in the assessment of cognitive function
  B. Consistent and appropriate documentation of cognitive assessment
  C. Consistent and appropriate care and follow-up in instances of impairment
  D. Timely and appropriate referral for diagnostic and treatment recommendations

VII. RELEVANT PRACTICE GUIDELINES
  A. The Registered Nurse Association of Ontario Best Practice Guideline for *Screening for Delirium, Dementia and Depression in Older Adults.* Retrieved from http://rnao.org/Page.asp?PageID=924&ContentID=818
  B. Guidelines and Protocols Advisory Committee (GPAC) guideline. Cognitive impairment in the elderly—recognition, diagnosis, management. Retrieved from http://www.bcguidelines.ca/gpac/guideline_cognitive.html
  C. National Institute for Health and Clinical Excellence (NICE) guideline. Delirium: diagnosis, prevention and management. Retrieved from http://guidance.nice.org.uk/CG103
  D. The National Guideline Clearinghouse. Delirium, dementia, amnestic, cognitive disorders. Retrieved from http://www.guideline.gov/browse/by-topic-detail.aspx?id=13949

RESOURCES

Recommended Instruments for Assessing Cognitive Functioning

Mini-Cog
http://www.nursingcenter.com/prodev/ce_article.asp?tid=756614

Mini-Mental State
http://www.minimental.com

Sweet 16
http://www.hospitalelderlifeprogram.org

Additional Online Information About Assessing Cognitive Functioning

The Iowa Index of Geriatric Assessment Tools (IIGAT)
http://www.healthcare.uiowa.edu/igec/tools/

"Try This"
A series of tips on various aspects of assessing and caring for older adults sponsored by the Hartford
    Institute for Geriatric Nursing at New York University College of Nursing.
http://www.consultgerirn.org

The Registered Nurse Association of Ontario Best Practice Guideline for *Screening for Delirium,
    Dementia and Depression in Older Adults.*
http://rnao.org/Page.asp?PageID=924&ContentID=818

Geriatric Toolkits
http://www.gericareonline.net/tools/index.html

ICU Delirium and Cognitive Impairment Study Group
http://www.icudelirium.org

Assessing care of vulnerable elders (ACOVE)
http://www.rand.org/health/projects/acove.html

REFERENCES

Alagiakrishnan, K., Marrie, T., Rolfson, D., Coke, W., Camicioli, R., Duggan, D., . . . Magee, B.
    (2007). Simple cognitive testing (Mini-Cog) predicts in-hospital delirium in the elderly. *Journal
    of the American Geriatrics Society, 55*(2), 314–316. Evidence Level IV.
American Psychiatric Association. (2000). *Diagnostic and statistical manual of mental disorders*
    (4th ed., text revision). Washington, DC: Author.
Borson, S., Scanlan, J. M., Brush, M., Vitaliano, P., & Dokmak, A. (2000). The Mini-Cog: A cogni-
    tive 'vital signs' measure for dementia screening in multi-lingual elderly. *International Journal of
    Geriatric Psychiatry, 15*(11), 1021–1027. Evidence Level IV.
Borson, S., Scanlan, J. M., Watanabe, J., Tu, S. P., & Lessiq, M. (2005). Simplifying detection of cogni-
    tive impairment: Comparison of the Mini-Cog and Mini-Mental state examination in a multieth-
    nic sample. *Journal of the American Geriatrics Society, 53*(3), 871–874. Evidence Level IV.
British Geriatrics Society Clinical Guidelines. (2005). *Guidelines for the prevention, diagnosis and
    management of delirium in older people in hospital.* Retrieved from http://www.bgs.org.uk/
    publications/Publications%20Downloads/Delirium-2006.DOC. Evidence Level I.
Brodaty, H., Low, L. F., Gibson, L., & Burns, K. (2006). What is the best dementia screening instru-
    ment for general practitioners to use? *American Journal of Geriatric Psychiatry, 14*(5), 391–400.
    Evidence Level I.

Chow, T. W., & MacLean, C. H. (2001). Quality indicators for dementia in vulnerable community-dwelling and hospitalized elders. *Annals of Internal Medicine, 135*(8 Pt. 2), 668–676. Evidence Level I.

Cole, M. G., McCusker, J., Bellavance, F., Primeau, F. J., Bailey, R. F., Bonnycastle, M. J., & Laplante, J. (2002). Systematic detection and multidisciplinary care of delirium in older medical inpatients: A randomized trial. *Canadian Medical Association Journal, 167*(7), 753–759. Evidence Level II.

Dellasega, C. (1998). Assessment of cognition in the elderly: Pieces of a complex puzzle. *Nursing Clinics of North America, 33*(3), 395–405. Evidence Level VI.

Ely, E. W., Stephens, R. K., Jackson, J. C., Thomason J. W., Truman B., Gordon S., . . . Bernard, G. R. (2004). Current opinions regarding the importance, diagnosis, and management of delirium in the intensive care unit: A survey of 912 healthcare professionals. *Critical Care Medicine, 32*(1), 106–112. Evidence Level IV.

Engberg, S. J., & McDowell, J. (2000). Comprehensive geriatric assessment. In J. T. Stone, J. F. Wyman, & S. A. Salisbury (Eds.), *Clinical gerontological nursing: A guide to advanced practice* (2nd ed., pp. 63–85). Philadelphia, PA: Saunders. Evidence Level VI.

Fick, D. M., Agostini, J. V., & Inouye, S. K. (2002). Delirium superimposed on dementia: A systematic review. *Journal of the American Geriatrics Society, 50*(10), 1723–1732. Evidence Level I.

Fick, D. M., & Foreman, M. D. (2000). Consequences of not recognizing delirium superimposed on dementia in hospitalized elderly individuals. *Journal of Gerontological Nursing, 26*(1), 30–40. Evidence Level IV.

Fletcher, K. (2007). Dementia. In E. Capezuti, D. Zwicker, M. Mezey, T. Fulmer (Eds.), *Evidence-based geriatric nursing protocols* (3rd ed., pp. 83–109). New York, NY: Springer Publishing. Evidence Level VI.

Folstein, M. F., Folstein, S. E., & McHugh, P. R. (1975). "Mini-Mental State": A practical method for grading the cognitive state of patients for the clinician. *Journal of Psychiatric Research, 12*(3), 189–198. Evidence Level IV.

Fong, T. G., Jones, R. N., Rudolph, J. L., Yang, F. M., Tommet, D., Habtemariam, D., . . . Inouye, S. K. (2010). Development and validation of a brief cognitive assessment tool: The Sweet 16. *Archives of Internal Medicine, 171*(5), 432–437. Evidence Level IV.

Foreman, M. D., Fletcher, K., Mion, L. C., & Trygslad, L. (2003). Assessing cognitive function. In M. Mezey, T. Fulmer, & I. Abraham (Eds.), D. Zwicker (Managing ed.), *Geriatric nursing protocols for best practice* (2nd ed., pp. 99–115). New York, NY: Springer Publishing Company. Evidence Level VI.

Foreman, M. D., & Milisen, K. (2004). Improving recognition of delirium in the elderly. *Primary Psychiatry, 11*(11), 46–50. Evidence Level I.

Foreman, M. D., & Vermeersch, P. E. H. (2004). Measuring cognitive status. In M. Frank-Stromborg & S. J. Olsen (Eds.), *Instruments for clinical health care research* (3rd ed., pp. 100–127). Sudbury, MA: Jones and Bartlett. Evidence Level I.

Hopkins, R. O., & Jackson, J. C. (2006). Assessing neurocognitive outcomes after critical illness: Are delirium and long-term cognitive impairments related? *Current Opinion in Critical Care, 12,*(5), 388–394. Evidence Level IV.

Inouye, S. K., Foreman, M. D., Mion, L. C., Katz, K. H., & Cooney, L. M., Jr. (2001). Nurses' recognition of delirium and its symptoms: Comparison of nurse and researcher ratings. *Archives of Internal Medicine, 161*(20), 2467-2473. Evidence Level IV.

Jorm, A. (1994). A short form of the Informant Questionnaire on Cognitive Decline in the Elderly (IQCODE): Development and cross-validation. *Psychological Medicine, 24*(1) 145–153. Evidence Level IV.

Lang, P. O., Heitz, D., Hédelin, G., Dramé, M., Jovenin, N., Ankri, J., . . . Blanchard, F. (2006). Early markers of prolonged hospital stays in older people: A prospective, multicenter study of 908 inpatients in French acute hospitals. *Journal of the American Geriatrics Society, 54*(7), 1031–1039. Evidence Level IV.

Lezak, M. D., Howieson, D. B., & Loring, D. W. (2004). *Neuropsychological assessment* (4th ed.). New York, NY: Oxford University Press. Evidence Level VI.

McEvoy, C. L. (2001). Cognitive changes in aging. In M .D. Mezey (Ed.), *The encyclopedia of elder care* (pp. 139–141), New York, NY: Springer Publishing. Evidence Level VI.

Persoon, A. (2010). *Development and validation of the Nurse Observation Scale for Cognitive Abilities – NOSCA* (Doctoral thesis, Radboud University, Nijmegen, The Netherlands). Evidence Level IV.

Registered Nurse Association of Ontario. (2003). *Screening for delirium, dementia and depression in older adults.*.Retrieved from http://rnao.org/Page.asp?PageID=924&ContentID=818.

Shekelle, P. G., MacLean, C. H., Morton, S. C., & Wenger, N. S. (2001). ACOVE quality indicators. *Annals of Internal Medicine, 135*(8 Pt 2) 653–667. Evidence Level I.

Tombaugh, T. N., & McIntyre, N. J. (1992). The Mini-Mental State Examination: A comprehensive review. *Journal of the American Geriatrics Society, 40*(9), 922–935. Evidence Level I.

Depression in Older Adults

9

Theresa A. Harvath and Glenise McKenzie

EDUCATIONAL OBJECTIVES

On completion of this chapter, the reader should be able to:

1. discuss the major risk factors for late-life depression
2. discuss the consequences of late-life depression
3. identify the core competencies of a systematic nursing assessment for depression with older adults
4. identify nursing strategies for older adults with depression

OVERVIEW

Contrary to popular belief, depression is not a normal part of aging. Rather, depression is a medical disorder that causes suffering for patients and their families, interferes with a person's ability to function, exacerbates coexisting medical illnesses, and increases use of health services (Lebowitz, 1996). Despite the efficacious treatments available for late-life depression, many older adults lack access to adequate resources; barriers in the health care reimbursement system are particular challenges for low income and ethnic minority older adults (Charney et al., 2003). In a comprehensive review of research on the prevalence of depression in later life, Hybels and Blazer (2003) found that although major depressive disorders are not prevalent in late life (1%–5%), the prevalence of clinically significant depressive symptoms is high (3%–30%). What is more, these depressive symptoms are associated with higher morbidity and mortality rates in older adults than in younger adults (Bagulho, 2002; Lyness et al., 2007).

The rates of depressive symptoms vary, depending on the population of older adults: community-dwelling older adults (3%–26%), primary care (10%), hospitalized older adults (23%), and nursing home residents (16%–30%; Hybels & Blazer, 2003).

Certain subgroups have higher levels of depressive symptoms, particularly those with more severe or chronic disabling conditions, such as those older people in acute

For description of Evidence Levels cited in this chapter, see Chapter 1, Developing and Evaluating Clinical Practice Guidelines: A Systematic Approach, page 7.

and long-term care settings. Depression also frequently coexists with dementia, specifically Alzheimer's disease, with prevalence rates ranging from 22% to 54% (Zubenko et al., 2003). Cognitive impairment may be a secondary symptom of depression, or depression may be the result of dementia (Blazer, 2002, 2003). It also should be noted that the prevalence of major depression has been increasing in those born more recently, so that it can be expected that the prevalence of depression in older adults will go up in the years to come.

Late-life depression often occurs within a context of medical illnesses, disability, cognitive dysfunction, and psychosocial adversity, frequently impeding timely recognition and treatment of depression, with subsequent unnecessary morbidity and death (Bagulho, 2002; Lyness et al., 2007). A substantial number of older patients encountered by nurses will have clinically relevant depressive symptoms. Nurses remain at the frontline in the early recognition of depression and the facilitation of older patients' access to mental health care. This chapter presents an overview of depression in older patients, with emphasis on age-related assessment considerations, clinical decision making, and nursing intervention strategies for older adults with depression. A standard of practice protocol for use by nurses in practice settings also is presented.

BACKGROUND AND STATEMENT OF PROBLEM

What is Depression?

In the broadest sense, depression is defined as a syndrome comprised of a constellation of affective, cognitive, and somatic or physiological manifestation (National Institutes of Health [NIH] Consensus Development Panel, 1992). Depression may range in severity from mild symptoms to more severe forms, both of which can persist over longer time with negative consequences for the older patient. Suicidal ideation, psychotic features (especially delusional thinking), and excessive somatic concerns frequently accompany more severe depression (NIH Consensus Development Panel, 1992). Symptoms of anxiety may also coexist with depression in many older adults (Cassidy, Lauderdale, & Sheikh, 2005; DeLuca et al., 2005). In fact, comorbid anxiety and depression have been associated with more severe symptoms, decreases in memory, poorer treatment outcomes (DeLuca et al., 2005; Lenze, et al., 2001), and increased rates of suicidal ideation (Sareen et al., 2005).

Major Depression

The *Diagnostic and Statistical Manual of Mental Disorders, fourth edition* (*DSM-IV-TR*) lists criteria for the diagnosis of major depressive disorder, the most severe form of depression. These criteria are frequently used as the standard by which older patients' depressive symptoms are assessed in clinical settings (American Psychiatric Association [APA], 2000). Five criteria from a list of nine must be present nearly every day during the same 2-week period and must represent a change from previous functioning: (a) depressed, sad, or irritable mood; (b) anhedonia or diminished pleasure in usually pleasurable people or activities; (c) feelings of worthlessness, self-reproach, or excessive guilt; (d) difficulty with thinking or diminished concentration; (e) suicidal thinking or attempts; (f) fatigue and loss of energy; (g) changes in appetite and weight; (h) disturbed sleep; and (i) psychomotor agitation or retardation. For this diagnosis, at least one of the five symptoms must include either depressed mood, by the patient's subjective account or observation of others, or markedly diminished pleasure in almost all people or activities. Concurrent medical conditions are frequently present in older patients and should not preclude a diagnosis of depression; indeed, there is a high incidence of medical comorbidity.

Major depression, as defined by the *DSM-IV-TR*, seems to be as common among older as younger cohorts. A recent review found diagnostic thresholds (number and type of symptoms) to be consistent between older adults (age 60 and older) and middle aged adults (age 40 and older; Anderson, Slade, Andrews, & Sachdev, 2009). However, older adults may more readily report somatic or physical symptoms than depressed mood (Pfaff & Almeida, 2005). The somatic or physical symptoms of depression, however, are often difficult to distinguish from somatic or physical symptoms associated with acute or chronic physical illness, especially in the hospitalized older patient, or the somatic symptoms that are part of common aging processes (Kurlowicz, 1994). For instance, disturbed sleep may be associated with chronic lung disease or congestive heart failure. Diminished energy or increased lethargy may be caused by an acute metabolic disturbance or drug response. Therefore, a challenge for nurses in acute care hospitals and other clinical settings is to not overlook or disregard somatic or physical complaints while also "looking beyond" such complaints to assess the full spectrum of depressive symptoms in older patients. In older adults with acute medical illnesses, somatic symptoms that persist may indicate a more serious depression, despite treatment of the underlying medical illness or discontinuance of a depressogenic medication (Kurlowicz, 1994). Older patients may link their somatic or physical complaints to a depressed mood or anhedonia.

In older adults with significant cognitive impairment, symptoms may differ from those who are cognitively intact. Depression may be expressed through repetitive verbalizations (e.g., calling out for help) or agitated vocalizations (e.g., screaming, yelling, or shouting), repetitive questions, expressions of unrealistic fears (e.g., fear of abandonment, being left alone), repetitive statements that something bad will happen, repetitive health-related concerns, and verbal and/or physical aggression (Cohen-Mansfield, Werner, & Marx, 1990). Based on the differences in presentation, Olin, Katz, Meyers, Schneider, and Lebowitz (2002) developed a set of provisional criteria (based on *DSM-IV-TR*) for the diagnosis of depression in Alzheimer's disease.

Minor Depression

Depressive symptoms that do not meet standard criteria for a specific depressive disorder are highly prevalent (15%–25%) in older adults. These symptoms are clinically significant and warrant treatment (Bagulho, 2002; Lyness et al., 2007). Such depressive symptoms have been variously referred to in the literature as "minor depression," "subsyndromal depression," "dysthymic depression," "subclinical depression," "elevated depressive symptoms," and "mild depression." The *DSM-IV-TR* also lists criteria for the diagnosis of "minor depressive disorder" and includes episodes of at least 2 weeks of depressive symptoms but with less than the five criteria required for major depressive disorder. Minor depression is two to four times as common as major depression in older adults and is associated with increased risk of subsequent major depression, greater use of health services, and has a negative impact on physical and social functioning and quality of life (Bagulho, 2002; Gaynes, Burns, Tweed, & Erickson, 2002; Lyness et al., 2007).

Course of Depression

Depression can occur for the first time in late life, or it can be part of a long-standing affective or mood disorder with onset in earlier years. Hospitalized older medical patients with depression are also more likely to have had a previous depression and experience higher rates of mortality than older patients without depression (von Ammon Cavanaugh, Furlanetto, Creech, & Powell, 2001). As in younger people, the course of depression in older adults is characterized by exacerbations, remissions, and chronicity (NIH Consensus Development Panel, 1992); however, older adults appear to be at increased risk for relapse (Mitchell & Subramaniam, 2005). Therefore, a wait-and-see approach with regard to treatment is not recommended.

Depression in Late Life is Serious

Depression is associated with serious negative consequences for older adults, especially for frail older patients, such as those recovering from a severe medical illness or those in nursing homes. Consequences of depression include heightened pain and disability, delayed recovery from medical illness or surgery, worsening of medical symptoms, risk of physical illness, increased health care use, alcoholism, cognitive impairment, worsening social impairment, protein–calorie subnutrition, loss of bone mineral density, functional decline, and increased rates of suicide- and non-suicide-related death (Bagulho, 2002; Hoogerduijn et al., 2007; Smalbrugge et al., 2006; von Ammon Cavanaugh et al., 2001; Wu Q, Magnus, Liu, Bencaz, & Hentz, 2009). The "amplification" hypothesis proposed by Katz, Streim, and Parmelee (1994) stated that depression can "turn up the volume" on several aspects of physical, psychosocial, and behavioral functioning in older patients ultimately accelerating the course of medical illness. For example, Gaynes et al. (2002) found that major depression and comorbid medical conditions interacted to adversely affect health-related quality of life in older adults, and Courtney, O'Reilly, Edwards, and Hassall (2009) identified depression as one of the factors most often associated with poorer quality of life for older adults in nursing homes. For older nursing home residents, depression is also associated with poor adjustment to the nursing home, resistance to daily care, treatment refusal, inability to participate in activities, and further social isolation (Achterberg et al., 2003).

Mortality by suicide is higher among older persons with depression than among their counterparts without depression (Juurlink, Herrmann, Szalai, Kopp, & Redelmeier, 2004). Rates of suicide among older adults (15–20 per 100,000) are the highest of any age group and even exceed rates among adolescents (McKeowen, Cuffe, & Schulz, 2006). This is, in large part, caused by the fact that White men older than the age of 85 are at greatest risk for suicide, where rates of suicide are estimated to be 80–113 per 100,000 (Erlangsen, Vach, & Jeune, 2005). In the oldest old (80 years and older), men and women had higher suicide rates than nonhospitalized older adults in the same age range, this age group had significantly higher rates of hospitalization than younger cohorts; three or more medical diagnoses were associated with increased suicide risk (Erlangsen et al., 2005). Among older psychiatric inpatients, increased risk for suicide was associated with affective disorders and first versus later admission (Erlangsen, Zarit, Tu, & Conwell, 2006).

Depressive symptoms, perception of lower health status, poor sleep quality, and absence of a confidant predicted late-life suicide (Turvey et al., 2002). Whereas physical illness and functional impairment increase risk for suicide in older adults, it appears that this relationship is strengthened by comorbid depression (Conwell, Duberstein, & Caine, 2002). Disruption of social support (Conwell et al., 2002), family conflict, and loneliness (Waern, Rubenowitz, & Wilhelmson, 2003) are also significantly associated with suicide in late life. Treatment of depression rapidly decreased suicidal ideation in older adults (Bruce et al., 2004; Szanto, Mulsant, Houck, Dew, & Reynolds, 2003). However, older adults in higher risk groups (male, older) needed a significantly longer response time to demonstrate a decrease in suicidal ideation (Szanto et al., 2003).

Studies have also shown that contact between suicidal older adults and their primary care provider is common (Luoma, Martin, & Pearson, 2002). Almost half of older suicide victims had seen their primary care provider within 1 month of committing suicide (Luoma et al., 2002), whereas 20% had seen a mental health provider. Most of the suicidal patients experienced their first episode of major depression, which was only moderately severe, yet the depressive symptoms went unrecognized and untreated. Older adults with clinically significant depressive symptomatology presented with physical rather than psychological symptoms, including patients who, when asked, admitted having suicidal ideation (Pfaff & Almeida, 2005).

Although the risk for suicide increases with advancing age (Hybels & Blazer, 2003), a growing body of evidence suggests that depression is also associated with higher rates of nonsuicide mortality in older adults (Kronish, Rieckmann, Schwartz, Schwartz, & Davidson, 2009; Schulz, Drayer, & Rollman, 2002); however, evidence is inclusive regarding depression as predictive of mortality in hospitalized older adults (Cole, 2007). Depression can also influence decision-making capacity and may be the cause of indirect life-threatening behavior such as refusal of food, medications, or other treatments in older patients (McDade-Montez, Christensen, Cvengros, & Lawton, 2006; Stapleton, Nielsen, Engelberg, Patrick, & Curtis, 2005). Furthermore, depressive symptoms in older adults have been associated with cognitive impairment and, in some cases, progression to dementia (Walker & Steffens, 2010). These observations suggest that accurate diagnosis and treatment of depression in older patients may reduce the mortality rate in this population. It is in the clinical setting, therefore, that screening procedures and assessment protocols have the most direct impact.

Depression in Late Life Is Misunderstood

Despite its prevalence, associated negative outcomes, and good treatment response, depression in older adults is highly underrecognized, misdiagnosed, and subsequently undertreated. According to a report by the Administration on Aging (2001), less than 3% of older adults receive treatment from mental health professionals. Use of mental health services is lower for older adults than any other age group (Administration on Aging, 2001). Barriers to care for older adults with depression exist at many levels. In particular, some older adults refuse to seek help because of perceived stigma of mental illness. Others may simply accept their feelings of profound sadness without realizing they are clinically depressed. Lack of care provider training in the identification and diagnosis of depression in older adults is also a barrier to timely recognition and treatment (Ayalon, Fialová, Areán, & Onder, 2010). Recognition of depression also is frequently obscured by anxiety and/or the various somatic or dementia-like symptoms manifest in older patients with depression, or because patient or providers believe that it is a "normal" response to medical illness, hospitalization, relocation to a nursing home, or other stressful life events. However, depression—major or minor—is not a necessary or normative consequence of life adversity (Snowdon, 2001). When depression occurs after an adverse life event, it represents pathology that should be treated.

Treatment for Late-Life Depression Works

The goals of treating depression in older patients are to decrease depressive symptoms, reduce relapse and recurrence, improve functioning and quality of life, improve medical health, and reduce mortality and health care costs. Depression in older patients can be effectively treated using either pharmacotherapy or psychosocial therapies, or both (Blazer, 2002, 2003; Mackin & Areán, 2005). If recognized, the treatment response for depression is good: 60%–80% of older adults remain relapse-free with medication maintenance for 6–18 months (NIH Consensus Development Panel, 1992). In addition, treatment of depression improves pain and functional outcomes in older adults (Lin et al., 2003). Recurrence of depression is a serious problem and has been associated with reduced responsiveness to treatment and higher rates of cognitive and functional decline (Driscoll et al., 2005). When compared to younger patients, older adults demonstrate comparable treatment response rates; however, they tend to have higher rates of relapse following treatment (Mitchell & Subramaniam, 2005). Therefore, continuation of treatment to prevent early relapse and longer term maintenance treatment to prevent later occurrences is important. Even in those patients with depression who have a comorbid medical illness or dementia, treatment response can be good (Iosifescu, 2007). Depressed older patients who have mild cognitive impairment are at greater risk for developing dementia if their depression goes untreated (Modrego & Ferrandez, 2004).

CAUSE AND RISK FACTORS

Several biologic and psychosocial factors have been associated with increased risk for late-life depression. Genetic factors or heredity seem to play more of a role when older adults have had depression throughout their life (Blazer & Hybels, 2005). Additional biologic causes associated with late-life depression include neurotransmitter or "chemical messenger" imbalance or dysregulation of endocrine function (Blazer, 2002, 2003). Elevated levels of homocysteine have also been associated with increased risk for depression in older adults (Almeida et al., 2008). Neuroanatomic correlates, cerebrovascular disease, brain metabolism alterations, gross brain disease, and the presence of apolipoprotein E have also been etiologically linked to late-life depression (Butters et al., 2003). Risk for depression in late life has been associated with physical disability, severe stroke, and cognitive impairment (Hackett & Anderson, 2005). Huang, Dong, Lu, Yue, and Liu (2010) found that depression was associated with arthritis, hypertension, diabetes, urologic problems, and severe stroke.

Psychosocial risk factors for depression in older adults include cognitive distortions, stressful life events (especially loss), chronic stress, low self-efficacy expectations (Blazer, 2002, 2003; Blazer & Hybels, 2005), poor self-perceived health, inadequate coping strategies, previous psychopathology (Vink, Aartsen, & Schoevers, 2008), narcissistic personality traits (Heisel, Links, Conn, van Reekum, & Flett, 2007), and a history of alcohol abuse (Hasin & Grant, 2002). (For more information, see Chapter 26, Substance Misuse and Alcohol Use Disorders.)

The social and demographic risk factors for depression in older adults include female sex, unmarried status, stressful life events, smaller network size, female gender, and the absence of a supportive social network (NIH Consensus Development Panel, 1992; Vink et al., 2008). Bereavement is also a risk factor for depression, especially in older women (Cole, 2007; Onrust & Cuijpers, 2006).

Interestingly, in a meta-analysis of the impact of negative life events on depression in older adults, Kraaij, Arensman, and Spinhoven (2002) found that while specific negative life events (e.g., death of significant others, illness in self or spouse, or negative relationship events) were moderately associated with increases in depression, the total number of negative life events and daily hassles had the strongest relationships with depression in older adults. The stress associated with family care giving has been repeatedly associated with higher rates of depression in older caregivers (Pinquart & Sorensen, 2004). In particular, caring for an older adult with dementia has been associated with higher rates of depression than other caregiving situations and with higher mortality rates (Pinquart & Sorensen, 2004). This suggests that clinicians should pay close attention to the accumulation of negative life events and daily hassles when developing programs and targeting interventions to mitigate depression in older adults who are at risk for developing depression.

In older adults, there is additional emphasis on the co-occurrence of specific physical conditions such as stroke, cancer, dementia, arthritis, hip fracture surgery, myocardial infarction, chronic obstructive pulmonary disease, and Parkinson's disease. Medical comorbidity is the hallmark of depression in older patients and this factor represents a major difference from depression in younger populations (Alexopoulos, Schultz, & Lebowitz, 2005). Several conditions have been associated with higher levels of depression in older adults, including heart failure (Johansson, Dahlström, & Broström, 2006) and other cardiovascular diseases (Van der Kooy et al., 2007), Alzheimer's disease, stroke, and Parkinson's disease (Hackett, Anderson, House, & Xia, 2008; Strober & Arnett, 2009). In an evidence-based review, Cole (2005) found that disability, older age, new medical diagnosis, and poor health status were among the most robust and consistent of all correlates of depression among older medical patients. Those with functional disabilities, especially those with new functional loss, are also at risk. For example, comorbid depression is common in older patients with hip fractures (Holmes & House, 2000; see Table 9.1).

Major depressive disorder has been found to be twice as common in community-dwelling older adults compared to primary care settings (Bruce et al., 2002). In a systematic review and meta-analysis, Cole and Dendukuuri (2003) found that depression in community-dwelling older adults was associated with bereavement, sleep disturbance, disability, prior depression, and female gender. Other significant factors included poor health status, poor self-perceived health, and new medical illness with disability (Cole, 2005; Cole & Dendukuuri, 2003).

Depression Among Minority Older Adults

Rates of depression among minority older adults are not well understood. Beals and colleagues (2005) found that the rates of major depressive episodes among older American Indians were 30% of the national average. In a review, Kales and Mellow (2006) found lower rates of depression and higher rates of psychotic diagnoses among African American older adults. In a systematic review of studies of older Asian immigrants, Kuo, Chong, and Joseph (2008) found that the prevalence of depression among Asian Americans ranged from 18% to 20% with significant variability between different Asian minority groups. For example, studies of Vietnamese older adults estimated depression at 50%, whereas studies of older Japanese Americans was at 3%. Depression was linked to gender, recency of immigration, English proficiency, acculturation, service barriers, and social support.

Baker and Whitfield (2006) reported that depressive symptoms were significantly associated with increased physical impairment among older Blacks. Williams and

TABLE 9.1

Physical Illnesses Associated with Depression in Older Patients*

Metabolic disturbances
- Dehydration
- Azotemia, uremia
- Acid-base disturbances
- Hypoxia
- Hyponatremia and hypernatremia.
- Hypoglycemia and hyperglycemia
- Hypocalcemia and hypercalcemia

Endocrine disorders
- Hypothyroidism and hyperthyroidism
- Hyperparathyroidism
- Diabetes mellitus
- Cushing's disease
- Addison's disease

Infections
- Viral
  - Pneumonia
  - Encephalitis
- Bacterial
- Pneumonia
- Urinary tract
- Meningitis
- Endocarditis
- Other
  - Tuberculosis
  - Brucellosis
  - Fungal meningitis
  - Neurosyphilis

Cardiovascular disorders
- Congestive heart failure
- Myocardial infarction, angina

Pulmonary disorders
- Chronic obstructive lung disease
- Malignancy

Gastrointestinal disorders
- Malignancy (especially pancreatic)
- Irritable bowel
- Other organic causes of chronic abdominal pain, ulcer, diverticulosis
- Hepatitis

Genitourinary disorders
- Urinary incontinence

Musculoskeletal disorders
- Degenerative arthritis

Osteoporosis with vertebral compression or hip fractures
- Polymyalgia rheumatica
- Paget's disease

Neurologic disorders
- Cerebrovascular disease
- Transient ischemic attacks
- Stroke
- Dementia (all types)
- Intracranial mass
- Primary or metastatic tumors
- Parkinson's disease

Other Illness
- Anemia (of any cause)
- Vitamin deficiencies
- Hematologic or other systemic malignancy
- Immune Disorders

Sources: Alexopoulos, G. S., Schultz, S. K., Lebowitz, B. D. (2005). Late-life depression: A model for medical classification. *Biological Psychiatry*, 58, 283–289; Cole, M. G. (2005). Evidence-based review of risk factors for geriatric depression and brief preventive interventions. *Psychiatric Clinics of North America*, 28(4), 785–803; Holmes, J. D., & House, A. O. (2000). Psychiatric illness in hip fracture. *Age and Ageing*, 29(6), 537–546. Evidence Level I.

colleagues (2007) found that when African American and Caribbean Blacks experience a major depressive disorder, it is usually untreated, more severe, and more disabling than for non-Hispanic Whites. Furthermore, significant disparities exist in the quality of mental health services received by minority older adults (Virnig et al., 2004). A study of Medicare + Choice plans enrollees revealed that minority older adults received substantially less follow-up for mental health problems following hospitalization (Virnig et al., 2004).

Although misdiagnosis and subsequent inappropriate treatment can lead to poor health outcomes for minority older adults (Kales & Mellow, 2006), it is not clear that "simple" bias alone can explain the disparities in depression management that exist. For example, Beals and colleagues (2005) point out that differences in the social construction of depressive experiences may confound the measurement of depression in ethnic older adults. Older American Indians may be reluctant to endorse symptoms of depression because cultural norms associate these complaints with weakness (Beals et al., 2005). In a thoughtful analysis of health disparities, Cooper, Beach, Johnson, and Inui (2006) explore the complex interactions and relationships between patients and providers that frame the context in which disparities can occur. They point out that many historical, cultural, and class-related factors can influence the development of therapeutic relationships between providers and patients. Until more research clarifies the symptom pattern of late-life depression in minority populations, it is important that clinicians be open to atypical presentations of depression that warrant closer scrutiny.

ASSESSMENT OF THE PROBLEM

Protocol 9.1 presents a standard of practice protocol for depression in older adults that emphasizes a systematic assessment guide for early recognition of depression by nurses in hospitals and other clinical settings. Early recognition of depression is enhanced by targeting high-risk groups of older adults for assessment methods that are routine, standardized, and systematic by use of both a depression screening tool and individualized depression assessment or interview (Piven, 2001).

It can be challenging to differentiate depression symptoms from dementia symptoms because cognitive impairment is frequently a symptom of depression and significant cognitive impairment in older depressed adults has been implicated in later development of dementia. Therefore, assessment for presenting symptoms indicative of both depression and dementia requires focused attention on the historical progression of symptoms, getting collateral information from a reliable informant (family or caregiver) and using a screening tool sensitive to change in mood symptoms in cognitively impaired individuals (Steffens, 2008).

Depression Screening Tools

Because many older adults do not present with obvious depressive symptoms (Pfaff & Almeida, 2005), it is important that screening for depression among older adults is incorporated into routine health assessments. Nursing assessment of depression in older patients can be facilitated by the use of a screening tool designed to detect symptoms of depression. Several depression screening tools have been developed for use with older adults. In a systematic review, Watson and Pignone (2003) evaluated the accuracy of different depression screening tools. They found that the Geriatric Depression Scale—Short Form (GDS-SF; Sheikh & Yesavage, 1986), the Center for Epidemiologic Studies Depression Scale (CES-D; Radloff, 1977), and the SelfCARE(D) (Banerjee, Shamash, MacDonald, & Mann, 1998) were the most accurate screening tools to detect major depression as well as subsyndromal depressive symptoms (Watson & Pignone, 2003).

In a more recent targeted review of evidence-based depression screening tools for older adults, the two most commonly cited were the GDS-SF and the CES-D. In addition, the Brief Patient Health Questionnaire-9 (BPHQ-9) and the Cornell Scale for Depression in Dementia (CSDD) were reviewed in depth because they are also evidence based and are being used with increasing regularity with older adults (Roman & Callen, 2008). The GDS-SF has been a reliable screening tool for depressive symptoms in mild cognitive impairment but not in older adults with Alzheimer's disease (Debruyne et al., 2009). The CSDD was developed specifically to detect symptoms of depression in older adults with dementia.

Individualized Assessment and Interview

Central to the individualized depression assessment and interview is a focused assessment of the full spectrum of symptoms (nine) for major depression as delineated by the *DSM-IV-TR* (APA, 2000). Furthermore, patients should be asked directly and specifically if they have been having suicidal ideation—that is, thoughts that life is not worth living—or if they have been contemplating or have attempted suicide. The number of symptoms, type, duration, frequency, and patterns of depressive symptoms, as well as a change from the patient's normal mood of functioning, should be noted. Additional components of the individualized depression assessment include evidence of psychotic thinking (especially delusional thoughts), anniversary dates of previous losses or nodal/stressful events, previous coping style (specifically alcohol or other substance abuse), relationship changes, physical health changes, a history of depression or other psychiatric illness that required some form of treatment, a general loss and crises inventory, and any concurrent life stressors. Subsequent questioning of the family or caregiver is recommended to obtain further information about the older adult's verbal and nonverbal expressions of depression.

DIFFERENTIATION OF MEDICAL OR IATROGENIC CAUSES OF DEPRESSION

Once depressive symptoms are recognized, medical and drug-related causes should be explored. As part of the initial assessment of depression in the older patient, it is important to obtain and review the medical history and physical and/or neurological examinations. Key laboratory tests should also be obtained and/or reviewed and include thyroid-stimulating hormone levels, chemistry screen, complete blood count, and medication levels if needed. An electrocardiogram, serum B_{12}, a urinalysis, and serum folate should also be considered to assess for coexisting medical conditions. These conditions may contribute to depression or might complicate treatment of the depression (Alexopoulos, Katz, Reynolds, Carpenter, & Docherty, 2001; see Table 9.2). In medically older patients, who frequently have multiple medical diagnoses and are prescribed with multiple medications, these "organic" factors in the cause of depression are a major issue in nursing assessment. In collaboration with the patient's physician, efforts should be directed toward treatment, correction, or stabilization of associated metabolic or systemic conditions. When medically feasible, depressogenic medications should be eliminated, minimized, or substituted with those that are less depressogenic (Dhondt et al., 1999). Even when an underlying medical condition or medication is contributing to the depression, treatment of that condition or discontinuation or substitution of the offending agent alone is often not sufficient to resolve the depression, and antidepressant medication is often needed.

INTERVENTIONS AND CARE STRATEGIES

Clinical Decision Making and Treatment

Regardless of the setting, older patients who exhibit the number of symptoms indicative of a major depression, specifically suicidal thoughts or psychosis, and who score *above* the established cutoff score for depression on a depression screening tool (e.g., 5 on the

TABLE 9.2

Drugs Used to Treat Physical Illness
That Can Cause Symptoms of Depression in Patients*

Antihypertensives	*Antiparkinsonian agents*
■ Reserpine	■ L-Dopa
■ Methyldope	*Antimicrobials*
■ Propranolol	■ Sulfonamides
■ Clonidine	■ Isoniazid
■ Hydralazine	*Cardiovascular agents*
■ Guanethidine	■ Digitals
■ Diuretics**	■ Lidocaine+
Analgesics	*Hypoglycemic agents+*
■ Narcotic	Steroids
■ Morphine	■ Corticosteroids
■ Codeine	■ Estrogens
■ Meperidine	*Others*
■ Pentazocine	■ Cimetidine
■ Propoxphene	■ Cancer chemotherapeutic agents
Nonnarcotic	
■ Indomethacin	

*Source: Dhondt, T., Derksen, P., Hooijer, C., Van Heycop Ten Ham, B., Van Gent, P. P., & Heeren, T. (1999). Depressogenic medication as an aetiological factor in major depression: An analysis in a clinical population of depressed elderly people. *International Journal of Geriatric Psychiatry, 14,* 875–881.
**By causing dehydration or electrolyte imbalance.
+Toxicity.
++By causing hypoglycemia.

GDS-SF) should be referred for a comprehensive psychiatric evaluation. Older patients with less severe depressive symptoms without suicidal thoughts or psychosis but who also score above the cutoff score on the depression screening tool (e.g., 5 on the GDS-SF) should be referred to available psychosocial services (i.e., psychiatric liaison nurses, geropsychiatric advanced practice nurses, social workers, psychologists, a clergy member) for psychotherapy or other psychosocial therapies, as well as to determine whether medication for depression is warranted. It is also important to note that older adults at risk for depression may benefit from brief interventions that focus on preventing the development of depression (Cole, 2008; Cole & Dendukuuri, 2003; Forsman, Jane-Llopis, Schierenbeck, & Wahlbeck, 2009).

The type and severity of depressive symptoms influence the type of treatment approach. In general, more severe depression, especially with suicidal thoughts or psychosis, requires intensive psychiatric treatment, including hospitalization, medication with an antidepressant or antipsychotic drug, electroconvulsive therapy (ECT), and intensive psychosocial support (Blazer, 2002, 2003). Less severe depression without suicidal thoughts or psychosis may require treatment with psychotherapy or medication, often on an outpatient basis. Collectively, these data also suggest that patients who have depression complicated by multiple medical and psychiatric comorbidities may benefit from a referral to an interdisciplinary treatment team with specific expertise in geropsychiatry.

The three major categories of treatment for depression in older adults are biologic therapies (e.g., pharmacotherapy, ECT, and exercise), psychosocial therapies (e.g., cognitive-behavioral, psychodynamic, and reminiscence therapy), and interdisciplinary team interventions. A compelling body of evidence supports the efficacy of these diverse treatment modalities for older adults with depression (Areán & Cook, 2002; Cuijpers, van Straten, & Smit, 2006; Hollon et al., 2005).

Biologic Therapies in Treatment of Late-Life Depression

In the past, tricyclic antidepressants (TCAs) were often contraindicated in older adults because of the anticholinergic side-effect profile (Mottram, Wilson, & Strobl, 2006). More recently, however, there has been a dramatic increase in the development and testing of different pharmacological agents used to treat depression in older adults. The most common classes of these newer medications include the selective serotonin reuptake inhibitors (SSRIs), serotonin-norepinephrine reuptake inhibitors (SNRIs), and TCA-related medications. These agents work selectively on neurotransmitters in the brain to alleviate depression. SSRIs have been effective in treating poststroke depression (Hackett et al., 2008; Chen, Guo, Zhan, & Patel, 2006) and depression in persons with Alzheimer's disease (Thompson, Herrmann, Rapoport, & Lanctôt, 2007).

When the SSRIs are compared to other classes of antidepressants to treat late-life depression (e.g., SNRIs, TCAs, TCA-related medications), they have similar treatment efficacy (Mottram et al., 2006; Mukai & Tampi, 2009; Salzman, Wong, & Wright, 2002; Shanmugham, Karp, Drayer, Reynolds, & Alexopoulos, 2005). However, SSRIs and SNRIs generally pose a lower treatment risk for older adults with depression (Chemali, Chahine, & Fricchione, 2009; Mottram et al., 2006; Mukai & Tampi, 2009; Shanmugham et al., 2005). Still, in a systematic review of the literature, Wilson, Mottram, and Vassilas (2008) found that although SSRIs are generally well tolerated in older adults, a significant minority experience serious side effects, including nausea, vomiting, dizziness, and drowsiness. In addition, serious hyponatremia has been associated with the use of SSRIs in older adults (Jacob & Spinler, 2006). Judicious use of TCA-related drugs may be an effective alternative for older adults who cannot tolerate SSRIs (Wilson et al., 2008).

Older patients should be closely monitored for therapeutic response to and potential side effects of antidepressant medication to assess whether dose adjustment of antidepressant medication may be warranted. Although, in general, it is necessary to start antidepressant medication at low doses in older patients, it is also necessary to ensure that older adults with persistent depressive symptoms receive adequate treatment (American Association of Geriatric Psychiatry, 1992; M. Buffum & J. Buffum, 2005).

Recent research that has suggested that the use of SSRIs in adolescents can increase suicidality has raised concerns about a similar dynamic with older adults. Several studies, however, have found that the use of SSRI antidepressants to treat late-life depression is not associated with increases in suicidal ideation (Barbui, Esposito, & Cipriani, 2009; Nelson, Delucchi, & Schneider, 2008; Stone et al., 2009). In fact, treatment of late-life depression with SSRIs has been shown to significantly reduce suicidal ideation and behavior in older adults (Barbui et al., 2009; Nelson et al., 2008; Stone et al., 2009).

Electroconvulsive Therapy

When older adults are not able to take antidepressants for treatment of late-life depression, clinicians are increasingly looking to the use of ECT to reduce symptoms of depression and improve function. For many individuals, the use of ECT conjures up images of barbaric treatments that leave patients severely cognitively impaired. Although the debate on the efficacy and appropriate use of ECT to treat late-life depression continues (Dombrovski & Mulsant, 2007), some research suggests that ECT can be an effective option for older adults with depression that is not responsive to other treatments (Navarro et al., 2008). Several studies have found that ECT does not cause increased cognitive impairment in older adults (Gardner & O'Connor, 2008).

Exercise Interventions

Physical exercise has been established as an effective treatment for depression in the general population, and evidence to support the use in older adults is building. In two recent systematic reviews of physical exercise, interventions concluded that exercise programs decrease depressive symptoms in older adults with major and minor depression (Sjosten & Kivela, 2006). Tai Chi and Qigong are specific meditative exercise methods that also may decrease depressive symptoms (Rogers, Larkey, & Keller, 2009).

PSYCHOSOCIAL APPROACHES

The term *psychosocial* encompasses a wide array of approaches. This section provides an overview of the three major psychosocial approaches used in the studies reviewed here: (a) cognitive behavioral, (b) psychodynamic, and (c) reminiscence or life review.

Cognitive behavioral therapies (CBT) seek to change the cognitive and/or behavioral context in which depression occurs through the use of various specific techniques such as providing new information, teaching problem-solving strategies, correcting skills deficits, modifying ineffective communication patterns, or changing the physical environment. Although specific treatment protocols vary, CBT approaches tend to be active and focused on solving specific, current day-to-day problems, rather than seeking global personality change in the client. Based on a large and growing evidence base, CBT has been shown effective in decreasing depression in clinically depressed older adults (Hill & Brettle, 2005; Laidlaw et al., 2008; Pinquart, Duberstein, & Lyness, 2007; Steinman et al., 2007; Wilson et al., 2008). Training caregivers (family or paid caregivers) to use CBT approaches (improved communication, increasing pleasant events, problem-solving behaviors) has also been shown to decrease depression and related behaviors in older adults with dementia (Teri, Mckenzie, & LaFazia, 2005). Gallagher-Thompson and Coon (2007) also identified CBT interventions as effective in decreasing depression in the older adults who are caregivers for family members with dementia.

Psychodynamic approaches focus on establishing a therapeutic relationship as a mechanism of change, as well as the historical causes of current client mood and behavior. The clients' psychological insight and ongoing emotional experience are considered critical for psychological progress. The evidence for effectiveness of psychodynamic approaches with older adults is limited. However, Pinquart and colleagues (2007) reported significant changes in depression with psychodynamic therapies based on three studies and nonsignificant changes in three studies of interpersonal therapy. Additionally, Bharucha, Dew, Miller, Borson, and Reynolds (2006) reviewed 18 studies of psychodynamic approaches ("talk therapy") with residents of long-term care settings and reported significant positive outcomes on measures of depression, hopelessness, and self-esteem. Marital and family therapy may also be beneficial in treating older adults with depression, especially older spouses engaged in caregiving (Buckwalter et al., 1999).

In reminiscence therapy, older adults are encouraged to remember the past and to share their memories, either with a therapist or with peers, as a way of increasing self-esteem and social intimacy. It is often highly directive and structured, with the therapist picking each session's reminiscence topic. In systematic reviews of the literature, reminiscence therapy was found to significantly reduce depression in older adults (Bohlmeijer, Smit, & Cuijpers, 2003; Hsieh & Wang, 2003; Mackin & Areán, 2005; Pinquart et al., 2007). Nursing interventions to encourage reminiscence include asking patients directly about their past or by linking events in history with the patient's life experience. The use of photographs, old magazines, scrapbooks, and other objects can also stimulate discussion.

In summary, psychosocial treatment has been found effective in decreasing depression in cognitively intact older adults. There is also empirical evidence for the efficacy of cognitive behavioral based therapies in decreasing depression in individuals with dementia and for the older adults who are caregivers for individuals with dementia. Current studies also demonstrate the utility of working closely with caregivers—whether family or staff—to reduce depression in persons with dementia. There is also a small but growing body of evidence related to the use of psychodynamic approaches aimed at decreasing depression in older adults associated with comorbid illnesses such as heart disease (Kang-Yi & Gellis, 2010; Lane, Chong Aun Yeong, & Gregory, 2005).

Interdisciplinary Team Models of Care

Several studies support the use of an interdisciplinary geriatric assessment team for late-life depression (Bao, Post, Ten, Schackman, & Bruce, 2009; Katon et al., 2005; Skultety & Zeiss, 2006). Interdisciplinary treatment teams improved physical functioning in older adults with major depressive disorder (Bao et al., 2009; Callahan et al., 2005; Katon et al., 2005; Skultety & Zeiss, 2006) and effectively reduced the depressive symptoms in community-dwelling older adults (age 70 years and older) who were at risk for hospitalization (Boult et al., 2001). Ethnic minority older adults experienced improved treatment of depression when treated by an interdisciplinary treatment team (Areán et al., 2005) as did low-income older adults (Areán, Gum, Tang, & Unützer, 2007). Similarly, patients with multiple comorbid medical conditions responded positively to an interdisciplinary approach to depression management (Harpole et al., 2005; Unützer et al., 2002). Although older adults with comorbid anxiety disorders took longer to respond to treatment, they experienced greater reductions in depression when treated by an interdisciplinary team than similar patients receiving usual primary care (Hegel et al., 2005).

Individualized Nursing Interventions for Depression

Psychosocial and behavioral nursing interventions can be incorporated into the plan of care, based on the patient's individualized need. Provision of safety precautions for patients with suicidal thinking is a priority. In acute medical settings, patients may require transfer to the psychiatric service when suicidal risk is high and staffing is not adequate to provide continuous observation of the patient. In outpatient settings, continuous surveillance of the patient should be provided while an emergency psychiatric evaluation and disposition is obtained.

Promotion of nutrition, elimination, sleep/rest patterns, physical comfort, and pain control has been recommended specifically for depressed medically ill older adult (Voyer & Martin, 2003). Relaxation strategies should be offered to relieve anxiety as an adjunct to pain management. Nursing interventions should also focus on enhancement of the older adult's physical function through structured and regular activity and exercise; referral to physical, occupational, and recreational therapies; and the development of a daily activity schedule (Barbour & Blumenthal, 2005). Enhancement of social support is also an important function of the nurse. This may be done by identifying, mobilizing, or designating a support person such as family, a confidant, friends, volunteers or other hospital resources, church member, support groups, patient or peer visitors, and particularly by accessing appropriate clergy for spiritual support.

Nurses should maximize the older adult's autonomy, personal control, self-efficacy, and decision making about clinical care, daily schedules, and personal routines (Lawton, Moss, Winter, & Hoffman, 2002). The use of a graded task assignment where a larger goal or task is subdivided into several small steps can be helpful in enhancing function, assuring successful experiences, and building older patients' confidence in their performance of various activities (Areán &, Cook, 2002). Participation in regular, predictable, and pleasant activities can result in more positive mood changes for older adults with depression (Koenig, 1991). A pleasant events inventory, elicited from the patient, can be used to incorporate pleasurable activities into the older patient's daily schedule (Koenig, 1991). Music therapy customized to the patient's preference is also recommended to reduce depressive symptoms (Siedliecki & Good, 2006).

Nurses should provide emotional support for depressed older patients by providing empathetic, supportive listening; encouraging patients to express their feelings in a focused manner on issues such as grief or role transition, supportive adaptive coping strategies; identifying and reinforcing strengths and capabilities; maintaining privacy and respect; and instilling hope. In particular, it is important to increase the patient's and family's awareness of the symptoms as part of a depression that is treatable and not the person's fault as a result of personal inadequacies.

CASE STUDY AND DISCUSSION

Ray Stimson is an 87-year-old man with multiple medical problems. He has a history of coronary artery disease (CAD) and had triple bypass surgery 4 years ago. He also has hypertension, Type II diabetes, and is hard of hearing. He was admitted to the hospital for surgical repair of a hip fracture following a fall in his home. Mr. Stimson is widowed (11 months) and has two adult children who do not live locally. Prior to his fall, he was living independently in the community; however, his children were growing increasingly concerned about his safety. Following surgery, Mr. Stimson was irritable and resisted efforts by the nursing staff to participate in self-care activities

(continued)

CASE STUDY *(continued)*

(e.g., walking, bathing). They often found him laying stoically in bed, staring into space. The nurses also observed that he was occasionally confused and would ask about his deceased wife.

A subsequent referral to the geropsychiatric consultation liaison nurse revealed that Mr. Stimson was experiencing a great deal of postoperative pain that was not well treated on his current medicine regimen. Nursing staff had charted concerns that his opioid analgesic was contributing to his mental confusion. The geropsychiatric evaluation also revealed that Mr. Stimson had been growing increasingly depressed over the past few months and was still actively grieving the loss of his wife of 62 years. As his health had failed and his independent living was threatened, he admitted he had contemplated suicide, stating, "Life is just not worth living anymore." Further assessment revealed that he did not have a specific plan in mind and admitted that he did not really think that was a solution to his problems, but that he could not see that he had many options.

The liaison nurse worked with the medical team to develop a more aggressive plan for pain management. She also arranged for a family conference to discuss discharge planning issues. During the family conference, the liaison nurse spoke to Mr. Stimson's children about long-term planning. She explained how important it was for Mr. Stimson to participate in any placement decisions they may be contemplating and to have a sense of control. Although his children were able to express their reservations and concerns about safety, they agreed to explore the kinds of community support services that could be activated to help support their father in his own home for as long as possible.

Mr. Stimson was able to participate in rehabilitation and gained enough strength to return to his home. Arrangements were made for follow-up with mental health services. He was started on an antidepressant and agreed to participate in the senior lunch program twice a week to increase the opportunity for socialization. Several months after his discharge, Mr. Stimson reported that he still missed his wife terribly and that he still was lonely at times. However, he had developed some friendships at the senior center and was getting out one to two times each week. His children called more often and had, for the time being, stopped sending him brochures for assisted living facilities. He acknowledged that he may need to move to a more supervised setting in the future, but for now, he was content to stay in the home where he had many pleasant memories to keep him company.

SUMMARY

Depression significantly threatens the personal integrity, health, and "experience of life" of many older adults. Depression is often reversible with prompt and appropriate treatment. Early recognition can be enhanced by training health care personnel in the use of a standardized protocol that outlines a systematic method for depression assessment adapted for older adults in various settings and with diverse comorbid conditions. Early identification of depression and successful treatment demonstrates to society that depression is the most treatable mental problem in late life. As Blazer (1989) stated, "When there is depression, hope remains" (pp. 164–166).

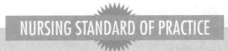

NURSING STANDARD OF PRACTICE

Protocol 9.1: Depression in Older Adults

I. BACKGROUND*

A. Depression—both major depressive disorders and minor depression—is highly prevalent in community-dwelling, medically ill, and institutionalized older adults.

B. Depression is not a natural part of aging or a normal reaction to acute illness hospitalization.

C. Consequences of depression include amplification of pain and disability, delayed recovery from illness and surgery, worsening of drug side effects, excess use of health services, cognitive impairment, subnutrition, and increased suicide- and non-suicide-related death.

D. Depression tends to be long lasting and recurrent. Therefore, a wait-and-see approach is undesirable, and immediate clinical attention is necessary. If recognized, treatment response is good.

E. Somatic symptoms may be more prominent than depressed mood in late-life depression.

F. Mixed depression and anxiety features may be evident among many older adults.

G. Recognition of depression is hindered by the coexistence of physical illness and social and economic problems common in late life. Early recognition, intervention, and referral by nurses can reduce the negative effects of depression.

II. ASSESSMENT PARAMETERS

A. Identify risk factors/high risk groups.
  1. Current alcohol/substance use disorder (Hasin & Grant, 2002).
  2. Specific comorbid conditions: dementia, stroke, cancer, arthritis, hip fracture, myocardial infarction, chronic obstructive pulmonary disease, and Parkinson's disease (Alexopoulos et al., 2005; Butters et al., 2003).
  3. Functional disability (especially new functional loss; Cole, 2003, 2005).
  4. Widow/widowers (NIH Consensus Development Panel, 1992).
  5. Caregivers (Pinquart & Sorensen, 2004).
  6. Social isolation/absence of social support (Kraaij et al., 2002).
  7. Diminished perception of light in one's environment (Friberg, Bremer, & Dickinsen, 2008).

B. Assess all at-risk groups using a standardized depression screening tool and documentation score. The GDS-SF is recommended because it takes approximately 5 minutes to administer, has been validated and extensively used with medically ill older adults, and includes *few* somatic items that may be confounded with physical illness (Pfaff & Almeida, 2005; Watson & Pignone, 2003).

C. Perform a *focused* depression assessment on all at-risk groups and document results. Note the number of symptoms; onset; frequency/patterns; duration (especially 2 weeks); change from normal mood, behavior, and functioning (APA, 2000).
  1. Depressive symptoms
  2. Depressed or irritable mood, frequent crying

(continued)

Protocol 9.1: Depression in Older Adults *(cont.)*

3. Loss of interest, pleasure (in family, friends, hobbies, sex)
4. Weight loss or gain (especially loss)
5. Sleep disturbance (especially insomnia)
6. Fatigue/loss of energy
7. Psychomotor slowing/agitation
8. Diminished concentration
9. Feelings of worthlessness/guilt
10. Suicidal thoughts or attempts, hopelessness
11. Psychosis (i.e., delusional/paranoid thoughts, hallucinations)
12. History of depression, current substance abuse (especially alcohol), previous coping style
13. Recent losses or crises (e.g., death of spouse, friend, pet; retirement; anniversary dates; move to another residence, nursing home); change in physical health status, relationships, roles

D. Obtain/review medical history and physical/neurological examination (Alexopoulos et al., 2001).
E. Assess for depressogenic medications (e.g., steroids, narcotics, sedative/hypnotics, benzodiazepines, antihypertensives, H_2 antagonists, beta-blockers, antipsychotics, immunosuppressive, cytotoxic agents).
F. Assess for related systematic and metabolic processes (e.g., infection, anemia, hypothyroidism or hyperthyroidism, hyponatremia, hypercalcemia, hypoglycemia, congestive heart failure, kidney failure).
G. Assess for cognitive dysfunction.
H. Assess level of functional disability.

III. CARE PARAMETERS
A. For severe depression (GDS score 11 or greater, five to nine depressive symptoms [must include depressed mood or loss of pleasure] plus other positive responses on individualized assessment [especially suicidal thoughts or psychosis and comorbid substance abuse], refer for psychiatric evaluation. Treatment options may include medication or cognitive behavioral, interpersonal, or brief psychodynamic psychotherapy/counseling (individual, group, family); hospitalization; or electroconvulsive therapy (Areán & Cook, 2002; Hollon et al., 2005).
B. For less severe depression (GDS score 6 or greater, less than five depressive symptoms plus other positive responses on individualized assessment), refer to mental health services for psychotherapy/counseling (see previous types), especially for specific issues identified in individualized assessment and to determine whether medication therapy may be warranted. Consider resources such as psychiatric liaison nurses, geropsychiatric advanced practice nurses, social workers, psychologists, and other community and institution-specific mental health services. If suicidal thoughts, psychosis, or comorbid substance abuse are present, a referral for a comprehensive psychiatric evaluation should always be made (Areán & Cook, 2002; Hollon et al., 2005).

(continued)

Protocol 9.1: Depression in Older Adults *(cont.)*

C. For all levels of depression, develop an *individualized* plan integrating the following nursing interventions:
  1. Institute safety precautions for suicide risk as per institutional policy (in outpatient settings, ensure continuous surveillance of the patient while obtaining an emergency psychiatric evaluation and disposition).
  2. Remove or control etiologic agents.
      a. Avoid/remove/change depressogenic medications.
      b. Correct/treat metabolic/systemic disturbances.
  3. Monitor and promote nutrition, elimination, sleep/rest patterns, physical comfort (especially pain control).
  4. Enhance physical function (i.e., structure regular exercise/activity; refer to physical, occupational, recreational therapies); develop a daily activity schedule.
  5. Enhance social support (i.e., identify/mobilize a support person(s) [e.g., family, confidant, friends, hospital resources, support groups, patient visitors]); ascertain need for spiritual support and contact appropriate clergy.
  6. Maximize autonomy/personal control/self-efficacy (e.g., include patient in active participation in making daily schedules, short-term goals).
  7. Identify and reinforce strengths and capabilities.
  8. Structure and encourage daily participation in relaxation therapies, pleasant activities (conduct a pleasant activity inventory), music therapy.
  9. Monitor and document response to medication and other therapies; readminister depression screening tool.
  10. Provide practical assistance; assist with problem solving.
  11. Provide emotional support (i.e., empathic, supportive listening, encourage expression of feelings, hope instillation), support adaptive coping, encourage pleasant reminiscences.
  12. Provide information about the physical illness and treatment(s) and about depression (i.e., that depression is common, treatable, and not the person's fault).
  13. Educate about the importance of adherence to prescribed treatment regimen for depression (especially medication) to prevent recurrence; educate about *specific* antidepressant side effects due to personal inadequacies.
  14. Ensure mental health community link up; consider psychiatric, nursing home care intervention.

IV. EVALUATION OF EXPECTED OUTCOMES
  A. Patient
  1. Patient safety will be maintained.
  2. Patients with severe depression will be evaluated by psychiatric services.
  3. Patients will report a reduction of symptoms that are indicative of depression. A reduction in the GDS score will be evident and suicidal thoughts or psychosis will resolve.
  4. Patient's daily functioning will improve.
  B. Health care provider
  1. Early recognition of patient at risk, referral, and interventions for depression, and documentation of outcomes will be improved.

(continued)

Protocol 9.1: Depression in Older Adults *(cont.)*

C. Institution
1. The number of patients identified with depression will increase.
2. The number of in-hospital suicide attempts will not increase.
3. The number of referrals to mental health services will increase.
4. The number of referrals to psychiatric nursing home care services will increase.
5. Staff will receive ongoing education on depression recognition, assessment, and interventions.

V. FOLLOW-UP TO MONITOR CONDITION
A. Continue to track prevalence and documentation of depression in at-risk groups.
B. Show evidence of transfer of information to postdischarge mental health service delivery system.
C. Educate caregivers to continue assessment processes.

*Somatic symptoms, also seen in many physical illnesses, are frequently associated with A and B; therefore, the full range of depressive symptoms should be assessed.

ACKNOWLEDGMENTS

This chapter is based partly on Chapter 5 of the third edition coauthored by Dr. Lenore H. Kurlowicz who died on September 21, 2007. The authors and coeditors acknowledge her tremendous contributions to the field of geropsychiatric nursing.

RESOURCES

Recommended Instruments for Screening for Depression

Geriatric Depression Scale-Short Form (GDS-SF)
Sheikh, J. I., & Yesavage, J. A. (1986). Geriatric depression scale (GDS) recent evidence and development of a shorter version. *Clinical Gerontologist, 5,* 165–173.

Center for Epidemiological Studies Depression Scale (CES-D)
Radloff, L. S. (1977). The CES-D scale: A self-report depression scale for research in the general population. *Applied Psychological Measurement, 1,* 385–401.

SelfCARE(D)
Banerjee, S., Shamash, K., Macdonald, A. J. D., & Mann, A. H. (1998). The use of SELFCARE(D) as a screening tool for depression in the clients of local authority home care services – a preliminary study. *International Journal of Geriatric Psychiatry, 13,* 695–699.

Additional Online Information About Assessing Depression

"Try This"
A series of tips on various aspects of assessing and caring for older adults sponsored by the Hartford Institute for Geriatric Nursing at New York University College of Nursing.
http://consultgerirn.org/resources

Portal of Geriatric Online Education
Provides resources for assessment and management of geriatric health issues.
http://www.pogoe.org/kmsearch

The Registered Nurse Association of Ontario Best Practice Guideline for Screening for Delirium, Dementia and Depression in Older Adults.
http://rnao.org/Page.asp?PageID = 924&ContentID = 818

Assessing Care of Vulnerable Elders (ACOVE)
http://www.rand.org/health/projects/acove.html

REFERENCES

Achterberg, W., Pot, A. M., Kerkstra, A., Ooms, M., Muller, M., & Ribbe, M. (2003). The effect of depression on social engagement in newly admitted Dutch nursing home residents. *The Gerontologist, 43*(2), 213–218. Evidence Level IV.

Administration on Aging. (2001). Older adults and mental health: Issues and opportunities. Retrieved from http://www.public-health.uiowa.edu/icmha/training/documents/Older-Adults-and-Mental-Health-2001.pdf

Alexopoulos, G. S., Katz, I. R., Reynolds, C. F., 3rd, Carpenter, D., & Docherty, J. P. (2001). The expert consensus guidelines series: Pharmacotherapy of depressive disorders in older patients (Special report). *Postgraduate Medicine*, 1–86. Evidence Level VI.

Alexopoulos, G. S., Schultz, S. K., Lebowitz, B. D. (2005). Late-life depression: A model for medical classification. *Biological Psychiatry, 58*, 283–289. Evidence Level IV.

Almeida, O. P., McCaul, K., Hankey, G. J., Norman, P., Jamrozik, K., & Flicker, L. (2008). Homocysteine and depression in later life. *Archives of General Psychiatry, 65*(11), 1286–1294. Evidence Level I.

American Association of Geriatric Psychiatry. (1992). Position statement: Psychotherapeutic medication in nursing homes. *Journal of the American Geriatrics Society, 40*, 946–949. Evidence Level VI.

American Psychiatric Association. (2000). *Diagnostic and statistical manual of mental disorders* (4th ed., text revision). Washington, DC: Author. Evidence Level IV.

Anderson, T. M., Slade, T., Andrews, G., & Sachdev, P. S. (2009). DSM-IV major depressive episode in the elderly: The relationship between the number and the type of depressive symptoms and impairment. *Journal of Affective Disorders, 117*(1–2), 55–62. Evidence Level IV.

Areán, P. A., Ayalon, L., Hunkeler, E., Lin, E. H., Tang, L., Harpole, L., . . . Unützer J. (2005). Improving depression care for older minority patients in primary care. *Medical Care, 43*(4), 381–390. Evidence Level VI.

Areán, P. A., & Cook, B. L. (2002). Psychotherapy and combined psychotherapy/pharmacotherapy for late life depression. *Biological Psychiatry, 52*(3), 293–303. Evidence Level VI.

Areán, P. A., Gum, A. M., Tang, L., & Unützer, J. (2007). Service use and outcomes among elderly persons with low incomes being treated for depression. *Psychiatric Services (Washington, D.C.), 58*(8), 1057–1064. Evidence Level II.

Ayalon, L., Fialová, D., Areán, P. A., & Onder, G. (2010). Challenges associated with the recognition and treatment of depression in older recipients of home care services. *International Psychogeriatrics, 22*(4), 514–522. Evidence Level V

Bagulho, F. (2002). Depression in older people. *Current Opinion in Psychiatry, 15*(4), 417–422. Evidence Level VI.

Baker, T. A., & Whitfield, K. E. (2006). Physical functioning in older blacks: An exploratory study identifying psychosocial and clinical predictors. *Journal of the National Medical Association. 98*(7), 1114–1120. Evidence Level IV.

Banerjee, S., Shamash, K., MacDonald, A. J., & Mann, A. H. (1998). The use of SELFCARE(D) as a screening tool for depression in the clients of local authority home care services—a preliminary study. *International Journal of Geriatric Psychiatry, 13*, 695–699. Evidence Level III.

Bao, Y., Post, E. P., Ten, T. R., Schackman, B. R., & Bruce, M. L. (2009). Achieving effective antidepressant pharmacotherapy in primary care: The role of depression care management in treating late-life depression. *Journal of the American Geriatrics Society, 57*(5), 895–900. Evidence Level IV.

Barbour, K. A., & Blumenthal, J. A. (2005). Exercise training and depression in older adults. *Neurobiology of Aging, 26*(Suppl. 1), S119–S123. Evidence Level VI.

Barbui, C., Esposito, E., & Cipriani, A. (2009). Selective serotonin reuptake inhibitors and risk of suicide: A systematic review of observational studies. *Canadian Medical Association Journal, 180*(3), 291–297. Evidence Level I.

Beals, J., Manson, S. M., Whitesell, N. R., Mitchell, C. M., Novins, D. K., Simpson, S., & Spicer, P. (2005). Prevalence of major depressive episode in two American Indian reservation populations: Unexpected findings with a structured interview. *American Journal of Psychiatry, 162*, 1713–1722. Evidence Level VI.

Bharucha, A. J., Dew, M. A., Miller, M. D., Borson, S., & Reynolds, C., III. (2006). Psychotherapy in long-term care: A review. *Journal of the American Medical Directors Association, 7*(9), 568–580. Evidence Level I.

Blazer, D. G. (1989). Depression in the elderly. *New England Journal of Medicine, 320*, 164–166.

Blazer, D. G. (2002). *Depression in late life* (3rd ed.). St. Louis, MO: Mosby. Evidence Level VI.

Blazer, D. G. (2003). Depression in late life: Review and commentary. *Journals of Gerontology: Series A: Biological Sciences and Medical Sciences, 58*(3), 249–265. Evidence Level VI.

Blazer, D. G., & Hybels, C. F. (2005). Origins of depression in late life. *Psychological Medicine, 35*(9), 1241–1252. Evidence Level VI.

Bohlmeijer, E., Smit, F., & Cuijpers, P. (2003). Effects of reminiscence and life review on late-life depression: A meta-analysis. *International Journal of Geriatric Psychiatry, 18*, 1088–1094. Evidence Level I.

Boult, C., Boult, L. B., Morishita, L., Dowd, B., Kane, R. L., & Urdangarin, C. F. (2001). A randomized clinical trial of outpatient geriatric evaluation and management. *Journal of the American Geriatrics Society, 49*, 351–359. Evidence Level II.

Bruce, M. L., McAvay, G. J., Raue, P. J., Brown, E. L., Meyers, B. S., Keohane, D. J., . . . Weber, C. (2002). Major depression in elderly home health care patients. *American Journal of Psychiatry, 159*(8), 1367–1374. Evidence Level VI.

Bruce, M. L., Ten Have, T. R., Reynolds, C. F., 3rd, Katz, I. I., Schulberg, H. C., Mulsant, B. H., . . . Alexopoulos, G. S. (2004). Reducing suicidal ideation and depressive symptoms in depressed older primary care patients: a randomized controlled trial. *Journal of the American Medical Association, 291*(9), 1081–1091.

Buckwalter, K. C., Gerdner, L., Kohout, F., Hall, G. R., Kelly, A., Richards, B., & Sime, M. (1999). A nursing intervention to decrease depression in family caregivers of persons with dementia. *Archives of Psychiatric Nursing, 13*(2), 80–88. Evidence Level IV.

Buffum, M. D., & Buffum, J. C. (2005). Treating depression in the elderly: An update on antidepressants. *Geriatric Nursing, 26*(3), 138–142. Evidence Level V.

Butters, M. A., Sweet, R. A., Mulsant, B. H., Ilyas Kamboh, M., Pollock, B. G., Begley, A.E., . . . DeKosky, S. T. (2003). APOE is associated with age-of-onset, but not cognitive functioning, in late-life depression. *International Journal of Geriatric Psychiatry, 18*, 1075–1081. Evidence Level IV.

Callahan, C. M., Kroenke, K., Counsell, S. R., Hendrie, H. C., Perkins, A. J., Katon, W., . . . Unützer, J. (2005). Treatment of depression improves physical functioning in older adults. *Journal of the American Geriatrics Society, 53*(3), 367–373. Evidence Level III.

Cassidy, E. L., Lauderdale, S., Sheikh, J. I. (2005). Mixed anxiety and depression in older adults: Clinical characteristics and management. *Journal of Geriatric Psychiatry and Neurology, 18*(2), 83–88. Evidence Level IV.

Charney, D. S., Reynolds, C. F., III, Lewis, L., Lebowitz, B. D., Sunderland, T., Alexopoulos, G. S., . . . Young, R. C. (2003). Depression and bipolar support alliance consensus statement on the unmet needs in diagnosis and treatment of mood disorders in late life. *Archives of General Psychiatry, 60*(7), 664–672. Evidence Level V.

Chemali, Z., Chahine, L. M., & Fricchione, G. (2009). The use of selective serotonin reuptake inhibitors in elderly patients. *Harvard Review of Psychiatry, 17*(4), 242–253. Evidence Level I.

Chen, Y., Guo, J. J., Zhan, S., Patel, N. C. (2006). Treatment effects of antidepressants in patients with post-stroke depression: A meta-analysis. *The Annals of Pharmacotherapy, 40*(12), 2115–2122. Evidence Level I.

Cohen-Mansfield, J., Werner, P., & Marx, M. S. (1990). Screaming in nursing home residents. *Journal of the American Geriatrics Society, 38*, 785–792. Evidence Level VI.

Cole, M. G. (2005). Evidence-based review of risk factors for geriatric depression and brief preventive interventions. *Psychiatric Clinics of North America, 28*(4), 785–803. Evidence Level I.

Cole, M. G. (2007). Does depression in older medical inpatients predict mortality? A systematic review. *General Hospital Psychiatry, 29*(5), 425–430. Evidence Level I.

Cole, M. G. (2008). Brief interventions to prevent depression in older subjects: A systematic review of feasibility and effectiveness. *The American Journal of Geriatric Psychiatry, 16*(6), 435–443. Evidence Level I.

Cole, M. G., & Dendukuuri, N. (2003). Risk factors for depression among elderly community subjects: A systematic review and meta-analysis. *American Journal of Psychiatry, 160*(6), 1147–1156. Evidence Level I.

Conwell, Y., Duberstein, P. R., & Caine, E. D. (2002). Risk factors for suicide in later life. *Biological Psychiatry, 52*(3), 193–204. Evidence Level VI.

Cooper, L. A., Beach, M. C., Johnson, R. L., & Inui, T. S. (2006). Delving below the surface: Understanding how race and ethnicity influence relationships in health care. *Journal of General Internal Medicine, 21*(Suppl. 1), S21–S27. Evidence Level VI.

Courtney, M., O'Reilly, M., Edwards, H., & Hassall, S. (2009). The relationship between clinical outcomes and quality of life for residents of aged care facilities. *Australian Journal of Advanced Nursing, 26*(4), 49–57. Evidence Level IV.

Cuijpers, P., van Straten, A., & Smit, F. (2006). Psychological treatment of late-life depression: A meta-analysis of randomized controlled trials. *International Journal of Geriatric Psychiatry, 21*(12), 1139–1149. Evidence Level I.

Debruyne, H., Van Buggenhout, M., Le Bastard, N., Aries, M., Audenaert, K., De Deyn, P. P., & Engelborghs, S. (2009). Is the geriatric depression scale a reliable screening tool for depressive symptoms in elderly patients with cognitive impairment? *International Journal of Geriatric Psychiatry, 24*(6), 556–562. Evidence Level IV.

DeLuca, A. K., Lenze, E. J., Mulsant, B. H., Butters, M. A., Karp, J. F., . . . Reynolds, C.F., III. (2005). Comorbid anxiety disorder in late life depression: Association with memory decline over four years. *International Journal of Geriatric Psychiatry, 20*, 848–854. Evidence Level III.

Dhondt, T., Derksen, P., Hooijer, C., Van Heycop Ten Ham, B., Van Gent, P. P., & Heeren, T. (1999). Depressogenic medication as an aetiological factor in major depression: An analysis in a clinical population of depressed elderly people. *International Journal of Geriatric Psychiatry, 14*, 875–881. Evidence Level IV.

Dombrovski, A. Y., & Mulsant, B. H. (2007). The evidence for electroconvulsive therapy (ECT) in the treatment of severe late life depression. ECT: The preferred treatment for severe depression in late life. *International Psychogeriatrics/IPA, 19*(1), 10–4, 27–35; discussion 24–26. Evidence Level I.

Driscoll, H. C., Basinski, J., Mulsant, B. H., Butters, M. A., Dew, M. A., Houck, P. R., . . . Reynolds, C. F., III. (2005). Late-onset major depression: Clinical and treatment-response variability. *International Journal of Geriatric Psychiatry, 20*, 661–667. Evidence Level IV.

Erlangsen, A., Vach, W., & Jeune, B. (2005). The effect of hospitalization with medical illnesses on the suicide risk in the oldest old: a population-based register study. *Journal of the American Geriatrics Society, 53*(5), 771–776. Evidence Level III.

Erlangsen, A., Zarit, S. H., Tu, X., & Conwell, Y. (2006). Suicide among older psychiatric inpatients: An evidence-based study of a high-risk group. *The American Journal of Geriatric Psychiatry*, *14*(9), 734–741. Evidence Level III.

Forsman, A., Jane-Llopis, E., Schierenbeck, I. & Wahlbeck, K. (2009). Psychosocial interventions for prevention of depression in older people (Protocol). *Cochrane Database of Systematic Reviews*, (2), CD007804. doi:10.1002/14651858.CD007804 Evidence Level I.

Friberg, T. R., Bremer, R. W., & Dickinsen, M. (2008). Diminished perception of light as a symptom of depression: Further studies. *Journal of Affective Disorders*, *108*(3), 235–240. Evidence Level IV.

Gallagher-Thompson, D., & Coon, D. W. (2007). Evidence-based psychological treatments for distress in family caregivers of older adults. *Psychology and Aging*, *22*(1), 37–51. Evidence Level I.

Gardner, B. K., & O'Connor, D. (2008). A review of the cognitive effects of electroconvulsive therapy in older adults. *Journal of ECT*, *24*(1), 68–80. Evidence Level I.

Gaynes, B. N., Burns, B. J., Tweed, D. L., & Erickson, P. (2002). Depression and health-related quality of life. *The Journal of Nervous and Mental Disease*, *190*(12), 799–806. Evidence Level III.

Hackett, M. L., & Anderson, C. S. (2005). Predictors of depression after stroke: A systematic review of observational studies. *Stroke: a Journal of Cerebral Circulation*, *36*(10), 2296–2301. Evidence Level I.

Hackett, M. L., Anderson, C. S., House, A., & Xia, J. (2008). Interventions for treating depression after stroke. *Cochrane Database of Systematic Reviews*, (4), CD003437. Evidence Level I.

Harpole, L. H., Williams, J. W., Jr., Olsen, M. K., Stechuchak, K. M., Oddone, E., Callahan, C. M., . . . Unützer, J. (2005). Improving depression outcomes in older adults with comorbid medical illness. *General Hospital Psychiatry*, *27*(1), 4–12. Evidence Level II.

Hasin, D. S., & Grant, B. F. (2002). Major depression in 6050 former drinkers: Association with past alcohol dependence. *Archives of General Psychiatry*, *59*, 794–800. Evidence Level III.

Hegel, M. T., Unützer, J., Tang, L., Areán, P. A., Katon, W., Noël, P. H., . . . Lin, E. H. (2005). Impact of comorbid panic and posttraumatic stress disorder on outcomes of collaborative care for late-life depression in primary care. *American Journal of Geriatric Psychiatry*, *13*(1), 48–58. Evidence Level II.

Heisel, M. J., Links, P. S., Conn, D., van Reekum, R., & Flett, G. L. (2007). Narcissistic personality and vulnerability to late-life suicidality. *The American Journal of Geriatric Psychiatry*, *15*(9), 734–741. Evidence Level IV.

Hill, A., & Brettle, A. (2005). The effectiveness of counselling with older people: Results of a systematic review. *Counselling & Psychotherapy Research*, *5*(4), 265–272. Evidence Level I.

Hollon, S. D., Jarrett, R. B., Nierenberg, A. A., Thase, M. E., Trivedi, M., & Rush, A. J. (2005). Psychotherapy and medication in the treatment of adult and geriatric depression: Which monotherapy or combined treatment? *Journal of Clinical Psychiatry*, *66*(4), 455–468. Evidence Level VI.

Holmes, J. D., & House, A. O. (2000). Psychiatric illness in hip fracture. *Age and Ageing*, *29*(6), 537–546. Evidence Level I.

Hoogerduijn, J. G., Schuurmans, M. J., Duijnstee, M. S., de Rooij, S. E., & Grypdonck, M. F. (2007). A systematic review of predictors and screening instruments to identify older hospitalized patients at risk for functional decline. *Journal of Clinical Nursing*, *16*(1), 46–57. Evidence Level I.

Hsieh, H., & Wang, J. (2003). Effect of reminiscence therapy on depression in older adults: A systematic review. *International Journal of Nursing Studies*, *40*(4), 335–345. Evidence Level I.

Huang, C. Q., Dong, B. R., Lu, Z. C., Yue, J. R., & Liu, Q. X. (2010). Chronic diseases and risk for depression in old age: A meta-analysis of published literature. *Ageing Research Reviews*, *9*(2), Evidence Level I.

Hybels, C. F., & Blazer, D. G. (2003). Epidemiology of late-life mental disorders. *Clinical Geriatric Medicine*, *15*, 663–696. Evidence Level IV.

Iosifescu, D. V. (2007). Treating depression in the medically ill. *Psychiatric Clinics of North America*, *30*, 77–99. Evidence Level V.

Jacob, S., & Spinler, S. A. (2006). Hyponatremia associated with selective serotonin-reuptake inhibitors in older adults. *The Annals of Pharmacotherapy, 40*(9), 1618–1622. Evidence Level I.

Johansson, P., Dahlström, U., & Broström, A. (2006). Consequences and predictors of depression in patients with chronic heart failure: Implications for nursing care and future research. *Progress in Cardiovascular Nursing, 21*(4), 202–211. Evidence Level V.

Juurlink, D. N., Herrmann, N., Szalai, J. P., Kopp, A., & Redelmeier, D. A. (2004). Medical illness and the risk of suicide in the elderly. *Archives of Internal Medicine,164*(11), 1179–1184. Evidence Level IV.

Kales, H. C., & Mellow, A. M. (2006). Race and depression: Does race affect the diagnosis and treatment of late-life depression? *Geriatrics, 61*(5), 18–21. Evidence Level VI.

Kang-Yi, C., & Gellis, Z. D. (2010). A systematic review of community-based health interventions on depression for older adults with heart disease. *Aging & Mental Health, 14*(1), 1–19. Evidence Level I.

Katon, W. J., Schoenbaum, M., Fan, M. Y., Callahan, C. M., Williams, J., Jr., Hunkeler, E., . . . Unützer, J. (2005). Cost-effectiveness of improving primary care treatment of late-life depression. *Archives of General Psychiatry, 62*(12), 1313–1320. Evidence Level II.

Katz, I. R., Streim, J., & Parmelee, P. (1994). Prevention of depression, recurrences, and complications in late life. *Preventive Medicine, 23*, 743–750. Evidence Level I.

Koenig, H. G. (1991). Depressive disorders in older medical inpatients. *American Family Practice, 44*, 1243–1250. Evidence Level VI.

Kraaij, V., Arensman, E., & Spinhoven, P. (2002). Negative life events and depression in elderly persons: A meta-analysis. *Journals of Gerontology: Series B: Psychological Sciences and Social Sciences, 57*(1), P87–P94. Evidence Level I.

Kronish, I. M., Rieckmann, N., Schwartz, J. E., Schwartz, D. R., & Davidson, K. W. (2009). Is depression after an acute coronary syndrome simply a marker of known prognostic factors for mortality? *Psychosomatic Medicine, 71*(7), 697–703. Evidence Level II.

Kuo, B., Chong, V., & Joseph, J. (2008). Depression and its psychosocial correlates among older Asian immigrants in North America: A critical review of two decades' research. *Journal of Aging & Health, 20*(6), 615–652. Evidence Level I.

Kurlowicz, L. H. (1994). Depression in hospitalized medically ill elders: Evolution of the concept. *Archives in Psychiatric Nursing, 8*, 124–126. Evidence Level VI.

Laidlaw, K., Davidson, K., Toner, H., Jackson, G., Clark, S., Law, J., . . . Cross, S. (2008). A randomised controlled trial of cognitive behaviour therapy vs treatment as usual in the treatment of mild to moderate late life depression. *International Journal of Geriatric Psychiatry, 23*(8), 843–850. Evidence Level II.

Lane, D. A., Chong Aun Yeong L., & Gregory, Y. (2005). Psychological interventions for depression in heart failure. *Cochrane Database of Systematic Reviews*, (1), CD003329. Evidence Level I.

Lawton, M. P., Moss, M. S., Winter, L., & Hoffman, C. (2002). Motivation in later life: Personal projects and well-being. *Psychology & Aging, 17*(4), 539–547. Evidence Level IV.

Lebowitz, B. D. (1996). Diagnosis and treatment of depression in late life an overview of the NIH consensus statement. *Journal of the American Geriatric Society, 4*(Suppl. 1), S3–S6. Evidence Level V.

Lenze, E. J., Mulsant, B. H., Shear, M. K., Alexopoulos, G. S., Frank, E., & Reynolds, C. F., III. (2001). Comorbidity of depression and anxiety disorders in later life. *Depression and Anxiety, 14*, 86–93. Evidence Level IV.

Lin, E. H., Katon, W., Von Korff, M., Tang, L., Williams, J. W., Jr., Kroenke, K., . . . Unützer, J. (2003). Effect of improving depression care on pain and functional outcomes among older adults with arthritis: A randomized controlled trial. *Journal of American Medical Association, 290*(18), 2428–2434. Evidence Level II.

Luoma, J. B., Martin, C. E., & Pearson, J. L. (2002). Contact with mental health and primary care providers before suicide: A review of the evidence. *American Journal of Psychiatry, 159*, 909–916. Evidence Level V.

Lyness, J. M., Kim, J., Tang, W., Tu, X., Conwell, Y., King, D. A., & Caine, E. D. (2007). The clinical significance of subsyndromal depression in older primary care patients. *American Journal of Geriatric Psychiatry, 15*(3), 214–223.

Mackin, R. S., & Areán, P. A. (2005). Evidence-based psychotherapeutic interventions for geriatric depression. *Psychiatric Clinics of North America, 28*(4), 805–820. Evidence Level VI.

McDade-Montez, E. A., Christensen, A. J., Cvengros, J. A., & Lawton, W. J. (2006). The role of depression symptoms in dialysis withdrawal. *Health Psychology, 25*(2), 198–204. Evidence Level IV.

McKeowen, R. E., Cuffe, S. P., & Schulz, R. M. (2006). US suicide rates by age group, 1970–2002: An examination of recent trends. *American Journal of Public Health, 96*(10), 1744–1751. Evidence Level V.

Mitchell, A. J., & Subramaniam, H. (2005). Prognosis of depression in old age compared to middle age: A systematic review of comparative studies. *American Journal of Psychiatry, 162*(9), 1588–1601. Evidence Level I.

Modrego, P. J., & Ferrandez, J. (2004). Depression in patients with mild cognitive impairment increases the risk of developing dementia of Alzheimer type: A prospective cohort study. *Archives in Neurology, 61*, 1290–1293. Evidence Level IV.

Mottram, P., Wilson, K., & Strobl, J. (2006). Antidepressants for depressed elderly. *Cochrane Database of Systematic Reviews*, (1), CD003491. Evidence Level I.

Mukai, Y., Tampi, R. R. (2009). Treatment of depression in the elderly: A review of the recent literature on the efficacy of single- versus dual-action antidepressants. *Clinical Therapeutics, 31*(5), 945–961. Evidence Level I.

National Institutes of Health Consensus Development Panel. (1992). Diagnosis and treatment of depression in late life. *The Journal of the American Medical Association, 268*, 1018–1024. Evidence Level I.

Navarro, V., Gastó, C., Torres, X., Masana, G., Penadés, R., Guarch, J., . . . Catalán, R. (2008). Continuation/maintenance treatment with nortriptyline versus combined nortriptyline and ECT in late-life psychotic depression: A two-year randomized study. *The American Journal of Geriatric Psychiatry, 16*(6), 498–505. Evidence Level II.

Nelson, J. C., Delucchi, K., & Schneider, L. S. (2008). Efficacy of second generation antidepressants in late-life depression: A meta-analysis of the evidence. *The American Journal of Geriatric Psychiatry, 16*(7), 558–567. Evidence Level I.

Olin, J. T., Katz, I. R., Meyers, B. S., Schneider, L. S., & Lebowitz, B. D. (2002). Provisional diagnostic criteria for depression of Alzheimer disease: Rationale and background. *American Journal of Geriatric Psychiatry, 10*, 129–141. Evidence Level V.

Onrust, S. A., & Cuijpers, P. (2006). Mood and anxiety disorders in widowhood: A systematic review. *Aging & Mental Health, 10*(4), 327–334. Evidence Level I.

Pfaff, J. J., & Almeida, O. P. (2005). Detecting suicidal ideation in older patients: Identifying risk factors within the general practice setting. *British Journal of General Practice, 55*(513), 261–262. Evidence Level IV.

Pinquart, M., Duberstein, P. R., & Lyness, J. M. (2007). Effects of psychotherapy and other behavioral interventions on clinically depressed older adults: A meta-analysis. *Aging & Mental Health, 11*(6), 645–657. Evidence Level I.

Pinquart, M., & Sorensen, S. (2004). Associations of caregiver stressors and uplifts with subjective well-being and depressive mood: A meta-analytic comparison. *Aging & Mental Health, 8*(5), 438–449. Evidence Level I.

Piven, M. L. S. (2001). Detection of depression in the cognitive intact older adult protocol. *Journal of Gerontological Nursing, 27*(6), 8–14. Evidence Level VI.

Radloff, L. S. (1977). The CES-D scale: A self-report depression scale for research in the general population. *Applied Psychological Measurement, 1*, 385–401. Evidence Level V.

Rogers, C. E., Larkey, L. K., & Keller, C. (2009). A review of clinical trials of tai chi and qigong in older adults. *Western Journal of Nursing Research, 31*(2), 245–279. Evidence Level I.

Roman, M. W., & Callen, B. L. (2008). Screening instruments for older adult depressive disorders: Updating the evidence-based toolbox. *Issues in Mental Health Nursing, 29*(9), 924–941. doi:10.1080/01612840802274578. Evidence Level I.

Salzman, C., Wong, E., & Wright, B. C. (2002). Drug and ECT treatment of depression in the elderly, 1996-2001: A literature review. *Biological Psychiatry, 52*(3), 265–284. Evidence Level V.

Sareen, J., Cox, B. J., Afifi, T. O., de Graaf, R., Asmundson, G. J., ten Have, M., & Stein, M. B. (2005). Anxiety disorders and risk for suicidal ideation and suicide attempts: A population-based longitudinal study of adults. *Archives of General Psychiatry, 62*(11), 1249–1257. Evidence Level IV.

Schulz, R., Drayer, R. A., & Rollman, B. L. (2002). Depression as a risk factor for non-suicide mortality in the elderly. *Biological Psychiatry, 52*(3), 205–225. Evidence Level IV.

Shanmugham, B., Karp, J., Drayer, R., Reynolds, C. F., 3rd, & Alexopoulos, G. (2005). Evidence-based pharmacologic interventions for geriatric depression. *Psychiatric Clinics of North America, 28*(4), 821–835. Evidence Level VI.

Sheikh, J. I., & Yesavage, J. A. (1986). Geriatric depression scale (GDS) recent evidence and development of a shorter version. *Clinical Gerontologist, 5*, 165–173. Evidence Level V.

Siedliecki, S. L., & Good, M. (2006). Effect of music on power, pain, depression, and disability. *Journal of Advanced Nursing*, 553–562. Evidence Level IV.

Sjosten, N., & Kivela, S. L. (2006). The effects of physical exercise on depressive symptoms among the aged: A systematic review. *International Journal of Geriatric Psychiatry, 21*(5), 410–418. Evidence Level I.

Skultety, K. M., & Zeiss, A. (2006). The treatment of depression in older adults in the primary care setting: An evidence-based review. *Health Psychology, 25*(6), 665–674. Evidence Level I.

Smalbrugge, M., Pot, A. M., Jongenelis, L., Gundy, C. M., Beekman, A. T., & Eefsting, J. A. (2006). The impact of depression and anxiety on well being, disability and use of health care services in nursing home patients. *International Journal of Geriatric Psychiatry, 21*(4), 325–332. Evidence Level IV.

Snowdon, J. (2001). Is depression more prevalent in old age? *Australian and New Zealand Journal of Psychiatry, 35*, 782–787. Evidence Level VI.

Stapleton, R. D., Nielsen, E. L., Engelberg, R. A., Patrick, D. L., Curtis JR. (2005). Association of depression and life-sustaining treatment. *Chest, 127*(1), 328–334. Evidence Level III.

Steffens, D. C. (2008). Separating mood disturbance from mild cognitive impairment in geriatric depression. *International Review of Psychiatry, 20*(4), 374–381. Evidence Level V.

Steinman, L. E., Frederick, J. T., Prohaska, T., Satariano, W. A., Dornberg-Lee, S., Fisher, R., . . . Snowden, M. (2007). Recommendations for treating depression in community-based older adults. *American Journal of Preventive Medicine, 33*(3), 175–181. Evidence Level I.

Stone, M., Laughren, T., Jones, M. L., Levenson, M., Holland, P. C., Hughes, A., . . . Rochester G. (2009). Risk of suicidality in clinical trials of antidepressants in adults: Analysis of proprietary data submitted to US food and drug administration. *British Medical Journal, 339*, b2880. doi:10.1136/bmj.b2880. Evidence Level I.

Strober, L. B., & Arnett, P. A. (2009). Assessment of depression in three medically ill, elderly populations: Alzheimer's disease, parkinson's disease, and stroke. *The Clinical Neuropsychologist, 23*(2), 205–230. Evidence Level I.

Szanto, K., Mulsant, B. H., Houck, P., Dew, M. A., & Reynolds, C. F., III. (2003). Occurrence and course of suicidality during short-term treatment of late-life depression. *Archives of General Psychiatry, 60*(6), 610–617. Evidence Level IV.

Teri, L., Mckenzie, G., & LaFazia, D. (2005). Psychosocial treatment of depression in older adults with dementia. *Clinical Psychology: Science and Practice, 12*(3), 303–316. Evidence Level I.

Thompson, S., Herrmann, N., Rapoport, M. J., & Lanctôt, K. L. (2007). Efficacy and safety of antidepressants for treatment of depression in Alzheimer's disease: A meta-analysis. *Canadian Journal of Psychiatry.Revue Canadienne De Psychiatrie, 52*(4), 248–255. Evidence Level I.

Turvey, C. L., Conwell, Y., Jones, M. P., Phillips, C., Simonsick, E., Pearson, J. L., & Wallace, R. (2002). Risk factors for late-life suicide: A prospective, community-based study. *American Journal of Geriatric Psychiatry, 10*(4), 398–406. Evidence Level III.

Unützer, J., Katon, W., Callahan, C. M., Williams, J. W., Jr., Hunkeler, E., Harpole, L., . . . Langston, C. (2002). Collaborative care management of late-life depression in the primary care setting: A randomized controlled trial. *The Journal of the American Medical Association, 288*(22), 2836–2845. Evidence Level II.

Van der Kooy, K., van Hout, H., Marwijk, H., Marten, H., Stehouwer, C., & Beekman, A. (2007). Depression and the risk for cardiovascular diseases: Systematic review and meta analysis. *International Journal of Geriatric Psychiatry, 22*(7), 613–626. Evidence Level I.

Vink, D., Aartsen, M. J., & Schoevers, R. A. (2008). Risk factors for anxiety and depression in the elderly: A review. *Journal of Affective Disorders, 106*(1–2), 29–44. Evidence Level I.

Virnig, B., Huang, Z., Lurie, N., Musgrave, D., McBean, A. M., & Dowd, B. (2004). Does Medicare managed care provide equal treatment for mental illness across races? *Archives of General Psychiatry, 61*, 201–205. Evidence Level IV.

von Ammon Cavanaugh, S., Furlanetto, L. M., Creech, S. D., & Powell, L. H. (2001). Medical illness, past depression, and present depression: A predictive triad for in-hospital mortality. *American Journal of Psychiatry, 158*(1), 43–48. Evidence Level III.

Voyer, P., & Martin, L. S. (2003). Improving geriatric mental health nursing care: making a case for going beyond psychotropic medications. *International Journal of Mental Health Nursing, 12*(1), 11–21. Evidence Level VI.

Waern, M., Rubenowitz, E., & Wilhelmson, K. (2003). Predictors of suicide in the old elderly. *Gerontology, 49*(5), 328–334. Evidence Level V.

Walker, E. M., & Steffens, D. C. (2010). Understanding depression and cognitive impairment in the elderly. *Psychiatric Annals, 40*(1), 29–40. Evidence Level IV.

Watson, L. C., & Pignone, M. P. (2003). Screening accuracy for late-life depression in primary care: A systematic review. *Journal of Family Practice, 52*(12), 956–964. Evidence Level I.

Williams, D. R., González, H. M., Neighbors, H., Nesse, R., Abelson, J. M., Sweetman, J., & Jackson, J. S. (2007). Prevalence and distribution of major depressive disorder in African Americans, Caribbean blacks, and non-Hispanic whites: Results from the National Survey of American Life. *Archives in General Psychiatry, 64*(3), 305–315. Evidence Level IV.

Wilson, K. C., Mottram, P. G., & Vassilas, C. A. (2008). Psychotherapeutic treatments for older depressed people. *Cochrane Database of Systematic Reviews,* (1), CD004853. Evidence Level I.

Wu, Q., Magnus, J. H., Liu, J., Bencaz, A. F., & Hentz, J. G. (2009). Depression and low bone mineral density: A meta-analysis of epidemiologic studies. *Osteoporosis International: A Journal Established as Result of Cooperation between the European Foundation for Osteoporosis and the National Osteoporosis Foundation of the USA, 20*(8), 1309–1320. Evidence Level I.

Zubenko, G. S., Zubenko, W. N., McPherson, S., Spoor, E., Marin, D. B., Farlow, M. R., . . . Sunderland, T. (2003). A collaborative study of the emergence and clinical features of the major depressive syndrome of Alzheimer's disease. *American Journal of Psychiatry, 160*, 857–866. Evidence Level I.

Dementia

10

Kathleen Fletcher

EDUCATIONAL OBJECTIVES

On completion of this chapter, the reader should be able to:

1. describe the spectrum of dementia syndromes
2. recognize the clinical features of dementia
3. discuss pharmacological and nonpharmacological approaches in the management of dementia
4. develop a nursing plan of care for an older adult with dementia

OVERVIEW

Dementia is most commonly defined as a clinical syndrome of cognitive deficits that involves both memory impairments and a disturbance in at least one other area of cognition (American Psychiatric Association, 2000). In addition to disruptions in cognition, dementia is associated with a gradual decline in function and changes in mood and behavior.

There are many causes of dementia and dementia-like presentations. Differentiating these changes early in the course of illness is important because condition-specific assessment, monitoring, and management strategies can be employed. Differential diagnoses among conditions that cause cognitive impairment are confounded by the fact that these conditions may coexist and disparate dementing disorders may be similarly clinically expressed.

Major goals in the clinical approach to a person presenting with cognitive impairments are identification and resolution of potentially reversible conditions (e.g., delirium, depression), recognition and control of comorbid conditions, early diagnosis and management of a dementing illness, and the provision of caregiver support. The focus of this chapter is on assessment and management of the progressive dementia syndromes.

For description of Evidence Levels cited in this chapter, see Chapter 1, Developing and Evaluating Clinical Practice Guidelines: A Systematic Approach, page 7.

BACKGROUND AND STATEMENT OF PROBLEM

Global estimates reflect that 24.3 million people have dementia today, with 4–6 million new cases every year (Ferri et al., 2005). The rapid growth of the older adult population in the United States is associated with a significant increase in the prevalence of dementia. Dementia affects about 5% of individuals aged 65 and older (Richie & Lovestone, 2002), and the prevalence increases exponentially with age rising to nearly 50% in individuals aged 85 and older (Evans et al., 1989). More than 4.5 million Americans have the most common form of dementia, Alzheimer's disease (AD), a number that is expected to triple by the middle of the 21st century (Hebert, Scherr, Bienias, Bennett, & Evans, 2003).

This chapter will discuss the most common forms of progressive dementia, AD, vascular dementia (VaD), and dementia with Lewy bodies (DLB). Less common, although not less significant, is progressive dementia associated with Parkinson's disease (PDD), frontotemporal dementia, dementias associated with HIV, and Creutzfeld-Jakob disease.

AD, the most common form of dementia, accounts for more than 60% of all cases. A chronic neurodegenerative disease, first described by Alois Alzheimer in 1907, AD is characterized by neurofibrillary plaques and "tangles" in the brain. The extracellular accumulation of amyloid beta-proteins in the neuritic plaques is one of the hallmarks of AD (Ariga, Miyatake, & Yu, 2010). The variation in the clinical presentation of the disease depends on the area of the brain that is affected. Classic features of AD include progressive loss of memory, deterioration of language and other cognitive functions, decline in the ability to perform activities of daily living (ADLs), and changes in personality and behavior and judgment dysfunction (Castellani, Rolston, & Smith, 2010). Mild cognitive impairment (MCI), a syndrome defined as cognitive decline greater than expected for an individual's age that minimally interferes with ADLs (Gauthier et al., 2006), may be a precursor of dementia. Incidence rates of MCI are 51–76.8 per 1,000 person-years, with a higher incidence in advanced age, lower education, and hypertension (Luck, Luppa, Briel, & Riedel-Heller, 2010). Individuals with MCI are nearly twice as likely to die and more than three times as likely to develop AD in a 5-year period as a cohort of individuals without MCI (Bennett et al., 2002).

VaD, sometimes referred to as vascular cognitive impairment and previously known as multi-infarct dementia (MID), refers to dementia resulting from cerebrovascular disease. It is the second most common cause of dementia among older adults and represents approximately 20% of all cases of dementia in the United States (Román, 2003). There are many types of VaD, and lumping them under a single rubric causes some diagnostic confusion (Kirshner, 2009). The diagnosis of VaD is based on the association between a cerebrovascular event and the onset of clinical features of dementia, including evidence of focal deficits, gait disturbances, and impairments in executive function. As compared with AD, memory may not be impaired or is more mildly affected. It is not uncommon that AD and VaD pathology coexist and this, often referred to as a mixed dementia, is likely to increase as the population ages (Langa, Foster, & Larson, 2004).

DLB is a neurodegenerative dementia that results when Lewy bodies form in the brain. Lewy bodies are pathological aggregations of alpha-synuclein found in the cytoplasma of neurons (McKeith et al., 2003). Clinical features include cognitive and behavioral changes in combination with features of parkinsonism. Disorders of executive function occur early. Hallucinations and visuospatial disturbances are prominent. Although rigidity and unsteady gait are common, tremors are not (Geldmacher, 2004).

Many, but not all, patients with Parkinson's disease develop a dementia years after the motor symptoms appear. Distinctions have been made clinically between the DLB and the PDD based on the sequence of the appearance of symptoms (McKeith et al., 2005). DLB and PDD may represent the same pathological process along a disease spectrum (Hanson & Lippa, 2009).

ASSESSMENT OF THE PROBLEM

Goals of Assessment

Early identification of cognitive impairment is the most important goal in assessment. Cognitive impairment resulting from conditions such as dementia, delirium, or depression represents critically serious pathology and requires urgent assessment and tailored interventions. Yet, diminished or altered cognitive functioning is often perceived by health care professionals as a normal consequence of aging, and opportunities for timely intervention are too often missed (Milisen, Braes, Fick, & Foreman, 2006). Although distinctions have been made comparing the clinical features of the common cognitive impairments associated with delirium, dementia, and depression, this is difficult to do clinically because these conditions often coexist and older adults can demonstrate atypical features in any of these conditions.

The second most important assessment goal is to identify a potentially reversible primary or contributing cause of a cognitive impairment. The common causes of reversible cognitive impairment (i.e., delirium) in the older adult are covered in the delirium chapter in this text.

History Taking

Complaints from the patient or observations made by others of memory loss, problems with decision making and/or judgment, or a decline in an ADL function should alert the health care professional that a progressive form of dementia might exist. Collecting an accurate history is the cornerstone to the assessment process, yet this obviously is a challenge in the individual presenting with cognitive impairment. The assessment domains covered in history taking include functional, cognitive, and behavioral queries and observations. The history-taking process involves first interviewing the patient followed, perhaps, by clarifying, elaborating, and validating information with the family or others familiar with the capabilities and expressions of the patient.

Even when a diagnosis of dementia has been made, it is often not communicated well across care settings. The easiest way to increase recognition of dementia in older hospital patients is to add the items "severe memory problems," "AD," and "dementia" to the list of diseases and conditions patients and families are routinely asked about on intake forms and in intake interviews.

Functional Assessment

AD is characterized by deterioration in the ability to perform ADLs. Because cognitive assessment can be embarrassing and/or threatening, it may be more respectful to initiate the conversation around the patient's functional domain. Asking the patient to elaborate on his or her functional abilities in ADLs as well as instrumental activities of daily living (IADLs) and eliciting any identified decline with specified chronology can provide some insight. The reader is referred to Chapter 6, Assessment of Physical Function, on function in this test for general approach and tools for functional assessment. Several functional tools have been tested specifically in individuals with dementia.

The Functional Activities Questionnaire (FAQ) is an informant-based measure of functional ability and has been recognized for its ability to discriminate early dementia (Pfeffer, Kurosaki, Harrah, Chance, & Filos, 1982). An informant, typically the primary caregiver, is asked to rate the performance of the patient in 10 different activities. The Modified Alzheimer's Disease Cooperative Study–Activities of Daily Living Inventory (ADCS-ADL) is a specific functional tool used primarily in clinical drug trials to assess and monitor patients with moderate-to-severe AD (Galasko et al., 1997). Clinical studies using this scale have indicated that cholinesterase inhibitors offer an effective approach to treating functional decline (Potkin, 2002). The patient's daily caregiver is asked to rate the older adult's usual performance on the more basic measures of function over the previous month to identify progression of functional decline.

Cognitive Assessment

The cognitive domain is assessed as part of a broader mental status evaluation, the components of which are listed in Table 10.1. Whereas some of the parameters of a mental status evaluation (such as memory or cognition) might be measured with a standardized tool such as the Mini-Mental State Examination (MMSE), others require specific inquiry or direct or indirect observation by the health care professional and/or caregiver. The measure of mood is totally subjective and is based on self-report status. The evaluation always provides the opportunity to identify sensory impairments (i.e., vision and hearing loss), which can further impact cognition, function, and behavior. There are a variety of tools for assessing cognitive impairment, some more sensitive to mild dementia and others to moderate-to-severe dementia.

The gold standard of tools that measure cognition is the MMSE developed more than 30 years ago (Folstein, Folstein, & McHugh, 1975). Used extensively in clinical trials as well as in a variety of clinical settings, it is relatively easy to administer and score and can be used to assess cognitive changes over time. The annual rate of decline on the MMSE in AD is 3.3 points annually (Han, Cole, Bellavance, McCusker, & Primeau, 2000). The MMSE has established validity and reliability, although concerns continue to be expressed by clinicians that it is time consuming and, in some circumstances, the

---

TABLE 10.1

Components of mental status evaluation.

Orientation: person, place, time

Attention and concentration: ability to attend and concentrate

Memory: ability to register, recall, retain

Judgment: ability to make appropriate decisions

Executive control functions: ability to abstract, plan, sequence, and use feedback to guide performance

Speech and language: ability to communicate ideas and receive and express a message

Presence of delusions, hallucinations

Mood and affect

relevancy of selected questions has been raised. The MMSE score is strongly related to education, with high false-positive rates for those with little education, and predictive power is also significantly influenced by language (Parker & Philp, 2004). It is insensitive to executive dysfunction and has been criticized for a lack of sensitivity in detecting early or mild dementia (Leifer, 2003). As has been suggested with other measures of cognitive testing, the MMSE may have a cultural bias (Manly & Espino, 2004). Clinicians must remain aware that a high score on the MMSE does not rule out cognitive decline or the possibility of dementia, particularly in high-functioning individuals with cognitive complaints (Manning, 2004). The tool is no longer in the public domain and copyright permission must be secured. A tool with comparable sensitivity and specificity for detecting dementia is the St. Louis University Medical Status (SLUMS) examination, and it is available free (Tariq, Tumosa, Chibnall, Perry, & Morley, 2006).

Unlike the more language-based tools described earlier, the Clock Drawing Test (CDT) assesses cognition focused on executive function. A systematic review of the literature identified the CDT's usefulness in predicting future cognitive impairment (Peters & Pinto, 2008). Scoring is based on the ability to free-hand draw the face of a clock, insert the hour numbers in the appropriate location, and then set the hands of the clock to the time designated by the examiner. The CDT is strongly correlated with executive function (i.e., the ability to execute complex behaviors and to solve problems) and is useful in the detection of mild dementia (Royall, Mulroy, Chiodo, & Polk, 1999). It also correlates moderately with driving performance—as the CDT score drops, the number of driving errors increases (Freund, Gravenstein, & Ferris, 2002; Freund, Gravenstein, Ferris, Burke, & Shaheen, 2005).

A clinically useful tool that combines the CDT with measures of cognition (i.e., three-word recall) is the Mini-Cognitive (Mini-Cog; Borson, Scanlan, Brush, Vitaliano, & Dokmak, 2000). The Mini-Cog detected cognitive impairment in a community sample of predominately ethnic minority better than primary care physician assessment (84% vs. 41%), particularly in milder stages of the disease (Borson, Scanlan, Watanabe, Tu, & Lessig, 2005).

A systematic review of the Mini-Cog for screening for dementia in primary care demonstrated that it was brief, easy to administer, clinically acceptable and effective, and minimally affected by education, gender, and ethnicity (Milne, Culverwell, Guss, Tuppen, & Whelton, 2008) with psychometric properties similar to the MMSE (Brodaty, Low, Gibson, & Burns, 2006).

Behavioral Assessment

Behavioral changes occur both early and throughout dementia (Kilik, Hopkins, Day, Prince, Prince, & Rows, 2008) and are also seen in MCI; commonly, these include depression, anxiety, and irritability (Monastero, Mangialasche, Camarda, Ercolani, & Camarda, 2009). Regular assessment and monitoring can help identify the triggers of disruptive behavior and early manifestations of the behavior. Timely interventions that result in de-escalation of the behavior can help decrease the level of distress experienced by both the patient and the caregiver. Behavioral management can help maintain functionality and safety. Commonly demonstrated behaviors are those associated with agitation and psychosis. Asking the patient about levels of restlessness, anxiety, and irritability is important because, at times, these emotional or behavioral states occur even earlier than cognitive changes. Aggression, wandering, delusions and hallucinations, and resistance to care are manageable with pharmacological and nonpharmacological treatment options.

The literature on the link between psychosis and aggression in people with dementia is mixed (Shub, Ball, Abbas, Gottumukkala, & Kunik, 2010). The Neuropsychiatric Inventory (NPI) measures frequency and severity of psychiatric symptoms and behavioral manifestations in individuals with dementias. The NPI takes about 10 minutes to administer, during which the caregiver is asked screening and probing questions related to the presence and degree of behaviors such as agitation, anxiety, irritability, apathy, and disinhibition. The NPI also includes a measure of caregiver stress. A briefer questionnaire version, the NPI-Q, also has established validity (Kaufer et al., 2000).

Because as many as 50% of individuals with dementia have coexisting depressive symptoms (Lee & Lyketsos, 2003), it is important to conduct an adjunctive assessment of depression. Recognizing depressive symptoms in older adults is challenging, and using an interviewer-rated instrument is recommended in addition to using clinical judgment (Onega, 2006). The Geriatric Depression Scale (GDS) is a screening instrument that takes only a few minutes to administer and is discussed along with appropriate depression management strategies in detail in Chapter 9, Depression in Older Adults.

Referral of the patient to a neuropsychologist for more extensive neuropsychological testing might be indicated to provide more specific diagnostic information associated with neurodegenerative disease states and areas of brain dysfunction. This kind of assessment can identify subtle cognitive impairments in higher functioning individuals, can distinguish MCI from dementia, and can provide direction and support for care providers and the family (Adelman & Daly, 2005).

Physical Examination and Diagnostics

Once the functional, cognitive, and behavioral domains in progressive dementia have been established through history taking of the patient and caregiver, a thorough review of systems is undertaken, followed by the physical examination. The history-taking process narrows the differential diagnosis of reversible and irreversible causes for dementia. A thorough neurological and cardiovascular examination will help to specify the etiology of a single type or combined dementia that will direct the need for laboratory and imaging tests. Cardiovascular findings such as hypertension, arrhythmias, and extra heart sounds or murmurs along with focal neurological findings such as weakness and sensory deficit may favor a diagnosis of VaD; pathological reflexes, gait disorders, and abnormal cerebellar findings may be indicative of AD; and parkinsonian signs might indicate dementia associated with either Lewy bodies or Parkinson's disease (Kane, Ouslander, Abrass, & Resnick, 2009).

There are no specific laboratory tests for the diagnosis of progressive dementia other than those that can primarily indicate a potentially reversible or contributing cause. The American Academy of Neurology (AAN) recommends two specific laboratory tests (i.e., thyroid function and B_{12}) in the initial evaluation of suspected dementia (Knopman et al., 2001). The AAN similarly recommends that all patients with suspected dementia have a magnetic resonance imaging (MRI) study or noncontrast computed tomography (CT) as part of the initial workup. Once dementia has become clinically relevant and a cause becomes apparent, there is no further diagnostic yield afforded by imaging.

Caregiver Assessment

It is important to remember that the caregiver is a patient, too, in that they suffer, as does the patient with dementia. Caregiver need and burden refers to the psychological, physical, and financial burden associated with caregiving. Caregivers are at risk for depression, physical illness, and anxiety (Cooper, Balamurali, & Livingston, 2007; Schoenmakers, Buntinx, & Delepeleire, 2010). The Zarit Burden Interview (ZBI) can be used to identify the degree of burden experienced by the caregiver. The ZBI is a four-item screening followed by an additional 12 items with good reliability and validity (Higginson, Gao, Jackson, Murray, & Harding, 2010). Administration of this tool to a community-dwelling caregiver can indicate the extent of impact caregiving has on the caregiver's health, social, and emotional well-being and finances. The Modified Caregiver Strain Index (CSI) is another tool that has been used to identify families with caregiving concerns (Onega, 2008). There is a growing body of literature that describes the relationship between people with dementia and the family members who care for them (Ablitt, Jones, & Muers, 2009).

INTERVENTIONS AND CARE STRATEGIES

There is no cure for progressive dementia. The management of individuals with dementia requires pharmacological and nonpharmacological interventions.

Pharmacological Interventions

The goals of pharmacological therapy in dementia include preserving what the disease destroys in cognitive and functional ability, minimizing what the disease imposes in the way of behavior disturbances, and slowing the progression of the disease effects brought on by the destruction of neurons (Geldmacher, 2003). Nurses, regardless of whether they are the prescribers of drug therapy, need to be informed about the variety of drugs used in managing dementia and the evidence supporting the pharmacological approaches. Although there is substantial evidence that adults with mild-to-moderate AD (and perhaps VaD and DLB) would benefit from drug therapy, there are no solid data in support for drug therapy into the advanced stage of the disease (Olsen, Poulsen, & Lublin, 2005).

Acetylcholinesterase inhibitors are the mainstay of treatment. Four are currently available in the United States: donepezil hydrochloride (Aricept), rivastigmine tartrate (Exelon), galantamine hydrobromide (Reminyl), and tacrine hydrochloride (Tacrine)—the oldest and less favored drug because of its adverse effect on the liver and multiple daily dosing. Cognitive improvements in patients with mild-to-moderate AD have been shown for each of the other three drugs (Birks, Grimley Evans, Iakovidou, & Tsolaki, 2000; Birks & Harvey, 2006; Loy & Schneider 2006). These drugs also provide cognitive and behavioral improvement in other forms of progressive dementia including VaD (Kavirajan & Schneider 2007) and DLB (Erkinjuntti et al., 2002; Wild, Pettit, & Burns, 2003). With the exception of Tacrine, the acetylcholinesterase inhibitors are safe and well tolerated; however, they may have gastrointestinal side effects (i.e., nausea, anorexia, and diarrhea). Dementia pharmacological therapy can improve the quality of life for the patient and the caregiver and delays nursing home placement (Geldmacher, Provenzano, McRae, Mastey, & Ieni, 2003; Lopez et al., 2002). Rivastigmine is also available as a transdermal patch.

Memantine (Namenda), approved for moderate-to-severe dementia, has a different mechanism of action than the acetylcholinesterase inhibitors. This N-methyl-D-aspartate receptor antagonist has neuroprotective effects that prevent excitatory neurotoxicity. Individuals with AD and VaD have improved cognition and behavior on this drug (McShane, Areosa Sastre, & Minakaran, 2006). Side effects of memantine, although uncommon, include diarrhea, insomnia, and agitation. Combined administration of cholinesterase inhibitors with memantine demonstrated increased efficacy in advanced AD as compared to cholinesterase inhibitors alone (Riepe et al., 2007).

Pharmacological Therapy for Problematic Behaviors

Behavior changes are common in the mid to later stages of progressive dementia and, although nonpharmacological interventions are preferred, supplementation with a tailored drug regimen is sometimes necessary. Psychotropic medications, primarily antipsychotics, can be administered to help the individual regain control and be less disruptive—positive outcomes for the caregiver as well as the patient. Drugs must be prescribed in the lowest effective dose for the shortest amount of time (Gray, 2004). The patient needs to be closely monitored for effectiveness and adverse side effects. Psychotropic medications have a high risk of adverse drug events and this is covered in the Chapter 17, Reducing Adverse Drug Events.

Psychotropic therapy for different behaviors is always short term (i.e., 3–6 months). Once the target symptoms are relieved or abbreviated, then consideration must be given to terminate therapy. Long-term psychotropic drug therapy should be considered only if the symptoms reoccur. Psychotic symptoms (such as delusions and hallucinations) frequently occur in the later stages of progressive dementia (Ropacki & Jeste, 2005) and are often associated with agitation and aggression (Holroyd, 2004). The conventional antipsychotic haloperidol (Haldol) has been used for decades and remains the most commonly used drug for control of psychotic symptoms in individuals with dementia. A Cochrane Review (Lonergan, Luxenberg, & Colford, 2002) validated the useful role of Haldol in managing aggression but did not find evidence for its role in managing agitation for patients with dementia. The side effects of conventional antipsychotics are considerable and include extrapyramidal symptoms, tardive dyskinesia, sedation, orthostatic hypotension, and falls.

Although not approved by the U.S. Food and Drug Administration (FDA), the atypical antipsychotics are often prescribed for use in patients with dementia. Evidence reflects that they may benefit people with dementia, but the risks of adverse events (e.g., cardiovascular, extrapyrimidal symptoms) may outweigh the benefit, especially with long-term treatment (Ballard & Waite, 2006). Agents available on the market include risperidone, olanzapine, quetiapine, ziprasidone, aripiprazole, and paliperidone. There is little to no published data on the efficacy and safety of the last three drugs listed earlier. Additional research is needed to determine when and how to use psychotropic medications to address behaviors in individuals with dementia. Other drug categories are sometimes used to control behavioral symptoms.

Benzodiazepines (e.g., lorazepam, oxazepam, alprazolam) are sometimes used to manage agitation and aggression; however, the risk–benefit ratio is often unsatisfactory. Although benzodiazepines may be useful in rapidly sedating the agitated patient with dementia, the potential for falls and worsening of cognition limit long-term use.

Although antidepressants and anticonvulsants are sometimes used to treat agitation in dementia, there is insufficient evidence to support their use. Behavioral disturbances should not necessarily be interpreted as depression.

Supplemental Drugs

Anti-inflammatory drugs and estrogen; herbals such as gingko; and vitamins such as B$_{12}$, folate, and vitamin E—although sometimes touted and commonly used—have no proven efficacy for dementia, although some isolated studies have demonstrated a benefit. Dementia associated with VaD requires appropriate control of hypertension, hyperlipidemia, and aspirin therapy. Parkinsonism (rigidity), seen with DLB, may benefit from dopaminergic therapy.

Nonpharmacological Strategies

Nonpharmacological strategies including those from the cognitive, behavioral, and environmental domains in combination with staff support and education are effective (Burgener & Twigg, 2002). Physical/functional, environmental, psychosocial, behavioral, and end-of-life (EOL) care interventions are discussed in the succeeding section.

Physical/Functional Interventions

Maintaining physical and functional well-being of the individual with progressive dementia facilitates independence, maintains health status, and can ease the caregiving burden. Interventions include adequate nutrition and hydration, regular exercise, maintenance of ADLs, proper rest and sleep, appropriate bowel and bladder routines, proper dental hygiene and care, and current vaccinations. Because comorbidities are common (Lyketsos et al., 2005), regular assessment, vigilant monitoring, and aggressive management of acute and chronic conditions are necessary. Vehicular driving safety might need to be examined because recent evidence indicates that individuals with dementia pose a risk in driving safety (Man-Son-Hing, Marshall, Molnar, & Wilson, 2007). There is insufficient evidence to support or refute the benefit of neuropsychiatric testing or intervention strategies for drivers with dementia (Iverson et al., 2010).

Environmental Interventions

A specialized ecological model of care, which facilitates interaction between the person and environment in a more home-like environment, has proven to be beneficial for individuals with dementia. This model affords greater privacy, encourages meaningful activities, and permits more choice than the traditional model of care. It also demonstrates that individuals with dementia experience less decline in ADLs and are more engaged with the environment with no measurable differences found in cognitive measures, depression, or social withdrawal (Reimer, Slaughter, Donaldson, Currie, & Eliasziw, 2004).

A systematic review reported inclusive results and suggested that more research is needed with regard to the use of bright light in fostering better sleep and reducing behavior problems in dementia (Forbes et al., 2009). The use of aromatherapy to reduce disturbed behavior, promote sleep, and stimulate motivation also shows promise but needs more study (Thorgrimsen, Spector, Wiles, & Orrell, 2003). Manipulation of the environment (e.g., alarms, circular hallways, visual or structural barriers) to minimize wandering has not conclusively demonstrated to be effective (Peatfield, Futrell, & Cox, 2002). There is a lack of robust evidence supporting nonpharmacological interventions for wandering (Robinson et al., 2007).

Psychosocial Interventions

Mental and social engagement is important to the well-being of all older adults. Meaningful activity and involvement is no less important in individuals with dementia. Although the effectiveness of counseling or procedural memory stimulation is not supported in mild-stage dementia, reality orientation does appear to be effective (Bates, Boote, & Beverley, 2004). The evidence suggests that cognitive therapy is more beneficial than no therapy at all, but it may be patient-specific (Forbes, 2004). Validation therapy, based on caregiver acceptance of the reality of the person with dementia's experience, may be of value but the evidence is lacking (Neal & Briggs, 2003).

Recreational therapies including music have shown to reduce psychological symptoms in dementia with limited efficacy and questionable duration of action (O'Connor, Ames, Gardner, & King, 2009), and more research is needed to explore the effects of music therapy on the behavior and well-being of individuals with dementia (Wall & Duffy, 2010).

Support groups, counseling, and education for individuals with early AD and their caregivers are essential. Caregivers often experience physical, financial, social, and emotional losses, and providing information through a structured education program and engaging them in the care planning process are essential (Jayasekara, 2009). Areas for caregiver education are detailed in Table 10.2.

Behavioral Interventions

Behavioral and psychosocial symptoms of dementia are common with every form of progressive dementia, particularly in the moderate stage. The three most troublesome symptoms are agitation, aggression, and wandering. Problematic behaviors that occur during meals or bathing can be particularly challenging. It is important to recognize and realize that any new behavior could be a sign of an acute illness or an environmental influence. Unrecognized pain can cause disruptive behavior. Short-term use of physical restraints may be necessary, but those selected should always be the least restrictive type and used for the shortest duration of time. The Progressively Lowered Stress Threshold (PLST) is a framework to optimize function, minimize disruption, and help the caregiver (Smith, Hall, Gerdner, & Buckwalter, 2006). The PLST model increases the positive appraisal and decreases the negative appraisal of the caregiving situation (Stolley, Reed, & Buckwalter, 2002) and helps

---

TABLE 10.2

Points to cover when educating caregivers.

Information about the disease and its progression

Strategies to maintain function and independence

Preservation of cognitive and physical vitality in dementia

Maintaining a safe and comfortable environment

Giving physical and emotional care

Communicating with the individual with dementia

Managing behavioral problems

Advance planning: health care and finances

Caregiver survival tips

Building a caregiver support network

the caregiver manage the aggressive behaviors demonstrated in AD (Lindsey & Buckwalter, 2009). By adapting the environment and routines, interventions are designed to help the patient with dementia use his or her functional skills and minimize potentially triggering reactions. There are six essential principles of care in the PLST:

1. *Maximize safe function*: Use familiar routines, limit choices, provide rest periods, reduce stimuli when stress occurs, and routinely identify and anticipate physical stressors (i.e., pain, urinary symptoms, hunger, or thirst).
2. *Provide unconditional positive regard*: Use respectful conversation, simple and under- standable language, and nonverbal expressions of touch.
3. *Use behaviors to gauge activity and stimulation*: Monitor for early signs of anxiety (e.g., pacing, facial grimacing) and intervene before behavior escalates.
4. *Teach caregivers to "listen" to the behaviors*: Monitor the language pattern (e.g., repeti- tion, jargon) and behaviors (e.g., rummaging) that might be showing how the person reduces stress when needs are not being met.
5. *Modify the environment*: Assess the environment to ensure safe mobility and promote way finding and orientation through cues.
6. *Provide ongoing assistance to the caregiver*: Assess and address the need for education and support.

Advance Planning and End-of-Life Care Interventions

Advanced planning and providing directives for care are important in guiding the types of interventions used at the end of life and can decrease the caregiver stress in proxy decision making. Nursing homes are common sites for EOL care for people with pro- gressive dementia; however, only 51% of all nursing home residents nationally have an advance directive (Mezey, Mitty, Bottrell, Ramsey, & Fisher, 2000). As many as 90% of the 4 million Americans with dementia will be institutionalized before death (Smith, Kokmen, & O'Brien, 2000), making this environment in particular an important focus for EOL care. There is a lack of research published on EOL care in nursing homes and most of it is descriptive (Oliver, Porock, & Zweig, 2004). The end stage of AD may last as long as 2–3 years (Brookmeyer, Corrada, Curriero, & Kawas, 2002) and frequently distressing signs and symptoms occur at this time.

Dementia itself or often-associated conditions can cause physical symptoms such as poor nutrition, urinary incontinence, skin breakdown, pain, infection, shortness of breath, fatigue, difficulty in swallowing, choking, and gurgling in addition to the behav- ioral symptoms mentioned earlier. There is no acceptable standard treatment for the consequences of advanced dementia and, where guidelines do exist, there is minimal to no palliative care content. Aggressive treatments such as antibiotics, tube feedings, psychotropic drugs, and physical restrains to address problematic behaviors appear to be prevalent, although there is no substantial evidence that these approaches are effective in end-stage dementia and that prognosis and life expectancy are improved by these strate- gies (Evers, Purohit, Perl, Khan, & Marin, 2002). Measuring quality of care at the end of life for those with dementia poses significant challenges because of the limitations in subjective reporting and therefore relies on the caregiver's analysis of cues to monitor the patient's condition and experience (Volicer, Hurley, & Blasi, 2001). Despite the clear recognition that significant improvements in EOL care for those with dementia is needed (Scherder et al., 2005), there is a lack of systematic evidence on how to approach palliative care for this population (Sampson, Ritchie, Lai, Raven, & Blanchard, 2005).

CASE STUDY

Mrs. P. is an 85-year-old Caucasian woman brought into the primary care clinic by her daughter for a geriatric consultation. She has a 4-year history of cognitive impairment that began with memory loss and impaired judgment that appears to be worsening; she is now experiencing some behavioral problems. Mrs. P. is high school educated, has been widowed for 10 years, and is a retired short-order cook. She currently lives with her daughter, son-in-law (both work full time), and grandson.

Her primary care physician completed a dementia workup at the time the symptoms appeared 4 years ago and started her on Donepezil, which was discontinued within a few days because of gastrointestinal side effects. She recently had paranoid ideation in which she accused her 15-year-old grandson of listening in on her phone conversations and taking some money from her purse. Her daughter reports that Mrs. P. has "a short fuse" and gets agitated easily. "She called me a moron and even took a swing at me the other day when I told her she smelled bad and needed to take a shower."

Mrs. P. performs her own personal hygiene, although she needs reminders and cueing at times; she is continent. She does not perform any IADLs (e.g., cooking, shopping), and it was unclear if she truly was no longer capable of performing these functions or no longer had the opportunity or desire to do them. Mrs. P. reports no desire to eat and had a weight loss resulting in a change in at least three clothing sizes that has occurred slowly over the past few years. When asked about her mood, she becomes tearful and says, "I get disgusted; no one cares about me anymore." Mrs. P. says she hates to be alone and that the family "just come and goes—they never talk with me." Her MMSE score is 18/30, with deficits in memory, calculation, and ability to copy the intersecting pentagons. She scores 10/15 on the GDS.

Past medical history includes thyroidectomy, left cataract extraction, cholecystectomy, and hysterectomy for benign disease. Her daughter thinks that Mrs. P. may have been on antihypertensives in the past. The only medication Mrs. P. takes at present is for her thyroid, but neither she nor her daughter knew the name of the drug.

On physical exam, she is afebrile; her blood pressure is 132/70, and she is about 10 lbs below her ideal body weight. Mrs. P. is alert, cooperative, and smiles at intervals during the examination and has slight hearing loss with clear canals—no thyromegaly. Cardiovascular exam reveals no murmur, edema, or discolorations of the extremities. Pulses are strong throughout. There are no focal neurological symptoms. Gait is slow but steady. Breasts are free of masses and abdomen is soft, nontender, and with no organ enlargement.

A diagnosis of depression and progressive dementia of the Alzheimer's type is made, and she is started on the combination of Donepezil and Memantine, both to be titrated slowly. Additional information from Mrs. P's primary care physician will be consulted about her thyroid function. Antidepressant therapy may be considered at a later date. Health teaching and additional resource information is provided to the family.

(continued)

CASE STUDY *(continued)*

Case Study Discussion

Depression is not uncommon in those with a progressive dementia. Severe anxiety, agitation, and aggression can occur; tearfulness and decreased appetite with weight loss may also be present. Using the PLST model, the nurse focuses on teaching the daughter to recognize triggers and prodromal signs of increasing anxiety and intervene appropriately when anxiety and agitation occur. Strategies are emphasized in each of the six PLST principles of care: maximize safe function, provide unconditional regard, use behaviors to gauge activity and stimulation, "listen" to the behaviors, modify the environment, and provide ongoing assistance to the caregiver. Less confrontational language and behaviors are emphasized in approaches and interactions with Mrs. P. The daughter is also provided with specific contact information of the geriatrician's office as well as the local and national resources available through the Alzheimer's Association (1-800-272-3900; www.alz.org) and the Alzheimer's Disease Education and Referral Center (ADEAR; 1-800-438-4380; http://www.nia.nih.gov/Alzheimers/). Additional instructions include dietary strategies to increase nutritional density, noting that additional resource information is available at the ADEAR site listed herein. Specific medication instructions with particular emphasis on how to use the titration packet are provided—*with the recommendation* to coadminister with food to reduce the likelihood of gastrointestinal side effects. The nurse plans a follow-up phone call for the next day and schedules a follow-up medical and health teaching appointment in 1 month to evaluate the effectiveness of the plan of care. The patient and family are instructed to call or return if new or changed behaviors or physical symptoms develop.

SUMMARY

It is important that health care professionals identify cognitive impairments in older adults early and differentiate a progressive from a reversible etiology, such as delirium. Comprehensive assessment, monitoring and pharmacological, and non-pharmacological management of physical, functional, cognitive, and behavioral problems are important, both in initial identification and in the ongoing care of the individual with progressive dementia. Education and support of the family and professional caregiver are essential. It is difficult to identify clearly what constitutes quality of life for the individual with progressive dementia, what interventions enhance this quality, and how this is accomplished. There is limited evidence in gerontological nursing to guide our care (Abraham, MacDonald, & Nadzam, 2006). It is imperative that geriatric nurses evaluate practice and generate new knowledge to ensure best practice in the care of individuals with progressive dementia as well as their caregivers.

Protocol 10.1: Recognition and Management of Dementia

I. GOALS
  A. Early recognition of dementing illness
  B. Appropriate management strategies in care of individuals with dementia

II. OVERVIEW
The rapid growth of the aging population is associated with an increase in the prevalence of progressive dementias. It is imperative that a differential diagnosis be ascertained early in the course of cognitive impairment and that the patient is closely monitored for coexisting morbidities. Nurses have a central role in assessment and management of individuals with progressive dementia.

III. BACKGROUND
  A. Definitions/Distinctions
    1. Dementia is a clinical syndrome of cognitive deficits that involves both memory impairments and a disturbance in at least one other area of cognition, such as aphasia, apraxia, agnosia, and disturbance in executive functioning.
    2. In addition to disruptions in cognition, dementias are commonly associated with changes in function and behavior.
    3. The most common forms of progressive dementia are Alzheimer's disease (AD), vascular dementia, and dementia with Lewy bodies; the pathophysiology for each is poorly understood.
    4. Differential diagnosis of dementing conditions is complicated by the fact that concurrent disease states (i.e., comorbidities) often coexist.
  B. Prevalence
    1. Dementia affects about 5% of individuals 65 years and older.
    2. Four to five million Americans have AD.
    3. Fourteen million are projected to have AD by the year 2040.
    4. Global prevalence of dementia is about 24.3 million, with 6 million new cases every year.
  C. Risk Factors
    1. Advanced age
    2. Mild cognitive impairment
    3. Cardiovascular disease
    4. Genetics: family history of dementia, Parkinson's disease, cardiovascular disease, stroke, presence of ApoE4 allele on chromosome 19
    5. Environment: head injury, alcohol abuse

IV. PARAMETERS OF ASSESSMENT
No formal recommendations for cognitive screening are indicated in asymptomatic individuals. Clinicians are advised to be alert for cognitive and functional decline in older adults to detect dementia and dementia-like presentation in early

(continued)

Protocol 10.1: Recognition and Management of Dementia *(cont.)*

stages. Assessment domains include cognitive, functional, behavioral, physical, caregiver, and environment.

  A. Cognitive Parameters
  1. Orientation: person, place, time
  2. Memory: ability to register, retain, recall information
  3. Attention: ability to attend and concentrate on stimuli
  4. Thinking: ability to organize and communicate ideas
  5. Language: ability to receive and express a message
  6. Praxis: ability to direct and coordinate movements
  7. Executive function: ability to abstract, plan, sequence, and use feedback to guide performance
  B. Mental Status Screening Tools
  1. Folstein Mini-Mental State Examination is the most commonly used test to assess serial cognitive change. The MMSE is copyrighted and a comparable tool called the St. Louis University Medical Status (SLUMS) Examination is in the public domain.
  2. Clock Drawing Test (CDT) is a useful measure of cognitive function that correlates with executive control functions.
  3. Mini-Cognitive (Mini-Cog) combines the Clock Drawing Test with the three-word recall.

When the diagnosis remains unclear, the patient may be referred for more extensive screening and neuropsychological testing, which might provide more direction and support for the patient and the caregivers.

  C. Functional Assessment
  1. Tests that assess functional limitations such as the Functional Activities Questionnaire (FAQ) can detect dementia. They are also useful in monitoring the progression of functional decline.
  2. The severity of disease progression in dementia can be demonstrated by performance decline in activity of daily living (ADL) and instrumental activity of daily living (IADL) tasks and is closely correlated with mental status scores.
  D. Behavioral Assessment
  1. Assess and monitor for behavioral changes, in particular, the presence of agitation, aggression, anxiety, disinhibitions, delusions, and hallucinations.
  2. Evaluate for depression because it commonly coexists in individuals with dementia. The Geriatric Depression Scale (GDS) is a good screening tool.
  E. Physical Assessment
  1. A comprehensive physical examination with a focus on the neurological and cardiovascular system is indicated in individuals with dementia to identify the potential cause and/or the existence of a reversible form of cognitive impairment.
  2. A thorough evaluation of all prescribed, over-the-counter, homeopathic, herbal, and nutritional products taken is done to determine the potential impact on cognitive status.

(continued)

Protocol 10.1: Recognition and Management of Dementia *(cont.)*

    3. Laboratory tests are valuable in differentiating irreversible from reversible forms of dementia. Structural neuroimaging with noncontrast computed tomography (CT) or magnetic resonance imaging (MRI) scans are appropriate in the routine initial evaluation of patients with dementia.

F. Caregiver/Environment

The caregiver of the patient with dementia often has as many needs as the patient with dementia; therefore, a detailed assessment of the caregiver and the caregiving environment is essential.

    1. Elicit the caregiver perspective of patient function and the level of support provided.

    2. Evaluate the impact that the patient's cognitive impairment and problem behaviors have on the caregiver (mastery, satisfaction, and burden). Two useful tools include the Zarit Burden Interview (ZBI) and the Caregiver Strain Index (CSI) tool.

    3. Evaluate the caregiver's experience and patient–caregiver relationship.

V. NURSING CARE STRATEGIES

The Progressively Lowered Stress Threshold (PLST) provides a framework for the nursing care of individuals with dementia.

A. Monitor the effectiveness and potential side effects of medications given to improve cognitive function or delay cognitive decline.

B. Provide appropriate cognitive enhancement techniques and social engagement.

C. Ensure adequate rest, sleep, fluid, nutrition, elimination, pain control, and comfort measures.

D. Avoid the use of physical and pharmacological restraints.

E. Maximize functional capacity: maintain mobility and encourage independence as long as possible; provide graded assistance as needed with ADL and IADL; provide scheduled toileting and prompted voiding to reduce urinary incontinence; encourage an exercise routine that expends energy and promotes fatigue at bedtime; and establish bedtime routine and rituals.

F. Address behavioral issues: identify environmental triggers, medical conditions, caregiver–patient conflict that may be causing the behavior; define the target symptom (i.e., agitation, aggression, wandering) and pharmacological (psychotropics) and nonpharmacological (manage affect, limit stimuli, respect space, distract, redirect) approaches; provide reassurance; and refer to appropriate mental health care professionals as indicated.

G. Ensure a therapeutic and safe environment: provide an environment that is modestly stimulating, avoiding overstimulation that can cause agitation and increase confusion and understimulation that can cause sensory deprivation and withdrawal. Utilize patient identifiers (name tags), medic alert systems and bracelets, locks, and wander guard. Eliminate any environmental hazards and modify the environment to enhance safety. Provide environmental cues or sensory aids that facilitate cognition, and maintain consistency in caregivers and approaches.

H. Encourage and support advance care planning: explain trajectory of progressive dementia, treatment options, and advance directives.

(continued)

Protocol 10.1: Recognition and Management of Dementia *(cont.)*

I. Provide appropriate end-of-life care in terminal phase: provide comfort measures including adequate pain management; weigh the benefits/risks of the use of aggressive treatment (e.g., tube feeding, antibiotic therapy).

J. Provide caregiver education and support: respect family systems/dynamics and avoid making judgments; encourage open dialogue, emphasize the patient's residual strengths; provide access to experienced professionals; and teach caregivers the skills of caregiving.

K. Integrate community resources into the plan of care to meet the needs for patient and caregiver information; identify and facilitate both formal (e.g., Alzheimer's association, respite care, specialized long-term care) and informal (e.g., churches, neighbors, extended family/friends) support systems.

VI. EVALUATION/EXPECTED OUTCOMES

A. Patient Outcomes: The patient remains as independent and functional in the environment of choice for as long as possible, the comorbid conditions the patient may experience are well managed, and the distressing symptoms that may occur at end of life are minimized or controlled adequately.

B. Caregiver Outcomes (lay and professional): Caregivers demonstrate effective caregiving skills; verbalize satisfaction with caregiving; report minimal caregiver burden; are familiar with, have access to, and utilize available resources.

C. Institutional Outcomes: The institution reflects a safe and enabling environment for delivering care to individuals with progressive dementia; the quality improvement plan addresses high-risk problem-prone areas for individuals with dementia, such as falls and the use of restraints.

VII. FOLLOW UP TO MONITOR CONDITION

A. Follow-up appointments are regularly scheduled; frequency depends on the patient's physical, mental, and emotional status and caregiver needs.

B. Determine the continued efficacy of pharmacological/nonpharmacological approaches to the care plan and modify as appropriate.

C. Identify and treat any underlying or contributing conditions.

D. Community resources for education and support are accessed and utilized by the patient and/or caregivers.

VIII. RELEVANT PRACTICE GUIDELINES

A. American Academy of Neurology: Detection of Dementia, Diagnosis of Dementia, Management of Dementia, and Encounter Kit for Dementia; http://www.aan.com/go/practice/guidelines

B. American Association of Geriatric Psychiatry: Position Statement: Principles of Care for Patients With Dementia Resulting From Alzheimer Disease; http://www.aagponline.org/prof/position_caredmnalz.asp

C. Alzheimer's Foundation of America (AFA): Excellence in Care; http://www.alzfdn.org

RESOURCES

Alzheimer's Association
http://www.alz.org

Alzheimer's Disease Education and Referral Center
http://www.alzheimers.nia.nih.gov

The National Family Caregiver's Association (NFCA)
http://www.nfcacares.org

American Association of Retired Persons (AARP)
http://www.aarp.org/caregiving

ElderWeb
http://www.elderweb.com

ConsultGeriRN
http://www.consultgerirn.org/resources

Hartford Institute for Geriatric Nursing
http://www.hartfordign.org/

National Conference of Gerontological Nurse Practitioners: Mental Health Toolkit
http://www.ncgnp.org/

REFERENCES

Ablitt, A., Jones, G. V., & Muers, J. (2009). Living with dementia: A systematic review of the influence of relationship factors. *Aging & Mental Health, 13*(9), 497–511. Evidence Level I.

Abraham, I. L., MacDonald, K. M., & Nadzam, D. M. (2006). Measuring the quality of nursing care to Alzheimer's patients. *The Nursing Clinics of North America, 41*(1), 95–104. Evidence Level VI.

Adelman, A. M., & Daly, M. P. (2005). Initial evaluation of the patient with suspected dementia. *American Family Physician, 71*(9), 1745–1750. Evidence Level VI.

American Psychiatric Association. (2000). *Diagnostic and statistical manual of mental disorders* (4th ed., text rev.).. Washington, DC: Author. Evidence Level VI.

Ariga, T., Miyatake, T., & Yu, R. K. (2010). Role of proteoglycans and glycosaminoglycans in the pathogenesis of Alzheimer's disease and related disorders: Amyloidogeneis and therapeutic strategies—a review. *Journal of Neuroscience Research, 88*(11), 2303–2315. Evidence Level IV.

Ballard, C., & Waite, J. (2006). The effectiveness of atypical antipsychotics for the treatment of aggression and psychosis in Alzheimer's disease. *Cochrane Database of Systematic Reviews*, (1), CD003476. Evidence Level I.

Bates, J., Boote, J., & Beverley, C. (2004). Psychosocial interventions for people with milder dementing illness: A systematic review. *Journal of Advanced Nursing, 45*(6), 644–658. Evidence Level I.

Bennett, D. A., Wilson, R. S., Schneider, J. A., Evans, D. A., Beckett, L. A., Aggarwal, N. T., . . . Bach, J. (2002). Natural history of mild cognitive impairment in older persons. *Neurology, 59*(2), 198–205. Evidence Level IV.

Birks, J., Grimley Evans, J., Iakovidou, V., & Tsolaki, M. (2000). Rivastigmine for Alzheimer's disease. *Cochrane Database of Systematic Reviews*. (4), CD001191. Evidence Level I.

Birks, J., & Harvey, R. J. (2006). Donepezil for dementia due to Alzheimer's disease. *Cochrane Database of Systematic Reviews* (Online). Retrieved from http://www.ncbi.nlm.nih.gov/pubmed/16437430. Evidence Level I.

Borson, S., Scanlan, J., Brush, M., Vitaliano, P., & Dokmak, A. (2000). The mini-cog: A cognitive 'vital signs' measure for dementia screening in multi-lingual elderly. *International Journal of Geriatric Psychiatry*, *15*(11), 1021–1027. Evidence Level IV.

Borson, S., Scanlan, J. M., Watanabe, J., Tu, S. P., & Lessig, M. (2005). Simplifying detection of cognitive impairment: Comparison of the Mini-Cog and Mini-Mental State Examination in a multiethnic sample. *Journal of the American Geriatrics Society*, *53*(5), 871–874. Evidence Level IV.

Brodaty, H., Low, L. F., Gibson, L., & Burns, K. (2006). What is the best dementia screening instrument for general practitioners to use? *The American Journal of Geriatric Psychiatry*, *14*(5), 391–400. Evidence Level I.

Brookmeyer, R., Corrada, M. M., Curriero, F. C., & Kawas, C. (2002). Survival following a diagnosis of Alzheimer disease. *Archives of Neurology*, *59*(11), 1764–1767. Evidence Level IV.

Burgener, S. C., & Twigg, P. (2002). Interventions for persons with irreversible dementia. *Annual Review of Nursing Research*, *20*, 89–124. Evidence Level I.

Castellani, R. J., Rolston, R. K., & Smith, M. A. (2010). Alzheimer disease. *Disease-a-month*, *56*(9), 484–546. Evidence Level IV.

Cooper, C., Balamurali, T. B., & Livingston, G. (2007). A systematic review of the prevalence and covariates of anxiety in caregivers of people with dementia. *International Psychogeriatrics*, *19*(2), 175–195. Evidence Level I.

Erkinjuntti, T., Kurz, A., Gauthier, S., Bullock, R., Lilienfeld, S., & Damaraju, C. V. (2002). Efficacy of galantamine in probable vascular dementia and Alzheimer's disease combined with cerebrovascular disease: A randomised trial. *Lancet*, *359*(9314), 1283–1290. Evidence Level II.

Evans, D. A., Funkenstein, H. H., Albert, M. S., Scherr, P. A., Cook, N. R., Chown, M. J., . . . Taylor, J. O. (1989). Prevalence of Alzheimer's disease in a community population of older persons. Higher than previously reported. *The Journal of the American Medical Association*, *262*(18), 2551–2556. Evidence Level IV.

Evers, M. M., Purohit, D., Perl, D., Khan, K., & Marin, D. B. (2002). Palliative and aggressive end-of-life care for patients with dementia. *Psychiatric Services*, *53*(5), 609–613. Evidence Level IV.

Ferri, C. P., Prince, M., Brayne, C., Brodaty, H., Fratiglioni, L., Ganguli, M., . . . Scazufca, M. (2005). Global prevalence of dementia: A Delphi consensus study. *Lancet*, *366*(9503), 2112–2117. Evidence Level IV.

Folstein, M. F., Folstein, S. E., & McHugh, P. R. (1975). "Mini-mental state." A practical method for grading the cognitive state of patients for the clinician. *Journal of Psychiatric Research*, *12*(3), 189–198. Evidence Level IV.

Forbes, D. (2004). Cognitive stimulation therapy improved cognition and quality of life in dementia. *Evidence-Based Nursing*, *7*(2), 54–55. Evidence Level II.

Forbes, D., Culum, I., Lischka, A. R., Morgan, D. G., Peacock, S., Forbes, J., & Forbes, S. (2009). Light therapy for managing cognitive, sleep, functional, behavioural, or psychiatric disturbances in dementia. *Cochrane Database of Systematic Reviews*, (4), CD003946. Evidence Level I.

Freund, B., Gravenstein, S., & Ferris, R. (2002). Use of the Clock Drawing Test as a screen for driving competency in older adults. *Journal of the American Geriatrics Society*, *50*(4), S3. Evidence Level IV.

Freund, B., Gravenstein, S., Ferris, R., Burke, B. L., & Shaheen, E. (2005). Drawing clocks and driving cars. *Journal of General Internal Medicine*, *20*(3), 240–244. Evidence Level IV.

Galasko, D., Bennett, D., Sano, M., Ernesto, C., Thomas, R., Grundman, M., & Ferris, S. (1997). An inventory to assess activities of daily living for clinical trials in Alzheimer's disease. The Alzheimer's Disease Cooperative Study. *Alzheimer Disease and Associated Disorders*, *11*(Suppl. 2), S33–S39. Evidence Level IV.

Gauthier, S., Reisberg, B., Zaudig, M., Petersen, R. C., Ritchie, K., Broich, K., . . . Winblad, B. (2006). Mild cognitive impairment. *Lancet*, *367*(9518), 1262–1270. Evidence Level VI.

Geldmacher, D. S. (2003). Alzheimer's disease: Current pharmacotherapy in the context of patient and family needs. *Journal of the American Geriatrics Society*, *51*(Suppl. 5), S289–S295. Evidence Level VI.

Geldmacher, D. S. (2004). Differential diagnosis of dementia syndromes. *Clinics in Geriatric Medicine, 20*(1), 27–43. Evidence Level VI.

Geldmacher, D. S., Provenzano, G., McRae, T., Mastey, V., & Ieni, J. R. (2003). Donepezil is associated with delayed nursing home placement in patients with Alzheimer's disease. *Journal of the American Geriatrics Society, 51*(7), 937–944. Evidence Level II.

Gray, K. F. (2004). Managing agitation and difficult behavior in dementia. *Clinics in Geriatric Medicine, 20*(1), 69–82. Evidence Level VI.

Han, L., Cole, M., Bellavance, F., McCusker, J., & Primeau, F. (2000). Tracking cognitive decline in Alzheimer's disease using the mini-mental state examination: A meta-analysis. *International Psychogeriatrics, 12*(2), 231–247. Evidence Level I.

Hanson, J. C., & Lippa, C. F. (2009). Lewy body dementia. *International Review of Neurobiology, 84*, 215–228. Evidence Level VI.

Hebert, L. E., Scherr, P. A., Bienias, J. L., Bennett, D. A., & Evans, D. A. (2003). Alzheimer disease in the US population: Prevalence estimates using the 2000 census. *Archives of Neurology, 60*(8), 1119–1122. Evidence Level IV.

Higginson, I. J., Gao, W., Jackson, D., Murray, J., & Harding, R. (2010). Short-form Zarit Caregiver Burden Interviews were valid in advanced conditions. *Journal of Clinical Epidemiology, 63*(5), 535–542. Evidence Level I.

Holroyd, S. (2004). Managing dementia in long-term care settings. *Clinics in Geriatric Medicine, 20*(1), 83–92. Evidence Level VI.

Iverson, D. J., Gronseth, G. S., Reger, M. A., Classen, S., Dubinsky, R. M., & Rizo, M. (2010). Practice parameter update: Evaluation and management of driving risk in dementia: Report of the Quality Standards Subcommittee of the American Academy of Neurology. *Neurology, 74*(16), 1316–1324. Evidence Level IV.

Jayasekara, R. (2009). Dementia: Family support following diagnosis. *Evidence Summaries - Joanna Briggs Institute.* Retrieved from http://www.jbiconnect.org/connect/docs/cis/es_html_viewer.php?SID=6786&lang=en&region=AU

Kane, R. L., Ouslander, J. G., Abrass, I. B., & Resnick, B. (2009). Confusion: Delirium and dementia. In *Essentials of clinical geriatrics* (6th ed., pp. 121–145). New York, NY: McGraw Hill. Evidence Level VI.

Kaufer, D. I., Cummings, J. L., Ketchel, P., Smith, V., MacMila, A., Shelley, T., . . . DeKosky, S. T. (2000). Validation of the NPI-Q, a brief clinical form of the Neuropsychiatric Inventory. *The Journal of Neuropsychiatry and Clinical Neurosciences, 12*(2), 233–239. Evidence Level IV.

Kavirajan, H., & Schneider, L. S. (2007). Efficacy and adverse effects of cholinesterase inhibitors and memantine in vascular dementia: A meta-analysis of randomised controlled trials. *Lancet Neurology, 6*(9), 782–792.

Kilik, L. A., Hopkins, R. W., Day, D., Prince, C. R., Prince, P. N., & Rows, C. (2008). The progression of behavior in dementia: An in-office guide for clinicians. *American Journal of Alzheimer's Disease and Other Dementias, 23*(3), 242–249. Evidence Level IV.

Kirshner, H. S. (2009). Vascular dementia: A review of recent evidence for prevention and treatment. *Current Neurology and Neuroscience Reports, 9*(6), 437–442. Evidence Level V.

Knopman, D. S., DeKosky, S. T., Cummings, J. L., Chui, H., Corey-Bloom, J., Relkin, N., . . . Stevens, J. C. (2001). Practice parameter: Diagnosis of dementia (an evidence-based review). Report of the Quality Standards Subcommittee of the American Academy of Neurology. *Neurology, 56*(9), 1143–1153. Evidence Level VI.

Langa, K. M., Foster, N. L., & Larson, E. B. (2004). Mixed dementia: Emerging concepts and therapeutic implications. *The Journal of the American Medical Association, 292*(23), 2901–2908. Evidence Level V.

Lee, H. B., & Lyketsos, C. G. (2003). Depression in Alzheimer's disease: Heterogeneity and related issues. *Biological Psychiatry, 54*(3), 353–362. Evidence Level IV.

Leifer, B. P. (2003). Early diagnosis of Alzheimer's disease: Clinical and economic benefits. *Journal of the American Geriatrics Society, 51*(Suppl. 5), S281–S288. Evidence Level VI.

Lindsey, P. L., & Buckwalter, K. C. (2009). Psychotic events in Alzheimer's disease: Application of the PLST model. *Journal of Gerontological Nursing, 35*(8), 20–27. Evidence Level V.

Lonergan, E., Luxenberg, J., & Colford, J. (2002). Haloperidol for agitation in dementia. *Cochrane Database of Systematic Reviews*, (2), CD002852. Evidence Level I.

Lopez, O. L., Becker, J. T., Wisniewski, S., Saxton, J., Kaufer, D. I., & Dekosky, S. T. (2002). Cholinesterase inhibitor treatment alters the natural history of Alzheimer's disease. *Journal of Neurology, Neurosurgery, and Psychiatry, 72*(3), 310–314. Evidence Level III.

Loy, C., & Schneider, L. (2006). Galantamine for Alzheimer's disease and mild cognitive impairment. *Cochrane Database of Systematic Reviews*, (1), CD001747.

Luck, T., Luppa, M., Briel, S., & Riedel-Heller, S. G. (2010). Incidence of mild cognitive impairment: A systematic review. *Dementia and Geriatric Cognitive Disorder, 29*(2), 164–175. Evidence Level I.

Lyketsos, C. G., Toone, L., Tschanz, J., Rabins, P. V., Steinberg, M., Onyike, C. U., . . . Williams, M. (2005). Population-based study of medical comorbidity in early dementia and cognitive impairment no dementia (CIND): Association with functional and "cognitive impairment, no dementia (CIND)": Association with functional and cognitive impairment: The Cache County Study. *The American Journal of Geriatric Psychiatry, 13*(8), 656–664. Evidence Level IV.

Manly, J. J., & Espino, D. V. (2004). Cultural influences on dementia recognition and management. *Clinics in Geriatric Medicine, 20*(1), 93–119. Evidence Level IV.

Manning, C. (2004). Beyond memory: Neuropsychologic features in differential diagnosis of dementia. *Clinics in Geriatric Medicine, 20*(1), 45–58. Evidence Level VI.

Man-Son-Hing, M., Marshall, S. C., Molnar, F. J., & Wilson, K. G. (2007). Systematic review of driving risk and the efficacy of compensatory strategies in persons with dementia. *Journal of the American Geriatric Society, 55*(6), 878–884. Evidence Level I.

McKeith, I. G., Burn, D. J., Ballard, C. G., Collerton, D., Jaros, E., Morris, C. M., . . . O'Brien, J. T. (2003). Dementia with Lewy bodies. *Seminars in Clinical Neuropsychiatry, 8*(1), 46–57. Evidence Level V.

McKeith, I. G., Dickson, D. W., Lowe, J., Emre, M., O'Brien, J. T., Feldman, H., . . . Yamada, M. (2005). Diagnosis and management of dementia with Lewy bodies: Third report of the DLB consortium. *Neurology, 65*(12), 1863–1872.

McShane, R., Areosa Sastre, A., & Minakaran, N. (2006). Memantine for dementia. Cochrane Database of Systematic Reviews, (2), CD003154, Evidence Level I.

Mezey, M. D., Mitty, E. L., Bottrell, M. M., Ramsey, G. C., & Fisher, T. (2000). Advance directives: Older adults with dementia. *Clinics in Geriatric Medicine, 16*(2), 255–268. Evidence Level VI.

Milisen, K., Braes, T., Fick, D. M., & Foreman, M. D. (2006). Cognitive assessment and differentiating the 3 Ds (dementia, depression, delirium). *The Nursing Clinics of North America, 41*(1), 1–22. Evidence Level VI.

Milne, A., Culverwell, A., Guss, R., Tuppen, J., & Whelton, R. (2008). Screening for dementia in primary care: A review of the use, efficacy and quality of measures. *International Psychogeriatrics, 20*(5), 911–926. Evidence Level I.

Monastero, R., Mangialasche, F., Camarda, C., Ercolani, S., & Camarda, R. (2009). A systematic review of neuropsychiatric symptoms in mild cognitive impairment. *Journal of Alzheimer's Disease, 18*(1), 11–30. Evidence Level I.

Neal, M., & Briggs, M. (2003). Validation therapy for dementia. *Cochrane Database of Systematic Reviews*, (3), CD001394. Evidence Level I.

O'Connor, D. W., Ames, D., Gardner, B., & King, M. (2009). Psychosocial treatments of psychological symptoms in dementia: A systematic review of reports meeting quality standards. *International Psychogeriatrics*, 21(2), 241–251.

Oliver, D. P., Porock, D., & Zweig, S. (2004). End-of-life care in U.S. nursing homes: A review of the evidence. *Journal of the American Medical Directors Association, 5*(3), 147–155. Evidence

Level I.

Olsen, C. E., Poulsen, H. D., & Lublin, H. K. (2005). Drug therapy of dementia in elderly patients. A review. *Nordic Journal of Psychiatry, 59*(2), 71–77. Evidence Level I.

Onega, L. L. (2006). Assessment of psychoemotional and behavioral status in patients with dementia. *The Nursing Clinics of North America, 41*(1), 23–41. Evidence Level VI.

Onega, L. L. (2008). Helping those who help others: The Modified Caregiver Strain Index. *The American Journal of Nursing, 108*(9), 62–69. Evidence Level V.

Parker, C., & Philp, I. (2004). Screening for cognitive impairment among older people in black and minority ethnic groups. *Age and Ageing, 33*(5), 447–452. Evidence Level VI.

Peatfield, J. G., Futrell, M., & Cox, C. L. (2002). Wandering: An integrative review. *Journal of Gerontological Nursing, 28*, 44–50. Evidence Level I.

Peters, R., & Pinto, E. M. (2008). Predictive value of the Clock Drawing Test. A review of the literature. *Dementia and Geriatric Cognitive Disorders, 26*(4), 351–355. Evidence Level I.

Pfeffer, R. I., Kurosaki, T. T., Harrah, C. H., Jr., Chance, J. M., & Filos, S. (1982). Measurement of functional activities in older adults in the community. *Journal of Gerontology, 37*(3), 323–329. Evidence Level IV.

Potkin, S. G. (2002). The ABC of Alzheimer's disease: ADL and improving day-to-day functioning of patients. *International Psychogeriatrics, 14*(Suppl. 1), 7–26. Evidence Level VI.

Reimer, M. A., Slaughter, S., Donaldson, C., Currie, G., & Eliasziw, M. (2004). Special care facility compared with traditional environments for dementia care: A longitudinal study of quality of life. *Journal of the American Geriatrics Society, 52*(7), 1085–1092. Evidence Level IV.

Richie, K., & Lovestone, S. (2002). The dementias. *Lancet, 360*(9347), 1759–1766. Evidence Level VI.

Riepe, M. W., Adler, G., Ibach, B., Weinkauf, B., Tracik, F., & Gunay, I. (2007). Domain-specific improvement of cognition on memantine in patients with Alzheimer's disease treated with rivastigmine. *Dementia and Geriatric Cognitive Disorders, 23*(5), 301–306.

Robinson, L., Hutchings, D., Dickinson, H. O., Corner, L., Beyer, F., Finch, T., . . . Bond, J. (2007). Effectiveness and acceptability of non-pharmacological interventions to reduce wandering in dementia: A systematic review. *International Journal of Geriatric Psychiatry, 22*(1), 9–22. Evidence Level I.

Román, G. C. (2003). Stroke, cognitive decline and vascular dementia: The silent epidemic of the 21st century. *Neuroepidemiology, 22*(3), 161–164. Evidence Level VI.

Ropacki, S. A., & Jeste, D. V. (2005). Epidemiology of and risk factors for psychosis of Alzheimer's disease: A review of 55 studies published from 1990 to 2003. *The American Journal of Psychiatry, 162*(11), 2022–2030. Evidence Level I.

Royall, D. R., Mulroy, A. R., Chiodo, L. K., & Polk, M. J. (1999). Clock drawing is sensitive to executive control: A comparison of six methods. *The Journals of Gerontology. Series B, Psychological Sciences and Social Sciences, 54*(5), 328–333. Evidence Level IV.

Sampson, E. L., Ritchie, C. W., Lai, R., Raven, P. W., & Blanchard, M. R. (2005). A systematic review of the scientific evidence for the efficacy of a palliative care approach in advanced dementia. *International Psychogeriatrics, 17*(1), 31–40. Evidence Level I.

Scherder, E., Oosterman, J., Swabb, D., Herr, K., Ooms, M., Ribbe, M., . . . Benedetti, F. (2005). Recent developments in pain in dementia. *British Medical Journal, 330*(7489), 461–464. Evidence Level V.

Schoenmakers, B., Buntinx, F., & Delepeleire, J. (2010). Factors determining the impact of caregiving on caregivers of elderly patients with dementia. A systematic review. *Maturitas, 66*(2), 191–200. Evidence Level I.

Shub, D., Ball, V., Abbas, A. A., Gottumukkala, A., & Kunik, M. E. (2010). The link between psychosis and aggression in persons with dementia: A systematic review. *The Psychiatric Quarterly, 81*(2), 97–110. Evidence Level I.

Smith, G. E., Kokmen, E., & O'Brien, P. C. (2000). Risk factors for nursing home placement in a population-based dementia cohort. *Journal of the American Geriatrics Society, 48*(5), 519–525.

Evidence Level IV.

Smith, M., Hall, G. R., Gerdner, L., & Buckwalter, K. C. (2006). Application of the Progressively Lowered Stress Threshold Model across the continuum of care. *The Nursing Clinics of North America, 41*(1), 57–81. Evidence Level V.

Stolley, J. M., Reed, D., & Buckwalter, K. C. (2002). Caregiving appraisal and interventions based on the progressively lowered stress threshold model. *American Journal of Alzheimer's Disease and Other Dementias,* 17(2), 110–20. Evidence Level II.

Tariq, S. H., Tumosa, N., Chibnall, J. T., Perry, M. H., III, & Morley, J. E. (2006). Comparison of the Saint Louis University mental status examination and the mini-mental state examination for detecting dementia and mild neurocognitive disorder—a pilot study. *The American Journal of Geriatric Psychiatry, 14*(11), 900–910. Evidence Level IV.

Thorgrimsen, L., Spector, A., Wiles, A., & Orrell, M. (2003). Aroma therapy for dementia. *Cochrane Database of Systematic Reviews,* (3), CD003150. doi:10.1002/14651858.CD003150 Evidence Level I.

Volicer, L., Hurley, A. C., & Blasi, Z. V. (2001). Scales for evaluation of end-of-life care in dementia. *Alzheimer Disease and Associated Disorders, 15*(4), 194–200. Evidence Level IV.

Wall, M., & Duffy, A. (2010). The effects of music therapy for older people with dementia. *British Journal of Nursing, 19*(2), 108–113. Evidence Level I.

Wild, R., Pettit, T., & Burns, A. (2003). Cholinesterase inhibitors for dementia with Lewy bodies. *Cochrane Database of Systematic Reviews,* (3), CD003672.

Delirium

11

*Dorothy F. Tullmann, Kathleen Fletcher, and
Marquis D. Foreman*

EDUCATIONAL OBJECTIVES

On completion of this chapter, the reader should be able to:

1. describe hospitalized older adults at risk for delirium
2. list four outcomes associated with delirium
3. discuss the importance of early recognition of delirium
4. develop a plan to prevent or treat delirium

OVERVIEW

Delirium is a common syndrome in hospitalized older adults and is one of the major contributors to poor outcomes of health care and institutionalization for older patients (Siddiqi, House, & Holmes, 2006). Delirium has been shown to be preventable by identifying modifiable risk factors and using a standardized nursing practice protocol (Milisen, Lemiengre, Braes, & Foreman, 2005) and involving a geriatric specialist (Siddiqi, Stockdale, Britton, & Holmes, 2007). If delirium does develop, early recognition is of paramount importance in order to treat the underlying pathology and minimize delirium's sequelae. Nurses play a key role in both the prevention and early recognition of this potentially devastating condition in older hospitalized adults (Milisen et al., 2005).

BACKGROUND AND STATEMENT OF PROBLEM

Definition

Delirium is a disturbance of consciousness with impaired attention and disorganized thinking that develops rapidly and with evidence of an underlying physiologic or medical condition (American Psychiatric Association [APA], 2000). Delirium is characterized by a reduced ability to focus, sustain, or shift attention; memory impairment;

For description of Evidence Levels cited in this chapter, see Chapter 1, Developing and Evaluating Clinical Practice Guidelines: A Systematic Approach, page 7.

disorientation and/or illusions; visual or other hallucinations; or misperceptions of stimuli. Delusional thinking may also occur. Unlike other chronic cognitive impairments, delirium develops over a short time and tends to fluctuate during the course of the day. A patient may present with either hyperactive, hypoactive, or mixed motoric subtypes of delirium (Meagher, 2009). Nurses typically associate delirium with hyperactivity and distressing, time-consuming, and harmful patient behaviors. However, the hypoactive subtype, with its lack of overt psychomotor activity, is also common (Meagher, 2009; Pandharipande, Cotton, et al., 2007) and has a higher risk of mortality, especially when superimposed on dementia (Yang et al., 2009).

Etiology and Epidemiology

Prevalence and Incidence

Among medical inpatients, delirium is present on admission to the hospital in 10%–31% of older patients, and during hospitalization, 11% to 42% of older adults develop delirium (Siddiqi et al., 2006). Among hip surgery patients, the incidence of delirium is 4%–53%. Those with hip fractures and cognitive impairment have the highest risk of delirium. (Bruce, Ritchie, Blizard, Lai, & Raven, 2007). Older adults admitted to medical intensive care units (ICUs) have both prevalent and incident delirium of 31% (McNicoll et al., 2003). In surgical (S) ICUs, the prevalence of delirium on admission is only 2.6%, but 28.3% develop delirium during their SICU stay (Balas et al., 2007). Up to 83% of mechanically ventilated patients in ICUs experience delirium (Ely, Inouye, et al., 2001), and more than half of older patients in medical ICUs still have delirium when transferred (Pisani, Murphy, Araujo, & Van Ness, 2010). The incidence of delirium superimposed on dementia ranges from 22% to 89% (Fick, Agostini, & Inouye, 2002). Delirium may persist for months after discharge (Cole, Ciampi, Belzile, & Zhong, 2009).

Pathophysiology

The pathogenesis of delirium is not well understood, but increasing evidence supports cholinergic deficiency and/or dopamine excess as well as cytokine activity as causes of delirium (Inouye, 2006). A genetic association between delirium and the apolipoprotein E epsilon 4 allele has also been identified (van Munster, Korevaar, Zwinderman, Leeflang, & de Rooji, 2009).

Risk Factors

The strongest predisposing risk factors for delirium are age (70 years and older), severity of illness, and cognitive impairment (Michaud et al., 2007). Other factors include depression, sensory impairment, fluid and electrolyte disturbances, and polypharmacy (especially psychotropics). Precipitating factors for delirium occurring during hospitalization include central nervous system pathology (such as stroke), metabolic, electrolyte and/or endocrine disturbances, and infection and drug toxicity or withdrawal. Pain, hypoperfusion/hypoxia, number of drugs (especially psychotropic and anticholinergic), and restraints have also been implicated. Finally, environmental factors such as ICU admission, multiple room changes, and an absence of a clock or glasses may also contribute to the development of delirium (Michaud et al., 2007). In older patients admitted for hip surgery, early cognitive impairment, such as memory impairments, incoherence, disorientation, as well as an underlying physical illness and age, are especially strong predictors of delirium (de Jonghe et al., 2007; Kalisvaart et al., 2006).

Outcomes

The outcomes of delirium are grave, especially in hospitalized older patients whose delirium persists postdischarge. Those with persistent delirium at 1, 3, and 6 months postdischarge consistently have increased mortality, nursing home placement, and decreased functional status and cognition than older adults who do not experience delirium (Cole, McCusker, Ciampi, & Belzile, 2008; Witlox et al., 2010).

Delirium also results in significant distress for the patient, their family members, and nurses (Bruera et al., 2009; Cohen, Pace, Kaur, & Bruera, 2009). Clearly, delirium is a high-priority nursing challenge for all who care for hospitalized older adults.

ASSESSMENT OF THE PROBLEM

The first critically important step in the assessment of delirium is identifying the risk factors for delirium (see discussed "Risk Factors") because eliminating or reducing these risk factors may prevent delirium in many cases (Milisen et al., 2005). Recognizing the features of delirium is important in order to further identify, eliminate, or reduce the precipitating factor(s) such as pain, infection, or other acute illnesses. This can best be done by routinely assessing patients at risk for delirium with a standardized screening tool for delirium (see "Resources" section), although this is currently occurring only in 17% of hospitals (Neuman, Speck, Karlawish, Schwartz, & Shea, 2010).

The Confusion Assessment Method (CAM) has high sensitivity and specificity in ICU, Emergency Department, acute and long-term care settings for detecting delirium (Wei, Fearing, Sternberg, & Inouye, 2008), and is the most widely used delirium screening instrument in hospitalized older adults. A version of the CAM for patients in intensive care units (CAM-ICU; Ely, Margolin, et al., 2001) is recommended for use with critically ill older adults (Jacobi et al., 2002; Schuurmans, Deschamps, Markham, Shortridge-Baggett, & Duursma, 2003). The CAM instrument identifies the key features of delirium—acute onset, inattention, disorganized thinking, altered level of consciousness, disorientation, memory impairment, perceptual disturbances, psychomotor agitation or retardation, and altered sleep–wake cycles (Inouye et al., 1990). For a diagnosis of delirium, there must be the presence of Feature 1 (acute onset or fluctuating course), Feature 2 (inattention), and either Feature 3 (disorganized thinking) or Feature 4 (altered level of consciousness).

It is important to remember that delirium may occur concurrently with dementia or depression. From 22% to 89% of older adults with dementia also have delirium superimposed on the dementia (Fick et al., 2002). As noted, patients with dementia are at increased risk for developing delirium and have worse outcomes when they do (Yang et al., 2009). Family and caregivers can be invaluable in helping to distinguish cognitive changes in those circumstances when the patient is not well known (see Chapter 8, Assessing Cognitive Function).

Bedside nurses are in the best position to recognize delirium because they possess the skill and responsibility of ongoing patient assessment and are in key positions to recognize risk factors for delirium and the earliest cognitive changes heralding the onset of delirium. Early identification of risk factors for and the earliest onset of delirium are critical to implement strategies to minimize the occurrence of this devastating pathology in hospitalized older adults.

INTERVENTIONS AND CARE STRATEGIES

According to the most recent Cochrane Review (Siddiqi et al., 2007), there is no strong evidence from delirium prevention studies to guide clinical practice. Only one of six randomized controlled trials (RCT) effectively prevented delirium with proactive geriatric consultation for older adults undergoing surgery for hip fracture (Marcantonio et al., 2001). Prophylactically administered low-dose haloperidol reduced the severity and duration of delirium but not its incidence (Kalisvaart et al., 2005). However, given the prevalence and seriousness of delirium, its complex and varied etiology, and the challenges associated with conduction RCTs, we strongly recommend the use of clinical practice guidelines based on other strong intervention studies for both prevention and treatment of delirium.

Once it has been determined that the patient is at risk for delirium, a standardized delirium protocol should be initiated immediately. Protocols tested in two multicomponent interventions effectively prevented delirium (Inouye et al., 1999; Marcantonio et al., 2001). The protocols varied somewhat, but two principles emerged from the research: Minimize the risk for delirium by preventing or eliminating the etiologic agent or agents and provide a therapeutic environment and general supportive nursing care (see Section V, Nursing Care Strategies, in Protocol 11.1). Older adults on a specialized geriatric unit receiving interprofessionally and protocol-guided care by a staff that had received specialized geriatric care education also developed significantly less delirium (Lundstrom et al., 2007).

Patients who developed delirium after hip surgery, when treated with a multicomponent intervention program had fewer days of delirium, complications, total days of hospitalization (Lundstrom et al., 2007), and improved health-related quality of life without incurring increased costs (Pitkala et al., 2008). Although multicomponent delirium-reduction interventions have yet to be tested in critical care settings, sedation interruption and early occupational and physical therapy in patients who are mechanically ventilated resulted in shorter duration of delirium (Schweickert et al., 2009).

Although nonpharmacologic interventions are preferred and should be used first (Michaud et al., 2007), antipsychotics (such as haloperidol) are used and are found to be efficacious in certain populations with agitated delirium (Breitbart et al., 1996; Devlin et al., 2010). Light propofol sedation my reduce severity and duration of delirium in hip surgery patients (Sieber et al., 2010).

Dexmedetomidine (dex; a γ-aminobutyric acid receptor agonist), a promising alternative for sedation, resulted in decreased delirium when compared with other commonly used sedation in ICU settings. When used for postoperative sedation after cardiac surgery, dex has been associated with lower rates of delirium and costs when compared with propofol and midazolam (Maldonado et al., 2009) and shorter duration of delirium when compared to morphine (Shehabi et al., 2009). In patients who are mechanically ventilated, dex is more efficacious than lorazepam in number of days at the targeted level of sedation and more days alive without coma or delirium (Pandharipande, Pun, et al., 2007). When compared to midazolam in patients who are mechanically ventilated, patients treated with dex have less delirium (Riker et al., 2009).

Alternative forms of pain management may also help reduce delirium. Hip fracture patients at low risk for delirium who received a prophylactic fascia iliac block developed significantly less delirium than those receiving traditional pain management regimens (Mouzopoulos et al., 2009).

CASE STUDY

Mr. Z is an 82-year-old patient admitted to your unit for prostate surgery. He is a retired accountant, lives with his wife, and is very active. He drives a car, plays golf, and regularly participates in activities at the senior center. His Type II diabetes is well controlled on Actoplus Met (pioglitazone hydrochloride and metformin hydrochloride). Mr. Z reports that he has decreased his fluid intake so he can avoid waking several times during the night to urinate. He also has a history of hypertension, moderate hearing loss (hearing aids bilaterally), and previous surgery for inguinal hernia repair. He wears bifocal glasses for distance and reading. He is alert, oriented, and expresses a good understanding of his upcoming surgery. His preoperative laboratory values are within normal limits except for a low hematocrit and a blood urea nitrogen/creatinine (BUN/Cr) ratio slightly elevated. His medications include Actoplus Met (pioglitazone hydrochloride and metformin hydrochloride) for his diabetes and Calan (verapamil) for hypertension.

What Factors Present on Admission to the Hospital Put Mr. Z at Risk for Developing Delirium?

- *Age.* Older adults are at greater risk for delirium, particularly if they have underlying dementia or depression. Physiologic changes that occur with aging can affect the ability of older adults to respond to physical and physiologic stress and to maintain homeostasis.
- *Dehydration.* An elevated BUN/Cr ratio indicates dehydration (from decreased fluid intake), a frequent contributing factor (along with electrolyte imbalance) to delirium of hospitalized older adults.
- *Anemia.* Because of a low hematocrit, the body has diminished ability to deliver adequate oxygen to the brain, making delirium more likely.
- *Sensory deficits.* Those with vision and hearing loss are more likely to misinterpret sensory input, which places them at increased risk for delirium.

It is important to understand that it might not be one particular factor but the interplay of patient vulnerability (predisposing factors) and precipitating factors—common during hospitalization—which place the older adult at risk for delirium.

What Can You Do to Help Prevent Delirium in Mr. Z?

- If possible, consult with a geriatric specialist (geriatrician or geriatric nurse practitioner) for a thorough geriatric assessment of Mr. Z.
- Make sure his glasses and hearing aids are on and functioning.
- Explore reasons for the low hematocrit.

(continued)

CASE STUDY *(continued)*

You provide care for Mr. Z again 2 days after surgery. He is confused and picking at the air and oriented to self only. An indwelling urinary catheter and peripheral intravenous line are in place. In his report, the day-shift nurse mentioned considering a physical restraint because Mr. Z was increasingly restless and was CAM positive, indicating he has delirium.

What Are the Clinical Features of Delirium?

- *Disturbance of consciousness* characterized by reduced clarity and awareness of the environment: reduced ability to focus, sustain, and shift attention. Patients have trouble following instructions or making sense of their environment, even with cues. They may also get "stuck" on a particular concern or thought.
- *Cognitive changes*: memory deficit, disorientation, language disturbance, and/ or perceptual disturbance.
- *Perceptual disturbances*: Hallucinations and delusions are common. Patients can be hyperactive and agitated or lethargic (hypoactive) and less active. The latter presentation is of particular concern because it is often not recognized by health care providers as delirium. The presentation may also be mixed, with the patient fluctuating from one to the other behavioral state.
- Delirium can be *characterized by* disturbances in the sleep–wake cycle and rapidly shifting emotional disturbances, with escalation of the disturbed behavior at night (sundowning).
- The cardinal sign of delirium is that the cited *changes occur rapidly* over several hours or days.

It is also important to consider that delirium may occur concurrently with dementia or depression. In fact, these patients are at increased risk for developing delirium. Family and caregivers can be invaluable in helping to identify or distinguish cognitive changes in circumstances when the patient is not well known to you.

What Additional Factors May Now Be Contributing to Mr. Z's Delirium?

- *Anesthesia and other medications.* It takes several hours for the body to clear the effects of anesthesia. Inasmuch as older adults have a larger percentage of body fat than younger persons do, and many drugs are fat-soluble, drug effects will last longer. Also, older adults tend to have less cellular water; hence, water-soluble drugs will be more concentrated and have a more pronounced effect. Nurses need to ask the patient or family if any new drugs other than pain medication have been added. What is the dose and frequency of the pain medications? Is the dose appropriate?
- *Pain.* What is Mr. Z's pain control regimen and status? Poor pain control contributes to restlessness and is associated with delirium. Is the current drug the best for good pain relief in this patient?
- *Hypoxemia.* Mr. Z is at risk because of limited mobility and possible atelectasis after surgery. What is his oxygen saturation (SpO_2)? Does he have crackles or diminished breath sounds?

(continued)

CASE STUDY *(continued)*

■ *Infection, inflammation, or other medical illness.* Postoperative infections, intra-operative myocardial infarctions (MIs), or strokes are possible causes of delir-ium in this case. Could Mr. Z have a urinary tract infection (UTI) since his postprostate surgery and particularly since he has a Foley catheter? An inflam-matory response to a new medical problem may be the cause of the delirium.

■ *Unfamiliar surroundings.* Particularly for those with sensory deficits, unfamil-iar environments can lead to misinterpretations of information, which may contribute to delirium.

What Steps Should Be Taken Now?

■ *Avoid the use of restraints,* which could worsen Mr. Z's agitation.

■ *Call the physician or nurse practitioner* immediately and report your findings; request that the patient be evaluated to determine the underlying cause of the delirium. If Mr. Z's delirium worsens, he may also need medication (e.g., low dose haloperidol) to control his symptoms.

■ *Frequent reality orientation.* Frequent orientation, reassurance, and helping Mr. Z interpret his environment and what is happening to him should be helpful. (Monitor the patient's reaction. If the patient becomes upset or angry, you will need to modify your approach to that of more reassurance and vali-dating the patient's experience rather than reorienting).

■ Are Mr. Z's *hearing aids and glasses* in place, and clean and functioning? Impaired sensory input contributes significantly to delirium. Also, he may seem more confused than he really is if he is not able to hear what you are saying.

■ Invite *family/significant others* to stay as much as they are able to assist with his orientation, reassurance, and sense of well-being. Monitor the effect of family visitation. If the patient has increased agitation or anxiety, then limit the visita-tion of the individual who seems to be triggering Mr. Z's upset.

■ *Mobilize the patient.* Mobility assists with orientation and helps prevent problems associated with immobility, such as atelectasis and deep venous thrombosis.

■ *Judicious use of medications* for pain, sleep, or anxiety. Drugs used to address these issues can exacerbate the delirium. Try nonpharmacologic approaches for sleep and anxiety first. If Mr. Z is having pain, are the drug and dose appropri-ate for him? A regular schedule of a smaller dose or non-narcotic pain medica-tion almost always is better than prn dosing.

■ Try to *provide for adequate sleep*: noise reduction at night; soft, relaxing music; warm milk; herbal tea; massage; and rescheduling care in order not to interrupt sleep.

■ Make sure the patient is well *hydrated.*

■ Talk to the doctor or NP about removing the *indwelling urinary catheter.* Because of his surgery, Mr. Z may need it immediately post-op, but it should be removed as soon as possible. Additionally, recommend a urinalysis to rule out UTI.

■ *Address safety concerns* (e.g., increase surveillance). Mr. Z is now also at risk for falls and/or pressure ulcers.

SUMMARY

Delirium is a common occurrence in hospitalized older adults and contributes to poor outcomes. Thus, it is important to promptly identify those patients at risk for delirium and implement preventive measures as well as promptly recognize delirium when it appears. Nursing assessments using validated delirium screening instruments must become routine. A standard of practice protocol provides concise information to guide nursing care of individuals at risk for or experiencing delirium.

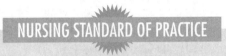

NURSING STANDARD OF PRACTICE

Protocol 11.1: Delirium

I. GOAL: To reduce the incidence of delirium in hospitalized older adults.

II. OVERVIEW:
  A. Delirium is a common syndrome in hospitalized older adults and is associated with increased mortality, hospital costs, and long-term cognitive and functional impairment (Siddiqi et al., 2006).
  B. Delirium can sometimes be prevented with the recognition of high-risk patients, implementation of a standardized delirium-reduction protocol, and proactive geriatric consultation (Bruera et al., 2009).
  C. Recognition of risk factors and routine screening for delirium should be part of comprehensive nursing care of older adults (Milisen et al., 2005).

III. BACKGROUND AND STATEMENT OF PROBLEM:
  A. Definition: Delirium is a disturbance of consciousness with impaired attention and disorganized thinking or perceptual disturbance that develops acutely, has a fluctuating course, and with evidence that there is an underlying physiologic or medical condition causing the disorder (APA, 2000).
  B. Etiology and Epidemiology
    1. *Prevalence and incidence:* Medical inpatients, prevalence is 10% to 31%; incidence is 3% to 29% (Siddiqi et al., 2006). Hip surgery patients, incidence of delirium is 4% to 53% with hip fractures and cognitive causing higher risk of delirium (Bruce et al., 2007). Medical ICUs, prevalence and incidence both 31% (McNicoll et al., 2003). Surgical ICUs, prevalence 2.6%, incidence 28.3% (Balas et al., 2007). Mechanically ventilated patients in ICU, up to 83% during ICU stay (Ely et al., 2001), more than 50% of medical ICU patients still have delirium when transferred (Pisani et al., 2010). Incidence of delirium superimposed on dementia, 22% to 89% (Fick et al., 2002).
    2. *Pathophysiology:* Unclear, may be cholinergic deficiency, dopamine excess, or cytokine activity (Inouye, 2006). A genetic association with apolipoprotein E epsilon 4 allele identified (van Munster et al., 2009).

(continued)

Protocol 11.1: Delirium *(cont.)*

3. *Risk factors:* Predisposing, age (70 years and older), severity of illness and cognitive impairment; also depression, sensory impairment, fluid and electrolyte disturbances and polypharmacy (especially psychotropics). Precipitating, central nervous system pathology (such as stroke), metabolic, electrolyte and/or endocrine disturbances, infection and drug toxicity or withdrawal; also pain, hypoperfusion/hypoxia, number of drugs, (especially psychotropic and anticholinergic) and restraints. Environmental factors, ICU admission, multiple room changes, and an absence of a clock or glasses (Michaud et al., 2007).

4. *Outcomes:* Increased mortality, nursing home placement, and decreased functional status and cognition (Cole et al., 2008; Witlox et al., 2010). Distress for the patient, their family members, and nurses (Cohen et al., 2009; Bruera et al., 2009).

IV. PARAMETERS OF ASSESSMENT

A. Assess for risk factors (Michaud et al., 2007)
  1. Baseline or pre-morbid cognitive impairment (see Chapter 8, Assessing Cognitive Function)
  2. Medications review (see Chapter 17, Reducing Adverse Drug Events)
  3. Pain (see Chapter 14, Pain Management)
  4. Metabolic disturbances (hypoglycemia, hypercalcemia, hyponatremia, hypokalemia)
  5. Hypoperfusion/hypoxemia (BP, capillary refill, SpO2)
  6. Dehydration (physical signs/symptoms, intake/output, Na1, BUN/Cr)
  7. Infection (fever, WBCs with differential, cultures)
  8. Environment (sensory overload or deprivation, restraints)
  9. Impaired mobility
  10. Sensory impairment (vision, hearing)

B. Features of delirium (APA, 2000; Inouye et al., 1990)—assess every shift (see "Resources" for validated instruments)
  1. Acute onset; evidence of underlying medical condition
  2. Alertness: Fluctuates from stuporous to hypervigilant
  3. Attention: Inattentive, easily distractible, and may have difficulty shifting attention from one focus to another; has difficulty keeping track of what is being said
  4. Orientation: Disoriented to time and place; should not be disoriented to person
  5. Memory: Inability to recall events of hospitalization and current illness; unable to remember instructions; forgetful of names, events, activities, current news, and so forth
  6. Thinking: Disorganized thinking; rambling, irrelevant, incoherent conversation; unclear or illogical flow of ideas; or unpredictable switching from topic to topic; difficulty in expressing needs and concerns; speech may be garbled
  7. Perception: Perceptual disturbances such as illusions and visual or auditory hallucinations; and misperceptions such as calling a stranger by a relative's name.

(continued)

Protocol 11.1: Delirium *(cont.)*

8. Psychomotor activity: May fluctuate between hypoactive, hyperactive, and mixed subtypes

V. NURSING CARE STRATEGIES (based on protocols in multicomponent delirium prevention studies [Inouye et al., 1999; Lundstrom et al., 2007; Marcantonio, Flacker, Wright, & Resnick, 2001])
A. Obtain geriatric consultation.
B. Eliminate or minimize risk factors.
  1. Administer medications judiciously; avoid high-risk medications (see Chapter 17, Reducing Adverse Drug Events).
  2. Prevent/promptly and appropriately treat infections.
  3. Prevent/promptly treat dehydration and electrolyte disturbances.
  4. Provide adequate pain control (see Chapter 14, Pain Management).
  5. Maximize oxygen delivery (supplemental oxygen, blood, and BP support as needed).
  6. Use sensory aids as appropriate.
  7. Regulate bowel/bladder function.
  8. Provide adequate nutrition (see Chapter 22, Nutrition).
C. Provide a therapeutic environment.
  1. Foster orientation: frequently reassure and reorient patient (unless patient becomes agitated); use easily visible calendars, clocks, caregiver identification; carefully explain all activities; communicate clearly.
  2. Provide appropriate sensory stimulation: quiet room; adequate light; one task at a time; noise reduction strategies.
  3. Facilitate sleep: back massage, warm milk or herbal tea at bedtime; relaxation music/tapes; noise reduction measures; avoid awaking patient.
  4. Foster familiarity: encourage family/friends to stay at bedside; bring familiar objects from home; maintain consistency of caregivers; minimize relocations.
  5. Maximize mobility: avoid restraints (see Chapter 13, Physical Restraints and Side Rails in Acute and Critical Care Settings) and urinary catheters; ambulate or active ROM three times daily.
  6. Communicate clearly, provide explanations.
  7. Reassure and educate family (see Chapter 24, Family Caregiving).
  8. Minimize invasive interventions.
  9. Consider psychotropic medication as a last resort for agitation.

VI. EVALUATION/EXPECTED OUTCOMES
A. Patient
  1. Absence of delirium or
  2. Cognitive status returned to baseline (prior to delirium)
  3. Functional status returned to baseline (prior to delirium)
  4. Discharged to same destination as prehospitalization
B. Health care provider
  1. Regular use of delirium screening tool
  2. Increased detection of delirium
  3. Implementation of appropriate interventions to prevent/treat delirium from standardized protocol

(continued)

Protocol 11.1: Delirium *(cont.)*

    4. Decreased use of physical restraints
    5. Decreased use of antipsychotic medications
    6. Increased satisfaction in care of hospitalized older adults
  C. Institution
    1. Staff education and interprofessional care planning
    2. Implementation of standardized delirium screening protocol
    3. Decreased overall cost
    4. Decreased length of stays
    5. Decreased morbidity and mortality
    6. Increased referrals and consultation to above-specified specialists
    7. Improved satisfaction of patients, families, and nursing staff

VII. FOLLOW-UP MONITORING OF CONDITION
  A. Decreased delirium to become a measure of quality care
  B. Incidence of delirium to decrease
  C. Patient days with delirium to decrease
  D. Staff competence in recognition and treatment of acute confusion/delirium
  E. Documentation of a variety of interventions for acute confusion/delirium

Na^+ = sodium; BUN/Cr = blood urea nitrogen/creatinine ratio; BP = blood pressure; Hgb/Hct = hemoglobin and hematocrit; SpO_2 = pulse oxygen saturation; WBCs = white blood cells; URI = upper respiratory infection; UTI = urinary tract infection; ROM = range of motion

RESOURCES

Recommended Delirium Screening Instruments

Confusion Assessment Method (CAM; Inouye et al., 1990; Wei et al., 2008)

Confusion Assessment Method for the Intensive Care Unit (CAM-ICU; Ely et al., 2001).

Other Delirium Screening Instruments

Delirium-O-Meter (de Jonghe, Kalisvaart, Timmers, Kat, & Jackson, 2005)
May be used for monitoring the different characteristics and the severity of delirium in geriatric patients.

Delirium Rating Scale (DRS)-98 (Trzepacz et al., 2001)
May be used to assess delirium severity.

Mini-Mental State Examination (MMSE; Folstein, Folstein, & McHugh, 1975; O'Keeffe, Mulkerrin, Nayeem, Varughese, & Pillay, 2005)
May be used to monitor course of delirium in hospitalized patients.

Additional Information About Delirium

Consult GeriRN
An online resources containing information regarding assessing and caring for older adults sponsored by the Hartford Institute for Geriatric Nursing at New York University College of Nursing.
http://consultgerirn.org/resources

ICU Delirium and Cognitive Impairment Study Group
http://www.icudelirium.org/delirium/

Hospital Elderlife Program
http://elderlife.med.yale.edu/public/pubs.php?pageid=01.03.07

REFERENCES

American Psychiatric Association. (2000). *Diagnostic and Statistical Manual of Mental Disorders: DSM-IV-TR* (4th ed.). Washington, DC: Author.

Balas, M. C., Deutschman, C. S., Sullivan-Marx, E. M., Strumpf, N. E., Alston, R. P., & Richmond, T. S. (2007). Delirium in older patients in surgical intensive care units. *Journal of Nursing Scholarship, 39*(2), 147–154. Evidence Level IV.

Breitbart, W., Marotta, R., Platt, M. M., Weisman, H., Derevenco, M., Grau, C., . . . Jacobson, P. (1996). A double-blind trial of haloperidol, chlorpromazine, and lorazepam in the treatment of delirium in hospitalized AIDS patients. *The American Journal of Psychiatry, 153*(2), 231–237. Evidence Level II.

Bruce, A. J., Ritchie, C. W., Blizard, R., Lai, R., & Raven, P. (2007). The incidence of delirium associated with orthopedic surgery: A meta-analytic review. *International Psychogeriatrics, 19*(2), 197–214. Evidence Level I.

Bruera, E., Bush, S. H., Willey, J., Paraskevopoulos, T., Li, Z., Palmer, J. L., . . . Elsayem, A. (2009). Impact of delirium and recall on the level of distress in patients with advanced cancer and their family caregivers. *Cancer, 115*(9), 2004–2012. Evidence Level IV.

Cohen, M. Z., Pace, E. A., Kaur, G., & Bruera, E. (2009). Delirium in advanced cancer leading to distress in patients and family caregivers. *Journal of Palliative Care, 25*(3), 164–171. Evidence Level IV.

Cole, M. G., Ciampi, A., Belzile, E., & Zhong, L. (2009). Persistent delirium in older hospital patients: A systematic review of frequency and prognosis. *Age and Ageing, 38*(1), 19–26. Evidence Level I.

Cole, M. G., McCusker, J., Ciampi, A., & Belzile, E., 2008. The 6- and 12-month outcomes of older medical inpatients who recover from subsyndromal delirium. *Journal of the American Geriatrics Society, 56*(11), 2093–2099. Evidence Level IV.

de Jonghe, J. F., Kalisvaart, K. J., Dijkstra, M., van Dis, H., Vreeswijk, R., Kat, M. G., . . . van Gool, W. A. (2007). Early symptoms in the prodromal phase of delirium: A prospective cohort study in elderly patients undergoing hip surgery. *The American Journal of Geriatric Psychiatry, 15*(2), 112–121. Evidence Level IV.

de Jonghe, J. F., Kalisvaart, K. J., Timmers, J. F., Kat, M. G., & Jackson, J. C. (2005). Delirium-O-Meter: A nurses' rating scale for monitoring delirium severity in geriatric patients. *International Journal of Geriatric Psychiatry, 20*(12), 1158–1166. Evidence Level IV.

Devlin, J. W., Roberts, R. J., Fong, J. J., Skrobik, Y., Riker, R. R., Hill, N. S., . . . Garpestad, E. (2010). Efficacy and safety of quetiapine in critically ill patients with delirium: A prospective, multicenter, randomized, double-blind, placebo-controlled pilot study. *Critical Care Medicine, 38*(2), 419–427. Evidence Level II.

Ely, E. W., Inouye, S. K., Bernard, G. R., Gordon, S., Francis, J., May, L., . . . Dittus, R. (2001). Delirium in mechanically ventilated patients: Validity and reliability of the confusion assessment method for the intensive care unit (CAM-ICU). *The Journal of the American Medical Association, 286*(21), 2703–2710. Evidence Level IV.

Ely, E. W., Margolin, R., Francis, J., May, L., Truman, B., Dittus, R., . . . Inouye, S. K. (2001). Evaluation of delirium in critically ill patients: Validation of the Confusion Assessment Method for the Intensive Care Unit (CAM-ICU). *Critical Care Medicine, 29*(7), 1370–1379. Evidence Level IV.

Fick, D. M., Agostini, J. V., & Inouye, S. K. (2002). Delirium superimposed on dementia: A systematic review. *Journal of the American Geriatrics Society, 50*(10), 1723–1732. Evidence Level IV.

Folstein, M. F., Folstein, S. E., & McHugh, P. R. (1975). "Mini-mental state." A practical method for grading the cognitive state of patients for the clinician. *Journal of Psychiatric Research, 12*(3), 189–198. Evidence Level IV.

Inouye, S. K. (2006). Delirium in older persons. *The New England Journal of Medicine, 354*(11), 1157–1165. Evidence Level VI.

Inouye, S. K., Bogardus, S. T., Jr., Charpentier, P. A., Leo-Summers, L., Acampora, D., Holford, T. R., Cooney, L. M., Jr. (1999). A multicomponent intervention to prevent delirium in hospitalized older patients. *The New England Journal of Medicine, 340*(9), 669–676. Evidence Level IV.

Inouye, S. K., van Dyck, C. H., Alessi, C. A., Balkin, S., Siegal, A. P., Horwitz, R. I. (1990). Clarifying confusion: The confusion assessment method. A new method for detection of delirium. *Annals of Internal Medicine, 113*(12), 941–948. Evidence Level IV.

Jacobi, J., Fraser, G. L., Coursin, D. B., Riker, R. R., Fontaine, D., Wittbrodt, E. T., . . . Lump, P. D. (2002). Clinical practice guidelines for the sustained use of sedatives and analgesics in the critically ill adult. *Critical Care Medicine, 30*(1), 119–141. Evidence Level VI.

Kalisvaart, K. J., de Jonghe, J. F., Bogaards, M. J., Vreeswijk, R., Egberts, T. C., Burger, B. J., . . . van Gool, W. A. (2005). Haloperidol prophylaxis for elderly hip-surgery patients at risk for delirium: A randomized placebo-controlled study. *Journal of the American Geriatrics Society, 53*(10), 1658–1666. Evidence Level II.

Kalisvaart, K. J., Vreeswijk, R., de Jonghe, J. F., van der Ploeg, T., van Gool, W. A., & Eikelenboom, P. (2006). Risk factors and prediction of postoperative delirium in elderly hip-surgery patients: Implementation and validation of a medical risk factor model. *Journal of the American Geriatrics Society, 54*(5), 817–822. Evidence Level IV.

Lundström, M., Olofsson, B., Stenvall, M., Karlsson, S., Nyberg, L., Englund, U., . . . Gustafson, Y. (2007). Postoperative delirium in old patients with femoral neck fracture: A randomized intervention study. *Aging Clinical and Experimental Research, 19*(3), 178–186. Evidence Level II.

Maldonado, J. R., Wysong, A., van der Starre, P. J., Block, T., Miller, C., & Reitz, B. A. (2009). Dexmedetomidine and the reduction of postoperative delirium after cardiac surgery. *Psychosomatics, 50*(3), 206–217. Evidence Level II.

Marcantonio, E. R., Flacker, J. M., Wright, R. J., & Resnick, N. M. (2001). Reducing delirium after hip fracture: A randomized trial. *Journal of the American Geriatrics Society, 49*(5), 516–522. Evidence Level II.

McNicoll, L., Pisani, M. A., Zhang, Y., Ely, E. W., Siegel, M. D., & Inouye, S. K. (2003). Delirium in the intensive care unit: Occurrence and clinical course in older patients. *Journal of the American Geriatrics Society, 51*(5), 591–598. Evidence Level IV.

Meagher, D. (2009). Motor subtypes of delirium: Past, present and future. *International Review of Psychiatry, 21*(1), 59–73. Evidence Level V.

Michaud, L., Büla, C., Berney, A., Camus, V., Voellinger, R., Stiefel, F., & Burnand, B. (2007). Delirium: Guidelines for general hospitals. *Journal of Psychosomatic Research, 62*(3), 371–383. Evidence Level V.

Milisen, K., Lemiengre, J., Braes, T., & Foreman, M. D. (2005). Multicomponent intervention strategies for managing delirium in hospitalized older people: Systematic review. *Journal of Advanced Nursing, 52*(1), 79–90. Evidence Level V.

Mouzopoulos, G., Vasiliadis, G., Lasanianos, N., Nikolaras, G., Morakis, E., & Kaminaris, M. (2009). Fascia iliaca block prophylaxis for hip fracture patients at risk for delirium: A randomized placebo-controlled study. *Journal of Orthopaedics and Traumatology, 10*(3), 127–133. Evidence Level II.

Neuman, M. D., Speck, R. M., Karlawish, J. H., Schwartz, J. S., & Shea, J. A. (2010). Hospital protocols for the inpatient care of older adults: Results from a statewide survey. *Journal of the American Geriatrics Society, 58*(10), 1959–1964. doi: 10.1111/j.1532-5415.2010.03056.x. Evidence Level IV.

O'Keeffe, S. T., Mulkerrin, E. C., Nayeem, K., Varughese, M., & Pillay, I. (2005). Use of serial Mini-Mental State Examinations to diagnose and monitor delirium in elderly hospital patients. *Journal of the American Geriatrics Society, 53*(5), 867–870. Evidence Level IV.

Pandharipande, P. P., Cotton, B. A., Shintani, A., Thompson, J., Costabile, S., Truman Pun B., . . . Ely, E. W. (2007). Motoric subtypes of delirium in mechanically ventilated surgical and trauma intensive care unit patients. *Intensive Care Medicine, 33*(10), 1726–1731. Evidence Level IV.

Pandharipande, P. P., Pun, B. T., Herr, D. L., Maze, M., Girard, T. D., Miller, R. R., . . . Ely, E. W. (2007). Effect of sedation with dexmedetomidine vs lorazepam on acute brain dysfunction in mechanically ventilated patients: The MENDS randomized controlled trial. *The Journal of the American Medical Association, 298*(22), 2644–2653. Evidence Level II.

Pisani, M. A., Murphy, T. E., Araujo, K. L., & Van Ness, P. H. (2010). Factors associated with persistent delirium after intensive care unit admission in an older medical patient population. *Journal of Critical Care, 25*(3), 540.e1–540.e7. Evidence Level IV.

Pitkala, K. H., Laurila, J. V., Strandberg, T. E., Kautiainen, H., Sintonen, H., & Tilvis, R. S. (2008). Multicomponent geriatric intervention for elderly inpatients with delirium: Effects on costs and health-related quality of life. *The Journal of Gerontology, 63*(1), 56–61. Evidence Level II.

Riker, R. R., Shehabi, Y., Bokesch, P. M., Ceraso, D., Wisemandle, W., Koura, F., . . . Rocha, M. G. (2009). Dexmedetomidine vs midazolam for sedation of critically ill patients: A randomized trial. *The Journal of American Medical Association, 301*(5), 489–499. Evidence Level II.

Schuurmans, M. J., Deschamps, P. I., Markham, S. W., Shortridge-Baggett, L. M., & Duursma, S. A. (2003). The measurement of delirium: Review of scales. *Research and Theory for Nursing Practice, 17*(3), 207–224. Evidence Level V.

Schweickert, W. D., Pohlman, M. C., Pohlman, A. S., Nigos, C., Pawlik, A. J., Esbrook, C. L., . . . Kress, J. P. (2009). Early physical and occupational therapy in mechanically ventilated, critically ill patients: A randomised controlled trial. *Lancet, 373*(9678), 1874–1882. Evidence Level II.

Shehabi, Y., Grant, P., Wolfenden, H., Hammond, N., Bass, F., Campbell, M., & Chen, J. (2009). Prevalence of delirium with dexmedetomidine compared with morphine based therapy after cardiac surgery: A randomized controlled trial (DEXmedetomidine compared to morphine-DEXCOM Study). *Anesthesiology, 111*(5), 1075–1084. Evidence Level II.

Siddiqi, N., House, A. O., & Holmes, J. D. (2006). Occurrence and outcome of delirium in medical in-patients: A systematic literature review. *Age and Ageing, 35*(4), 350–364. Evidence Level V.

Siddiqi, N., Stockdale, R., Britton, A. M., & Holmes, J. (2007). Interventions for preventing delirium in hospitalised patients. *Cochrane Database of Systematic Reviews.*(2), CD005563. Evidence Level I.

Sieber, F. E., Zakriya, K. J., Gottschalk, A., Blute, M. R., Lee, H. B., Rosenberg, P. B., & Mears, S. C. (2010). Sedation depth during spinal anesthesia and the development of postoperative delirium in elderly patients undergoing hip fracture repair. *Mayo Clinic Proceedings, 85*(1), 18–26. Evidence Level II.

Trzepacz, P. T., Mittal, D., Torres, R., Kanary, K., Norton, J., & Jimerson, N. (2001). Validation of the Delirium Rating Scale-revised-98: Comparison with the delirium rating scale and the cognitive test for delirium. *The Journal of Neuropsychiatry and Clinical Neurosciences, 13*(2), 229–242. Evidence Level IV.

van Munster, B. C., Korevaar, J. C., Zwinderman, A. H., Leeflang, M. M., & de Rooij, S. E. (2009). The associ ation between delirium and the apolipoprotein E epsilon 4 allele: New study results and a meta-analysis. *The American Journal of Geriatric Psychiatry, 17*(10), 856–862. Evidence Level I.

Wei, L. A., Fearing, M. A., Sternberg, E. J., & Inouye, S. K. (2008). The Confusion Assessment Method: A systematic review of current usage. *Journal of the American Geriatrics Society, 56*(5), 823–830. Evidence Level I.

Witlox, J., Eurelings, L. S., de Jonghe, J. F., Kalisvaart, K. J., Eikelenboom, P., & van Gool, W. A. (2010). Delirium in elderly patients and the risk of postdischarge mortality, institutionalization, and dementia: A meta-analysis. *The Journal of the American Medical Association, 304*(4), 443–451. Evidence Level I.

Yang, F. M., Marcantonio, E. R., Inouye, S. K., Kiely, D. K., Rudolph, J. L., Fearing, M. A., & Jones, R., N. (2009). Phenomenological subtypes of delirium in older persons: Patterns, prevalence, and prognosis. *Psychosomatics, 50*(3), 248–254. Evidence Level IV.

Iatrogenesis: The Nurse's Role in Preventing Patient Harm

12

Deborah C. Francis and Jeanne M. Lahaie

EDUCATIONAL OBJECTIVES

On completion of this chapter, the reader will be able to:

1. define iatrogenesis
2. describe the common iatrogenic problems affecting older adults
3. describe the nurse's role in preventing iatrogenic harm in hospitalized older adults

OVERVIEW

Iatrogenesis is a common and serious hazard of hospitalization that is associated with increased patient morbidity and mortality, prolonged hospital stays, and nursing home placement, at significant cost to patients and health care organizations alike. From the Greek word *iatros*, *iatrogenesis* means harm brought forth by a healer or any unintended adverse patient outcome because of a health care intervention, not considered the natural course of the illness or injury. Common well-known iatrogenic problems affecting older adults include adverse drug events (ADE), complications of diagnostic and therapeutic interventions, nosocomial or hospital-acquired infections (HAI), pain, and a variety of geriatric syndromes (e.g., falls, delirium, functional decline, pressure ulcers). Less well recognized are the potentially harmful influences of the knowledge, values, beliefs, and attitudes of well-intentioned health care providers and patients themselves, upon patient outcomes. The purpose of this chapter is to describe common iatrogenic problems affecting older adults and to describe the role of the nurse in preventing iatrogenic harm.

Iatrogenesis is not new to modern medicine. In the 1840s, Semmelweis noted that deaths from puerperal sepsis were lower in those patients treated by midwives who were working only with laboring mothers (Hani, 2010). These low death rates contrasted sharply with high death rates in those mothers treated by medical students who were also dissecting cadavers and performing surgery. Semmelweis introduced a hand-washing

For description of Evidence Levels cited in this chapter, see Chapter 1, Developing and Evaluating Clinical Practice Guidelines: A Systematic Approach, page 7.

program that lowered the cases of fatal puerperal fever from 12.84% to 2.38%, leading to his development of germ theory and the critical role of hand hygiene in the prevention of infection. In 1981, Steel, Gertman, Crescenzi, and Anderson (2004) raised the alarm after reporting that, even with very conservative inclusion criteria, 36% of patients suffered at least one iatrogenic event during a hospital stay.

BACKGROUND AND STATEMENT OF PROBLEM

Iatrogenesis became a commonly used term when medical errors causing patient harm made headlines with the release of the landmark Institute of Medicine (IOM; Kohn, Corrigan, & Donaldson, 1999) report, *To Err is Human: Building a Safer Health System*. It reported that errors made by medical practitioners caused between 44,000 and 98,000 deaths per year at a cost of up to $29 billion in unnecessary health care expenses, disability, and lost income. The report strongly urged immediate, vast, and comprehensive systemwide changes, including both voluntary and mandatory reporting programs by health care organizations, jump-starting the patient safety movement of today. In 2004, a national study of 37 million Medicare patients in 5,000 hospitals found that an average of 195,000 people die every year because of potentially preventable patient safety incidents (Health Grades, Inc., 2004). Although *To Err is Human* called for cutting medical errors by half, iatrogenesis persists. The Agency for Healthcare Research and Quality (AHRQ) reported to Congress in 2008 that preventable medical injuries were increasing by 1% annually (Agency for HealthCare Research and Quality, 2008). Further, in November 2010, the U.S. Department and Health and Human Services' Office of the Inspector General reported an alarming increase in the number of deaths from adverse events—180,000 patients each year—associated with $4.4 billion to government costs. In addition, it is estimated that one in seven Medicare beneficiaries (13.5%)—some 134,000 patients a month—experience at least one adverse event, many preventable (Wilson, 2010).

The patients at greatest risk for experiencing an adverse event while in the hospital are older (Rothschild, Bates, & Leape, 2000), critically ill (Garrouste et al., 2008), or represent an ethnic or racial minority group (Johnstone & Kanitsaki, 2006), and up to 70% of the events are considered preventable (Soop, Fryksmark, Köster, & Haglund, 2009; Zegers et al., 2009). The true extent of the problem remains poorly understood because of a host of factors. Lack of standardization in the literature as to what constitutes iatrogenesis and different methods of data collection and analysis hinders knowledge of the issue. In addition, there is both a lack of recognition of the problem and standardized procedures for investigating and reporting adverse events by hospitals and providers, who are known to disagree about what constitutes a complication and quality of care (Weingart et al., 2006). Patients themselves, especially older adults, are hesitant to formally identify and report iatrogenic harm, if they even recognize it. Many are too ill or do not understand sophisticated medical care enough to recognize an adverse event (Bismark, Brennan, Paterson, Davis, & Studdert, 2006). As such, it is difficult to estimate the true human and financial cost of this problem, and what we know of iatrogenesis may be the tip of the iceberg.

Iatrogenesis in the Older Adult

The risk of an iatrogenic event is highest among patients 65 years and older (Rothschild et al., 2000; Rowell, Nghiem, Jorm, & Jackson, (2010), with evidence suggesting it affects between 10.6% and 58.3 % of hospitalized older adults (Rowell et al., 2010; Steel et al., 2004; Marengoni et al., 2010; Thornlow, Anderson, & Oddone, 2009). A landmark Harvard Medical Practice Study in 2000 found that older adults suffered twice as many diagnostic complications, two-and-one-half times as many medication reactions, four times as many therapeutic mishaps, and nine times as many falls as compared to younger patients (Rothschild & Leape, 2000). A more recent review of the national Healthcare Cost and Utilization Project (HCUP) scores found that for 11 of 13 safety indicators, older patients, especially those older than 85 years, were more likely than younger patients to experience higher rates of adverse events (Thornlow, 2009). The diagnosis of heart failure in combination with either chronic renal failure or chronic obstructive pulmonary disease significantly increases the risk of adverse event-related, in-hospital death (Marengoni et al., 2010). Patients admitted from a skilled nursing facility (SNF) are at a significantly greater risk for developing complications in the hospital (Malone & DantoNocton, 2004).

Endogenous Risk Factors for Iatrogenesis

Normal age-related changes and diminished physiological reserve capacity, especially in hepatic, renal, and cognitive function, and impaired homeostatic and compensatory mechanisms impede the ability of the older patient to respond to the physiological and psychological stressors related to acute illness, and make the older adult more vulnerable to iatrogenesis. Age-associated physiological changes tend to exaggerate the effects of medications, leading to more adverse side effects, which are often treated with the addition of more medications, compounding the risk of iatrogenic harm. This risk is potentiated by the presence of multiple comorbid conditions and drug–drug and drug–disease interactions from resulting polypharmacy (Robinson & Weitzel, 2008).

Aging is associated with an increased risk of infection caused by immune senescence. This age-related blunting of the febrile response and the decreased physiological ability of many older adults to mount an immune response or a fever can delay diagnosis and treatment, and may result in inappropriate care (McElhaney, 2005). A diminished thirst sensation dramatically increases the risk of dehydration in the older patient who, for functional or cognitive reasons, may also be unable to independently drink adequate amounts of fluids. The older adult with age-associated decline in cardiac reserve who is receiving continuous intravenous fluids is also at increased risk for iatrogenic congestive heart failure (CHF).

Another important consideration is the atypical presentation of disease in the older adult. Early symptoms of acute medical conditions tend to be vague, more insidious, and atypical, and so are often missed or misinterpreted by clinicians, family, caregivers, and patients alike. This impairs accurate diagnosis and timely treatment, and subsequently results in a greater frequency of emergent, higher risk interventions. For example, an acute appendicitis in the older adult may present as nonlocalized abdominal discomfort or may not manifest symptoms until perforation occurs. An older person with a myocardial infarction may have no pain at all. Older adults with a urinary tract infection (UTI) or pneumonia commonly present with confusion, falls, or functional impairment, rather than the typical symptoms of infection seen in younger persons. Lack of awareness of atypical presentation can lead to delay in treatment and to patients being inappropriately treated with high-risk medications or labeled as "demented," rather than assessing for and treating unmet needs, such as delirium-related infection or pain.

Exogenous Risk Factors for Iatrogenesis

The hospital environment and the complex interrelationships of hospital and provider practice patterns influence patient safety outcomes. For example, inadequate nurse staffing has consistently been associated with adverse patient outcomes (Frith et al., 2010), and interruptions during clinical care are known to cause more nursing errors (Westbrook, Woods, Rob, Dunsmuir, & Day, 2010). The hospital environment itself can also be hazardous to vulnerable elders with sensory, functional, and cognitive deficits, leading to more falls and fall-related injury. To further complicate matters, physicians and nurses are typically not adequately trained in geriatric care, and so are not prepared to manage the complex, chronic care needed by frail older patients (IOM, 2008). Without a solid understanding of the special needs of the geriatric patient and the factors within an organization that can increase risk, nurses may inadvertently cause more harm to patients during the course of treatment.

The hospitalized older adult is at particularly high risk for cascade iatrogenesis, which occurs when an initial medical or nursing intervention triggers a series of complications, initiating a cascade of decline that is often irreversible (Robinson & Weitzel, 2008). For example, the cognitively impaired surgical patient who is inappropriately treated for pain may develop delirium, be medicated for agitated behaviors, become lethargic from oversedation, and subsequently develop aspiration pneumonia. Deconditioning caused by prolonged bed rest increases fall risk and could lead to a fractured hip when the patient falls while trying to get to the bathroom. This prolongs the hospital stay, increasing the risk of further complications and adverse outcomes. Iatrogenic cascades have been found to occur most frequently among the oldest, most functionally impaired patients, and those with a higher severity of illness upon admission (Robinson & Weitzel, 2008).

ASSESSMENT OF THE PROBLEM

Adverse Drug Events

Adverse effects of medications are the most common type of iatrogenesis in hospitalized older adults. These include not only any adverse outcome that occurs during the course of routine, appropriate medication use, but also adverse outcomes caused by inappropriate prescribing, administration errors, and suboptimal adherence by the patient. It is estimated that 35% of older persons experience ADE every year, almost half of which are preventable (Safran et al., 2005). On average, patients with ADE experience longer hospital stays and have greater in-hospital and 30-day mortality. Some 10%–20% of older adults are prescribed nonsteroidal anti-inflammatory drugs (NSAIDs) in spite of known gastrointestinal side effects, including ulcerations and bleeding, and the increased risk of impaired renal function, resulting in an estimated 3,300 excess deaths and 41,000 excess hospitalizations annually (Arnstein, 2010). Still, many nurses and other health care practitioners are not aware of the risks, with some hospital protocols continuing to use NSAIDs as a first-line agent to treat pain in older adults, in spite of the 2009 guidelines from the American Geriatric Society (2009) to the contrary.

Polypharmacy, which is prevalent among older patients, increases the risk of drug–drug interactions, whose effect on this population is more dramatic. It has been shown to be a significant predictor of hospitalization, nursing home placement, death, hypoglycemia, fractures, impaired mobility, pneumonia, and malnutrition (Frazier, 2005).

A 2004 national study estimated that 888,000 ADE occurred in hospitalized Medicare patients from high-risk medications alone, including warfarin, hypoglycemic agents, digoxin, and antibiotics (Classen, Jaser, & Budnitz, 2010). The nurse needs to closely monitor the patient for adverse side effects of medication and be aware of the need for age-adjusted doses especially with high-risk medications. Anticoagulation dosing based on creatinine clearance and weight, for example, is critical in order to avoid further harm to the patient (Jaffer & Brotman, 2006). Medication reconciliation upon admission, transfer, and discharge is another key strategy needed to maintain geriatric patient safety. The reader is referred to Chapter 17, Reducing Adverse Drug Events for assessment and interventions to prevent ADE.

Adverse Effects of Diagnostic, Medical, Surgical, and Nursing Procedures

Acutely ill older patients are at greatest risk for iatrogenic harm, due in part to the need for more diagnostic, prophylactic, and therapeutic medical, surgical, or nursing procedures and interventions

Diagnostic procedures involve some degree of risk based on whether they are invasive or administer a pharmacological or radiological agent, such as contrast material. Contrast dye, commonly used in CT scans and myelography, can produce both allergic and nonallergic reactions ranging from urticaria, angioedema, and anaphylaxis. Radiocontrast infusion in patients with renal impairment can cause acute renal failure (ARF) or an exacerbation of CHF. Gadolinium, used as a contrast agent for magnetic resonance imaging (MRI), has been associated with nephrogenic systemic sclerosis in patients with impaired renal function. In addition, patients with preexisting renal impairment exposed to nephrotoxins such as aminoglycosides or a radiocontrast agent and patients with CHF given NSAIDs are at significantly greater risk for ARF (Cheung, Ponnusamy, & Anderton, 2008). Exposure to iodinated radiocontrast material should be avoided or minimized in patients with renal insufficiency, and nursing staff must closely monitor the patient's hydration status before and after the use of contrast dye in diagnostic studies. Particular attention needs to be paid to the patient's orthostatic blood pressure, urine output, and jugular venous pressure (Cheung et al., 2008). Administering age-adjusted, appropriate medications to premedicate prior to procedures is critical, as is the ability of the nurse to question what may be a high-risk drug or dose for the older adult. For example, the anticholinergic antihistamine, diphenhydramine, which is routinely prescribed before a blood transfusion to prevent minor transfusion reactions, can precipitate delirium in older patients.

Medical procedures such as thoracentesis and cardiac catheterization have also been linked to significantly more preventable adverse effects in the older adult, such as cardiac arrhythmias, bleeding, infection, and pneumothorax (Dumont, Keeling, Bourguignon, Sarembock, & Turner, 2006). The literature is full of case reports of iatrogenic injuries and deaths due to medical or nursing procedures such as venous embolism caused by the injection of CT contrast (Imai, Tamada, Gyoten, Yamashita, & Kajihara, 2004); aspiration deaths caused by barium, emollient laxatives, and contrast medium (Hunsaker & Hunsaker, 2002); colonic perforations caused by endoscopy or enema (Bobba & Arsura, 2004); and complications associated with percutaneous endoscopic gastrostomy tubes (Ghevariya, Paleti, Momeni, Krishnaiah, & Anand, 2009).

Risk for injurious falls is higher in older adults with devices or lines that tether the patient to the bed. As such, proactive assessment of when to discontinue tethering devices, and ongoing evaluation of the potential safety hazard is important. Restraints, including full hospital bed rails, once a cornerstone of fall prevention programs, have increasingly been recognized as harmful and potentially fatal to patients. It is the older adult who is at greatest risk for being restrained in an effort to prevent a fall or to manage agitated behaviors associated with delirium, so every effort must be made to implement nonpharmacological, restraint-free behavior management and fall prevention interventions as noted in the protocol chapters. Restraining the patient with physical devices or medication often exacerbates agitated behavior and may contribute to falls, aspiration, skin breakdown, deconditioning, and other complications, especially when applied without addressing pain, elimination, or other care needs.

Medical and nursing interventions, even those that are considered relatively risk free, such as the administration of intravenous therapy, can be dangerous in the older patient. Excessive venipuncture (e.g., from laboratory tests ordered daily in stable patients) places the vulnerable older patient at increased risk not only for infection, but also for phlebitis, venous thrombotic embolism (VTE), and unnecessary suffering. Given the age-related reduced cardiac reserve, intravenous fluids can lead to preventable CHF or electrolyte abnormalities. Sherman (2005) identifies three forms of geriatric iatrogenesis, referred to as the *hypo's of hospitalization*, that can delay discharge, increase costs, and lead to adverse patient outcomes. Iatrogenic-induced *hypokalemia* occurs when intravenous fluids are given without potassium, whereas orthostatic *hypotension* can be induced when an antihypertensive medication is given based exclusively on supine blood pressures. Transient decreases in oral intake in patients receiving oral hypoglycemic agents, or standing insulin orders can cause preventable *hypoglycemia*.

Bed rest, in and of itself, can have serious negative effects on older patients, including functional decline, VTE, pressure ulcers, delirium, orthostatic hypotension, falls, anorexia, constipation, and fecal impaction, among other adverse outcomes. Older adults are at greatest risk for VTE, which is both preventable and common in hospitalized older adults, due in part to underuse of prophylactic anticoagulation (Jacobs, 2003). Aggressive pharmacological thromboprophylaxis is necessary unless there is a contraindication such as active bleeding, when mechanical prophylaxis with sequential compression devices is warranted (Jaffer & Brotman, 2006).

Perioperative complications in older patients can be as high as twice that of younger patients, and mortality can be three to seven times higher (Saver, 2010). Bentrem, Cohen, Hynes, Ko, and Bilimoria (2009) found that older adults were more likely to experience the following surgical complications: cardiac (acute myocardial infarction and cardiac arrest), pulmonary (pneumonia, pulmonary embolism, and respiratory failure), and urological (UTI and renal failure). On a positive note, the authors found that surgical site infections (SSIs), postoperative bleeding events, VTE, and rates of return to the OR were not significantly different than those of younger adults.

Nurses are called upon to take a more active role in identifying older patients at higher risk of surgical complications, given the evidence that only a small percentage of surgeons and anesthetists recognize these age-associated risks and routinely order commensurate postoperative monitoring in older patients (Pirret, 2003). A simple preoperative nursing assessment tool used in more than 7,000 patients over a 2-year period identified the higher risk patients in need of improved postoperative monitoring and reduced acute admissions to the ICU from 40% to 19% (Pirret, 2003). Saver (2010) recommends a multipronged approach to reduce surgical complications in the older adult that includes tracking clinical indicators, performing a thorough assessment, protecting patients intraoperatively, and providing patient education. The assessment should review six preoperative markers that have been linked to 6-month mortality in older adults: impaired cognition, recent falls, low serum albumin, anemia, functional dependence, and multiple comorbidities. Functional dependence in activities of daily living (ADLs) is the biggest predictor of mortality, and having four or more of the pre-operative markers predicted mortality with high sensitivity and specificity. Assessment findings can be used to target post-op interventions including prevention of delirium, falls, and functional decline. Also, nurses can collaborate with nutrition services to increase postoperative monitoring and management (Barbosa-Silva & Barros, 2005).

Postoperative nursing care that focused on preventing infection, reducing tension at the surgical site, and optimizing nutritional status effectively prevents *surgical wound dehiscence*, a serious complication with up to 50% mortality (Hahler, 2006). The older adult's oral intake needs to be carefully monitored and reported, and insulin adjusted to prevent hypoglycemia and optimize glycemic control (Sherman, 2005). It is also important to monitor the geriatric patient for *atrial fibrillation*, a potentially preventable condition that occurs in about one-third of patients after coronary artery bypass surgery and has been associated with other complications, including cognitive changes, renal impairment, infection (Mathew et al., 2004), and stroke (Lip & Edwards, 2006).

Safe nursing processes of care must be adopted and well integrated into the hospital and nursing culture. Westbrook et al. (2010) demonstrated that interruption of a nurse during a medication pass resulted in a 12.1% increase in failure to follow a standard procedure and a 12.7% increase in clinical errors. Hospital initiatives now include efforts to ensure nurses who are passing medications are not disturbed and to expect more involvement by the patient in care decisions and treatment planning so as to mitigate this risk.

Given the plethora of evidence that communication and other systems problems cause iatrogenic patient harm, The Joint Commission (TJC) mandates more involvement of patients in their care and formal time outs and other verification procedures at high-risk times to prevent wrong-site surgeries and other errors. Prior to any invasive procedure, nurses must also ensure the patient clearly understands the inherent risks and benefits before giving informed consent. Although health care professionals (HCPs) are trained to weigh the risks and benefits, it is critical to heighten one's assessment of the situation and to err on the side of caution in the geriatric patient. Potentially harmful diagnostic and therapeutic procedures may well be contraindicated if the potential benefit does not clearly increase the potential for improving patient outcomes. This is particularly important, given the strong evidence that the older population tends to have lower rates of understanding the risks and benefits of the procedure for which they are providing written or verbal consent (Mahon, 2010).

Given the age-associated increase in sensory deficits, it is critical to identify and address any visual or hearing deficits that may impede patient understanding. Several discussions over time to evaluate and ensure that the patient understands the situation may be warranted. If a difference of professional opinion occurs, nurses are encouraged to bring significant issues of potential harm up the chain of command.

Hospital-Acquired Infection

HAI, first defined in 1970 by the Centers for Disease Control and Prevention (CDC) as one that develops in a patient after hospital admission, is a serious risk for any patient. Like other iatrogenic harm, the risk and potential for poor outcomes related to HAIs rises dramatically with age (Duffy, 2002). HAIs are one of the leading causes of morbidity and mortality in hospitalized patients (World Health Organization [WHO], 2002). It is estimated that HAIs affect more than 2 million patients in the United States every year and cause at least 90,000 deaths (Leape & Berwick, 2005), at a cost exceeding $4.5 billion (Hollenbeak et al., 2006). Although the true incidence is difficult to determine, evidence suggests that 5%–10% of patients develop HAI, which increases morbidity, mortality, length of stay, and cost of care (Gordts, Vrijens, Hulstaert, Devriese, & Van de Sande, 2010; Lanini et al., 2009). In addition, a disturbing increase in risk has been noted in recent decades (Burke, 2003). The rate of HAI is highest among older (Rothschild et al., 2000) and critically ill patients, who tend to be the most sick and most immunocompromised, undergo more invasive procedures, and receive more intravascular devices, which significantly increases the risk of secondary infection.

UTIs are the most common HAIs, accounting for 30% to 40% of all nosocomial infections (Brosnahan, Jull, & Tracy, 2004). The risk is directly related to the use and duration of indwelling urethral catheters, accounting for approximately 80% of hospital-acquired UTIs. In one series, 9% of older patients who received an indwelling catheter developed a UTI during the acute hospital stay; 50% of catheters used were determined not to be clinically justified (Hazelett, Tsai, Gareri, & Allen, 2006). A systematic review of the effects of duration of indwelling catheters on patient outcomes revealed both a significant increase in UTIs when the catheter was left in for more than 48 hours and a reduction in hospital length of stay when it was removed within 48 hours (Fernandez & Griffiths, 2006). Even without a catheter, the older patient is at increased risk for a UTI because of age-related physiological changes, functional abnormalities (prostate enlargement), the use of medications that promote urinary retention, and chronic diseases that increase infection risk or impair bladder function (e.g., diabetes; see Chapter 19, Catheter-Associated Urinary Tract Infection Prevention).

Hospital-acquired pneumonia (HAP) is the second most common type of nosocomial infection after UTI, with an estimated mortality rate of 20%–46% (Arozullah, Khuri, Henderson, Paley, & Daley, 2001), and is the third most common postoperative complication after urinary tract and wound infections. Patients receiving continuous mechanical ventilation have a six- to twenty-one-fold increased risk of developing bacterial HAP (CDC, 2003). Pulmonary aspiration of secretions from the oropharyngeal or gastrointestinal tract is the most common cause of HAP and is considered preventable in the majority of cases (Weitzel, Robinson, & Holmes, 2006).

Hospital-acquired bloodstream infections are common, serious, and costly infections that are a leading cause of death in this country (Wenzel & Edmond, 2001). These infections are most often related to the use of an invasive device, and more than 50% occur in the critically ill patient. Catheter-associated bloodstream infections (CABSI) are serious infections in ICU patients, occurring in 3%–7% of all patients with central venous catheters (Warren, Zack, Cox, Cohen, & Fraser, 2003), associated with increased mortality and cost (Shannon et al., 2006).

SSI are the most common type of nosocomial infection in patients undergoing surgery, and are associated with prolonged and more costly hospitalizations (Malone, Genuit, Tracy, Gannon, & Napolitano, 2002). Patients with SSIs are also twice as likely to die, 60% more likely to be admitted to the ICU, and five times more likely to be rehospitalized than patients who do not develop SSI (Kirkland, Briggs, Trivette, Wilkinson, & Sexton, 1999). Gram-positive organisms account for the majority of bacterial infections (Malone et al., 2002). Although the risk of SSI varies according to type of surgery and patient-specific factors, evidence demonstrates that factors related to the hospital itself, such as practice patterns and the environment of care, significantly increase the risk of patient harm (Hollenbeak et al., 2006).

Other infections that commonly affect hospitalized older patients include those affecting the gastrointestinal tract, such as *Clostridium difficile* (*C. difficile*) *colitis* and the skin, such as methicillin-resistant *Staphylococcus aureus* (MRSA). *C. difficile* infections are affecting significant numbers of hospitalized older patients. It is estimated that 20% –40% of hospitalized patients are colonized with the *C. difficile* toxin as compared to 2%–3% of healthy adults (Bartlett, 2006). Fifteen percent to 25% of patients with anti-biotic-associated diarrhea, and more than 95% with pseudomembranous colitis carry the *C. difficile* toxin, which is becoming more refractory to treatment and more apt to relapse (Freeman et al., 2010; Dubberke et al., 2010).

The alarming increase in antimicrobial-resistant organisms, such as MRSA and van-comycin-resistant enterococcus (VRE) is of great concern. Patients older than 80 years of age are at significantly greater risk for being carriers of MRSA (Eveillard, Mortier, et al., 2006). MRSA increased in prevalence from 2% of *S. aureus* infections in 1974 to 63% in 2004, whereas VRE has steadily increased from less than 1% in 1990 to 28.5% of enterococcol isolates in 2003 (CDC, 2006). On a positive note, a more recent review from nine U.S. hospitals suggests that MRSA decreased 9.4% per year from 2005 to 2008 (Kallen et al., 2010). Vancomycin resistance has been shown to be an independent risk factor for death and is associated with poor patient outcomes, including longer length of stay, increased mortality, and higher costs of care (Salgado & Farr, 2003). More recently, the increase in multiple drug-resistant organisms has been associated with significantly longer hospital stays, increased cost, and higher mortality.

INTERVENTIONS AND CARE STRATEGIES

Nursing Strategies for Hospital-Acquired Infections

Reducing the rate of HAI comprises one of TJC's National Patient Safety Goals and three of the six goals of the Institute of Healthcare Improvement (IHI) 5 Million Lives Campaign. The WHO and the CDC have published numerous guidelines for the pre-vention of health care infections with recommendations based on levels of evidence from the literature. Adherence to these evidence-based best practices, such as hand hygiene and infection control, is key to preventing iatrogenic infections. The reader is referred to the list of evidence-based CDC guidelines at the end of this chapter.

Infection control staff must be actively involved in implementing guidelines, train-ing staff and performing ongoing surveillance, and reporting processes with support from hospital leadership. Infection control efforts need to address strict adherence to appropriate cleansing of equipment and the environment, isolation of colonized patients, and appropriate surveillance programs as outlined in CDC guidelines. Hospitals par-ticipating in the CDC's National Nosocomial Infections Surveillance (NNIS) system significantly reduced bloodstream infections, UTIs, and pneumonia in ICU patients, as well as SSIs. Success was attributed to the use of standardized definitions and surveil-lance protocols and risk stratification for calculation of infection rates, combined with an active prevention program (Jarvis, 2003).

Nurses play an important role in monitoring immunizations as well as antibiotic stewardship, critical to slowing the emergence of bacterial resistance. Nurses also have a voice in the formulation of policy as well as clinical decision making. They can educate other clinicians about a hospital's antibiotic prescribing policies, including reserving newer or broader-spectrum antibiotics and vancomycin for cases of proven drug resistance or life-threatening emergencies.

Given the increased risk in patients who are mechanically ventilated, implementation of bundled evidence-based interventions for ventilator-associated pneumonia (VAP) prevention, such as those proposed by IHI, is imperative (Wip & Napolitano, 2009). Avoidance of the supine position is critical in preventing aspiration pneumonia, especially in patients receiving enteral feeding (Li Bassi & Torres, 2011). Placing the patient in the prone position to promote drainage of oropharyngeal and airway secretions has also been noted to be beneficial, and more research is warranted in the use of the lateral Trendelenburg position (Li Bassi & Torres, 2011). Although the evidence suggests that elevating the head of the bed between 30 and 45 degrees decreases the incidence of VAP, adherence to the optimal 45-degree level is problematic and increases the risk of a sacral pressure ulcer. Unfortunately, there is limited evidence to recommend the safest, lowest head-of-bed (HOB) elevation (Li Bassi & Torres, 2011).

Besides adherence to hand hygiene and HOB elevation, there is good evidence that routine oral care effectively reduces the rate of HAP in critical care patients (Simmons-Trau, Cenek, Counterman, Hockenbury, & Litwiller, 2004). Unfortunately, oral hygiene continues to be a nursing function of "low priority" in most health care settings (Wenzel & Edmond, 2001). A review of the evidence on subglottal secretion aspiration revealed it consistently and significantly reduced the incidence of VAP, yet the practice is limited in clinical settings (Scherzer, 2010). Systematic review of the factors associated with enteral feeding in preventing VAP found appropriate enteral feeding to be the most important factor (Chen, 2009). In addition, intermittent enteral feeding and ensuring small residual volume is recommended to reduce gastroesophageal reflux, and early feeding and increased total volume intake can prevent ICU mortality. Use of an antiseptic oral rinse for cardiac-surgery patients, noninvasive positive pressure ventilation, condensate collection, subglottal secretion drainage, early extubation, and avoiding gastric overdistension and unplanned extubation have also been found to be effective preventive measures for VAP (Hsieh & Tuite, 2006). Tolentino-DelosReyes, Ruppert, and Shiao (2007) demonstrated a significant improvement in critical care nurses' knowledge and adherence to evidence-based practice after an educational program on the ventilator "bundle," or set of interventions, to decrease VAP. The implementation of an evidence-based guideline in five U.S. hospitals that included five nursing interventions (HOB elevation, oral care, ventilator tubing condensate removal, hand hygiene, and glove use) reduced the rates of VAP and length of ICU stay, although not significantly (Abbott, Dremsa, Stewart, Mark, & Swift, 2006).

Central venous catheter infections can be significantly reduced using nontechnological strategies such as strict hand washing, maximal sterile barrier precautions, use of antiseptic solutions, insertion and management by trained personnel, and continuing quality improvement programs (Gnass et al., 2004). It has been suggested that cleansing the access port with either 70% alcohol or 3.15% chlorhexidine/70% alcohol for 15 seconds is effective in disinfecting the port (Kaler & Chinn, 2007), and that nursing staff must be diligent in this practice to protect the patient.

Patients with malnutrition, diabetes, postoperative anemia, and ascites are known to be at increased risk for SSI, so nurses need to closely monitor those patients and collaborate with nutrition services to intervene as indicated (Malone et al., 2002). Multiple evidence-based guidelines for SSI prevention have been developed and include antibiotic prophylaxis within 1 hour of incision with discontinuation within 24 hours. As such, the timing of antibiotic administration must be a nursing priority, and attention paid to processes of care to ensure adherence (Gagliardi, Fenech, Eskicioglu, Nathens, & McLeod, 2009).

Encouraging early mobilization and lung expansion interventions, such as coughing and deep breathing exercises, incentive spirometry, and chest physiotherapy, are critical nursing interventions to prevent atelectasis, secretion retention, and pneumonia. Unfortunately, there is a clear lack of evidence in specifically which surgical patients most benefit from perioperative lung expansion interventions (Freitas, Soares, Cardoso, & Atallah, 2007; Lawrence, Cornell, & Smetana, 2006).

Close monitoring and effective glycemic control in critically ill patients can effectively reduce nosocomial infection rates (Grey & Perdrizet, 2004), as well as in-hospital mortality and length of stay in the ICU (Krinsley, 2004). Tight glycemic control of older adults, however, does not lower the risk of mortality in the inpatient setting and, in fact, can put seniors at risk for hypoglycemia and its complications (Alagiakrishnan & Mereu, 2010).

Besides active prevention measures, maintaining a high degree of vigilance for infection throughout the hospital stay is critical. Although assessment of vital signs and white blood cell counts provide important information, the more atypical presentation of infection requires that nursing staff closely monitor the geriatric patient for any cognitive and functional changes that could reflect the presence of infection. Nursing staff must be aware of the increased vulnerability of the frail, older patient due to immune senescence, which reduces the T cell response to an infectious agent. Fever can be absent in 30%–50% of older adults with infection, and any two-point increase from baseline needs to be considered a fever equivalent. Infection may present as confusion, falls, decline in self-care ability, reduced food and/or fluid intake, re-emergence of previously resolved stroke symptoms, new incontinence, generalized asthenia, new-onset atrial fibrillation, worsened glycemic control, or a host of other subtle findings. The development of any of these conditions should prompt suspicion for occult infection. Thus, the role of the nurse as patient advocate is crucial—one that demands ongoing vigilance.

Quality Improvement Initiatives to Minimize Infection

Processes of care need to be reviewed and interdisciplinary quality improvement efforts initiated to minimize infection, as well as any patient harm. Gagliardi et al. (2009) found that individual knowledge, attitudes, and beliefs, along with systems issues, such as team communication, allocation of resources, and organizational support for promoting and monitoring care processes, highly influence practice regarding antibiotic prophylaxis for the prevention of SSI infection. They recommend written order sets, multidisciplinary pathways, and quality improvement strategies to ensure adherence to SSI prophylaxis.

A 5-year nurse-led interdisciplinary patient safety initiative used a systems approach to improve nurse-identified issues by addressing human factors, staff education, and no-blame reporting systems and successfully reduced the rate of serious ADEs by 45% (Luther et al., 2002). In addition, it effectively reduced (a) VAP (from 47.8 to 10.9/1000 ventilator days), (b) CABSI (from 90th to 50th percentile), (c) length of hospital stay (from 8.1 to 4.5 days), (d) RN vacancy rate, and (e) the use of contracted nurses by more than half (50% ICU, 65% medical–surgical units). Strong organizational commitment was noted as key to success (Luther et al., 2002).

Another study found monthly feedback of infection rates to staff and training resulted in a 66% reduction in CABSIs in the ICU (Coopersmith et al., 2002). Providing nursing staff with quarterly unit-specific data on catherter-associated UTI rates reduced the overall rate of catheter patient days from 32 to 17.4/1000 at a cost savings of $403,000 for more than an 18-month period (Goetz, Kedzuf, Wagener, & Muder, 1999). Gastmeier et al. (2002) demonstrated that nosocomial infection rates can be reduced by quality improvement efforts such as quality circles and continuous surveillance. These findings demonstrate the importance of staff education and quality improvement efforts using a multidisciplinary approach and close interdepartmental collaboration and communication with organizational support at all levels.

GERIATRIC SYNDROMES

Overview

Geriatric syndromes are health conditions associated with aging and frailty, with a variety of causes that fail to fall into discrete disease categories (Inouye, Studenski, Tinetti, & Kuchel, 2007). These syndromes are increasingly being recognized as serious and preventable iatrogenic complications that increase risk for adverse outcomes, including prolonged length of stay and discharge to a more dependent level of care, loss of function and independence, and even death (Anpalahan & Gibson, 2008). They are highly prevalent, especially among the frail elder, multifactorial in nature, and associated with significant disability and diminished quality of life. Geriatric syndromes include, but are not limited to delirium, functional decline, falls, malnutrition, pressure ulcers, depression, incontinence, and pain that occur in the course of receiving medical and nursing care. The reader is referred to the appropriate book chapters in this book that address the assessment and management of these common iatrogenic geriatric syndromes.

It has been suggested that geriatric syndromes need to be recognized as a valuable theoretical framework,and used to train nurses (Stierle et al.,2006) and medical students (Olde Rikkert, Rigaud, van Hoeyweghen, & de Graaf, 2003). Tsilimingras, Rosen, and Berlowitz (2003) contend that the patient safety initiatives sparked by *To Err Is Human* do not go far enough to address the unique needs of the older patient who is at greatest risk for iatrogenic harm. They recommend that geriatric syndromes need to be recognized as distinct iatrogenic events, going so far as to call them medical errors, and urge major system reform to address these preventable and costly problems. They propose the need to routinely identify and report all geriatric syndromes and, when they occur, proactively identify and address system failures, reduce ADEs, improve the continuity of care, improve geriatric training programs, and establish dedicated geriatric units (Tsilimingras et al., 2003).

Nursing Management of Geriatric Syndromes

Evidence-based standards of practice for HAI, falls, functional decline, pressure ulcers, delirium, and other geriatric syndromes, as outlined in this book, need to be adopted in targeted high-risk patients to prevent iatrogenesis. Nurses are also encouraged to use risk assessment tools and best practice interventions, such as the ones described at the *How to Try This* series on the Hartford Center for Geriatric Nursing website (http://consultgerirn.org/resources). Clinical pathways of evidence-based interventions designed to reduce complications in older adults have achieved measurable success in acute care hospitals. For example, a clinical pathway significantly reduced the postoperative morbidity in patients with hip fractures by reducing postoperative CHF and cardiac arrhythmias from 5% to 1%, and reducing postoperative delirium from 51% to 22% (Beaupre et al., 2006). In addition, nurses identifying the at-risk older adult and implementing delirium prevention best practice interventions is key to preventing this serious and costly complication (Fick, Agostini, & Inouye, 2002). Vigilant nurses competent in geriatrics will use the knowledge of the concept of diminishing physiological reserve capacity to identify the need to balance diagnostic and therapeutic interventions with the need for rest and sleep. Closely monitoring sleep patterns in order to prevent sleep deprivation and scheduling tests and therapy only after the patient has adequate rest is critical to prevent delirium and promote healing.

A nurse-driven mobility protocol has been shown to decrease functional decline and length of stay in hospitalized older adults (Padula, Hughes, & Baumhover, 2009). Nurses also have a responsibility to optimize nutritional status in order to prevent iatrogenic complications. The older adult's oral intake needs to be carefully monitored and reported and insulin adjusted to prevent hypoglycemia and optimize glycemic control (Sherman, 2005).

Nursing staff should routinely take orthostatic vital signs or at least measure the blood pressure of the older patient in the sitting position to ensure that significant orthostatic hypotension is not induced by treating supine hypertension (Sherman, 2005). Older adults tend to be at greatest risk for falling caused by a variety of intrinsic and extrinsic factors that are well documented in the literature. Proactive identification and management of risk factors is critical, and the reader is referred to Chapter 15, Fall Prevention: Assessment, Diagnoses, and Intervention Strategies.

Pain, in and of itself, can be a form of iatrogenic harm. Pain management is a key nursing responsibility from an ethical, legal, and regulatory standpoint, and every effort must be implemented to ensure the patient is not suffering needlessly because of acute or chronic pain (Pasero & McCaffery, 2001). A 2010 study of older adults with pain on an acute medical unit found that (a) 70% of the patients had pain, although their nurses did not ask them if they had pain in 75% of these cases; (b) nurses documented pain assessment or management in only 33% of cases; (c) nearly 50% of patients did not receive a prescribed analgesic for their pain; (d) 14% of patients with pain did not have any analgesia ordered; and (e) more than 50% of the patients did not receive appropriate pain management (Coker et al., 2010).

Undertreatment of pain in older adults may lead to the iatrogenic condition known as *pseudoaddiction*, where the HCP may confuse relief-seeking requests for more pain medication as the "drug-seeking behavior" of an addict (Pergolizzi et al., 2008). Undertreated pain limits function in older adults and has been shown to lead to disability and it can lead to decreased quality of life, depression, and diminished socialization (D'Arcy, 2009; Reid, Williams, & Gill, 2005). Iatrogenic disturbance pain (IDP), the presence of day-to-day pain that accompanies routine nursing caregiving activities, has also been described as a significant source of suffering impacting quality of life (Mentes, Teer, & Cadogan, 2004). The reader is referred to Chapter 14, Pain Management for a more comprehensive discussion of this topic.

In summary, nurses are in a unique role to prevent geriatric syndromes and cascade iatrogenesis (Robinson & Weitzel, 2008) and must use their knowledge of aging to proactively advocate for safe, quality geriatric patient care to members of the health care team. Moore and Duffy (2007) argue that the main reason why older adults are in the hospital is the need for nursing vigilance, whereby the nurse has the knowledge to understand what is happening, the ability to anticipate what can happen, to weigh the risks and benefits, and to intervene to minimize the risk and to monitor outcomes.

INTERVENTIONS RELATED TO CHANGING PROVIDER AND PATIENT KNOWLEDGE, BELIEFS, AND ATTITUDES

Nurses' Knowledge, Attitudes, and Beliefs

Although the majority of the literature focuses on iatrogenic illness and injuries that result from either the commission or omission of a physical act, arguments can be made that equally detrimental effects to patients can occur as a direct result of the knowledge, values, attitudes, beliefs, fears, and biases of nurses and other HCPs. A nurse's perception of older adults as chronically ill and frail may foster increasing dependence and functional decline if the patient is not provided the opportunity or assistance to routinely ambulate or engage in self-care skills.

A nurse who fails to place the patient's values ahead of his or her own may cause undue suffering and harm when these values are in conflict. Failure to treat pain in dying patients for fear of hastening death increases suffering, lowers quality of life remaining, and conflicts with evidence that treatment of pain in dying patients can prolong life and provide a higher quality of the life that remains. Conversely, nurses who participated in programs such as the End-of-Life Nursing Education Consortium (ELNEC) have reported an improvement in their knowledge, confidence, and attitudes regarding palliative care for dying patients as well as a decrease in their anxiety regarding death of patients (Barrere, Durkin, & LaCoursiere, 2008). Likewise, outdated myths and attitudes of aging can interfere with a nurse's role in protecting the vulnerable older adult, including effective pain management (D'Arcy, 2009). It is well known that a significant number of nursing home patients suffer needlessly in pain due in part to fear of addiction that takes precedence over comfort. Older adults, more than any other age group, tend to be undertreated for pain (Robinson, 2007) and other conditions, including osteoporosis (Davis, Ashe, Guy, & Khan, 2006) and depression (Harman et al., 2002). The assumption that the quality of life of the demented person is "poor" may lead the nurse to assume that institutionalization or palliation is the most appropriate goal of care, regardless of the values of the elder (Kenny, 1990).

Kenny (1990) asserts that the current and traditional system of hospital care not only perpetuates dependency and iatrogenesis among geriatric patients, but also "erodes" their identity, self-esteem, and individuality. In addition, prolonged hospital stays are known to increase social isolation, decrease function, and foster dependence (Graf, 2008). One is left to wonder how much this may contribute to the high rates of depression seen in the hospitalized older patient. Nurses must be careful to distinguish between "care as discipline" and the *gift of care*, defined by Fox as the relationship between the patient and the provider that is mediated by love, generosity, trust, and delight (Greenwood, 2007). The danger lies in labeling a recipient of care who has impaired cognition as a "dementia patient," or a patient with multiple admissions as a "frequent flier," thus diminishing sensitivity to the humanity of the individual who is hospitalized (Greenwood, 2007). A diagnosis of dementia may lead an uneducated or age-biased nurse to expect less of a patient, and inadvertently promote functional decline, or to inaccurately assess for pain and undermedicate, promoting patient suffering and more complications (D'Arcy, 2009).

Nurses have a responsibility to educate themselves in order to act responsibly and safely. In addition, it is important to carefully examine one's values and beliefs systems, so as not to unwittingly contribute to the patient's suffering because of ignorance or biases against older patients that can compromise clinical objectivity and patient care.

Patient Knowledge, Attitudes, and Beliefs

To make matters worse, older patients are known to underreport or deny symptoms (Coker et al., 2010), in part because they have grown accustomed to living with chronic aches and pains and may interpret new symptoms as the presentation of a long-standing health problem. They may believe the symptom is a normal part of aging or fear a loss of independence or, worse, institutionalization, if they admit to a physical or cognitive deficit. Underreporting of pain is particularly common and problematic among older adults. Some 40% of fatalities following hip replacement surgeries in seniors are caused by pulmonary embolism (Morrison et al., 2003). Researchers posit that this is related to immobility and could be because of seniors' reluctance to take needed pain medication that allows them to ambulate and participate in therapy, as well as providers' lack of knowledge that severe pain is associated with a ninefold increased risk of delirium in cognitively intact patients (Morrison et al., 2003) means to prevent error and patient harm (Sherwood, Thomas, Bennett, & Lewis, 2002; Wallace, Spurgeon, Benn, Koutantji, & Vincent, 2009).

INTERVENTIONS RELATED TO NATIONAL AND ORGANIZATIONAL PRIORITIES

In 2010, the National Council of the State Boards of Nursing in the United States recognized the need to improve the educational preparation of nurses in geriatrics and, at the time of this publication, is in the planning stages to require all nurses to have training in the care of geriatric patients. In addition, the U.S. Department of Health and Human Services (USDHHS, 2010) has included training in geriatric care by physicians, nurses, and other health care providers in its *Healthy People 2020* goals. These goals aim to increase the number of physicians and nurses certified in geriatric care from 2.7% to 3% for physicians and 1.4% to 1.5% for nurses—a 10% improvement for both disciplines.

National geriatric nursing leaders have been promoting the geriatric nursing skills and competence of all nurses, including those in subspecialty nursing. Wakefield et al. (2005) argue that nursing and medical school must integrate patient safety principles into their curricula in order to teach HCPs to more effectively prevent and manage errors, and to ease the burden on an already overstretched health care system. More emphasis placed on teaching the "aviation" model derived from high-risk industries, which emphasizes feedback, teamwork, and communication is recommended.

The IOM's *To Err Is Human* report increased provider awareness to the dangers of diagnostic and therapeutic interventions and led to a significant increase in patient safety research, literature, and initiatives (Stelfox, Palmisani, Scurlock, Orav, & Bates, 2006). Continued funding for patient safety research and major patient safety initiatives such as those provided by the AHRQ, the IHI, Leapfrog Group, and the IOM will continue to support hospitals in their efforts to create safe care environments (Leape & Berwick, 2005).

Organizational Imperatives to Prevent Iatrogenesis

It is now well recognized that a significant proportion of iatrogenic complications are directly related to the complex interplay of organizational and human factors that create opportunities for patient harm (Leape, 2009). Hospitals and nursing leadership are urged to comply with not only regulatory mandates, but also to embrace patient safety as an explicit organizational goal, actively promoting a just culture of safety in which everyone is aware of the significance of iatrogenesis. This goal is supported by practices that enforce, recognize, and reward safety behaviors at the individual, unit, and organizational levels (Dennison, 2005).

Nurses at all levels play a pivotal role in promoting patient safety. They are not only the largest workforce of health care providers, providing the final safety checkpoint at the bedside (Hughes & Clancy, 2005). Ensuring nurse competence in geriatric nursing is critical to preventing iatrogenesis in vulnerable older patients, and hospitals that are committed to implementing geriatric best practices have been shown to positively influence patient care (Boltz et al., 2008). Organizations that ensure coordinated and effective training in both patient safety and geriatric patient care, well integrated into staff orientation and ongoing training programs, are poised to be effective. Collaboration between nursing education and risk management, quality improvement, infection control, and medicine will help to identify an institution's educational priorities and the most appropriate training strategies.

Although it is the lack of systems such as those for decision support and medication reconciliation that is often the cause of patient harm (Morris, 2004), hospitals have been known to assign culpability, punishment, and blame to individuals involved in the errors, rather than encouraging the reporting of these errors to conduct a root cause analysis (Dennison, 2005; Morris, 2004). Accordingly, a national survey of nurses in 25 U.S. hospitals found that a large percentage of iatrogenic harm is not reported by nurses; a mere 36% felt near misses should be reported (Blegen et al., 2004). Hospitals need to recognize both what constitutes high-risk situations and those patients most at risk of adverse outcomes, and implement effective patient safety and performance improvement strategies designed to minimize harm. Nursing peer review and other audit functions are important processes that promote the understanding of the factors involved in patient safety incidents (Diaz, 2008).

Nurses need to be at the forefront and engaged in interdisciplinary efforts to improve the safety culture of an organization (Blegen et al., 2010). Significant strides in improving patient care have been made with nurses actively involved in identifying care-related problems. For example, the IHI and the Robert Wood Johnson Foundation sponsored national initiative, *Transforming Care at the Bedside* (TCAB) creates, tests, and implements nurse-generated practice changes to improve patient care and safety (Viney, Batcheller, Houston, & Belcik, 2006). A nationwide study of the effect of nursing rounds at least every 2 hours, with specific attention to patient comfort, positioning, and toileting, demonstrated a significant decrease in call light use, and a subsequent reduction in patient falls and increase in patient satisfaction (Meade, Bursell, & Ketelsen, 2006). A nurse-led project to improve medication administration reliability using strategies that addressed process improvement and nursing leadership skills led to a sustained accuracy rate of 96% at 18 months, from 85% at baseline (Kliger, Blegen, Gootee, & O'Neil, 2009). The critical need for optimal implementation of, and adherence to, evidence-based practice, including adoption of nursing protocols, to minimize the risk of error and patient harm cannot be overemphasized.

Safety-Promoting Structures and Processes

Nursing leadership has the responsibility to ensure that hospital structure and processes of care maximize staff effectiveness and minimize the risk of harm for vulnerable patients. Safe patient care cannot be ensured without the appropriate organizational systems that promote a positive work environment and efficient communication of pertinent information. Appropriate nurse staffing and nursing competence is imperative given strong evidence that both staffing levels and educational preparation inversely affect patient care and outcomes (Frith et al., 2010; Kendall-Gallagher & Blegen, 2010). The groundbreaking AHRQ report entitled *Keeping Patients Safe: Transforming the Work Environment of Nurses* demonstrated that staffing and workflow design clearly impact errors and patient safety outcomes (Page, 2004). A study of HAIs in the ICU confirmed previous data that nurse staffing is directly related to infection rate. The authors noted an increase in infection several days after heavy workload and advocate maintaining staffing at higher levels to minimize the risk of infection (Hugonnet, Chevrolet, & Pittet, 2007). Lower nurse staffing correlates with increased mortality (Aiken, Clarke, Sloane, Lake, & Cheney, 2008), and Loan, Jennings, Brosch, Depaul, and Hildreth (2003) call for the need to develop databases to further examine the effect on staffing data and patient outcomes. Scott, Rogers, Hwang, & Zhang (2006) surveyed critical care nurses in the United States and found evidence that longer work hours not only decreased nurse's vigilance but also increased the risk of errors and near misses, supporting the IOM recommendations to limit nurse's work hours to a maximum of 12 hours in a 24-hour period. Yet, in spite of increased attention and major research done in this area, lack of standardized data and other problems continue to hinder attempts to find a clear solution to the optimal staffing needed to minimize error (Blegen, 2006). Research must continue in this area so that improvements in nurse staffing, work areas, and transfer of knowledge both between providers and within the organization is optimized in order to maintain patient safety (Blegen, 2006).

Communication and collaboration is vital to ensure appropriate exchange of information and coordination of care (IOM, 2001) because lack of communication is considered a major contributor to iatrogenic complications. TJC recognized that communication breakdown is the cause of nearly 70% of all sentinel events, whereas a study to elicit stories of preventable physical or psychological harm caused by medical error found breakdown in communication was a far greater problem than technical error (Kuzel et al., 2004). It is critical to evaluate and optimize what patient information is communicated during any hand-off report, especially at high-risk times, and create evidence-based guidelines as to what needs to be included during this process (Alvarado et al., 2006). Inaccurate or absent information can dramatically increase the risk of harmful effects on older patients. The plan of care for the older patient that lacks critical baseline functional and cognitive data can hamper recognition of subtle changes in condition and may contribute to functional decline and other adverse outcomes, including cascade iatrogenesis. Nurses need to include daily functional priorities and goals that have been developed with the patient and/or family into every shift or hand off report.

Patient transfer or any hand off presents opportunities for increased harm to patients. Patient transfer from either another unit or hospital has been found to be independently associated with the development of nosocomial infections (Eveillard, Quenon, Rufat, Mangeol, & Fauvelle, 2001), whereas patient transfer from hospital to a SNF is a significant risk factor for ADEs (Boockvar et al., 2004). Every effort must be made to also address the communication of appropriate data during any transfer of patient care. Posthospital medication management strategies using interdisciplinary teams, information technology, and transitional care models need to be considered to minimize the risk of ADEs postdischarge (Foust, Naylor, Boling, & Cappuzzo, 2005). Phone calls to recently discharged patients can be an effective intervention to minimize adverse events and prevent unnecessary readmissions (Forster et al., 2004).

Information technology has the potential to significantly improve our ability to provide safe patient care by enhancing communication and providing decision support. The electronic medical record (EMR) needs to be considered a priority by the organization as a means to ensure evidence-based patient care is implemented and monitored (IOM, 2001), yet a mere 1.5% of U.S. hospitals have even basic EMR keeping in place, and only 9.1% have computerized physician order entry (CPOE; Landrigan et al., 2010). A well-designed EMR with CPOE has been shown to reduce the number of medication errors by 81% (Koppel et al., 2005). Not only are prescription errors caused by illegible handwriting prevented, but also the EMR can ensure best-practice prescribing using standardized order sets and preprogrammed medication alerts to prevent adverse drug–drug interactions. The EMR also has the capability to provide decision support, promote continuity of care and decrease adverse events with more efficient communication among care providers, especially at high-risk times such as during cross-coverage (Petersen, Orav, Teich, O'Neil, & Brennan, 1998) and any handoff. Computerized prompts to use a nonpharmacological sleep protocol, which is as effective and far less harmful than sedative-hypnotic medications and promotes higher quality sleep, has decreased the use of higher risk sleeping medications among hospitalized patients (Agostini, Zhang, & Inouye, 2007).

Koppel et al. (2005) warns, however, that attention needs to be paid to the role of the EMR in facilitating medication errors and every measure taken to reduce this risk after identifying 22 types of error risks with the CPOE system. Nurses need to be aware of the limitations of CPOE and remain vigilant partners in care to ensure patient safety. It is also important that health care providers with geriatric expertise be involved from the onset with the building of the EMR to ensure that best-practice geriatric assessment and management protocols are included.

Environmental safety needs to be an organizational priority and should involve all staff and physicians. Routine safety rounds that include leadership and encourage open discussions of safety at the unit level can be successful in promoting a culture of safety (Reinertsen & Johnson, 2010). Regularly scheduled safety inspections of the environment and equipment need to occur and include clinicians with geriatric expertise to assist in identifying potential safety hazards related to aging changes such as lighting and seating heights. Standardization of equipment is important to minimize the risk of error, although mechanisms need to be in place to ensure prompt reporting and removal from service of any malfunctioning equipment. In addition, considering normal changes of aging is important when planning hospital construction and renovation, so that architectural design promotes geriatric patient safety and function.

Partnering With Patients

Nurses can effectively encourage patients to be vigilant and proactive partners in care in order to prevent unnecessary harm (Hibbard, Peters, Slovic, & Tusler, 2005). Providing patient education about medical errors has been shown to increase self-advocacy behaviors and satisfaction in patients (Hibbard et al., 2005). Berntsen (2006) calls for the implementation of a patient-centered philosophy as a way of minimizing patient harm. Patient-centeredness espouses that the needs, wants, and preferences of the patient should drive health care interventions (Berntsen, 2006). Nurses providing patient-centered care compassionately and empathetically respond to the needs of the patient and offer ample opportunities for patients and families to direct their care through involved and informed decision making (Berntsen, 2006). A collaborative relationship between the nurse and the patient to attain mutually agreed upon goals can foster more patient control, self-care, autonomy, and prevent iatrogenesis (Messmer, 2006). In older patients with cognitive impairment or language barriers, family members should become integral partners in this process.

SUMMARY

Significant progress has been made in better understanding and addressing the problem of iatrogenesis with the work of agencies such as the AHRQ, IHI, TJC, IOM, National Patient Safety Foundation, Leapfrog Group, and others. Major strides have been made in the Veterans Administration heath system, which has emerged as a leader in this area by implementing systemwide patient safety training initiatives and creating multiple patient safety research centers. Yet, there remains much work to be done, especially in the area of preventing harm to the vulnerable older adult patient.

Nurses must recognize their critical role in preventing iatrogenic complications, which far too often can and do trigger a cascade of physical and cognitive decline that could have been prevented. Nurses have a responsibility to maintain vigilance and advocate for their patients, especially for patients who cannot do so for themselves, such as cognitively impaired elders and those without family support. Hospitalized older adults depend on the nurse's knowledge of their baseline functional and cognitive status and risk factors in order to implement individualized and function-promoting treatment plans. They rely on the nursing staff's ability to recognize subtle changes and to proactively intervene to keep older patients safe while hospitalized. They also depend on nurses to be actively engaged in monitoring safety, conducting problem solving, and leading quality initiatives to promote the best possible hospital experience and outcomes.

Involving patients, family, and caregivers as much as possible, and providing predischarge training and referral to community resources can help discharge at-risk patients in a timelier manner and prevent unnecessary hospital readmissions. No longer should iatrogenic harm be the unfortunate price patients pay for medical progress, nor should we accept the fact that random, unfortunate events happen in a chaotic environment. Rather, nurses need to take a stand to understand their role as patient advocates and educate themselves and others to the problem of iatrogenesis, and to take every precaution necessary to ensure a culture of patient safety.

RESOURCES

Patient Safety

Agency for Health Care Research and Quality (AHRQ)
Patient Safety Network: http://www.psnet.ahrq.gov/
http://healthit.ahrq.gov/portal/server.pt?open=512&objID=653&PageID=5583&cached=false&mode=2
Medical error: http://www.ahrq.gov/qual/errorsix.htm

Institute for Healthcare Improvement
http://www.ihi.org/IHI/

Institute of Medicine
http://www.iom.edu/

IOM Crossing the Quality Chasm
http://www.iom.edu/CMS/8089.aspx

The Joint Commission
http://www.jointcommission.org/PatientSafety

National Patient Safety Foundation
http://www.npsf.org/

United States Department of Veterans Affairs National Center for Patient Safety
http://www.patientsafety.gov/

World Health Organization World Alliance on Patient Safety
http://www.who.int/patientsafety/en/

Healthy People 2020, Objectives for Older Adults
http://www.healthypeople.gov/2020/topicsobjectives2020/objectiveslist.aspx?topicid=31

Infection Control

Centers for Disease Control and Prevention (CDC)
http://www.cdc.gov

Association for Professionals in Infection Control and Epidemiology (APIC), Society of Healthcare
    Epidemiology of America (SHEA),
http://www.apic.org/Content/NavigationMenu/GovernmentAdvocacy/MandatoryReporting/Position
    Papers/mr_position_papers.htm

National Nosocomial Infection Surveillance System:
http://www.cdc.gov/ncidod/dhqp/nnis.html

Handwashing Guidelines
http://www.mrw.interscience.wiley.com/cochrane/clsysrev/articles/CD005186/frame.html

World Health Organization's World Alliance for Patient Safety
Guidelines on Hand Hygiene in Health Care (Advanced Draft, 2005)
http://www.who.int/patientsafety/events/05/HH_en.pdf

Clinical Practice

AHRQ (Agency for Healthcare Research and Quality) Clinical Practice Guidelines
http://www.ahrq.gov/clinic/cpgsix.htm

EPIQ (Effective Practice, Informatics and Quality Improvement)
Supports effective, evidence-based practice, health informatics, and quality improvement initiatives
http://www.health.auckland.ac.nz/population-health/epidemiology-biostats/epiq/

National Guideline Clearinghouse: a public resource for evidence-based clinical practice guidelines
http://www.guideline.gov/

Joanna Briggs Institute (Promote and Support Best Practice): International, interdisciplinary
    evidence-based resources.
http://www.joannabriggs.edu.au/about/home.php

American Geriatrics Society
http://www.adgapstudy.uc.edu/

Hartford Institute for Geriatric Nursing
http://hartfordign.org/uploads/File/hcr_geriatric_nursing_tips.pdf

American Geriatrics Society Clinical Practice Guidelines
http://www.americangeriatrics.org/health_care_professionals/clinical_practice/clinical_guidelines_
recommendations/

Geriatric and Palliative Care Weblogs
http://www.geripal.org/

Clinical Geriatrics
http://www.americangeriatrics.org/health_care_professionals/clinical_practice/clinical_guidelines_
recommendations/

Workforce Development

Institute of Medicine
http://www.iom.edu/Reports/2008/Retooling-for-an-Aging-America-Building-the-Health-Care-
Workforce.aspx
http://www.iom.edu/~/media/Files/Report%20Files/2008/Retooling-for-an-Aging-America-
Building-the-Health-Care-Workforce/ReportBriefRetoolingforanAgingAmericaBuilding
theHealthCareWorkforce.pdf

REFERENCES

Abbott, C. A., Dremsa, T., Stewart, D. W., Mark, D. D., & Swift, C. C. (2006). Adoption of a ventilator-associated pneumonia clinical practice guideline. *Worldviews on Evidence-Based Nursing*, *3*(4), 139–152. Evidence Level III.

Agency for HealthCare Research and Quality. (2008). National Health Quality Report 2008. Retrieved from http://www.ahrq.gov/qual/nhqr08/nhqr08.pdf

Agostini, J. V., Zhang, Y., & Inouye, S. K. (2007). Use of a computer-based reminder to improve sedative-hypnotic prescribing in older hospitalized patients. *Journal of the American Geriatrics Society*, *55*(1), 43–48. Evidence Level III.

Aiken, L. H., Clarke, S. P., Sloane, D. M., Lake, E. T., & Cheney, T. (2008). Effects of hospital care environment on patient mortality and nurse outcomes. *Journal of Nursing Administration*, *38*(5), 223–229. Evidence Level IV.

Alagiakrishnan, K., & Mereu, L. (2010). Approach to managing hypoglycemia in elderly patients with diabetes. *Postgraduate Medicine*, *122*(3), 129–137. Evidence Level V.

Alvarado, K., Lee, R., Christoffersen, E., Fram, N., Boblin, S., Poole, N., . . . Forsyth, S. (2006). Transfer of accountability: Transforming shift handover to enhance patient safety. *Healthcare Quarterly*, (Spec No. 9), 75–79. Evidence Level IV.

American Geriatrics Society. (2009). Pharmacological management of persistent pain in older persons. *Journal of the American Geriatrics Society*, *57*(8), 1331–1346. Evidence Level I.

Anpalahan, M., & Gibson, S. J. (2008). Geriatric syndromes as predictors of adverse outcomes of hospitalization. *Internal Medicine Journal*, *38*(1), 16–23. Evidence Level IV.

Arnstein, P. (2010). Balancing analgesic efficacy with safety concerns in the older patient. *Pain Management Nursing*, *11*(Suppl. 2), S11–S22. doi:10.1016/j.pmn.2010.03.003. Evidence Level V.

Arozullah, A. M., Khuri, S. F., Henderson, W. G., & Daley, J. (2001). Development and validation of a multifactorial risk index for predicting postoperative pneumonia after major noncardiac surgery. *Annals of Internal Medicine*, *135*(10), 847–857. Evidence Level IV.

Barbosa-Silva, M. C., & Barros, A. J. (2005). Bioelectric impedance and individual characteristics as prognostic factors for post-operative complications. *Clinical Nutrition*, *24*(5), 830–838. Evidence Level IV.

Barrere, C. C., Durkin, A., & LaCoursiere, S. (2008). The influence of end-of-life education on attitudes of nursing students. *International Journal of Nursing Education Scholarship*, 5, Article 11. Evidence Level III.

Bartlett, J. G. (2006). Narrative review: The new epidemic of Clostridium difficile-associated enteric disease. *Annals of Internal Medicine*, *145*(10), 758–764. Evidence Level V.

Beaupre, L. A., Cinats, J. G., Senthilselvan, A., Lier, D., Jones, C. A., Scharfenberger, A., . . . Saunders, L. D. (2006). Reduced morbidity for elderly patients with a hip fracture after implementation of a perioperative evidence-based clinical pathway. *Quality & Safety in Health Care*, *15*(5), 375–379. doi:10.1136/qshc.2005.017095. Evidence Level IV.

Bentrem, D. J., Cohen, M. E., Hynes, D. M., Ko, C. Y., & Bilimoria, K. Y. (2009). Identification of specific quality improvement opportunities for the elderly undergoing gastrointestinal surgery. *Archives of Surgery*, *144*(11), 1013–1020. Evidence Level IV.

Berntsen, K. J. (2006). Implementation of patient centeredness to enhance patient safety. *Journal of Nursing Care Quality*, *21*(1), 15–19. Evidence Level VI.

Bismark, M. M., Brennan, T. A., Paterson, R. J., Davis, P. B., & Studdert, D. M. (2006). Relationship between complaints and quality of care in New Zealand: A descriptive analysis of complainants and non-complainants following adverse events. *Quality & Safety in Health Care*, *15*(1), 17–22. Evidence Level IV.

Blegen, M. A. (2006). Patient safety in hospital acute care units. *Annual Review of Nursing Research*, 24, 103–125. Evidence Level V.

Blegen, M. A., Sehgal, N. L., Alldredge, B. K., Gearhart, S., Auerbach, A. A., & Wachter, R. M. (2010). Improving safety culture on adult medical units through multidisciplinary teamwork and communication interventions: The TOPS project. *Quality & Safety in Health Care*, *19*(4), 346–350. Evidence Level III.

Blegen, M. A., Vaughn, T., Pepper, G., Vojir, C., Stratton, K., Boyd, M., & Armstrong. G. (2004). Patient and staff safety: Voluntary reporting. *American Journal of Medical Quality*, *19*(2), 67–74. Evidence Level V.

Bobba, R. K., & Arsura, E. L. (2004). Septic shock in an elderly patient on dialysis: Enema-induced rectal injury confusing the clinical picture. *Journal of the American Geriatrics Society*, *52*(12), 2144. Evidence Level V.

Boltz, M., Capezuti, E., Bowar-Ferres, S., Norman, R., Secic, M., Kim, H., . . . Fulmer, T. (2008). Hospital nurses' perception of the geriatric nurse practice environment. *Journal of Nursing Scholarship*, *40*(3), 282–289. Evidence Level IV.

Boockvar, K., Fishman, E., Kyriacou, C. K., Monias, A., Gavi, S., & Cortes, T. (2004). Adverse events due to discontinuations in drug use and dose changes in patients transferred between acute and long-term care facilities. *Archives of Internal Medicine*, *164*(5), 545–550. Evidence Level IV.

Brosnahan, J., Jull, A., & Tracy, C. (2004). Types of urethral catheters for management of short-term voiding problems in hospitalised adults. *Cochrane Database of Systematic Reviews*, (1), CD004013. Evidence Level I.

Burke, J. P. (2003). Infection control—a problem for patient safety. *New England Journal of Medicine*, *348*(7), 651–656. Evidence Level V.

Centers for Disease Control and Prevention. (2003). *Guidelines for preventing health-care-associated pneumonia*. Retrieved from http://www.cdc.gov/ncidod/dhqp/gl_hcpneumonia.html. Evidence Level I.

Centers for Disease Control and Prevention. (2006). *Management of multi-drug resistant organisms in healthcare settings*. Evidence Level I.

Chen, Y. C. (2009). Critical analysis of the factors associated with enteral feeding in preventing VAP: A systematic review. *Journal of the Chinese Medical Association*, *72*(4), 171–178. Evidence Level V.

Cheung, C. M., Ponnusamy, A., & Anderton, J. G. (2008). Management of acute renal failure in the elderly patient: A clinician's guide. *Drugs & Aging*, *25*(6), 455–476. Evidence Level V.

Classen, D. C., Jaser, L., & Budnitz, D. S. (2010). Adverse drug events among hospitalized Medicare patients: Epidemiology and national estimates from a new approach to surveillance. *Joint Commission Journal on Quality and Patient Safety*, *36*(1), 12–21. Evidence Level IV.

Coker, E., Papaioannou, A., Kaasalainen, S., Dolovich, L., Turpie, I., & Taniguchi, A. (2010). Nurses' perceived barriers to optimal pain management in older adults on acute medical units. *Applied Nursing Research*, *23*(3), 139–146. Evidence Level IV.

Coopersmith, C. M., Rebmann, T. L., Zack, J. E., Ward, M. R., Corcoran, R. M., Schallom, M. E., . . . Fraser, V. J. (2002). Effect of an education program on decreasing catheter-related bloodstream infections in the surgical intensive care unit. *Critical Care Medicine*, *30*(1), 59–64. Evidence Level V.

D'Arcy, Y. (2009). Overturning barriers to pain relief in older adults. *Nursing*, *39*(10), 32–39. Retrieved from https://auth.lib.unc.edu/ezproxy_auth.php?url=http://search.ebscohost.com/login.aspx?direct=true&db=c8h&AN=2010431004&site=ehost-live&scope=site. Evidence Level V.

Davis, J. C., Ashe, M. C., Guy, P., & Khan, K. M. (2006). Undertreatment after hip fracture: A retrospective study of osteoporosis overlooked. *Journal of the American Geriatrics Society*, *54*(6), 1019–1020. Evidence Level IV.

Dennison, R. D. (2005). Creating an organizational culture for medication safety. *Nursing Clinics of North America*, *40*(1), 1–23. Evidence Level VI.

Diaz, L. (2008). Nursing peer review: Developing a framework for patient safety. *Journal of Nursing Administration*, *38*(11), 475–479. doi:10.1097/01.NNA.0000339473.27349.28. Evidence Level V.

Dubberke, E. R., Butler, A. M., Yokoe, D. S., Mayer, J., Hota, B., Mangino, J. E., . . . Fraser, V. J. (2010). Multicenter study of Clostridium difficile infection rates from 2000 to 2006. *Infection Control and Hospital Epidemiology*, *31*(10), 1030–1037. Evidence Level IV.

Duffy, J. R. (2002). Nosocomial infections: Important acute care nursing-sensitive outcomes indicators. *AACN Clinical Issues*, *13*(3), 358–366. Evidence Level V.

Dumont, C. J., Keeling, A. W., Bourguignon, C., Sarembock, I. J., & Turner, M. (2006). Predictors of vascular complications post diagnostic cardiac catheterization and percutaneous coronary interventions. *Dimensions of Critical Care Nursing*, *25*(3), 137–142. Evidence Level IV.

Eveillard, M., Mortier, E., Lancien, E., Lescure, F. X., Schmit, J. L., Barnaud, G., . . . Joly-Guillou, M. L. (2006). Consideration of age at admission for selective screening to identify methicillin-resistant Staphylococcus aureus carriers to control dissemination in a medical ward. *American Journal of Infection Control*, *34*(3), 108–113. Evidence Level IV.

Eveillard, M., Quenon, J. L., Rufat, P., Mangeol, A., & Fauvelle, F. (2001). Association between hospital-acquired infections and patients' transfers. *Infection Control and Hospital Epidemiology*, *22*(11), 693–696. Evidence Level IV.

Fernandez, R. S., & Griffiths, R. D. (2006). Duration of short-term indwelling catheters—a systematic review of the evidence. *Journal of Wound, Ostomy, and Continence Nursing*, *33*(2), 145–153. Retrieved from http://search.ebscohost.com/login.aspx?direct=true&db=c8h&AN=2009148467&site=ehost-live&scope=site. Evidence Level I.

Fick, D. M., Agostini, J. V., & Inouye, S. K. (2002). Delirium superimposed on dementia: A systematic review. *Journal of the American Geriatrics Society*, *50*(10), 1723–1732. Evidence Level I.

Forster, A. J., Clark, H. D., Menard, A., Dupuis, N., Chernish, R., Chandok, N., . . . van Walraven, C. (2004). Adverse events among medical patients after discharge from hospital. *Canadian Medical Association Journal*, *170*(3), 345–349. Evidence Level IV.

Foust, J. B., Naylor, M. D., Boling, P. A., & Cappuzzo, K. A. (2005). Opportunities for improving post-hospital home medication management among older adults. *Home Health Care Services Quarterly*, *24*(1–2), 101–122. Evidence Level VI.

Frazier, S. C. (2005). Health outcomes and polypharmacy in elderly individuals: An integrated literature review. *Journal of Gerontological Nursing*, *31*(9), 4–11. Evidence Level V.

Freeman, J., Bauer, M. P., Baines, S. D., Corver, J., Fawley, W. N., Goorhuis, B., . . . Wilcox, M. H. (2010). The changing epidemiology of Clostridium difficile infections. *Clinical Microbiology Reviews*, *23*(3), 529–549. Evidence Level VI.

Freitas, E. R., Soares, B. G., Cardoso, J. R., & Atallah, A. N. (2007). Incentive spirometry for preventing pulmonary complications after coronary artery bypass graft. *Cochrane Database of Systematic Reviews*, (3), CD004466. Evidence Level I.

Frith, K. H., Anderson, E. F., Caspers, B., Tseng, F., Sanford, K., Hoyt, N. G., & Moore, K. (2010). Effects of nurse staffing on hospital-acquired conditions and length of stay in community hospitals. *Quality Management in Health Care, 19*(2), 147–155. Evidence Level IV.

Gagliardi, A. R., Fenech, D., Eskicioglu, C., Nathens, A. B., & McLeod, R. (2009). Factors influencing antibiotic prophylaxis for surgical site infection prevention in general surgery: A review of the literature. *Canadian Journal of Surgery, 52*(6), 481–489. Evidence Level V.

Garrouste Orgeas, M., Timsit, J. F., Soufir, L., Tafflet, M., Adrie, C., Philippart, F., . . . Carlet, J. (2008). Impact of adverse events on outcomes in intensive care unit patients. *Critical Care Medicine, 36*(7), 2041–2047. Evidence Level IV.

Gastmeier, P., Bräuer, H., Forster, D., Dietz, E., Daschner, F., & Rüden, H. (2002). A quality management project in 8 selected hospitals to reduce nosocomial infections: A prospective, controlled study. *Infection Control and Hospital Epidemiology, 23*(2), 91–97. Evidence Level II.

Ghevariya, V., Paleti, V., Momeni, M., Krishnaiah, M., & Anand, S. (2009). Complications associated with percutaneous endoscopic gastrostomy tubes. *Annals of Long Term Care, 17*(12), 36–41. Retrieved from https://auth.lib.unc.edu/ezproxy_auth.php?url=http://search.ebscohost.com/login.aspx?direct=true&db=c8h&AN=2010534613&site=ehost-live&scope=site. Evidence Level V.

Gnass, S. A., Barboza, L., Bilicich, D., Angeloro, P., Treiyer, W., Grenóvero, S., & Basualdo, J. (2004). Prevention of central venous catheter-related bloodstream infections using non-technologic strategies. *Infection Control and Hospital Epidemiology, 25*(8), 675–677. Evidence Level IV.

Goetz, A. M., Kedzuf, S., Wagener, M., & Muder, R. R. (1999). Feedback to nursing staff as an intervention to reduce catheter-associated urinary tract infections. *American Journal of Infection Control, 27*(5), 402–404.

Gordts, B., Vrijens, F., Hulstaert, F., Devriese, S., & Van de Sande, S. (2010). The 2007 Belgian national prevalence survey for hospital-acquired infections. *Journal of Hospital Infection, 75*(3), 163–167. Evidence Level IV.

Graf, C. L. (2008). The hospital admission risk profile: The HARP helps to determine a patient's risk of functional decline. *American Journal of Nursing, 108*(8), 62–71. Evidence Level V.

Greenwood, D. (2007). Relational care: Learning to look beyond intentionality to the 'non-intentional' in a caring relationship. *Nursing Philosophy, 8*(4), 223–232. Retrieved from https://auth.lib.unc.edu/ezproxy_auth.php?url=http://search.ebscohost.com/login.aspx?direct=true&db=c8h&AN=2009680988&site=ehost-live&scope=site. Evidence Level V.

Grey, N. J., & Perdrizet, G. A. (2004). Reduction of nosocomial infections in the surgical intensive-care unit by strict glycemic control. *Endocrine Practice, 10*(Suppl. 2), 46–52. Evidence Level II.

Hahler, B. (2006). Surgical wound dehiscence. *Medsurg Nursing, 15*(5), 296–300.

Hani, D. (2010). Semmelweis' germ theory: The introduction of hand washing. Retrieved from http://www.experiment-resources.com/semmelweis-germ-theory.html. Evidence Level VI.

Harman, J. S., Brown, E. L., Have, T. T., Mulsant, B. H., Brown, G., & Bruce, M. L. (2002). Primary care physicians attitude toward diagnosis and treatment of late-life depression. *CNS Spectrums, 7*(11), 784–790. Evidence Level IV.

Hazelett, S. E., Tsai, M., Gareri, M., & Allen, K. (2006). The association between indwelling urinary catheter use in the elderly and urinary tract infection in acute care. *BMC Geriatrics, 6*, 15. Evidence Level IV.

Health Grades, Inc. (2004). *Patient safety in American hospitals*. Retrieved from www.healthgrades.com/media/english/pdf/hg_patient_safety_study_final.pdf. Evidence Level V.

Hibbard, J. H., Peters, E., Slovic, P., & Tusler, M. (2005). Can patients be part of the solution? Views on their role in preventing medical errors. *Medical Care Research and Review, 62*(5), 601–616. Evidence Level III.

Hollenbeak, C. S., Lave, J. R., Zeddies, T., Pei, Y., Roland, C. E., & Sun, E. F. (2006). Factors associated with risk of surgical wound infections. *American Journal of Medical Quality, 21*(Suppl. 6), 29S–34S. Evidence Level IV.

Hsieh, H. Y., & Tuite, P. K. (2006). Prevention of ventilator-associated pneumonia: What nurses can do. *Dimensions of Critical Care Nursing, 25*(5), 205–208. Evidence Level V.

Hughes, R. G., & Clancy, C. M. (2005). Working conditions that support patient safety. *Journal of Nursing Care Quality, 20*(4), 289–292. Evidence Level V.

Hugonnet, S., Chevrolet, J. C., & Pittet, D. (2007). The effect of workload on infection risk in critically ill patients. *Critical Care Medicine, 35*(1), 76–81. Evidence Level IV.

Hunsaker, D. M., & Hunsaker, J, C., III. (2002). Therapy-related café coronary deaths: Two case reports of rare asphyxial deaths in patients under supervised care. *American Journal of Forensic Medicine and Pathology, 23*(2), 149–154. Evidence Level V.

Imai, S., Tamada, T., Gyoten, M., Yamashita, T., & Kajihara, Y. (2004). Iatrogenic venous air embolism caused by CT injector—from a risk management point of view. *Radiation Medicine, 22*(4), 269–271. Evidence Level V.

Inouye, S. K., Studenski, S., Tinetti, M. E., & Kuchel, G. A. (2007). Geriatric syndromes: Clinical, research, and policy implications of a core geriatric concept. *Journal of the American Geriatrics Society, 55*(5), 780–791. Evidence Level VI.

Institute of Healthcare Improvement. Protecting 5 million lives from harm. Retrieved from http://www.ihi.org/offerings/Initiatives/PastStrategicInitiatives/5MillionLivesCampaign/Pages/default.aspx

Institute of Medicine. (2001). *Crossing the quality chasm: A new health system for the 21st century.* Washington, DC: National Academy Press. Evidence Level V.

Institute of Medicine. (2008). Retooling for an Aging America: Building the Health Care Workforce. Evidence Level V.

Jacobs, L. G. (2003). Prophylactic anticoagulation for venous thromboembolic disease in geriatric patients. *Journal of the American Geriatrics Society, 51*(10), 1472–1478. Evidence Level V.

Jaffer, A. K., & Brotman, D. J. (2006). Prevention of venous thromboembolism in the geriatric patient. *Clinics in Geriatric Medicine, 22*(1), 93–111. Retrieved from https://auth.lib.unc.edu/ezproxy_auth.php?url=http://search.ebscohost.com/login.aspx?direct=true&db=c8h&AN=2009159700&site=ehost-live&scope=site. Evidence Level V.

Jarvis, W. R. (2003). Benchmarking for prevention: The Centers for Disease Control and Prevention's National Nosocomial Infections Surveillance (NNIS) system experience. *Infection, 31*(Suppl. 2), 44–48. Evidence Level V.

Johnstone, M. J., & Kanitsaki, O. (2006). Culture, language, and patient safety: Making the link. *International Journal for Quality in Health Care, 18*(5), 383–388. Evidence Level VI.

Kaler, W., & Chinn, R. (2007). Successful disinfection of needleless access ports: A matter of time and friction. *Journal of the Association for Vascular Access, 12*(3), 140–142. Retrieved from http://www.ingentaconnect.com/search/article?title=successful+disinfection+of+needleless+ports&title_type=tka&year_from=1998&year_to=2009&database=1&pageSize=20&index=1. doi:10.2309/java.12-3-9. Evidence Level III.

Kallen, A. J., Mu, Y., Bulens, S., Reingold, A., Petit, S., Gershman, K., . . . Fridkin, S. K. (2010). Health care-associated invasive MRSA infections, 2005–2008. *Journal of the American Medical Association, 304*(6), 641–648. Evidence Level IV.

Kendall-Gallagher, D., & Blegen, M. A. (2010). Competence and certification of registered nurses and safety of patients in intensive care units. *Journal of Nursing Administration, 40*(Suppl. 10), S68–S77. Evidence Level IV.

Kenny, T. (1990). Erosion of individuality in care of elderly people in hospital—an alternative approach. *Journal of Advanced Nursing, 15*(5), 571–576. Evidence Level VI.

Kirkland, K. B., Briggs, J. P., Trivette, S. L., Wilkinson, W. E., & Sexton, D.J. (1999). The impact of surgical-site infections in the 1990s: Attributable mortality, excess length of hospitalization, and extra costs. *Infection Control and Hospital Epidemiology, 20*(11), 725–730. Evidence Level IV.

Kliger, J., Blegen, M. A., Gootee, D., & O'Neil, E. (2009). Empowering frontline nurses: A structured intervention enables nurses to improve medication administration accuracy. *Joint Commission Journal on Quality and Patient Safety, 35*(12), 604–612. Evidence Level V.

Kohn, L. T., Corrigan, J. M., & Donaldson, M. S. (Eds.) (1999). *To err is human: Building a safer health system.* Washington, DC: National Academy Press. Evidence Level V.

Koppel, R., Metlay, J. P., Cohen, A., Abaluck, B., Localio, A. R., Kimmel, S. E., & Strom, B. L. (2005). Role of computerized physician order entry systems in facilitating medication errors. *Journal of the American Medical Association, 293*(10), 1197–1203. Evidence Level IV.

Krinsley, J. S. (2004). Effect of an intensive glucose management protocol on the mortality of critically ill adult patients. *Mayo Clinic Proceedings, 79*(8), 992–1000. Evidence Level II.

Kuzel, A. J., Woolf, S. H., Gilchrist, V. J., Engel, J. D., LaVeist, T. A., Vincent, C., & Frankel, R. M. (2004). Patient reports of preventable problems and harms in primary health care. *Annals of Family Medicine, 2*(4), 333–340. Evidence Level IV.

Landrigan, C. P., Parry, G. J., Bones, C. B., Hackbarth, A. D., Goldmann, D. A., & Sharek, P. J. (2010). Temporal trends in rates of patient harm resulting from medical care. *New England Journal of Medicine, 363*(22), 2124–2134. Evidence Level IV.

Lanini, S., Jarvis, W. R., Nicastri, E., Privitera, G., Gesu, G., Marchetti, F., . . . Ippolito, G. (2009). Healthcare-associated infection in Italy: Annual point-prevalence surveys, 2002–2004. *Infection Control and Hospital Epidemiology, 30*(7), 659–665. Evidence Level IV.

Lawrence, V. A., Cornell, J. E., & Smetana, G. W. (2006). Strategies to reduce postoperative pulmonary complications after noncardiothoracic surgery: Systematic review for the American College of Physicians. *Annals of Internal Medicine, 144*(8), 596–608. Evidence Level I.

Leape, L. L. (2009). Errors in medicine. *Clinica Chimica Acta, 404*(1), 2–5. Evidence Level V.

Leape, L. L., & Berwick, D. M. (2005). Five years after To Err Is Human: What have we learned? *Journal of the American Medical Association, 293*(19), 2384–2390. Evidence Level VI.

Li Bassi, G., & Torres, A. (2011). Ventilator-associated pneumonia: Role of positioning. *Current Opinion in Critical Care, 17*(1), 57–63. Evidence Level V.

Lip, G. Y., & Edwards, S. J. (2006). Stroke prevention with aspirin, warfarin and ximelagatran in patients with non-valvular atrial fibrillation: A systematic review and meta-analysis. *Thrombosis Research, 118*(3), 321–333. Evidence Level I.

Loan, L. A., Jennings, B. M., Brosch, L. R., DePaul, D., & Hildreth, P. (2003). Indicators of nursing care quality. Findings from a pilot study. *Outcomes Management, 7*(2), 51–58. Evidence Level IV.

Luther, K. M., Maguire, L., Mazabob, J., Sexton, J. B., Helmreich, R. L., & Thomas, E. (2002). Engaging nurses in patient safety. *Critical Care Nursing Clinics of North America, 14*(4), 341–346. Evidence Level VI.

Mahon, M. M. (2010). Advanced care decision making: Asking the right people the right questions. *Journal of Psychosocial Nursing and Mental Health Services, 48*(7), 13–19. doi: 10.3928/02793695-20100528-01. Evidence Level VI.

Malone, D. L., Genuit, T., Tracy, J. K., Gannon, C., & Napolitano, L. M. (2002). Surgical site infections: Reanalysis of risk factors. *Journal of Surgical Research, 103*(1), 89–95. Evidence Level IV.

Malone, M. L., & DantoNocton, E. S. (2004). Improving the hospital care of nursing facility residents. *Annals of Long Term Care, 12*(5), 42–49. Evidence Level V.

Marengoni, A., Bonometti, F., Nobili, A., Tettamanti, M., Salerno, F., Corrao, S., . . . Mannucci, P. M. (2010). In-hospital death and adverse clinical events in elderly patients according to disease clustering: The REPOSI study. *Rejuvenation Research, 13*(4), 469–477. Evidence Level IV.

Mathew, J. P., Fontes, M. L., Tudor, I. C., Ramsay, J., Duke, P., Mazer, C. D., . . . Mangano, D. T. (2004). A multicenter risk index for atrial fibrillation after cardiac surgery. *Journal of the American Medical Association, 291*(14), 1720–1729. Evidence Level IV.

McElhaney, J. E. (2005). The unmet need in the elderly: designing new influenza vaccines for older adults. *Vaccine, 23*(Suppl. 1), S10–S25. Evidence Level V.

Meade, C. M., Bursell, A. L., & Ketelsen, L. (2006). Effects of nursing rounds: On patients' call light use, satisfaction, and safety. *American Journal of Nursing, 106*(9), 58–70. Evidence Level V.

Mentes, J. C., Teer, J., & Cadogan, M. P. (2004). The pain experience of cognitively impaired nursing home residents: Perceptions of family members and certified nursing assistants. *Pain Management Nursing, 5*(3), 118–125. Evidence Level IV.

Messmer, P. R. (2006). Professional model of care: Using King's theory of goal attainment. *Nursing Science Quarterly, 19*(3), 227–229. Evidence Level VI.

Moore, S. M., & Duffy, E. (2007). Maintaining vigilance to promote best outcomes for hospitalized elders. *Critical Care Nursing Clinics of North America, 19*(3), 313–319. Evidence Level V.

Morris, A. H. (2004). Iatrogenic illness: A call for decision support tools to reduce unnecessary variation. *Quality & Safety in Health Care, 13*(1), 80–81. Evidence Level VI.

Morrison, R. S., Magaziner, J., Gilbert, M., Koval, K. J., McLaughlin, M. A., Orosz, G., . . . Siu, A. L. (2003). Relationship between pain and opioid analgesics on the development of delirium following hip fracture. *Journals of Gerontology. Series A, Biological Sciences and Medical Sciences, 58*(1), 76–81. Evidence Level IV.

Olde Rikkert, M. G., Rigaud, A. S., van Hoeyweghen, R. J., & de Graaf, J. (2003). Geriatric syndromes: Medical misnomer or progress in geriatrics? *Netherlands Journal of Medicine, 61*(3), 83–87. Evidence Level VI.

Padula, C. A., Hughes, C., & Baumhover, L. (2009). Impact of a nurse-driven mobility protocol on functional decline in hospitalized older adults. *Journal of Nursing Care Quality, 24*(4), 325–331. Evidence Level V.

Page, A. (2004). *Keeping patients safe: Transforming the work environment of nurses.* Washington, DC: National Academy Press. Evidence Level V.

Pasero, C., & McCaffery, M. (2001). The undertreatment of pain. *American Journal of Nursing, 101*(11), 62–65. Evidence Level V.

Pergolizzi, J., Böger, R. H., Budd, K., Dahan, A., Erdine, S., Hans, G., . . . Sacerdote, P. (2008). Opioids and the management of chronic severe pain in the elderly: Consensus statement of an International Expert Panel with focus on the six clinically most often used World Health Organization Step III opioids (buprenorphine, fentanyl, hydromorphone, methadone, morphine, oxycodone). *Pain Practice, 8*(4), 287–313. Evidence Level VI.

Petersen, L. A., Orav, E. J., Teich, J. M., O'Neil, A. C., & Brennan, T. A. (1998). Using a computerized sign-out program to improve continuity of inpatient care and prevent adverse events. *Joint Commission Journal on Quality Improvement, 24*(2), 77–87. Evidence Level IV.

Pirret, A. M. (2003). A preoperative scoring system to identify patients requiring postoperative high dependency care. *Intensive & Critical Care Nursing, 19*(5), 267–275. Evidence Level IV.

Reid, M. C., Williams, C. S., & Gill, T. M. (2005). Back pain and decline in lower extremity physical function among community-dwelling older persons. *The Journals of Gerontology. Series A, Biological Sciences and Medical Sciences, 60*(6), 793–797. Evidence Level IV.

Reinertsen, J. L., & Johnson, K. M. (2010). Rounding to influence. Leadership method helps executives answer the "hows" in patient safety initiatives. *Healthcare Executive, 25*(5), 72–75. Evidence Level V.

Robinson, C. L. (2007). Relieving pain in the elderly. *Health Progress, 88*(1), 48–53, 70.

Robinson, S., & Weitzel, T. (2008). Going downhill: Preventing cascade iatrogenesis. *Nursing, 38*(4), 62–63. Retrieved from https://auth.lib.unc.edu/ezproxy_auth.php?url=http://search.ebscohost.com/login.aspx?direct=true&db=c8h&AN=2009888603&site=ehost-live&scope=site. Evidence Level V.

Rothschild, J. M., Bates, D. W., & Leape, L. L. (2000). Preventable medical injuries in older patients. *Archives of Internal Medicine, 160*(18), 2717–2728. Evidence Level V.

Rothschild, J. M., & Leape, L. L. (2000). *The Nature and Extent of Medical Injury in Older Patients.* Washington, DC: American Association of Retired Persons.

Rowell, D., Nghiem, H. S., Jorm, C., & Jackson, T. J. (2010). How different are complications that affect the older adult inpatient? *Quality & Safety in Health Care, 19*(6), e34. Evidence Level IV.

Safran, D. G., Neuman, P., Schoen, C., Kitchman, M. S., Wilson, I. B., Cooper, B., . . . Rogers, W. H. (2005). Prescription drug coverage and seniors: Findings from a 2003 national survey. *Health Affairs (Millwood).* Suppl. Web Exclusives, W5-152–W5-166. Evidence Level IV.

Salgado, C. D., & Farr, B. M. (2003). Outcomes associated with vancomycin-resistant enterococci: A meta-analysis. *Infection Control and Hospital Epidemiology, 24*(9), 690–698. Evidence Level IV.

Saver, C. (2010). High complication rate in older adults calls for well-planned care. *OR Manager*, *26*(6),10–13. Evidence Level V.

Scherzer, R. (2010). Subglottic secretion aspiration in the prevention of ventilator-associated pneumonia: A review of the literature. *Dimensions of Critical Care Nursing*, *29*(6), 276–280. Evidence Level V.

Scott, L. D., Rogers, A. E., Hwang, W. T., & Zhang, Y. (2006). Effects of critical care nurses' work hours on vigilance and patients' safety. *American Journal of Critical Care*, *15*(1), 30–37. Evidence Level V.

Shannon, R. P., Patel, B., Cummins, D., Shannon, A. H., Ganguli, G., & Lu, Y. (2006). Economics of central line—associated bloodstream infections. *American Journal of Medical Quality*, *21*(Suppl. 6), 7S–16S. Evidence Level IV.

Sherman, F. T. (2005). The 3 "hypo's" of hospitalization. *Geriatrics*, *60*(5), 9–10. Evidence Level VI.

Sherwood, G., Thomas, E., Bennett, D. S., & Lewis, P. (2002). A teamwork model to promote patient safety in critical care. *Critical Care Nursing Clinics of North America*, *14*(4), 333–340. Evidence Level V.

Simmons-Trau, D., Cenek, P., Counterman, J., Hockenbury, D., & Litwiller, L. (2004). Reducing VAP with 6 Sigma. *Nursing Management*, *35*(6), 41–45. Evidence Level V.

Soop, M., Fryksmark, U., Köster, M., & Haglund, B. (2009). The incidence of adverse events in Swedish hospitals: A retrospective medical record review study. *International Journal for Quality in Health Care*, *21*(4), 285–291. doi:10.1093/intqhc/mzp025. Evidence Level IV.

Steel, K., Gertman, P. M., Crescenzi, C., & Anderson, J. (2004). Iatrogenic illness on a general medical service at a university hospital. 1981. *Quality & Safety in Health Care*, *13*(1), 76–80. Evidence Level IV.

Stelfox, H. T., Palmisani, S., Scurlock, C., Orav, E. J., & Bates, D. W. (2006). The "To Err is Human" report and the patient safety literature. *Quality & Safety in Health Care*, *15*(3), 174–178. Evidence Level VI.

Stierle, L. J., Mezey, M., Schumann, M. J, Esterson, J., Smolenski, M. C., Horsley, K. D., . . . Gould, E. (2006). The nurse competence in aging initiative: Encouraging expertise in the care of older adults. *American Journal of Nursing*, *106*(9), 93–96. Evidence Level VI.

Thornlow, D. K. (2009). Increased risk for patient safety incidents in hospitalized older adults. *Medsurg Nursing*, *18*(5), 287–291. Evidence Level IV.

Thornlow, D. K., Anderson, R., & Oddone, E. (2009). Cascade iatrogenesis: Factors leading to the development of adverse events in hospitalized older adults. *International Journal of Nursing Studies*, *46*(11), 1528–1535. Evidence Level IV.

Tolentino-DelosReyes, A. F., Ruppert, S. D., & Shiao, S. Y. (2007). Evidence-based practice: Use of the ventilator bundle to prevent ventilator-associated pneumonia. *American Journal of Critical Care*, *16*(1), 20–27. Evidence Level V.

Tsilimingras, D., Rosen, A. K., & Berlowitz, D. R. (2003). Patient safety in geriatrics: A call for action. *Journals of Gerontology. Series A, Biological Sciences and Medical Sciences*, *58*(9), M813–M819. Evidence Level V.

U.S. Department of Health and Human Services. (2010). Healthy People 2020: Topics & Objectives, Older Adults, Prevention, OA-7. Increase the proportion of the health care workforce with geriatric certification. Retrieved from http://healthypeople.gov/2020/topicsobjectives2020/objectiveslist.aspx?topicid=31

Viney, M., Batcheller, J., Houston, S., & Belcik, K. (2006). Transforming care at the bedside: Designing new care systems in an age of complexity. *Journal of Nursing Care Quality*, *21*(2), 143–150. Evidence Level V.

Wakefield, A., Attree, M., Braidman, I., Carlisle, C., Johnson, M., & Cooke, H. (2005). Patient safety: Do nursing and medical curricula address this theme? *Nurse Education Today*, *25*(4), 333–340. Evidence Level V.

Wallace, L. M., Spurgeon, P., Benn, J., Koutantji, M., & Vincent, C. (2009). Improving patient safety incident reporting systems by focusing upon feedback-lessons from English and Welsh trusts. *Health Services Management Research*, *22*(3), 129–135. Evidence Level IV.

Warren, D. K., Zack, J. E., Cox, M. J., Cohen, M. M., & Fraser, V. J. (2003). An educational intervention to prevent catheter-associated bloodstream infections in a nonteaching, community medical center. *Critical Care Medicine, 31*(7), 1959–1963. Evidence Level III.

Weingart, S. N., Pagovich, O., Sands, D. Z., Li, J. M., Aronson, M. D., Davis, R. B., . . . Bates, D. W. (2006). Patient-reported service quality on a medicine unit. *International Journal for Quality in Health Care, 18*(2), 95–101. doi:10.1093/intqhc/mzi087. Evidence Level IV.

Weitzel, T., Robinson, S., & Holmes, J. (2006). Preventing nosocomial pneumonia: Routine oral care reduced the risk of infection at one facility. *American Journal of Nursing, 106*(9), 72A–72E. Evidence Level IV.

Wenzel, R. P., & Edmond, M. B. (2001). The impact of hospital-acquired bloodstream infections. *Emerging Infectious Diseases, 7*(2), 174–177. Evidence Level V.

Westbrook, J. I., Woods, A., Rob, M. I., Dunsmuir, W. T., & Day, R. O. (2010). Association of interruptions with an increased risk and severity of medication administration errors. *Archives of Internnal Medicine, 170*(8), 683–690. doi:10.1001/archinternmed.2010.65 Evidence Level IV.

Wilson, D. (2010, November 24). Mistakes chronicled on Medicare patients. *The New York Times.* Retrieved from http://www.nytimes.com/2010/11/16/business/16medicare.html

Wip, C., & Napolitano, L. (2009). Bundles to prevent ventilator-associated pneumonia: How valuable are they? *Current Opinion in Infectious Diseases, 22*(2), 159–166. Evidence Level V.

World Health Organization. (2002). *Prevention of hospital-acquired infection: A practical guide* (2nd ed.). Geneve, Switzerland: Author. Evidence Level V.

Zegers, M., de Bruijne, M. C., Wagner, C., Hoonhout, L. H., Waaijman, R., Smits, M., . . . van der Wal, G. (2009). Adverse events and potentially preventable deaths in Dutch hospitals: Results of a retrospective patient record review study. *Quality & Safety in Health Care, 18*(4), 297–302. Evidence Level IV.

Physical Restraints and Side Rails in Acute and Critical Care Settings

13

Cheryl M. Bradas, Satinderpal K. Sandhu, and
Lorraine C. Mion

EDUCATIONAL OBJECTIVES

On completion of this chapter, the reader should be able to:

1. describe the consequences of physical restraint use, including side rails in older adults
2. describe the characteristics of an effective restraint reduction program
3. develop individualized care plan strategies that promote alternatives to restraint use through evidence-based care for falls, delirium, nutrition, medications, sleep, pain, and function
4. evaluate educational needs of patients and families related to restraint reduction
5. facilitate interdisciplinary team collaboration to ensure all aspects of restraint reduction program are addressed

OVERVIEW

The Centers for Medicare and Medicaid Services (CMS) defines physical restraint as "any manual method, physical or mechanical device, material, or equipment that immobilizes or reduces the ability of the patient to move his or her arms, legs, body or head freely" (U. S. Department of Health and Human Services [HHS], 2007). Examples include wrist or leg restraints, hand mitts, Geri-chairs, and, in certain situations, full side rails and reclining chairs. Despite the federal regulations placed on hospitals since 1999, eliminating the use of physical restraints for the management of patients in acute nonpsychiatric settings has remained challenging. Typically, health care professionals utilize physical restraints and/or side rails to protect the patient or others (Evans & FitzGerald, 2002). However, the use of physical restraints or side rails for the involuntary immobilization of the patient may not only be an infringement of the patient's rights, but can also result in patient harm, including soft tissue injury, fractures, delirium, and

For description of Evidence Levels cited in this chapter, see Chapter 1, Developing and Evaluating Clinical Practice Guidelines: A Systematic Approach, page 7.

even death (Bower, McCullough, & Timmons, 2003; Evans, Wood, & Lambert, 2003; Miles, 1993).

The standards from The Joint Commission (TJC) and regulations from CMS have raised concerns among hospital professionals about the feasibility and safety of eliminating use of physical restraints and side rails in hospitals. The almost nonexistent use of physical restraint in the United Kingdom in comparable settings provides evidence that this can be achieved (O'Keeffe, Jack, & Lye, 1996; Williams & Finch, 1997). This chapter focuses on the issues of physical restraint in acute, nonpsychiatric hospital settings with particular attention to older adult patients.

BACKGROUND AND LEGAL ISSUES

Regulations and Accrediting Standards

In 1992, the U.S. Food and Drug Administration (FDA) issued a medical alert on the potential hazards of restraint devices (FDA, 2006a). Any harm that arises from the use of a restraining device, which now includes bedside rails, must be reported to the FDA. TJC hospital standards began to address the use of physical restraints in the early 1990s. Over the ensuing years, the standards have become increasingly prescriptive.

In 1999, CMS established an interim rule for hospitals and, in December 2006, finalized the Patients' Rights Condition of Participation (HHS, 2007). These conditions establish the minimum protections of patients' rights and safety and may be superseded by state regulations or accrediting agencies. In brief, use of physical restraint should be used as a last resort; only used when less restrictive mechanisms have been determined to be ineffective; the use of restraint must be in accordance with a written modification to the patient's plan of care; used in accordance with the order of a physician or licensed independent practitioner; must never be written as a PRN order; each order must be renewed every 24 hours for reasons of violent or self-destructive behavior; each order for restraint use for nonviolent reasons must be renewed according to hospital policy; and restraint must be discontinued at the earliest possible time.

Risks of Liability

A major obstacle in reducing clinicians' use of physical restraint or side rails is the fear of liability if restraints are not used. Case law has been mixed; hospitals have been found liable both for the use of physical restraints and for not using physical restraints (Kapp, 1994; Kapp, 1996). Although hospitals have a clear duty to protect patients from harm, they do not have a duty to restrain patients. As the practice in hospitals becomes one of reduced restraints because of changing legal and accrediting standards, it will become easier for hospitals to justify nonuse of restraints in instances of patient injury where use of nonrestraint interventions were clearly demonstrated (Kapp, 1999).

Professional Standards of Care

A number of organizations have established guidelines for the use of physical restraints, including the American Nurses Association and the Society for Critical Care Medicine (American Nurses Association, 2001; Maccioli et al., 2003). The National Quality Forum has designated physical restraint as a nursing-sensitive measure to be monitored in hospitals and nursing facilities. Lastly, as part of the condition for participation as a *magnet facility*, hospitals must examine the use of physical restraint in relation to nursing skill mix and hours. These guidelines have become the standard for customary practice and are used as an appropriate legal standard that defines the parameters of liability. Furthermore, these guidelines in combination with TJC and CMS requirements are used to establish hospital-based policies and procedures and quality of performance activities.

PREVALENCE AND RATIONALE OF STAFF

Extent of Use

These standards and guidelines have led to an overall decrease in physical restraint use in acute care and a change in practice patterns. In the 1980s, the overall prevalence rate of physical restraint use on general floors ranged from 6% to 13%, with higher rates (18%–22%) among older adult patients (Frengley & Mion, 1998). In the late 1990s, the overall hospital restraint prevalence decreased but varied as much as three-fold, with rates ranging from 39 restraint days/1,000 patient days to 82 restraint days/1,000 patient days (Minnick, Mion, Leipzig, Lamb, & Palmer, 1998; Mion et al., 2001). For the first time, restraint use was examined in critical care units and was noted to be as high as 500 restraint days/1,000 patient days. Intensive care unit (ICU) rates varied markedly, between units in the same hospital setting as well as matched units between hospitals.

A national prevalence study involving 434 units in 40 acute care hospitals selected at random from five geographic areas was completed in 2005 (Minnick, Mion, Johnson, Catrambone, & Leipzig, 2007). Findings from this study revealed overall hospital prevalence of 50 restraint days/1,000 patient days but with a 10-fold variation among hospitals from a rate of 9–94 restraint days/1,000 patient days. The majority of use was accounted for in ICUs. The pattern of differences by type of unit was again present (e.g., medical versus surgical and adult versus pediatric). However, even when controlling by type of unit, more than 10-fold variation existed among similar settings. For example, overall prevalence among the 41 general ICUs was 202.6 restraint days/1,000 patient days with a range of 9–351/1,000 patient days. Further, analyses revealed that variation in practice persisted even when controlling for size of hospital, academic or nonacademic status, geographic region, type of hospital (e.g., nonprofit, profit, and government), staffing ratios, and nursing skill mix. Clearly, there are major practice differences *even when controlling for patient population.*

Decision to Use Physical Restraint

Today's hospital nurses cite prevention of patient therapy disruption as the primary reason for restraint use (reported for 75% of restraint days), presence of "confusion" (25.4% of the restraint days), and fall prevention (17.6% of the restraint days; Minnick et al., 2007). Other less commonly voiced reasons included management of agitation or violent behavior, wandering, and positioning. Although most nurses cite patient care issues as the rationale to use physical restraint, a small proportion of nurses have cited insufficient staffing for restrained patients (Evans & FitzGerald, 2002; Minnick et al., 1998).

The CMS regulations mandate that physicians or licensed independent practitioners must order physical restraint. Similar to nurses, physicians vary in their decisions to order physical restraint (Mion et al., 2010; Sandhu et al., 2010). Factors associated with physicians' decisions to order restraint include (a) lack of knowledge of physical restraint and hospital policy, (b) higher appraisal of patient harm, (c) specialty (family practice or general surgery), (d) trusting the nurse, (e) patient behavior, and (f) presence of dementia. Given the variation in actual use of restraint, it appears that the decision to use physical restraint continues to be one based on individual judgment and beliefs rather than on scientifically validated guidelines or protocols.

ETHICAL ISSUES IN THE USE OF PHYSICAL RESTRAINT

The primary ethical dilemma resulting from physical restraint is the clinician's value or emphasis of beneficence versus the patient's autonomy (Schafer, 1985; Slomka, Agich, Stagno, & Smith, 1998). Clinicians believe that physical restraint prevents patient falls and patient disruption of therapy (Frengley & Mion, 1998; Lamb, Minnick, Mion, Palmer, & Leipzig, 1999). The presence of a physical restraint, by its very nature, is applied against a patient's wishes and inevitably compromises the individual's dignity and diminishes respect for the person. Beneficence requires that at least no harm should arise from the use of physical restraint and that, optimally, a good outcome would result from use. The lack of beneficial results from the use of physical restraints has been well documented in many health care settings. Little is known, however, of the risk-to-benefit ratio of use or nonuse of physical restraint in patients who are critically ill (Maccioli et al., 2003).

The discussion of physical restraints from an ethical viewpoint must also incorporate the sociocultural and political contexts. For example, clinicians have reported on low to nonexistent use of physical restraint in the United Kingdom, stemming perhaps from a legal mandate existing since the 1800s prohibiting their use. It has been suggested that in the United States, the domination of risk in geriatric assessment (e.g., prevent harm, prevent falls) shapes much of clinicians' understanding of old age (Kaufman, 1994). If one's primary focus is on the likelihood of patient risk resulting in harm, one is less likely to see self-esteem or dignity as the more important value or model to guide clinical decisions (Slomka et al., 1998). Interestingly, Slomka and associates point out the contradictory nature of the frequent use of physical restraint in the United States—that is, a society that places a high value on autonomy yet so willing to violate that autonomy in the interest of perceived patient benefit (Slomka et al., 1998).

The discussion of ethics in clinical practice must also acknowledge the realities of reduced resources and escalating costs (Minnick et al., 2007; Slomka et al., 1998). Decisions and protocols about the use of physical restraints and methods to reduce and/ or eliminate restraints will be impacted by cost-containment efforts, and clinicians and administrators alike may be reluctant to minimize or eliminate restraints. If alternatives to physical restraints in acute care settings can be shown to contribute to quality outcomes (e.g., patient safety, patient dignity, or satisfaction) and within existing cost-containment efforts, then there is an increased likelihood of successfully implementing and maintaining practice guidelines. There is a chance, however, that if restraint reduction efforts are seen as too expensive (e.g., use of "sitters"), then the emphasis on cost constraint may trump other considerations (Slomka et al., 1998).

ADMINISTRATIVE RESPONSIBILITIES

Changing established practices and philosophies of care can be a daunting task. Although education and training is important, the single most important factor in affecting a major shift in the present paradigm of care to one that is restraint-free care is the commitment by administrators and key clinical leaders (Mion et al., 2001; Williams & Finch, 1997). Indeed, the huge variation seen in the rates among 40 hospitals that cannot be explained by size of hospital, type of hospital, or geographic location lends support to this observation. Administrators, including nurse managers, set the tone for the practice on the unit. Reducing health care providers' reliance on physical restraint in managing confused or agitated patients, especially in the critical care units, is a major shift that leaves many staff uneasy. Clinical staff, especially the frontline care providers, must feel supported during the transition period. The goal set and supported by administration of a restraint-free environment would establish the presence of a physical restraint as an outlier that requires a full analysis as for a sentinel event. The outcome of such analyses may well lead to the recognition of system problems and organizational arrangements that can be improved, which, in turn, lead to even fewer restraints in use.

INTERVENTIONS AND CARE STRATEGIES

The studies of the prevalence of the use of physical restraints for nonpsychiatric purposes in hospitals have shown that there is great discrepancy between general medical and surgical units and ICUs in terms of the extent and rationale. Therefore, the use of physical restraints and approaches to possible alternatives can be considered separately for general hospital units and critical care units.

General Medical and Surgical Units

Although rates of physical restraint use on general medical and surgical units have declined in the past 20 years, wide variation exists: from 3 to 123 restraint days/1,000 patient days on medical units and from 0 to 65 restraint days/1,000 patient days on surgical units (Minnick et al., 2007). It is apparent there are units that demonstrate best practices, but also that further efforts are needed to eliminate this practice as a national standard. Otherwise, significant numbers of patients will continue to be restrained.

Many hospitals provide care for acutely ill, frail older adults in settings that are not designed environmentally for the care of such older people (Catrambone, Johnson, Mion, & Minnick, 2009; Mion et al., 2006; Palmer, Landefeld, Kresevic, & Kowal, 1994). Environmental structure can either facilitate or inhibit monitoring and surveillance, noise control, appropriate lighting, socialization, cognition, and function (Catrambone et al., 2009; Palmer et al., 1994). Studies in long-term care settings have demonstrated that the use of environmental strategies can enhance function among those suffering from dementia; similar strategies need to be considered in acute care settings.

Besides environmental strategies, organizational factors such as systems to determine staffing numbers and mix, models of care delivery, and transmission or communication of the plan of care among multiple disciplines and departments are gaining increased recognition in the patient safety movement (Leape & Berwick, 2005). Many health care providers lack the knowledge, skills, and sensitivity in providing appropriate care to older adults. TJC standard to ensure age-specific education and training is a step in the right direction, but further efforts are required.

No single approach to eliminating physical restraints on general medical and surgical units can be successful. Studies in a variety of settings have shown that the use of advanced practice nurses, comprehensive interdisciplinary approaches to enhance cognitive and physical function, staff education, organizational strategies, and environmental interventions can eliminate or reduce physical restraints in a cost-effective manner while promoting other patient outcomes, such as reduced fall rates (Amato, Salter, & Mion, 2006; Inouye et al., 1999; Landefeld, Palmer, Kresevic, Fortinsky, & Kowal, 1995; Mion et al., 2001).

Critical Care Units

The practice of physical restraints is now predominantly within ICUs to maintain needed life-sustaining therapies or life-maintaining therapies (Minnick et al., 2007). Strategies that have been used with success in long-term care settings, rehabilitation settings, and general hospital units are not as successful in critical care environments (Mion et al., 2001). The severity of illness of patients, the intensity and delivery of care, the pace of activity, and the consequences of interruptions, delays, or disruptions of therapeutic devices differ significantly between non-ICUs and ICUs. The thought of delirious patients dislodging external ventricular drains with subsequent brain damage, pulling out central lines with threat of hemorrhage, or self-extubation from mechanical ventilation with subsequent respiratory arrest is one that heavily influences critical care nurses' decisions to use physical restraints (Frengley & Mion, 1998; Happ, 2000).

Efforts to limit physical restraint use in the ICU are hampered by lack of information regarding the extent of therapy disruption in these units or the resulting immediate and subsequent harm to patients (Maccioli et al., 2003). A number of studies, mostly single site, have examined self-extubation from mechanical ventilation (Frengley & Mion, 1998). Rates have ranged from 0.3% to 14.3%, with higher rates in medical ICUs. Reintubation after self-extubation ranged from 11% to 76%. *Importantly, 33%–91% of those who self-extubated did so while physically restrained.* As part of the national prevalence study described earlier, the authors also examined the prevalence of patient-initiated device removal, patient contexts, patient risk-adjusted factors, and consequences (Mion, Minnick, Leipzig, Catrambone, & Johnson, 2007). In 49 ICUs in 39 hospitals, the authors collected data on 49,482 patient days. Patients removed 1,623 devices on 1,097 occasions for an overall rate of 22.1 episodes/1,000 patient days. Similar to results on physical restraint prevalence, wide variation in rates were noted: from none to 102.4 episodes/1,000 patient days. Approximately, half the episodes occurred on day shift, and 44% were in physical restraint at the time of the episode. Patient harm occurred in 250 (23%) events, mostly minor in nature. In 10 (0.9%) episodes, patients incurred major harm. No deaths occurred. The authors examined rates of reinsertion and found these varied by type of device. Devices that are easily applied, such as monitor lead or oxygen masks, had much higher reinsertion rates than devices that are more complex and difficult to insert (such as endotracheal tubes or surgical drains). It may be that devices are utilized too long, which could contribute to prolonged use of physical restraint. In turn, physical restraint may contribute to agitation and delirium (Inouye & Charpentier, 1996). Additional hospital resources (e.g., x-rays, laboratory tests) were utilized in slightly more than half the episodes; thus, a potentially costly problem (Fraser, Riker, Prato, & Wilkins, 2001).

Information gathered on staffing levels and mix showed little variation among these ICUs; hence, there was no association between staffing ratios and therapy disruptions. Of the three studies on self-extubation that examined relationship to staffing levels, two also showed no association (Boulain, 1998; Chevron et al., 1998; Marcin et al., 2005). The authors found *no* association between a unit's restraint rate and rate of therapy disruption, a finding similar to some studies (Kapadia, Bajan, & Raje, 2000; Mion et al., 2001) but not others (Carrión et al., 2000; Tominaga, Rudzwick, Scannell, & Waxman, 1995).

Finally, the pattern of sedation and analgesia in these units was unclear, and 30% of the patients had received no analgesia or sedation in the 24 hours prior to the episode. Others have reported on inconsistent sedation and analgesia practices in ICUs (Bair et al., 2000; Egerod, Christensen, & Johansen, 2006; Mehta et al., 2006). In an earlier cohort study, the authors examined medical intensive care unit (MICU) patient outcomes after implementing sedation and analgesia guidelines and found that those cared for with the guidelines had less self-extubation events and use of physical restraints (Bair et al., 2000). Examining appropriate strategies for sedation and analgesia in critically ill patients may well result in improved clinical outcomes while providing care in a more humane fashion.

Attention to the environment of the ICU is as important as any other setting. Indeed, the environment can affect more strongly persons whose personal competence is low and who are unable to exert control over the environment. Inouye and Charpentier (1996) exquisitely demonstrated the inverse relationship of the individual's level of vulnerability with that of environmental or process insults on subsequent development of delirium among hospitalized older adults. Environmental features such as noise, light, and unit design have been shown to be associated with agitation, anxiety, and disorientation of ICU patients (Frengley & Mion, 1998).

Lack of communication with ICU patients by care providers has been documented and results in distress, anxiety, and confusion (Fontaine, 1994). Attention to the physical environment, use of communication techniques with seemingly noncommunicative patients, encouragement of collaborative practice among ICU disciplines, and non-pharmacologic approaches to relieve patient distress, anxiety, and agitation have been suggested but largely untested (Maccioli et al., 2003). Nevertheless, a multipronged approach to optimize physical and cognitive function, address onset, as well as management of delirium, and appropriate and adequate pain control are likely to affect nurses' and physicians' reliance on physical restraint.

ALTERNATIVES TO PHYSICAL RESTRAINTS

Overview

This book has provided the reader with a number of protocols addressing care issues such as falls, delirium, sleep, nutrition, medications, and function. The reader is encouraged to review these protocols closely. Implementing best practices aimed at these areas will in itself reduce the use of physical restraints. A brief overview of an approach that the authors have found successful is presented herein.

The two major reasons for using physical restraints to prevent therapy disruption and falls require comprehensive yet targeted approaches. The act of self-terminating therapy among hospitalized, acutely ill older adults is most likely a manifestation of delirium and less likely a desire to enact a clinical decision, as with advanced directives. Both falls and delirium are well-known syndromes with significant morbidity and mortality among older adults. Both are complex syndromes with multiple underlying etiologies that require a combination of individual-, environmental-, and organizational-specific strategies (Tinetti, Inouye, Gill, & Doucette, 1995). Inouye and colleagues (1999) have demonstrated a multicomponent approach to preventing delirium in a randomized controlled trial and subsequently implemented in a number of hospitals (Bradley, Webster, Schlesinger, Baker, & Inouye, 2006). Fall prevention also requires a multicomponent approach (Oliver, Healey, & Haines, 2010). Given the complexity of falls and delirium, it is unlikely that any single intervention would suffice as an alternative to physical restraint. Rather, attention to the environment and organization of the unit, as described in the two previous sections, combined with patient-specific approaches provides the most successful approach to eliminating restraint use (Amato et al., 2006; Mion et al., 2001).

Fall Prevention

Falls are well-known, serious events in hospitalized older patients. Although nurses perceive that physical restraint prevents falls from occurring, the reality is that physical restraints have not been shown to prevent falls and can actually contribute to fall injury (Frengley & Mion, 1998). The goal is to minimize the risk or probability of falling without compromising the older individual's mobility and functional independence. Using a systematic or standardized approach, the nurse and physician assess the patient for intrinsic (personal), extrinsic (environment), and situational (activity) factors. Common intrinsic risk factors include impaired gait or balance, sedating medications, vision and hearing impairments, and cognitive impairment including impaired memory, impulsiveness, or poor judgment; a number of fall risk assessment guidelines are available (Oliver et al., 2010). The reader is referred to Chapter 15, Fall Prevention: Assessment, Diagnoses, and Intervention Strategies, for a more in depth discussion. What is important to note is that the evaluation for intrinsic factors need not be complex or time consuming. For instance, the nurse can do a simple evaluation of gait and balance by simply observing the person's ability to transfer in and out of bed or chair and ability to walk to and from the bathroom. The nurse can quickly note any difficulty with steadiness, ability to stand up independently without using a rocking motion or use of upper extremities, ability to sit down without "plopping" onto the surface of the chair, and the ability to walk steadily to the bathroom without holding onto objects or the wall. At this time, notation can be made of lightheadedness or dizziness, presence of orthostatic hypotension, and use of sedating medications.

Extrinsic factors include clothing and footwear. Shoes or slippers should be nonskid, but rubber-soled footwear is not recommended because this material can "grip" the floor causing the person to pitch forward. Furniture design, such as beds at a proper height and chairs with extended armrests for easier leverage, can facilitate mobility. Reclining chairs are helpful for those with poor trunk control and who slide out of chairs with a 90-degree seating angle. On the other hand, reclining chairs could be a type of restraint if used for patients with general deconditioning or weakened states who subsequently struggle to rise out of the chair. Although beds low to floor assist with preventing fall injury, they may actually contribute to a fall in a person with weak quadriceps muscle strength who struggles to stand upright from a very low position (Capezuti et al., 2008; Tominaga et al., 1995; Tzeng & Yin, 2008); hence, the nurse must use clinical judgment of whether the intervention is to prevent a fall or prevent a fall injury. These goals do not necessarily result in similar interventions. Hospital equipment can also contribute to falls such as legs collapsing on bedside commodes, wheelchairs tipping when a patient leans forward, or tubing from lower extremity intermittent compression devices that are left on when a patient stands up from bed.

The findings of either intrinsic or extrinsic factors should lead to targeted interventions. There are some fall-prevention strategies that one could consider as "universal,"—that is, be implemented for all patients regardless of the risk level. For instance, all patients should have beds at appropriate heights for ease of exiting and entering, have call bells within reach, and have clear pathways. Depending on the type of unit, some units may elect to incorporate universal interventions that other floors would consider a targeted intervention. For example, an acute stroke unit may elect to automatically place all patients on a toileting schedule at time of admission and reevaluate continually whether this intervention is required, whereas the other units in the hospital would elect to use this as a targeted intervention only for those patients with cognitive impairment and incontinence. An important fall prevention strategy in any setting is mobilization and exercise. Even in critical care settings, there is a growing body of literature that demonstrates the physiologic and physical benefits of early mobilization and rehabilitation (Truong, Fan, Brower, & Needham, 2009).

Protection of Medical Devices

Disruption of therapy or self-termination of devices can be dealt with by first identifying the underlying reason for the patient's attempts to terminate therapies. In many cases, the nurse will identify "confusion" as the underlying cause. As discussed in earlier chapters, the nurse needs to differentiate dementia, delirium, or delirium superimposed on dementia. Additionally, the interdisciplinary team must discern the underlying causes of delirium, including pain. A systematic approach to determine the cause of the behavior is necessary for treatment. For example, if an older adult is suffering from alcohol withdrawal, it is unlikely that interventions such as increased surveillance or pain relief will have much impact on the person's agitation and delirium. Refer to Chapter 10, Dementia; Chapter 11, Delirium; and Chapter 8, Assessment of Cognitive Function, for further protocols to identify cognitive impairments and to prevent and manage delirium.

Historically, the options for managing agitation in the critical care unit have been sedation and/or physical restraint. The type and amount of sedation, however, may actually contribute to delirium and agitation (Wunsch & Kress, 2009). Multiple studies suggest that limiting the use of benzodiazepines and use of an alternative medication dexmedetomidine can decrease ventilator time, length of stay, and long-term brain dysfunction (Wunsch & Kress, 2009). The use of physical restraint in critical care settings has been associated with delirium as well as posttraumatic stress disorder (Jones et al., 2007; Micek, Anand, Laible, Shannon, & Kollef, 2005; Nirmalan, Dark, Nightingale, & Harris, 2004; Wallen, Chaboyer, Thalib, & Creedy, 2008).

As the health care team works to address the patient's behavior, nonpharmacologic approaches to protecting the device from self-termination can be made. First, evaluate daily whether the device is absolutely necessary. Since the occurrence of the CMS designation of nonpayment of nosocomial catheter infections (e.g., urinary tract infections from indwelling catheters, ventilator-related pneumonia), many ICUs have implemented multidisciplinary daily mandatory checklists that incorporates assessment for compliance to infection control and timely discontinuation of devices (Byrnes et al., 2009; DuBose et al., 2010). Even in the critical care environment, major therapy devices may not be reinserted once a patient pulls it out. Thus, always question whether the device is absolutely necessary or whether a less noxious device or approach may be used instead. For example, if a nasogastric tube is used for nutrition, request the assessment of other disciplines, such as speech or occupational therapists, to determine whether oral feeding could be introduced. If long-term enteral feeding is required, an interdisciplinary team plan with the patient and family is warranted given the known deleterious effects of tube feedings with certain conditions.

Some therapeutic devices cannot be altered or discontinued, for example, use of endotracheal tubes, nasal cannula, or oxygen masks. A second approach is to use anchoring techniques to secure the device against the patient's attempts to dislodge the device or to use camouflage to "hide" the device from the patient. Proper anchoring addresses comfort as well as stabilization of the device(s). For example, it is not unusual for pressure ulcers to develop on nares or behind ears and neck because of undue pressure from the device; clearly a source of discomfort for the patient. Proper stabilization of the tube or device with secure anchoring can minimize accidental dislodgment as well as deter more purposeful removal. For instance, a nasogastric tube can be placed so as to not interfere with or interrupt the person's visual field. Seeing the tube dangling in front of one's eyes or pulling on one's nares is an obvious irritant. If a gastrostomy tube is determined to be appropriate in the person's plan of care, abdominal binders can aid in reducing the person's ability to pull it out. There are a number of commercial products available to secure various tubes, including nasogastric tubes, endotracheal tubes, intravenous lines, and indwelling bladder catheters. Although none of these devices is likely to prevent a determined person from pulling out a device, they do provide anchoring and stability of the device that are probably more secure than taping methods.

Side Rails

A discussion on physical restraints in hospitals would not be complete without mentioning side rails. Side rails, in and of themselves, are not considered a restraining device by either TJC or CMS. It is the nurse's intent of their use that determines whether side rails are a restraining device or a protective device. This has led to some confusion by nurses. Full side rails to transfer patients in carts, during procedures (e.g., conscious sedation), or protect a sedated or lethargic patient from rolling out of the bed can be considered as protective devices. A number of specialty beds, such as ICU pulmonary beds or bariatric beds, require full side rails in use. Many bed manufacturers have bed controls and call systems embedded in the side rail frames, resulting in patients requesting the side rails be kept raised for ease of control. Hospital patients have also been observed to request partial to full side rails to be raised because of the narrowness of the beds or to facilitate movement (e.g., transfers, repositioning).

In ICU settings, full side rails are used predominantly because of bed equipment specification (e.g., pulmonary beds) or because of procedural considerations (e.g., sedation protocols; Minnick, Mion, Johnson, Catrambone, & Leipzig, 2008). In non-ICUs, nurses use full side rails primarily for fall prevention (46%), especially for older patients (Minnick et al., 2008). Full side rails to keep patients in bed who *desire* to leave bed are restraints. It does not matter what the cognitive level of the person is. If a severely demented patient wishes to leave the bed, full side rails are considered a restraint, even if the nurse believes the side rails are for "patient safety." Side rails have been shown to increase fall injuries because patients either try to squeeze through rails or climb over the foot of the bed or are not a recommended strategy for fall prevention for the conscious but cognitively impaired patient (Braun & Capezuti, 2000). Indeed, the FDA has received reports of more than 400 deaths as a direct result of side rail entrapment from a variety of health care settings, including hospitals (FDA, 2006b). The reader is referred to Braun and Capezuti (2000) for an excellent review of the legal and medical aspects of side rail use.

SUMMARY

The pattern and rationale for physical restraint use has changed over the past two decades. Focusing on assessment and prevention of delirium and falls will likely minimize their use. Further work is needed in the ICU settings for best strategies to identify, prevent, and manage delirium that would include nonpharmacologic as well as pharmacologic approaches. To avoid the use of physical restraints, practical and cost-effective strategies need to be devised and tested. This would best be done in an interdisciplinary patient-centered fashion.

NURSING STANDARD OF PRACTICE

Protocol 13.1: Physical Restraints and Side Rails in Acute and Critical Care Settings

I. GOAL: To eliminate the use of physical restraints and side rails in acute and critical care settings.

II. OVERVIEW

A. The use of physical restraints or side rails for the involuntary immobilization of the patient may not only be an infringement of the patient's rights, but can also result in patient harm, including soft tissue injury, fractures, delirium, and even death (Bower et al., 2003; Evans et al., 2003; Miles, 1993).

B. The primary ethical dilemma resulting from physical restraint is the clinician's value or emphasis of beneficence versus the patient's autonomy.

C. Use of physical restraint should be used as a last resort; only used when less restrictive mechanisms have been determined to be ineffective; the use of restraint must be in accordance with a written modification to the patient's plan of care; used in accordance with the order of a physician or licensed independent practitioner (LIP); must never be written as a PRN order; each order must be renewed every 4 hours, for adults up to 24 hours at which time a reevaluation by a LIP is required for reasons of violent or self-destructive behavior; each order of restraint use for nonviolent reasons must be renewed according to hospital policy; and restraint must be discontinued at the earliest possible time (HHS, 2007).

III. BACKGROUND AND STATEMENT OF PROBLEM

A. Definition: The Centers for Medicare and Medicaid Services (CMS) defines physical restraint as "any manual method, physical or mechanical device, material, or equipment that immobilizes or reduces the ability of the patient to move his or her arms, legs, body or head freely" (HHS, 2007). Examples include wrist or leg restraints, hand mitts, Geri-chairs, and, in certain situations, full side rails and reclining chairs.

B. Etiology: Hospital nurses' reasons for use of physical restraint are prevention of patient disruption of medical devices and therapy (75%), confusion (25%), and fall prevention (18%; Minnick et al., 2007).

C. Epidemiology

1. Prevalence of physical restraint use on individual non-ICU rates range from 0 to 123 restraint days/1,000 patient days, with overall rates ranging among types of units from 3.6 (pediatric units) to 49.2 (neuroscience units; Minnick et al., 2007).

2. Individual ICU rates range from 0 to 267.9 restraint days/1,000 patient days with overall rates ranging by types from 50.6 (pediatric ICUs) to 267 (neurology and neurosurgery ICUs; Minnick et al., 2007).

IV. PARAMETERS OF ASSESSMENT

A. Assess for underlying cause(s) of agitation and cognitive impairment leading to patient-initiated device removal (refer to Chapter 8, Assessing Cognitive

(continued)

Function; Chapter 9, Depression in Older Adults; Chapter 10, Dementia; and Chapter 11, Delirium).
1. If abrupt change in perception, attention, or level of consciousness:
   a. Assess for life-threatening physiologic impairments
   b. Respiratory, neurologic, fever and sepsis, hypoglycemia and hyperglycemia, alcohol or substance withdrawal, and fluid and electrolyte imbalance
   c. Notify physician of change in mental status and compromised physiologic status
2. Differential assessment (interdisciplinary)
   a. Obtain baseline or premorbid cognitive function from family and caregivers
   b. Establish whether the patient has history of dementia or depression
   c. Review medications to identify drug–drug interactions, adverse effects
   d. Review current laboratory values
B. Assess fall risk: intrinsic, extrinsic, and situational factors (refer to Chapter 15, Fall Prevention: Assessment, Diagnoses, and Intervention Strategies)
C. Assess for medications that may cause drug–drug interactions and adverse drug effects (refer to Chapter 17, Reducing Adverse Drug Events).

V. NURSING CARE STRATEGIES
A. Interventions to Minimize or Reduce Patient-Initiated Device Removal
   1. Disruption of any device
      a. Reassess daily to determine whether it is medically possible to discontinue device; try alternative mode of therapy (DuBose et al., 2010; Mion et al., 2001; Nirmalan et al., 2004).
      b. For mild-to-moderate cognitive impairment, explain device and allow patient to feel under nurse's guidance.
   2. Attempted or actual disruption: ventilator
      a. Determine underlying cause of behavior for appropriate medical and/or pharmacologic approach
      b. More secure anchoring
      c. Appropriate sedation and analgesia protocol
      d. Start with less restrictive means: mitts, elbow extenders
   3. Attempted or actual disruption: nasogastric tube
      a. If for feeding purposes, consult with nutritionist and speech or occupational therapist for swallow evaluation.
      b. Consider gastrostomy tube for feeding as appropriate if other measures are ineffective.
      c. Anchoring of tube, either by taping techniques or commercial tube holder
      d. If restraints are needed, start with least restrictive: mitts, elbow extenders
   4. Attempted or actual disruption: intravenous (IV) lines
      a. Commercial tube holder for anchoring
      b. Long-sleeved robes, commercial sleeves for arms
      c. Consider Hep-Lock and cover with gauze
      d. Taping, securement of IV line under gown, sleeves
      e. Keep IV bag out of visual field
      f. Consider alternative therapy: oral fluids, drugs

(continued)

Protocol 13.1: Physical Restraints and Side Rails in Acute and Critical Care Settings *(cont.)*

5. Treatment (Interdisciplinary)
   a. Treat underlying disorder(s)
   b. Judicious, low dose use of medication if warranted for agitation
   c. Communication techniques: low voice, simple commands, reorientation
   d. Frequent reassurance and orientation
   e. Surveillance and observation: Determine whether family member(s) willing to stay with patient; move patient closer to nurses' station; perform safety checks more frequently; redeploy staff to provide one-on-one observation if other measure is ineffective
6. Attempted or actual disruption: bladder catheter
   a. Consider intermittent catheterization if appropriate
   b. Proper securement, anchoring to leg. Commercial tube holders available

B. Interventions to Reduce Fall Risk
   1. Patient-centered interventions
      a. Supervised, progressive ambulation even in ICUs (Inouye et al., 1999; Truong et al., 2009)
      b. Physical therapist/occupational therapist (PT/OT) consultation: weakened or unsteady gait, trunk weakness, upper arm weakness
      c. Provide physical aids in hearing, vision, walking
      d. Modify clothing: skidproof slippers, slipper socks, robes no longer than ankle length
      e. Bedside commode if impaired or weakened gait
      f. Postural hypotension: behavioral recommendations such as ankle pumps, hand clenching, reviewing medications, elevating head of bed
   2. Organizational interventions (Mion, 2001)
      a. Examine pattern of falls on unit (e.g., time of day, day of week)
      b. Examine unit factors that can contribute to falls that can be ameliorated (e.g., report in back room versus walking rounds to improve surveillance)
      c. Restructure staff routines to increase number of available staff throughout the day
      d. Set and maintain toilet schedules
      e. Install electronic alarms for wanderers
      f. Consider bed and chair alarms (note: no to little evidence on effectiveness)
      g. Moving patient closer to nurse station
      h. Increased checks on high-risk patients
   3. Environmental interventions (Amato et al., 2006; Landefeld et al., 1995)
      a. Keep bed in low, locked position
      b. Safety features, such as grab bars, call bells, bed alarms, are in good working order
      c. Ensure bedside tables and dressers are in easy reach
      d. Clear pathways of hazards
      c. Bolster cushions to assist with posture, maintain seat in chair
      d. Adequate lighting, especially bathroom at night
      e. Furniture to facilitate seating: reclining chairs (note: may be considered restraint in some instances), extended arm rests, high back

C. Review medications using Beers Criteria for potentially inappropriate medications

(continued)

**Protocol 13.1: Physical Restraints and Side Rails in
Acute and Critical Care Settings** *(cont.)*

VI. EVALUATION AND EXPECTED OUTCOMES
A. Patient
   1. Patient will remain free of restraints
   2. Physical restraints will be used only as a last resort
B. Nursing Staff
   1. Will be able to accurately assess patients who are at risk for use of physical restraint
   2. Will only use physical restraints when less restrictive mechanisms have been determined to be ineffective
   3. Will have an increased use of nonrestraint, safety alternatives
C. Organization
   1. Will have a decrease in incidence and/or prevalence of restraints
   2. Will not have an increase of falls, agitated behavior, and patient-initiated removal of medical devices

VII. FOLLOW-UP MONITORING OF CONDITION
A. Monitor restraint incidence comparing benchmark rates over time by unit
B. Document prevalence rate of restraint use on an ongoing basis
C. Focus education on assessment and prevention of delirium and falls
D. Consult with interdisciplinary members to identify additional safety alternatives

VIII. RELEVANT PRACTICE GUIDELINES
A. American Nurses Association. (2001). *Position statement: Reduction of patient restraint and seclusion in health care settings.* Retrieved from NursingWorld website: http://www.nursingworld.org/MainMenuCategories/EthicsStandards/Ethics-Position-Statements/prtetrestrnt14452.aspx
B. Maccioli, G. A., Dorman, T., Brown, B. R., Mazuski, J. E., McLean, B. A., Rosenbaum, S. H., . . . Society of Critical Care Medicine. (2003). Clinical practice guidelines for the maintenance of patient physical safety in the intensive care unit: Use of restraining therapies—American College of Critical Care Medicine Task Force 2001–2002. *Critical Care Medicine*, *31*(11), 2665–2676.

RESOURCES

Additional Information About Restraints

Consult GeriRN

An online resources containing information regarding assessing and caring for older adults sponsored by the Hartford Institute for Geriatric Nursing at New York University College of Nursing.
http://consultgerirn.org/resources

The Joint Commission: Sentinel Event Alert
http://www.jointcommission.org/sentinel_event_alert_issue_8_preventing_restraint_deaths/

REFERENCES

Amato, S., Salter, J. P., & Mion, L. C. (2006). Physical restraint reduction in the acute rehabilitation setting: A quality improvement study. *Rehabilitation Nursing, 31*(6), 235–241. Evidence Level III.

American Nurses Association. (2001). *Position statement: Reduction of patient restraint and seclusion in health care settings*. Retrieved from NursingWorld website: http://www.nursingworld.org/MainMenu Categories/EthicsStandards/Ethics-Position-Statements/prtetrestrnt14452.aspx. Evidence Level VI.

Bair, N., Bobek, M., Hoffman-Hogg, L., Mion, L. C., Slomka, J., & Arroliga, A. C. (2000). Introduction of sedative, analgesic, and neuromuscular blocking agent guidelines in a medical intensive care unit: Physician and nurse adherence. *Critical Care Medicine, 28*(3), 707–713. Evidence Level III.

Boulain, T. (1998). Unplanned extubations in the adult intensive care unit: A prospective multi-center study. Association des Réanimateurs du Centre-Ouest. *American Journal Respiratory and Critical Care Medicine, 157*(4 Pt. 1), 1131–1137. Evidence Level IV.

Bower, F. L., McCullough, C. S., & Timmons, M. E. (2003). A synthesis of what we know about the use of physical restraints and seclusion with patients in psychiatric and acute care settings: 2003 update. *The Online Journal of Knowledge Sysnthesis for Nursing, 10*, 1. Evidence Level V.

Bradley, E. H., Webster, T. R., Schlesinger, M., Baker, D., & Inouye, S. K. (2006). Patterns of diffusion of evidence-based clinical programmes: A case study of the Hospital Elder Life Program. *Quality & Safety in Health Care, 15*(5), 334–338. Evidence Level IV.

Braun, J. A., & Capezuti, E. (2000). The legal and medical aspects of physical restraints and bed siderails and their relationship to falls and fall-related injuries in nursing homes. *DePaul Journal of Healthcare Law, 3*(1), 1–72. Evidence Level I.

Byrnes, M. C., Schuerer, D. J., Schallom, M. E., Sona, C. S., Mazuski, J. E., Taylor, B. E., . . . Coopersmith, C. M. (2009). Implementation of a mandatory checklist of protocols and objectives improves compliance with a wide range of evidence-based intensive care unit practices. *Critical Care Medicine, 37*(10), 2775–2781. Evidence Level III.

Capezuti, E., Wagner, L., Brush, B., Boltz, M., Renz, S., & Secic, M. (2008). Bed and toilet height as potential environmental risk factors. *Clinical Nursing Research, 17*(1), 50–66. Evidence Level IV.

Carrión, M. I., Ayuso, D., Marcos, M., Paz Robles, M., de la Cal, M. A., Alía, I., & Esteban, A. (2000). Accidental removal of endotracheal and nasogastric tubes and intravascular catheters. *Critical Care Medicine, 28*(1), 63–66. Evidence Level III.

Catrambone, C., Johnson, M. E., Mion, L. C., & Minnick, A. F. (2009). The design of adult acute care units in U.S. hospitals. *Journal of Nursing Scholarship, 41*(1), 79–86. Evidence Level IV.

Chevron, V., Ménard, J. F., Richard, J. C., Girault, C., Leroy, J., & Bonmarchand, G. (1998). Unplanned extubation: Risk factors of development and predictive criteria for reintubation. *Critical Care Medicine, 26*(6), 1049–1053. Evidence Level IV.

Department of Health and Human Services. (2007). Medicare program; proposed changes to the hospital inpatient prospective payment systems and fiscal year 2008 rates; correction. *Federal Register, 72*(109), 31507–31540.

DuBose, J., Teixeira, P. G., Inaba, K., Lam, L., Talving, P., Putty, B., . . . Belzberg, H. (2010). Measurable outcomes of quality improvement using a daily quality rounds checklist: One-year analysis in a trauma intensive care unit with sustained ventilator-associated pneumonia reduction. *The Journal of Trauma, 69*(4), 855–860. Evidence Level III.

Egerod, I., Christensen, B. V., & Johansen, L. (2006). Trends in sedation practices in Danish intensive care units in 2003: A national survey. *Intensive Care Medicine, 32*(1), 60–66. Evidence Level IV.

Evans, D., & FitzGerald, M. (2002). Reasons for physically restraining patients and residents: A systematic review and content analysis. *International Journal of Nursing Studies, 39*(7), 735–743. Evidence Level I.

Evans, D., Wood, J., & Lambert, L. (2003). Patient injury and physical restraint devices: A systematic review. *Journal of Advanced Nursing, 41*(3), 274–282.

Fontaine, D. K. (1994). Nonpharmacologic management of patient distress during mechanical ventilation. *Critical Care Clinics, 10*(4), 695–708. Evidence Level VI.

Fraser, G. L., Riker, R. R., Prato, B. S., & Wilkins, M. L. (2001). The frequency and cost of patient-initiated device removal in the ICU. *Pharmacotherapy, 21*(1), 1–6. Evidence Level IV.

Frengley, J. D., & Mion, L. C. (1998). Physical restraints in the acute care setting: Issues and future direction. *Clinics in Geriatric Medicine, 14*(4), 727–743. Evidence Level V.

Happ, M. B. (2000). Preventing treatment interference: The nurse's role in maintaining technologic devices. *Heart & Lung: The Journal of Critical Care, 29*(1), 60–69. Evidence Level IV.

Inouye, S. K., Bogardus, S. T., Jr., Charpentier, P. A., Leo-Summers, L., Acampora, D., Holford, T. R., & Cooney, L. M., Jr. (1999). A multicomponent intervention to prevent delirium in hospitalized older patients. *The New England Journal of Medicine, 340*(9), 669–676. Evidence Level II.

Inouye, S. K., & Charpentier, P. A. (1996). Precipitating factors for delirium in hospitalized elderly persons. Predictive model and interrelationship with baseline vulnerability. *The Journal of American Medical Association, 275*(11), 852–857. Evidence Level IV.

Jones, C., Bäckman, C., Capuzzo, M., Flaaten, H., Rylander, C., & Griffiths, R. D. (2007). Precipitants of post-traumatic stress disorder following intensive care: A hypothesis generating study of diversity of care. *Intensive Care Medicine, 33*(6), 978–985. Evidence Level IV.

Kapadia, F. N., Bajan, K. B., & Raje, K. V. (2000). Airway accidents in intubated intensive care unit patients: An epidemiological study. *Critical Care Medicine, 28*(3), 659–664. Evidence Level IV.

Kapp, M. B. (1994). Physical restraints in hospitals: Risk management's reduction role. *Journal of Healthcare Risk Management, 14*(1), 3–8. Evidence Level VI.

Kapp, M. B. (1996). Physical restraint use in critical care: Legal issues. *AACN Clinical Issues, 7*(4), 579–584. Evidence Level VI.

Kapp, M. B. (1999). Physical restraint use in acute care hospitals: Legal liability issues. *Elder's Advisor, 1*(1), 1–10. Evidence Level VI.

Kaufman, S. R. (1994). Old age, disease, and the discourse on risk: Geriatric assessment in U.S. health care. *Medical Anthropology Quarterly, 8*(4), 430–447. Evidence Level VI.

Lamb, K. V., Minnick, A., Mion, L. C., Palmer, R., & Leipzig, R. (1999). Help the health care team release its hold on restraint. *Nursing Management, 30*(12), 19–23. Evidence Level IV.

Landefeld, C. S., Palmer, R. M., Kresevic, D. M., Fortinsky, R. H., & Kowal, J. (1995). A randomized trial of care in a hospital medical unit especially designed to improve the functional outcomes of acutely ill older patients. *The New England Journal of Medicine, 332*(20), 1338–1344. Evidence Level II.

Leape, L. L., & Berwick, D. M. (2005). Five years after To Err Is Human: What have we learned? *The Journal of American Medical Association, 293*(19), 2384–2390. Evidence Level VI.

Maccioli, G. A., Dorman, T., Brown, B. R., Mazuski, J. E., McLean, B. A., Kuszaj, J. M., . . . Society of Critical Care Medicine. (2003). Clinical practice guidelines for the maintenance of patient physical safety in the intensive care unit: Use of restraining therapies—American College of Critical Care Medicine Task Force 2001–2002. *Critical Care Medicine, 31*(11), 2665–2676. Evidence Level VI.

Marcin, J. P., Rutan, E., Rapetti, P. M., Brown, J. P., Rahnamayi, R., & Pretzlaff, R. K. (2005). Nurse staffing and unplanned extubation in the pediatric intensive care unit. *Pediatric Critical Care Medicine, 6*(3), 254–257. Evidence Level IV.

Mehta, S., Burry, L., Fischer, S., Martinez-Motta, J. C., Hallett, D., Bowman, D., . . . Canadian Critical Care Trials Group. (2006). Canadian survey of the use of sedatives, analgesics, and neuromuscular blocking agents in critically ill patients. *Critical Care Medicine, 34*(2), 374–380. Evidence Level IV.

Micek, S. T., Anand, N. J., Laible, B. R., Shannon, W. D., & Kollef, M. H. (2005). Delirium as detected by the CAM-ICU predicts restraint use among mechanically ventilated medical patients. *Critical Care Medicine, 33*(6), 1260–1265. Evidence Level IV.

Miles, S. H. (1993). Restraints and sudden death. *Journal of the American Gerietrics Society, 41*(9), 1013. Evidence Level V.

Minnick, A. F., Mion, L. C., Johnson, M. E., Catrambone, C., & Leipzig, R. (2007). Prevalence and variation of physical restraint use in acute care settings in the US. *Journal of Nursing Scholarship, 39*(1), 30–37. Evidence Level IV.

Minnick, A. F., Mion, L. C., Johnson, M. E., Catrambone, C., & Leipzig, R. (2008). The who and why's of side rail use. *Nursing Management, 39*(5), 36–44. Evidence Level IV.

Minnick, A. F., Mion, L. C., Leipzig, R., Lamb, K., & Palmer, R. M. (1998). Prevalence and patterns of physical restraint use in the acute care setting. *The Journal of Nursing Administration, 28*(11), 19–24. Evidence Level IV.

Mion, L. C., Fogel, J., Sandhu, S., Palmer, R. M., Minnick, A. F., Cranston, T., . . . Leipzig, R. (2001). Outcomes following physical restraint reduction programs in two acute care hospitals. *The Joint Commission Journal on Quality Improvement, 27*(11), 605–618. Evidence Level III.

Mion, L. C., Hazel, C., Cap, M., Fusilero, J., Podmore, M. L., & Szweda, C. (2006). Retaining and recruiting mature experienced nurses: A multicomponent organizational strategy. *The Journal of Nursing Administration, 36*(3), 148–154. Evidence Level IV.

Mion, L. C., Minnick, A. F., Leipzig, R., Catrambone, C. D., & Johnson, M. E. (2007). Patient-initiated device removal in intensive care units: A national prevalence study. *Critical Care Medicine, 35*(12), 2714–2720. Evidence Level IV.

Mion, L. C., Sandhu, S. K., Khan, R. H., Ludwick, R., Claridge, J. A., Pile, J., . . . Winchell, J. (2010). Effect of situational and clinical variables on the likelihood of physicians ordering physical restraint. *Journal of the American Geriatrics Society, 58*(7), 1279–1288. Evidence Level III.

Nirmalan, M., Dark, P. M., Nightingale, P., & Harris, J. (2004). Editorial IV: Physical and pharmacological restraint of critically ill patients: Clinical facts and ethical considerations. *British Journal of Anesthesia, 92*(6), 789–792. Evidence Level V.

O'Keeffe, S., Jack, C. L., & Lye, M. (1996). Use of restraints and bedrails in a British hospital. *Journal of the American Geriatrics Society, 44*(9), 1086–1088. Evidence Level IV.

Oliver, D., Healey, F., & Haines, T. P. (2010). Preventing falls and fall-related injuries in hospitals. *Clinics in Geriatric Medicine, 26*(4), 645–692. Evidence Level I.

Palmer, R. M., Landefeld, C. S., Kresevic, D., & Kowal, J. (1994). A medical unit for the acute care of the elderly. *Journal of the American Geriatrics Society, 42*(5), 545–552. Evidence Level VI.

Sandhu, S. K., Mion, L., Khan, R. H., Ludwick, R., Claridge, J., Pile, J. C., . . . Dietrich, M. S. (2010). Likelihood of ordering physical restraints: Influence of physician characteristics. *Journal of the American Geriatrics Society, 58*(7), 1272–1278. Evidence Level III.

Schafer, A. (1985). Restraints and the elderly: When safety and autonomy conflict. *Canadian Medical Association Journal, 132*(11), 1257–1260. Evidence Level VI.

Slomka, J., Agich, G. J., Stagno, S. J., & Smith, M. L. (1998). Physical restraint elimination in the acute care setting: Ethical considerations. *HEC Forum, 10*(3–4), 244–262. Evidence Level VI.

Tinetti, M. E., Inouye, S. K., Gill, T. M., & Doucette, J. T. (1995). Shared risk factors for falls, incontinence, and functional dependence. Unifying the approach to geriatric syndromes. *The Journal of the American Medical Association, 273*(17), 1348–1353. Evidence Level VI.

Tominaga, G. T., Rudzwick, H., Scannell, G., & Waxman, K. (1995). Decreasing unplanned extubations in the surgical intensive care unit. *American Journal of Surgery, 170*(6), 586–590. Evidence Level III.

Truong, A. D., Fan, E., Brower, R. G., & Needham, D. M. (2009). Bench-to-bedside review: Mobilizing patients in the intensive care unit—from pathophysiology to clinical trials. *Critical Care, 13*(4), 216. Evidence Level I.

Tzeng, H. M., & Yin, C. Y. (2008). Heights of occupied patient beds: A possible risk factor for inpatient falls. *Journal of Clinical Nursing, 17*(11), 1503–1509. Evidence Level IV.

U.S. Food and Drug Adminstration. (2006a). *A guide for modifying bed systems and using accessories to reduce the reisk of entrapment.* Retrieved from http://www.fda.gov/MedicalDevices/Productsand MedicalProcedures/GeneralHospitalDevicesandSupplies/HospitalBeds/ucm123673.htm

U.S. Food and Drug Adminstration. (2006b). FDA News: FDA issues guidance on hospital bed design to reduce patient entrapment2006.; *PO-36:FDA News.* Retrieved from http://www.fda .gov/bbs/topics/NEWS/2006/NEW01331.html

Wallen, K., Chaboyer, W., Thalib, L., & Creedy, D. K. (2008). Symptoms of acute posttraumatic stress disorder after intensive care. *American Journal of Critical Care, 17*(6), 534–544. Evidence Level IV.

Williams, C. C., & Finch, C. E. (1997). Physical restraint: Not fit for woman, man, or beast. *Journal of the American Geriatrics Society, 45*(6), 773–775. Evidence Level VI.

Wunsch, H., & Kress, J. P. (2009). A new era for sedation in ICU patients. *The Journal of the American Medical Association, 301*(5), 542–544. Evidence Level VI.

Pain Management

14

Ann L. Horgas, Saunjoo L. Yoon, and Mindy Grall

EDUCATIONAL OBJECTIVES

On completion of this chapter, the reader will be able to:

1. discuss the importance of effective pain management for older adults
2. describe best methods of assessing pain
3. discuss pharmacological and nonpharmacological strategies for managing pain
4. state at least two key points to include in education for patients and families

OVERVIEW

Pain is a very common experience among older adults. The prevalence of pain in older adults ranges from 50% to 86% (Horgas, Elliott, & Marsiske, 2009). Across all care settings and most specialty areas, nurses will interact with older adults (Herr, 2010). By the year 2030, it is projected that one in five US residents will be older than 65 years of age (Rosenthal & Kavic, 2004), and those older than age 85 represent the fastest growing segment of the population. In 2000, adults older than the age of 65 accounted for half of all hospital inpatient days (Rosenthal & Kavic, 2004). Furthermore, approximately 50% of admissions to the intensive care unit (ICU) are adults older than the age of 65 (McNicoll et al., 2003; Pisani, McNicoll, & Inouye, 2003). Thus, care of older adults is no longer restricted to nurses working in long-term care. Nurses in the acute care setting also need to be knowledgeable about the most effective strategies for assessing and managing pain in this population (Herr, 2010).

BACKGROUND AND STATEMENT OF PROBLEM

There are many causes of pain in older adults. *Acute pain* is typically associated with surgery, fractures, or trauma (Herr, Bjoro, Steffensmeier, & Rakel, 2006). *Persistent pain* (i.e.., pain that continues for more than 3–6 months) is most frequently associated

---

For description of Evidence Levels cited in this chapter, see Chapter 1, Developing and Evaluating Clinical Practice Guidelines: A Systematic Approach, page 7.

with musculoskeletal conditions such as osteoarthritis (The American Geriatrics Society [AGS] Panel on the Pharmacological Management of Persistent Pain in Older Persons, 2009). In 2000, it was estimated that almost 9 million surgeries were performed on older adults, including 1.25 million musculoskeletal surgeries (Herr, Titler, & Schilling, 2004). In addition, cancer is associated with significant pain for one third of patients with active disease and for two thirds of those with advanced disease (Reiner & Lacasse, 2006). In the acute care setting, older adults are therefore likely to have acute pain superimposed on persistent pain.

Pain has major implications for older adults' health, functioning, and quality of life (Wells, Pasero, & McCaffery, 2008). Pain is associated with depression, social withdrawal, sleep disturbances, impaired mobility, decreased activity engagement, and increased health care use (AGS Panel on the Pharmacological Management of Persistent Pain in Older Persons, 2009). Other geriatric conditions that can be exacerbated by pain include falls, cognitive decline, deconditioning, malnutrition, gate disturbances, and slowed rehabilitation (AGS Panel on the Pharmacological Management of Persistent Pain in Older Persons, 2009). In the hospital setting, older adults suffering from acute pain have been reported to be at increased risk for thromboembolism, hospital-acquired pneumonia, and functional decline (Wells et al., 2008). Unrelieved acute pain has also been implicated in the development of subsequent persistent pain (Desbiens, Mueller-Rizner, Connors, Hamel, & Wenger, 1997; Desbiens, Wu, et al., 1997). Unrelieved pain, thus, has important implications for physical, functional, and mental health among older adults.

Over the past decade, a substantial number of clinical and empirical efforts have been undertaken to improve the assessment and management of pain in older adults. For instance, in 2001, the Joint Commission on Accreditation of Healthcare Organizations (JCAHO) addressed pain assessment and management as part of the survey and accreditation process. The Joint Commission (2001) asserted that patients have the right to appropriate assessment and management of pain and declared pain as the fifth vital sign. This mandate exposed some of the challenges associated with assessing and managing pain in older adults in general, and in persons with dementia in particular. This, in part, spurred clinical and research activity to develop measures for assessing pain in older adults, particularly those with cognitive impairment. These behavioral measures have been reviewed in several published reports (Herr, Bjoro, & Decker, 2006; Herr, Bursch, Ersek, Miller, & Swafford, 2010), including a comprehensive chapter focusing specifically on pain assessment tools in the classic reference by Pasero and McCaffery (2011). In addition, there have been multiple clinical guidelines by leading scientific and clinical organizations including the AGS (AGS Panel on the Pharmacological Management of Persistent Pain in Older Persons, 2009; Hadjistavropoulos et al., 2007), the American Pain Society (Hadjistavropoulos et al., 2007), and the American Society for Pain Management Nursing (Herr, Coyne, et al., 2006). Links to these resources are included at the end of this chapter. Despite the Joint Commission mandate and the dissemination of clinical guidelines aimed at improving pain management, there is persistent evidence that pain remains ineffectively assessed and poorly managed in older adults across care settings (Herr, 2010; Herr et al., 2004; Horgas et al., 2009; Morrison, Magaziner, McLaughlin, et al., 2003; Titler et al., 2009).

The purpose of this chapter is to provide the best evidence on the assessment and treatment of pain in older adults, especially those with cognitive impairment. It is hoped that the information here can be used to establish, implement, and evaluate protocols in the acute care setting that will improve pain management for older adults.

ASSESSMENT OF PAIN

Pain is defined as a complex, multidimensional subjective experience with sensory, cognitive, and emotional dimensions (AGS Panel on the Pharmacological Management of Persistent Pain in Older Persons, 2009; Melzack & Casey, 1968). For clinical practice, Margo McCaffery's classic definition of pain is perhaps the most relevant. She states Pain is whatever the experiencing person says it is, existing whenever he says it does (McCaffery, 1968). This definition serves as a reminder that pain is highly subjective and that patients' self-report and description of pain is paramount in the pain assessment process. This definition, however, also highlights the difficulty inherent in pain assessment. There is no objective measure of pain; the sensation and experience of pain are completely subjective. As such, there is a tendency for clinicians to doubt patients' reports of pain. Pasero and McCaffery (2011) provided a comprehensive chapter on biases, misconceptions, and misunderstandings that hampered clinicians' assessment and treatment of patients who reported pain. These issues apply to patients across the life span, and led the authors to conclude the following:

> A veritable mountain of literature published during the past three decades attests to the undertreatment of pain. Much of this literature is consistent with the hypothesis that human beings, including health care providers in all societies, have strong tendencies or motivations to deny or discount pain, especially severe pain, and to avoid relieving the pain. Certainly we should struggle to identify and correct personal tendencies that lean to inadequate pain management, but this may not be a battle that can be won. Perhaps it is best to assume that there are far too many biases to overcome and that the best strategy is to establish policies and procedures that protect patients and ourselves from being victims of these influences. (p. 48)

Among older adults, there is persistent evidence that pain is underdetected and poorly managed among older adults (Herr, 2010; Horgas et al., 2009; Horgas & Tsai, 1998; Smith, 2005). There are a number of factors that contribute to this situation, including individual-based, caregiver-based, and organizational-based factors. Individual-based factors that may impair pain assessment include the following: (a) belief that pain is a normal part of aging, (b) concern of being labeled a hypochondriac or complainer, (c) fear of the meaning of pain in relation to disease progression or prognosis, (d) fear of narcotic addiction and analgesics, (e) worry about health care costs, and (f) a belief that pain is not important to health care providers (AGS Panel on Persistent Pain in Older Persons, 2002; Gordon et al., 2002). In addition, cognitive impairment is an important factor in reducing older adults' ability to report pain (Horgas et al., 2009; Smith, 2005).

Pain detection and management are also influenced by provider-based factors. Health care providers have been found to share the mistaken belief that pain is a part of the normal aging process and to avoid using opioids due to fear about potential addiction and adverse side effects (Pasero & McCaffery, 2011). Similarly, cognitive status influences providers' assessment and treatment of pain. Several studies have documented that cognitively impaired older adults were prescribed and administered significantly less analgesic medication than were cognitively intact older adults (Horgas & Tsai, 1998; Morrison, Magaziner, Gilbert, et al., 2003). This finding may reflect cognitively impaired adults' inability to recall and report the presence of pain to their health care providers. It may also reflect caregivers' inability to detect pain, especially among frail older adults. Health care providers should face the challenge of pain assessment by first systematically examining their own biases, beliefs, and behaviors about pain, and eliciting and understanding the challenges and beliefs their patients bring to the situation as well (Pasero & McCaffery, 2011).

Self-Reported Pain

There is no objective biological marker or laboratory test for the presence of pain. Thus, the patients' self-report is considered the gold standard for pain assessment (AGS Panel on Persistent Pain in Older Persons, 2002, AGS Panel on the Pharmacological Management of Persistent Pain in Older Persons, 2009). The first principle of pain assessment is to *ask* about the presence of pain in regular and frequent intervals (Pasero & McCaffery, 2011). It is important to allow older adults sufficient time to process the questions and formulate answers, especially when working with cognitively impaired older adults. It is also important to explore different words that patients may use synonymously with pain, such as discomfort or aching.

Pain intensity can be measured in various ways. Some commonly used tools include the numerical rating scale, the verbal descriptor scale, and the faces scale (Herr, 2002a). The *numerical rating scale* (NRS) is widely used in hospital settings. Patients are asked to rate the intensity of their pain on a 0–10 scale. The NRS requires the ability to discriminate differences in pain intensity and may be difficult for some older adults to complete. The *verbal descriptor scale*, however, has been specifically recommended for use with older adults (Herr, 2002a). This tool measures pain intensity by asking participants to select a word that best describes their present pain (e.g., no pain to worst pain imaginable). This measure has been found to be a reliable and valid measure of pain intensity and is reported to be the easiest to complete and the most preferred by older adults (Herr, Bjoro, & Decker, 2006). Pictures of faces are also used to measure pain intensity, especially among cognitively impaired older adults. The *Faces Pain Scale* (FPS), initially developed to assess pain intensity in children, consists of seven facial depictions, ranging from the least pain to the most pain possible (Herr, Bjoro, & Decker, 2006). Among adults, the FPS is considered more appropriate than other pictorial scales because the cartoon faces are not age-, gender-, or race-specific. However, the FPS has relatively low reliability and validity when used among older adults with cognitive impairment and is not recommended for use in this population (Herr, Bjoro, & Decker, 2006). See the Resources section for information on accessing these measurement tools.

Observed Pain Indicators

Dementia compromises older adults' ability to self-report pain. In patients with dementia, and other patients who cannot provide self-report, other assessment approaches must be used to identify the presence of pain. A hierarchical pain assessment approach is recommended that includes four steps:

1. attempt to obtain a self-report of pain;
2. search for an underlying cause of pain, such as surgery or a procedure;
3. observe for pain behaviors; and
4. seek input from family and caregivers (Herr, Coyne, et al., 2006; Wells et al., 2008).

If any of these steps are positive, the nurse should assume that pain is present and a trial of analgesics can be initiated. Pain behaviors should be observed before and after the analgesic trial in order to evaluate if the analgesic was effective or if a stronger dose is needed.

Observational techniques for pain assessment focus on behavioral or nonverbal indicators of pain (Hadjistavropoulos et al., 2007; Herr, Coyne, et al., 2006; Horgas et al., 2009). Behaviors such as guarded movement, bracing, rubbing the affected area, grimacing, painful noises or words, and restlessness are often considered pain behaviors (Horgas & Elliott, 2004; Horgas et al., 2009). In the acute care setting, vital signs are often considered physiological indicators of pain. It is important to note, however, that elevated vital signs are not considered a reliable indicator of pain, although they can be indicative of the need for pain assessment (Herr, Coyne, et al., 2006; Pasero & McCaffery, 2011).

A number of observational measures have been developed over the past decade. These behavioral tools are typically either pain behavior scales (scored by identifying the number and intensity of behaviors) or pain checklists (identifying the number and types of behaviors that individuals display, without intensity ratings; Wells et al., 2008). Although there is no perfect behavioral measure of pain, three specific tools have been recommended for use in patients who cannot self-report (Pasero & McCaffery, 2011). These are the Checklist of Nonverbal Pain Indicators (CNPI; Feldt, 2000), the Pain Assessment in Advanced Dementia (PAINAD) scale (Warden, Hurley, & Volicer, 2003), and the Pain Assessment Checklist for Seniors With Severe Dementia (PACSLAC; Fuchs-Lacelle & Hadjistavropoulos, 2004). A comprehensive review of these measures, as well as other similar tools, is available on the City of Hope website (see Resources section). In addition, the Hartford Institute for Geriatric Nursing provides online resources for pain assessment in older adults with dementia that include information on the PAINAD tool, and an instructional video on how to use it (see Resources section for link). Several caveats about observational tools must be noted: (a) the presence of these behaviors is suggestive of pain but is not always a reliable indicator of pain, and (b) the presence of pain behaviors does not provide information about the intensity of pain (Pasero & McCaffery, 2011; Wells et al., 2008). As such, pain behavior tools are one part of a comprehensive pain assessment.

In summary, pain assessment is a clinical procedure that can be hampered by many factors. Systematic and thorough assessment, however, is a critical first step in appropriately managing pain in older adults. Assessment issues are summarized in the recommended pain management protocol. The use of a standardized pain assessment tool is important in measuring pain. It enables health care providers to document their assessment, measure change in pain, evaluate treatment effectiveness, and communicate to other health care providers, the patient, and the family. Comprehensive pain assessment includes measures of self-reported pain and pain behaviors. Information from family and caregivers should also be obtained, although these data should be considered supplemental rather than definitive (Horgas & Dunn, 2001).

INTERVENTIONS AND CARE STRATEGIES

Managing pain in older adults can be a challenging process. The main goal is to maximize function and quality of life by minimizing pain whenever possible (Herr, 2010; Wells et al., 2008). Optimal pain treatment uses a multimodal approach, tailored to the patient, that combines pharmacological and nonpharmacological strategies (Wells et al., 2008). Pharmacological interventions are an integral component of pain management in older adults (Pasero & McCaffery, 2011). Important considerations regarding the use of pharmacological pain management must be taken into account, given the physiological changes that occur with aging. It should be emphasized that pharmaceutical pain management is often more imperative in older adults with dementia because their ability to participate in nonpharmacological pain management strategies may be limited by their cognitive capacity (Buffum, Hutt, Chang, Craine, & Snow, 2007).

When choosing pain strategies, consideration should be given to severity of pain because moderate and severe pain often require different modalities in order to provide adequate pain relief. Additionally, cognitive impairments are often confounded by visual and hearing impairments in older adults. Therefore, to optimize pain relief while minimizing the potential for poor outcomes, careful consideration should be given to an individual's ability to adhere to treatment (Pergolizzi et al., 2008).

Several excellent pain management guidelines and protocols have been developed for use in the management of pain in older adults. For instance, the AGS has recently updated their clinical practice guidelines for managing persistent pain in older adults (AGS Panel on the Pharmacological Management of Persistent Pain in Older Persons, 2009). The consensus statement by the World Health Organization (WHO) on the use of Step III opioids for chronic, severe pain in older adults provides detailed guidelines pertaining to the assessment of pain and use of opioids for cancer and non-cancer-related pain (Pergolizzi et al., 2008). In addition, there are other published guidelines for the assessment and management of pain in specific diseases, such as osteoarthritis (American Pain Society, 2002; American Pain Society Quality of Care Committee, 1995). Pasero and McCaffery (2011) also provide one of the most comprehensive guides for pain management, including a recently updated edition that addresses pain management in older adults. See Resources section of Protocol 14.1 for more information on accessing these resources.

Pharmacological Pain Treatment

Pain treatment with medications involves decision making based on multiple considerations. Ideally, it is a mutual process among health care providers, patients, and caregivers, with the goal of optimizing quality of life and functioning (Wells et al., 2008). An effective pain management strategy includes a careful discussion of risks versus benefits, frequent reviews of drug regimens used by older adults, and the establishment of clear goals of therapy with the patient. It is often a process of trial and error that aims to balance medication effectiveness with management of side effects.

Guiding principles for optimal pain management in older adults include the following components (Buffum et al., 2007; Gordon et al., 2005). First, the treatment of pain should be initiated immediately upon the detection of pain. Secondly, regularly scheduled (rather than "as-needed") dosing of pain medications should be employed. Additionally, multiple modalities for the evaluation of pain control should be used, including verbal, behavioral, and functional responses to pain medication. Pain medication should be titrated according to these responses, and a pain medication regimen should be chosen based on what is known about each individual patient. This includes the severity of cognitive impairment and how this affects the patient's ability to express pain, interaction of pain medications with other medications, and knowledge of pain medication side effects, such as constipation.

For individuals with cancer-related pain, the WHO provides a three-step analgesic ladder that has been widely used as a guide for treating pain in this population. Choices are made from three drug categories based on pain severity: the nonopioids, opioids, and adjuvant agents. Combinations of drugs are used because two or more drugs can treat different underlying pain mechanisms, different types of pain, and allow for smaller doses of each analgesic to be used, thus minimizing side effects. In 2008, the WHO established guidelines for the use of Step III opioids (buprenorphine, fentanyl, hydromorphone, methadone, morphine, and oxycodone) in older adults with cancer and noncancer pain (Pergolizzi et al., 2008). Their criteria for the selection of analgesics in older adults with cancer are based on the type of pain, efficacy of the medication, side-effect profile, potential for abuse, and interactions with other medications (Pergolizzi et al., 2008). These guidelines make clear that Step III opioids are the gold standard of treatment for cancer pain and are also efficacious in noncancer diseases. The authors point out, however, a dearth of specific studies investigating the use of these drugs in older adults.

Special Considerations for Administering Analgesics

When considering the addition of pain medication to an older, and potentially frail person's medication regimen, several issues must be evaluated. Confounding factors for medication side effects include comorbidities, the use of multiple medications, and drug-to-drug interactions (Klotz, 2009). Normal physiological changes that occur with aging, superimposed on comorbidities, place older adults at higher risk for side effects. Specific age-related changes influence the pharmacodynamics (mechanisms of drug action in the body) and pharmacokinetics (processes of drug absorption, distribution, metabolism, and elimination in the body; Klotz, 2009). Specific side effects to consider when prescribing and/or administering pain medications to the older adult include risks for sedation, mental status changes and cognition, balance, and gastrointestinal side effects—including bleeding and constipation (Buffum et al., 2007).

Recommendations for beginning pain medication treatment include starting at low doses and gradually titrating upward, while monitoring and managing side effects. The adage "start low and go slow" is often used. Titrate doses upward to desired effect using short-acting medications first, and consider using longer duration medications for long-lasting pain, once drug tolerability has been established. For most older adults, choose a drug with a short half-life and the fewest side effects if possible (Pasero & McCaffery, 2011; Wells et al., 2008).

Multiple drug routes are available for administration of pain medications. As long as patients are able to swallow safely, the oral route is the first choice because it is the least invasive and very effective. The onset of action is within 30 minutes to 2 hours. For more immediate pain relief, intravenous administration is recommended, particularly in the immediate postoperative period. Intramuscular injections should be avoided in older adults because of the potential for tissue injury and unpredictable absorption, and because they produce pain. Overall, adopting a preventive approach to pain management, whenever possible, is recommended. By treating pain before it occurs, less medication is required than to relieve it (Wells et al., 2008). Examples of pain prevention are around-the-clock dosing and dosing prior to a painful treatment or event.

Types of Analgesic Medications

The AGS has recently published updated guidelines for pain management in older adults (AGS Panel on the Pharmacological Management of Persistent Pain in Older Persons, 2009). Information on accessing these guidelines is included in the Resources section at the end of this chapter. The guidelines provide comprehensive information about managing persistent pain, but the recommendations apply to acute pain management as well. Thus, the reader is referred to these guidelines for more comprehensive information.

Nonopioid Medications. Acetaminophen is considered the drug of choice for mild-to-moderate pain in older adults (Herr, Bjoro, Steffensmeier, et al., 2006). It is recommended that the total daily dose should not exceed 4 g per day (maximum 3 g/day in frail elders). Because of the potential for hepatic toxicity, the maximum dosage should be reduced by 50%–75% in adults with impaired hepatic metabolism, renal disease, or a history of alcohol abuse (Herr, Bjoro, Steffensmeier, et al., 2006).

Nonsteroidal anti-inflammatory drugs (NSAIDs), commonly used to treat pain in the general population, are not recommended for use in persons older than the age of 75 (Kuehn, 2009). There are two types of NSAIDs: nonselective (e.g., ibuprofen, naproxen) and cyclooxygenase (COX)-2 selective inhibitors. Several of the COX-2 drugs have been removed from the market because of serious, life-threatening cardiovascular side effects, and those that remain available should be used with caution and only within the recommended dosages (AGS Panel on the Pharmacological Management of Persistent Pain in Older Persons, 2009).

NSAIDs are associated with serious cardiovascular and gastrointestinal side effects, and gastric damage is the most common side effect. All adults older than the age of 65 are considered to be at moderate risk for gastrointestinal side effects and should receive gastric protective therapy with proton pump inhibitor (Kuehn, 2009).

Opioid Medications. Opioid drugs (e.g., codeine and morphine) are effective at treating moderate-to-severe pain from multiple causes. According to the AGS (AGS Panel on the Pharmacological Management of Persistent Pain in Older Persons, 2009), opioid analgesics can be used safely and effectively in older adults if they are properly selected and monitored. All providers caring for older patients should prescribe opioids based on clearly defined therapeutic goals. Prescribing should occur based on serial attempts to reach these goals, with the lowest doses chosen based on efficacy and side effects.

Many older adults and health care providers are reluctant to use opioids because of fears of addiction, side effects, and intolerance. Potential side effects include nausea, pruritus, constipation, drowsiness, cognitive effects, and respiratory depression. The most serious side effect, respiratory depression, is rare and can be mitigated by slow dose escalation and careful monitoring for signs of sedation (AGS Panel on the Pharmacological Management of Persistent Pain in Older Persons, 2009; Wells et al., 2008). To prevent constipation, preventive measures should be initiated when the opioid is started (e.g., stool softeners, adequate fluid intake, moderate activity; AGS Panel on Persistent Pain in Older Persons, 2002).

Adjuvant Drugs. Adjuvant drugs are those drugs administered in conjunction with analgesics to relieve pain. They are often administered with nonopioids and opioids to achieve optimal pain control through additive analgesic effects or to enhance response to analgesics, especially for neuropathic pain (AGS Panel on Persistent Pain in Older Persons, 2002; Wells et al., 2008). Although tricyclic antidepressants (e.g., nortriptyline, desipramine) have shown dual effects on both pain and depression, they are inappropriate for pain management in older adults because of high rates of serious anticholinergic side effects (AGS Panel on the Pharmacological Management of Persistent Pain in Older Persons, 2009; Fick et al., 2003). With the advent of antidepressants that exert serotonin reuptake inhibition, and mixed serotonin and norepinephrine uptake inhibition, pain management with these types of medications has become more common in older adults because they are effective in the treatment of neuropathic pain and have a better side-effect profile (AGS Panel on the Pharmacological Management of Persistent Pain in Older Persons, 2009). Anticonvulsants (e.g., gabapentin) may be used as adjuvant drugs for neuropathic pain, such as trigeminal neuralgia and postherpetic neuralgia, and they have fewer side effects than tricyclic antidepressants (AGS Panel on the Pharmacological Management of Persistent Pain in Older Persons, 2009). Local anesthetics, such as lidocaine as a patch, gel, or cream, can be used as an additional treatment for the pain of postherpetic neuralgia.

Equianalgesia refers to equivalent analgesia effects. Understanding equianalgesic dosing (e.g., dose conversion chart, conversion ratio) improves prescribing practices for managing pain in older adults. Equianalgesic dosing charts provide lists of drugs and doses of commonly prescribed pain medications that are approximately equal in providing pain relief and can provide practical information for selecting appropriate starting doses when changing from one drug to another or finding optimal drug combinations (AGS Panel on the Pharmacological Management of Persistent Pain in Older Persons, 2009; Pasero & McCaffery, 2011; Pasero, Portenoy, McCaffery, 1999).

Drugs to Avoid in Older Adults

Some medications should be generally avoided in older adults because they are either ineffective for them or cause higher risk of having side effects. Meperidine (Demerol), ketorolac (Toradol), and pentazocine (Talwin) are considered inappropriate analgesic medications for older adults. These medications cause central nervous system side effects, including confusion or hallucinations, and may not be effective enough when administered at the commonly prescribed dose or may produce more side effects than positive analgesic effect (Fick et al., 2003). Additionally, sedatives, antihistamines, and antiemetics should be used with caution because of long duration of action, risk of falls, hypotension, anticholinergic effects, and sedating effects (Gordon et al., 2005).

Nonpharmacological Pain Treatment

Nondrug strategies are an important component of pain management. Many older adults report using several nonpharmacological modalities to manage pain (AGS Panel on Persistent Pain in Older Persons, 2002; Barry, Gill, Kerns, & Reid, 2005; Herr, 2002b). The most commonly reported nonpharmacological strategies used in the acute care setting were relaxation (e.g., breathing, meditation, imagery, music), activity modification, massage, and heat or cold application (Wells et al., 2008). Older adult patients should be encouraged to use nonpharmacological treatment in combination with pharmacological treatment.

Types of Nonpharmacological Treatment Strategies

Nonpharmacological pain treatment strategies generally fall into two major categories: physical pain relief modalities and psychological pain relief modalities. Physical pain relief modalities include, but are not limited to, transcutaneous electrical nerve stimulation (TENS), physical therapies, use of heat and cold, massage, and movement. Psychological pain relief modalities focus on changes in the person's perception of the pain and improvement of coping strategies (Rudy, Hanlon, & Markham, 2002). These include relaxation, distraction, guided imagery, and hypnosis. Cognitive behavioral treatment, meditation, and biofeedback are strategies used for persistent pain. Various types of dietary supplements are also commonly used nonpharmacological pain treatments among older adults. To date, a few of these nonpharmacological strategies have been empirically evaluated for their effectiveness in pain management (Wells et al., 2008).

For persistent pain, several physical strategies such as exercise, electrical stimulation (e.g., TENS), and low-level laser therapy have been evaluated, but the results are equivocal (Furlan, Imamura, Dryden, & Irvin, 2009). The AGS Panel on Exercise and Osteoarthritis (2001) provided guidelines of exercise prescriptions for older adults with osteoarthritis pain. Recommendations should be individualized based on the person's comorbidities, adherence, personal preference, and feasibility of exercise. Massage therapy may be effective to manage chronic low back pain and can be more beneficial when it is combined with education and exercise (Furlan et al., 2009). Despite many trials of tai chi, the effectiveness of this intervention for chronic pain in older adults is still inconclusive because of methodological issues in the studies (Hall, Maher, Latimer, & Ferreira, 2009). Electrical stimulation, including TENS, has shown significant benefits for shoulder pain after stroke (Price & Pandyan, 2001).

Psychological pain relief modalities, such as cognitive behavioral therapy, biofeedback, and meditation, are commonly used for persistent pain (Middaugh & Pawlick, 2002). Cognitive behavioral treatments, including relaxation, guided imagery, and meditation, have also shown significant improvement in pain and mobility due to osteoarthritis among older adults (Baird, Murawski, & Wu, 2010). In the acute care setting, relaxation, massage, and music are often used to help manage acute pain (Wells et al., 2008). Each of these nondrug approaches has demonstrated mixed results, largely because of individual patient preferences and methodological differences in how the studies were conducted. Thus, there is no conclusive evidence that these modalities relieve pain. Instead, they should be considered on an individualized basis, depending on patient preference and response, and as an adjunct to pharmacological treatment.

In summary, nonpharmacological treatments are widely used comfort measures to help manage pain. These approaches are challenging to study because it is difficult to find a convincing placebo and to control the dose of the treatment. In addition, studies have contributed inconsistent findings because of differences in study designs, inconsistent measures, and mixed intervention durations. Despite the lack of rigorous support for these nondrug approaches, older adults express interest in using these strategies to manage their pain (Dunn & Horgas, 2000; Herr, 2002b; Horgas & Elliott, 2004). Thus, nurses should consider all possible options for managing pain and discuss these approaches with their older adult patients.

Special Considerations of Using Nonpharmacological Treatment for Older Adults

Individuals vary widely in their preferences for and ability to use nonpharmacological interventions to manage pain. Spiritual and/or religious coping strategies, for instance, must be consistent with individual values and beliefs. Other strategies, such as guided imagery, biofeedback, or relaxation, may not be feasible for cognitively impaired older adults. Therefore, it is important for health care providers to consider a broad array of nonpharmacological pain management strategies and to tailor selections to the individual. It is also important to gain individual and family input about the use of home and folk remedies because use of herbals or home remedies is often not disclosed to health care providers and may result in negative drug–herb interactions (Yoon & Horne, 2001; Yoon, Horne, & Adams, 2004; Yoon & Schaffer, 2006).

IMPROVING PAIN MANAGEMENT IN CARE SETTINGS

Nurses have a critical role in assessing and managing pain. The promotion of comfort and relief of pain is fundamental to nursing practice and, as integral members of interdisciplinary health care teams, nurses must work collaboratively to effectively assess and treat pain. Given the prevalence of pain in older adults and the burgeoning aging population seeking care in our health care systems, this nursing role is vitally important. In addition, nurses have the primary responsibility to teach the patient and family about pain and how to manage it both pharmacologically and nonpharmacologically. As such, nurses must be knowledgeable about pain management in general, and about managing pain in older adults in particular. Moreover, nurses are responsible for basing their practice on the best evidence available, and helping to bridge the gap between evidence, recommendations, and clinical practice.

Nurses, however, must work within an organizational climate that supports and encourages efforts to improve pain management. These efforts must go beyond simply distributing guidelines and recommendations because this approach has not been effective (Dirks, 2010). Some quality improvement processes that should be considered in promoting improved pain management include the following (Dirks, 2010):

1. Facilities/institutions must demonstrate and maintain strong institutional commitment and leadership to improve pain management.
2. Facilities/institutions will establish an internal pain team of committed and knowledgeable staff who can lead quality improvement efforts to improve pain management practices.
3. Facilities/institutions must establish evidence of documentation of pain assessment, intervention, and evaluation of treatment effectiveness. This includes adding pain assessment and reassessment questions to flow sheets and electronic forms.
4. Facilities/institutions will provide evidence of using a multispecialty approach to pain management. This includes referral to specialists for specific therapies (e.g., psychiatry, psychology, physical therapy, interdisciplinary pain treatment specialists). Clinical pathways and decision support tools will be developed to improve referrals and multispecialty consultation.
5. Facilities/institutions will provide evidence of pain management resources for staff (e.g., educational opportunities; print materials, access to web-based guidelines and information).

CASE STUDY

Mrs. B. is a 93-year-old woman, living with her daughter in the community. She has been diagnosed with anxiety disorder, hypertension, and diabetes, and has a severe hearing problem. Recently, Mrs. B. fell in her bathroom and broke her right leg, which resulted in admission to the hospital. Prior to the fall, she typically walked around the neighborhood daily with her daughter. She now stays in her hospital bed with bruising, swelling, and pain in her right lower extremity. Her daughter has stayed with Mrs. B. at the bedside and is worried about her anxiety and pain. Mrs. B. is ordered oxycodone hydrochloride 5–10 mg every 6 hours orally or morphine sulfate 1 mg intravenously every 4 hours for pain as needed.

The nurse conducted an assessment of vital signs and completed a thorough pain assessment and mental status assessment, starting with self-report questions and asking the daughter for observations about her mother's response. The nurse explained the analgesic choices, including the types, routes, dosages, and potential side effects, to the patient and her daughter. When the nurse asked Mrs. B. and her daughter about their perspective of pain medications and their acceptable level of pain (pain goal), both expressed fear of taking opioid medications. After further discussions with the nurse, Mrs. B. and her daughter agreed to oxycodone 5 mg (instead of 10 mg) to manage Mrs. B.'s pain. They expressed that this was an informed decision—that Mrs. B.'s anxiety about pain medication was relieved, and that they felt relieved to be part of the pain treatment decision. Follow-up pain evaluation revealed that 5 mg of oxycodone did not relieve Mrs. B.'s pain. Another 5 mg of oxycodone was given to Mrs. B. for pain. Afterward, Mrs. B. rested comfortably. Her daughter was relieved to see her mother resting comfortably and felt more knowledgeable about her mother's pain experience and how to manage it.

SUMMARY

Pain is a significant problem for older adults, which has the potential to negatively impact independence, functioning, and quality of life. In the acute care setting, pain can negatively affect healing. In order for pain to be effectively managed, it must first be carefully and systematically assessed. Pain assessment in older adults should start with self-reported pain. It should also incorporate assessment of nonverbal pain behaviors and family input about usual pain responses and patterns, particularly in patients unable to communicate their pain. The use of established pain assessment/measurement tools is recommended. Pain treatment in older adults should be tailored to the type and severity of pain, with medications that can be safely used in older adults, or combined with nonpharmacological treatment for heightened effectiveness. Older adults, their families, and their care providers should be knowledgeable about pain and how to manage it. Thus, education is an important part of the process and should not be overlooked. Health care settings must emphasize the importance of effective pain management and empower their staff through resources, education, committed leadership, and organizational policies to provide high quality pain management to older adults. Pain management is a critical nursing role that can improve the health care experience and quality of life for older adults.

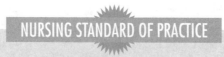

Protocol 14.1: Pain Management in Older Adults

I. STANDARD: All older adults will either be pain free or their pain will be controlled to a level that is acceptable to the patient and allows the person to maintain the highest level of functioning possible.

II. OVERVIEW: Pain, a common, subjective experience for many older adults, is associated with a number of acute (e.g., surgery, trauma) and chronic (e.g., osteoarthritis) conditions. Despite its prevalence, evidence suggests that pain is often poorly assessed and poorly managed, especially in older adults. Cognitive impairment due to dementia represents a particular challenge to pain management because older adults with these conditions may be unable to verbalize their pain. Nurses, an integral part of the interdisciplinary care team, need to understand the myths associated with pain management, including addiction and belief that pain is a normal result of aging, to provide optimal care and to educate patients and families about managing pain. Nurses must also examine their personal biases about pain and its management.

III. BACKGROUND
  A. Definitions
    1. *Pain*: Pain is defined as "an unpleasant sensory and emotional experience" (AGS, 2002, 2009) and also as "whatever the experiencing person says it is, existing whenever he says it does" (McCaffery, 1968). These definitions highlight the multidimensional and highly subjective nature of pain. Pain is usually characterized according to the duration of pain (e.g., acute vs. persistent) and the cause of pain (e.g., nociceptive vs. neuropathic). These definitions have implications for pain management strategies.
    2. *Acute pain*: Defines pain that results from injury, surgery, or trauma. It may be associated with autonomic activity such as tachycardia and diaphoresis. Acute pain is usually time limited and subsides with healing.
    3. *Persistent pain*: Defines pain that lasts for a prolonged period (usually more than 3–6 months) and is associated with chronic disease or injury (e.g., osteoarthritis; AGS, 2009). Persistent pain is not always time dependent, however, and can be characterized as pain that lasts longer than the anticipated healing time. Autonomic activity is usually absent, but persistent pain is often associated with functional loss, mood disruptions, behavior changes, and reduced quality of life.
    4. *Nociceptive pain*: The term refers to pain caused by stimulation of specific peripheral or visceral pain receptors. This type of pain results from disease processes (e.g., osteoarthritis), soft-tissue injuries (e.g., falls), and medical treatment (e.g., surgery, venipuncture, and other procedures). It is usually localized and responsive to treatment.
    5. *Neuropathic pain*: Refers to pain caused by damage to the peripheral or central nervous system. This type of pain is associated with diabetic neuropathies, postherpetic and trigeminal neuralgias, stroke, and chemotherapy treatment for cancer. It is usually more diffuse and less responsive to analgesic medications.

(continued)

Protocol 14.1: Pain Management in Older Adults *(cont.)*

B. Epidemiology
1. Approximately 50% of community-dwelling older adults and 85% of nursing home residents experience persistent pain.
2. More than one half of all inpatient hospital days are occupied by older adults, and more than 9 million surgeries are performed on older adults annually (Rosenthal & Kavic, 2004). Thus, pain is a common experience among older adults in the acute care setting (Herr, 2010).

C. Etiology
1. More than 80% of older adults have chronic medical conditions that are typically associated with pain, such as osteoarthritis and peripheral vascular disease.
2. Older adults often have multiple medical conditions, both chronic and/or acute, and may suffer from multiple types and sources of pain.

D. Significance
1. Pain has major implications for older adults' health, functioning, and quality of life. If unrelieved, pain is associated with the following (Pasero & McCaffery, 2011; Wells et al., 2008):
   a. Impaired immune function and healing
   b. Impaired mobility
   c. Postoperative complications related to immobility (e.g., thrombosis, embolus, pneumonia)
   d. Sleep disturbances
   e. Mental health symptoms (e.g., depression, anxiety)
   f. Withdrawal and decreased socialization
   g. Functional loss and increased dependency
   h. Exacerbation of cognitive impairment
   i. Increased health care utilization and costs
2. Nurses have a key role in pain management. The promotion of comfort and relief of pain is fundamental to nursing practice. Nurses need to be knowledgeable about pain in late life in order to provide optimal care, to educate patients and families, and to work effectively in interdisciplinary health care teams.
3. The Joint Commission requires regular and systematic assessment of pain in all hospitalized patients. Since older adults constitute a significant portion of the patient population in many acute care settings, nurses need to have the knowledge and skill to address specific pain needs of older adults.

IV. ASSESSMENT PARAMETERS
A. Assumptions (AGS, 2002, 2009; Herr, Coyne, et al., 2006; Pasero & McCaffery, 2011)
1. Most hospitalized older patients suffer from both acute and persistent pain.
2. Older adults with cognitive impairment experience pain but are often unable to verbalize it.
3. Both patients and health care providers have personal beliefs, prior experiences, insufficient knowledge, and mistaken beliefs about pain and pain management that (a) influence the pain management process, and (b) must be acknowledged before optimal pain relief can be achieved.

(continued)

Protocol 14.1: Pain Management in Older Adults *(cont.)*

4. Pain assessment must be regular, systematic, and documented in order to accurately evaluate treatment effectiveness.
5. Self-report is the gold standard for pain assessment.
6. Effective pain management requires an individualized approach.

B. Strategies for Pain Assessment
   1. Initial, quick pain assessment (Herr, Bjoro, Steffensmeier, et al., 2006)
      a. Assess older adults who present with acute pain of moderate-to-severe intensity or who appear to be in distress.
      b. Assess pain location, intensity, duration, quality, and onset.
      c. Assess vital signs. If changes in vital signs are absent, do not assume that pain is absent (Herr, Coyne, et al. 2006).
   2. Comprehensive pain assessment (AGS, 2009; Herr, Coyne, et al., 2006; Pasero & McCaffery, 2011)
      a. Review medical history, physical exam, and laboratory and diagnostic tests in order to understand sequence of events contributing to pain.
      b. Assess cognitive status (e.g., dementia, delirium), mental state (e.g., anxiety, agitation, depression), and functional status. If there is evidence of cognitive impairment, do not assume that the patient cannot provide a self-report of pain. Be prepared to augment self-report with observational measures and proxy report using the hierarchical approach.
      c. Assess present pain, including intensity, character, frequency, pattern, location, duration, and precipitating and relieving factors.
      d. Assess pain history, including prior injuries, illnesses, and surgeries; pain experiences; and pain interference with daily activities.
      e. Review medications, including current and previously used prescription drugs, over-the-counter drugs, and complementary therapies (including home remedies). Determine what pain control methods have previously been effective for the patient. Assess patient's attitudes and beliefs about pain and the use of analgesics, adjuvant drugs, and nonpharmacological treatments. Assess history of medication or alcohol abuse.
      f. Assess self-reported pain using a standardized measurement tool. Choose from published measurement tools and recall that older adults may have difficulty using 10-point numerical rating scales. Vertical verbal descriptor scales or faces scales may be more useful with older adults.
      g. Assess pain regularly and frequently, but at least every 4 hours. Monitor pain intensity after giving medications to evaluate effectiveness.
      h. Observe for nonverbal and behavioral signs of pain, such as facial grimacing, withdrawal, guarding, rubbing, limping, shifting of position, aggression, agitation, depression, vocalizations, and crying. Also watch for changes in behavior from the patient's usual patterns.
      i. Gather information from family members about the patient's pain experiences. Ask about the patient's verbal and nonverbal/behavioral expressions of pain, particularly in older adults with dementia.
      j. When pain is suspected but assessment instruments or observation is ambiguous, institute a clinical trial of pain treatment (i.e., in persons with dementia). If symptoms persist, assume pain is unrelieved and treat accordingly.

(continued)

Protocol 14.1: Pain Management in Older Adults *(cont.)*

V. NURSING CARE STRATEGIES (AGS, 2009; Hadjistavropoulos et al., 2007; Herr, Bjoro, Steffensmeier, et al., 2006; Herr, Coyne, et al., 2006, Wells et al., 2008)

A. General Approach
  1. Pain management requires an individualized approach.
  2. Older adults with pain require comprehensive, individualized plans that incorporate personal goals, specify treatments, and address strategies to minimize the pain and its consequences on functioning, sleep, mood, and behavior.

B. Pain Prevention
  1. Develop a written pain treatment plan upon admission to the hospital, or prior to surgery or treatments. Help the patient to set realistic pain treatment goals, and document the goals and plan.
  2. Assess pain regularly and frequently to facilitate appropriate treatment.
  3. Anticipate and aggressively treat for pain before, during, and after painful diagnostic and/or therapeutic treatments. Administer analgesics 30 minutes prior to activities.
  4. Educate patients, families, and other clinicians to use analgesic medications prophylactically prior to and after painful procedures.
  5. Educate patients and families about pain medications, their side effects, adverse effects, and issues of addiction, dependence, and tolerance.
  6. Educate patients to take medications for pain on a regular basis and to avoid allowing pain to escalate.
  7. Educate patients, families, and other clinicians to use nonpharmacological strategies to manage pain, such as relaxation, massage, and the use of heat and cold.

C. Treatment Guidelines
  1. Pharmacological (AGS, 2009; Pasero & McCaffery, 2011)
     a. Administer pain drugs on a regular basis to maintain therapeutic levels. Use PRN (as needed) medications for breakthrough pain.
     b. Document treatment plan to maintain consistency across shifts and with other care providers.
     c. Use equianalgesic dosing to obtain optimal pain relief and to minimize side effects.
     d. For postoperative pain, choose the least invasive route. Intravenous analgesics are the first choice after major surgery. Avoid intramuscular injections. Transition from parenteral medications to oral analgesics when the patient has oral intake.
     e. Choose the correct type of analgesic. Use opioids for treating moderate-to-severe pain and nonopioids for mild-to-moderate pain. Select the analgesic based on thorough medical history, comorbidities, other medications, and history of drug reactions.
     f. Among nonopioid medications, acetaminophen is the preferred drug for treating mild-to-moderate pain. Guidelines recommend not exceeding 4 g per day (maximum 3 g/day in frail elders). The maximum dose should be reduced to 50%–75% in adults with reduced hepatic function or history of alcohol abuse.

(continued)

Protocol 14.1: Pain Management in Older Adults *(cont.)*

    g. The other major class of nonopioid medications, nonsteroidal anti-inflammatory drugs (NSAIDs), should be used with caution in older adults. Monitor for gastrointestinal (GI) bleeding and consider giving with a proton pump inhibitor to reduce gastric irritation. Also monitor for bleeding, nephrotoxicity, and delirium.

    h. Older adults are at increased risk for adverse drug reactions due to age- and disease-related changes in pharmacokinetics and pharmacodynamics. Monitor medication effects closely to avoid overmedication or undermedication and to detect adverse effects. Assess hepatic and renal functioning.

  2. Nonpharmacological (Pasero & McCaffery, 2011; Wells et al., 2008)

    a. Investigate older patients' attitudes and beliefs about, preference for, and experience with nonpharmacological pain treatment strategies.

    b. Tailor nonpharmacological techniques to the individual.

    c. Cognitive behavioral strategies focus on changing the person's perception of pain (e.g., relaxation therapy, education, distraction) and may not be appropriate for cognitively impaired persons.

    d. Physical pain relief strategies focus on promoting comfort and altering physiologic responses to pain (e.g., heat, cold, TENS units) and are generally safe and effective.

D. Follow-up Assessment

  1. Monitor treatment effects within 1 hour of administration, and at least every 4 hours.

  2. Evaluate patient for pain relief and side effects of treatment.

  3. Document patient's response to treatment effects.

  4. Document treatment regimen in patient care plan to facilitate consistent implementation.

VI. EXPECTED OUTCOMES

A. Patient

  1. Patient will be either pain free or pain will be at a level that the patient judges as acceptable.

  2. Patient maintains highest level of self-care, functional ability, and activity level possible.

  3. Patient experiences no iatrogenic complications, such as falls, GI upset/bleeding, or altered cognitive status.

B. Nurse

  1. The nurse will demonstrate evidence of ongoing and comprehensive pain assessment.

  2. The nurse will document evidence of prompt and effective pain management interventions.

  3. The nurse will document systematic evaluation of treatment effectiveness.

  4. The nurse will demonstrate knowledge of pain management in older patients, including assessment strategies, pain medications, nonpharmacological interventions, and patient/family education.

(continued)

Protocol 14.1: Pain Management in Older Adults *(cont.)*

C. Institution (Dirks, 2010)
  1. Facilities/institutions will maintain strong institutional commitment and leadership to improve pain management. Evidence of institutional commitment include:
      a. Providing adequate resources (including compensation for staff education and time; necessary materials)
      b. Clear communication of how better pain management is congruent with organizational goals
      c. Establishment of policies and standard operating procedures for the organization
      d. Requiring clear accountability for outcomes
  2. Facilities/institutions will establish an internal pain team of committed and knowledgeable staff who can lead quality improvement efforts to improve pain management practices.
  3. Facilities/institutions will require evidence of documentation of pain assessment, intervention, and evaluation of treatment effectiveness. This includes adding pain assessment and reassessment questions to flow sheets and electronic forms.
  4. Facilities/institutions will provide evidence of using a multispecialty approach to pain management. This includes referral to specialists for specific therapies (e.g., psychiatry, psychology, physical therapy, interdisciplinary pain treatment specialists). Clinical pathways and decision support tools will be developed to improve referrals and multispecialty consultation.
  5. Facilities/institutions will provide evidence of pain management resources for staff (e.g., educational opportunities; print materials, access to web-based guidelines and information).

RESOURCES

Pain Assessment and Management

Hartford Institute for Geriatric Nursing: Try This Series: Assessing Pain in Older Adults.
http://www.consultgerirn.org/resources

American Geriatrics Society Guideline on the Management of Persistent Pain in Older Adults.
http://www.americangeriatrics.org/files/documents/2009_Guideline.pdf

Agency for Healthcare Research and Quality National Clinical Guideline Clearinghouse.
http://www.guideline.gov/content.aspx?id=10198

American Association of Pain Management Nurses (ASPMN): Geriatric Pain Assessment: Self-Directed Learning.
https://www.commercecorner.com/aspmn/productlist1.aspx

American Pain Society: Pain Guidelines and Online Resource Centers.
http://www.ampainsoc.org/library/principles.htm
http://www.ampainsoc.org/resources/clinician1.htm

American Medical Directors Association (AMDA: Clinical Practice Guideline: Pain Management in the Long-Term Care Setting.
http://www.amda.com/tools/cpg/chronicpain.cfm

City of Hope: State of the Art Review of Tools for Assessing Pain in Nonverbal Older Adults.
http://prc.coh.org//elderly.asp

American Association of Pain Management Nurses (ASPMN: Pain Assessment in the Non-verbal Patient: Position Statement with Clinical Practice Recommendations.
http://aspmn.org/Organization/position_papers.htm

Medical College of Wisconsin: Improving Pain Management in Long-Term Care Facilities
http://www2.edc.org/lastacts/archives/archivesJan01/featureinn.asp

Measurement Tools

See City of Hope website listed previously for comprehensive review of tools for persons with dementia.

REFERENCES

American Geriatrics Society Panel on Exercise and Osteoarthritis. (2001). Exercise prescription for older adults with osteoarthritis pain: Consensus practice recommendations. A supplement to the AGS Clinical Practice Guidelines on the management of chronic pain in older adults. *Journal of the American Geriatrics Society, 49*(6), 808–823. Evidence Level I.

American Geriatrics Society Panel on Persistent Pain in Older Persons. (2002). The management of persistent pain in older persons. *Journal of the American Geriatrics Society, 50,* S205–S224. Evidence Level V.

American Geriatrics Society Panel on the Pharmacological Management of Persistent Pain in Older Persons. (2009). Pharmacological management of persistent pain in older persons. *Journal of the American Geriatriatrics Society, 57*(8), 1331–1346. Evidence Level I.

American Pain Society. (2002). *Guideline for the management of pain in osteoarthritis, rheumatoid arthritis, and juvenile chronic arthritis.* Glenview, IL: American Pain Society. Evidence Level I.

American Pain Society Quality of Care Committee. (1995). Quality improvement guidelines for the treatment of acute pain and cancer pain. *Journal of the American Medical Association, 274*(23), 1874–1880. Evidence Level I.

Baird, C. L., Murawski, M. M., & Wu, J. (2010). Efficacy of guided imagery with relaxation for osteoarthritis symptoms and medication intake. *Pain Management Nursing, 11*(1), 56–65. Evidence Level III.

Barry, L. C., Gill, T. M., Kerns, R. D., & Reid, M. C. (2005). Identification of pain-reduction strategies used by community-dwelling older persons. *The Journals of Gerontology, Series A: Medical Sciences, 60*(12), 1569–1575. Evidence Level IV.

Buffum, M. D., Hutt, E., Chang, V. T., Craine, M. H., & Snow, A. L. (2007). Cognitive impairment and pain management: Review of issues and challenges. *Journal of Rehabilitation Research and Development, 44*(2), 315–330. Evidence Level V.

Desbiens, N. A., Mueller-Rizner, N., Connors, A. F., Jr., Hamel, M. B., & Wenger, N. S. (1997). Pain in the oldest-old during hospitalization and up to one year later. HELP Investigators. Hospitalized Elderly Longitudinal Project. *Journal of the American Geriatrics Society, 45*(10), 1167–1172. Evidence Level IV.

Desbiens, N. A., Wu, A. W., Alzola, C., Mueller-Rizner, N., Wenger, N. S., Connors, A. F., Jr., . . . Phillips, R. S. (1997). Pain during hospitalization is associated with continued pain six months later in survivors of serious illness. The SUPPORT Investigators. Study to Understand Prognoses and Preferences for Outcomes and Risks of Treatments. *American Journal of Medicine, 102*(3), 269–276. Evidence Level IV.

Dirks, F. (2010). A national framework for geriatric home care excellence. *American Journal of Nursing, 110*(8), 64. Evidence Level VI.

Dunn, K. S., & Horgas, A. L. (2000). The prevalence of prayer as a spiritual self-care modality in elders. *Journal of Holistic Nursing, 18*(4), 337–351. Evidence Level IV.

Feldt, K. S. (2000). The checklist of nonverbal pain indicators (CNPI). *Pain Management Nursing, 1*(1), 13–21. Evidence Level V.

Fick, D. M., Cooper, J. W., Wade, W. E., Waller, J. L., Maclean, J. R., & Beers, M. H. (2003). Updating the Beers criteria for potentially inappropriate medication use in older adults: Results of a US consensus panel of experts. *Archives of Internal Medicine, 163*(22), 2716–2724. Evidence Level I.

Fuchs-Lacelle, S., & Hadjistavropoulos, T. (2004). Development and preliminary validation of the pain assessment checklist for seniors with limited ability to communicate (PACSLAC). *Pain Management Nursing, 5*(1), 37–49. Evidence Level IV.

Furlan, A. D., Imamura, M., Dryden, T., & Irvin, E. (2009). Massage for low back pain: An updated systematic review within the framework of the Cochrane Back Review Group. *Spine, 34*(16), 1669–1684. Evidence Level I.

Gordon, D. B., Dahl, J. L., Miaskowski, C., McCarberg, B., Todd, K. H., Paice, J. A. . . . Carr, D. B. (2005). American pain society recommendations for improving the quality of acute and cancer pain management: American Pain Society Quality of Care Task Force. *Archives of Internal Medicine, 165*(14), 1574–1580. Evidence Level I.

Gordon, D. B., Pellino, T. A., Miaskowski, C., McNeill, J. A., Paice, J. A., Laferriere, D., & Bookbinder, M. (2002). A 10-year review of quality improvement monitoring in pain management: Recommendations for standardized outcome measures. *Pain Management Nursing, 3*(4), 116–130. Evidence Level I.

Hadjistavropoulos, T., Herr, K.; Turk, D. C., Fine, P. G., Dworkin, R. H., Helme, R., . . . Williams, J. (2007). An interdisciplinary expert consensus statement on assessment of pain in older persons. *The Clinical Journal of Pain, 23*(Suppl 1):S1–S43. Evidence Level I.

Hall, A., Maher, C., Latimer, J., & Ferreira, M. (2009). The effectiveness of Tai Chi for chronic musculoskeletal pain conditions: A systematic review and meta-analysis. *Arthritis and Rheumatism, 61*(6), 717–724. Evidence Level I.

Herr, K. (2002a). Chronic pain: Challenges and assessment strategies. *Journal of Gerontological Nursing, 28*(1), 20–27. Evidence Level V.

Herr, K. (2002b). Chronic pain in the older patient: Management strategies. 2. *Journal of Gerontological Nursing, 28*(2), 28–34. Evidence Level V.

Herr, K. (2010). Pain in the older adult: An imperative across all health care settings. *Pain Management Nursing, 11*(2 Suppl), S1–S10. Evidence Level VI.

Herr, K., Bjoro, K., & Decker, S. (2006). Tools for assessment of pain in nonverbal older adults with dementia: A state-of-the-science review. *Journal of Pain and Symptom Management, 31*(2), 170–192. Evidence Level I.

Herr, K., Bjoro, K., Steffensmeier, J. J., & Rakel, B. (2006). *Acute pain management in older adults.* Iowa City, IA: University of Iowa Gerontological Nursing Interventions Research Center, Research Translation and Dissemination Core. Evidence Level I.

Herr, K., Bursch, H., Ersek, M., Miller, L. L., & Swafford, K. (2010). Use of pain-behavioral assessment tools in the nursing home: Expert consensus recommendations for practice. *Journal of Gerontological Nursing, 36*(3), 18–29; quiz 30–11. Evidence Level VI.

Herr, K., Coyne, P. J., Key, T., Manworren, R., McCaffery, M., Merkel, S., . . . Wild, L.; American Society for Pain Management Nursing. (2006). Pain assessment in the nonverbal patient: Position statement with clinical practice recommendations. *Pain Management Nursing, 7*(2):44–52. Evidence Level I.

Herr, K., Titler, M. G., Schilling, M. L., Marsh, J. L., Xie, X., Ardery, G., . . . Everett, L. Q. (2004). Evidence-based assessment of acute pain in older adults: Current nursing practices and perceived barriers. *The Clinical Journal of Pain, 20*(5), 331–340. Evidence Level V.

Horgas, A. L., & Dunn, K. (2001). Pain in nursing home residents: Comparison of residents' self-report and nursing assistants' perceptions. *Journal of Gerontological Nursing, 27*(3), 44–53. Evidence Level IV.

Horgas, A. L., & Elliott, A. F. (2004). Pain assessment and management in persons with dementia. *The Nursing Clinics of North America, 39*(3), 593–606. Evidence Level V.

Horgas, A. L., Elliott, A. F., & Marsiske, M. (2009). Pain assessment in persons with dementia: Relationship between self-report and behavioral observation. *Journal of the American Geriatrics Society, 57*(1), 126–132. Evidence Level III.

Horgas, A. L., & Tsai, P. F. (1998). Analgesic drug prescription and use in cognitively impaired nursing home residents. *Nursing Research, 47*(4), 235–242. Evidence Level IV.

Joint Commission on Accreditation of Healthcare Organizations. (2001). *Accreditation manual or hospitals.* Oakbrook Terrace, IL: Author. Evidence Level VI.

Klotz, U. (2009). Pharmacokinetics and drug metabolism in the elderly. *Drug Metabolism Reviews, 41*(2), 67–76. Evidence Level V.

Kuehn, B. M. (2009). New pain guideline for older patients: Avoid NSAIDs, consider opioids. *The Journal of American Medical Association, 302*(1), 19. Evidence Level V.

McCaffery, M. (1968). *Nursing practice theories related to cognition, bodily pain, and man-environmental interaction.* Los Angeles, CA: UCLA Students Store. Evidence Level V.

McNicoll, L., Pisani, M. A., Zhang, Y., Ely, E. W., Siegel, M. D., & Inouye, S. K. (2003). Delirium in the intensive care unit: Occurrence and clinical course in older patients. *Journal of the American Geriatrics Society, 51*(5):591–598. Evidence Level IV.

Melzack, R., & Casey, K. L. (1968). Sensory, motivational, and central control determinants of pain: A new conceptual model. In D. R. Kenshalo (Ed.), *The skin senses* (pp. 423–443). Springfield, IL: Charles C. Thomas Press. Evidence Level IV.

Middaugh, S. J., & Pawlick, K. (2002). Biofeedback and behavioral treatment of persistent pain in the older adult: A review and a study. *Applied Psychophysiology and Biofeedback, 27*(3), 185–202. Evidence Level III.

Morrison, R. S., Magaziner, J., Gilbert, M., Koval, K. J., McLaughlin, M. A., Orosz, G., . . . Siu, A. L. (2003). Relationship between pain and opioid analgesics on the development of delirium following hip fracture. *The Journals of Gerontology Series A: Biological Sciences and Medical Sciences, 58*(1), 76–81. Evidence Level IV.

Morrison, R. S., Magaziner, J., McLaughlin, M. A., Orosz, G., Silberzweig, S. B., Koval, K. J., & Siu, A. L. (2003). The impact of post-operative pain on outcomes following hip fracture. *Pain, 103*(3), 303–311. Evidence Level IV.

Pasero, C., & McCaffery, M. (2011). *Pain assessment and pharmacologic management.* St. Louis, MO: Mosby Elsevier. Evidence Level VI.

Pasero, C., Portenoy, R. K., & McCaffery, M. (1999). Opioid analgesics. In M. McCaffery & C. Pasero (Eds.), *Pain clinical manual* (2nd ed., pp. 161–299). St. Louis, MO: Mosby. Evidence Level V.

Pergolizzi, J., Böger, R. H., Budd, K., Dahan, A., Erdine, S., Hans, G., . . . Sacerdote, P. (2008). Opioids and the management of chronic severe pain in the elderly: Consensus statement of an International Expert Panel with focus on the six clinically most often used World Health Organization Step III opioids (buprenorphine, fentanyl, hydromorphone, methadone, morphine, oxycodone). *Pain Practice, 8*(4), 287–313. Evidence Level I.

Pisani, M. A., McNicoll, L., & Inouye, S. K. (2003). Cognitive impairment in the intensive care unit. *Clinics in Chest Medicine, 24*(4), 727–737. Evidence Level V.

Price, C. I., & Pandyan, A. D. (2001). Electrical stimulation for preventing and treating post-stroke shoulder pain: A systematic Cochrane review. *Clinical Rehabilitation, 15*(1), 5–19. Evidence Level I.

Reiner, A., & Lacasse, C. (2006). Symptom correlates in the gero-oncology population. *Seminars in Oncology Nursing, 22*(1), 20–30. Evidence Level IV.

Rosenthal, R. A., & Kavic, S. M. (2004). Assessment and management of the geriatric patient. *Critical Care Medicine, 32*(4 Suppl), S92–S105. Evidence Level V.

Rudy, T. E., Hanlon, R. B., & Markham, J. R. (2002). Psychosocial issues and cognitive-behavioral therapy: From theory to practice. In D. K. Weiner, K. Herr, & T. E. Rudy (Eds), *Persistent pain in older adults: An interdisciplinary guide for treatment* (58–94). New York, NY: Springer. Evidence Level V.

Smith, M. (2005). Pain assessment in nonverbal older adults with advanced dementia. *Perspective in Psychiatric Care, 41*(3), 99–113. Evidence Level I.

Titler, M. G., Herr, K., Brooks, J. M., Xie, X. J., Ardery, G., Schilling, M. L., . . . Clarke W. R. (2009). Translating research into practice intervention improves management of acute pain in older hip fracture patients. *Health Services Research, 44*(1), 264–287. Evidence Level V.

Warden, V., Hurley, A. C., & Volicer, L. (2003). Development and psychometric evaluation of the Pain Assessment in Advanced Dementia (PAINAD) scale. *Journal of the American Medical Directors Association, 4*(1), 9–15. Evidence Level IV.

Wells, N., Pasero, C., & McCaffery, M. (2008). Improving the quality of care through pain assessment and management. In R. G. Hughes (Ed), *Patient safety and quality: An evidence-based handbook for nurses* (Vol. 1, pp. 469–489). Rockville, MD: Agency for Healthcare Research and Quality.

Yoon, S. J., & Horne, C. H. (2001). Herbal products and conventional medicines used by community-residing older women. *Journal of Advance Nursing, 33*(1), 51–59. Evidence Level IV.

Yoon, S. L., Horne, C. H., & Adams, C. (2004). Herbal product use by African American older women. *Clinical Nursing Research, 13*(4), 271–288. Evidence Level IV.

Yoon, S. L., & Schaffer, S. D. (2006). Herbal, prescribed, and over-the-counter drug use in older women: prevalence of drug interactions. *Geriatric Nursing, 27*(2), 118–129. Evidence Level IV.

Fall Prevention: Assessment, Diagnoses, and Intervention Strategies

15

Deanna Gray-Miceli and Patricia A. Quigley

EDUCATIONAL OBJECTIVES

On the completion of this chapter, the reader should be able to:

1. evaluate the older adult patient who is unsafe and at risk for fall and injury, as well as corresponding nursing interventions to minimize risks for injury among fall-prone hospitalized older adults
2. design nursing plans of care aimed at reducing serious injuries among older adults prone to falls based on the suspected fall type
3. use findings from a comprehensive postfall assessment to develop an individualized plan of nursing care for the secondary prevention of recurrent falls
4. mobilize institutional resources to provide a collaborative interprofessional falls or safety team
5. use the latest evidence innovations in practice to champion a nurse-led fall prevention intervention to prevent recurrent falls

OVERVIEW

Two specific aims of any effort in acute care institutions to reduce falls among older adults are (a) to reduce risk of injury from falls including fatal falls and (b) to champion an interprofessional fall prevention program to prevent patient falls. Both aims seek to promote improvements in patient safety by reducing preventable falls through system-wide solutions whenever possible (Joint Commission National Patient Safety Goals, 2006).

Overall, across *all* patient settings, evidence exists that fall prevention programs are effective. The RAND report cites, from a meta-analysis of 20 randomized clinical trials (among all patient settings, but mostly long-term care), that fall prevention programs reduced either the number of older adults who fell or the monthly rate of falling (U.S. Department of Health and Human Services, 2004). Hospital-based studies are emerging to provide solid scientific evidence of the effect of fall prevention programs on fall rates and, more importantly, fall-related injuries.

Oliver and colleagues (2007) have produced a compilation of the best evidence of practice innovations used by hospitals across the United States and the United Kingdom, and their outcome effect on falls and injury reduction. After careful scrutiny (Oliver et al., 2007), they have identified the key components guiding multifactorial interventions used to prevent falls in hospitals (i.e., education, use of toileting schedules, and alarm devices). Oliver et al.'s (2007) approach has analyzed and weighed the individual intervention—within the multifactorial intervention—into its constitute parts, thereby minimizing any methodological design issues (Oliver, Healy, & Haines, 2010). Many of these multifactorial interventions are targeted to education initiatives, environmental issues, or seek to improve equipment implicated in falls.

Before beginning any discussion on specific individual fall prevention intervention, the acute care nurse must realize one's role in championing a team effort in fall and injury prevention. Professional nurses are uniquely poised because they know the biopsychosocial and functional needs of their patients and situational contexts of how patients respond to the acute care environment. Such individual knowledge of each patient they care for positions the professional nurse, along with leadership skill, in a unique position to champion teamwork on their acute care unit.

BACKGROUND AND STATEMENT OF PROBLEM

The Importance of Fall and Injury Prevention in Acute Care

Many of the health care outcomes from falls, such as injury and/or functional decline, typically strike those patients older than age 85 years *and* can be prevented. The most serious outcome is a *fatality*. The National Center for Injury Prevention and Control (NCIPC) tabulates fatal falls across the ages averaging more than 14,000 fatalities among seniors. Fatal falls rank as the seventh leading cause of unintentional injury–fatality among older adults (Centers for Disease Control and Prevention [CDC], NCIPC, 2007). The fatal fall incidence increases with age—those older than age 85 years being the most vulnerable. Hospital in-patient falls are estimated to vary according to the unit, with one study reporting 3.1 falls per 1,000 patient-days (Fischer et al., 2005). In this study, bleeding or laceration occurred in 53.6%, fracture or dislocation in 15.9%, and hematoma or contusion in 13%. Other serious injuries documented from falls included hip fracture and traumatic brain injury (TBI), among others.

ASSESSMENT OF THE PROBLEM

Deciding Risk for a Serious Fall-Related Injury

"One look is worth a thousand words, but don't forget to look more than once"

Diagnosis: Impaired consciousness

Important characteristics of level of alertness are the patient's ability to sustain attention, and in determining if they are awake or not. If impairment exists in level of consciousness, the patient is at risk for injury; thus, any postoperative surgical patient is at greatest risk for injury from a fall. An important factor in determining a patient's safety within his or her environment will be if he or she can process information and execute simple one-, two-, and/or three-stage commands. The ability to execute a command is contingent on level of consciousness, behavior, and cognition.

Traditionally, level of consciousness is assessed and written as alert and oriented x 3, referring to person, place, and time. The ability of the person to sustain attention can be gauged by observation of his or her ability (or not) to execute a command, for instance, following instructions. This type of assessment is typically routine when the nurse first greets the patient and is beyond a simple assessment of whether or not the patient is awake, "alert," and oriented and can say, "Hello." All of these determinations are critical factors in the nurse's judgment of patient safety. After the first assessment, the nurse should reassess the older patient frequently because level of consciousness can change quickly.

Critical Thinking Points

How many times do nurses reassess their own judgment and make changes accordingly to their original impressions? Typically, in fall risk assessments, the reassessment is made each shift and at the time of transition to another unit. Although a patient may "look to be safe" resting in bed, they may be totally unsafe when they sit up on the side of the bed or take a step to walk. Therefore, the situational context is very important to note.

Consider these points: While patients are safe in bed, are they also safe to be unsupervised alone? Are they safe to sit, transfer, or walk unassisted?

All of these nursing observations and ultimate clinical determination of patient safety hinge on the older patient's level of consciousness, level of alertness, as well as behavior and current cognitive capabilities.

Level of consciousness is formally measured by use of standardized assessment tools such as the Confusion Assessment Method and other such tools (see http://consultgerirn. org/resources).

Diagnosis: Impaired Behavior, Affect, or Cognition

Observation of a patient's behavior includes the patient's affect, demeanor, and ability to process stimuli in the environment. Agitated older adults are at risk for falls and injury because attention to the normal environmental cues is blunted or lost altogether. Depressed older adults may be at risk for impaired safety awareness and management because of blunted responses or apathy as well as centrally acting medications used to treat the depressants. Cognitive impairment should be evaluated because dementia is an independent risk factor of falls (van Doorn et al., 2003).

For each of these four factors—consciousness, affect, behavior, and cognition— nurses work with physicians to evaluate underlying causes and find treatable solutions wherever possible. Note that the root of many of the disturbances of *consciousness, behavior,* and *affect* are due to some classic acute medical events such as hypotension, profound blood loss, or toxicity from medications (see Table 15.1). If no identifiable solution exists, prudent and standard care (i.e., best practice) requires nurses to ensure the safety of patients by instituting interventions related to improved monitoring and assistance with activities. In the order of least to most restrictive, nurses employ various solutions until the patient is no longer judged by the nurse to be at risk for a safety issue or in danger for a serious fall-related injury (see Table 15.2). Note that research on these best practices for fall prevention is slowly emerging, and the absence of research in this area does not justify not using the intervention, because it may be a best practice intervention accepted as standard care.

Assess and Diagnose the Older Adult Patient's Risk for Serious Injury

Fractures

There are a few commonsense questions the acute care nurse must ask when determining whether an elderly patient is at risk for serious injury (see Table 15.3). Serious injury is

TABLE 15.1

Medical Factors Associated With Risk to Fall Due to Impaired Safety Judgment

Summary of acute medical events, which can impair cognition, level of consciousness, or behavior predisposing to impaired patient judgment and safety
  Impaired level of consciousness
    Volume depletion disorders
    Dehydration
    Acute internal bleeding
    Medication toxicity
  Infection/sepsis
    Urinary track infections
    Pneumonia
  Intracranial mass/hemorrhage
    Electrolyte imbalances
    Diabetic ketoacidosis
    Cerebral hypoxia
  Impaired cognition (memory, short-term attention span)
    Dementia
    Untreated depression
    Medication toxicity
    Mental illness/developmental disability/mental retardation
  Behavior agitation
    Acute or chronic unmanaged pain
    Medication toxicity
    Depression

defined as broken bones such as vertebral fractures, pelvic fractures, internal bleeding, or fatality. All of the items listed in Table 15.3 are acute or chronic medical illnesses or conditions giving rise to the possibility that an acute injury could result. One of the most prevalent conditions increasing risk for serious injury in older patients, such as a fracture, is the presence of osteoporosis. For many reasons, the true incidence of osteoporosis is unknown in the older population, especially in men (Kaufman et al., 2000) who comprise a large percentage of the acute care hospital and long-term care beds.

TABLE 15.2

Best Practice "Protective" Interventions for Patients With Impaired Level of Consciousness, Cognition, or Behavior

Examples of best practice standard of care interventions (least to most restrictive)
  Relocate patient bed to be near an observational port
  Use of a personal or chair alarm
  Dangle at bedside for 5 minutes before rising with assistance
  Use of a sitter service, volunteer, or caregiver for one-on-one observation
  Use of a bedpan as opposed to a bedside commode
  Physicians orders for out of bed only with standby assistance
  Physician orders for arm in arm assistance with ambulation
  Physician orders for cane, walker, and standby assistance with ambulation
  Out of bed for limited time with assistance only
  Use of hipsters or protective hip wear
  Use of helmets for the head, if at risk for head injury

TABLE 15.3

Medical Conditions Raising the Risk of Serious Injury/Internal Bleeding

Medical Conditions
 Underlying osteoporosis
 Current hip or vertebral fracture
 Thrombocytopenia
 Acute lymphocytic leukemia
 Acute anemia or loss of blood volume
 Any state of alerted level of consciousness "delirium," lethargy, obtunded or comatose

Medications
 Blood thinners
 Thrombocytopenic agents

Therefore, it is entirely conceivable that the older adult will fracture an extremity or vertebrae with a fall, even though there is no documented diagnosis of osteoporosis. This is because osteoporosis can be present, even though it has not formally been diagnosed. Most older individuals with hip fractures have osteoporosis, yet findings from a retrospective analysis of records of patients receiving hip fracture surgery appears that the frequency of treating these high-risk older patients for osteoporosis is less than optimal; women are offered treatment more than men (Kamel, 2004).

If osteoporosis has been diagnosed, then certain protective interventions should be considered such as the use of hip protectors (Applegarth et al., 2009; Bulat, Applegarth, Quigley, Ahmed, & Quigley, 2008). As indicated for those older persons without safety judgment and are unable to transfer and ambulate independently, the use of low-height beds and/or floor mats placed around the bedside will lessen the height of the fall, or padding a hard surface to reduce the chance for injury. Treatment for osteoporosis needs to be discussed, ranging from the use of medication agents to supplemental calcium and vitamin D, although research findings show a controversial association between vitamin D and physical performance improvements in gait and balance (Annweiler, Schott, Berrut, Fantino, & Beauchet, 2009). However, a recent meta-analysis found vitamin D to be the only intervention shown to be effective in reducing falls among female stroke survivors in an institutional setting (Batchelor, Hill, Mackintosh, & Said, 2010).

Other medical comorbidities that increase the risk of serious injury include bleeding disorders and use of blood-thinning medications to prevent stroke. A risk versus benefit analysis should always be part of fall management decision making for patient safety and prevention of injury (Quigley & Goff, 2011). Those with thrombocytopenia require monitoring of neurological status postfall in an effort to early identify a patient with a looming internal bleed or developing hematoma. These clinical conditions are very serious and can be fatal if not assessed early.

Best Practice Interventions for Suspected Serious Injury

Head Trauma

Frequent neurological checks are done for several days following head injury in older patients who are on blood thinners or who have coexisting medical conditions to detect the development of serious conditions such as a subdural hematoma. In addition, vital signs, assessing behavior, affect, cognition, and level of consciousness are all part of any assessment

TABLE 15.4
Best Practice Interventions for Patients Suspected of a Serious Injury

Interventions

Notify the physician or health care professional immediately

Apply supplemental oxygen if indicated

Assess vital signs and pulse oximetry every 15 minutes

Prepare the patient for an x-ray of the extremity or CT scan of the head

Pad side rails if there is altered level of consciousness among those bedridden

Do not leave the patient alone; obtain a sitter or one-on-one assistance

Lower the height of the bed, use tab alarms or personal alarms

Maintain bed rest

Assess and maintain airway, breathing, and circulation

Assess and monitor pain (Does it increase over time or is it unrelieved?)

Maintain an NPO status unless ordered otherwise

For suspected injury to soft tissue, apply ice for swelling, follow the RICE principle

Prepare the patient for laboratory data, frequently a serum blood count, type and cross match, bleeding time and serum electrolytes is ordered

Observe and monitor the injured site: Does the swelling increase? Is there an open fracture? Does the tissue discolor is there loss of circulation?

Are there any coexisting symptoms, which worsen over time, such as headache, backache, pain in the extremity, or experiences of dizziness or shortness of breath?

---

of the patient with head injury. Changes in speech, such as slurred speech, or subtle diminution in cognitive abilities (i.e., they no longer recognize you after recalling your name) are significant findings postfall head injury that requires immediate attention.

Older patients who have unwitnessed falls or do not recall falling despite evidence to the contrary should be monitored for head injury following the CDC guidelines for head injury (see Resources). Traumatic brain injury caused by head injuries is a condition that is preventable and, more importantly, readily recognizable. Subtle changes in cognition, level of consciousness, or behavior postfall indicate underlying head trauma. Table 15.4 details best practice interventions in cases in which a head injury is suspected postfall.

Of all causes, falls are the leading cause of TBI (CDC, NCIPC, 2007), with older adults age 75 and older having the highest rate of TBI-related hospitalization and death (Langlois, Rutland-Brown, & Thomas, 2006). Groups at risk for the development of TBI include men who are twice as likely to sustain a TBI—adults age 75 or older; African Americans have the highest death rate from TBI (CDC, NCIPC, 2007). There is strong clinical reason to suspect that older adults in anticoagulants are at higher risk for TBI, should then sustain a fall with head injury, but empiric research in this age-group is lacking. Still, best practice approaches to care of older adults must include a risk–benefit evaluation of medications, such as Coumadin, Plavix, and/or aspirin, among others, that place the older adult at increased risk for bleeding following a fall. Additionally, use of helmets may be considered because they absorb trauma and reduce impact to the head (Quigley & Goff, 2011).

Why Do Older Adult Patients in an Acute Care Setting Fall and Who Is at Greatest Risk

The Value of Identifying Fall Type

Reasons for patient falls are tied directly to impairments in consciousness, cognition, behavior, and acute and chronic types of medical conditions. Some of these risks are due to *intrinsic* factors, whereas others are due to *extrinsic* factors. The standard of care calls for assessment of fall risk factors and then to develop intervention plan targeted toward these factors.

Environmental falls are potentially preventable because they encompass foreseeable events, such as spills or improper shoe wear, which is correctable (Connell, 1996). Important intrinsic risks to fall among older adults are summarized in Table 15.5, while Table 15.6 lists some examples of age-related and associated conditions that cause falls. Positive predictive validity of falls has also been used as evidence by the patient's underlying history of falls, visual impairment, requiring toileting assistance, dependency in transfer/mobility, balance disturbance, and cognitive impairment (Blahak et al., 2009; Papaioannou, 2004; Tinetti, Williams, & Mayewski, 1986). Last, common extrinsic or environmental factors, which represent preventable falls, are highlighted in Table 15.7.

Fall risk is formally assessed through administration of fall risk tools (see Table 15.8). The National Center for Patient Safety recommends the Morse Falls Scale, but *not* for long-term use (available at: http://www.va.gov/ncps/CogAids/FallPrevention/Index .html#topofpage&page=page-4). The Stratify tool has also been widely used but

TABLE 15.5

Examples of Intrinsic Risks to Fall

Intrinsic Risks

Lower extremity weakness
History of falls
Gait deficit
*Balance deficit
Use of an assistive device
Visual deficit
Arthritis
Impaired activity of daily living (ADL)
   Dependency in transferring/mobility
Depression
Cognitive impairment
   *Delirium
   Agitated confusion
   *Older than age 80 years
   Urinary incontinence/frequency
   *Diabetes
   Culprit medications: benzodiazepines, sedatives/hypnotics, alcohol, antidepressants, neuroleptics, antiarrhythmics, digoxin, and diuretics.
   *Polypharmacy

Note: * Indicates independent predictor of falls with prolonger lengths of stay and increased nursing home placement (Corsinovi et al., 2009).

Sources: Corsinovi, L., Bo, M., Aimonino, N. R.., Marinello, R., Gariglio, F., Marchetto, C., . . . Molaschi, M. (2009). Predictors of fall s and hospitalization outcomes in elerly patients admitted to an acute geriatric unit. *Archives of Gerontology and Geriatrics, 49*(1), 142–145.

ECRI Institute. (2006). *Falls prevention strategies in healthcare settings guide.* Plymouth Meeting, PA: ECRI Publishers.

Oliver, D., Daly, F., Martin, F. C., McMurdo, M. E. (2004). Risk factors and risk assessment tools for falls in hospital inpatients: A systematic review. *Age and Ageing, 33*(2), 122–130.

Papaioannou, A., Parkinson, W., Cook, R., Ferko, N., Coker, E., & Adachi, J. D. (2004). Prediction of falls using a risk assessment tool in the acute care setting. *BMC Medicine, 2,* 1.

Rubenstein, L. Z., & Josephson, K. R. (2002). The epidemiology of falls and syncope. *Clinics of Geriatric Medicine, 18*(2), 141–58.

TABLE 15.6

Medical Events and Diseases Associated with Falls in Older Adults

Age-related
Dizziness with standing from physiological age-related changes
Dizziness with head rotation from physiological age-related changes

Accidental/Environmental (see Table 15.7)
Slipping or tripping on a wet/slippery surface
Trip/slip
Lack of support from equipment or assistive device

Acute (Treatable) Sudden Symptoms
Mental confusion/delirium
Heart racing or skipping beats (arrhythmia)
Dizziness with standing up (orthostatic hypotension)
Dizziness with room spinning (vertigo)
Generalized weakness (infection, sepsis)
Involuntary movement of limbs accompanied by confusion, unresponsiveness, or absent facial features (seizure)
Lower extremity weakness (electrolyte imbalance)
Gait ataxia associated with acute alcohol ingestion
Feeling faint or dizzy or unable to sustain consciousness (hypoglycemia)
Blacking out or loss of recall of fall event (syncope)
Unilateral weakness, sudden speech change, and/or facial droop (TIA/CVA)

Chronic (Manageable) Gradual or Recurrent Symptoms
Lower extremity numbness (neuropathy, diabetes, PVD, B^{12} deficiency)
Lower extremity weakness (arthritis, CVA, thyroid disease)
Fatigue (anemia, CHF)
Dyspnea on exertion (emphysema, pneumonia)
Weakness (frailty, disuse, anemia)
Lightheadedness (carotid stenosis, cerebrovascular disease, emphysema)
Dizziness with standing (OH secondary to diabetes)
Dizziness with head rotation (carotid stenosis, hypersensitivity)
Dizziness with movement (labyrinthitis)
Forgetting the fall (dementia)
"I don't know" responses (depression)
Lower extremity joint pain (arthritis)
Unsteadiness with walking (dementia, CVA/MID)
Poor balance (Parkinson's disease)

Notes: TIA = transient ischemic attack; CVA = cerebrovascular accident; PVD = peripheral vascular disease; CHF = congestive heart failure; OH = orthostatic hypotension; MID = multi-infarct dementia.
Sources: Gray-Miceli, D., Johnson, J. C., & Strumpf, N. E. (2005). A stepwise approach to a comprehensive post fall assessment. *Annals of Long-Term Care: Clinical Care and Aging, 13*(12), 16–24.
Rubenstein, L. Z., & Josephson, K. R. (2006). Falls and their prevention in the elderly: What does the evidence show? *Medical Clinics of North American, 90*(5), 807–824.

researchers report its use offers no added benefit over nursing staff's clinical judgment. Oliver et al. (2010) recommend the Morse Fall Scale and the Stratify tool as the two screening tools with best predictive properties for anticipated physiological falls.

The Veterans Administration VISN 8 Patient Safety Center has defined "intentional falls" as those occurring from patients being pushed or falling to the ground deliberately and these falls are usually not preventable. In other empirical research directed at determining the various types of falls occur among older adults using a

TABLE 15.7

Extrinsic Risks to Fall

Floor surfaces that are slippery, wet, extrashiny or uneven or cracked

Equipment that is faulty, nonsupportive, or collapsing when used, laden with debris

IV poles, stretchers, or beds that are unsturdy or move away from the patient when used for support

Poor lighting or extraglaring "blinding" bright lights

Bathrooms lacking grab rails, bars, or nonskid appliqués or mats

Physical restraints

Inappropriate shoe wear

comprehensive postfall assessment (PFA) tool as the basis for determination, a broader classification scheme has emerged consisting of eight different fall types observed: falls due to acute illness, chronic diseases, medications, behavior, unknown, environment, misjudgment, or poor patient safety awareness (Gray-Miceli, Ratcliffe, & Johnson, 2010). Fall risk screening tools identify the likelihood of an anticipated physiological fall with known intrinsic and extrinsic fall risk factors. These screening tools provide first level of assessment data as the basis for comprehensive assessment. Only through comprehensive PFA can multifactorial, complex fall, and injury risk factors are defined (Quigley, Neily, Watson, Wright, & Strobel, 2007). Fall risk assessment and PFA are

TABLE 15.8

Listing of Some Empirically Tested Fall Assessment Tools

Name of Tool	Author	Setting	Training	Time to Administer	Sensitivity
Assessment of high risk to fall	Spellbring	IP	Y	17 minutes	UK
Berg Balance Test	Berg	OP	Y	15 minutes	77
Patient Fall Questionnaire	Rainville	IP	Y	UK	UK
STRATIFY	Oliver	IP	N	UK	93
Fall Prediction Index	Nyberg	IP-CVA	UK	UK	100
Resident Assessment Instrument	Morris	NH	Y	80 minutes	UK
Post-Fall Index	Gray-Miceli	NH	Y	22 minutes	UK
Morse Fall Scale	Morse	IP	Y	< 1 minute	78
Fall Risk Assessment Tool	MacAvoy	IP	N	UK	93
Hendrich Fall Risk Model	Hendrich	IP	N	<1 minute	77
Timed Get Up and Go	Shumway-Cook	OP	Y	<1 minute	87
Tinetti Performance Oriented Mobility	Tinetti	IP	Y	20 minutes	80

Note. IP = inpatient; CVA = cerebrovascular accident; OP = outpatient; NH = nursing home; Y = yes; N = no; UK = unknown.

Source: Adapted from ECRI Institute. (2006). *Falls prevention strategies in healthcare settings.* Plymouth Meeting, PA: ECRI Publisher; Perell, K., Nelson, A., Goldman, R., Luther, S. L., Prieto-Lewis, N., & Rubenstein, L. Z. (2001). Fall risk assessment measures: An analytic review. *Journal of Gerontology, 56*(12), 761–766.

two very different and distinct approaches for falls prevention. Fall risk assessment tools offer limited types of inquiry typically streamlined focusing on five or six areas of inquiry, which are not a substitution or replacement for a comprehensive postfall inquiry or assessment . Critical information is missing in these streamlined fall risk assessment tools.

Patient-Specific Factors Linked to Fall Risk

Evidence from systematic reviews of fall risk factors in hospital inpatients supports the following risk factors to be linked to falls: a recent fall, muscle weakness, behavioral disturbance, agitation or confusion, urinary incontinence or frequency, use of "culprit" medications(especially sedative/hypnotics), postural hypotension, syncope, and those older than age 85 years (Oliver et al., 2010). In the acute care setting, fall risk tools have been summarized in an analytic review by Perell and colleagues (2001; Scott, Votova, Scanlan, & Close, 2007)

The nursing assessment of the older adult patient who falls does not stop with administration of these assessment tools or other types of assessment. Rather, the assessment is a dynamic and continuous process of quality improvement, which extends to formulate an analysis of the information and situational context of the patient so that corrective plans of action can unfold.

Physical Restraint Use Contributing to Fall Risk

Capezuti and colleagues (2002) cite physical restraint use as a contributor to risk for falling, not a solution for fall prevention. Also noted by Capezuti et al. (2002), neither physical restraints nor side rails have ever been shown to reduce falls or associated injury. In fact, in the last 20 years, there have been numerous reports of restraint-related injuries reported in the professional literature, by the U.S. Food and Drug Administration, and The Joint Commission. Many of these injuries are due to patient attempts to remove restraints or to ambulate while restrained (Agostini, Baker, & Bogardus, 2001). The injuries include neurological injuries (DiMaio, Dana, & Bux, 1985), stress-induced complications (related to agitation secondary to restraint), and strangulation (Dube, & Mitchell, 1986; Miles, 2002). The most common mechanism of restraint-related death is by asphyxiation—the person is suspended by a restraint from a bed/chair and the ability to inhale is inhibited by gravitational chest compression (DiNunno, Vacca, Costantinedes, & Di Nunno, 2003). Clearly, the risk of serious injury or fatality due to physical restraint is substantial and must be considered when deciding about using restraints. Serious direct injury from bedrails is usually related to use of outmoded designs and incorrect assembly rather (Healey, Oliver, Milne, & Connelly, 2008).

Medications Contributing to Fall Risk in Older Adults

"Culprit" drugs or medications implicated in increasing fall risk are those causing potentially dangerous side effects including drowsiness, mental confusion, problems with balance or loss of urinary control, and sudden drops in blood pressure with standing (postural hypotension; Ensrud et al., 2002; Neutel, Perry, & Maxwell, 2002; Smith,

2003). Classifications of medications implicated in falls for older adults include psychotropic agents (benzodiazepines, sedatives/hypnotics, antidepressants, and neuroleptics), antiarrhythmics, digoxin, and diuretics (Leipzig, Cumming, & Tinetti, 1999). The risk of falls alone should not automatically disqualify a person from being treated with warfarin (Garwood, & Corbett, 2008).

Postfall Assessment

Determination of why the fall occurred is of vital. The value of postfall assessment, if performed properly and comprehensively using appropriately empirically tested tools, is that underlying fall etiologies can be discerned so that appropriate plans of care can be instituted. To simply perform a fall risk assessment or perform a PFA and document the findings without linking the risk or actual fall cause to a strategy is *useless*. Once the type of fall is determined using a comprehensive postfall evaluation tool, the nurse can put into motion an appropriate plan of care.

The purpose of the PFA is to identify the clinical status of the older adult, verify and treat injuries, and to identify underlying causes of the fall whenever possible. Components of the PFA are typically routinely performed by professional nurses in all patient settings, although this evaluation may be skeletal or limited according to the completeness of questions and examination included on the tool used. Few empirically published tools for PFA exist, and previous research has shown that fall risk determination, using short forms, asking 5–8 questions about risk, often replace (inappropriately) PFA in institutionalized settings (Gray-Miceli, Strumpf, Reinhard, Zanna, & Fritz, 2004; Ray et al., 1997; Rubenstein, Robbins, Josephson, Schulman, & Osterweil, 1990).

Evidence shows comprehensive PFA tools are useful and available to assist professional registered nurses in performing a PFA, especially in institutionalized settings (Gray-Miceli, Strumpf, Johnson, Draganescu, & Ratcliffe, 2006). In institutional settings where teams are unavailable, comprehensive PFA may be carried out through consultation with specialty-trained providers.

The PFA is a comprehensive, yet fall-focused history and physical examination of the present problem (falling), coupled with a functional assessment, review of past medical problems, and medications. Clinical fall prevention guidelines are very clear about all of the necessary components for inclusion for patients who have fallen, which include fall history; fall circumstance; medical problems; medication review; mobility assessment; vision assessment; neurological examination, including mental status; and cardiovascular assessment. In addition to this information, data are collected about the patient's physical status. Performing a comprehensive PFA allows the clinician to identify intrinsic risks and recent causes of a fall such as orthostatic hypotension and/or bradyarrhythmia or tachyarrhythmia associated with dizziness (Gray-Miceli et al., 2006). In the hospital setting, certain components of a PFA can be elicited immediately following a patient fall, with the decision to ask certain questions immediately depends on the medical stability of the patient and nursing judgment.

The Immediate Postfall Assessment

As soon as possible, an assessment is made to determine the extent of any sustained injuries. Before any intervention is taken, any staff member should remain with the patient and call for help. During this time, the older adult patient is verbally reassured and kept warm (but not moved) until help arrives. There are many key observations to be noted about the fallen individual's medical and psychological condition, as well as condition of the environment. The medical stability of the patient determines the sequence of information gathered either immediately or in the interim period, according to current standards of practice followed by licensed professionals. For instance, if unconscious from a head injury sustained during the fall, neurological checks, vital signs with apical pulse rate, and pulse oxygenation are assessed first. Other assessments of gait or functional status are conducted after the patient has stabilized. While this is being performed, or if shoes/slippers are worn, other staff members can assess environmental spills. Information about the lighting and use of assistive devices can be gathered. Any verbalizations made by the patient should be noted about his or her condition. Critical observations made during the immediate PFA (see Table 15.9) that should be communicated to the primary care provider include observation or verbalizations of pain, extremity swelling, unstable vital signs, discolored skin, temperature, laceration or contusions of the skin, loss of consciousness, decreased range of motion, evidence of head or neck injury and abnormal or erratic neurological responses, uncontrollable bleeding, and incontinence of bowel or bladder at the time of the fall.

Interim Postfall Assessment

During the interim period of PFA and monitoring (anywhere from several hours to days), the nurses continue to review, determine, and communicate pertinent findings from this assessment and its progression or resolution. Once the patient is medically stable, fall risk assessment can be reassessed by the interdisciplinary team, revaluating intrinsic and extrinsic risks so that a plan of care can be determined. Developing a plan of care and requesting a change in physician orders for level of supervision required by

---

TABLE 15.9

Immediate Postfall Assessment

Actions Taken by Professional Nurses and Nursing Staff

If the older adult patient is found on the floor, remain with patient, summons additional help, proceed to:

   Ask the older adult to explain what happened if possible

   Ask the older adult how he or she is feeling and if there is pain

   Control any bleeding (follow unit protocol) from injured site

   Assess level of consciousness and perform neurological assessment including and pupillary checks (according to unit protocol)

   Gather and document vital signs: note the apical pulse rate and the supine blood pressure

   Examine for signs of external injury to the head, spine, neck, and extremities

   Determine oxygenation status

   Determine finger stick glucose if hypoglycemia is suspected

   If stable, sit the patient up with support and assess sitting blood pressure

   Gather and review pertinent symptoms at the time of the fall

   Immobilize an extremity if fracture is suspected

   Reassure the older patient

   If stable, assist with transfer to be or appropriate area for further evaluation

   Diagnosis and treatment

Source: Reprinted with permission from ECRI. Gray-Miceli, D. (2006). *Falls prevention strategies in healthcare settings,* Chapter 5, Patient Post fall Assessment: Plymouth Meeting: ECRI Publishing; Copyright Deanna Gray-Miceli, 2005.

nursing staff of the older patient or specific activity restrictions depending on the fall assessment findings.

Longitudinal Postfall Assessment

Following a patient fall, the presence of injury may not be apparent until days or even weeks later. When cognitive impairment exists, the accuracy of the historical accounts of pain obtained immediately after the fall may be questioned. Observations of functional status with attention to any subtle or blatant changes in mobility can signal an underlying fracture or a looming unstable joint that was not previously reported. Likewise, during a patient fall in which the older adult is cognitively intact, and then later develops, an acute delirium should signal to the professional nurse the possibility of injury. In these two instances, the standard of care warrants as part of the ongoing postfall assessment, to monitor vital signs and neurological status for a period of several days or more, as clinically indicated. Fall policy and procedures should reflect this provision because any change in patient condition warrants follow-through, documentation, and communication to senior level providers, other nursing staff, and family (see Table 15.10).

Overview of Effective Fall and Injury Prevention in Hospitals

Effective fall prevention programs in acute care hospitals are championed by nurses using one or more approaches. Moving beyond traditional measures of fall rates to assessing and measuring patient injury from falls provides more information and segmentation of vulnerable patients so that a new level of intervention is applied. This process advances the evidence related to falls into the quality management program for falls prevention. Assessing risk for injury provides the evidence for nurses to provide specific interventions to reduce injury (e.g., hip protectors, floor mats, and helmets) based on using existing tools. The evidence is strong to support the benefit of multifactorial fall prevention programs for injurious falls in acute care. System-level interventions with emerging evidence of effectiveness emerge from the work of innovation: nurse champions, safety huddles, teach-back strategies, postfall huddles, and interventions to reduce fall-related trauma.

TABLE 15.10

Critical Observations Made During the Immediate Postfall Assessment

Expressions or verbalizations of pain (facial grimacing, crying, screaming, agitation)

Changes in behavior or function, which may indicate pain

Swelling of an extremity (writs, arm leg) or head (hematoma, skull pain)

Unstable vital signs

Discolored cyanotic skin

Skin temperature (cold, clammy, diaphoretic)

Skin lacerations, contusions

Loss of consciousness (LOC), no response to stimuli or significant change in LOC

Changed range of motion of extremities

Evidence of neck, head, or spinal cord injury

Abnormal or erratic neurological responses, such as absent pupil response, fixed or dilated pupils, seizures, or abnormal changes in posture

---

Source: Reprinted with permission from ECRI Institute. (2006). *Fall prevention strategies in healthcare settings,* Chapter 5, Patient Post fall Assessment: ECRI Publishing.

Nurse Champions

Embracing nurse champions at the point of care, the Institute for Healthcare Improvement's (IHI) Transforming Care at the Bedside has partnered with the VISN 8 Patient Safety Center to focus on acute care fall and injury prevention for the last 5 years. Dedicated to building program capacity, infrastructure, and expertise, fall experts have mentored and coached nurses from across acute care settings to address vulnerable older adults are at greatest risk for loss of function or loss of life if any type of fall occurs. This approach to nursing practice has been transformational (Boushon et al., 2008).

Teach Backs

Health literacy requires that providers evaluate the degree to which individuals learn by assessing their capacity to obtain information, process, and understand basic health information and services so that they can make informed health decisions (Institute of Medicine, 2004). Teach backs identifies what the patient learned by a return demonstration or feedback, and more importantly, what the patient had difficulty learning, so that the provider can fill that gap through ongoing education.

Comfort Care and Safety Rounds. Nursing staff are completing comfort care and safety rounds as one of their tests of change. This intervention has emerging evidence of effectiveness based on the results of researchers Meade, Bursell, and Ketelsen (2006), hourly rounds in acute care reduced falls ($p = 0.01$), and by 60% 1 year later in the follow-up hospitals.

Safety Huddle Postfall

Safety huddles were patterned after the military's "After Action Review" (AAR) process. Safety huddles provide a mechanism for immediate knowledge transfer for learning from errors and close calls. In a safety huddle, staff are instructed to immediately assess a situation or event to understand what happened, what should have happened, what accounted for the difference, and what corrective action could be implemented to prevent a similar event. This AAR mimics a modified root cause analysis. All staff received a brochure explaining the AAR process and are instructed to perform a safety huddle as soon as possible after becoming aware of a fall. Nurse managers or advanced practice nurses coach staff in the safety huddle process through role playing and use of a brochure and presentation that describes the process. The nurse managers lead the initial huddles, and staff followed thereafter. Over time, staff begin to use safety huddles to examine other patient safety situations and to ensure that falls precautions are consistently applied in the shift-to-shift hand-off process. Incorporation into the hand-off process also provided the opportunity for staff to reassess a patient's status (Quigley et al., 2009).

Interventions to Reduce Trauma

Patients with risk factors for serious injury (osteoporosis or osteoporosis risk factors; anticoagulants for postoperative patients) should be automatically placed on *high-risk* falls precautions and interventions to reduce risk for serious injury should be implemented. Interventions to reduce the risk trauma and prevent injury include the following: place a bedside mat on floor at side of bed unless contraindicated; use height-adjustable bed (low-bed position to reduce distance from bed to floor); helmet use for patients at risk for head injury (those on anticoagulants, patients with severe seizure disorder, and history of falling and hitting head); and dress with hip protectors for patients at risk for hip fracture. These interventions when combined create protective bundles. For example, those patients at risk for hip fracture should be placed at high risk for falls and in height-adjustable beds, wear hip protectors, have floor mats at bedside when in bed, and receive comfort and safety rounds. Those patients at risk for hemorrhagic bleed should be placed at high risk for falls and in height-adjustable beds, have floor mats at bedside when in bed, and receive comfort and safety rounds. Helmets should be considered for patients with history of head injury and falls, and on anticoagulants. All patients should receive education about their fall and injury risks.

Program Evaluation

Many health systems use a specifically designed incident report form for falls that collects detailed literature-based data about fall occurrences (Elkins et al., 2004). For example, these data might include time of day, location, activity, orthostasis, and incontinence. From the analysis of the data, one can determine the type of fall, such as accidental, anticipated physiological, and unanticipated physiological fall and severity of injury— minor, moderate, or major/severe (Donaldson, Brown, Aydin, Bolton, & Rutledge, 2005). Analysis of data of this depth and scope enables clinicians, administrators, and risk managers to profile the level of fall risk of their patients along with actual factors contributing to the fall, as well as identifying overall patterns and trends surrounding fall occurrence.

Fall Prevention Program

Fall prevention begins with an integrated/coordinated approach inclusive of fall risk determination and PFA to identify risk factors. Accurate documentation should be provided in the plan of care, nursing and interdisciplinary notes, and other aspects of the medical record such as the problem-list help to ensure communication and ongoing monitoring. Review of fall-related information collected about a fall event or a person deemed at risk for fall by the interdisciplinary team adds an important dimension to fall care. The team offers input from their unique perspective of the fall circumstance and how to best manage a fall or a patient at high risk for falls. The interdisciplinary team consists of the medical provider, nurse, physical or occupational therapist, risk manager, pharmacist, and other direct health care providers.

Hospital-based fall prevention programs have been described in the literature, but few clinical trials have been conducted, demonstrating their effectiveness due to methodological limitations associated with this complex fast-paced setting. One study examined the effect of a program of fall prevention that includes multifactorial components of fall risk assessment, a choice of interventions, patient education, and staff education, as well as labels or "graphics alerting others to at risk patients." Use of this model and its outcomes were examined prospectively for 5 years by Dempsey (2004) who reported a significant reduction in fall rates. However, over time compliance deteriorated warranting further nursing inquiry considering use of a process approach to increase nurse autonomy in fall prevention.

Exemplary models of care also exist through the National Center for Patient Safety at the United States Department of Veterans Affairs (available at: http://www.va.gov/ncps/SafetyTopics/fallstoolkit/index.html). The Veterans Affairs, VISN 8 Patient Safety Center of Inquiry, under the direction of an advanced nurse practitioner–nurse scientist, spearheads an impressive program of fall prevention through its health care network of inpatient hospitals. Fall prevention through best practice approaches are evaluated and translated into standard practices among general falls prevention, interventions for high-risk patients, and education of staff, patients, and families.

Models of care, serving as exemplars of the geriatric nurse-centered approach, realize improvements in hospital lengths of stay and health outcomes as well as fewer iatrogenic geriatric syndromes such as inpatient falls. Use of the Acute Care of the Elderly (ACE) units; Nurses Improving Care for Healthsystem Elders (NICHE) program; and the Geriatric Resource Nurse (GRN) model, which use a system-level quality improvement approach, including educational programs for staff, realized a decrease fall rate by 5.8% (Smyth, Dubin, Restrepo, Nueva-Espana, & Capezuti, 2001).

INTERVENTIONS FOR FALL PREVENTION AND MANAGEMENT

Instituting General Safety Measures

Hospitals and their staff have a legal responsibility and due diligence to ensure freedom from environmental hazards and safety for all patients, staff, and visitors. Routine environmental assessment using a checklist should include the unit, corridors, entrance, and exits, as well as patient holding areas, patient rooms, and areas where patients are transported to (radiology, nuclear imaging, operating room). In each of these areas, an environmental assessment is performed focusing on floor surfaces, furniture, hallways, steps, device safety such as stretchers, wheelchairs, and other types of chairs, free of clutter, bathrooms with appropriate grab rails, and routine assessment of equipment. Use of a checklist signed by the designated employee allows for audit review of compliance, serving as an internal benchmark of compliance.

As part of general safety, some facilities designate any older adult age 65 years and older admitted to be on "safety precautions," which can include various other safety measures (presented in the succeeding text). Clinically, it is important to recognize, in advance whenever possible, that if instructions are given to the patient for general safety precautions, that the older adult is actually able to hear, understand, and demonstrate that he or she can follow instructions. Simply "telling the older adult" to be careful or to not get up without assistance is insufficient in the face of an ongoing or new onset of delirium or cognitive impairment. Rather, other safety measures need to be immediately instituted, discussed with the team and the family caregiver, and incorporated as part of the plan of care. Immediate options always include (a) increasing surveillance by either staying with the patient continuously; (b) moving the patient to a closer location (provided there is staff constantly observing the patient); (c) providing a one-on-one type of sitter service for continual surveillance; or (d) engaging the older patient in diversional activities or other forms of therapeutic recreation. Sitter type services can be provided by hospital staff, volunteers, or through private duty services. Discussion with family caregivers and the interdisciplinary team are essential in these cases.

Early Mobility for Older Patients Who Fall

Early mobility, whenever the older patient is medically stable, is a fundamental and basic aspect of care for all older adult patients to receive during their hospitalization. It is a step toward the prevention of deconditioning, reduced mobility and immobility, and other cascading problems that can result when less sedentary (for instance, orthostatic pneumonia or atelectasis). Early mobility as an intervention begins with the simple and conscious decision by nursing to assist the patient out of bed to walk to the bathroom whenever possible, rather than to use a bedpan or even a bedside commode that offers little opportunity for mobility. Wearing proper footwear, corrective lenses, and clearing a path that is clutter- and spill-free are essential. Use of a walking aid such as a standard cane or walker may also be required; appropriate assistive devices can be ascertained through an occupational or physical therapist consultation (Quigley & Goff, 2011).

Another essential aspect for the older adult with comorbidities is for nurses to preemptively ask the older patient, who is transitioning with your assistance, from sitting to standing and then while walking, "How are you feeling"? Of concern is the detection of symptoms such as lightheadedness, vertigo with rotational movement, or muscular stiffness. These symptoms can be managed and monitored, if significant enough to prohibit mobility, once they are detected. Another concern exists for the older adult patient with orthostatic hypotension. In this instance, gradual upright incline with assistance while monitoring for symptoms of lightheadedness are important. Should an older adult experience symptoms or develop acute physiological evidence of a problem (for instance, near syncope, syncope, or changes in heart rate or blood pressure), slowly easing him or her back to a recumbent position and notifying the physician for further evaluation is warranted.

Mobility programs build upon the positive feedback that the patient is feeling and objectively gaining strength each day is instituted. Checklist can monitor progress and serve to validate to the patient his or her clinical progression. Care must be taken, however, to remind persons who are restricted from independent mobility to always wait for assistance. Recommendations are to set a similar time each day and to use consistent staff. An integral component of any mobility program is footwear of patients. A recent study found patients who wore their own footwear significantly improved participants' balance compared to being barefoot; in fact, the greatest benefit was seen in those individuals with the poorest balance (Horgan et al., 2009).

Some Best Practice Exemplars Used by Acute Care Hospitals

The difference between environmental safety assessment and safety rounds is that safety rounds are a regular, systematic observation by one or two key personnel of the hospital unit; when assumed by the same personnel, hazards may be more quickly appreciated. Further, they occur at regular points in time, such as every 2 or 4 hours around the clock and also detect patients in need of assistance. This level of frequency is likely to detect problems early so that intervention can ensure the prevention of environmental type of falls. Use of checklist can help to ensure compliance and monitor for patterns of hazards and types of hazards that need correction.

Many hospital-based fall prevention programs include toileting rounds. Toileting rounds use nurse's aides to regularly assess older adult patients for the need to urinate and to provide the patient with assistance. The purpose of toileting rounds is to prevent patients from incurring urinary accidents (and potential falls) by encouraging regular voiding. In many circumstances, urinary accidents can lead to falls. Scenarios include the older adult sensing a need to urinate, getting up out of bed unassisted, and incurring a fall by an unrecognized physiologic mechanism (e.g., orthostatic hypotension). Another scenario is in route to the bathroom; the older adult has a urinary accident on the floor and slips and falls on the wet floor. By offering toileting rounds on a regular basis, the potential for these occurrences are minimized, reducing fall rates as well as the iatrogenic complications (e.g., hip fracture). Toileting is a fundamental element of basic care that has an important place in the prevention of patient falls, but its importance is underrecognized. In a study by Brown et al. (2000), urge incontinence (and not stress), especially if occurring weekly or more often, increased risk of falls and nonspinal, non-traumatic fractures in older White women living in the community.

Specific Nursing Interventions

Personal alarms are routinely used to alert nursing staff about impending falls or changes in patient mobility status. Care should be taken when deciding to use these devices, because they do not prevent a fall from occurring (Oliver et al., 2010); rather, they heighten staff's awareness by sounding an alarm, indicating a change in position has occurred. There are many commercial products available, but generally, they are of two types, personal alarms clipped to the patient's gown or chair and bed-chair pressure sensors. Despite their widespread use, there is little evidence regarding their effectiveness in reducing falls in an acute care hospital setting. Use of a bed sensor alarm was studied in a geriatric rehabilitation unit with older adult patients, deemed by nurses to be at increased fall for falling (Kwok, Mok, Chien, & Tam, 2006). In this study, the availability of bed sensor devices neither reduced physical restraint use nor improved the clinical outcomes of older adults with perceived fall risk. In a nursing home–based study, however, use of the "NOC WATCH," a nonintrusive monitor used with older adults at high risk for falling (Kelly, Phillips, Cain, Polissar, & Kelly, 2002), reduced fall rate by 91%, thereby supporting other clinical trials using a randomized design. Falls may not be the best indicator of the effectiveness of alarms, rather timeliness of rescue (Quigley, & Goff, 2011). Further, greater nurse surveillance capacity was significantly associated with better quality care and fewer adverse events (Kutney-Lee, Lake, & Aiken, 2009).

Both floor mats and use of low-rise beds have an important place in the armamentarium of clinical interventions to prevent the occurrence of serious injury when a bed fall occurs. Floor mats are simply placed surrounding the bed and serve to cushion the impact of the fall. They vary in thickness, and if portions of an area are uncovered, substantial injury could still occur if a patient attempts to get out of bed and a bed fall ensues. Little, if any, empirical research evidence exists regarding their effectiveness in preventing falls from bed causing fractures to the hip or traumatic brain injury in acute care settings. However, one observational cluster randomized trial in 18 nursing homes found that both types of hip protectors (soft and hard), when worn correctly, had the potential to reduce the risk of a hip fracture in falls by nearly 60% (Bentzen, Bergland, & Forsen, 2008).

A recent meta-analysis, however, reported that hip protectors are an ineffective intervention for those living at home and that their effectiveness in the institutional setting is uncertain (Parker, Gillespie, & Gillespie, 2006).

Technological advances have occurred, offering staff and patients a greater variety of solutions to the problem of falling. Improvements realized have occurred with walking aides such as canes that "talk" and provide feedback to the user, balance retraining that help patients learn about where their body is in space and to help learn how to compensate for muscular impairments, and other types of equipment used at the bedside when transitioning patients. Although these devices are available, research is evolving and limited in terms of their effectiveness in fall prevention (Nelson et al., 2004).

An integral component of any fall prevention educational intervention for hospitalized older adults or preparing for discharge home concerns their working knowledge of what their fall was due to and what can be done about it. Exploring the older adult's beliefs and attitudes are important and can lead to dispelling myths they may hold about falling; for instance, they may believe it is a normal part of aging or that nothing can be done about it. An older person's view and conceptualization about their falling is a starting point for a tailored educational intervention. A systematic review of the literature of many studies examining older adults preferences, views, and experiences in relation to fall prevention strategies reported several important findings (McInnes, & Askie, 2004): (a) In clinical practice, it is important to consult with individuals to find out what they are willing to modify; and (b) what changes they are prepared to make to reduce their risk of falling, otherwise they may not attend fall prevention programs.

CASE STUDY

Mrs. S. is an 80-year-old White female admitted to the step-down rehabilitation unit at the hospital following a 3-week admission for treatment of a community-acquired pneumonia. Mrs. S. received intravenous (IV) antibiotics and fluids for management of the infiltrate and associated dehydration. Mrs. S.'s hospitalization was complicated by development of acute confusion, which escalated following use of IV theophylline and use of Ventolin nebulizers. Mrs. S. also developed a deep vein thrombosis of the leg, which was treated with IV heparin, and she now receives Coumadin. Mrs. S.'s fall risk score was significant for visual impairment due to a cataract, delirium, focal lower extremity weakness due to osteoarthritis, chronic obstructive lung disease, osteoporosis, and forgetfulness with short-term memory loss.

Prior to this hospitalization, Mrs. S. was functioning independently in her home, until her son and daughter found her on the floor, mildly confused and disoriented, complaining of dizziness. Mrs. S. was transported to the emergency room for further evaluation. She was diagnosed with a right lung infiltrate via chest x-ray; moderate-to-severe dehydration. An IV line was started and she was treated with antibiotics and admitted for observation. A 12-lead electrocardiogram showed a sinus bradycardia at 54 beats per minute. A CAT scan of the head was not performed; rather, Mrs. S. was placed on observation and admitted to a medical–surgical unit.

After the 3-week long hospitalization, Mrs. S. is transferred via wheel chair to the rehabilitation unit. During the admission assessment, you note Mrs. S.'s total fall risk score increased by 4 points due to increased confusion/disorientation, periods of restlessness, and reduced mobility. Mrs. S.'s vital signs are stable. You learn in the nursing report that Mrs. S. needs constant supervision or she wanders off the unit. During the physical examination, you are paged overhead and respond by going to the nursing station. When you return to examine Mrs. S., she is gone. A second overhead page is called "stat" for assistance on your unit. Apparently, Mrs. S. was found sitting on the floor outside of the elevator, complaining of pain in her right hip and right ankle.

The immediate PFA shows possible loss of consciousness as Mrs. S. was observed unresponsive for a few seconds. There is evidence of a head injury with a laceration and hematoma to the scalp as well as right lower leg pain and swelling. Mrs. S.'s blood pressure sitting is 80/50, and her pulse rate is 60—regular, but weak. Ice is applied to her scalp and her leg is immobilized. The physician is notified immediately and a stat

(continued)

CASE STUDY *(continued)*

CAT scan of the head is ordered, later confirming an acute intracranial bleed. Mrs. S. is prepared for cranial surgery and then hip fracture repair the following day.

Case Study Discussion

1. What nursing actions should have been taken to prevent the fall and serious injury?

   Mrs. S. is at high risk for serious injury due to her fall risk screen score and use of an anticoagulation medication, Coumadin. The standard of practice for caring for an older adult hospitalized with increased risk for falls with serious injury requires the nurse to recognize that this patient is likely to have impaired judgment and inability to follow direction due to her disorientation, relocation to a new unit, and evidence of restlessness. Because she is ambulatory, but forgetful, this creates a situation where the patient needs constant supervision. Mrs. S. should be allowed to ambulate, but only with 1:1 supervision and/or physical assistance whenever possible. The nurse failed to recognize the importance of providing constant supervision to the patient. Actions that should have been undertaken include constant supervision by support staff, such as volunteers and/or a special assignment of a nurse's aide to stay with the patient. Family would need to be notified of this decision and to enlist their support for considering a private duty nurses assistant. Acute confusion or delirium renders Mrs. S. unsafe to make the necessary decisions or judgments about her care.

   In terms of preventing serious injury, Mrs. S. could be offered a hip protector, because they are indicated for older adults who are deemed at high risk for fracture. Osteoporotic older adults who fall are likely to fracture an extremity or incur serious injury. Use of a low-rise bed and floor mats should be used because she is at high risk for falling from bed again. Her needs can be anticipated by regular rounds and by offering the use of toilet that can help prevent urinary accidents and/or falls walking toward the bathroom.

   It is imperative that Mrs. S.'s mobility be allowed to continue to move freely and ambulate provided she is supervised and/or assisted due to the disorientation. Daily walking on the unit, in the patient's room, and whenever possible to increase mobility is essential.

2. How should the nursing assessment be focused?

   Further assessment for reversible causes of delirium is warranted. Since the Ventolin has precipitated acute confusion, this drug should be used sparingly and possibly substituted with less "anticholinergic agents." A pharmacy consultation, as part of the interdisciplinary assessment, would be appropriate. Alternative respiratory interventions for increased pulmonary secretions such as clapping, postural drainage deep breathing, and the use of an inspirometry could be instituted.

   Further assessment of Mrs. S.'s falls (i.e., a fall evaluation) is clinically indicated. She has had two falls recently: one at home and one at the hospital. The etiology of these falls is not clear. The history of "being dazed" occurring in both falls warrants additional workup. In the emergency room, the patient did not receive a CT scan of her head. The fall evaluation includes, among other tests, a 24-hour Holter monitor. A consultation with a geriatrician and/or neurologist is clinically warranted.

SUMMARY

Fall and serious injury prevention is a shared responsibility by all health care providers and professionals caring for older adult patients. National recommendations exist to guide practice and should be routinely incorporated into any fall prevention program and practice policy. Some of the evidence-based research presented here can help clinicians make choices about which interventions may be the most efficacious or effective, bearing in mind that this choice changes with changes in the patient's condition. Therefore, selecting the most appropriate intervention will always depend on what the nursing and medical assessment determine the likely cause of the fall to be and the medical stability of the patient at that time. Among older adults with advanced years of age with complex illness and multiple comorbidities and geriatric syndromes, this determination becomes increasingly more challenging, but not impossible to determine. The safety of older adults in the hospital and continuing upon discharge home depends on continual assessment and reevaluation of their condition coupled with education, the use of the most effective and safest technology, and the older adult's knowledge and willingness to participate in evidenced-based care.

NURSING STANDARD OF PRACTICE

Protocol 15.1: Fall Prevention

I. GOALS
    A. Prevent falls and serious injury outcomes in hospitalized older adults.
    B. Recognize multifactorial risks and causes of falls in older adults.
    C. Institute recommendations for fall prevention and management consistent with clinical practice guidelines and standards of care.

II. OVERVIEW. Falls among older adults are not a normal consequence of aging; rather, they are considered a geriatric syndrome most often due to discrete multifactorial and interacting, predisposing (intrinsic and extrinsic risks), and precipitating (dizziness, syncope) causes (Gray-Miceli, Johnson, & Strumpf, 2005; Rubenstein, & Josephson, 2006). Fall epidemiology varies according to clinical setting. In acute care, fall incidence ranges from 2.3 to 7 falls per 1,000 patient days depending on the unit. Nearly one-third of older adults living in community fall each year in their home. The highest fall incidence occurs in the institutional long-term care setting (nursing home), where 50%–75% of the 1.63 million nursing home residents experience a fall yearly. Falls rank as the 8th leading cause of unintentional injury for older Americans and are responsible for over 16,000 deaths last year (Oliver et al., 2010).

III. BACKGROUND/STATEMENT OF THE PROBLEM
    A. Definition
        1. Fall: A fall is an unexpected event in which the participant comes to rest on the ground, floor, or lower level (Prevention of Falls Network Europe, 2006).

(continued)

Protocol 15.1: Fall Prevention *(cont.)*

B. Fall Etiology
  1. Fall risk factors include intrinsic risks of cognitive, vision, gait, or balance impairment, high-risk/contraindicated medications, and/or the extrinsic risks of assistive devices, inappropriate footwear, restraint, use of unsturdy furniture or equipment, poor lighting, uneven or slippery surfaces (Chang et al., 2004).
  2. Fall causes include, among others, orthostatic hypotension, arrhythmia, infection, generalized or focal muscular weakness, syncope, seizure, hypoglycemia, neuropathy, medication.

IV. PARAMETERS OF ASSESSMENT
  A. Assess and document all older adult patients for intrinsic risk factors to fall:
  1. Advancing age- especially if over age 75
  2. History of a recent fall
  3. Specific comorbidities: dementia, hip fracture, Type 2 diabetes, Parkinson's disease, arthritis, and depression
  4. Functional disability: use of assistive device
  5. Alteration in level of consciousness or cognitive impairment
  6. Gait, balance, or visual impairment
  7. Use of high-risk medications (Chang et al., 2004)
  8. Urge urinary incontinence (Brown et al., 2000)
  9. Physical restraint use (Capezuti et al., 2002)
  10. Bare feet or inappropriate shoe wear
  11. Identify risks for significant injury due to current use of anticoagulants such as Coumadin, Plavix, or aspirin and/or those with osteoporosis or risks for osteoporosis (John A. Hartford Foundation Institute for Geriatric Nursing, 2003)
  B. Assess and document patient-care environment routinely for extrinsic risk factors to fall and institute corrective action:
  1. Floor surfaces for spills, wet areas, unevenness
  2. Proper level of illumination and functioning of lights (night light works)
  3. Table tops, furniture, beds are sturdy and in good repair
  4. Grab rails and bars are in place in the bathroom
  5. Use of adaptive aides work properly and in good repair
  6. Bed rails do not collapse when used for transitioning or support
  7. Patient gowns/clothing do not cause tripping .
  8. IV poles are sturdy if used during mobility and tubing does
  C. Perform a PFA following a patient fall to identify possible fall causes (if possible, begin the identification of possible causes within 24 hours of a fall) as determined during the immediate, interim, and longitudinal postfall intervals. Because of known incidences of delayed complication of falls, including fractures, observe all patients for about 48 hours after an observed or suspected fall (ECRI Institute, 2006; Gray-Miceli et al., 2006; Panel on Prevention of Falls in Older Persons, 2011).
  1. Perform a physical assessment of the patient at the time of the fall, including vital signs (which may include orthostatic blood pressure readings), neurological assessment, and evaluation for head, neck, spine, and/or extremity injuries.

(continued)

Protocol 15.1: Fall Prevention *(cont.)*

2. Once the assessment rules out any significant injury:
   a. obtain a history of the fall by the patient or witness description and document
   b. note the circumstances of the fall, location, activity, time of day and any significant symptoms
   c. review of underlying illness and problems
   d. review medications
   e. assess functional, sensory, and psychological status
   f. evaluate environmental conditions
   g. review risk factors for falling (American Medical Directors Association, 2003; ECRI Institute, 2006; John A. Hartford Foundation Institute for Geriatric Nursing, 2003; Panel on Prevention of Falls in Older Persons, 2011).

D. In the acute care setting, an integrated multidisciplinary team (comprised of the physician, nurse, health care provider, risk manager, physical therapist, and other designated staff) plans care for the older adult, at risk for falls or who has fallen, hinged upon findings from an individualized assessment (Joint Commission National Patient Safety Goals, 2006; ECRI Institute, 2006).

E. The process approach to an individualized PFA includes use of standardized measurement tools of patient risk in combination with a fall-focused history and physical examination, functional assessment, and review of medications (American Medical Directors Association, 2003; John A. Hartford Foundation Institute for Geriatric Nursing, 2003; Panel on Prevention of Falls in Older Persons, 2011) When plans of care are targeted to likely causes, individualized interventions are likely to be identified. If falling continues despite attempts at individualized interventions, the standard of care warrants a reexamination of the older adult and their fall.

V. NURSING CARE STRATEGIES

A. General safety precaution and fall prevention measures that apply to all patients especially older adults:

1. Assess the patient care environment routinely for extrinsic risk factors and institute appropriate corrective action.
   a. Use standardized environmental checklists to screen; document findings
   b. Communicate findings to risk managers, housekeeping, maintenance department, all staff and hospital administration if needed
   c. Re-evaluate environment for safety (ECRI Institute, 2006)

2. Assess/screen older adult patient for multifactorial risk factors to fall on admission, following a change in condition, upon transfer to a new unit, and following a fall (ECRI Institute, 2006):
   a. Use standardized or empirically tested fall risk tools in conjunction with other assessment tools to evaluate risk for falling (Panel on Prevention of Falls in Older Persons, 2011; Tinetti, Williams, & Mayewski, 1986)
   b. Document findings in nursing notes, interdisciplinary progress notes, and the problem list.
   c. Communicate and discuss findings with interdisciplinary team members.
   d. In the interdisciplinary discussion, include review and reduction or elimination of high risk medications associated with falling.

(continued)

Protocol 15.1: Fall Prevention *(cont.)*

    e. As part of fall protocol in the facility, flag the chart of use graphic or color display of the patients risk potential to fall

    f. Communicate to the patient, the family caregiver identified risk to fall, and specific interventions chosen to minimize the patients risk

    g. Include patient and family members in the interdisciplinary plan of care and discussion about fall prevention measures.

    h. Promote early mobility and incorporate measures to increase mobility, such as daily walking, if medically stable and not otherwise contraindicated.

    i. Upon transfer to another unit, communicate the risk assessment and interventions chosen and their effectiveness in fall prevention.

    j. Upon discharge, review fall risk factors and measures to prevent falls in the home with the older patient and/or family caregiver. Provide patient literature/brochures if available. If not readily available, refer to the Internet for appropriate websites/resources.

    k. Explore with the older patient and/or family caregiver avenues to maintain mobility and functional status; consider referral to home-based exercise or group exercises at community senior centers. If discharge is planned to a subacute or rehabilitation unit, label on the transfer form the older adults mobility status at the time of discharge functional or other forms of physical activity in the home to strength lower extremities or assist with gait/balance problems.

3. Institute general safety precautions according to facility protocol, which may include:

    a. Referral to a fall prevention program

    b. Use of a low rise bed that measures 14″ from floor

    c. Use of floor mats if patient is at risk for serious injury such as osteoporosis

    d. Easy access to call light

    e. Minimization and/or avoidance of physical restraints

    f. Use of personal or pressure sensors alarms

    g. Increased observation/surveillance

    h. Use of rubber-soled heeled shoes or nonskid slippers

    i. Regular toileting at set intervals and/or continence program; provide easy access to urinals and bedpans

    j. Observation during walking rounds or safety rounds

    k. Use of corrective glasses for walking

    l. Reduction of clutter in traffic areas

    m. Early mobility program (ECRI Institute, 2006).

4. Provide staff with clear, written procedures describing what to do when a patient fall occurs.

B. Identify specific patients requiring additional safety precautions and/or evaluation by a specialist or:

    1. those with impaired judgment or thinking due to acute or chronic illness (delirium, mental illness)

    2. those with osteoporosis, at risk for fracture

    3. those with current hip fracture

    4. those with current head or brain injury (standard of care)

(continued)

Protocol 15.1: Fall Prevention *(cont.)*

C. Review and discuss with interdisciplinary team findings from the individualized assessment and develop a multidisciplinary plan of care to prevent falls (Chang et al., 2004).
1. Communicate to the physician significantly postfall assessment findings (ECRI Institute, 2006).
2. Monitor the effectiveness of the fall prevention interventions instituted.
3. Following a patient fall observe for serious injury due to a fall and follow facility protocols for management (standard of care).
4. Following a patient fall monitor vital signs, level of consciousness, neurological checks and functional status as per facility protocol. If significant changes in patient condition occurs, consider further diagnostic tests such as plain film x-rays, CT scan of the head/spine/extremity, neurological consultation and /or transfer to a specialty unit for further evaluation (standard of care).

VII. EVALUATED/EXPECTED OUTCOMES
A. Patients
1. Patient safety will be maintained.
2. Patient falls will be avoided.
3. Patients will not develop serious injury outcomes from a fall if it occurs.
4. Patients will know their risks for falling.
5. Patients will be prepared upon discharge to prevent falls in their homes.
6. Patient prehospitalization level of mobility will continue.
7. Patients who develop fall related complications such as injury, change in cognition function will be promptly assess and treated appropriately as well to reverse these aftermaths.
B. Nursing Staff
1. Nursing staff will be able to accurately detect, refer, and manage older adults at risk for falling or who have experienced a fall
2. Nursing staff will integrate into their practice comprehensive assessment and management approaches for fall prevention in the institution
3. Nursing staff will gain appreciation for older adults unique experience of falling and how it influencing their daily living, functional, physical and emotional status
4. Nurses will educate older adult patients anticipating discharge about fall prevention strategies
C. Family Caregivers
1. Family caregivers will benefit from added knowledge about fall prevention to become sensitized and more aware of simple strategies to prevent falls.
D. Health Care Organization
1. Health care organizations will realize reduced fall and injurious fall rates.
2. Health care organizations will realize the benefits of fall prevention programs that minimize liability.
3. Health care organizations will support budgetary lines for fall prevention interventions directed to patients and health care staff.

(continued)

Protocol 15.1: Fall Prevention *(cont.)*

VIII. FOLLOW-UP MONITORING OF CONDITION
A. Monitor fall incidence and incidences of patient injury due to a fall, comparing rates on the same unit over time.
B. Compare falls per patient month against national benchmarks available in the National Database of Nursing Quality Indicators.
C. Incorporate continuous quality improvement criteria into fall prevention program
D. Identify fall team members and roles of clinical and nonclinical staff (ECRI Institute, 2006).
E. Educate patient and family caregivers about fall prevention strategies so they are prepared for discharge.

IX. RELEVANT PRACTICE GUIDELINES
A. Panel on Prevention of Falls in Older Persons, Summary of the Updated American Geriatrics Society/British Geriatrics Society Clinical Practice Guideline for Prevention of Falls in Older Persons, JAGS 59:148-157, 2011 Evidence Level I.
B. American Medical Directors Association. (2003). Falls and fall risk. Columbia, MD: American Medical Directors Association;2003 Evidence Level VI.
C. University of Iowa Gerontological Nursing Interventions Research Center (UIGN). Fall prevention for older adults. Iowa City, Iowa: University of Iowa Gerontological Nursing Interventions Research Center, Research Dissemination Core; 2004. Evidence Level VI.
D. ECRI Institute. (2006). *Falls prevention strategies in healthcare settings,*: Plymouth Meeting, PA. 2006. Evidence Level VI.

RESOURCES

Evidenced-based clinical practice guidelines for falls prevention
http://www.americangeriatrics.org/files/documents/health_care_pros/JAGS.Falls.Guidelines.pdf

Centers for Disease Control Guidelines for Head Injury
http://www.cdc.gov/concussion/pdf/TBI_Clinicians_Factsheet-a.pdf

Falls Prevention Strategies in Healthcare Settings
http://www.ecri.org

VISN 8 Patient Safety Center of Inquiry/Fall
http://www.patientsafety.gov/SafetyTopics/fallstoolkit/index.html

REFERENCES

Agostini, J. V., Baker, D. I., & Bogardus, S. T. (2001). Prevention of falls in hospitalized and institutionalized older people. In *Making health care safer: A critical analysis of patient safety practices.* Agency for Healthcare Research and Quality. File Inventory, Evidence Report/Technology

Assessment Number 43 (AHRQ Publication No. 01-E058). Rockville, MD. Retrieved from http://archive.ahrq.gov/clinic/ptsafety/. Evidence Level VI.

American Medical Directors Association. (2003). *Falls and fall risk*. Columbia, MD: AMDA. Evidence Level VI.

Annweiler, C., Schott, A. M., Berrut, G., Fantino, B., & Beauchet, O. (2009). Vitamin D-related changes in physical performance: A systematic review. *The Journal of Nutrition, Health & Aging, 13*(10), 893–898.

Applegarth, S. P., Bulat, T., Wilkinson, S., Fitzgerald, S. G., Ahmed, S., & Quigley, P. (2009). Durability and residual moisture effects on the mechanical properties of external hip protectors. *Gerontechnology, 8*(1), 26–34.

Batchelor, F., Hill, K., Mackintosh, S., & Said, C. (2010). What works in falls prevention after stroke? A systematic review and meta-analysis. *Stroke, 41*(8), 1715–1722.

Bentzen, H., Bergland, A., & Forsen, L. (2008). Risk for hip fractures in soft protected, hard protected, and unprotected falls. *Injury Prevention: Journal of the International Society for Child and Adolescent Injury Prevention, 14*(5), 306–310.

Blahak, C., Baezner, H., Pantoni, L., Poggesi, A., Chabriat, H., Erkinjuntti, T., . . . LADIS Study Group. (2009). Deep frontal and periventricular age related white matter changes but not basal ganglia and infratentorial hyperintensities are associated with falls: Cross sectional results from the LADIS study. *Journal of Neurology, Neurosurgery, and Psychiatry, 80*(6), 608–613.

Boushon, B., Nielsen, G., Quigley, P., Rutherford, P., Taylor, J., & Shannon, D. (2008). *Transforming care at the bedside how-to guide: Reducing patient injuries from falls*. Retrieve from http://www.ihi .org/IHI/Topics/PatientSafety/ReducingHarmfromFalls/Tools/TCABHowToGuideReducing PatientInjuriesfromFalls.htm

Brown, J. S., Vittinghoff, E., Wyman, J.F., Stone, K. L., Nevitt, K. E., & Grady, D. (2000). Urinary incontinence: Does it increase risk for falls and fractures? Study of osteoporotic fractures research group. *Journal of the American Geriatric Society, 48*(7), 721–725. Evidence Level III.

Bulat, T., Applegarth, S., Quigley, P., Ahmed, S., & Quigley, P. (2008). The effect of multiple impacts on hip protector force attenuation properties. *Clinical Interventions in Aging, 3*(3), 567–571.

Capezuti, E., Maislin, G., Strumpf, N., & Evans, L. K. (2002). Side rail use and bed-related fall outcomes among nursing home residents. *Journal of the American Geriatrics Society, 50*(1), 90–96. Evidence Level III.

Centers for Disease Control and Prevention, National Center for Injury Prevention and Control. (2007). Preventing falls among older adults. Retrieved from http://www.cdc.gov/ncipc/duip/ preventadultfalls.htm. Evidence Level VI.

Chang, J. T., Morton, S. C., Rubsenstein, L. Z., Mojica, W. A., Maglione, M., Suttorp, M. J., . . . Shekelle, P. G. (2004). Interventions for the prevention of falls in older adults: Systematic review and meta-analysis of randomized controlled trial. *British Medical Journal, 328*(7441), 680. Evidence Level I.

Connell, B. R. (1996). Role of the environment in falls prevention. *Clinics in Geriatric Medicine, 12*(4), 859–880. Evidence Level VI.

Dempsey, J. (2004). Falls prevention revisited. A call for a new approach. *Journal of Clinical Nursing, 13*(4), 479–485. Evidence Level IV.

DiMaio, V. J. M., Dana, S. E., & Bux, R. C. (1985). Deaths caused by vest restraint. *Journal of the American Medical Association, 255*, 906. Evidence Level V.

DiNunno, N., Vacca, M., Costantinedes, F., & Di Nunno, C. (2003). Death following atypical compression of the neck. *American Journal of Forensic Medicine and Pathology, 24*(4), 364–368. Evidence Level V.

Donaldson, N., Brown, D. S., Aydin, C. E., Bolton, M. L., & Rutledge, D. N. (2005). Leveraging nurse-related dashboard benchmarks to expedite performance improvement and document excellence. *Journal of Nursing Administration, 35*(4), 163–172.

Dube, A. H., & Mitchell, E. K. (1986). Accidental strangulation from vest restraints. *Journal of the American Medical Association, 256*(19), 2725–2726. Evidence Level VI.

ECRI Institute. (2006). *Falls prevention strategies in healthcare settings.* Plymouth Meeting, PA: ECRI Publishers. Evidence Level VI.

Elkins, J., Williams, L., Spehar, A., Marano-Perez, J., Gulley, T., & Quigley, P. (2004). Successful redesign: Fall incident report—A safety initiative. *Federal Practitioner, 21*(3), 29–44.

Ensrud, K. E., Blackwell, T. L., Mangione, C. M., Bowman, P. J., Whooley, M. A., Bauer, D. C., . . . Study of Osteoporotic Fractures Research Group. (2002). Central nervous system-active medications and risk for falls in older women. *Journal of the American Geriatrics Society, 50*(10), 1629–1637. Evidence Level II.

Fischer, I. D., Krauss, M. J., Dunagan, W. C., Birge, S., Hitcho, E., Johnson, S., . . . Fraser, V. J., (2005). Patterns and predictors of inpatient falls and fall related injuries in a large academic hospital. *Infection Control Hospital Epidemiology, 26*(10), 822–827. Evidence Level IV.

Garwood, C. L., & Corbett, T. L. (2008). Use of anticoagulation in elderly patients with atrial fibrillation who are at risk for falls. *The Annals of Pharmacolotherpay, 42*(4), 523–532. Evidence Level I.

Gray-Miceli, D., Johnson, J. C., & Strumpf, N. E. (2005). A stepwise approach to a comprehensive post fall assessment. *Annals of Long-Term Care: Clinical Care and Aging, 13*(12), 16–24. Evidence Level VI.

Gray-Miceli, D., Ratcliffe, S. J., & Johnson, J. C. (2010). Use of a postfall assessment tool to prevent falls. *Western Journal of Nursing Research, 32*(7), 932–948.

Gray-Miceli, D., Strumpf, N. E., Johnson, J. C., Draganescu, M., & Ratcliffe, S. J. (2006). Psychometric properties of the Post-Fall Index. *Clinical Nursing Research, 15*(3), 157–176. Evidence Level III.

Gray-Miceli, D., Strumpf, N. E., Reinhard, S. C., Zanna, M. T., & Fritz, E. (2004). Current approaches to postfall assessment in nursing homes. *Journal of the American Medical Directors Association, 5*(6), 16–24. Evidence Level IV.

Healey, F., Oliver, D., Milne, A., & Connelly, J. B. (2008). The effect of bedrails on falls and injury: A systematic review of clinical studies. *Age & Aging, 37*(4), 368–378. Evidence Level I.

Horgan, N. F., Crehan, F., Bartlet, E., Keogan, F., O'Grady, A. M., Moore, A. R., . . . Curran M. (2009). The effects of usual footwear on balance amongst elderly women attending a day hospital. *Age & Aging, 38*(1), 62–67.

Institute of Medicine. (2004). *Health literacy: A prescription to end confusion.* Retrieved from http://www.ama-assn.org

John A. Hartford Foundation Institute for Geriatric Nursing. (2003). Preventing falls in acute care. In M. Mezey, T. Fulmer, I. Abraham, D. Zwicker (Eds.), *Geriatric nursing protocols for best practice* (2nd ed., pp. 141–164). New York, NY: Springer Publishing. Evidence Level VI.

The Joint Commission. (2006). *National patient safety goals.* Retrieved from http://www.jointcommission.org. Evidence Level VI.

Kamel, H. K. (2004). Secondary prevention of hip fractures among hospitalized elderly: Are we doing enough? *The Internet Journal of Geriatrics and Gerontology, 1*(1), 1–5. Retrieved from http://www.ispub.com/ostia/index.php?xmlFilePath=journals/ijgg/vol1n1/hip.xml. Evidence Level IV.

Kaufman, J. M., Johnell, O., Abadie, E., Adami, S., Audran, M., Avouac, B., . . . Reginster, J. Y. (2000). Background for studies on the treatment of male osteoporosis: State of the art. *Annals of the Rheumatic Diseases, 59*(10), 765–772,

Kelly, K. E., Phillips, C. L., Cain, K. C., Polissar, N. L., & Kelly, P. B. (2002). Evaluation of a non-intrusive monitor to reduce falls in nursing home patients. *Journal of the American Medical Directors Association, 3*(6), 377–382. Evidence Level IV.

Kutney-Lee, A., Lake, E. T., & Aiken, L. H. (2009). Development of the hospital nurse surveillance capacity profile. *Research in Nursing & Health, 32*(2), 217–228. Level IV.

Kwok, T., Mok, F., Chien, W. T., & Tam, E. (2006). Does access to bed-chair pressure sensors reduce physical restraint use in the rehabilitation setting. *Journal of Clinical Nursing, 15*(5), 581–587. Evidence Level II.

Langlois, J. A., Rutland-Brown, W., & Thomas, K. E. (2006). *Traumatic brain injury in the United States: Emergency department visits, hospitalization and deaths.* Atlanta, GA: CDC and the National Center for Injury Prevention and Control. Evidence Level V.

Leipzig, R. M., Cumming, R. G., & Tinetti, M. E. (1999). Drugs and falls in older people: A systematic review and meta-analysis: II. Cardiac and analgesic drugs. *Journal of the American Geriatrics Society, 47*(1), 40–50. Evidence Level I.

McInnes, E., & Askie, L. (2004). Evidence review on older people's views and experiences of falls prevention strategies. *Worldviews on Evidenced-Based Nursing, 1*(1), 20–37. Evidence Level I.

Meade, C., Bursell, M., & Ketelsen, L. (2006). Effects of nursing rounds on patients' call light use, satisfaction and safety. *American Journal of Nursing, 106*(9), 58–70.

Miles, S. H. (2002). Deaths between bedrails and air pressure mattresses. *Journal of the American Geriatrics Society, 50*(6), 1124–1125. Evidence Level VI.

Nelson, A., Powell-Cope, G., Gavin-Dreschnack, D., Quigley, P., Bulat, T., Baptiste, A. S., . . . Friedman, Y. (2004). Technology to promote safe mobility in the elderly. *Nursing Clinics of North America, 39*(3), 649–671. Evidence Level VI.

Neutel, C. I., Perry, S., & Maxwell, C. (2002). Medication use and risk of falls. *Pharmacoepidemiological and Drug Safety, 11*(2), 97–104. Evidence Level VI.

Oliver, D, Connelly, J. B., Victor, C. R., Shaw, F. E., Whitehead, A., Genc, Y., . . . Gosney, M. A. (2007). Strategies to prevent falls and fractures in hospitals and care homes and effect of cognitive impairment: Systematic review and meta-analysis. *British Medical Journal, 334*(7584), 53–4. Evidence Level I.

Oliver, D., Healy, F., & Haines, T. P. (2010). Preventing falls and fall-related injuries in hospitals. *Clinic Geriatric Medicine, 26*(4), 645–692.

Panel on Prevention of Falls in Older Persons. (2011). Summary of the Updated American Geriatrics Society/British Geriatrics Society Clinical Practice Guideline for prevention of falls in older persons. *Journal of the American Geriatrics Society, 59*, 148–157. doi:10.1111/j.1532-5415.2010.03234.x. Evidence Level I.

Papaioannou, A., Parkinson, W., Cook, R., Ferko, N., Coker, E., & Adachi, J. D. (2004). Prediction of falls using a risk assessment tool in the acute care setting. *BMC Medicine, 21*(2), 1. Evidence Level III.

Parker, M. J. Gillespie, W. J. & Gillespie, L. D. (2006). Effectiveness of hip protectors for preventing hip fractures in elderly people. *BMJ, 332*(7541), 571–574. Evidence Level I.

Perell, K., Nelson, A., Goldman, R., Luther, S. L., Prieto-Lewis, N., & Rubenstein, L. Z. (2001). Fall risk assessment measures: An analytic review. *Journal of Gerontology, 56*(12), 761–766. Evidence Level V.

Prevention of Falls Network Europe. (2006). Retrieved from http://www.profane.eu.org. Evidence Level VI.

Quigley, P., & Goff, L. (2011). Current and emerging innovations to keep patients safe. Technological innovations play a leading role in fall-prevention programs. Special Report: Best Practices for Fall Reduction. A Practice Guide. *American Nurse Today*, March, 14–17.

Quigley, P., Hahm, B., Collazo, S., Gibson, W., Janzen, S., Powell-Cope, G., . . . White, S. V. (2009). Reducing serious injury from falls in two veterans' acute medical-surgical units. *Journal of Nursing Care Quality, 24*(1), 33–41.

Quigley, P., Neily, J., Watson, M., Wright, M., & Strobel, K. (2007). Measuring fall program outcomes. *Online Journal of Issues in Nursing, 12*(2). doi:10.3912/OJIN.Vol12No02PPT01

Ray, W. A., Taylor, J. A., Meador, K. G., Thapa, P. B., Brown, A. K., Kajihara, H. K., . . . Griffin, M. R. (1997). A randomized trial of a consultation service to reduce falls in nursing homes. *Journal of the American Medical Association, 278*, 557–562. Evidence Level II.

Rubenstein, L. Z., & Josephson, K. R. (2006). Falls and their prevention in the elderly: What does the evidence show? *Medical Clinics of North American, 90*(5), 807–824. Evidence Level I.

Rubenstein, L .Z., Robbins, A.S., Josephson, K.R., Schulman, B. L., & Osterweil, D. (1990). The value of assessing falls in an elderly population: A randomized clinical trial. *Annals of Internal Medicine, 113*(4), 308–316. Evidence Level II.

Scott, V., Votova, K., Scanlan, A., & Close, J. (2007). Multifactorial and functional mobility assessment tools for fall risk among older adults in community, home-support, long-term and acute care settings. *Age and Aging, 36*(2), 130–139.

Smyth, C., Dubin, S., Restrepo, A., Nueva-Espana, H. & Capezuti, E, (2001). Creating order out of chaos: Models of GNP practice with hospitalized older adults. *Clinical Excellence for Nurse Practitioners, 5*(2), 88–95. Evidence Level IV.

Smith R. G. (2003). Fall-contributing adverse effects of the most frequently prescribed drugs. *Journal of the American Podiatric Medical Association*; *93*(1), 42–50. Evidence Level VI.

Tinetti, M. E., Williams, T. S., & Mayewski, R. (1986). Fall risk index for elderly patients based on number of chronic disabilities. *American Journal of Medicine, 80*(3), 429–434. Evidence Level II.

U.S. Department of Health and Human Services Centers for Medicare and Medicaid Services. (2004). *Evidence Report and Evidenced-based Recommendations: Fall Prevention Interventions in the Medicare Population* (RAND Contract No. 500-98-0281). Period September 30, 1998 to September 29, 2003. Evidence Level I.

van Doorn, C., Gruber-Baldini, A. L., Zimmerman, S., Hebel, J. R., Port, C. L., Baumgarten, M., . . . Epidemiology of Dementia in Nursing Homes Research Group. (2003). Dementia as a risk factor for falls and fall injuries among nursing home residents. *Journal of the American Geriatrics Society, 51*(9), 1213–1218.

Preventing Pressure Ulcers and Skin Tears

16

Elizabeth A. Ayello and R. Gary Sibbald

EDUCATIONAL OBJECTIVES

On completion of this chapter, the reader should be able to:

1. complete a comprehensive pressure ulcer risk assessment
2. classify pressure ulcers using the correct staging definitions (check for applicability in your clinical care setting or country)
3. develop a comprehensive, holistic plan to prevent pressure ulcers in individuals at risk
4. identify older adults at risk for skin tears
5. classify skin tears using the Payne–Martin classification system
6. develop a plan to prevent and treat skin tears

OVERVIEW

The skin is the largest external organ, so preserving its integrity is an important aspect of nursing care. Performing a risk assessment and implementing a consistent prevention protocol may avoid some losses of skin integrity including pressure ulcers or skin tears. Although pressure ulcers and skin tears may look similar, they are different types of skin injury; skin tears are acute traumatic wounds, whereas pressure ulcers are chronic wounds. It is important, therefore, to assess the wound and to determine the correct etiology so that the proper individualized treatment plan can be implemented.

BACKGROUND AND STATEMENT OF PROBLEM

Pressure Ulcers

Pressure ulcers are a significant health care problem worldwide (Bolton, 2010). They have a significant impact on health-related quality of life (HRQL; Gorecki et al., 2009). In February 2009, the National Pressure Ulcer Advisory Panel (NPUAP; European Pressure Ulcer Advisory Panel [EPUAP] & NPUAP, 2009), in conjunction with the EPUAP, revised the classic 1989 pressure ulcer definition ("Pressure ulcers prevalence," 1989) to eliminate the word friction in the definition (see Table 16.1). Pressure ulcers

For description of Evidence Levels cited in this chapter, see Chapter 1, Developing and Evaluating Clinical Practice Guidelines: A Systematic Approach, page 7.

TABLE 16.1

2009 International NPUAP-EPUAP Pressure Ulcer Definition and Classification System

Pressure ulcer definition

A pressure ulcer is localized injury to the skin and/or underlying tissue, usually over a bony prominence, as a result of pressure, or pressure in combination with shear. A number of contributing or confounding factors are also associated with pressure ulcers; the significance of these factors is yet to be elucidated.

NPUAP/EPUAP pressure ulcer classification system

Category/Stage 1: Nonblanchable redness of intact skin

Intact skin with nonblanchable erythema of a localized area, usually over a bony prominence. Discoloration of the skin, warmth, edema, hardness, or pain may also be present. Darkly pigmented skin may not have visible blanching.

Further description

The area may be more painful, firmer or softer, or warmer or cooler than adjacent tissue. Category 1 may be difficult to detect in individuals with dark skin tones. This may indicate an "at-risk" individual.

Category/Stage 2: Partial thickness skin loss or blister

Partial thickness, loss of dermis presenting as a shallow, open ulcer with a red or pink wound bed, without slough. It may also present as an intact or open or ruptured serum-filled blister.

Further description

Presents as a shiny or dry shallow ulcer without slough or bruising. This category should not be used to describe skin tears, tape burns, incontinence-associated dermatitis, maceration, or excoriation.

Category/Stage 3: Full thickness skin loss (fat visible)

Full thickness tissue loss, subcutaneous fat may be visible but bone, tendon, or muscle are *not* exposed. Some slough may be present. It may include undermining and tunneling.

Further description

The depth of a Category 3 pressure ulcer varies by anatomical location. The bridge of the nose, ear, occiput, and malleolus do not have (adipose) subcutaneous tissue and Category 3 ulcers can be shallow. In contrast, areas of significant adiposity can develop extremely deep Category 3 pressure ulcers. Bone or tendon is not visible or directly palpable.

Category/Stage 4: Full thickness tissue loss (muscle and bone are visible)

Full thickness tissue loss with exposed bone, tendon, or muscle. Slough or eschar may be present. It often includes undermining and tunneling.

Further description

The depth of a Category 4 pressure ulcer varies by anatomical location. The bridge of the nose, ear, occiput, and malleolus do not have (adipose) subcutaneous tissue and these ulcers can be shallow. Category 4 ulcers can extend into muscle and/or supporting structures (e.g., fascia, tendon, or joint capsule) making osteomyelitis or osteitis likely to occur. Exposed bone or muscle is visible or directly palpable.

Additional Categories for the United States

Unstageable/Unclassified: Full thickness skin or tissue loss depth unknown

Full thickness tissue loss in which actual depth of the ulcer is completely obscured by slough (yellow, tan, gray, green, or brown) and/or eschar (tan, brown, or black) in the wound bed.

Further description

Until enough slough and/or eschar are removed to expose the base of the wound, the true depth cannot be determined, but it will be either a Category 3 or 4. Stable (dry, adherent, intact, without erythema, or fluctuance) eschar on the heels serves as "the body's natural (biological) cover" and should not be removed.

Suspected deep tissue injury—depth unknown

Purple or maroon localized area of discolored, intact skin or blood-filled blister caused by damage of underlying soft tissue from pressure and/or shear.

(continued)

TABLE 16.1

2009 International NPUAP-EPUAP Pressure Ulcer Definition and Classification System *(continued)*

Further description

The area may be preceded by tissue that is painful, firm, mushy, boggy, warmer, or cooler as compared to adjacent tissue. Deep tissue injury may be difficult to detect in individuals with dark skin tones. Evolution may include a thin blister over a dark wound bed. The wound may further evolve and become covered by thin eschar. Evolution may be rapid exposing additional layers of tissue even with optimal treatment.

Note. NPUAP = National Pressure Ulcer Advisory Panel; EPUAP = European Pressure Ulcer Advisory Panel. Adapted from *Treatment of Pressure Ulcers: Quick Reference Guide*, by European Pressure Ulcer Advisory Panel, & National Pressure Ulcer Advisory Panel, 2009, Washington, DC: National Pressure Ulcer Advisory Panel. Copyright 2009 by the National Pressure Ulcer Advisory Panel. Reprinted with permission.

are believed to develop as a result of the tissues' internal response to external mechanical loading (EPUAP & NPUAP, 2009).

The exact combination of pressure, ischemia, muscle deformation, and reperfusion injury that leads to a pressure ulcer remains unclear (EPUAP & NPUAP, 2009). Most pressure ulcers on adults are found on the sacrum, with heels being the second most common site (VanGilder, Amlung, Harrison, & Meyer, 2009). Data in 2009 from 92,408 U.S. facilities reported an overall prevalence rate of 12.3%, with facility acquired rate of 5.0% and 3.2% when Stage 1 ulcers are excluded (VanGilder, Amlung, Harrison, & Meyer, 2009). This same study of 86,932 U.S. acute care facilities reported an overall prevalence rate of 11.9%, with facility acquired rate of 5.0% and 3.1% when Stage 1 ulcers were excluded (VanGilder et al., 2009).

Table 16.2 summarizes the number of pressure ulcers by stages from this study (VanGilder et al., 2009). The distribution of pressure ulcers has changed over the past years, with the number of Stage 1 ulcers decreasing and the number of unstageable pressure ulcers increasing to 15% as well as suspected deep tissue injury (sDTI) to 9% (VanGilder, MacFarlane, Harrison, Lachenbruch, & Meyer, 2010). Device-related pressure ulcers account for 9.1% of ulcers, with ears being the most common location (see Table 16. 3; VanGilder et al., 2009). In hospice patients, besides sacrum and heels, elbows were a common site for ulcers with most ulcers occurring within 2 weeks prior to death (Hanson et al., 1991). In one hospital's 10-bed palliative care unit, 5% of their patients

TABLE 16.2

2009 Pressure Ulcer Prevalence by Stages in Acute Care

Type of Pressure Ulcer	Number of Pressure Ulcers
Stage 1 or 2	4,985
Stage 3 or 4, eschar or unable to stage	876
DTI	642
Stage unspecified	86
Device-related	1,631

Note. DTI = deep tissue injury. Adapted from VanGilder, C., Amlung, S., Harrison, P., & Meyer, S. (2009). Results of the 2008–2009 International Pressure Ulcer Prevalence Survey and a 3-year, acute care, unit-specific analysis. *Ostomy/Wound Management, 55*(11), 39–45, (data p. 42).

TABLE 16.3

Location of Device-Related Pressure Ulcers

Location	Location Percentage of Device-Related Pressure Ulcer
Ears	20%
Sacral/Coccyx	17%
Heel	12%
Buttocks	10%

Adapted from VanGilder, C., Amlung, S., Harrison, P., & Meyer, S. (2009). Results of the 2008–2009 International Pressure Ulcer Prevalence Survey and a 3-year, acute care, unit-specific analysis. *Ostomy/Wound Management, 55*(11), 39–45, (data on page 42).

developed a Kennedy terminal pressure ulcer (shaped like a pear, over the sacrum, bruise-like discoloration with yellow and brown black; Brennan & Trombley, 2010).

Pressure Ulcer Risk Factors

No single factor puts a patient at risk for pressure ulcer skin breakdown. Nonnemacher et al. (2009) are addressing the question of what combination of factors increase the risk and they are exploring 12 factors that seem to have the most impact on predicting pressure ulcer risk. Historically, pressure ulcers occur from a combination of intensity and duration of pressure as well as from tissue tolerance (Bergstrom, Braden, Laguzza, & Holman, 1987; Braden & Bergstrom, 1987, 1989). Immobility as seen in bedbound or chairbound patients and those unable to change positions leading to shear, under-nourishment or malnutrition, incontinence, friable skin, impaired cognitive ability, and decreased ability to respond to one's environment are some of the important identified risk factors for pressure ulcers (Braden, 1998). True pressure ulcers need to be distinguished from moisture-associated dermatitis or surface injury in the buttocks region caused by the contact irritation of local friction and moisture factors.

A study of 20 hospitals of patients waiting for surgery determined a higher incidence of pressure ulcers for longer surgery waiting times or time in an intensive care unit (ICU; Baumgarten et al., 2003). Most pressure ulcers, in one study of 84 surgical patients, occurred within the first three postoperative days (Karadag & Gümüskaya, 2006).

Patients With Hip Fracture and Pressure Ulcer Risk

In a study of nine hospitals, the cumulative incidence of Stage 2 or higher pressure ulcer in older adults with hip fractures was 36.1% (Baumgarten et al., 2009). The less time that patients waited to go to the operating room (OR) for their repair of a hip fracture, the fewer the number of associated Level 4 pressure ulcers (Hommel, Ulander, & Thorngren, 2003). The length of time on the OR table also increased the risk for pressure ulcers in patients with hip fracture (Houwing et al., 2004). Campbell, Woodbury, and Houghton (2010b) found that one-third of their sample of patients with hip fracture developed Stage 2 or higher pressure ulcers. Implementation of a heel pressure ulcer prevention program (HPUPP) for orthopedic patients in Canada resulted in complete elimination of heel pressure ulcers compared to preimplementation level of 13.8% (Baumgarten et al., 2008). However, this was not designed for sustainability after the original study of a wedge-shaped lower leg positioner to lift the heel off the bed.

Critically Ill, Intensive Care Unit Patients and Pressure Ulcer Risk

In a case control study of medical patients in two hospitals, Baumgarten and colleagues (2008) found that the odds of developing a pressure ulcer were twice as high for those having an ICU stay. In contrast, Shalin, Dassen, and Halfens (2009) found a low incidence of pressure ulcers in their 121 ICU patients that they concluded were caused by using foam and alternating air pressure mattresses. APACHE II scores, physiological criteria and Glasgow Coma Scale to predict ICU outcomes with higher scores having poorer outcomes, were higher in patients who developed pressure ulcers. In contrast, other researchers found no relationship between pressure ulcer development and APACHE II scores (Kaitani, Tokunaga, Matsui, & Sanada, 2010). Shanks, Kleinhelter, and Baker (2008) found that despite the consistent implementation of pressure ulcer prevention protocols in their critically ill patients, the patients that developed more hypotensive episodes were more likely to develop subsequent pressure ulcers.

Regulatory and Government Initiatives

Recent regulatory and government initiatives continuously support the importance of pressure ulcer prevention. Beginning October 1, 2008, the Centers for Medicare and Medicaid Services (CMS) no longer pay a higher diagnosis-related group (DRG) for pressure ulcers acquired during hospitalization (CMS Hospital Acquired Conditions, 2011). Recording of location and stage of any stage 3 and 4 pressure ulcers present on admission (POA) is now holding clinicians legally responsible for establishing the medical diagnosis accountable for documenting this information in the patient's medical record; otherwise, the hospital will not be reimbursed (Russo, Steiner, & Spector, 2006). Data from the Healthcare Cost and Utilization Project (HCUP) statistical review reveal that over the past 11 years, pressure ulcers have increased in hospitalized patients by 80%, even though the number of hospitalizations during this period of 1993–2006 only increased by 15% (CMS Hospital Acquired Conditions, 2011). In the state of New Jersey (NJ), pressure ulcers, Stage 3 or 4, are now reportable in acute care (NJ Department of Health and Senior Services, 2004). Pressure ulcers are one of the 12 targeted areas to reduce harm to hospitalized patients in the United States as part of the Institute for Healthcare Improvement's (IHI) "5 Million Lives Campaign" launched in December 2006 (IHI, 2006). The former head of IHI is now the head of CMS. Thus, at the beginning of the 21st century, appropriate risk assessment and preventative care take on even more important meaning. Several successful initiatives to decrease pressure ulcer incidence are reported in the literature (Lyder & Ayello, 2009; McInerney, 2008). Nurses will find the Agency for Healthcare Research and Quality (AHRQ) toolkit helpful in developing quality initiatives to decreased pressure ulcer incidence (Pancorbo-Hidalgo, Garcia-Fernandez, Lopez-Medina, & Alvarez-Nieto, 2006).

ASSESSMENT OF THE PROBLEM

When To Do an Assessment

The assessment of the relative pressure ulcer risk is the first step of any individual patient or health care system plan for prevention. Some pressure ulcer clinical guidelines recommend that patients are assessed for pressure ulcer development on admission to a facility, on discharge, whenever the patient's condition changes, then reassessed periodically (EPUAP & NPUAP, 2009; Norton, McLaren, & Exton-Smith, 1962). The IHI recommends daily pressure ulcer risk assessment (IHI, 2006).

Pressure Ulcer Risk Assessment Tools

Guidelines recommend that a comprehensive assessment for pressure ulcer risk include a history and physical exam, skin inspection, and a pressure ulcer risk assessment calculation using a valid and reliable assessment tool. Both the Braden (Norton et al., 1962) and Norton scale (Norton et al., 1962; Norton, McLaren, & Exton-Smith, 1975) are considered reliable and valid. A study of 429 patients in acute care found the modified Braden scale to be a better predictor than the Norton scale (Kwong et al., 2005). Although Kottner and Dassen (2010) found that the Braden scale was more valid and reliable than the Waterlow scale, they do not recommend either of these scales for ICU patients. Research to create new scales specific to ICU patients continues (Suriadi, Sanada, Sugama, Thigpen, & Subuh, 2008).

The Braden scale created in 1987 (Bergstrom et al., 1987) as part of a research study has six factors and is the most widely used in the United States. Sensory perception, mobility, and activity address clinical situations that predispose the patient to intense and prolonged pressure. Moisture, nutrition, and friction and shear address factors that alter tissue tolerance for pressure. Each of the six categories is ranked with a numerical score, with 1 representing the lowest possible subscore with the greatest risk. The sum of the six subscores is the final Braden scale score, which can range from 6 to 23.

A low Braden scale score indicates that a patient is at risk for pressure ulcers. The original onset of risk score on the Braden scale was 16 or less (Braden & Bergstrom, 1987). Further research in older adults (Bergstrom & Braden, 1992) and in persons with darkly pigmented skin (Lyder et al., 1998, 1999) support a score of 18 or less. Research by Chan, Tan, Lee, and Lee (2005) also found that the total Braden scale score was the only significant predictor of pressure ulcers in hospitalized patients. In 2009, Chan, Pang, and Kwong (2009) found that using a modified Braden scale, with a cutoff score of 19 in 107 bed orthopedic department of an acute care hospital in Hong Kong, 9.1% of patients developed pressure ulcers. In a retrospective study of intensive care patients in Korea using a cutoff score of 13, the Braden scale had low-to-moderate positive predictive performance without a more comprehensive approach to patient-risk assessment (Cho & Noh, 2010). Risk was associated with pressure ulcer development in ICU patients where they had low Braden scale scores on the first day of hospitalization and low Glasgow scale scores (Fernances & Caliri, 2008).

Once risk is identified, either for overall score or in *any* low subscales (CMS, 2004), prevention interventions need to be implemented. However, one study found that despite identification of pressure ulcer risk using the Norton scale, only 51% of the sample of the 792 patients, 65 years and older hospitalized patients, had a preventive device in place (Rich, Shardell, Margolis, & Baumgarten, 2009).

DOES RACE MAKE A DIFFERENCE?

When it comes to severity of pressure ulcers, race may make a difference. Ayello and Lyder (2001) analyzed and summarized the existing data about pressure ulcers across the skin pigmentation spectrum. Blacks have the lowest incidence (19%) of superficial tissue damage classified as Stage 1 pressure ulcers, and Whites have the highest incidence at 46% (Barczak, Barnett, Childs, & Bosley, 2007). The more severe tissue injury seen in Stages 2–4 pressure ulcers is higher in persons with darkly pigmented skin (Barczak et al., 2007; Meehan, 1990, 1994). Three national surveys showed that Blacks had 39% (Barczak et al., 2007), 16% (Meehan, 1990), and 41% (Meehan, 1994) higher incidence of Stage 2 pressure ulcers compared to Caucasians. Subsequent studies by Lyder and colleagues (1998, 1999) continue to support a higher incidence of pressure ulcers in persons with darkly pigmented skin. Fogerty, Guy, Barbul, Nanney, and Abumrad (2009) found that not only was there a higher prevalence of pressure ulcers, but also that they occurred in younger African Americans as compared to Caucasians.

Inadequate detection of Stage 1 pressure ulcers in persons with darkly pigmented skin may be because clinicians erroneously believe that dark skin tolerates pressure better than light skin (Bergstrom, Braden, Kemp, Champagne, & Ruby, 1996), or that only color changes indicate an ulcer (Bennett, 1995; Henderson et al., 1997; Lyder, 1996; Lyder et al., 1998, 1999; Rich et al., 2009). Research has begun to validate these assessment characteristics in the Stage 1 definition. In 2001, Lyder and colleagues (2001) reported a higher diagnostic accuracy rate of 78% using the revised definition compared with 58% with the original definition. Sprigle, Linden, McKenna, Davis, and Riordan (2001) found changes in skin temperature; in particular, that warmth then coolness accompanied most Stage 1 pressure ulcers.

Clinicians should pay careful attention to a variety of factors when assessing a client with darkly pigmented skin for Stage 1 pressure ulcers. Differences in skin over bony prominences (e.g., the sacrum and the heels) as compared with surrounding skin may be indicators of a Stage 1 pressure ulcer. The skin should be assessed for alterations in pain or local sensation. In addition, a change of skin color should be noted by being familiar with the range of skin pigmentation that is normal for your particular patient (Bennett, 1995; Henderson et al., 1997).

INTERVENTIONS AND CARE STRATEGIES

Determining a patient's risk for developing a pressure ulcer is only the first step in providing best practice care. Once risk is identified, implementing a consistent protocol to prevent the development of a pressure ulcer is essential. A nursing standard of practice protocol for pressure ulcer prevention is presented to facilitate proactive interventions to prevent pressure ulcers. A change in attitudes of health care professionals may be required to facilitate prevention (Buss, Halfens, Abu-Saad, & Kok, 2004). Educating nursing students (Holst et al., 2010) as well as nurses in an ICU unit resulted in decrease in pressure ulcers (Uzun, Aylaz, & Karadag, 2009). Several clinical guidelines on preventing and treating pressure ulcers exist (EPUAP & NPUAP, 2009; Wound, Ostomy, and Continence Nurses Society, 2010). Components of a pressure ulcer prevention protocol should minimally include interventions targeting the following: skin care (including addressing moisture and friction), pressure redistribution, repositioning, and nutrition.

Skin Care

Skin that is too dry or too wet has been associated with pressure ulcers. Although there is limited research, dry skin is believed to predispose ulcer formation (Allman, Goode, Patrick, Burst, & Bartolucci, 1995; Reddy, Gill, & Rochon, 2006). The type of cream used on the skin for different parts of the body may make a difference as evidenced by a study of 79 patients treated with dimethyl sulfoxide cream who had an increase in pressure ulcers when this cream was used on the heels as compared to the buttocks (Houwing, Van der Zwet, van Asbeck, Halfens, & Arends, 2008). Other researchers (Stratton et al., 2005) found that a silicone-based dermal nourishing cream reduced the proportion of hospital-acquired pressure ulcers to zero after 8 months. Each of these creams are lubricating, adding an external ointment type of layer preventing insensible losses. The stratum corneum has 10% moisture content and when this level goes below a critical level, the skin integrity is lost with defects between the keratin layers (dry skin, winter itch, eczema craquelé). The second way to moisturize the skin is with urea or lactic acid preparations. These are humectants that actually bind water to the stratum corneum but will sting or burn when applied to open skin because of their hydroscopic properties. Skin can also be too wet with macerated stratum corneum, decreasing the cutaneous barrier and subjecting affected individuals to increase risk of yeast and bacterial infections.

Use of a soft silicone dressing on the sacrum of critically ill patients resulted in zero pressure ulcers in one ICU (Brindle, 2010). Hydrocolloid dressings decreased pressure ulcers from nasotracheal intubation (Huang, Tseng, Lee, Yeh, & Lai, 2009). When hydrocolloid or film dressings were applied to the skin under face masks, there were fewer pressure ulcers (Weng, 2008).

Repositioning and Pressure Redistribution

Because immobility is a risk factor in the development of pressure ulcers in hospitalized patients (Lindgren, Unosson, Fredrikson, & Ek, 2004), efforts must be implemented to address pressure. Although repositioning patients is a key intervention to redistribute the pressure and prevent pressure ulcers, the best frequency for turning and repositioning as well as which support surface to use remains a challenge (Defloor, De Bacquer, & Grypdonck, 2005; Norton et al., 1975; Young, 2004). Patients on a particular support surface may not have to be repositioned every 2 hours, depending on the persons' tolerance to pressure. There is no one repositioning timetable for all, it needs to be individualized (EPUAP & NPUAP, 2009). The use of a wedge-shaped cushion rather than a pillow may be more effective in decreasing pressure ulcers in some patients (Heyneman, Vanderwee, Grypdonck, & Defloor, 2009).

Redistributing pressure is a key component of preventing pressure ulcers. When compared to alternating pressure overlays, alternating pressure mattresses reduced length of stay for hospitalized patients, thus, decreasing costs as well as the added benefit of delaying the time to when a pressure ulcer appeared (Iglesias et al., 2006; Nixon et al., 2006). The incidence of heel pressure ulcers have been decreased when the appropriate heel suspending device has been used to relieve pressure (Gilcreast et al., 2005). In 2010, a prospective 150-patient, 6-month study by Campbell, Woodbury, and Houghton (2010a), pressure ulcer incidence was 16% being significantly lower ($p = .016$) for those who received help with pressure relief interventions. In a single study, when persons with a body mass index (BMI) greater than 35 were placed on appropriate size low air loss equipment, no new pressure ulcers developed (Pemberton, Turner, & Van Gilder, 2009). In Australia where real medical sheepskin is available, one study that had some questionable methodology demonstrated that patients randomly assigned to the real sheepskin mattress overlay during their hospital stay had a 9.6% incidence risk of pressure ulcers compared to the control group that had 16.6% (Jolley et al., 2004). A similar increased attention to pressure redistribution also needs to be brought into the OR.

Nutrition

There is lack of consensus about the best way to assess nutritional impairment but, generally, consultation by a dietician for nutritional status, determination of any unintended weight loss, and evaluation of laboratory values such as serum albumin or prealbumin should be considered. Cordeiro and colleagues (2005) found that the concentrations of ascorbic acid and alpha-tocopherol were significantly decreased in patients with pressure ulcers or infection. In a randomized double blind study on the effect of daily supplement with protein, arginine, zinc, and antioxidants versus water-based placebo supplement in patients with hip fractures, the incidence of Stage 2 pressure ulcers demonstrated a 9% difference between the nutritionally supplemented group and the placebo group (Houwing et al., 2003). The Cochrane Database reviewed the role of nutrition in pressure ulcer prevention and treatment. The analysis of the database was inconclusive because of the lack of high-quality trials (Langer, Schloemer, Knerr, Kuss, & Behrens, 2003). When and how patients should be nutritionally supplemented to prevent pressure ulcers remains unclear (Houwing et al., 2003; Reddy et al., 2006; Stratton et al., 2005), but at times the literature is contradictory. The NPUAP nutritional recommendations (EPUAP & NPUAP, 2009) for pressure ulcer prevention are included in Protocol 16.1.

SKIN TEARS

Skin tears are traumatic wounds caused by shear and friction (O'Regan, 2002). This skin injury occurs when the epidermis is separated from the dermis (Malone, Rozario, Gavinski, & Goodwin, 1991). Because aging skin has a thinner epidermis, a flatter dermal-epidermal junction and decreased dermal collagen, older persons are more prone to skin injury from mechanical trauma (Baranoski, 2000; Payne & Martin, 1993; White, Karam, & Cowell, 1994). Therefore, skin tears are common in older adults, with more than 1.5 million occurring annually in institutionalized adults in the United States (Thomas, Goode, LaMaster, Tennyson, & Parnell, 1999), although the incidence in acute care is unknown. Skin tears are frequently located at areas of age-related purpura (Malone et al., 1991; White et al., 1994).

Assessment of Skin Tears

The following areas should be assessed for skin tears: shins, face, dorsal aspect of hands, and plantar aspect of the foot (Malone et al., 1991). Besides older adults, others with thinning skin who are at risk for skin tears are patients on long-term steroid therapy, women with decreased hormone levels, persons with peripheral vascular disease or neuropathy (the decreased sensation making them more susceptible to injury), and those with inadequate nutritional intake (O'Regan, 2002).

The three-group risk assessment tool was developed during a research study by White and colleagues (1994). Because of its length, it is not always used clinically to assess for risk of skin tears (White et al., 1994). Within the tool, there are three groups delineated by level of risk: Groups 1, 2, and 3. Group 1 refers to a positive history of skin tears within the last 90 days or skin tears that are already present. A positive score in this group requires that the patient be put on a skin tear prevention protocol. Group 2 requires four of the next six criteria to identify an increased risk: (a) decision-making skills are either impaired or slightly impaired, or extensive assistance and total dependence for activities of daily living (ADLs) is noted; (b) wheelchair assistance needed; (c) loss of balance; (d) bed or chair confined; (e) unsteady gait; and (f) bruises. If a patient has a score of 4 or more items in Group 2, then implement a skin tear prevention protocol. Group 3 includes the following 14 items requiring any five for an increased risk: (a) physically abusive; (b) resists ADL care; (c) agitation; (d) hearing impaired; (e) decreased tactile stimulation; (f) wheels self; (g) manually or mechanically lifted; (h) contractures of arms, legs, shoulders, and/or hands; (i) hemiplegia and hemiparesis; (j) trunk, partial, or total inability to balance or turn body; (j) pitting edema of legs; (k) open lesions on extremities; (l) three or four discrete senile purpura lesions on extremities; and (m) dry, scaly skin. An increased risk has also been identified in individuals with a combination of three items in Group 2 and three items in Group 3. Positive responses to five or more items in Group 3 or three items in both Groups 2 and 3 should also trigger the implementation of a skin tear prevention protocol (White et al., 1994).

Several authors have suggested protocols to prevent skin tears (Baranoski, 2000; Battersby, 1990; Mason, 1997; O'Regan, 2002; White et al., 1994). Lacking research in acute care, some nursing home research supports the value of skin ulcer care protocols to reduce the incidence of skin tears (Bank, 2005; Birch & Coggins, 2003; Hanson, Anderson, Thompson, & Langemo, 2005). After changing from soap and water to a no-rinse, one step bed product, skin tears declined from 23.5% to 3.5% in one nursing home (Birch & Coggins, 2003). Hanson and colleagues (2005) also found that skin tears could be reduced in two different nursing homes when staff was educated in appropriate skin cleaning and protection strategies. A reduction in monthly average of skin tears from 18 to 11 after using longer lasting moisturizer lotion sleeves to protect the arms, and padded side rails was reported in yet another nursing home study (Bank, 2005). One study claims a decrease in skin tears when skin is treated with cream (Groom, Shannon, Chakravarthy, & Fleck, 2010).

Interventions for Skin Tears

If a skin tear does occur, it is important to correctly identify it and begin an appropriate plan of care. The Payne–Martin classification system (Payne & Martin, 1993) may be used to describe skin tears. The three categories are the following:

- Category 1: A skin tear without tissue loss
- Category 2: A skin tear with partial tissue loss
- Category 3: A skin tear with complete tissue loss where the epidermal flap is absent

The usual healing time for skin tears is 3–10 days (Krasner, 1991). Although skin tears are prevalent in the older adult patient, there is no consistent approach to managing these skin injuries (Baranoski, 2000; O'Regan, 2002). Research is just beginning to provide evidence on which dressing is best to use for skin tears. One study (Edwards, Gaskill, & Nash, 1998) compared the use of four different types of dressings in treating skin tears in a nursing home: three occlusive (transparent film, hydrocolloid, and polyurethane foam) and one nonocclusive dressing of Steristrips covered by a nonadhesive cellulose-polyester material. The nonocclusive dressing facilitated healing at a faster rate than the occlusive dressings. Another study by Thomas and colleagues (1999) studied older adult skin tears in three nursing homes and identified that there was a higher rate of complete healing that occurred with foam dressings compared to transparent films.

Goals of care for skin tears include retaining the skin flap if present, providing a moist, nonadherent dressing, and protecting the site from further injury (O'Regan, 2002). A consensus protocol for treating skin tears based on suggested plans of care have been developed by several authors (Baranoski, 2000; Baranoski & Ayello, 2008; Edwards et al., 1998; O'Regan, 2002) and can be found in Protocol 16.2.

CASE STUDY 1

Mr. Randy Gonnagetawound, age 70, has diabetes mellitus with several microvascular and macrovascular complications. He was admitted to the hospital after a right-sided cerebral vascular accident. Past history includes retinal hemorrhages, a previous myocardial infarction, peripheral vascular disease, and a neuroischemic foot ulcer (healed after a left femoral popliteal bypass, intravenous antibiotics, and plantar pressure redistribution with deep toed shoe and orthotic). He is incontinent of feces and urine and responds by nodding to verbal commands. The left arm and leg are paralyzed. He has a gag reflex but cannot swallow. His Braden score is 10.

Current Data

Physical exam: There is an area of persistent erythema with bruising on the left buttock along with a number of superficial nonpalpable purpuric lesions on the arms and legs.

Physical Assessment and Pertinent Admission History

General: Responds to verbal questioning but he cannot move his left side. Over the past 3 days, he has been increasingly fatigued, completely bedridden. He can change position only with movement of the right side.

Vital signs: Temperature = 39.2 °C

Respiration: 10 per minute and regular Pulse: 88 and irregular

Blood pressure: 162/94

Weight: 195 lbs.

Height: 5 ft 9 in.

Abdominal: Intake has been limited to half bowl of cereal twice a day and piece of toast and tea for lunch for the past 3 days. Last bowel movement was 3 days ago; + bowel sounds.

Cardiovascular: Irregular heartbeat, no S_3S_4 at apex, +1 pedal edema, faintly palpable pedal pulses; capillary refill prolonged at 8 seconds

Respiratory: Crackles over right lower lobe, coughing periodically, nonproductive of mucous

Renal: Episodes of urinary incontinence for the past 3 days prior to admission

(continued)

CASE STUDY 1 *(continued)*

Integumentary: Skin is warm, dry, and translucent; tenting noted

Laboratory data: Hg 10, HCT 28, RBC: 3.2, WBC: 11,000 shift to the left. Albumin 3.0 g/dl, K: 3.1, BUN: 32 mg/100 ml, glucose and/or HbA1c not available

Medical Orders

D_5W 1/2 NS with 10 mEq KCl at 100 cc/hr

Colace 100 mg PO tid

Pulse oximetry monitoring continuously

Metamucil 1 package QD

Bed rest

Multivitamin 1 tablet QD

Daily weights

Soft diet as tolerated

Mr. Gonnagetawound is a prime candidate for developing a pressure ulcer. His low numerical score on the Braden scale (10) puts him at high risk. Immediate strategies to prevent the occurrence of an ulcer are needed. Immobility is a leading risk factor for pressure ulcer development, so a major part of his plan of care needs to first be directed to initiate moving as much as possible. A physiotherapy consult is needed to evaluate and recommend a plan of progressive exercise and activity. The plan should be to get him out of bed and moving within the constraints of his limitations from the stroke, as well as being in the chair rather than the bed. When in the chair, he should have a gel cushion for pressure redistribution. He will need to be repositioned every hour when in the chair. A Group 2, alternating low-air-loss mattress needs to be placed on his bed. For the limited time, when he is in bed, he needs to be turned and positioned. His skin should be assessed every shift to evaluate signs for early skin injury.

A consult to a speech therapist is essential. A swallowing study is warranted to determine his ability to safely take an oral diet. A nutritional consult with a dietician will address his needs for appropriate calories, protein, and vitamins or minerals. A toileting regimen needs to be implemented to address the fecal and urinary incontinence. A discussion with the prescribing health care provider can explore whether he should continue on the Colace and Metamucil. His skin needs cleansing after each episode of incontinence. Use of a no-rinse bathing system is preferred here rather than soap and water. This vulnerable skin needs protection by using one of the many skin barriers available on the market.

Both Mr. Gonnagetawound and his family need instruction on why it is so important to get him moving and why nutrition, skin care, turning, and repositioning are so critical to his skin health.

Considering his general health, low hemoglobin, possibility of sepsis, and increase capillary refill must also be monitored and addressed. It would be beneficial to know the HbA1c to determine blood sugar control and prevent long-term complications.

CASE STUDY 2

Mrs. Keri Sight, 88 years old, is admitted to the hospital from a long-term care facility with a primary diagnosis of pneumonia, and secondary diagnosis of senile dementia of the Alzheimer's type with impaired communication skills. She has a history of congestive heart failure and osteoporosis. She spends most of the day in a wheelchair and needs two-person assistance for ambulation. Her skin is thin and dry, resembling an onion; each arm and leg has a purpura area. She is 15 lbs. less than her ideal body weight and has difficulty swallowing. Laboratory values are as follows: total protein, 5.5 g/dl; albumin, 2.6 g/dl; and BUN, 28. She is verbally aggressive to the staff on which she depends for assistance for her ADLs.

Assessment of Mrs. Sight on admission for skin integrity as well as pressure ulcer risk needs to be done. Because she has four of the criteria from Group 2 of the skin tear risk assessment tool developed by White and colleagues (1994; impaired decision-making skills caused by senile dementia, dependence for ADLs, wheelchair or bed confined, unsteady gait), she is at risk for developing skin tears. Other factors that would put her at risk are her thin, dry skin with four purpura present and poor nutritional status. Her dependence on staff for ADLs and assistance coupled with her dementia predispose her to skin injury during bathing and other ADLs. A comprehensive pressure ulcer risk assessment including her skin assessment, comorbidities, and Braden scale score puts her at very high risk for developing pressure ulcers. A pressure ulcer prevention protocol such as in Protocol 16.2 is implemented. The rest of this case discussion will focus on her skin tear risk needs.

A skin tear prevention protocol needs to be implemented for Mrs. Sight immediately. In order to achieve a safe environment for her, the staff must know how to approach her with her dementia. To address her nutrition and hydration risk factors, a dietary consultation should be performed. Her ability to safely swallow needs to be evaluated by a speech therapist. After the swallowing evaluation, a plan to encourage frequent fluids and assist with eating should be implemented. To protect Mrs. Sight's skin from additional injury, avoid using hot water to bathe her and, instead, use one of the nonrinse, soapless bathing products. Her family can be asked to bring in a soft fleece jogging suit for her to wear. The purpura areas on her arms and legs should be covered with stockinet or some other soft nonadherent dressing or skin-protective barrier product to further protect these areas. Her bed rails and the arms and legs of her wheelchair should be padded. Staff should use the palm of their hands and a turn sheet when repositioning Mrs. Sight in bed. Lotion can be applied twice a day to her dry skin. Daily assessment of her skin including the five minimal characteristics proposed by CMS should be done (Rich et al., 2009).

SUMMARY

The skin is the largest organ, so pay attention to it. Although the research into prevention strategies is limited, there is support for doing the appropriate risk assessment for these two types of skin injuries: pressure ulcers and skin tears.

General skin assessment is important for the early breakdown, protecting the skin by using appropriate bathing techniques, products to minimize the effects of friction and shear on the skin, and paying attention to nutritional status. In the case of pressure ulcers, redistributing the pressure by turning and repositioning and appropriate use of support surfaces is also critical. Immediate initiation of prevention protocols after risk identification is key with each major abnormal risk factor correction part of the treatment protocol. By doing so, you can prevent and treat skin integrity problems such as skin tears and pressure ulcers.

NURSING STANDARD OF PRACTICE

Protocol 16.1: Pressure Ulcer Prevention

I. GOALS
A. Prevention of pressure ulcers (PU)
B. Early recognition of PU development and skin changes

II. BACKGROUND AND STATEMENT OF PROBLEM
A. Pressure ulcer 2009: Occurrence data reported for 2009 (VanGilder et al., 2009)
  1. All U.S. facilities
     Overall Prevalence: 12.3%
     Facility acquired (FA) prevalence: 5.0 %
     Prevalence excluding Stage 1: 9.0%
     FA prevalence excluding Stage 1: 3.2%
  2. Acute care
B. Etiology and/or Epidemiology
  1. Risk factors (immobility, undernutrition or malnutrition, incontinence, friable skin, impaired cognitive ability)
  2. Higher incidence of Stage 2 and higher in persons with darkly pigmented skin

III. PARAMETERS OF ASSESSMENT
A. Perform a complete skin assessment as part of the risk assessment policy and practices (EPUAP & NPUAP, 2009, p. 27)
  1. Inspect skin regularly for color changes such as redness in lightly pigmented persons and discoloration in darkly pigmented persons (EPUAP & NPUAP, 2009, p. 28)
  2. Look at the skin under any medical device (e.g., catheters, oxygen, airway or ventilator tubing, face masks, braces, collars).
  3. Palpate skin for changes in temperature (warmth) edema or hardness
  4. Ask the patient if they have any areas of pain or discomfort over bony prominences
B. Assess for intrinsic and extrinsic risk factors
C. Braden scale risk score—18 or less for older adults and persons with darkly pigmented skin

(continued)

Protocol 16.1: Pressure Ulcer Prevention *(cont.)*

IV. NURSING CARE STRATEGIES AND INTERVENTIONS

A. Risk Assessment Documentation
  1. On admission to acute care
  2. Reassessment intervals whenever the client's condition changes and based on patient care setting:
      a. Based on patient acuity every 24–48 hours general units
      b. Critically ill patients every 12 hours
  3. Use a reliable and standardized tool for doing a risk assessment, such as the Braden scale as part of a comprehensive risk assessment (available at http://www.bradenscale.com/braden.PDF)
  4. Document risk assessment scores and implement prevention protocols based on overall scores, low subscores, and the comprehensive assessment of other risk factors.
  5. Assess risk of surgical patients for increased risk of pressure ulcers including the following factors: length of operation, number of hypotensive episodes, and/or low-core temperatures intraoperatively, reduced mobility on first day postoperatively.
B. General Care Issues and Interventions
  1. Culturally sensitive early assessment for Stage 1 pressure ulcers in clients with darkly pigmented skin
      a. Use a halogen light to look for skin color changes—may be purple hues or other discoloration based on patient's skin tone.
      b. Compare skin over bony prominences to surrounding skin—may be boggy or stiff, warm or cooler.
  2. Prevention recommendations:
      a. Skin care (EPUAP & NPUAP, 2009)
          i. Assess skin regularly.
          ii. Clean skin at time of soiling—avoid hot water and irritating cleaning agents.
          iii. Use emollients on dry skin.
          iv. Do not massage bony prominences as a pressure ulcer prevention strategy as well as do not vigorously rub skin at risk for pressure ulcers.
          v. Protect skin from moisture-associated damage (e.g., urinary and/or fecal incontinence, perspiration, wound exudates) by using barrier products.
          vi. Use lubricants, protective dressings, and proper lifting techniques to avoid skin injury from friction and shear during transferring and turning of clients. Avoid drying out the patient's skin; use lotion after bathing.
          vii. Avoid hot water and soaps that are drying when bathing older adults. Use body wash and skin protectant (Hunter et al., 2003).
          viii. Teach patient, caregivers, and staff the prevention protocol
          ix. Manage moisture by determining the cause; use absorbent pad

(continued)

Protocol 16.1: Pressure Ulcer Prevention *(cont.)*

that wicks moisture.

    x. Protect high-risk areas such as elbows, heels, sacrum, and back of head from friction injury.

b. Repositioning and support surfaces

    i. Keep patients off the reddened areas of skin

    ii. Repositioning schedules should be individualized based on the patient's condition, care goals, vulnerable skin areas, and type of support surface being used (EPUAP & NPUAP, 2009).

    iii. Communicate the repositioning schedule to all the patient's caregivers.

    iv. Raise heels of bedbound clients off the bed using either pillows or heel-protection devices; do not use donut-type devices (Gilcreast et al., 2005).

    v. Use a 30 degree tilted side lying position; do not place clients directly in a 90 degree side lying position on their trochanter

    vi. Keep head of the bed at lowest height possible.

    vii. Use transfer and lifting devices (trapeze, bed linen) to move patients rather than dragging them in bed during transfers and position changes.

    viii. Use pressure-reducing devices (static air, alternating air, gel, or water mattresses; Iglesias et al., 2006; Hampton & Collins, 2005). Use higher specification foam mattresses rather than standard hospital mattress for patients at risk for pressure ulcers. If the patient cannot be frequently repositioned manually, use an active support surface (overlay or mattress).

    ix. Use pressure redistributing mattresses on the operating table for patients identified at risk for developing pressure ulcers.

    x. Reposition chairbound or wheelchair-bound clients every hour. In addition, if client is capable, have him or her do small weight shifts every 15 minutes.

    xi. Use a pressure-reducing device (not a donut) for chairbound clients.

    xii. Keep the patient as active as possible; encourage mobilization

    xiii. Avoid positioning the patient directly on his or her trochanter

    xiv. Avoid using donut-shaped devices

    xv. Offer a bedpan or urinal in conjunction with turning schedules

    xvi. Manage friction and shear:

        a) Elevate the head of the bed no more than 30 degrees.

        b) Have the patient use a trapeze to lift self up in bed.

        c) Staff should use a lift sheet or mechanical lifting device to move *patient.*

c. Nutrition

    i. Assess nutritional status of patients at risk for pressure ulcers.

    ii. For at-risk patient, follow nutritional guidelines for hydration

(continued)

Protocol 16.1: Pressure Ulcer Prevention *(cont.)*

  (1 ml/kcal of fluid per day) and calories (30–35 kcal/kg of body weight per day), protein 1.25–1.5 g/kg per day). Give high-protein supplements or tube feedings in addition to the usual diet in persons at nutritional and pressure ulcer risk (EPUAP & NPUAP, 2009).
 iii. Manage nutrition
 iv. Consult a dietitian and correct nutritional deficiencies by increasing protein and calorie intake and A, C, or E vitamin supplements as needed (CMS, 2004; Houwing et al., 2003)
 v. Offer a glass of water with turning schedules to keep patient hydrated.
C. Interventions Linked to Braden Risk Scores (Adapted from Ayello & Braden [2001])
  Prevention protocols linked to Braden risk scores are as follows:
  1. At risk: score of 15–18
 a. Frequent repositioning turning; use a written schedule
 b. Maximize patient's mobility
 c. Protect patient's heels
 d. Use a pressure-reducing support surface if patient is bedbound or chairbound.
  2. Moderate risk: score of 13–14
 a. Same as cited, but provide foam wedges for 30 degree lateral position.
  3. High risk: score of 10–12
 a. Same as cited, but add the following b and c.
 b. Increase the turning frequency
 c. Do small shifts of position
  4. Very high risk: score of 9 or less
 a. Same as cited but use a pressure-relieving surface.
 b. Manage moisture, nutrition, and friction and shear.

V. EVALUATION AND EXPECTED OUTCOMES
A. Patient
  1. Skin will remain intact.
  2. Pressure ulcer will heal.
B. Provider or Nurse
  1. Nurses will accurately perform PU risk assessment using standardized tool.
  2. Nurses will implement PU prevention protocols for clients interpreted as at risk for PU.
  3. Nurses will perform a skin assessment for early detection of pressure ulcers.
C. Institution
  1. Reduction in development of new pressure ulcers.
  2. Increased number of risk assessments performed.
  3. Cost-effective prevention protocols developed.

VI. FOLLOW-UP MONITORING OF CONDITION
A. Monitor effectiveness of prevention interventions.
B. Monitor healing of any existing pressure ulcers.

NURSING STANDARD OF PRACTICE

Protocol 16.2: Skin Tear Prevention

I. GOALS
A. Prevent skin tears in older adult clients.
B. Identify clients at risk for skin tears (Mason, 1997)
C. Foster healing of skin tears by:
   1. Retaining skin flap
   2. Providing a moist, nonadherent dressing (Edwards et al., 1998; Thomas et al., 1999)
   3. Protecting the site from further injury

II. BACKGROUND AND STATEMENT OF THE PROBLEM
A. Traumatic wounds from mechanical injury of skin
B. Need to clearly differentiate etiology of skin tears from pressure ulcers
C. Common in the older adult, especially over the areas of age-related purpura

III. PARAMETERS OF ASSESSMENT
A. Use the three-group risk assessment tool (White et al., 1994) to assess for skin tear risk.
B. Use the Payne–Martin (Payne & Martin, 1993) classification system to assess clients for skin tear risk.
   1. Category 1: a skin tear without tissue loss
   2. Category 2: a skin tear with partial tissue loss
   3. Category 3: a skin tear with complete tissue loss where the epidermal flap is absent

IV. NURSING CARE STRATEGIES AND INTERVENTIONS (Baranoski, 2000; Baranoski & Ayello, 2008)
A. Preventing Skin Tears
   1. Provide a safe environment:
      a. Do a risk assessment of older adult patients on admission.
      b. Implement prevention protocol for patients identified as at risk for skin tears.
      c. Have patients wear long sleeves or pants to protect their extremities (Bank, 2005).
      d. Have adequate light to reduce the risk of bumping into furniture or equipment.
      e. Provide a safe area for wandering.
   2. Educate staff or family caregivers in the correct way of handling patients to prevent skin tears. Maintain nutrition and hydration:
      a. Offer fluids between meals.
      b. Use lotion, especially on dry skin on arms and legs, twice daily (Hanson et al., 1991).
      c. Obtain a dietary consultation.

(continued)

3. Protect from self-injury or injury during routine care:
    a. Use a lift sheet to move and turn patients.
    b. Use transfer techniques that prevent friction or shear.
    c. Pad bed rails, wheelchair arms, and leg supports (Bank, 2005).
    d. Support dangling arms and legs with pillows or blankets.
    e. Use nonadherent dressings on frail skin.
        i. Apply skin protective products (creams, ointments, liquid sealants, etc.) or a nonadherent wound dressing such as hydrogel dressing with gauze as a secondary dressing, silicone, or Telfa-type dressings.
        ii. If you must use tape, be sure it is made of paper, and remove it gently. In addition, you can apply the tape to hydrocolloid strips placed strategically around the wound rather than taping directly onto fragile surrounding skin around the skin tear.
    f. Use gauze wraps, stockinettes, flexible netting, or other wraps to secure dressings rather than tape.
    g. Use no-rinse, soapless bathing products (Birch & Coggins, 2003; Mason, 1997)
    h. Keep skin from becoming dry, apply moisturizer (Bank, 2005; Hanson et al., 1991)
B. Treating Skin Tears (Baranoski & Ayello, 2008)
    1. Gently clean the skin tear with normal saline.
    2. Let the area air dry or pat dry carefully.
    3. Approximate the skin tear flap.
    4. Use caution if using adherent dressings, as skin damage can occur when removing dressings.
    5. Consider putting an arrow to indicate the direction of the skin tear on the dressing to minimize any further skin injury during dressing removal.
        a. Skin sealants, petroleum-based products, and other water-resistant products such as protective barrier ointments or liquid barriers may be used to protect the surrounding skin from wound drainage or dressing, or tape removal trauma.
        b. Always assess the size of the skin tear; consider doing a wound tracing.
        c. Document assessment and treatment findings.

V. EVALUATION AND EXPECTED OUTCOMES
A. No skin tears will occur in at-risk clients.
B. Skin tears that do occur will heal.

VI. FOLLOW-UP MONITORING OF CONDITION
A. Continue to reassess for any new skin tears in older adults.

RESOURCES

Tools

Agency for Healthcare Research and Quality. (2011). *Preventing pressure ulcers in hospitals: A toolkit for improving quality of care.*
http://www.ahrq.gov/research/ltc/pressureulcertoolkit/

Ayello, E. A. (2007). *Try this: Best practices in nursing care to older adults. Predicting pressure ulcer risk.* Retrieved from the Hartford Institute for Geriatric Nursing, College of Nursing website; http://www.consultgerirn.org/resources

Braden, B., & Bergstrom, N. (1988). *Braden Scale for predicting pressure sore risk.*
http://www.bradenscale.com/braden.PDF

Authoritative Sites

Agency for Healthcare Research and Quality. (2011). *USDHHS supported clinical guidelines: Pressure ulcers.*
http://www.guideline.gov

National Pressure Ulcer Advisory Panel (NPUAP)
Pressure ulcer prevention and treatment, research, and policy information.
http://www.npuap.org/

Wound, Ostomy, and Continence Nursing Society (WOCN)
Guidelines, position statements, best practices, and much more.
http://www.wocn.org/

Other Related Professional Organizations

American Professional Wound Care Association (APWCA)
http://www.apwca.org/

European Pressure Ulcer Advisory Panel (EPUAP)
http://www.epuap.org/

World Council of Enterostomal Therapists (WCET)
http://www.wcetn.org/

World Union of Wound Healing Societies (WUWHS)
http://www.wuwhs.org/

Wound Healing Society (WHS)
http://www.woundheal.org/

REFERENCES

Allman, R. M., Goode, P. S., Patrick, M. M., Burst, N., & Bartolucci, A. A. (1995). Pressure ulcer risk factors among hospitalized patients with activity limitations. *Journal of the American Medical Association, 273*(11), 865–870. Evidence Level IV.

Ayello, E. A., & Braden, B. (2001). Why is pressure ulcer risk so important? *Nursing, 31*(11), 74–79. Evidence Level V.

Ayello, E. A., & Lyder, C. H. (2001). Pressure ulcers in persons of color: Race and ethnicity. In J. G. Cuddigan, E. A. Ayello, & C. Sussman (Eds.), *Pressure ulcers in America: Prevalence, incidence, and implications for the future* (pp. 153–162). Reston, VA: National Pressure Ulcer Advisory Panel. Evidence Level V.

Bank, D. (2005). Decreasing the incidence of skin tears in a nursing and rehabilitation center. *Advances in Skin and Wound Care, 18*, 74–75. Evidence Level IV.

Baranoski, S. (2000). Skin tears: The enemy of frail skin. *Advances in Skin and Wound Care, 13*(3 Pt. 1), 123–126. Evidence Level V.

Baranoski, S., & Ayello, E. A. (2008). *Wound care essentials: Practice principles* (2nd ed.). Springhouse, PA: Lippincott, Williams, & Wilkins. Evidence Level V.

Barczak, C. A., Barnett, R. I., Childs, E. J., & Bosley, L. M. (1997). Fourth national pressure ulcer prevalence survey. *Advances in Wound Care, 10*(4), 18–26. Evidence Level IV.

Battersby, L. (1990). Exploring best practice in the management of skin tears in older people. *Nursing Times, 105*(16), 22–26. Evidence Level V.

Baumgarten, M., Margolis, D. J., Berlin, J. A., Strom, B. L., Garino, J., Kagan, S. H., . . . Carson, J. L. (2003). Risk factors for pressure ulcers among older hip fracture patients. *Wound repair and regeneration, 11*(2), 96–103. Evidence Level IV.

Baumgarten, M., Margolis, D. J., Localio, A. R., Kagan, S. H., Lowe, R. A., Kinosian, B., . . . Mehari, T. (2008). Extrinsic risk factors for pressure ulcers early in the hospital stay: A nested case-control study. *Journals of Gerontology. Series A, Biological Sciences and Medical Sciences, 63*(4), 408–413. Evidence Level IV.

Baumgarten, M., Margolis, D. J., Orwig, D. L., Shardell, M. D., Hawkes, W. G., Langenberg, P., . . . Magaziner, J. (2009). Pressure ulcers in elderly patients with hip fracture across the continuum of care. *Journal of the American Geriatrics Society, 57*(5), 863–870. Evidence Level V.

Bennett, M. A. (1995). Report of the task force on the implications for darkly pigmented intact skin in the prediction and prevention of pressure ulcers. *Advances in Wound Care, 8*(6), 34–35. Evidence Level V.

Bergstrom, N., & Braden, B. J. (1992). A prospective study of pressure sore risk among institutionalized elderly. *Journal of the American Geriatrics Society, 40*(8), 747–758. Evidence Level III.

Bergstrom, N., Braden, B. J., Kemp, M., Champagne, M., & Ruby, E. (1996). Multi-site study of incidence of pressure ulcers and the relationship between risk level, demographic characteristics, diagnoses, and prescription of preventive interventions. *Journal of the American Geriatrics Society, 44*(1), 22–30. Evidence Level IV.

Bergstrom, N., Braden, B. J., Laguzza, A., & Holman, V. (1987). The Braden Scale for predicting pressure sore risk. *Nursing Research, 36*(4), 205–210. Evidence Level III.

Birch, S., & Coggins, T. (2003). No-rinse, one-step bed bath: The effects on the occurrence of skin tears in a long-term care setting. *Ostomy/Wound Management, 49*(1), 64–67. Evidence Level IV.

Bolton, L. (2010). Pressure ulcers. In J. M. Macdonald & M. J. Geyer (Eds.), *Wound and lymphedema management* (pp. 95–101). Geneva, Switzerland: World Health Organization. Evidence Level V.

Braden, B. J. (1998). The relationship between stress and pressure sore formation. *Ostomy/Wound Management, 44*(3A Suppl.), 26S–36S. Evidence Level IV.

Braden, B. J., & Bergstrom, N. (1987). A conceptual schema for the study of the etiology of pressure sores. *Rehabilitation Nursing, 12*(1), 8–12. Evidence Level II.

Braden, B. J., & Bergstrom, N. (1989). Clinical utility of the Braden Scale for predicting pressure sore risk. *Decubitus, 2*(3), 44–51. Evidence Level III.

Brennan, M. R., & Trombley, K. (2010). Kennedy terminal ulcers—a palliative care unit's experience over a 12 month period of time. *World Council of Enterostomal Therapists Journal, 30*(3), 20–22.

Brindle, C. T. (2010). Outliers to the Braden Scale: Identifying high-risk ICU patients and the results of prophylactic dressing use. *World Council of Enterostomal Therapists Journal, 30*(1), 11–18. Evidence Level IV.

Buss, I. C., Halfens, R. J., Abu-Saad, H. H., & Kok, G. (2004). Pressure ulcer prevention in nursing homes: Views and beliefs of enrolled nurses and other health care workers. *Journal of Clinical Nursing, 13*(6), 668–676. Evidence Level III.

Campbell, K. E., Woodbury, M. G., & Houghton, P. E. (2010a). Heel pressure ulcers in orthopedic patients: A prospective study of incidence and risk factors in an acute care hospital. *Ostomy/ Wound Management, 56*(2), 44–54. Evidence Level V.

Campbell, K. E., Woodbury, M. G., & Houghton, P. E. (2010b). Implementation of best practice in the prevention of heel pressure ulcers in the acute orthopedic populations. *International Wound Journal, 7*(1), 28–40. Evidence Level V.

Centers for Medicare and Medicaid Services. (2004). *Guidance for surveyors in long term care. Tag F 314. Pressure ulcers.* Retrieved from http://www.cms.hhs.gov/manuals/downloads/som107ap_pp_guidelines_ltcf.pdf. Evidence Level V.

Centers for Medicare and Medicaid Services Hospital Acquired Conditions. (2011). *Present on admission indicator.* Retrieved from https://www.cms.gov/hospitalacqcond/06_hospital-acquired_conditions.asp

Chan, E. Y., Tan, S. L., Lee, C. K., & Lee, J. Y. (2005). Prevalence, incidence and predictors of pressure ulcers in a tertiary hospital in Singapore. *Journal of Wound Care, 14*(8), 383–384, 386–388. Evidence Level IV.

Chan, W. S., Pang, S. M., & Kwong, E. W. (2009). Assessing predictive validity of the modified Braden scale for prediction of pressure ulcer risk of orthopaedic patients in an acute care setting. *Journal of Clinical Nursing, 18*(11), 1565–1573. Evidence Level IV.

Cho, I., & Noh, M. (2010). Braden Scale: Evaluation of clinical usefulness in an intensive care unit. *Journal of Advanced Nursing, 66*(2), 293–302. Evidence Level III.

Cordeiro, M. B., Antonelli, E. J., da Cunha, D. F., Júnior, A. A., Júnior, V. R., & Vannucchi, H. (2005). Oxidative stress and acute-phase response in patients with pressure sores. *Nutrition, 21*(9), 901–907. Evidence Level IV.

Defloor, T., De Bacquer, D., & Grypdonck, M. (2005). The effect of various combinations of turning and pressure reducing devices on the incidence of pressure ulcers. *International Journal of Nursing Studies, 42*(1), 37–46. Evidence Level III.

Edwards, H., Gaskill, D., & Nash, R. (1998). Treating skin tears in nursing home residents: A pilot study comparing four types of dressings. *International Journal of Nursing Practice, 4*(1), 25–32. Evidence Level III.

European Pressure Ulcer Advisory Panel, & National Pressure Ulcer Advisory Panel. (2009). *Treatment of pressure ulcers: Quick reference guide.* Washington, DC: National Pressure Ulcer Advisory Panel. Evidence Level I.

Fernances, L. M., & Caliri, M. H. (2008). Using the Braden and Glasgow scales to predict pressure ulcer risk in patients hospitalized at intensive care units. *Revista Latino-Americana De Enfermagem, 16*(6), 973–978. Evidence Level V.

Fogerty, M., Guy, J., Barbul, A., Nanney, L. B., & Abumrad, N. N. (2009). African Americans show increased risk for pressure ulcers: A retrospective analysis of acute care hospitals in America. *Wound Repair and Regeneration, 17*(5), 678–684. Evidence Level IV.

Gilcreast, D. M., Warren, J. B., Yoder, L. H., Clark, J. J., Wilson, J. A., & Mays, M. Z. (2005). Research comparing three heel ulcer-prevention devices. *Journal of Wound, Ostomy, and Continence Nursing, 32*(2), 112–120. Evidence Level II.

Gorecki, C., Brown, J. M., Nelson, E. A., Briggs, M., Schoonhoven, L., Dealey, C., . . . European Quality of Life Pressure Ulcer Project group. (2009). Impact of pressure ulcers on quality of life in older patients: A systematic review. *Journal of the American Geriatrics Society, 57*(7), 1175–1183. Evidence Level I.

Groom, M., Shannon, R. J., Chakravarthy, D., & Fleck, C. A. (2010). An evaluation of costs and effects of a nutrient-based skin care program as a component of prevention of skin tears in an extended convalescent center. *Journal of Wound, Ostomy, and Continence Nursing, 37*(1), 46–51. Evidence Level V.

Hampton, S., & Collins, F. (2005). Reducing pressure ulcer incidence in a long-term setting. *British Journal of Nursing, 14*(15 Suppl.), S6–S12. Evidence Level II.

Hanson, D., Langemo, D. K., Olson, B., Hunter, S., Sauvage, T. R., Burd, C., & Cathcart-Silberberg, T. (1991). The prevalence and incidence of pressure ulcers in the hospice setting: Analysis of two methodologies. *American Journal of Hospice & Palliative Care, 8*(5), 18–22. Evidence Level IV.

Hanson, D. H., Anderson, J., Thompson, P., & Langemo, D. (2005). Skin tears in long term care: Effectiveness on skin care protocols on prevalence. *Advances in Skin and Wound Care, 18*, 74. Evidence Level III.

Henderson, C. T., Ayello, E. A., Sussman, C., Leiby, D. M., Bennett, M. A., Dungog, E. F., . . . Woodruff, L. (1997). Draft definition of stage I pressure ulcers: Inclusion of persons with darkly pigmented skin. NPUAP Task Force on Stage I Definition and Darkly Pigmented Skin. *Advances in Wound Care, 10*(5), 16–19. Evidence Level IV.

Heyneman, A., Vanderwee, K., Grypdonck, M., & Defloor, T. (2009). Effectiveness of two cushions in the prevention of heel pressure ulcers. *Worldviews on Evidenced-base Nursing/Sigma Theta Tau International, Honor Society of Nursing, 6*(2), 114–120. Evidence Level III.

Holst, G., Willman, A., Fagerström, C., Borg, C., Hellström, Y., & Borglin, G. (2010). Quality of care: Prevention of pressure ulcers—Nursing students as facilitators of evidence-based practice. *Vård i Norden, 30*(1), 40–42. Evidence Level V.

Hommel, A., Ulander, K., & Thorngren, K. (2003). Improvements in pain relief, handling time and pressure ulcers through internal audits of hip fracture patients. *Scandinavian Journal of Caring Sciences, 17*(1), 78–83. Evidence Level IV.

Houwing, R. H., Rozendaal, M., Wouters-Wesseling, W., Beulens, J. W., Buskens, E., & Haalboom, J. R. (2003). A randomized, double-blind assessment of the effect of nutritional supplementation on the prevention of pressure ulcers in hip-fracture patients. *Clinical Nutrition, 22*(4), 401–405. Evidence Level II.

Houwing, R. H., Rozendaal, M., Wouters-Wesseling, W., Beulens, J. W., Buskens, E., & Haalboom, J. R. (2003). A randomised, double-bind assessment of the effect of nutritional supplementation on the prevention of pressure ulcers in hip-fracture patients. *Clinical Nutrition, 22*(4), 401–405. Evidence Level II.

Houwing, R. H., Rozendaal, M., Wouters-Wesseling, W., Buskens, E., Keller, P., & Haalboom, J. (2004). Pressure ulcer risk in hip fracture patients. *Acta Orthopaedica Scandinavica, 75*(4), 390–393. Evidence Level IV.

Houwing, R., van der Zwet, W., van Asbeck, S., Halfens, R., & Arends, J. W. (2008). An unexpected detrimental effect on the incidence of heel pressure ulcers after local 5% DMSO cream application: A randomized, double-blind study in patients at risk for pressure ulcers. *Wounds: A Compendium of Clinical Research and Practice, 20*(4), 84–88. Evidence Level II.

Huang, T. T., Tseng, C. E., Lee, T. M., Yeh, J. Y., & Lai, Y. Y. (2009). Preventing pressure sores of the nasal ala after nasotracheal tube intubation: From animal model to clinical application. *Journal of Oral and Maxillofacial Surgery, 67*(3), 543–551. Evidence Level III.

Hunter, S., Anderson, J., Hanson, D., Thompson, P., Langemo, D., & Klug, M. G. (2003). Clinical trial of a prevention and treatment protocol for skin breakdown in two nursing homes. *Journal of Wound, Ostomy, and Continence Nursing, 30*(5), 250–258. Evidence Level III.

Iglesias, C., Nixon, J., Cranny, G., Nelson, E. A., Hawkins, K., Phillips, A., . . . PRESSURE Trial Group. (2006). Pressure relieving support surfaces (PRESSURE) trial: Cost effectiveness analysis. *British Medical Journal, 332*(7555), 1416. Evidence Level II.

Institute for Healthcare Improvement. (2006). *5 million lives saved campaign: Pressure ulcers*. Retrieved from http://www.ihi.org/IHI/Programs/Campaign/. Evidence Level V.

Jolley, D. J., Wright, R., McGowan, S., Hickey, M. B., Campbell, D. A., Sinclair, R. D., & Montgomery K. C. (2004). Preventing pressure ulcers with the Australian Medical Sheepskin: An open-label randomized controlled trial. *The Medical Journal of Australia, 180*(7), 324–327. Evidence Level II.

Kaitani, T., Tokunaga, K., Matsui, N., & Sanada, H. (2010). Risk factors related to the development of pressure ulcers in the critical care settings. *Journal of Clinical Nursing, 19*(3–4), 414–421. Evidence Level IV.

Karadag, M., & Gümüskaya, N. (2006). The incidence of pressure ulcers in surgical patients: A sample hospital in Turkey. *Journal of Clinical Nursing, 15*(4), 413–421. Evidence Level IV.

Kottner, J., & Dassen, T. (2010). Pressure ulcer risk assessment in critical care: Interrater reliability and validity studies of the Braden and Waterlow scales and subjective rating in two intensive care units. *International Journal of Nursing Studies, 47*(6), 671–677. Evidence Level III.

Krasner, D. (1991). An approach to treating skin tears. *Ostomy/Wound Management, 32,* 56–58. Evidence Level VI.

Kwong, E., Pang, S., Wong, T., Ho, J., Shao-ling, X., & Li-jun, T. (2005). Predicting pressure ulcer risk with the modified Braden, Braden, and Norton scales in acute care hospitals in Mainland China. *Applied Nursing Research, 18*(2), 122–128. Evidence Level IV.

Langer, G., Schloemer, G., Knerr, A., Kuss, O., & Behrens, J. (2003). Nutritional interventions for preventing and treating pressure ulcers. *Cochrane Database of Systematic Reviews,* (4), CD003216. Evidence Level I.

Lindgren, M., Unosson, M., Fredrikson, M., & Ek, A. C. (2004). Immobility—A major risk factor for development of pressure ulcers among adult hospitalized patients: A prospective study. *Scandinavian Journal of Caring Sciences, 18*(1), 57–64. Evidence Level VI.

Lyder, C. H. (1996). Examining the inclusion of ethnic minorities in pressure ulcer prediction studies. *Journal of Wound, Ostomy, and Continence Nursing, 23*(5), 257–260. Evidence Level IV.

Lyder, C. H., & Ayello, E. A. (2009). Annual checkup: The CMS pressure ulcer present-on-admission indicator. *Advances in Skin & Wound Care, 22*(10), 476–484.

Lyder, C. H., Preston, J., Grady, J. N., Scinto, J., Allman, R., Bergstrom, N., & Rodeheaver, G. (2001). Quality of care for hospitalized medicare patients at risk for pressure ulcers. *Archives of Internal Medicine, 161*(12), 1549–1554. Evidence Level III.

Lyder, C. H., Yu, C., Emerling, J., Mangat, R., Stevenson, D., Empleo-Frazier, O., & McKay, J. (1999). The Braden Scale for pressure ulcer risk: Evaluating the predictive validity in Black and Latino/Hispanic elders. *Applied Nursing Research, 12*(2), 60–68. Evidence Level IV.

Lyder, C. H., Yu, C., Stevenson, D., Mangat, R., Empleo-Frazier, O., Emerling, J., & McKay, J. (1998). Validating the Braden Scale for the prediction of pressure ulcer risk in Blacks and Latino/Hispanic elders: A pilot study. *Ostomy/Wound Management, 44*(3A Suppl.), 42S–49S. Evidence Level IV.

Malone, M. L., Rozario, N., Gavinski, M., & Goodwin, J. (1991). The epidemiology of skin tears in the institutionalized elderly. *Journal of the American Geriatrics Society, 39*(6), 591–595. Evidence Level IV.

Mason, S. R. (1997). Type of soap and the incidence of skin tears among residents of a long-term care facility. *Ostomy/Wound Management, 43*(8), 26–30. Evidence Level IV.

McInerney, J. A. (2008). Reducing hospital-acquired pressure ulcer prevalence through a focused prevention program. *Advances in Skin & Wound Care, 21*(2), 75–78. Evidence Level V.

Meehan, M. (1990). Multisite pressure ulcer prevalence survey. *Decubitus, 3*(4), 14–17. Evidence Level IV.

Meehan, M. (1994). National pressure ulcer prevalence survey. *Advances in Wound Care, 7*(3), 27–30, 34. Evidence Level IV.

New Jersey Department of Health and Senior Services. (2004). *Interim mandatory patient safety reporting requirements for general hospitals. Patient safety reporting initiative.* Retrieved from http://www.state.nj.us/health/ps/documents/irr.pdf

Nixon, J., Cranny, G., Iglesias, C., Nelson, E. A., Hawkins, K., Phillips, A., . . . Cullum, N. (2006). Randomised, controlled trial of alternating pressure mattresses compared with alternating pressure overlays for the prevention of pressure ulcers: PRESSURE (pressure relieving support surfaces) trial. *British Medical Journal, 332*(7555), 1413. Evidence Level II.

Nonnemacher, M., Stausberg, J., Bartoszek, G., Lottko, B., Neuhaeuser, M., & Maier, I. (2009). Predicting pressure ulcer risk: A multifactorial approach to assess risk factors in a large university hospital population. *Journal of Clinical Nursing, 18*(1), 99–107. Evidence Level V.

Norton, D., McLaren, R., & Exton-Smith, A. N. (1962). *An investigation of geriatric nursing problems in hospitals*. London, UK: Corporation for the Care of Old People. Evidence Level IV.

Norton, D., McLaren, R., & Exton-Smith, A. N. (1975). *An investigation of geriatric nurse problems in hospitals*. Edinburgh, UK: Churchill Livingstone. Evidence Level IV.

O'Regan, A. (2002). Skin tears: A review of the literature. *Journal of Wound, Ostomy, and Continence Nursing, 39*(2), 26–31. Evidence Level V.

Pancorbo-Hidalgo, P. L., Garcia-Fernandez, F. P., Lopez-Medina, I. M., & Alvarez-Nieto, C. (2006). Risk assessment scales for pressure ulcer prevention: A systematic review. *Journal of Advanced Nursing, 54*(1), 94–110. Evidence Level I.

Payne, R. L., & Martin, M. L. (1993). Defining and classifying skin tears: Need for common language. *Ostomy/Wound Management, 39*(5): 16–26. Evidence Level IV.

Pemberton, V., Turner, V., & VanGilder, C. (2009). The effect of using a low-air-loss surface on the skin integrity of obese patients: Results of a pilot study. *Ostomy/Wound Management, 55*(2), 44–48. Evidence Level IV.

Pressure ulcers prevalence, cost, and risk assessment: Consensus development conference statement—The National Pressure Ulcer Advisory Panel. (1989). *Decubitus, 2*(2), 24–28. Evidence Level I.

Reddy, M., Gill, S. S., & Rochon, P. A. (2006). Preventing pressure ulcers: A systematic review. *Journal of the American Medical Association, 296*(8), 974–984. Evidence Level I.

Rich, S. E., Shardell, M., Margolis, D., & Baumgarten, M. (2009). Pressure ulcer preventive device use among elderly patients early in the hospital stay. *Nursing Research, 58*(2), 95–104. Evidence Level IV.

Russo, C. A., Steiner, C., & Spector, W. (2006). *Hospitalizations related to pressure ulcers among adults 18 years and older, 2006.* Retrieved from at http://www.hcup-us.ahrq.gov/reports/statbriefs/sb64.jsp. Evidence Level IV.

Shahin, E. S., Dassen, T., & Halfens, R. (2009). Incidence, prevention and treatment of pressure ulcers in intensive care patients: A longitudinal study. *International Journal of Nursing Studies, 46*(4), 413–421. Evidence Level III.

Shanks, H. T., Kleinhelter, P., & Baker, J. (2008). Skin failure: A retrospective review of patients with hospital-acquired pressure ulcers. *World Council of Enterostomal Therapists Journal, 29*(1), 6–10. Evidence Level IV.

Sprigle, S., Linden, M., McKenna, D., Davis, K., & Riordan, B. (2001). Clinical skin temperature measurement to predict incipient pressure ulcers. *Advances in Skin & Wound Care, 14*(3), 133–137. Evidence Level IV.

Stratton, R. J., Ek, A. C., Engfer, M., Moore, Z., Rigby, P., Wolfe, R., & Elia, M. (2005). Enteral nutritional support in prevention and treatment of pressure ulcers: A systematic review and meta-analysis. *Ageing Research Reviews, 4*(3), 422–450. Evidence Level I.

Suriadi, Sanada, H., Sugama, J., Thigpen, B., & Subuh, M. (2008). Development of a new risk assessment scale for predicting pressure ulcers in an intensive care unit. *Nursing in Critical Care, 13*(1), 34–43. Evidence Level IV.

Thomas, D. R., Goode, P. S., LaMaster, K., Tennyson, T., & Parnell, L. K. (1999). A comparison of an opaque foam dressing versus a transparent film dressing in the management of skin tears in institutionalized subjects. *Ostomy/Wound Management, 45*(6), 22–28. Evidence Level III.

Uzun, O., Aylaz, R., & Karadağ, E. (2009). Prospective study: Reducing pressure ulcers in intensive care units at a Turkish medical center. *Journal of Wound, Ostomy, & Continence Nursing, 36*(4), 404–411. Evidence Level V.

VanGilder, C., Amlung, S., Harrison, P., & Meyer, S. (2009). Results of the 2008–2009 International Pressure Ulcer Prevalence Survey and a 3-year, acute care, unit-specific analysis. *Ostomy/Wound Management, 55*(11), 39–45. Evidence Level IV.

VanGilder, C., MacFarlane, G. D., Harrison, P., Lachenbruch, C., & Meyer, S. (2010). The demographics of suspected deep tissue injury in the United States: An analysis of the International Pressure Ulcer Prevalence Survey 2006–2009. *Advances in Skin & Wound Care*, *23*(6), 254–261. Evidence Level IV.

Weng, M. H. (2008). The effect of protective treatment in reducing pressure ulcers for non-invasive ventilation patients. *Intensive & Critical Care Nursing*, *24*(5), 295–299. Evidence Level III.

White, M. W., Karam, S., & Cowell, B. (1994). Skin tears in frail elders: A practical approach to prevention. *Geriatric Nursing*, *15*(2), 95–98. Evidence Level IV.

Wound, Ostomy, and Continence Nurses Society. (2010). *Guideline for prevention and management of pressure ulcers*. Mt. Laurel, NJ: Author. Evidence Level I.

Young, T. (2004). The 30 degree tilt position vs the 90 degree lateral and supine positions in reducing the incidence of non-blanching erythema in a hospital inpatient population: A randomized controlled trial. *Journal of Tissue Viability*, *14*(3), 88–96. Evidence Level IV.

Reducing Adverse Drug Events

17

DeAnne Zwicker and Terry Fulmer

EDUCATIONAL OBJECTIVES

On completion of this chapter, the reader should be able to:

1. conduct a comprehensive medication assessment
2. specify four medications or medication classes having a high potential for toxicity in older adults
3. describe five reasons that older adults experience adverse drug events
4. delineate strategies to prevent common medication-related problems in older adults

OVERVIEW

One in seven Medicare beneficiaries experienced an adverse event while hospitalized in 2008. Of those, 31% of the adverse events were related to medications (Levinson, 2010). Nearly 1.9 million adverse drug events (ADEs) occur each year in older adults enrolled in Medicare and 180,000 of those are life threatening or fatal (Gurwitz et al., 2003). ADEs are common in older adults yet are potentially preventable (Safran et al., 2005).

Persons older than the age of 65 years experience medication-related events for seven major reasons: (a) alteration in pharmacokinetics (i.e., reduced ability to metabolize and excrete medications) and pharmacodynamics (Mangoni & Jackson, 2004; Rochon, 2010); (b) polypharmacy (Gallagher, Barry, & O'Mahony, 2007; Hajjar & Kotchen, 2003); (c) incorrect doses of medications (more than or less than therapeutic dosage; Doucette, McDonough, Klepser, & McCarthy, 2005; Hanlon, Schmader, Ruby, & Weinberger, 2001; Sloane, Zimmerman, Brown, Ives, & Walsh, 2002); (d) using medication for treatment of symptoms that are not disease-dependent or -specific (i.e., self-medication or prescribing cascades; Neafsey & Shellman, 2001; Rochon & Gurwitz, 1997); (e) iatrogenic causes such as ADEs and inappropriate prescribing (Fick et al., 2003; Pirmohamed et al., 2004; Rothberg et al., 2008); (f) problems with medication adherence (Steinman & Hanlon, 2010); and (g) medication errors (Agency for Healthcare Research and Quality [AHRQ], 2001; Doucette et al., 2005).

For description of Evidence Levels cited in this chapter, see Chapter 1, Developing and Evaluating Clinical Practice Guidelines: A Systematic Approach, page 7.

Intrinsic factors such as advanced age, frailty, and polypharmacy place older adults at greater risk for adverse outcomes. Older adults are the largest consumers of medications with 82% taking at least one medication, 29%–39% taking five or more drugs, and up to 90% taking over-the-counter (OTC) drugs (Hanlon, Fillenbaum, Ruby, Gray, & Bohannon, 2001; Kohn, Corrigan, & Donaldson, 2000). Older adults often combine OTC medications with prescription medications yet do not report their OTC use to health care providers. Likewise, providers often do not inquire about OTCs or herbal remedies. Underreporting may lead to unrecognized adverse drug–disease or drug–drug interactions (Astin, Pelletier, Marie, & Haskell, 2000; Rochon, 2010). These factors make it paramount that nurses identify older adults at risk for adverse events.

BACKGROUND AND STATEMENT OF PROBLEM

Adverse Drug Events

An ADE is an adverse outcome that occurs during normal use of medicine, inappropriate use, inappropriate or suboptimum prescribing, poor adherence or self-medication, or harm caused by a medication error. It is estimated that 35% of older persons experience ADEs, almost half of which are preventable (Safran et al., 2005). Older adults are also at significant risk for further ADEs while in the hospital and after discharge. Acute drug toxicity represents 2.5% of emergency department (ED) visits for unintentional injuries, of which 42% resulted in a hospital admission (Budnitz et al., 2006; Hanlon et al., 2006). Significant morbidity and mortality are associated with ADEs, with the cost estimated to be approximately $75–$85 billion annually (Budnitz et al., 2006; Fick et al., 2003; Hanlon et al., 2001). ADEs are also associated with preventable adverse outcomes such as depression, constipation, falls, immobility, confusion, hip fractures, rehospitalization, anorexia, and death (Aspden, Wolcott, Bootman, & Cronenwett, 2007).

Iatrogenic Causes of Adverse Drug Events

Older adults' susceptibility to ADEs is well documented in the literature on iatrogenic events and medication errors (Gurwitz et al., 2003; Hohl et al., 2005). The term *iatrogenic*, as it relates to ADEs, means any undesirable condition in a patient occurring as the result of treatment by a health care professional, specifically pertaining to an illness or injury resulting from a medication/drug or treatment. An iatrogenic medication event is one that is preventable, such as the wrong dose of a medication given resulting in an adverse outcome. Adverse drug reactions (ADRs), inappropriate prescribing of high-risk medication to older adults, and medication errors are also considered iatrogenic ADEs. In a systematic review, the most common preventable ADEs included antiplatelet medications, diuretics, and anticoagulants. Prescribing problems, adherence problems, and monitoring problems have been associated with preventable admissions as well (Howard et al., 2007; Steinman & Hanlon, 2010). Frail older adults with multiple medical problems, memory issues, and multiple prescribed and nonprescribed medications are at highest risk for ADEs (Rochon, 2010).

Adverse Drug Reactions

An ADR, a type of ADE, is any toxic or unintended response to a medication (Committee of Experts [COE] on Safe Medication Practices, 2005). The prevalence rate of hospital admissions caused by ADRs has been reported between 5% and 35% (Gurwitz et al.,

2003; Kohn et al., 2000). A recent systematic review reported 10.7% prevalence rate of hospital admissions caused by ADRs in older adults; however, a confounding factor in the accuracy is the different methods and studies employ to gather the data (Kongkaew, Noyce, & Ashcroft, 2008). Among a community-dwelling population of older adults, 38% of ADRs were considered serious, life threatening, or fatal and 27% were considered preventable (Gurwitz et al., 2005). Pirmohamed et al. (2004) reported that 70% of ADRs were either possibly avoidable or definitely avoidable in a study of 18,820 older adults.

Twenty-nine percent of ADEs require evaluation by a physician, evaluation in the emergency room, or hospitalization for clinical management (Hohl et al., 2005; Petrone & Katz, 2005). A meta-analysis revealed that ADRs accounted for 6.7% of hospital admissions and in-hospital ADRs; when extrapolated, they would be the fourth–sixth leading cause of in-hospital mortality for all causes of death, which does not include ADRs related to errors, nonadherence, overdose, or therapeutic failures (Lazarou, Pomeranz, & Corey, 1998; Steinman & Hanlon, 2010). Drug–drug and drug–disease interactions are the most common ADRs (Hansten, Horn, & Hazlet, 2001; Juurlink, Mamdani, Kopp, Laupacis, & Redelmeier, 2003; Zhan et al., 2005). Drug–drug interactions occur when one therapeutic agent either alters the concentration (i.e., pharmacokinetic interactions) or the biological effect of another agent—pharmacodynamic interactions (Leucuta & Vlase, 2006). Gray and Gardner (2009) reported that polypharmacy and multiple prescribers tend to be key factors in these adverse reactions. Older adults with multiple chronic medical problems requiring multiple medications are at high risk for these interactions (Rochon, 2010).

Medication Errors

The Institute of Medicine (IOM) reported in 1999 that almost 7,000 hospital deaths were associated with medication errors (Kohn et al., 2000). Medication errors occur frequently, yet many hospitals still lack automated physician order entry systems that are reported to decrease the number of medication errors (National Coordinating Council for Medication Errors Reporting and Prevention [NCC MERP], 2001).

A *medication error* is defined by the COE on Management of Safety and Quality in Health Care (COE, 2005) as any preventable event that may cause or lead to inappropriate medication use or patient harm while the medication is in the control of the health care professional, patient, or consumer. Such events may be related to professional practice, health care products, procedures, and systems, including prescribing; order communication, product labeling, packaging, and nomenclature; compounding, dispensing, and distribution; administration, education, and use. A large percentage of errors are caused by administration of the wrong medication or the correct medication with the wrong dose or at the wrong time interval between dosing (Rochon, 2010). There are many reasons medication errors occur; however, it is beyond the scope of this chapter. Information regarding the immense literature on medication errors is provided in the Resources section of this chapter.

Adherence

Medication adherence (or compliance) with a medication regimen is generally defined as "the extent to which a person's medication-taking behavior corresponds with agreed recommendations of a health care provider" (Sabaté, 2003, pp. 3). Seventy percent of patients who begin taking a prescribed drug discontinue it within 1 year, with the greatest drop-off rate at 6 months (Osterberg & Blaschke, 2005). A national survey of 17,685 Medicare beneficiaries older than age 65 years found that 52% do not take medications as prescribed (Safran et al., 2005). Nonadherence was primarily associated with a belief that the drug made them feel worse or was not helping (25%), or cost of the medicine, resulting in a decision to skip or take a smaller dose (26%). Prescription drug coverage significantly impacted adherence, with 37% nonadherence among those without coverage compared with 22% nonadherence beneficiaries with coverage. Patients are often reluctant to admit nonadherence; however, pill counts and refill history can aid in determining this issue (Osterberg & Blaschke, 2005; Steinman & Hanlon, 2010).

Acute care nurses are ideally positioned to identify and aid in preventing ADEs in hospitalized older adults and in transitions to other levels of care. Areas in which nurses must be familiar are iatrogenic causes of ADEs such as ADRs, inappropriate medications, identifying system issues to reduce medicine errors, and risk of nonadherence in older adults. Education of patient and families, recognizing inappropriate medications, and reinforcing the need for drug monitoring are areas where nurses can make a difference in aging persons (Fick et al., 2003; Rochon, 2010). Nurses must take a proactive role in assuring patient safety through interdisciplinary collaboration with patient and family, doctors, advance practice nurses, and pharmacists to prevent adverse medication outcomes.

ASSESSMENT OF THE PROBLEM

Assessment Tools

Assessment tools are used to evaluate an older adult's ability to self-administer medications (i.e., functional capacity assessment); assessment of the medication list for potential inappropriate medications, drug–drug or drug–disease interactions; and assessment of renal function in collaboration with interdisciplinary team members. Commonly used tools include the following:

- *2002 Criteria for Potentially Inappropriate Medication Use in Older Adults: Independent of Diagnoses or Condition* (Fick et al., 2003). Used to assess medication list for medications that should generally be avoided in older adults. (See http:// www.consultgerirn.org/resources, "Try This" series, issue number 16.1.)
- *2002 Criteria for Potentially Inappropriate Medication Use in Older Adults: Considering Diagnoses or Condition* (Fick et al., 2003; see "Try This" series, issue number 16.2). Used to assess for the presence of medications that may interact adversely with a disease or condition a person has.
- *Drug–Drug Interactions* (Table 17.1). List of medications known to interact with other medications. This may be performed by a computer or personal digital assistant (PDA) program, such as *Facts and Comparisons* PDA program to identify drug–drug and drug–disease interactions or "Physician Order Entry (POE)" programs.
- *Cockroft–Gault Formula* (Table 17.2). Useful for estimating creatinine clearance based on age, weight, and serum creatinine levels (Terrell, Heard, & Miller, 2006).
- *Functional Capacity (activity of daily living [ADL], independent activity of daily living [IADL], Mini-Cog/Mini-Mental State Exam [MMSE]).* Used to assess physical and cognitive ability to self-administer medications. (See Chapter 6, Assessment of Physical Function, and Chapter 10, Dementia, respectively in this text or visit http://www.consultgerirn.org.)

TABLE 17.1

Common Drug–Drug Interactions

Drug 1	Drug 2	Interaction	Adverse Effect(s)
Warfarin (Coumadin)	Diltiazem[1] Verapamil[1] Metronidazole[1,3]	Inhibits drug metabolism	↑ anticoagulation Potential bleeding
Warfarin	NSAID*[2,3] ASA[2]	NSAID ↓ prostaglandin Increases GI erosion ↓ platelet aggregation	GI bleed
	Sulfa drugs[3] Macrolides[2]	Unknown Inhibits metabolism and clearance	↑ effects of warfarin, potential GI bleed
	Acetaminophen[3] combined with narcotic Fluconazole[3] Cipro[2] Biaxin[2]	↑ INR	Bleeding
Digoxin	Amiodarone[1,2]	↓ renal or nonrenal clearance of digoxin	Digoxin toxicity
	Clarithromycin[1,2]	Inhibits renal clearance of digoxin	
	Verapamil[1,2]	↓ Impulse conduction and muscle contraction	Potential bradycardia or heart block
Levothyroxine	Calcium carbonate[1]	L-thyroxine absorbs calcium carbonate in acidic environment	Reduced absorption of T_4 (L-thyroxin)
Glyburide	Co-trimoxazole[2]	Potentiates effect of sulfonylureas	Hypoglycemia
ACE inhibitors	Potassium-sparing[2] diuretics	Unknown	Life-threatening hyperkalemia
Diuretic	NSAID*[1]	↓ renal perfusion	Renal impairment
Phenytoin4	Cimetidine, erythromycin,	Not specified	Increases levels
(Dilantin)	clarithromycin, fluconazole		of Dilantin within 1 week
Theophylline	Quinolones	↓ liver metabolism of theophylline	Theophylline toxicity
Acetylcholinesterase inhibitor	Anticholinergics[1]	↓ ability to augment acetylcholine level	Therapy less effective

Note. ASA = aspirin; GI = gastrointestinal; INR = international normalized ratio; ACE = angiotensin-converting enzyme. There are many other common drug–drug interactions; this table is not intended to be all inclusive. Use of computer devices is typically the best method for determining drug–drug interactions (see Resources section). *NSAID = nonsteroidal anti-inflammatory agents: prescription and over-the-counter such as Toradol or ibuprofen respectively.

Adapted from

[1] Cusak, B., & Vestal, R. E. (2000). Clinical pharmacology. In M. H. Beers & R. Berkow (Eds.), *The Merck manual of geriatrics* (3rd ed., pp. 54–74). Whitehouse Station, NJ: Merck Research Laboratories. Evidence Level VI.

[2] Feldstein, A. C., Smith, D. H., Perrin, N., Yang, X., Simon, S. R., Krall, M., . . . Soumerai, S. B. (2006). Reducing warfarin medication interactions: An interrupted time series evaluation. *Archives of Internal Medicine, 166*(9), 1009–1015.

[3] Ament, P. W., Bertolino, J. G., & Liszewski, J. L. (2000). Clinically significant drug interactions. *American Family Physician, 61*(6), 1745–1754. Evidence Level VI.

TABLE 17.2

Cockroft–Gault formula for estimation of creatinine clearance (CrCl).

Formula for Men:

CrCl in milliliters per minute* =

$$\frac{(140 - \text{age in years}) (\text{weight in kilograms})}{72(\text{serum creatinine in milligrams per deciliter})}$$

Formula for Women: *Use above formula and multiply by 0.85

A creatinine clearance of < 50 ml/min places older adults at risk for adverse drug events and virtually all people older than age 70 have a creatinine clearance of < 50 (Fouts, Hanlon, Pieper, Perfetto, & Feinberg, 1997).

- *Brown Bag Method* (Nathan, Goodyer, Lovejoy, & Rashid, 1999). Method used to assess all medications an older adult has at home including prescription from all providers, OTCs, and herbal remedies. All medications at home are placed in a bag and brought to hospital or other care setting. Should be used in conjunction with a complete medication history. (See Interventions and Nursing Care Strategies or Protocol 17.1 for details on taking a complete medication history and Table 17.3, which outlines medication history questions.)
- *Drugs Regimen Unassisted Grading Scale (DRUGS) Tool.* Standardized method for assessing potential medication adherence problems. Used at transfer to other levels of care (Edelberg, Shallenberger, & Wei, 1999; Hutchison, Jones, West, & Wei, 2006).

ASSESSMENT STRATEGIES

Changes With Aging

Aging changes in pharmacokinetics and pharmacodynamics are important to consider when assessing medications in older adults (Mangoni & Jackson, 2004; Rochon, 2010). *Pharmacokinetics* is best defined as the time course of absorption, distribution across compartments, metabolism, and excretion of drugs in the body. As the body ages, the metabolism and excretion of many drugs declines and physiological changes require dosage adjustment for some drugs (Cusak & Vestal, 2000). *Pharmacodynamics* is defined as the response of the body to the drug that is affected by receptor binding, postreceptor effects, and chemical interactions (Cusak & Vestal, 2000). Pharmacodynamic problems occur when two drugs act at the same or interrelated receptor sites, resulting in additive, synergistic, or antagonistic effects. Many interactions of drugs are multifactorial, with sequence of events that are both pharmacokinetic and pharmacodynamic (Spina & Scordo, 2002). The following are changes that may occur with aging:

- Changes in drug *absorption* (i.e., increase gastric pH and decreased gastrointestinal [GI] motility in an absorptive surface) once thought to be caused mainly by aging changes are now thought to be caused by underlying disease states (Mangoni & Jackson, 2004). There may, however, be a change of absorption rate in persons taking many medications, for example, fluoroquinolones taken with iron may impair absorption (Semla & Rochon, 2004).

TABLE 17.3

Complete Medication History*

Date Performed

Patient Name

Medication allergies and type of reaction (e.g., hives)

Prescription medications

    Specifically ask about eye drops, topical creams, B^{12} injections, or other injections (at home or at medical office, how often). Recently discontinued medications and why.

Medication reconciliation performed and verified

    Discrepancies found and reason(s)

Over-the-counter drugs

    How often do you exceed the recommended dose on package?

    Do you read the labels? Why or why not?

    Do you ask a pharmacist or your provider about interactions with your prescriptions?

    Ask specifically what patient is taking in the following classes:

Pain relievers

    What have you tried, what works, and what does not? What pain do you take it for? How often?

Allergy medications

    When do you take them? Year round? What season? Or When symptoms develop?

Sinus congestion/cold or cough medications (combined products with more than one ingredient?)

Heart burn medications, how often?

Diarrhea or constipation treatments, how often?

Sleeping medications, ask specifically diphenhydramine (Benadryl)

Eye drops—how often what do you take them for?

Herbal remedies (orally or as a tea) or *Chinese medicine*

      - ginkgo biloba

      - ginseng

      - glucosamine

      - St. John's wort

      - echinacea

Nutritional supplements

    Ask how often?

    Ask specifically about:

      Calcium with vitamin D, vitamin E, C, or B's

      Megavitamins

      Protein supplements such as Ensure, Boost, or protein bars

      Vitamin drinks

Medications that have been stopped and why? (Did you discontinue or provider?)

    Alcohol

      Ask about type/amount per day

    Smoking (what and how much; e.g., cigarette packs per day, how many years)

    Past or annual immunizations, date last received

      Pneumonia vaccine

      Flu vaccine

      Other

Regular lab tests—performed to evaluate medication levels or side effects (e.g., potassium level, digoxin level, INR, liver toxicity, renal function). Inquire about those not drawn that should be based on aforementioned medical list.

Use of memory aids—reminders to take medications (e.g., pill dispenser box)

Assess adherence: Consider using DRUGS tool (Edelberg et al., 1999; Hutchison et al., 2006).

*Note.** Use in conjunction with brown bag method (see assessment tools). INR = international normalized ratio; DRUGS = Drug Regimen Unassisted Grading Scale.

- Drug *distribution* changes associated with aging include decreased cardiac output, reduced total body water, decreased serum albumin (which is more likely to be related to malnutrition or acute illness than aging), and increased body fat. Reduced total body water creates a potential for higher serum drug levels because of a low volume of distribution and occurs with water-soluble drugs (hydrophilic) such as alcohol or lithium. Decreased serum albumin results in higher unbound drug levels with protein-bound drugs such as warfarin, phenytoin, digoxin, and theophylline. Lipophilic drugs (e.g., long-acting benzodiazepines [BZDs]) are stored in the body fat of older persons and slowly leech out, resulting in increased half-life and resulting in the drug staying around longer (Gallagher et al., 2007).
- A significant change in *drug metabolism* is a reduction in the cytochrome p-450 system, which affects metabolism of many drugs cleared by this enzyme system (Cusak & Vestal, 2000; Mangoni & Jackson, 2004; Tune, 2001). Many classes of drugs are cleared by the cytochrome p-450 enzyme system including cardiovascular drugs, analgesics, nonsteroidal anti-inflammatory drugs (NSAIDs), antibiotics, diuretics, psychoactive drugs, and others (Mangoni & Jackson, 2004). Drugs such as beta-blockers that have a first pass effect in the liver may be effective in lower doses in older adults (Gallagher et al., 2007). For a list of drugs cleared by this enzyme system see *The Merck Manual of Geriatrics* at http://www.merckmanuals.com/mm_geriatrics. Metabolism may be affected by disease states common in older individuals (e.g., thyroid disease, congestive heart failure [CHF], and cancer) or drug-induced metabolic changes (Cusak & Vestal, 2000). Several drugs are cleared by multistage hepatic metabolism, which is more likely to be prolonged in older persons (Mangoni & Jackson, 2004). Some drugs undergo hepatic metabolism then renal clearance. Such drugs (diazepam) have enormously longer half-lives in the older adult because both systems are impaired.
- *Elimination or clearance* of medications from the body may be slowed because of decline in glomerular filtration rate, renal tubular secretion, and renal blood flow that naturally decreases with age (Semla & Rochon, 2004). Decrease in clearance prolongs drug half-life and leads to increase plasma concentrations (Gallagher et al., 2007). A decrease in glomerular filtration is usually not accompanied by an increase in serum creatinine because of decreasing lean muscle mass with age and subsequent decline in creatinine production. Lack of dosage adjustment for renal insufficiency is a common reason for ADEs (Rochon, 2010). Therefore, serum creatinine is not an accurate measure of renal function in the older adult. Instead, assessment of renal function using the Cockroft–Gault formula (Table 17.2) should be calculated prior to initiation of renal clearing medications (Mangoni & Jackson, 2004; Semla & Rochon, 2004).

Beers Criteria

In 1999, the Centers for Medicare and Medicaid Services (CMS) incorporated the Beers criteria into regulatory guidelines in long-term care (Lapane, Hughes, & Quilliam, 2007). Long-term care facilities can be cited if any of the drugs on the list are prescribed. The Joint Commission (TJC) also adopted the criteria as a potential sentinel event (2007) in hospitals.

The Beers criteria address two key areas: (a) medications or medication classes that should generally be avoided in persons aged 65 years and older; and (b) medications that should be avoided in older persons with specific medical conditions. A severity rating of *high* or *low* is given to each medication based on its potential negative impact on older adults. The most recent Beers criteria, updated in 2003 by Fick et al., identifies 48 medications or classes that should generally be avoided in persons older than 65 years, as well as 20 specific medications that should not be used in the presence of specific conditions. Inappropriate medications on the Beers list that resulted in ED visit for ADEs included insulin, warfarin, and digoxin (Fu, Liu, & Christensen, 2004); these drugs are commonly reported as high risk in other studies (see High-Risk Medications section). See "Try This" series, issue numbers 16.1 and 16.2 at http://www.consultgerirn.org for Beers criteria.

Medications on the Beers inappropriate list have been shown to be associated with poor health outcomes. Fick and colleagues (2003) reported that ambulatory older adults prescribed with medications from the Beers list were more likely to be hospitalized or evaluated in an emergency room than those not taking such medications. Other studies report a positive association between potentially inappropriate drug prescribing and ADRs in first-visit older adult outpatients (Chang et al., 2005; Fu et al., 2004). Although the Beers criteria for inappropriate medications are an excellent guideline for assessing *potential* inappropriate medications, they need to be used in conjunction with patient-centered care (Swagerty, Brickley, American Medical Directors Association [AMDA], & American Society of Consultant Pharmacists [ASCP], 2005). A joint position statement by the AMDA and ASCP points out that the Beers criteria are based on consensus data (e.g., lower level of evidence) rather than on higher levels of evidence such as systematic reviews or randomized controlled trials. Jano and Aparasu (2007) found that use of inappropriate medications (Beers list) was associated with an increase in ADRs and increased costs across settings; however, they suggest the predictive ability of the criteria needs to improve.

Assessment for Potential Adverse Drug Reactions

ADRs commonly occur because of the number of medications taken (polypharmacy) by older persons and their concomitant medical conditions. The severity of adverse reactions increases because of changes in pharmacokinetics and pharmacodynamics in older adults. Assessment for older adults' risk of ADRs and potential drug–disease and drug–drug interactions must be considered before initiating medications in the older adult.

Potential medication-related and patient-related risk factors for ADRs in older persons were examined and reported by Hajjar and Kotchen (2003). A consensus panel of four geriatric pharmacists and geriatric physician experts reviewed a list of evidence-based risk factors compiled by two experts from the literature to ascertain older adult risk factors for ADRs. The most prevalent risk factors identified are presented in Table 17.4.

The most preventable ADRs in the *outpatient* setting reported by Gurwitz and colleagues (2003) are cardiovascular medications followed by diuretics, nonopioids analgesics, hypoglycemics, and anticoagulants. In 2005, the largest number of preventable ADRs occurred at the prescribing or monitoring stages and includes wrong drug choices or dosages, inadequate patient education, or clinically important drug–drug interactions (Gurwitz et al., 2005). Monitoring for errors include inadequate evaluation of drug levels and failure to respond to signs, symptoms, or abnormal lab levels indicative of toxicity. Nurses can help to prevent ADRs in the acute care setting by monitoring

TABLE 17.4
Risk Factors for Potential Adverse Drug Reactions in Older Adults

Medication-related factors
  Class of medication
    Anticholinergics
    Benzodiazepines
    Antipsychotics
    Sedative/hypnotics
    Non-ASA, non-COX-2 NSAIDs
    TCAs
    Opioid analgesics
    Corticosteroids
  Specific medication
    Chlorpropamide
    Theophylline salts
    Warfarin salts
    Lithium salts

Patient characteristics
  Polypharmacy
  Dementia
  Multiple chronic medical problems
  Renal insufficiency (CrCl ~50 ml/min)
  Recent hospitalization
  Advanced age (= 85 years of age)
  Multiple prescribers
  Regular use of alcohol (~1 fl oz/d)
  Prior ADR

Note. ASA = acetylsalicylic acid; COX = cyclooxygenase; NSAIDs = nonsteroidal anti-inflammatory drugs; TCAs = tricarboxylic acid; CrCl = creatinine clearance; ADR = adverse drug reaction. From Hajjar, E. R., Hanlon, J. T., Artz, M. B., Lindblad, C. I., Pieper, C. F., Sloane, R. J., . . . Schmader, K. E. (2003). Adverse drug reaction risk factors in older outpatients. *The American Journal of Geriatric Pharmacotherapy*, 1(2), 82–89. Reprinted with permission from Elsevier. 61251.

or recommending lab values, determining appropriateness of drugs and doses when orders are written, and monitoring for signs and symptoms of toxicity. It is important for nurses to understand that ADRs may be difficult to recognize as they often present as atypical symptoms such as confusion, falls, lethargy, constipation, and depression (Hanlon et al., 1997).

Drug–Drug Interactions

Concurrent use of more than one drug simultaneously, particularly those with similar properties, can result in serious toxicities in older adults resulting in synergistic, additive, or antagonistic effects. For example, concurrent use of any two of the following drugs: antiparkinsonian drugs, tricyclic antidepressants (e.g., amitriptyline), antipsychotics (e.g., Haldol), antiarrhythmics (e.g., disopyramide), and OTC antihistamines (e.g., diphenhydramine, chlorpheniramine) may cause or worsen dry mouth, gum disease, blurred vision, constipation, urinary retention, and/or cognitive deficits (Cusak & Vestal, 2000).

Little is known about the epidemiology of drug–drug interactions in clinical practice (Juurlink et al., 2003); however, studies indicate that drug–drug interactions are a common cause of predictable ADEs (Hansten et al., 2001). Drug–drug interactions have resulted in serious adverse events among several classes of medications. For example, hypoglycemia resulted in around 900 patients out of 179,000 older patients treated with glyburide along with co-trimoxazole, and 12 patients died. Digoxin toxicity was experienced by more than 1,000 out of 230,000 patients admitted and 33 died while hospitalized (Juurlink et al., 2003). Those with digoxin toxicity were 13 times more likely to have received clarithromycin 1 week prior to hospitalization; suggesting avoidance of concomitant use of digoxin and clarithromycin may have prevented the toxicity. In the same study, concomitant prescribing of angiotensin-converting enzyme (ACE) inhibitors and potassium-sparing diuretics 1 week before admission were observed in 622,285 older persons with ADRs. The researchers estimated that 7.8% of hospitalizations for hyperkalemia could have been prevented if addition of potassium-sparing diuretics had been avoided (Juurlink et al., 2003). In a retrospective review of the National Hospital Ambulatory Medical Care Survey, Zhan and colleagues (2005) reported that older adults with two or more prescriptions had at least one inappropriate drug–drug combination present, and 6.6% of patients on warfarin were prescribed a drug with a potentially harmful interaction. Other common drug–drug interactions reported in other research are shown in Table 17.1.

Interactions With Over-The-Counter and Herbal Remedies

Drug interactions between prescription medications and herbal remedies or OTC medications are often not reviewed during medication reconciliation, hospital admission, or office visits, yet 40% of all OTCs are consumed by older adults (Astin et al., 2000; Kohn et al., 2000). In a survey of 1,001 older adults, up to 75% reported using OTCs that increased as age increased. Twenty-three percent reported use of two or more OTCs for chronic conditions in the past month; OTC use has increased over the last decade as well as polypharmacy (Hanlon et al., 2001; Radimer et al., 2004; Sloane et al., 2002).

Community-dwelling older adults in the United States consume approximately 1.8 OTC medications per day (Hanlon et al., 2001). Herbal or dietary supplement use such as ginseng, ginkgo biloba extract, and glucosamine is on the rise among older adults, increasing from 14% in 1998 to 26% in 2002 (Kaufman, Kelly, Rosenberg, Anderson, & Mitchell, 2002; Kelly et al., 2005). In a study examining community-dwelling older adults' use of prescription, OTC, and dietary supplements, 68% of older adults used prescription medications concurrently with OTCs, dietary supplements, or both (Qato et al., 2008). More than 50% of older adults used five or more prescriptions, OTC, or dietary supplements, concurrently. The prevalence rate of 5 or more prescription medications increased steadily with age, and 1 in 8 older adults regularly used five or more dietary supplements. This substantially increases the risk of drug–drug interactions in older adults (Qato et al., 2008). The researchers also reported 46 potential drug–drug interactions with 11 classified as potentially of major severity, 28 classified as moderate severity, and 7 as minor severity. Overall, 1 in 25 older adults (2.2 million) were at risk for potential major drug–drug interactions. Half of all potential major drug–drug interactions involved nonprescription medications (Qato et al., 2008).

The most commonly reported prescription or OTC medications, according to Qato et al. (2008), included single or multicomponent products that were cardiovascular drugs such as antihyperlipidemics, aspirin, hydrochlorothiazide, lisinopril, metoprolol, and others; dietary supplements were primarily multivitamins or minerals. Alternative therapies included garlic, coenzyme Q, omega-3 fatty acids, and glucosamine-chondroitin. In a review of herbal products and potential interactions with cardiovascular (CV) diseases, Tachjian, Maria, and Jahangir (2010) described herbal remedies that produce adverse effects on the CV system. These include St. John's wort, motherwort, ginseng, ginkgo biloba, garlic, grapefruit juice, hawthorn, saw palmetto, danshen, echinacea, tetrandrine, aconite, yohimbine, gynura, licorice, and black cohosh. Herbal agents that interfere with digoxin levels include Chan Su, danshen, Asian and Siberian ginseng, licorice, and uzara root. Those that may adversely interact with warfarin include St. John's wort, ginseng, ginkgo biloba, and garlic. Motherwort and BZDs together have a synergistic sedative effect and can result in coma. Ginseng may have either a hypotensive or hypertensive effect. Several other interactions are presented in this review.

St. John's wort was reported as being in the top selling herbs in the United States yet could potentially result in serious adverse reactions. Its effect on drug metabolism induces the cytochrome p-450 enzyme system where many prescription medications are metabolized. OTC and herbal supplements are typically not reported to medical providers as most consumers do not consider them medication and many health care providers do not ask about herbal remedies and OTC drugs (Astin et al., 2000; Gardiner, Graham, Legedza, Eisenberg, & Phillips, 2006; Tachjian et al., 2010). Other concerns are herbal products that lack scientific evidence of safety, lack regulatory oversight, and there is an abundance of public misinformation (Tachjian et al., 2010). The implications for unidentified drug–drug and drug–disease interactions are astounding.

Medication Adherence

As individuals age, they may encounter difficulties that decrease their ability to adhere to medication regimens (e.g., vision impairment, arthritis, economics). Medication adherence with older adults is complex and needs careful nursing assessment. There are a number of ways to assess for potential adherence-related problems (Bergman-Evans, 2006; Edelberg et al., 1999) as well as to ascertain if a patient is adhering to recommended treatment (Rohay, Dunbar-Jacob, Sereika, Kwoh, & Burke, 1996). Barriers to medication adherence include forgetting to take or limited organizational skills; belief that the drug is either not needed, is ineffective, or too many drugs are being taken; patient has difficulty taking such as opening bottles or swallowing; and cost (Steinman & Hanlon, 2010). Several interventions are available in this systematic review but are beyond the scope of this chapter. An array of devices can assist in enhancing adherence behavior (Fulmer et al., 1999; Haynes et al., 2005; Steinman & Hanlon, 2010). See Resources section for further information.

Reconciliation of Medications

Medication reconciliation (MR) confirms the patient's current medication regimen and compares this against the physician's admission, transfer, and discharge orders to identify and resolve discrepancies. Discrepancies between physician-acquired prescription medication histories and comprehensive medication histories at the time of hospital admission were common, occurring in up to 67% of cases (Tam et al., 2005). Around 22% of medication discrepancies could have resulted in patient harm during their hospitalization and

59% of the discrepancies could have resulted in patient harm if the discrepancy continued after discharge (Sullivan, Gleason, Rooney, Groszek, & Barnard, 2005).

Poor communication of medical information at transition points of care (at admission, transfer, and discharge) often results in medication errors, but appropriate strategies can reduce the likelihood of errors (Santell, 2006). Adverse events were seen on transfer from hospital to a nursing home in 20% of patients, particularly those readmitted to the nursing home (Boockvar et al., 2004). TJC has recommended standards for communicating drug therapies to other levels of care and across the continuum (Nickerson, MacKinnon, Roberts, & Saulnier, 2005). MR is often performed by pharmacists or nurses; however, MR can be performed by a nurse with pharmacist collaboration or computer-based programs (Doucette et al., 2005; Gleason et al., 2004; Nickerson et al., 2005). Accuracy of the list can mean the difference between patient safety and patient harm.

The MR process includes comparison of medications on patient and family report or admission and transfer documents with medication orders at the time of admission, time of transfer to other units, or discharge to other levels of care. Barriers for nurses performing MR reported in one study included lack of confidence in existing institutional safety systems, inconsistent practices (whether pharmacists are consulted or not), lack of communication between health professionals, and staffing concerns (MR is time consuming; Chevalier, Parker, MacKinnon, & Sketris, 2006). The brown bag method can be used for corroborating medications (Nathan et al., 1999) with community-dwelling older adults, when used in conjunction with a good medication or admission history.

At discharge, the pharmacist has been involved in identifying problems with drug therapy and communicating with the community pharmacy, medical provider, or admitting staff at the transitional site of care (Hanlon et al., 2001; Nickerson et al., 2005). A systematic review across many health care settings and at home found that interventions by clinical pharmacist showed a considerable reduction in drug-related problems as well as reduced morbidity, mortality, and health care costs (Hanlon, Lindblad, & Gray, 2004). Many hospital pharmacies are now linked electronically to health care providers and/or local pharmacies. Finally, discharge education and counseling to patients including assessment of factors that might affect adherence has shown to reduce ADEs (Hanlon et al., 2001) and methodologies known to enhance understanding such as "teach back" especially low-literacy populations (Schillinger et al., 2003). See Resources section for evidence-based information on medication reconciliation.

High-Risk Medications

Many studies have revealed common high-risk medications in older adults. Special attention should be paid to drugs that carry a high risk of serious adverse effects such as warfarin, hypoglycemic drugs, and digoxin that result in one-third of all emergency room visits for ADEs (Steinman & Hanlon, 2010). Additionally, taking BZDs is an independent risk factor for falls; diphenhydramine (Benadryl) may lead to impaired cognition or urinary retention (in men); and antipsychotics may lead to falls, death, or pneumonia (Steinman & Hanlon, 2010). Antipsychotics and other psychotropics are also associated with an increased risk for falls (Rochon et al., 2007). Nurses should become familiar with high-risk medications and medication classes prescribed for older adults in order to aid in preventing ADEs. Many tools are available for the nurse to assess for high-risk medications, for potential drug–drug, drug–disease, or drug–herbal interactions. Common high-risk medications are discussed in the following sections.

Warfarin

Warfarin has been identified throughout many research studies as among the highest risk medications taken by older persons (Gaddis, Holt, & Woods, 2002; Hanlon et al., 2006). Warfarin leads to ED visits, preventable hospital readmission, and adverse events after discharge (Alexopoulou et al., 2008; Budnitz et al., 2006; Howard et al., 2007; Pirmohamed et al., 2004). Together, polypharmacy and warfarin use consistently increases the risk of ADRs (Hanlon et al., 2006).

Warfarin is highly bound (approximately 97%) to plasma protein, mainly albumin. The high degree of protein binding is one of several mechanisms whereby other drugs interact with warfarin (Olson et al., 2010). Those with malnutrition and low albumin levels are at risk for unbound warfarin in the bloodstream and higher risk of bleeding. Warfarin is metabolized by hepatic cytochrome P450 isoenzymes predominately to inactive metabolites excreted in the bile; it is also excreted by the kidneys. Warfarin metabolism may be changed in advanced age and in the presence of liver problems. Drug interactions are extensive and includes (a) drugs that inhibit warfarin metabolism and prolong prothrombin time (e.g., Cipro, phenytoin, amiodarone); (b) drugs that inhibit vitamin K activity (e.g., cephalosporins and high-dose penicillins); (c) additive effects with other anticoagulants such as aspirin, Lovenox, and others; and (d) drugs that reduce the effectiveness of warfarin such as phenytoin, barbiturates, cholestyramine, and others (Olson et al., 2010).

Fifty-eight percent of older persons do not report use of herbal supplements. Commonly used herbal remedies (ginkgo biloba and garlic) interact with warfarin to augment its anticoagulant effect and may lead to serious bleeding problems (Astin et al., 2000; Miller, 1998). Many foods may interact with warfarin, specifically those with high vitamin K content such as chickpeas, spinach, and green tea (Miller, 1998). It is imperative to identify older adults on warfarin who fall or are at risk for falling as their risk of serious injury increases on warfarin. The risk of harm versus the benefit must be weighed and the nurse should clarify the risk versus benefit with the primary prescriber (Steinman & Hanlon, 2010).

Antihypertensive Agents

Hypertension affects approximately two thirds of individuals older than age 65 years but only 27% of people have adequate control. Physiological changes of aging can alter the pharmacokinetics and pharmacodynamics of cardiovascular drugs in older persons, thus increasing the risk of ADEs (Nolan & Marcus, 2000). The antihypertensives, as a class, tend to produce a variety of unintended effects including orthostatic hypotension (associated with diuretics and alpha-blockers), sedation and depression (associated with some beta-blockers), confusion (associated with alpha-blockers), impotence, and constipation (e.g., verapamil). Comprehensive and ongoing assessment for potential adverse effects (e.g., routinely checking orthostatic blood pressure) is key to monitoring drug efficacy and safety while hospitalized. Nurses should monitor for symptoms such as dizziness and lightheadedness on standing. The use of four or more medications should prompt the measurement of postural blood pressure (Tinetti & Kumar, 2010). Particular attention should be given to the possible discontinuation or dose reduction of medications known to increase orthostasis or fall risk.

Dose for dose, water-soluble compounds are more potent in aging persons, whereas fat-soluble drugs (such as propranolol and carvedilol) can be expected to have an extended half-life because of their higher volume of distribution. Because of changes in fat or lean body mass, older adults may require an increase in dosing intervals of fat-soluble beta-blockers. Additionally, because of age-related changes that decrease the integrity of the blood–brain barrier, it predisposes older adults to untoward events with alpha-agonists. Bronstein and colleagues (2008) reported lipid soluble beta-blockers that have marked antidysrhythmic effects more lethal (e.g., propranolol, oxprenolol). The lethality significantly increases when given with calcium channel blockers, cyclic antidepressants, and/or psychotropics, even if the amount of beta-blocker is relatively small (Bronstein et al., 2008).

Orthostatic hypotension is a serious problem that can affect older adults on continuous antihypertensive therapy. Sustained treatment renders them more susceptible to diuretic-induced dehydration and orthostatic changes. Orthostasis may also be caused by concomitant illness (e.g., infection). The known sequelae of orthostatic hypotension in older adults include falls that is a true trauma and a medical emergency in physically frail, anticoagulated, or functionally compromised older adults. Orthostatic hypotension is an independent risk factor for recurrent falls in nursing home residents (Ooi, Hossain, & Lipsitz, 2000).

Psychoactive Drugs

Mental health disorders are not part of normal aging. Nearly 20% of persons older than age 55 years experience mental disorders with the most common prevalence being anxiety, severe cognitive impairment, and mood disorders, respectively. Mental disorders are underreported and suicide rates are highest among older adults compared to younger adults. Adults older than age 85 years have the highest suicide rates of all—more than twice the national rate.

Sedative–hypnotic drugs significantly increase risk for adverse events in older adults and should generally be used sparingly and monitored very closely. BZDs, regardless of half-life, have been associated with cognitive impairment, hip fractures, and falls (Bloch et al., 2011; Hajjar et al., 2003). In a prospective study of 9,093 patients, older adults who take BZDs are at greater risk for mobility problems and ADL disability, and short-acting BZDs did not appear to improve safety benefits over long-acting agents (Gray et al., 2006). Higher plasma concentrations of sedatives and hypnotic are seen because of increased volume of distribution as well as increased sensitivity, including BZDs and opioids (Rochon, 2010). The likelihood of falls with fractures is more than twice as high for the long-acting BZDs than short-acting agents. Likewise, Tamblyn, Abrahamowicz, du Berger, McLeod, and Bartlett (2005) reported that 17.7% of older persons given at least one prescription for BZDs at hospital discharge were treated for at least one injury on follow-up visit of which fractures were the most common. In a study of intubated ICU patients, lorazepam was identified as an independent risk factor for development of delirium (Pandharipande et al., 2006). Oversedation, respiratory depression, confusion, and other alterations in cognitive capacity, as well as falls, are frequently associated with sedative-hypnotic drug use. (See Chapter 15, Fall Prevention: Assessment, Diagnoses, and Intervention Strategies.)

Psychoactive medications include antidepressants (tricyclics, selective serotonin reuptake inhibitors [SSRIs]), anxiolytic agents (e.g., diazepam, lorazepam), antipsychotics (also referred to as *neuroleptics*), mood-stabilizing compounds (lithium), and psychoactive stimulants. Psychoactive compounds are prescribed to stabilize mood, agitated behaviors, and for therapeutic effects in clinical depression. Mood stabilizers and psychoactive stimulants are known to have a relatively narrow therapeutic window even in younger adults. Lithium, in particular, requires very close monitoring of levels and signs of toxicity in older adults; it also interacts with many other drugs. Some unintended interactions may be prevented if age-related changes are considered and careful surveillance is part of routine care (Budnitz et al., 2006).

The half-life of psychoactive drugs is prolonged in older adults and, in general, this class of drugs must be used with extreme caution to avoid inducing delirium, falls, and other traumatic events. In a systematic review, medications strongly linked with falls included sedatives, hypnotics, BZDs, and antidepressants (Woolcott et al., 2009). A significant association between falls and psychotropic medications has also been reflected in two other meta-analyses (Bloch et al., 2011; Leipzig, Cumming, & Tinetti, 1999). Drug classes determined to be a risk factor for falls included psychotropics, antidepressants, BZDs, hypnotics, neuroleptics, and tranquilizers. Risk seemed to be more significant for adults older than age 80 years in each of the classes. Drug classes that had double the odds of traumatic falls included neuroleptics, antidepressants, and BZDs. An extensive list of specific drugs for each class is listed in the review by Bloch et al. (2011). Although antianxiety agents such as BZDs and sedative-hypnotics are generally overprescribed for older adults, the antidepressants are generally considered to be underprescribed. It is estimated that almost 15% of older persons living in the community, 5% in primary care, and 15%–25% in nursing homes have significant depressive symptoms (Spina & Scordo, 2002).

The SSRIs, as a class of antidepressants, have strikingly different side effects than other antidepressants (e.g., tricyclics). This class does not cause cardiotoxicity or orthostatic hypotension and does not have anticholinergic effects as do tricyclic antidepressants. In general, these drugs tend to be a better choice of antidepressants in older adults. The most common side effects are GI related (nausea, anorexia) that may be ameliorated by starting with a low dose (half that for younger adults; e.g., fluoxetine 5 mg) and slowly increasing (e.g., to 10 mg) after 1 week. A serious but uncommon sequelae of SSRIs is serotonin syndrome. This syndrome may occur if more than one antidepressant is prescribed with an SSRI or if concurrent use of St. John's wort, a commonly self-administered OTC herbal remedy for depression.

The antipsychotics are often used inappropriately as first-line treatment for persons older than age 65 years presenting with agitation and behavioral problems associated with dementia (Kindermann, Dolder, Bailey, Katz, & Jeste, 2002). Evidence-based recommendations suggest the underlying cause of agitation should be determined (may be caused by delirium or pain) and nonpharmacological interventions attempted prior to administering antipsychotics such as Haldol (Zwicker & Fletcher, 2009).

Most antipsychotics are not U. S. Food and Drug Administration (FDA) approved for agitation (without a psychotic diagnosis) and data on their effectiveness suggest that the risk is greater than the benefit (Leipzeig et al., 1999; Woolcott et al., 2009). Antipsychotics must be used with extreme caution in this population, largely because of the potential for development of abnormal, and often irreversible, involuntary movements (extrapyramidal symptoms) associated with their administration and increased risk for falls. The newer antipsychotics present a much lower risk of extrapyramidal movement disorders than conventional antipsychotics. Unlike conventional antipsychotics, the newer atypical ones (e.g., clozapine, risperidone, olanzapine, and quetiapine) apparently provide several advantages with respect to both efficacy and safety.

A major study examining the effectiveness of antipsychotic use in Alzheimer's disease concluded that the adverse effects are greater than the advantages of these therapies (Schneider et al., 2006). In 2004, the FDA issued a warning against off-label use of antipsychotics for dementia-related psychotic symptoms because of potential adverse effects. Data from the CMS indicate that newer atypical antipsychotic medications, compared to older antipsychotics, do not appear to be associated with an increased risk of ventricular arrhythmias or cardiac arrest (Liperoti et al., 2005). Psychotropic medications are associated with an increased risk for falls (Gurwitz et al., 2005). Drug–drug interactions with antipsychotics are common.

Anticholinergics

Medications with high anticholinergic properties must be used with great caution in older adults because of adverse effects such as inability to concentrate to frank delirium, agitation, hallucinations, blurred vision, slowed GI motility, decreased secretions, urinary retention, tachycardia, impaired sweating, and constipation (Rochon, 2010; Spina & Scordo, 2002; Terrell et al., 2006; Tune, 2001). Studies have reported that patients with dementia are at higher risk for delirium associated with anticholinergics; however, a recent study indicates that use of anticholinergic drugs is "independently and specifically" associated with a subsequent increase in delirium symptom severity in older medical inpatients (Han et al., 2001).

Urinary retention, resulting from an anticholinergic, can be a lethal side effect in a male with benign prostatic hypertrophy (BPH) and a history of UTIs; urosepsis and death may result in men. Catterson and colleagues (1997) discussed the vicious cycle of treatment and/or iatrogenesis that may occur with administration of anticholinergic drugs. An illustrative example is an older adult with dementia and BPH who is administered diphenhydramine (Benadryl) for sleep and who is also taking oxybutynin (Ditropan), both of which have anticholinergic properties. The additive effects of the two medications may lead to urinary retention and agitation that may, in turn, lead to treatment of the agitation with antipsychotics (which also have anticholinergic effects) and exacerbate the problem and cascade of events further. Rochon (2010) refered to this as the "prescribing cascade" that leads to cascade iatrogenesis.

Anticholinergic properties occur not only in antidepressant and antipsychotic medications, as previously mentioned, but are also properties of most OTC antihistamines and sleep aids, intestinal and bladder relaxants, corticosteroids, antihypertensives, antiarrythmics and other cardiovascular drugs, and some antibiotics. See Tune (2001) or Kemper, Steiner, Hicks, Pierce, and Iwuagwu (2007) for a list of medications with anticholinergic effects. An anticholinergic risk scale (ARS) has been developed by Rudolph, Salow, Angelini, and McGlinchey (2008) to identify older adults at highest risk for adverse effects from anticholinergic drugs.

Cardiotonics

Digoxin is useful in treating CHF because of *systolic* dysfunction in the older adult but is not the recommended treatment for CHF from underlying *diastolic* dysfunction in older adults. Digoxin toxicity occurs more frequently in older adults, presents atypically, and may result in death. Juurlink and colleagues (2003) reported that about 2.3% of cases of digoxin toxicity could have been prevented in hospitalized older adults. Ahmed, Allman, and Delong (2002) reported that digoxin is often prescribed inappropriately in hospital patients. Classic symptoms of digoxin toxicity (nausea, anorexia, visual disturbance) may occur; however, symptomatic cardiac disturbance and arrhythmias are more common in the older adult and are not often thought to be caused by digoxin toxicity. Older adults may experience toxicity symptoms even with normal plasma levels of digoxin (Flaherty, Perry, Lynchard, & Morley, 2000). Many older people will have some reduction in renal function with aging; therefore, monitoring for symptoms, especially atypical symptoms of digoxin toxicity, and monitoring renal function and potassium levels is important.

Particular caution must be exercised when digoxin is prescribed with diuretics; this combination can cause hypokalemia and exacerbate renal impairment that can potentiate digoxin toxicity. Because the therapeutic window for digoxin is narrow and because it is water-soluble (e.g., the drug has a smaller volume of distribution and, thus, higher plasma concentration), correct and safe dosing of older adults is challenging. The maximum recommended dose in older persons for treating systolic heart failure is 0.125 mg (Fick et al., 2003). Debilitated older adults who often have low serum albumin levels are at risk for higher plasma level and digoxin toxicity.

Despite the recommendation that ACE inhibitors (ACEIs) should be prescribed for all patients with heart failure because of left ventricular or systolic dysfunction and who have normal renal function (Packer et al., 1999), Sloane and colleagues (2002) found that 62% of adults in assisted living residents (*n* = 2,014) were not on an ACEI. Monitoring of renal function and serum potassium should continue as the ACEI dose is titrated up. Rarely do older patients on an ACE inhibitor need potassium supplementation, the combination of which can be lethal. Juurlink and colleagues (2003) reported that 523 out of 1,222,093 patients on ACEIs were hospitalized with hyperkalemia; of these patients, 21 died while hospitalized.

Hypoglycemic Agents

Hypoglycemic agents carry a high risk of serious adverse effects in older adults. Control of blood glucose level is paramount to prevent microvascular and macrovascular complications of diabetes. However, the use of general disease-specific evidence guidelines for diabetic control can lead to overmedication in older adults. Tight glycemic control in advance age or in older person with multiple comorbidities can result in greater harm than benefit (Greenfield et al., 2009; Steinman & Hanlon, 2010).

The American Geriatrics Society (AGS) has issued guidelines for improving the care of older people with diabetes (Brown, Mangione, Saliba, Sarkisian, & California Healthcare Foundation [CHF]/American Geriatrics Society [AGS] Panel on Improving Care for Elders with Diabetes, 2003). They suggest that the risks of intensive glycemic control, including hypoglycemia, polypharmacy, and drug–drug and drug–disease interactions, may significantly alter the risk–benefit equation. For frail older adults, persons with limited life expectancy, and others in whom the risks of intensive glycemic control appear to outweigh the potential benefits, a less stringent target than the American Diabetes Association (ADA) recommendation of 7% or 8% in frail older adult is appropriate. Oral agents with shorter half-life are also recommended and insulin is less often recommended because of vision changes and common arthritic conditions, unless it is provided in pre-filled syringes. Metformin is not recommended for those older than age 80 years because it may lead to metabolic acidosis. Blood pressure and lipid control, however, are recommended to help reduce microvascular and macrovascular problems along with a daily low-dose of aspirin (Greenfield et al., 2009; Steinman & Hanlon, 2010).

Over-The-Counter Medications

Self-medication with OTC medications, herbal remedies, and dietary supplements may lead to adverse drug–disease interactions and drug–drug interactions (Astin et al., 2000; Rochon, 2010). Neafsey and Shellman (2001) found that 86% of sample of 168 older adults attending a hypertension clinic reported at least two or more self-medication practices that could result in an adverse drug interaction. In the United States, community-dwelling older adults take about as many OTC drugs as prescription drugs (Hanlon et al., 2001). Salicylates, such as aspirin, are a significant concern regarding ADRs in older persons. In a study of 18,820 patients, 18% of all ADR hospital admissions were aspirin-related and low dose aspirin was implicated most often (Pirmohamed et al., 2004). In combination with alcohol, because of its water solubility, age-related renal insufficiency can worsen and result in chronic salicylate intoxication. Cold remedies that include alcohol are a significant source of drug potentiation in aging adults. Indeed, alcohol consumption is frequently omitted from history taking of older adults, even though it interacts with OTC and prescription medications in frank and subtle ways to produce unintended drug harm.

The OTCs most commonly implicated in hospital admissions are low dose aspirin and nonsteroidal anti-inflammatory drugs (NSAIDs; Pirmohamed et al., 2004). The FDA has been evaluating OTC ingredients and labeling of OTCs; however, it is a long-range project and yet to be seen if the FDA will be more specific on safety issues that relate to older adults. Astin and colleagues (2000) reported that 24% of seniors use herbal remedies (the most common being ginkgo biloba and garlic), and 58% did not report usage to their primary provider. Ginkgo biloba and garlic interact with warfarin to augment its anticoagulant effect and may lead to bleeding (Miller, 1998); the potential adverse consequences are staggering.

INTERVENTIONS AND CARE STRATEGIES

Comprehensive Medication Assessment and Management

Medication assessment begins with a thorough drug history and assessment obtained from the older adult or a reliable informant. Medication history errors occur in up to 67% of patients at the time of admission to the hospital and increased up to 83% when nonprescription drugs were included (Tam et al., 2005). This suggested a need for systematic approach to accurate medication histories at the time of admission. No studies provide a systematic approach to history taking, although specific aspects of the medication assessment include the following evidence-based activities:

■ Obtain a *complete medical history* and validate that the medication history is true (Lau, Florax, Porsius, & De Boer, 2000), ascertaining the numbers and types of medications typically consumed, as well as an estimate of how long it has been taken.

■ Nathan and colleagues (1999) recommended that older adults bring all their medications and OTCs to provider or hospital or other health care setting in a brown bag in order to document medication types, instructions for self-administration, dates, and duration of the drug regimen. This method fosters identification of multiple prescribers and dispensing pharmacies and can signal polypharmacy and/or possible substance abuse, particularly regarding analgesics, anxiolytics, and sedative hypnotics.

- Focused questions by the clinician should address nicotine and alcohol use, as well as vitamins, herbal remedies, and OTC medications that are routinely used (Astin et al., 2000; Lau et al., 2000). This information should be included in the medication profile. (See Table 17.3 for a suggested medication history or visit http://www.consumermedsafety.org/tools/Keeping_Track_of_Your_Medications.pdf.)

- Ask detailed questions about OTC and "recreational" drugs, alcohol use, and herbal or other folk remedies. Provide a list of herbal remedies and folk medicines to choose from (Tachjian et al., 2010). Be specific about the actual amount and under what circumstances these substances are used. Accurate information can help explain symptoms that otherwise may not make sense. Evaluate for duplicate medications or classes that occur because of unrecognized trade names versus generic names, and OTCs with the same active ingredients in them, especially acetaminophen (Astin et al., 2000).

- Perform *MR* to verify actual medication regimen at hospital admission and discharge and across the continuum of care (Gleason et al., 2004; Nickerson et al., 2005; Tangalos & Zarowitz, 2006).

- Patients are often reluctant to admit to nonadherence; however, pill counts and refill history can aid in determining this issue (Steinman & Hanlon, 2010). Employ a medication discrepancy tool to facilitate discrepancy across settings (University of Colorado Health Sciences Center, 2005).

- Monitor new symptoms and consider their likelihood of being caused by an ADR before adding new medications to treat the symptom (Petrone & Katz, 2005; Rochon, 2010) prior to requesting a new medication to treat symptoms; avoid the prescribing cascade.

- Attempt a trial of nonpharmacological interventions and treatments prior to requesting medication for new symptoms (e.g., agitation). Nurses often make these recommendations when notifying primary provider for a new problem or symptom.

- Continually monitor for possible toxicity to those drugs with high prevalence rate of toxicity (see Beers criteria; Beers, 1997; Beers et al., 1992). PDA technology can help nurses assess high-risk medications such as *facts and comparisons*.

- Consider medications as the underlying cause when falls occur. Particularly, consider recently added medications that are high risk for causing falls such as diuretics and psychotropics.

- Collaborate with the interdisciplinary team to effect change in reducing the numbers of ADEs and ADRs, many of which are preventable (Hanlon et al., 2001). Although many studies describe and recommend an interdisciplinary approach as the best method for improving drug treatment outcomes, most do not delineate the specific role or function of the individual team members nor do they measure outcomes of the team (Lam & Ruby, 2005; Williams et al., 2004). Recommendations to consider for an interdisciplinary approach include a medication care team (nurse, pharmacist, primary physician/nurse practitioner, social worker) with specific functions assigned to review medications at admission and discharge utilizing evidence-based recommendations. Discharge interventions may be performed by various team members including the following:
  - Reminder systems may be instituted by pharmacists in collaboration with nurses as reported effective by Muir, Sanders, Wilkinson, and Schmader (2001). A visual intervention (medication grid) was delivered to physicians to

see if it could reduce medication regimen complexity, and researchers report that the simple intervention had a significant impact on medication regimen complexity in older adults.

o Pharmacist may also review (preferably using a computer-based program) medication list at admission, when new medications are added and prior to discharge for potential drug–drug interactions, drug–disease interactions, and/or inappropriate medications for older adults.

o Age-specific alerts sustained the effectiveness of drug-specific alerts to reduce potentially inappropriate prescribing in older people and resulted in a considerably decreased burden of the alerts (Simon et al., 2006).

o Computerized physician order entry system has the potential to prevent an estimated 84% of dose, frequency, and route errors. Anywhere from 28% to 95% of ADEs can be prevented by reducing medication errors through computerized monitoring systems (AHRQ, 2001).

o Medication interaction alerts may reduce the frequency of coprescribing of interacting medications (Feldman et al., 2006).

o Pharmacist may also function as the communicator of the hospital drug regimen to community pharmacy, primary care provider, and/or other levels of care.

o Social worker may review issues at home such as access to medications, costs, caregiver support, and barriers to discharge interventions.

■ Nurses and other interdisciplinary members need to be proactive participants in reducing rehospitalization related to ADEs and implement discharge education and counseling to patients including the following:

o *Assess cognitive and affective status* to assure that memory problems or vegetative symptoms associated with depression are not interfering with the safe use of prescription drugs (see Chapter 8, Assessing Cognitive Function, and Chapter 9, Depression in Older Adults).

o *Assess abilities and limitations* such as functional ability, including the ability to read the medication label, to open the medication container, and consume or self-administer the prescribed medication as intended (Curry, Walker, Hogstel, & Burns, 2005; see Chapter 6, Assessment of Physical Function, and Chapter 8, Assessing Cognitive Function). The plan of care should address actual and potential problems and the need for reassessment at regular intervals and after major medical events (e.g., cerebrovascular accident [CVA] or delirium).

o *Devices to accommodate* some impairments or barriers may be recommended. For example, tamperproof lids are often difficult for older adults to remove, particularly if there are arthritic changes. A simple request to the pharmacist to provide a nonchildproof lid may improve the safe and effective use of prescribed medication. Consult with occupational therapy.

o *Assess health literacy* (Curry et al., 2005). Query whether the older person understands what the drug is to be used for, how often it is to be taken, circumstances of ingestion (e.g., with food), and other aspects of drug self-administration that signal intelligent drug use; use teach-back method to verify understanding (Hutchison et al., 2006; Schillinger et al., 2003).

o *Assess for ability to recognize generic* versus brand name medication and their use (Curry et al., 2005). Ask the older adult to describe circumstances in which the medication was not used or was used differently than prescribed. If the older adult cannot describe medication use, consider removing the drug or provide written instruction for the home (Muir et al., 2001).

   ○ *Assess beliefs, concerns, and problems* related to the medication regimen. Ask older adult if she or he believes that the drug is actually doing what it is intended to do. If the medication is not useful, not creating symptom relief, or causing adverse effects, consider removing it or replacing it with a more acceptable substitute.

   ○ *Discuss the impact of medication expenses.* Many medications particularly those that are new to the market can be prohibitively expensive, particularly for persons on fixed incomes. Discuss influence of TV ads. Ask the older adult what concerns they have about the costs and risks of administration (Curry et al., 2005). In addition, discuss Medicare Part D concerns or confusion. Where economic problems are identified, generic drugs and other avenues should be explored to manage the cost issue.

   ○ *Consider instrumental issues* related to drug use, such as availability of family members or other social supports to facilitate medication adherence, and who monitors the need to change specific medications dictated by third-party reimbursement and medication coverage plans.

  ■ Patients should be given the *necessary information* and the opportunity to exercise the degree of control they choose over health care decisions that affect them and the necessary information to effectuate this. Patients who are informed and are involved in decision making are less likely to make decisions that may lead to ADRs, such as abruptly discontinuing a medication that should be tapered off slowly (NCC MERP, 2001).

CASE STUDY

Mr. Jones is an 82-year-old male admitted 2 days ago for a surgical repair of a left hip fracture he sustained when he fell as he was getting dressed at home. He is currently preoperative on the surgery schedule for tomorrow morning. He has a history of multi-infarct dementia, atrial fibrillation, hypertension, and was noted to have intermittent runs of premature ventricular contractions on his last admission 3 months ago, but has had no further cardiac symptoms since then. He was transferred to the orthopedic unit yesterday from the ED at 6 a.m. after having spent the night for nursing observation. While in the ED, he received both Haldol 5 mg and Ativan 2 mg IV for severe agitation. His wife says that when he is at home, he is usually able to make his needs known but was "out of sorts" yesterday, very tired, and in noticeable pain after he fell. She tells you he is now "out of his mind" compared to how he was when she first brought him to the ED and has become progressively worse cognitively.

The staff nurse from the day shift—giving you report—tells you he has not slept at all, refused to eat anything, and that during her shift, he has become increasingly agitated and combative. He was given Haldol 5 mg at 2 p.m. and is currently restrained. She reports he was so agitated that they had to get security to help the staff. It is now 4:00 p.m. and you are doing your assessment of Mr. Jones. You first awaken him and assess his mental status,

(continued)

CASE STUDY *(continued)*

talking to him in a calm, gentle voice. You note he is lethargic with an inability to sustain attention. He is disoriented to place and time and cannot remember how old he is. He is afebrile, with a blood pressure (BP) of 140/72, heart rate (HR) of 45 beats per minute (bpm), and respiratory rate (RR) of 22 breaths per minute. Both of his upper extremities are in soft restraints. He is on a cardiac monitor that indicates he has bradycardia with a rate of 48 bpm; however, his rate increases to 57 bpm when he begins to wake up.

What Would You Do Next?

You decide to re-review his medication list and see what he is taking. His medications are as follows:

> Carvedilol CR 20 mg daily
> Digoxin 0.125 mg daily
> Amiodarone 400 mg daily
> Warfarin 5 mg daily × 5 years with normal INR
> Aricept and Namenda (dose unknown) daily

You also look at his lab results and find his blood counts and fluid and electrolytes are within normal limits except for potassium of 3.2 mEq/L.

You quickly notify the hospitalist and ask her to come and see the patient immediately because of his low heart rate and change in mental status. When she gets to the unit, you also ask her to discontinue the restraints and PRN Haldol and Ativan. As you suspect, he is now overmedicated and, further, your calm voice seems to be enough to prevent agitation. You are not only concerned that his agitation is caused by untreated pain from his hip fracture but are also concerned about giving any pain medication that he has not received since admission because of his lethargy. At present, the patient is not showing nonverbal signs of pain.

CASE STUDY DISCUSSION

Initial Nursing Assessment and Interventions

You are on the right track, performing baseline vital signs, looking at a rhythm strip, and comparing Mr. Jones's vital sign results to prior readings. Your assessment, including a review of his medications, lab results, considering a change in baseline mental status, and considering pain as a reason for mental status change were the correct assessment parameters, and each give clues about the potential underlying causes of his current mental state. Untreated pain can cause delirium exhibited by agitation and may cause a cancellation of the surgery—something that nobody wants. Had the gentleman been treated for pain rather than agitation, he might have presented as comfortable and oriented, given that the correct medication and dosage were given. The dose of Haldol was too high, and should be initiated at 0.5 mg (not 5 mg), although it is not FDA approved for agitation nor beneficial unless the patient is psychotic or trying to harm another person or himself. The maximum dose is 3 mg/day for older

(continued)

CASE STUDY *(continued)*

adults. Demerol is contraindicated in older adults for pain and the best choice would be morphine or a small dose of Dilaudid if morphine allergic.

You are also correct in your approach to a patient who is or has been agitated—using a calm, soothing approach and removing the restraints that can exacerbate agitation and are most often unacceptable in the practice setting and considered a poor substitute for nursing care. Had his blood pressure been significantly lower than his baseline, calling rapid response would have been indicated and may still be depending on how Mr. Jones presents over the next several hours.

Interventions

While waiting for the hospitalist to arrive on the unit, you continue to assess his vital signs and mental status. Next, you access the bedside computer for the internet to try to determine what the potential underlying causes are for Mr. Jones's presentation. You review the potential side effect of the medicines and discover that Carvedilol has both alpha- and beta-blocking effects and was probably prescribed to address both his hypertension as well as for rate control of the atrial fibrillation. Taking this drug with digoxin and amiodarone can lead to a drug–drug interaction by an additive effect and, therefore, lower the heart rate; fortunately, it is not seriously affecting his blood pressure while he is in bed. Once he is stabilized, orthostatic blood pressure should be checked, knowing that his pressure may drop upon standing, which could provoke an additional fall. In addition, you learn that a common unknown side effect of the dementia medications (e.g., Namenda and Aricept) is bradycardia. Finally, you realize his low potassium may also affect cardiac conduction. You remind the team that Mr. Jones fell at home, and that is what brought him in for surgery. You suggest to the hospitalist that she may want to ask the primary care physician about the risk and benefits of continuing the warfarin while Mr. Jones is at risk for falls. You also suggest that the surgeon be alerted to Mr. Jones's condition, in the event that Mr. Jones is not able to tolerate the surgical intervention in his current state of agitation, exhaustion, and with his potassium depleted. You also determine a need to reconcile with his wife whether he was taking any medications that may lower his potassium that may have been missed on the initial reconciliation. You will ask her to bring his medications and OTCs in a brown bag.

Many nurses may say "this is the physician's job" or "this is up to the pharmacist" to determine the potential adverse effects of the drugs. However, nurses are at the bedside 24 hours a day, and have a more comprehensive picture of how the patient is responding to nursing care, medication, and therapies while admitted. Armed with knowledge about geriatric syndromes and atypical presentation in older adults, nurses can be pivotal and instrumental in the early identification of patients at risk. Additionally, the patient advocate that the role nurses play is a major component of the safety and quality movement underway in care settings nationally. Of course, reaching out for expert consultation from other team members will always enhance the plan of care, but the more nurses learn about best practices for geriatric patients and the geriatric resources available, the more it becomes a routine to identify risk factors for ADEs and other geriatric syndromes discussed in this text. Nurses are key members of the interdisciplinary team promoting a safe environment for patients.

SUMMARY

Nurses have the unique opportunity to intervene and improve safety by focusing on the prevention of ADEs in older adults. Traditionally focused on "caring," nurses have taken the lead in implementing preventive strategies on behalf of the patient. Although acute care nurses are not typically prescribers, unless they are advanced practice nurses (APNs) with prescriptive authority, they have always reviewed and confirmed medication orders, carried them out, and alerted the primary provider of concerns or problems with medications. Nurses have always ensured a culture of safety by advocating for their patients and must continue to be proactive in doing so. Nurses are also responsible for identifying wrong drugs, dosages, and so on prior to administering them. Given that nurses are at the bedside 24/7, they can make medication suggestions to prescribers based on their holistic knowledge of the patient and recognition of new symptoms. Nurses are the primary source for providing discharge education and counseling to older adults at discharge; therefore, they play a key role in preventing medication-related consequences after discharge, including prevention of rehospitalization because of medication-related problems. Consulting with experts on the interdisciplinary team and/or use of computer programs can facilitate provision of accurate discharge information. Nurses are in a pivotal position to take the lead in patient safety.

NURSING STANDARD OF PRACTICE

Protocol 17.1: Reducing Adverse Drug Events in Older Adults

I. GOAL: To proactively identify older adults at risk for adverse drug events (ADEs) and reduce the likelihood of it.

II. OVERVIEW: ADEs whether from drug–drug or drug–disease interactions, inappropriate prescribing, poor adherence, or medication errors lead to serious or potentially fatal outcomes for older adults. Around 31% of all adverse events in hospitals are caused by medication-related problems. More than half of ADEs are potentially preventable (Levinson, 2010; Rochon, 2010; Safran et al., 2005).

III. BACKGROUND
   A. Definitions
      1. *Adverse drug event*: Injury occurring during the patient's drug therapy whether resulting from appropriate care or from unsuitable or suboptimum care. ADEs include adverse drug reactions (ADRs) during normal use of medicine and any harm secondary to a medication error (COE Medication Practices, 2007, pp. 1).
      2. *Iatrogenic ADEs*: Any undesirable condition in a patient occurring as the result of treatment by a health care professional; pertaining to an illness or injury resulting from a medication.
      3. *Adverse drug reaction*: Any noxious or unintended and undesired effect of a drug that occurs at normal human doses for prophylaxis, diagnosis, or therapy.

(continued)

Protocol 17.1: Reducing Adverse Drug Events in Older Adults *(cont.)*

4. *Drug–drug interactions*: When one therapeutic agent alters either the concentration (pharmacokinetic interactions) or the biological effect of another agent (pharmacodynamic interactions; Leucuta & Vlase, 2006; Levinson, 2010).

5. *Medication adherence*: The extent to which a person's medication-taking behavior corresponds with agreed recommendations of a health care provider (Sabaté, 2003).

6. *Drug–disease interactions*: Undesired drug effects (exacerbation of a disease or condition caused by a drug) that occur in patients with certain disease states (e.g., beta-blocker given to patient with bronchospasm).

7. *Pharmacokinetics*: The time course of absorption, distribution across compartments, metabolism, and excretion of drugs in the body. The metabolism and excretion of many drugs decrease and the physiological changes of aging require dose adjustment for some drugs (Levinson, 2010).

8. *Pharmacodynamics*: The response of the body to the drug that is affected by receptor binding, postreceptor effects, and chemical interactions. Pharmacodynamic problems occur when two drugs act at the same or interrelated receptor sites, resulting in additive, synergistic, or antagonistic effects. The effects of two or more drugs together can be either *additive* (combination of drugs "add up" to increase effect), *synergistic* (one agent magnifies the effect of the other), or *antagonistic* (one medication inhibits the effect of the other).

9. *Medication reconciliation*: The process of comparing a patient's medication orders to all of the medications that the person has been taking (Santell, 2006).

B. Epidemiology

1. It is estimated that the majority of older adults older than age 65 years (79%) are on medications, with 39% taking five or more prescription drugs and up to 90% taking over-the-counter (OTC) drugs (Hanlon et al., 2001). Persons older than age 65 years consume more than one-third of all prescription drugs and purchase 40% of all OTC medicines (Kohn et al., 2000).

2. An estimated 35% of older persons experience ADEs and almost half of these are preventable (Safran et al., 2005).

3. Prevalence of ADR-related hospitalizations ranges from 5% to 35% (Gurwitz et al., 2005; Kongkaew et al., 2008). Drug toxicity admission was 2.5% in the emergency department (ED) with 42% being admitted to the hospital for ADEs (Budnitz et al., 2006).

4. ADEs are estimated to cost the health care system $75–$85 billion annually (Fick et al., 2003).

C. Etiology

Adults become increasingly susceptible to ADEs as they age. Physiological changes characteristic of aging predispose older adults to experience ADEs resulting in four times more hospitalizations in older versus younger persons. Persons older than age 65 years experience medication-related problems for seven major reasons:

1. Age-related physiological changes that result in altered pharmacokinetics and pharmacodynamics (Mangoni & Jackson, 2004; Rochon, 2010).

(continued)

Protocol 17.1: Reducing Adverse Drug Events in Older Adults *(cont.)*

2. Multiple medications (i.e., polypharmacy) that are often prescribed by multiple providers (Hajjar et al., 2003; Hanlon et al., 2001; Rochon, 2010).
3. Incorrect doses of medications (more than or less than a therapeutic dosage; Astin et al., 2000; Hanlon et al., 2001; Sloane et al., 2002).
4. Medication consumption for the treatment of symptoms that are not disease dependent or specific (self-medication or prescribing cascades; Neafsey & Shellman, 2001; Rochon, 2010).
5. Iatrogenic causes such as
   a. ADRs including drug–drug or drug–disease interactions (Gurwitz et al., 2005; Hohl et al., 2005; Petrone & Katz, 2005; Rothberg et al., 2008)
   b. Inappropriate prescribing for older adults (Fick et al., 2003; Rochon, 2010)
   c. Problems with medication adherence (Fulmer et al., 1999; Haynes et al., 2005)
   d. Medication errors (Doucette et al., 2005; Kohn et al., 2000; Rochon, 2010)

IV. ASSESSMENT TOOLS AND STRATEGIES

A. Assessment Tools
   1. Use appropriate assessment tools as indicated for each individual's needs and specific setting:
      a. "Beers Criteria for Potentially Inappropriate Medication Use in Older Adults. Part I: 2002 Criteria Independent of Diagnoses or Conditions." "Beers Criteria for Potentially Inappropriate Medication Use in Older Adults Part II: 2002 Criteria Considering Diagnoses or Conditions" (Fick et al., 2003; see "Try This" series, issue numbers 16.1 and 16.2 at http://www.consultgerirn.org/resources)
      b. Common drug–drug interactions (see Table 17.1). List of some common known interactions.
      c. Cockroft–Gault formula to estimate renal function (see Table 17.2).
      d. Functional capacity (activity of daily living [ADL], independent activity of daily living [IADL], Mini-Cog, or Mini-Mental State Exam [MMSE]): assess ability to self-administer medications. (See Chapter 6, Assessment of Physical Function, and Chapter 8, Assessing Cognitive Function; or Resources section at http://www.consultgerirn.org/resources.)
      e. Brown bag method (Nathan et al., 1999). Method used to assess all medications an older adult has at home including prescriptions from all providers, OTC medications, and herbal remedies (all medications are to be brought in a brown bag). Should be used in conjunction with a complete medication history (Table 17.3).
      f. Drugs Regimen Unassisted Grading Scale (DRUGS) tool. Assessment of self-administration ability (Edelberg et al., 1999; Hutchison et al., 2006).

B. Assessment Strategies
   1. Comprehensive medication assessment should be performed at admission, discharge, and intervals in between (Petrone & Katz, 2005; Shekelle, MacLean, Morton, & Wenger, 2001). Obtain a detailed medication history and confirm its accuracy (Brown et al., 2003) detailing the type and amount

(continued)

Protocol 17.1: Reducing Adverse Drug Events in Older Adults *(cont.)*

of prescriptions; OTCs, vitamins, supplements, and herbal remedies (Hanlon et al., 2001; Kaufman et al., 2002); and alcohol and illicit drugs using appropriate assessment tool (e.g., brown bag method; Nathan et al., 1999).

2. Asses for medication- and patient-related risk factors for ADRs (Table 17.4).

3. Assess renal function using Cockroft–Gault formula prior to administering renal clearing drugs (Table 17.2).

4. Reconciliation of medications from home or other levels of care with medications ordered at admission and at discharge in consultation with a pharmacist, geriatric expert, or computer-based program (Gleason, 2004; Joanna Briggs Institute [JBI], 2006; Santell, 2006; Simon et al., 2006).

5. Review medication list using Beers criteria for potentially inappropriate medications, particularly those with *high severity* and for potential drug–drug and drug–disease interactions (Fick et al., 2003; Rochon, 2010; Zhan et al., 2005).

6. At discharge from hospital, use appropriate tools to assess individual's ability to self-administer medications:

   a. Assess functional capacity: ADLs, IADLs, Mini-Cog. (See Chapter 6, Assessment of Physical Function, and Chapter 8, Assessing Cognitive Function, in this text.)

   b. Assess individuals (at admission or initial encounter and at discharge) who administer their own medicines with DRUGS tool to identify potential areas of self-administration difficulty (Edelberg et al., 1999; Hutchison, et al., 2006).

V. INTERVENTIONS

A. Reducing ADEs (during and posthospitalization)

1. *Patient empowerment.* Patients should be given the necessary information and the opportunity to exercise the degree of control they choose over health care decisions that affect them. If patients are involved in decision making, they are less likely to make decisions that may lead to ADRs such as abruptly discontinuing a medication that should be tapered off (Aspden et al., 2007; NCC MERP, 2001).

2. *Comprehensive medication history* on admission as indicated (Table 17.3).

3. *Collaborate with the interdisciplinary team* to effect change in reducing the numbers of ADEs and ADRs, many of which are preventable (Hanlon et al., 2001).

4. *Prescribing principles.* Although bedside nurses are not involved in prescribing, they are involved in reviewing and signing off medications, thus should be aware of prescribing principles. Monitoring for appropriate prescribing and alerting the prescriber to potential problem areas helps reduce medication-related problems. Prescribing a medication is multifaceted: deciding that a drug is truly indicated; choosing the best drug; determining appropriate dose for the individual; monitoring for toxicity and effectiveness; and seeking consultation when necessary (Rochon, 2010). These principles support recommendations to:

   a. *Reduce the dose.* "Start Low and Go Slow" or give the lowest possible dose when starting a medication and slow upward titration to obtain clinical

(continued)

Protocol 17.1: Reducing Adverse Drug Events in Older Adults *(cont.)*

benefit; many ADEs are dose-related (Petrone & Katz, 2005; Rochon, 2010). Primary provider should be notified if the dosage ordered is higher than the recommended starting dose (e.g., digoxin maximum dose < 0.125 mg for treatment of *systolic* heart failure; Fick et al., 2003).

b. *Discontinue unnecessary therapy.* Prescribers are often reluctant to stop medications, especially if they did not initiate the treatment. This practice increases the risk for an adverse event (Rochon, 2010).

c. Attempt a *trial of nonpharmacological interventions* and treatments prior to requesting medication for new symptoms (Rochon, 2010).

d. *Recommend safer drugs.* Avoid drugs that are likely to be associated with adverse outcomes (review Beers criteria; Petrone & Katz, 2005).

e. *Assess renal function* using Cockroft–Gault formula (for renally cleared drugs) to determine accurate dosage prior to prescribing such as many routinely prescribed intravenous (IV) antibiotics. Dosage recommendations are available based on this formula are presented in common prescribing resources.

f. *Optimize drug regimen.* When prescribing medications, the focus should be on risk versus benefit where the expected health benefit (e.g., relief of agitation in dementia with psychosis) exceeds the expected negative consequences (e.g., morbidity and mortality from falls that result in hip fracture; Leipzig et al., 1999; Ooi et al., 2000; Rochon, 2010).

g. *Initiation of new medication.* Assess risk factors for ADRs, potential drug–disease and drug–drug interactions, and correct drug dosages (Doucette et al., 2005; NCC MERP, 2001; Petrone & Katz, 2005). See Table 17.1 and Table 17.4.

h. *Avoid the prescribing cascade.* Avoid the prescribing cascade by *first* considering any new symptom as being an adverse effect of a current medication prior to adding a new medication (Rochon, 2010; Rochon & Gurwitz, 1997).

i. *Avoid inappropriate medications.* Review criteria for potential inappropriate medications, drug–disease interactions, and potential drug–drug interactions (Fick et al., 2003).

j. *Employ nonpharmacological approaches* for symptoms (e.g., therapeutic activity kit for agitation; Zwicker & Fletcher, 2009).

B. Specific interventions for prevention of iatrogenic ADR (in hospital and after discharge)

1. Consider any new symptom as a possible ADR before requesting or administering new medication for the symptom, avoiding the prescribing cascade (Gurwitz et al., 2005).

2. Monitor medication orders for wrong drug choices (high-risk inappropriate medications, drug–disease, and drug–drug interactions), wrong dosages, or administration errors (Doucette et al., 2005; Gurwitz et al., 2005; Hanlon et al., 1997). Consider use of technological handheld devices such as personal digital assistant (PDA) for quick access to Beers criteria, drug–drug or drug–disease interactions, and geriatric assessment tools. (See Resources section.)

(continued)

Protocol 17.1: Reducing Adverse Drug Events in Older Adults *(cont.)*

3. Improve prescribing practices by documenting indication for initiation of new drug therapy, maintaining a current medication list, documenting response to therapy as well as the need for ongoing treatment, and evaluating comorbidities (Merle, Laroche, Dantoine, & Charmes, 2005).

4. Institutional implementation of computer-assisted technology for medication order entry (AHRQ, 2001). Identifying and reporting ADRs can also be performed using computer-assisted national surveillance system.

5. Institutions must facilitate a culture of safety to reduce ADRs or ADEs (Kohn et al., 2000).

C. Interventions at Discharge

1. *Reconciliation* of medications at admission and discharge helps to reduce ADR or ADEs and rehospitalization (Gleason et al., 2004; Nickerson et al., 2005).

2. *Assess abilities and limitations* and health literacy in self-administration of medications using appropriate tools at discharge and recognize that self-administration and nonadherence can induce ADRs (Curry et al., 2005; Merle et al., 2005).

3. *Assess for adherence* issues that may develop after discharge, which can help to reduce ADEs and rehospitalization (Bergman-Evans, 2006; Edelberg et al., 1999; Fulmer, Kim, Montgomery, & Lyder, 2000; Nickerson et al., 2005). Recommend devices that can assist in enhancing adherence, behavior, and interventions to address cost and other adherence issues.

4. *Patient/Caregiver education.* Provide patient and caregiver education using relevant nursing content and principles including assessment of factors that might affect compliance. Nurses are the primary source for providing education to patients at discharge; therefore, their role is key to preventing medication-related consequences after hospitalization, including rehospitalization (Curry et al., 2005). Discharge education and counseling includes the following:

   a. Education tailored to the age group and needs of the individual (Bergman-Evans, 2006).

   b. Educate the patient and caregiver about benefits and risks and potential medication side effects (Rochon, 2010; Shekelle et al., 2001).

   c. Teach safe medication management; use teach-back as a methodology (Curry et al., 2005; Schillinger et al., 2003).

   d. Consider an interactive computer program (personal education program) designed for the learning styles and psychomotor skills of older adults to teach about potential drug interactions that can result from self-medication with OTC agents and alcohol (Neafsey, Strickler, Shellman, & Chartier, 2002).

VI. EXPECTED OUTCOMES

A. Patients will

1. Experience fewer iatrogenic outcomes from medication-related events.

2. Demonstrate understanding of their medication regimens upon discharge from the hospital.

B. Health care providers will

1. Use a range of interventions to prevent, alleviate, or ameliorate medication problems with older adults.

(continued)

Protocol 17.1: Reducing Adverse Drug Events in Older Adults *(cont.)*

2. Improve prescribing practices by documenting indication for initiation of new drug therapy, maintaining a current medication list, and documenting response to therapy as well as the need for ongoing treatment.
3. Evaluate nature and origins of medication-related problems in a timely manner.
4. Increase their knowledge about medication safety in older adults.
5. Increase referrals to appropriate practitioners for collaboration and medication safety (e.g., pharmacist, geriatrician, geriatric/gerontological or psychiatric clinical nurse specialist, nurse practitioner, or consultation-liaison service).

C. Institution will
  1. Provide a culture of safety that encourages safe medication practices (Kohn et al., 2000).
  2. Provide education to health care providers regarding prevention, identification, and reporting of ADRs (Gurwitz et al., 2003).
  3. Make information on ADRs accessible to patients (Gurwitz et al., 2003).
  4. Enhance surveillance and reporting of ADRs using a national surveillance system (Gurwitz et al., 2003). Consider use of computerized physician order entry system (Gurwitz et al., 2003; JBI, 2006).
  5. Track and report decreased morbidity and mortality caused by medication-related problems.
  6. Provide a system for medication reconciliation and follow-up its effectiveness regarding rehospitalization rates caused by ADRs.
  7. Review for careful documentation of iatrogenic medication and other iatrogenic events for continuous quality improvement (CQI).
  8. Provide ongoing education related to safe medication management for physicians, other licensed independent providers, pharmacists, and nursing staff.

VII. FOLLOW-UP
A. Health care providers will
  1. Provide consistent and appropriate care and follow-up in presence of a medication-related problem.
  2. Monitor and evaluate with physical exam and/or laboratory tests (as appropriate) on regular basis to ensure that the older adult is responding to therapy as expected (Edelberg et al., 1999).
B. Institutions will
  1. Provide ongoing assessment of staff competence in assessing and intervening for prevention of ADEs.
  2. Embed reduction of ADEs in the institution's culture of safety.

VII. RELEVANT PRACTICE GUIDELINES
A. Bergman-Evans, B. (2004). *Improving medication management for older adult clients* (NGC Guideline No. 003993). Iowa City, IA: University of Iowa Gerontological Nursing Interventions Research Center, Research Dissemination Core. Retrieved from http://www.guideline.gov
B. Health Care Association of New Jersey. (2006). *Medication management guideline.* Hamilton, NJ: Author. Retrived from http://www.guideline.gov. Note: Geared for posthospital institutions for adult patients.

RESOURCES

Medication Complexity

Steinman, M. A., & Hanlon, J. T. (2010). Managing medications in clinically complex elders: "There's got to be a happy medium." *Journal of the American Medical Association, 304*(14), 1592–1601. Evidence Level I.

Medication Reconciliation

Bayoumi, I., Howard, M., Holbrook, A. M., & Schabort, I. (2009). Interventions to improve medication reconciliation in primary care. *The Annals of Pharmacotherapy, 43*(10), 1667–1675. Evidence Level I.

Jennings, B. (2008). Patient acuity. In R. G. Hughes (Ed.), *Patient safety and quality: An evidence-based handbook for nurses*. Rockville, MD: Agency for Healthcare Research and Quality. http://www.ncbi.nlm.nih.gov/books/NBK2648/

Medication and Medical Error Prevention

Joanna Briggs Institute. (2006). Strategies to reduce medication errors with reference to older adults. *Nursing Standard, 20*(41), 5.3–57.

National Coordinating Council for Medication Errors Reporting and Prevention. (2011). *Medication error reporting and prevention*. http://www.nccmerp.org/councilRecs.html

Herbal Remedies

Huang, S. M., Hall, S. D., Watkins, P., Love, L. A., Serabjit-Singh, C., Betz, J. M., . . . Center for Drug Evaluation and Research and Office of Regulatory Affairs. (2004). Drug interactions with herbal products and grapefruit juice: A conference report. *Clinical Pharmacology and Therapeutics, 75*(1), 1–12. http://www.ascpt.org

Huang, S. M., & Lesko, L. J. (2004). Drug-drug, drug-dietary supplement, and drug-citrus fruit and other food interactions: What have we learned? *Journal of Clinical Pharmacology, 44*(6), 559–569. http://www.jclinpharm.org

Medication Adherence

Haynes, R. B., Ackloo, E., Sahota, N., McDonald, H. P., & Yao, X. (2008). Interventions for enhancing medication adherence [Audio podcast]. *Cochrane Database of Systematic Reviews*, (2), CD000011. www.cochrane.org/reviews/en/ab000011.html

Williams, A., Manias, E., & Walker, R. (2008). Interventions to improve medication adherence in people with multiple chronic conditions: A systematic review. *Journal of Advanced Nursing, 63*(2), 132–143.

REFERENCES

Agency for Healthcare Research and Quality. (2001). *Reducing and preventing adverse drug events to decrease hospital costs* (Research in Action, Issue No. 1, AHRQ Publication No. 01-0020). Rockville, MD: Author. Retrieved from http://www.ahrq.gov/qual/aderia/aderia.htm. Evidence Level I.

Ahmed, A., Allman, R. M., & DeLong, J. F. (2002). Inappropriate use of digoxin in older hospital-ized heart failure patients. *The Journals of Gerontology. Series A, Biological Sciences and Medical Sciences, 57*(2), M138–M143. Evidence Level III.

Alexopoulou, A., Dourakis, S. P., Mantzoukis, D., Pitsariotis, T., Kandyli, A., Deutsch, M., & Archimandritis, A. J. (2008). Adverse drug reactions as a cause of hospital admissions: A 6-month experience in a single centre in Greece. *European Journal of Internal Medicine, 19*(7), 505–510.

Aspden, P., Wolcott, J. A., Bootman, J. L., & Cronenwett, L. R. (Eds). (2007). *Preventing medication errors*. Washington, DC: The National Academies Press.

Astin, J. A., Pelletier, K. R., Marie, A., & Haskell, W. L. (2000). Complementary and alternative medicine use among elderly persons: One-year analysis of a Blue Shield Medicare supplement. *Journals of Gerontology. Series A, Biological Sciences and Medical Sciences, 55*(1), M4–M9. Evidence Level IV.

Beers, M. H. (1997). Explicit criteria for determining potentially inappropriate medication use by the elderly: An update. *Archives of Internal Medicine, 157*(14), 1531–1536. Evidence Level VI.

Beers, M. H., Ouslander, J. G., Fingold, S. F., Morgenstern, H., Reuben, D. B., Rogers, W., . . . Beck, J. C. (1992). Inappropriate medication prescribing in skilled-nursing facilities. *Annals of Internal Medicine, 117*(8), 684–689.

Bergman-Evans, B. (2006). AIDES to improving medication adherence in older adults. *Geriatric Nursing, 27*(3), 174–182. Evidence Level V.

Bloch, F., Thibaud, M., Dugué, B., Brèque, C., Rigaud, A. S., & Kemoun, G. (2011). Psychotropic drugs and falls in the elderly people: Updated literature review and meta-analysis. *Journal of Aging and Health, 23*(2), 329–346.

Boockvar, K., Fishman, E., Kyriacou, C. K., Monias, A., Gavi, S., & Cortes, T. (2004). Adverse events due to discontinuations in drug use and dose changes in patients transferred between acute and long-term care facilities. *Archives of Internal Medicine, 164*(5), 545–550.

Bronstein, A. C., Spyker, D. A., Cantilena, L. R., Jr., Green, J. L., Rumack, B. H., Heard, S. E., & American Association of Poison Control Centers. (2008). 2007 Annual Report of the American Association of Poison Control Centers' National Poison Data System (NPDS): 25th Annual Report. *Clinical Toxicology, 46*(10), 927–1057.

Brown, A. F., Mangione, C. M., Saliba, D., Sarkisian, C. A., California Healthcare Foundation/American Geriatrics Society Panel on Improving Care for Elders With Diabetes. (2003). Guide-lines for improving the care of the older person with diabetes mellitus. *Journal of the American Geriatrics Society, 51*(5 Suppl. Guidelines), S265–S280. Evidence Level VI.

Budnitz, D. S., Pollock, D. A., Weidenbach, K. N., Mendelsohn, A. B., Schroeder, T. J., & Annest, J. L. (2006). National surveillance of emergency department visits for outpatient adverse drug events. *Journal of the American Medical Association, 296*(15), 1858–1866. Evidence Level V.

Catterson, M. L., Preskorn, S. H., & Martin, R. I. (1997). Pharmodynamic and pharmokinetic considerations in geriatric psychophamacology. *The Psychiatric Clinics of North America, 20*(1), 205–218.

Chang, C. M., Liu, P. Y., Yang, Y. H., Yang, Y. C., Wu, C. F., & Lu, F. H. (2005). Use of the Beers criteria to predict adverse drug reactions among first-visit elderly outpatients. *Pharmacotherapy, 25*(6), 831–838. Evidence Level IV.

Chevalier, B. A., Parker, D. S., MacKinnon, N. J., & Sketris, I. (2006). Nurses' perceptions of medication safety and medication reconciliation practices. *Nursing Leadership, 19*(3), 61–72. Evidence Level V.

Committee of Experts (COE) on Safe Medication Practice. (2005). *Glossary of terms related to patient and medication safety*. Retrieved August 23, 2011 from http://www.bvs.org.ar/pdf/seguridadpaciente.pdf

Curry, L. C., Walker, C., Hogstel, M. O., & Burns, P. (2005). Teaching older adults to self-manage medications: Preventing adverse drug reactions. *Journal of Gerontological Nursing, 31*(4), 32–42. Evidence Level VI.

Cusak, B., & Vestal, R. E. (2000). Clinical pharmacology. In M. H. Beers & R. Berkow (Eds.), *The Merck manual of geriatrics* (3rd ed., pp. 54–74). Evidence Level VI.

Doucette, W. R., McDonough, R. P., Klepser, D., & McCarthy, R. (2005). Comprehensive medication therapy management: Identifying and resolving drug-related issues in a community pharmacy. *Clinical Therapeutics, 27*(7), 1104–1111. Evidence Level V.

Edelberg, H. K., Shallenberger, E., & Wei, J. Y. (1999). Medication management capacity in highly functioning community-living older adults: Detection of early deficits. *Journal of the American Geriatrics Society, 47*(5), 592–596. Evidence Level IV.

Feldman, P. H., McDonald, M., Rosati, R. J., Murtaugh, C., Kovner, C., Goldberg, J. D., & King, L. (2006). Exploring the utility of automated drug alerts in home healthcare. *Journal for Healthcare Quality, 28*(1), 29–40. Evidence Level IV.

Fick, D. M., Cooper, J. W., Wade, W. E., Waller, J. L., Maclean, J. R., & Beers, M. H. (2003). Updating the Beers criteria for potentially inappropriate medication use in older adults: Results of a US consensus panel of experts. *Archives of Internal Medicine, 163*(22), 2716–2724. Evidence Level VI.

Flaherty, J. H., Perry, H. M., III, Lynchard, G. S., & Morley, J. E. (2000). Polypharmacy and hospitalization among older home care patients. *The Journals of Gerontology. Series A, Biological Sciences and Medical Sciences, 55*(10), M554–M559.

Fouts, M., Hanlon, J. T., Pieper, C. F., Perfetto, E. M., & Feinberg, J. L. (1997). Identification of elderly nursing facility residents at high risk for drug-related problems. *The Consultant Pharmacist, 12*, 1103–1111.

Fu, A. Z., Liu, G. G., & Christensen, D. B. (2004). Inappropriate medication use and health outcomes in the elderly. *Journal of the American Geriatrics Society, 52*(11), 1934–1939. Evidence Level IV.

Fulmer, T., Kim, T. S., Montgomery, K., & Lyder, C. (2000). What the literature tells us about the complexity of medication compliance in the elderly. *Generations, 24*(4), 43–48.

Fulmer, T. T., Feldman, P. H., Kim, T. S., Carty, B., Beers, M., Molina, M., & Putnam, M. (1999). An intervention study to enhance medication compliance in community-dwelling elderly individuals. *Journal of Gerontological Nursing, 25*(8), 6–14.

Gaddis, G. M., Holt, T. R., & Woods, M. (2002). Drug interactions in at-risk emergency department patients. *Academic Emergency Medicine, 9*(11), 1162–1167. Evidence Level IV.

Gallagher, P., Barry, P., & O'Mahony, D. (2007). Inappropriate prescribing in the elderly. *Journal of Clinical Pharmacy and Therapeutics, 32*(2), 113–121. Evidence Level V.

Gardiner, P., Graham, R. E., Legedza, A. T., Eisenberg, D. M., & Phillips, R. S. (2006). Factors associated with dietary supplement among prescription medication users. *Archives of Internal Medicine, 166*(18), 1968–1974. Evidence Level IV.

Gleason, K. M., Groszek, J. M., Sullivan, C., Rooney, D., Barnard, C., & Noskin, G. A. (2004). Reconciliation of discrepancies in medication histories and admission orders of newly hospitalized patients. *American Journal of Health-System Pharmacy, 61*(16), 1689–1695. Evidence Level IV.

Gray, C. L., & Gardner, C. (2009). Adverse drug events in the elderly: An ongoing problem. *Journal of Managed Care Pharmacy, 15*(7), 568–571. Evidence level VI.

Gray, S. L., LaCroix, A. Z., Hanlon, J. T., Penninx, B. W., Blough, D. K., Leveille, S. G., . . . Buchner, D. M. (2006). Benzodiazepine use and physical disability in community-dwelling older adults. *Journal of the American Geriatrics Society, 54*(2), 224–230. Evidence Level II.

Greenfield, S., Billimek, J., Pellegrini, F., Franciosi, M., De Berardis, G., Nicolucci, A., & Kaplan, S. H. (2009). Comorbidity affects the relationship between glycemic control and cardiovascular outcomes in diabetes: A cohort study. *Annals of Internal Medicine, 151*(12), 854–860. Evidence Level IV.

Gurwitz, J. H., Field, T. S., Harrold, L. R., Rothschild, J., Debellis, K., Seger, A. C., . . . Bates, D. W. (2003). Incidence and preventability of adverse drug events among older persons in the ambulatory setting. *Journal of the American Medical Association, 289*(9), 1107–1116. Evidence Level IV.

Gurwitz, J. H., Field, T. S., Judge, J., Rochon, P., Harrold, L. R., Cadoret, C., . . . Bates, D. W. (2005). The incidence of adverse drug events in two large academic long-term care facilities. *The American Journal of Medicine, 118*(3), 251–258. Evidence Level II.

Hajjar, E. R., Hanlon, J. T., Artz, M. B., Lindblad, C. I., Pieper, C. F., Sloane, R. J., . . . Schmader, K. E. (2003). Adverse drug reaction risk factors in older outpatients. *The American Journal of Geriatric Pharmacotherapy, 1*(2), 82–89.

Hajjar, I., & Kotchen, T. A. (2003). Trends in prevalence, awareness, treatment, and control of hypertension in the United States, 1988–2000. *Journal of the American Medical Association, 290*(2), 199–206. Evidence Level IV.

Han, L., McCusker, J., Cole, M., Abrahamowicz, M., Primeau, F., & Elie, M. (2001). Use of medications with anticholinergic effect predicts clinical severity of delirium symptoms in older medical inpatients. *Archives of Internal Medicine, 161*(8), 1099–1105.

Hanlon, J. T., Fillenbaum, G. G., Ruby, C. M., Gray, S., & Bohannon, A. (2001). Epidemiology of over-the-counter drug use in community dwelling elderly: United States perspective. *Drugs & Aging, 18*(2), 123–131. Evidence Level V.

Hanlon, J. T., Lindblad, C. I., & Gray, S. L. (2004). Can clinical pharmacy services have a positive impact on drug-related problems and health outcomes in community-based older adults? *The American Journal of Geriatric Pharmacotherapy, 2*(1), 3–13. Evidence Level I.

Hanlon, J. T., Pieper, C. F., Hajjar, E. R., Sloane, R. J., Lindblad, C. I., Ruby, C. M., & Schmader, K. E. (2006). Incidence and predictors of all and preventable adverse drug reactions in frail elderly persons after hospital stay. *Journals of Gerontology. Series A, Biological Sciences and Medical Sciences, 61*(5), 511–515. Evidence Level II.

Hanlon, J. T., Schmader, K. E., Koronkowski, M. J., Weinberger, M., Landsman, P. B., Samsa, G. P., & Lewis, I. K. (1997). Adverse drug events in high risk older outpatients. *Journal of the American Geriatrics Society, 45*(8), 945–948. Evidence Level IV.

Hanlon, J. T., Schmader, K. E., Ruby, C. M., & Weinberger, M. (2001). Suboptimal prescribing in older inpatients and outpatients. *Journal of the American Geriatrics Society, 49*(2), 200–209. Evidence Level V.

Hansten, P. D., Horn, J. R., & Hazlet, T. K. (2001). ORCA: OpeRational ClassificAtion of drug interactions. *Journal of the American Pharmaceutical Association, 41*(2), 161–165. Evidence Level IV.

Haynes, R. B., Yao, X., Degani, A., Kripalani, S., Garg, A., & McDonald, H. P. (2005). Interventions for enhancing medication adherence. *Cochrane Database of Systematic Reviews,* (4), CD000011.

Hohl, C. M., Robitaille, C., Lord, V., Dankoff, J., Colacone, A., Pham, L., . . . Afilalo, M. (2005). Emergency physician recognition of adverse drug-related events in elder patients presenting to an emergency department. *Academic Emergency Medicine, 12*(3), 197–205. Evidence Level IV.

Howard, R. L., Avery, A. J., Slavenburg, S., Royal, S., Pipe, G., Lucassen, P., & Pirmohamed, M. (2007). Which drugs cause preventable admissions to hospital? A systematic review. *British Journal of Clinical Pharmacology, 63*(2), 136–147.

Hutchison, L. C., Jones, S. K., West, D. S., & Wei, J. Y. (2006). Assessment of medication management by community-living elderly persons with two standardized assessment tools: A cross-sectional study. *The American Journal of Geriatric Pharmacotherapy, 4*(2), 144–153. Evidence Level IV.

Jano, E., & Aparasu, R. R. (2007). Healthcare outcomes associated with beers' criteria: A systematic review. *The Annals of Pharmacotherapy, 41*(3), 438–447. Evidence Level I.

Joanna Briggs Institute. (2006). Strategies to reduce medication errors with reference to older adults. *Nursing Standard, 20*(41), 53–57. Evidence Level I.

Juurlink, D. N., Mamdani, M., Kopp, A., Laupacis, A., & Redelmeier, D. A. (2003). Drug-drug interactions among elderly patients hospitalized for drug toxicity. *Journal of the American Medical Association, 289*(13), 1652–1658. Evidence Level III.

Kaufman, D. W., Kelly, J. P., Rosenberg, L., Anderson, T. E., & Mitchell, A. A. (2002). Recent patterns of medication use in the ambulatory adult population of the United States: The Slone survey. *Journal of the American Medical Association, 287*(3), 337–344. Evidence Level IV.

Kelly, J. P., Kaufman, D. W., Kelley, K., Rosenberg, L., Anderson, T. E., & Mitchell, A. A. (2005). Recent trends in use of herbal and other natural products. *Archives of Internal Medicine, 165*(3), 281–286. Evidence Level IV.

Kemper, R. F., Steiner, V., Hicks, B., Pierce, L., & Iwuagwu, C. (2007). Anticholinergic medications: Use among older adults with memory problems. *Journal of Gerontological Nursing, 33*(1), 21–29. Evidence Level IV.

Kindermann, S. S., Dolder, C. R., Bailey, A., Katz, I. R., & Jeste, D. V. (2002). Pharmacological treatment of psychosis and agitation in elderly patients with dementia: Four decades of experience. *Drugs & Aging, 19*(4), 257–276. Evidence Level V.

Kohn, L. T., Corrigan, J. M., & Donaldson, M. S. (2000). *To err is human: Building a safer health system*. Washington, DC: National Academy Press. Evidence Level VI.

Kongkaew, C., Noyce, P. R., & Ashcroft, D. M. (2008). Hospital admissions associated with adverse drug reactions: A systematic review of prospective observational studies. *The Annals of Pharmacotherapy, 42*(7), 1017–1025. Evidence Level I.

Lam, S., & Ruby, C. M. (2005). Impact of an interdisciplinary team on drug therapy outcomes in a geriatric clinic. *American Journal of Health-System Pharmacy, 62*(6), 626–629. Evidence Level II.

Lapane, K. L., Hughes, C. M., & Quilliam, B. J. (2007). Does incorporating medications in the surveyors' interpretive guidelines reduce the use of potentially inappropriate medications in nursing homes? *Journal of the American Geriatrics Society, 55*(5), 666–673.

Lau, H. S., Florax, C., Porsius, A. J., & De Boer, A. (2000). The completeness of medication histories in hospital medical records of patients admitted to general internal medicine wards. *British Journal of Clinical Pharmacology, 49*(6), 597–603. Evidence Level IV.

Lazarou, J., Pomeranz, B. H., & Corey, P. N. (1998). Incidence of adverse drug reactions in hospitalized patients: A meta-analysis of prospective studies. *Journal of the American Medical Association, 279*(15), 1200–1205. Evidence Level I.

Leipzig, R. M., Cumming, R. G., & Tinetti, M. E. (1999). Drugs and falls in older people: A systematic review and meta-analysis: I. Psychotropic drugs. *Journal of the American Geriatrics Society, 47*(1), 30–39. Evidence Level I.

Leucuta, S. E., & Vlase, L. (2006). Pharmacokinetics and metabolic drug interactions. *Current Clinical Pharmacology, 1*(1), 5–20.

Levinson, D. R. (2010). *Adverse events in hospitals: National incidence among medicare beneficiaries*. Retrieved from http://oig.hhs.gov/oei/reports/oei-06-09-00090.pdf

Liperoti, R., Gambassi, G., Lapane, K. L., Chiang, C., Pedone, C., Mor, V., & Bernabei, R. (2005). Conventional and atypical antipsychotics and the risk of hospitalization for ventricular arrhythmias or cardiac arrest. *Archives of Internal Medicine, 165*(6), 696–701. Evidence Level III.

Mangoni, A. A., & Jackson, S. H. (2004). Age-related changes in pharmacokinetics and pharmacodynamics: Basic principles and practical applications. *British Journal of Clinical Pharmacology, 57*(1), 6–14. Evidence Level VI.

Merle, L., Laroche, M. L., Dantoine, T., & Charmes, J. P. (2005). Predicting and preventing adverse drug reactions in the very old. *Drugs & Aging, 22*(5), 375–392. Evidence Level VI.

Miller, L. G. (1998). Herbal medicinals: Selected clinical considerations focusing on known or potential drug-herb interactions. *Archives of Internal Medicine, 158*(20), 2200–2211. Evidence Level V.

Muir, A. J., Sanders, L. L., Wilkinson, W. E., & Schmader, K. (2001). Reducing medication regimen complexity: A controlled trial. *Journal of General Internal Medicine, 16*(2), 77–82. Evidence Level III.

Nathan, A., Goodyer, L., Lovejoy, A., & Rashid, A. (1999). 'Brown bag' medication reviews as a means of optimizing patients' use of medication and of identifying potential clinical problems. *Family Practice, 16*(3), 278–282. Evidence Level IV.

National Coordinating Council for Medication Errors Reporting and Prevention. (2001). *Taxonomy of medication errors*. Retrieved from http://www.nccmerp.org/pdf/taxo2001-07-31.pdf. Evidence Level IV.

Neafsey, P. J., & Shellman, J. (2001). Adverse self-medication practices of older adults with hypertension attending blood pressure clinics: Adverse self-medication practices. *The Internet Journal of Advanced Nursing Practice, 5*(1), 15. Evidence Level IV.

Neafsey, P. J., Strickler, Z., Shellman, J., & Chartier, V. (2002). An interactive technology approach to educate older adults about drug interactions arising from over-the-counter self-medication practices. *Public Health Nursing, 19*(4), 255–262. Evidence Level II.

Nickerson, A., MacKinnon, N. J., Roberts, N., & Saulnier, L. (2005). Drug-therapy problems, inconsistencies and omissions identified during a medication reconciliation and seamless care service. *Healthcare Quarterly, 8*(Spec. No.), 65–72. Evidence Level II.

Nolan, P. E., Jr., & Marcus, F. I. (2000). Cardiovascular drug use in the elderly. *The American Journal of Geriatric Cardiology, 9*(3), 127–129. Evidence Level VI.

Olson, D. R., Trichey, D., Miller, M., et al. (2010). *Emedicine.* Retrieved from http://emedicine.medscape.com/article. Evidence Level V.

Ooi, W. L., Hossain, M., & Lipsitz, L. A. (2000). The association between orthostatic hypotension and recurrent falls in nursing home residents. *The American Journal of Medicine, 108*(2), 106–111. Evidence Level II.

Osterberg, L., & Blaschke, T. (2005). Adherence to medication. *The New England Journal of Medicine, 353*(5), 487–497.

Packer, M., Poole-Wilson, P. A., Armstrong, P. W., Cleland, J. G., Horowitz, J. D., Massie, B. M., . . . Uretsky, B. F. (1999). Comparative effects of low and high doses of the angiotensin-converting enzyme inhibitor, lisinopril, on morbidity and mortality in chronic heart failure. ATLAS Study Group. *Circulation, 100*(23), 2312–2318. Evidence Level II.

Pandharipande, P., Shintani, A., Peterson, J., Pun, B. T., Wilkinson, G. R., Dittus, R. S., . . . Ely, E. W. (2006). Lorazepam is an independent risk factor for transitioning to delirium in intensive care unit patients. *Anesthesiology, 104*(1), 21–26. Evidence Level III.

Petrone, K., & Katz, P. (2005). Approaches to appropriate drug prescribing for the older adult. *Primary Care, 32*(3), 755–775. Evidence Level IV.

Pirmohamed, M., James, S., Meakin, S., Green, C., Scott, A. K., Walley, T. J., . . . Breckenridge, A. M. (2004). Adverse drug reactions as cause of admission to hospital: Prospective analysis of 18 820 patients. *British Medical Journal, 329*(7456), 15–19. Evidence Level IV.

Qato, D. M., Alexander, G. C., Conti, R. M., Johnson, M., Schumm, P., & Lindau, S. T. (2008). Use of prescription and over-the-counter medications and dietary supplements among older adults in the United States. *Journal of the American Medical Association, 300*(24), 2867–2878. Evidence level V.

Radimer, K., Bindewald, B., Hughes, J., Ervin, B., Swanson, C., & Picciano, M. F. (2004). Dietary supplement use by US adults: Data from the National Health and Nutrition Examination Survey, 1999–2000. *American Journal of Epidemiology, 160*(4), 339–349.

Rochon, P. A. (2010). *Drug prescribing for older adults.* Retrieved from http://www.utdol.com. Evidence Level V.

Rochon, P. A., & Gurwitz, J. H. (1997). Optimising drug treatment for elderly people: The prescribing cascade. *British Medical Journal, 315*(7115), 1096–1099. Evidence Level V.

Rochon, P. A., Stukel, T. A., Bronskill, S. E., Gomes, T., Sykora, K., Wodchis, W. P., . . . Anderson, G. M. (2007). Variation in nursing home antipsychotic prescribing rates. *Archives of Internal Medicine, 167*(7), 676–683. Evidence Level IV.

Rohay, J., Dunbar-Jacob, J., Sereika, S., Kwoh, K., & Burke, L. E. (1996). The impact of method of calculation of electronically monitored adherence data. *Controlled Clinical Trials, 17* (82S–83S), A76.

Rothberg, M. B., Pekow, P. S., Liu, F., Korc-Grodzicki, B., Brennan, M. J., Bellantonio, S., . . . Lindenauer, P. K. (2008). Potentially inappropriate medication use in hospitalized elders. *Journal of Hospital Medicine, 3*(2), 91–102. Evidence Level V.

Rudolph, J. L., Salow, M. J., Angelini, M. C., & McGlinchey, R. E. (2008). The anticholinergic risk scale and anticholinergic adverse effects in older persons. *Archives of Internal Medicine, 168*(5), 508–513.

Sabaté, E. (2003). *Adherence to long-term therapies: Evidence for action*. Geneva, Switzerland: World Health Organization. Retrieved from http://whqlibdoc.who.int/publications/2003/9241545992.pdf

Safran, D. G., Neuman, P., Schoen, C., Kitchman, M. S., Wilson, I. B., Cooper, B., . . . Rogers, W. H. (2005). *Prescription drug coverage and seniors: Findings from a 2003 national survey*. Retrieved from http://content.healthaffairs.org/cgi/content/abstract/hlthaff.w5.152. Evidence Level IV.

Santell, J. P. (2006). Reconciliation failures lead to medication errors. *Joint Commission Journal on Quality and Patient Safety, 32*(4), 225–229.

Schillinger, D., Piette, J., Grumbach, K., Wang, F., Wilson, C., Daher, C., . . . Bindman, A. B. (2003). Closing the loop: Physician communication with diabetic patients who have low health literacy. *Archives of Internal Medicine, 163*(1), 83–90.

Schneider, L. S., Tariot, P. N., Dagerman, K. S., Davis, S. M., Hsiao, J. K., Ismail, M. S., . . . CATIE-AD Study Group. (2006). Effectiveness of atypical antipsychotic drugs in patients with Alzheimer's disease. *The New England Journal of Medicine, 355*(15), 1525–1538.

Semla, T., & Rochon, P. A. (2004). Pharmacotherapy. In E. L. Cobbs & E. H. Duthie (Eds.), *Geriatrics review syllabus: A core curriculum in geriatric medicine* (5th ed.). Malden, MA: Blackwell Publishing. Level of Evidence VI.

Shekelle, P. G., MacLean, C. H., Morton, S. C., & Wenger, N. S. (2001). Acove quality indicators. *Annals of Internal Medicine, 135*(8 Pt. 2), 653–667.

Simon, S. R., Smith, D. H., Feldstein, A. C., Perrin, N., Yang, X., Zhou, Y., . . . Soumerai, S. B. (2006). Computerized prescribing alerts and group academic detailing to reduce the use of potentially inappropriate medications in older people. *Journal of the American Geriatrics Society, 54*(6), 963–968. Evidence Level II.

Sloane, P. D., Zimmerman, S., Brown, L. C., Ives, T. J., & Walsh, J. F. (2002). Inappropriate medication prescribing in residential care/assisted living facilities. *Journal of the American Geriatrics Society, 50*(6), 1001–1011. Evidence Level II.

Spina, E., & Scordo, M. G. (2002). Clinically significant drug interactions with antidepressants in the elderly. *Drugs & Aging, 19*(4), 299–320. Evidence Level VI.

Steinman, M. A., & Hanlon, J. T. (2010). Managing medications in clinically complex elders: "There's got to be a happy medium." *Journal of the American Medical Association, 304*(14), 1592–1601. Evidence Level I.

Sullivan, C., Gleason, K. M., Rooney, D., Groszek, J. M., & Barnard, C. (2005). Medication reconciliation in the acute care setting: Opportunity and challenge for nursing. *Journal of Nursing Care Quality, 20*(2), 95–98.

Swagerty, D., Brickley, R., American Medical Directors Association, & American Society of Consultant Pharmacists. (2005). American Medical Directors Association and American Society of Consultant Pharmacists joint position statement on the Beers List of Potentially Inappropriate Medications in Older Adults. *Journal of the American Medical Directors Association, 6*(1), 80–86. Evidence Level VI.

Tachjian, A., Maria, V., & Jahangir, A. (2010). Use of herbal products and potential interactions in patients with cardiovascular disease. *Journal of the American College of Cardiology, 55*(6), 515–525. Evidence Level V.

Tam, V. C., Knowles, S. R., Cornish, P. L., Fine, N., Marchesano, R., & Etchells, E. E. (2005). Frequency, type and clinical importance of medication history errors at admission to hospital: A systematic review. *Canadian Medical Association Journal, 173*(5), 510–515. Evidence Level I.

Tamblyn, R., Abrahamowicz, M., du Berger, R., McLeod, P., & Bartlett, G. (2005). A 5-year prospective assessment of the risk associated with individual benzodiazepines and doses in new elderly users. *Journal of the American Geriatrics Society, 53*(2), 233–241. Evidence Level II.

Tangalos, E. G., & Zarowitz, B. J. (2006). Medication management in the elderly. *Annals of Long-Term Care, 14*(8), 27–31. Evidence Level VI.

Terrell, K. M., Heard, K., & Miller, D. K. (2006). Prescribing to older ED patients. *The American Journal of Emergency Medicine, 24*(4), 468–478. Evidence Level V.

Tinetti, M. E., & Kumar, C. (2010). The patient who falls: "It's always a trade-off." *Journal of the American Medical Association, 303*(3), 258–266.

Tune, L. E. (2001). Anticholinergic effects of medication in elderly patients. *The Journal of Clinical Psychiatry, 62*(Suppl. 21), 11–14. Evidence Level V.

University of Colorado Health Sciences Center. (2005). *Medication management . . . Be safe & take. Clinician enrichment program.* Quality Insights of Pennsylvania, the Medicare Quality Improvement Organization Support Center for Home Health, under contract with the Centers for Medicare & Medicaid Services. Retrieved August 23, 2011 from http://www.homecareforyou.com/exam/papers/medmgt.pdf

Williams, M. E., Pulliam, C. C., Hunter, R., Johnson, T. M., Owens, J. E., Kincaid, J., . . . Koch, G. (2004). The short-term effect of interdisciplinary medication review on function and cost in ambulatory elderly people. *Journal of the American Geriatrics Society, 52*(1), 93–98. Evidence Level II.

Woolcott, J. C., Richardson, K. J., Wiens, M. O., Patel, B., Marin, J., Khan, K. M., & Marra, C. A. (2009). Meta-analysis of the impact of 9 medication classes on falls in elderly persons. *Archives of Internal Medicine, 169*(21), 1952–1960.

Zhan, C., Correa-de-Araujo, R., Bierman, A. S., Sangl, J., Miller, M. R., Wickizer, S. W., & Stryer, D. (2005). Suboptimal prescribing in elderly outpatients: Potentially harmful drug-drug and drug-disease combinations. *Journal of the American Geriatrics Society, 53*(2), 262–267. Evidence Level IV.

Zwicker, D., & Fletcher, K. (2009). *Evidence based nonpharmacologic interventions for agitation.* Retrieved from http://www.consultgerirn.org

Urinary Incontinence

18

Annemarie Dowling-Castronovo and Christine Bradway

EDUCATIONAL OBJECTIVES

On completion of this chapter, the reader should be able to:

1. discuss transient and established etiologies of urinary incontinence (UI)
2. describe the core components of a nursing assessment for UI in hospitalized older adults
3. discuss the importance of nurse collaboration within the interdisciplinary team in an effort to best assess and document type of UI
4. develop an individualized plan of care for an older adult with UI

OVERVIEW

Despite evidence supporting urinary incontinence (UI) management strategies (DuBeau et al., 2010; Fantl et al., 1996), nursing staff and laypersons often use containment strategies, such as adult briefs or other absorbent products, to manage UI. In addition, individuals with UI erroneously believe that containing UI is a normal consequence of aging (Bush, Castelluci, & Phillips, 2001; Dowd, 1991; Kinchen et al., 2003; Milne, 2000; Mitteness, 1987a, 1987b), feel that UI is a difficult-to-discuss personal problem (Bush et al., 2001), and prefer self-help strategies rather than seeking professional advice (Milne, 2000). Personal care strategies are often the result of information gained through lay media and personal contacts, not necessarily from health care professionals (Cochran, 2000; Jeter & Wagner, 1990; Miller, Brown, Smith, & Chiarelli, 2003; Milne, 2000). In comparison to nurses in other health care settings, nurses in hospitals view incontinent patients more negatively (Vinsnes, Harkless, Haltbakk, Bohm, & Hunskaar, 2001). Therefore, attitudes and beliefs regarding UI are important for the nurse to consider in an effort to best assess and manage UI.

For description of Evidence Levels cited in this chapter, see Chapter 1, Developing and Evaluating Clinical Practice Guidelines: A Systematic Approach, page 7.

BACKGROUND AND STATEMENT OF PROBLEM

UI affects more than 17 million adults in the United States and is most often defined as the involuntary loss of urine sufficient to be a problem (Fantl et al., 1996; National Association for Continence, 1998; Resnick & Ouslander, 1990). Prevalence and incidence rates of UI are viewed cautiously due to inconsistencies with definitions and measurements of both these epidemiological statistics. In addition, variable or poorly articulated UI definitions (Abrams et al., 2003; Palmer, 1988) as well as underreporting and underassessment of UI (Schultz, Dickey, & Skoner, 1997) in the hospital setting can render data of questionable reliability. Prevalence of UI in community-dwelling adult populations ranges from 8% to 46% (Anger, Saigal, & Litwin, 2006; Diokno, Brock, Brown, & Herzog, 1986; Du Moulin, Hamers, Ambergen, Janssen, & Halfens, 2008; Herzog & Fultz, 1990; T. M. Johnson et al., 1998; Lee, Cigolle, & Blaum, 2009). For individuals with dementia, UI prevalence rates range from 11% to 90%; higher prevalence rates reflect institutionalized cognitively impaired older adults (Brandeis, Baumann, Hossain, Morris, & Resnick, 1997; Skelly & Flint, 1995). Although the highest prevalence rate occurs in institutionalized older adults, 15%–53% of homebound older adults and 10%–42% of older adults admitted to acute care also suffer from UI (Dowd & Campbell, 1995; Fantl et al., 1996; McDowell et al., 1999; Palmer, Bone, Fahey, Mamon, & Steinwachs, 1992; Schultz et al., 1997). Twelve percent to 36% of older hospitalized adults develop acute UI (e.g., new-onset UI, meaning that these individuals were continent on hospital admission; Kresevic, 1997; Sier, Ouslander, & Orzeck, 1987); for patients undergoing hip surgery, the incidence of acute UI ranges from 19% to 32 % (Palmer, Baumgarten, Langenberg, & Carson, 2002; Palmer, Myers, & Fedenko, 1997).

In addition to being a common geriatric syndrome, UI significantly affects health-related quality of life (HRQOL; DuBeau, Simon, & Morris, 2006; Shumaker, Wyman, Uebersax, McClish, & Fantl, 1994). The consequences of UI may be characterized physically, psychosocially, and economically. For example, an episode of urge UI occurring once weekly, or more frequently, has been associated with falls or fracture (Brown, Sawaya, Thom, & Grady, 2000; Chiarelli, Mackenzie, & Osmotherly, 2009; Hasegawa, Kuzuya, & Iguchi, 2010). Other physical consequences associated with UI include skin irritations or infections, urinary tract infections (UTIs), pressure ulcers, and limitation of functional status (Fantl et al., 1996; T. M. Johnson et al., 1998). UI is associated with psychological distress (Bogner et al., 2002) including depression, poor self-rated health, and social isolation or condition-specific functional loss (Bogner et al., 2002; Fantl et al., 1996; T. M. Johnson et al., 1998), and poststroke UI is risk factor for poor outcomes (Pettersen, Saxby, & Wyller, 2007). Therefore, it is essential that nurses assess and treat UI when addressing other health problems such as depression or falls.

Although there is conflicting evidence regarding the role of UI as a predictor for nursing home placement, UI has been identified as a marker of frailty in community-dwelling older adults (Holroyd-Leduc, Mehta, & Covinsky, 2004) and a predictor of 1-year mortality among older adults hospitalized for an acute myocardial infarction (Krumholz, Chen, Chen, Wang, & Radford, 2001). The negative psychosocial impact of UI affects not only the individual but also family caregivers (CGs; Brittain & Shaw, 2007; Cassells & Watt, 2003; Gotoh et al., 2009). Economically, the total direct cost for all incontinent individuals is estimated to be more than $16 billion annually in the United States (Landefeld et al., 2008; Wilson, Brown, Shin, Luc, & Subak, 2001; Wyman, 1997).

Nurses are in a key position to identify and treat UI, a quality indicator ("Assessing Care," 2007), in hospitalized older adults. This chapter reviews the etiologies and consequences of UI, with emphasis on the most common types of UI encountered in the acute care setting. Assessment parameters and care strategies for UI are highlighted and a nursing standard of practice protocol focused on comprehensive assessment and management of UI for hospitalized older adults is included.

ASSESSMENT OF THE PROBLEM

Adverse physiological consequences of UI commonly encountered in acute care settings include an increased potential for UTIs and indwelling urinary catheter use, dermatitis, skin infections, and pressure ulcers (Sier et al., 1987). Moreover, UI that results in functional decline predisposes older individuals to complications associated with bed rest and immobility (Harper & Lyles, 1988).

Etiologies of Urinary Incontinence

Continence is a complex, multidimensional phenomenon influenced by anatomical, physiological, psychological, and cultural factors (Gray, 2000). Thus, continence requires intact lower urinary tract function, as well as cognitive and functional ability to recognize voiding signals and use a toilet or commode, the motivation to maintain continence, and an environment that facilitates the process (Jirovec, Brink, & Wells, 1988). Physiologically, continence is a result of urethral pressure being equal to or greater than bladder pressure (C. P. Hodgkinson, 1965), of which angulation of the urethra, supported by pelvic muscles, plays a role (DeLancey, 1994, 2010). Continence also requires the ability to suppress auto-contractility of the detrusor (C. P. Hodgkinson, 1965). Micturition (urination) involves voluntary as well as reflexive control of the bladder, urethra, detrusor muscle, and urethral sphincter. When the bladder volume reaches approximately 400 ml, stretch receptors in the bladder wall send a message to the brain and an impulse for voiding is sent back to the bladder. The detrusor muscle then contracts and the urethral sphincter relaxes to allow urination (Gray, Rayome, & Moore, 1995). Normally, the micturition reflex can be voluntarily inhibited (at least for a time) until an individual desires to void or finds an appropriate place for voiding. UI occurs as the result of a disruption at any point during this process. For a comprehensive review, Gray (2000) provided a detailed analysis of voiding physiology. Common age-associated changes, including a decrease in bladder capacity, benign prostatic hyperplasia (BPH) in men, and menopausal loss of estrogen in women, can affect lower urinary tract function and predispose older individuals to UI (Bradway & Yetman, 2002). Despite these aging changes, UI is not considered a normal consequence of aging.

The two major types of UI are transient (or acute/reversible) and established (or chronic/persistent; Newman & Wein, 2009). Transient UI is characterized by the sudden onset of potentially reversible symptoms. Causes of transient UI include delirium, infections (e.g., untreated UTI), atrophic vaginitis, urethritis, pharmaceuticals, depression or other psychological disorders that affect motivation or function, excessive urine production, restricted mobility, and stool impaction or constipation (e.g., that creates additional pressure on the bladder and can cause urinary urgency and frequency). Hospitalized older adults are at risk of developing transient UI. Complicated by shorter hospital stays, these individuals may also be at risk of being discharged without resolution of transient UI and, thus, urine leakage persists and may become established UI. However, transient UI is often preventable, or at least reversible (e.g., transient UI precipitated by a UTI that resolves with successful treatment, or acute UI related to diuretic therapy for heart failure exacerbation), if the underlying cause for the UI is identified and treated (Ding & Jayaratnam, 1994; Fantl et al., 1996; Palmer, 1996).

Kresevic (1997) reported that hospitalized older adults with new-onset UI were more likely to be on bed rest, restrained, depressed, dehydrated, malnourished, and dependent in ambulation when compared with their continent counterparts. Furthermore, the relative risk of developing new-onset UI was twofold for older adults with depression (*OR* = 2.28), malnutrition (*OR* = 2.29), and dependent ambulation (*OR* = 2.55). Study participants identified that being able to walk, having use of a bedpan or commode, and nursing assistance fostered continence (Kresevic, 1997). Likewise, Palmer et al. (2002) determined that in addition to mobility dependency, other risk factors for new-onset UI, specific to a hip fracture population included: institutionalization prior to hospital, the presence of confusion (identified by a retrospective chart review) preceding hip fracture, and being an African American woman.

Established UI has either a sudden or gradual onset and is often present prior to hospital admission; however, health care providers or family CGs may first identify UI during the course of an acute illness, hospitalization, or abrupt change in environment or daily routine (Palmer, 1996). Types of established UI include stress, urge, mixed, overflow, and functional UI.

Stress UI is defined as an involuntary loss of urine associated with activities that increase intra-abdominal pressure. Symptomatically, individuals with stress UI usually present with complaints of small amounts of daytime urine loss that occurs during physical effort or exertion (e.g., position change, coughing, sneezing) that result in increased intra-abdominal pressure. Stress UI is more common in women; however, stress UI may also occur in men postprostatectomy (Abrams et al., 2003; Fantl et al., 1996; Hunter, Moore, Cody, & Glazener, 2004; Jayasekara, 2009).

Urge UI is characterized by an involuntary urine loss associated with a strong desire to void (urgency). Individuals with urge UI often complain of being unable to hold the urge to urinate and leak on the way to the bathroom. This history is most helpful to the identification of urge UI (Holroyd-Leduc, Tannenbaum, Thorpe, & Straus, 2008). In addition to urinary urgency, signs and symptoms of urge UI most often include urinary frequency, nocturia and enuresis, and UI of moderate to large amounts. Bladder changes common in aging make older adults particularly prone to this type of UI (Abrams et al., 2003; Fantl et al., 1996; Jayasekara, 2009). Individuals with overactive bladder (OAB) may complain of urgency, with or without UI, as well as urinary frequency and nocturia. Assessment should focus on pathological or metabolic conditions that may explain these symptoms (Abrams et al., 2003).

Mixed UI is defined as involuntary urine loss as a result of both increased intra-abdominal pressure and detrusor instability (Fantl et al., 1996; Jayasekara, 2009). On history, individuals describe symptoms of stress UI in combination with symptoms of urge UI and OAB.

Overflow UI is an involuntary loss of urine associated with overdistention of the bladder, and may be caused by an underactive detrusor muscle or outlet obstruction leading to overdistention of the bladder and leakage of urine. Individuals with overflow UI often describe dribbling, urinary retention or hesitancy, urine loss without a recognizable urge, an uncomfortable sensation of fullness or pressure in the lower abdomen, and incomplete bladder emptying. Clinically, suprapubic palpation may reveal a distended or painful bladder as a result of urine retention, which may be acute or chronic. A common condition associated with this type of UI is BPH. Neurological conditions such as multiple sclerosis and spinal cord injuries or diabetes mellitus, which result in bladder muscle denervation, may also cause overflow UI (Abrams et al., 2003; Doughty, 2000; Fantl et al., 1996; Jayasekara, 2009).

Functional UI is caused by nongenitourinary factors such as cognitive or physical impairments that result in an inability for the individual to be independent in voiding. For example, acutely ill hospitalized individuals may be challenged by a combination of an acute illness and environmental changes. This, in turn, makes the voiding process even more complex, resulting in a functional type of UI (Fantl et al., 1996; B. Hodgkinson, Synnott, Josephs, Leira, & Hegney, 2008).

ASSESSMENT PARAMETERS

Nurse continence experts suggest that entry-level nurses demonstrate the ability to collect and organize data surrounding urine control, and implement nursing interventions that promote continence (Jirovec, Wyman, & Wells, 1998). Nurses play a critical role in the basic assessment and management of UI in hospitalized older adults. Because UI is an interdisciplinary issue, collaboration with other members of the health care team is essential. It is not sufficient for nurses to only identify and document the presence of UI. Instead, the type of UI should be determined and documented based on a careful history and focused assessment; urodynamic tests are not required as part of the initial assessment of UI (DuBeau et al., 2010). Basic history and examination techniques are presented here to assist the nurse in identifying the type of UI along with a nursing standard of practice protocol (see Protocol 18.1) to guide UI assessment and management.

History

When a patient is admitted to the hospital, nursing history should include questions to determine if the individual has preexisting UI or risk factors (see Table 18.1) for UI. The nurse should be alert for the following UI-associated risk factors specific to the hospital setting: depression, malnourishment, dependent ambulation, being a resident of a long-term care institution, confusion, and being an African American woman (Kresevic, 1997; Palmer et al., 2002). Therefore, the nurse should screen for depression, determine body mass index (BMI), monitor albumin and total protein levels if available, consult with a dietitian, and perform a validated assessment of both cognitive and functional status.

The nurse should include screening questions such as "Have you ever leaked urine? If yes, how much does it bother you?" for all older adult patients. Although not validated in the hospital setting, examples of screening instruments used in other settings include the Urinary Distress Inventory-6 (UDI-6) and the Male Urinary Distress Inventory (MUDI). The UDI-6 is a self-report symptom inventory for UI that is reliable and valid for identifying the type of established UI in community-dwelling females (Lemack & Zimmern, 1999; Uebersax, Wyman, Shumaker, McClish, & Fantl, 1995). The MUDI is a valid and reliable measure of urinary symptoms in the male population (Robinson & Shea, 2002). Determining the degree of "bother" and the effect on HRQOL is important and should include the perspective of both the patient and CG or significant other. Various instruments for quantifying bother and HRQOL exist (Abrams et al., 2003; Bradway, 2003; Robinson & Shea, 2002; Shumaker et al., 1994).

Historical questions should focus on the characteristics of UI: time of onset, frequency, and severity of the problem. Questions also should review past health history and address possible precipitants of UI such as coughing, uncontrollable urinary urgency, functional decline, and acute illness (e.g., UTI, hip fracture). Nurses should inquire about lower urinary tract symptoms such as nocturia, hematuria, and urinary

TABLE 18.1

Risk Factors Associated With Urinary Incontinence

- Age (B. Hodgkinson et al., 2008; Holroyd-Leduc et al., 2004; Shamliyan et al., 2007)

- Caffeine intake (Holroyd-Leduc et al., 2004)

- Immobility/functional limitations (Fantl et al., 1996; Holroyd-Leduc & Straus, 2004; Kresevic, 1997; Offermans et al., 2009; Palmer et al., 2002; Shamliyan et al., 2007)

- Impaired cognition (Fantl et al., 1996; Palmer et al., 2002; Shamliyan et al., 2007)

- Medications (Fantl et al., 1996; Newman & Wein, 2009; Offermans et al., 2009)

- Obesity (Fantl et al., 1996; Subak et al., 2005; Subak et al., 2009)

- Diuretics (Fantl et al., 1996)

- Smoking (Fantl et al., 1996)

- Fecal impaction; fecal incontinence(Fantl et al., 1996; Offermans et al., 2009)

- Malnutrition (Kresevic, 2007)

- Depression (Kresevic, 2007)

- Delirium (Fantl et al., 1996; Offermans et al., 2009)

- Pregnancy/vaginal delivery/episiotomy (DeLancey, 2010; Fantl et al., 1996; Holroyd-Leduc & Straus, 2004; Nygaard, 2006; Shamliyan et al., 2007)

- Treatment of prostate cancer including radical prostatectomy and radiation therapy (Hunter et al., 2004; Shamliyan et al., 2007)

- Hearing and/or visual impairment (Holroyd-Leduc & Straus, 2004)

- Low fluid intake (Fantl et al., 1996)

- Environmental barriers (Fantl et al., 1996; Offermans et al., 2009)

- High-impact physical activities (Fantl et al., 1996)

- Diabetes mellitus (Fantl et al., 1996; Holroyd-Leduc & Straus., 2004; Shamliyan et al., 2007)

- Parkinson's disease (Holroyd-Leduc & Straus, 2004)

- Stroke (Fantl et al., 1996; Holroyd-Leduc & Straus, 2004; Meijer et al., 2003; Shamliyan et al., 2007; Thomas et al., 2005)

- Chronic obstructive pulmonary disease (Dowling-Castronovo, 2004; Holroyd-Leduc & Straus, 2004)

- Estrogen depletion (Fantl et al., 1996; Holroyd-Leduc & Straus, 2004)

- Pelvic organ prolapse (Shamliyan et al., 2007)

- Pelvic muscle weakness (DeLancey, 1994; Fantl et al., 1996; Holroyd-Leduc & Straus, 2004; Kegel, 1956)

- Childhood nocturnal enuresis (Fantl et al., 1996)

- Race (Fantl et al., 1996; Holroyd-Leduc et al., 2004; Palmer et al., 2002)

- Institutionalization prior to hospitalization (Palmer et al., 2002)

- Arthritis and/or back problems (Holroyd-Leduc & Straus, 2004)

hesitancy, as well as current management strategies for UI. The presence and rationale for an indwelling urinary catheter should be documented (see Chapter 19, Catheter-Associated Urinary Tract Infection Prevention).

A bladder diary or voiding record is recommended as a tool for obtaining objective information about the patient's voiding pattern, incontinent episodes, and UI severity (Lau, 2009). There are numerous voiding records available; for example, visit http://consultgerirn.org/resources. Although the 7-day voiding record is the most evaluated and recommended tool used to quantify UI and identify activities associated with unwanted urine loss (Jeyaseelan, Roe, & Oldham, 2000), a 3-day voiding record has been recommended as more feasible in outpatient and long-term care settings (DuBeau et al., 2010; Fantl et al., 1996). A voiding record completed for even 1 day may help identify patients with bladder dysfunction or those requiring further referral. Advanced practice nurses or urologic/continence specialists can assist nursing staff with interpretation and offer suggestions regarding nursing interventions based on information from the voiding record.

Comprehensive Assessment

A wide variety of medications can adversely affect continence. Diuretics are the most commonly known class of medications that contribute to UI due to polyuria, frequency, and urgency. Medications with anticholinergic and antispasmodic properties may cause mental status changes, urinary retention with or without overflow incontinence, and stool impaction. Various psychotropic medications (e.g., tricyclic antidepressants, antipsychotics, sedative-hypnotics) have anticholinergic effects, contribute to immobility, and cause sedation and possibly delirium—each of which negatively affects bladder control. Alpha-adrenergic blockers may cause urethral relaxation, whereas alpha-adrenergic agonists may cause urinary retention. Calcium channel blockers also may cause urinary retention (Newman & Wein, 2009).

Nurses should document all over-the-counter, herbal, and prescription medications on admission. Additionally, nurses must closely scrutinize new medications as possible causes if UI suddenly develops during the patient's hospital stay. Medications that may contribute to iatrogenic (i.e., hospital-caused) UI include diuretics and sedative-hypnotics. Essentially, when a hospitalized patient develops transient UI, the nurse must ask the question: Could a new medication be affecting this patient's bladder control? If the answer is yes, then the nurse reviews this finding with the prescribing practitioner to learn if the contributing medication may be discontinued or modified.

Important components of a comprehensive examination include abdominal, genital, rectal, and skin examinations. In particular, the abdominal examination should assess for suprapubic distention indicative of urinary retention. Inspection of male and female genitalia can be completed during bathing or as part of the skin assessment. The nurse should observe the patient for signs of perineal irritation, lesions, or discharge. In women, a Valsalva maneuver (if not medically contraindicated) or voluntary cough may identify pelvic prolapse (e.g., cystocele, rectocele, uterine prolapse) or stress UI as a result of increased intra-abdominal pressure with bearing down (Burns, 2000). Postmenopausal women are especially prone to atrophic vaginitis. Significant findings for atrophic vaginitis include perineal inflammation, tenderness (and, on occasion, trauma as a result of touch), and thin, pale genital tissues. During the genital examination, patients should be instructed to cough or perform the Valsalva maneuver (sometimes referred to as a bladder stress test) to determine if there is urine leakage, again caused by increased intra-abdominal pressure, which may be attributed to stress UI (Holroyd-Leduc et al., 2008).

Digital rectal and skin examinations are essential in identifying transient causes of UI such as constipation, fecal impaction, and the presence of fungal rashes. The "anal wink" (contraction of the external anal sphincter) indicates intact sacral nerve innervation and is assessed by lightly stroking the circumanal skin. Absence of the anal wink may suggest sphincter denervation (Burns, 2000) and risk of stress UI. In men, the prostate gland should be palpated during the rectal examination because BPH may contribute to urge or overflow UI. A normal prostate gland is symmetrically heart-shaped,

TABLE 18.2
Postvoid Residual (PVR; Shinopulos, 2000)
Instruct the patient to void. Postvoid (ideally within 15 minutes or less); measure the residual urine remaining in the bladder by either: ▪ Bladder sonography (Scan): Noninvasive ultrasound of the suprapubic area identifies the residual amount of urine, or   ▪ Sterile catheterization A PVR of greater than 100 cc is considered abnormal and requires further evaluation by a urology specialist.

about the size of a large chestnut, and often described as "rubbery" or similar to the tip of the nose. When enlarged, as with BPH, the examiner may palpate symmetrical enlargement. Pain on palpation or asymmetrical borders may be indicative of prostatitis or prostate cancer, respectively (Gray & Haas, 2000).

In some cases, diagnostic testing may provide additional information. The most common diagnostic tests include urinalysis, urine culture and sensitivity, and postvoid residual (PVR) urine (Dubeau et al., 2010). Urinalysis and urine cultures are used to identify the presence of a UTI and bacterial agent responsible, which may contribute to acute UI. A measurement of PVR may reveal incomplete bladder emptying. Two methods for accurately evaluating PVR are bladder sonography and sterile catheter insertion after the patient has voided (see Table 18.2).

An additional diagnostic test such as a simple bedside urodynamic test, which provides information regarding detrusor activity, may be warranted in some cases (Burns, 2000; Newman & Wein, 2009). A simple bedside urodynamic test is most likely to be performed by an advanced practice nurse or physician. It is done after a PVR has been performed and measured via the sterile catheterization method. After the bladder is emptied, the catheter is maintained in the bladder, and a 50-ml syringe (without plunger) is connected to the catheter, with the center of the syringe in alignment with the symphysis pubis. Sterile water is then instilled to fill the bladder. The fluid level is monitored for evidence of bladder contractions, which are reflected in movement of the fluid level.

Functional, environmental, and mental status assessments are essential components of the UI evaluation in older adults. The nurse should observe the patient voiding, assess mobility, note any use of assistive devices, and identify any obstacles that interfere with appropriate use of toilets or toilet substitutes such as bedside commode.

INTERVENTIONS AND CARE STRATEGIES

Evidence demonstrates hospital nurses lack the knowledge necessary for evidence-based incontinence care (Coffey, McCarthy, McCormack, Wright, & Slater, 2007; Connor & Kooker, 1996; Cooper & Watt, 2003); therefore, adapting this for the acute care environment includes staff education. A brief, unit-based in-service followed by patient rounds may be instrumental in identifying patients at risk for UI and those actually experiencing UI. The North American Nursing Diagnosis Association (NANDA), Nursing Interventions Classification (NIC), and Nursing Outcomes Classification (NOC) provide structure for planning and evaluating UI assessment and management (M. Johnson, Bulechek, McCloskey-Dochterman, Maas, & Moorhead, 2001).

However, there is no structured guidance for the assessment and management of transient UI. Nurses are likely to be the first to identify, and perhaps prevent, transient UI. Research is needed to understand the role nurses play in preventing UI (Sampselle, Palmer, Boyington, O'Dell, & Wooldridge, 2004).

Treating Transient and Functional Causes of Urinary Incontinence

First, transient causes of UI should be investigated, identified, and treated. Individuals with a history of established UI should have usual voiding routines and continence strategies immediately incorporated into the acute care plan, whenever possible. Nurses play an essential role in the initiation of discharge planning and patient or CG teaching regarding all aspects of UI. Teaching and discharge planning should begin at admission as appropriate, reviewed continually, and revised as necessary.

The environment is vital in managing UI, particularly functional UI. Incontinent older adults are often dependent on adaptive devices (e.g., walker) or CGs for assistance with voiding, making them "dependently continent." Call bells should be identified and within easy reach. If limited mobility is anticipated, nursing staff should consider using an elevated toilet or commode seat, male or female urinal, or bedpan. Nurses should obtain referrals to physical and occupational therapy for ambulation aids, gait training, further assessment of activities of daily living associated with continence, and improved muscle strength. Physical and chemical restraints should be avoided including side rails (see Case Study). Patients should be encouraged and assisted to void before leaving the unit for tests (Fantl et al., 1996; Jirovec, 2000; Jirovec et al., 1988; Palmer, 1996).

Toileting programs (e.g., individualized, scheduled toileting programs including timed voiding; prompted voiding) have varied success rates (Colling, Ouslander, Hadley, Eisch, & Campbell, 1992; Eustice, Roe, & Paterson, 2000; Ostaszkiewicz, Johnston, & Roe, 2004; Rathnayake, 2009c). Timed voiding has been promoted as a strategy for managing UI in individuals who are not cognitively or physically able to participate in independent toileting (Rathnayake, 2009c). A voiding record is essential for developing an individualized scheduled toileting or timed voiding program, which mimics the patient's normal voiding patterns and requires continual assessment and reevaluation for successful outcomes. For example, if the initial scheduled toileting time is set for 8:00 a.m., yet at 6:30 a.m., the patient consistently attempts to independently void or is noted to be incontinent, then the toileting time should be adjusted to 6:00 a.m. Evidence is lacking regarding the effectiveness of timed voiding as a primary management strategy for UI; however, it may be used based on the nurse's judgment of the clinical situation (Rathnayake, 2009c).

Prompted voiding requires the CG to ask if the patient needs to void, offer assistance, and then offer praise for successful voiding (Eustice et al., 2000; Jirovec, 2000; Ostaszkiewicz et al., 2004). In nursing home residents with UI, prompted voiding may achieve short-term improvement in daytime UI and may be effective in reducing UI in cognitively intact older adults (B. Hodgkinson et al., 2008; Rathnayake, 2009b). Prompted voiding has not been studied in hospitalized patients.

Healthy Bladder Behavior Skills

Traditionally, nursing interventions for UI focus on containment strategies by means of receptacles (e.g., bedpan, urinal, commode, urinary catheters) or by various absorbent products (e.g., sanitary napkin, adult brief, incontinent pad; Harmer & Henderson, 1955; Henderson & Nite, 1978; Palese et al., 2007). Various treatments beyond containment strategies include dietary management, pelvic floor muscle exercises (PFMEs; Kegel, 1956), urge inhibition and bladder training (retraining) strategies, toileting programs (e.g., individualized, scheduled toileting programs/timed voiding; prompted voiding), pharmacological therapy, and surgical options (Fantl et al., 1996; B. Hodgkinson et al., 2008). These treatments (excluding pharmacological and surgical options) are viewed as healthy bladder behavior skills (HBBS). Although the recommendation is to offer HBBS to all older adults with UI (Fantl et al., 1996; Teunissen, de Jonge, van Weel, & Lagro-Janseen, 2004), it is unclear how to best incorporate HBBS in the care of hospitalized older adults. Despite the fact that contemporary nursing practice textbooks list and describe HBBS as nursing interventions (Kozier, Erb, Berman, & Snyder, 2004; Newman & Wein, 2009; Taylor, Lillis, & LeMone, 2005), many of these interventions have not been adequately examined in the acute care setting, and nurses do not routinely implement these interventions in the acute care setting (Bayliss, Salter, & Locke, 2003; Schnelle et al., 2003; Watson, Brink, Zimmer, & Mayer, 2003). Underreporting and underassessment are barriers to optimally addressing UI in the hospital setting as reflected in the study by Schultz et al. (1997), which reported that only 0.1% of medical records captured the problem of UI present at the time of hospital admission. Accurate assessment and identification of type of UI is needed before care strategies are initiated.

Prior to instituting HBBS, the nurse needs to assess the motivation of the patient, informal CG, and nursing staff because behavior modification is a premise of HBBS (Palmer, 2004). Examples of dietary management strategies include avoiding certain foods and beverages known to be bladder irritants such as caffeine, acidic foods or fluids, and NutraSweet (Gray & Haas, 2000). Some individuals with a BMI greater than 27 may benefit from a weight-loss program. For example, in one study, a weight loss of 5%–10% significantly decreased UI episodes for some obese women (Subak et al., 2005).

If not contraindicated, the nurse recommends adequate fluid intake, specifically water, and an increased intake of dietary fiber to maintain bowel regularity. It is important to work closely with older adults who fear that unwanted urine loss is a result of increased fluid intake. Education should focus on the adverse consequence of inadequate fluid intake such as volume depletion or potential for dehydration, and that too little fluid intake may result in concentrated urine, which, in turn, may cause increased bladder contractions and increased feelings of urinary urgency. Lastly, to manage and limit nocturia, patients may be advised to limit fluid intake a few hours before bedtime (Doughty, 2000; Fantl et al., 1996); however, this is questionable for older adults who do not have easy access to fluids or have diminished thirst sensation (DuBeau et al., 2010). In the hospital setting, the nurse must note the schedule of diuretics. For example, many institutions schedule every 12-hour diuretic dose times at 10 a.m. and 10 p.m. For some patients, it will be extremely important that nurses navigate organizational processes to reschedule diuretic doses to an alternate time such as 6 a.m. and 4 p.m. or 6 p.m. This simple strategy may decrease nocturia, which, in turn, will likely decrease the risk of falls. Research that examines which UI interventions best modify fall risk is needed (Wolf, Riolo, & Ouslander, 2000).

For community-dwelling, cognitively intact older adults, PFME is at least as effective as pharmacological therapies in treating stress and urge UI (B. Hodgkinson et al., 2008). PFME holds promise for the primary prevention of UI but requires additional research (Hay-Smith, Herbison, & Morkved, 2002), particularly in the acute care setting. PFMEs were developed to augment the strength, endurance, and coordination of the pelvic muscles, which play a role in maintaining continence.

Integrating PFMEs into the plan of care requires an assessment of the patient's baseline understanding of PFMEs to identify knowledge deficits. Ideally, PFMEs are taught during a vaginal or rectal examination when the clinician manually assists the patient to identify the pelvic muscles by instructing the patient to squeeze around the gloved examination finger. This method allows for performance appraisal (Hay-Smith et al., 2002); and together with weekly phone consults and monthly performance appraisal, this method is known to improve UI outcomes for community-dwelling individuals (Tsai & Liu, 2009). Alternately, PFMEs may be verbally taught by instructing the patient to gently squeeze or contract the rectal or vaginal muscles. Either teaching method includes instructions to not squeeze the stomach, buttocks, or thigh muscles (because this only increases intra-abdominal pressure) but to isolate the contraction of the pelvic muscles.

Preferably, each exercise should consist of contracting for 10 seconds and relaxing for 10 seconds. Some patients may need to start with 3 or 5 seconds, and then increase as their muscle becomes stronger. There is no set "exercise dose" (Du Moulin, Hamers, Paulus, Berendsen, & Halfens, 2005); however, it is usual practice to recommend 15 PFMEs three times per day. For community-dwelling women with stress, urge, or mixed UI, PFMEs (at least 24 per day for at least 6 weeks) should be included in first-line conservative management programs (Choi, Palmer, & Park, 2007; Syah, 2010). Patients may notice improvement in 2–4 weeks but not immediately. Nurses should reinforce compliance and other HBBS and initiate a referral for discharge follow-up with a continence specialist for PFME reinforcement via biofeedback, if available (Bradway & Hernly, 1998). In a study of community-dwelling adults, PFME instruction and reinforcement using biofeedback improved both UI outcomes and concurrent depressive symptoms (Tadic et al., 2007); therefore, hospitalized patients may benefit from a referral to a continence nurse or other provider specializing in care of individuals with UI (e.g., urologist, gynecologist, urogynecologist) for follow-up after discharge.

Urge inhibition is based on behavioral theory and is another recommended HBBS for treatment of urge UI (Teunissen et al., 2004), although the mechanism of how urge inhibition works is not well understood (Gray, 2005; Smith, 2000). Urge inhibition includes distraction techniques (e.g., reciting a favorite poem or song), relaxation techniques, and rapid pelvic floor muscle contractions with the goal being to suppress the urge to void until desirable (Smith, 2000).

Bladder training (retraining) is another behavioral technique used to treat urge UI (DuBeau et al., 2010; Teunissen et al., 2004) and OAB, is often used in conjunction with urge-inhibition techniques and Functional Incontinence Training (FIT; DuBeau et al., 2010; Schnelle et al., 2003), and may be more effective if used in combination with PFMEs or anticholinergic drugs (Rathnayake, 2009a). Bladder training requires a baseline voiding record to determine the timing of voids and UI episodes. If urinary frequency is present, the patient is instructed to lengthen the time between voids in an effort to retrain the bladder. When a strong urge to void occurs, the patient is instructed to use urge-inhibition techniques to suppress urinary urgency. For example, if the patient is not in a position to empty the bladder in a socially appropriate manner, the nurse instructs the patient to quickly squeeze and relax pelvic floor muscles several times to suppress the urge to void. This technique is sometimes referred to as "quick flicks" (Gray, 2005). Relaxation and distraction and urge inhibition techniques are also beneficial during bladder training.

In some instances (e.g., for patients experiencing incomplete bladder emptying or overflow UI), patients and staff can use Crede's maneuvers (i.e., deep suprapubic palpation) to facilitate bladder emptying. The Crede's maneuver is used with caution and requires manual compression over the suprapubic area during bladder emptying. The Crede's maneuver should be avoided if vesicoureteral reflux (i.e., abnormal flow of urine from the bladder back up the ureters) or overactive sphincter mechanisms are suspected because it may dangerously elevate pressure within the bladder (Doughty, 2000). In some cases, instructing patients to double void (i.e., after an initial void, instruct patients to stand or reposition for a second void) also facilitates bladder emptying.

Additional Nursing Interventions

A causal link between UI and skin breakdown has not been adequately supported; however, maintaining skin integrity is a goal of nursing care. Decomposition of urinary urea by microorganisms releases ammonia and forms ammonium hydroxide, an alkali. This alkali makes the protective "acid mantle" of the skin vulnerable and jeopardizes skin integrity. If UI episodes persist despite management strategies, perineal skin care interventions should focus on maintaining the integrity of the protective acid mantle of the skin (Ersser, Getliffe, Voegeli, & Regan, 2005; see Chapter 16, Preventing Pressure Ulcers and Skin Tears).

Although absorbent products are commonly used for UI containment, there is little evidence available to guide product selection and no evidence of how absorbent products may interact with the acid mantle (Fader, Cottenden, & Getliffe, 2008). Community-dwelling women with light UI reported important characteristics of absorbent pads including the ability to hold and hide UI and ease of use (Getliffe, Fader, Cottenden, Jamieson, & Green, 2007). In hospitals, nursing staff reported problems with quality and availability of absorbent products (Clayman, Thompson, & Forth, 2005). Pertaining to reusable versus disposable absorbent products, there is no demonstrable risk of cross-infection with reusable absorbent products when appropriate laundering protocols are followed, and there are no clear cost savings with using one over the other. Reusable products have limited acceptability among users (Fader et al., 2008), and use of adult briefs is significantly associated with an increased risk of infection (Zimakoff, Stickler, Pontoppidan, & Larsen, 1996). Although bed pads contain urine, consumer satisfaction is questionable, and there are no studies on the use of chair pads. Although limited evidence exists, suggesting that disposable insert pads may be more effective for women with UI than other absorbent products (Rathnayake, 2009d), there is no clear evidence to suggest one absorbent product being superior to another, particularly in the acute care setting. Evidence does support pilot testing of absorbent products according to individual circumstances, including patient, family, and institutional preferences, and offering a choice of products to women with UI (Dunn, Kowanko, Paterson, & Pretty, 2002; Fader et al., 2008; Rathnayake, 2009d).

A student nurse received report on Mr. G, an 86-year-old man with history of Alzheimer's dementia who is hospitalized for delirium. The nurse was told that Mr. G. was "pleasantly confused," required full assistance with personal care, and spent most of the day in a Geri-chair. The student nurse performed an assessment that revealed the following:

Patient sleeping in bed with all side rails up, call bell within reach, no urinal in sight.

PMH-CAD, Mild HTN, Mild osteoarthritis

PSH: None

Medications: diphenhydramine (Benadryl) 25 mg PRN for sleep, enalapril (Vasotec) 5 mg PO OD for HTN, MVI 1 tab PO OD, donepezil (Aricept) 10 mg PO OD for Alzheimer's dementia

VS: 114/60, 72, 14, 98.0F

Alert and oriented to self; sleepy; no focal deficits

Heart Rate: Regular

Breath sounds clear, slightly decreased at the bases

Abdomen: +BS in all quadrants, soft, nontender, no suprapubic tenderness; left quadrant slightly dull to percussion; no palpable masses

Dry adult brief in place

The student nurse learns from the patient's wife (i.e., the primary CG at home) that the patient has experienced occasional urinary leaking in the past but not to the extent of needing "diapers." He has a history of chronic constipation. With the nursing instructor's guidance, the student nurse assisted Mr. G. to a dangling position at the side of the bed. After assessing and evaluating that the patient's muscular strength was strong, ambulation was attempted. The patient ambulated to the bathroom, the adult brief was removed, and Mr. G. was prompted to void. He successfully voided and had a bowel movement. He proceeded to wash his hands and returned to the bedside chair (not the Geri-chair) and enjoyed breakfast. The adult brief was left off during the time the student nurse was there to assist him. During this time, Mr. G. made one attempt to initiate voiding and was successfully assisted by the student nurse.

The importance of ongoing nursing assessment was stressed as being vital to quality of care. Had the student nurse just transferred the patient to the Geri-chair, he may not have effectively emptied his bowel and bladder. Mr. G.'s constipation was addressed by providing appropriate fluid and fiber intake and by continuing with an individualized toilet schedule as tolerated. The avoidance of diphenhydramine for the older adults was also discussed because it is known to cause anticholinergic effects including urinary retention. Diphenhydramine raises concerns about sedation as well, which may alter Mr. G.'s response to the need to void.

Evidence suggests that prompted voiding and individualized toileting schedules reduce the number of UI episodes (Eustice et al., 2000; Fink, Taylor, Tacklind, Rutks, & Wilt, 2008; Ostaszkiewicz et al., 2004). In addition, prompted voiding in cognitively impaired long-term care residents has demonstrated an increase in self-initiative toileting activities (Holroyd-Leduc & Straus, 2004). These strategies have not been studied in the hospital setting; however, this case study demonstrates that nursing interventions used in other settings may also be beneficial for acutely hospitalized older adults.

SUMMARY

Although acute care stays are generally short, UI is a significant health problem that should not be overlooked. Behavioral and supportive therapies and patient education should be initiated by nurses if the patient is cognitively, physically, and emotionally able to participate. Evidence from long-term care and community settings suggests that nurse continence experts play an essential role in improving the quality of continence care (Du Moulin et al., 2005; McDowell et al., 1999; Watson, 2004). Therefore, if patients remain incontinent at discharge, hospital nurses have the responsibility to design a plan that includes referral to a continence nurse specialist or other continence expert for follow-up.

Other than identifying UI as a risk for falls, there are no requirements specific to UI from The Joint Commission (http://www.jointcommission.org/). Nevertheless, it is recommended that a continuous quality improvement (CQI) criterion should encompass critical elements in an effective and successful urinary continence program. For example, quality indicators for UI in the vulnerable older adult population that may be used in the hospital setting include documentation of (a) the presence of UI, (b) the bothersome nature for the older adult and significant other, (c) focused history and physical examination, (d) documentation of urinalysis and/or culture, (e) PVR and, if elevated to more than 300 cc, referral for evaluation of renal function; (f) type of UI; (g) discussion of HBBS; (h) interdisciplinary evaluation for urodynamic evaluation and pharmacological/surgical treatments; and (i) response to treatment ("Assessing Care," 2007; Fung, Spencer, Eslami, & Crandall, 2007).

Nurses have a significant role in improving the assessment and treatment of UI in hospitalized older adults. It is recommended that nurses are particularly vigilant for patients who are "admitted dry and become wet" during a hospitalization. These patients will particularly benefit from evidence-based assessment and management. Moreover, nurses can help to promote changes in attitudes toward UI and provide education on individual, facility-wide, community, and national levels.

NURSING STANDARD OF PRACTICE

Protocol 18.1: Urinary Incontinence in Older Adults Admitted to Acute Care

I. GOAL

A. Nursing staff will utilize comprehensive assessments and implement evidence-based management strategies for patients identified with urinary incontinence (UI).

B. Nursing staff will collaborate with interdisciplinary team members to identify and document type of UI.

C. Patients with UI will not have UI-associated complications.

II. OVERVIEW

UI affects approximately 17 million Americans (Fantl et al., 1996; Landefeld et al., 2008; National Association for Continence, 1998; Resnick & Ouslander,

(continued)

**Protocol 18.1: Urinary Incontinence in Older Adults
Admitted to Acute Care** *(cont.)*

1990). More than 35% of older adults admitted to the hospital develop UI (Kresevic, 1997). In addition to medications, constipation/fecal impaction, low fluid intake, environmental barriers, diabetes mellitus, and stroke (Fantl et al., 1996; Holroyd-Leduc & Straus, 2004; Meijer et al., 2003; Offermans, Du Moulin, Hamers, Dassen, & Halfens, 2009; Shamliyan, Wyman, Bliss, Kane, & Wilt, 2007; Thomas et al., 2005), immobility, impaired cognition, malnutrition, and depression are additional factors specific to identifying older adults at risk for UI in the hospital setting (Kresevic, 1997). Complications of UI include falls, skin irritation leading to pressure ulcers, social isolation, and depression (Bogner et al., 2002; Brown et al., 2000; Fantl et al., 1996; T. M. Johnson et al., 1998; Morris & Wagg, 2007). Nurses play a key role in the assessment and management of UI.

III. BACKGROUND
A. Definitions
   UI is the involuntary loss of urine sufficient to be a problem (Fantl et al., 1996). UI may be transient (acute) or established (chronic). Types of established UI include:
   1. *Stress UI* is defined as an involuntary loss of urine associated with activities that increase intra-abdominal pressure (Abrams et al., 2003; Fantl et al., 1996; Hunter et al., 2004).
   2. *Urge UI* is characterized by an involuntary urine loss associated with a strong desire to void (urgency; Abrams et al., 2003; Fantl et al., 1996). An individual with overactive bladder (OAB) may complain of urinary urgency, with or without UI (Abrams et al., 2003).
   3. *Mixed UI* is defined as a combination of stress UI and urge UI (Jayasekara, 2009).
   4. *Overflow UI* is an involuntary loss of urine associated with overdistention of the bladder, and may be caused by an underactive detrusor muscle or outlet obstruction leading to overdistention of the bladder and overflow of urine (Abrams et al., 2003; Doughty, 2000; Fantl et al., 1996; Jayasekara, 2009).
   5. *Functional UI* is caused by nongenitourinary factors, such as cognitive or physical impairments that result in an inability for the individual to be independent in voiding (Fantl et al., 1996; B. Hodgkinson et al., 2008).
B. Epidemiology
   UI affects approximately 17 million Americans (Fantl et al., 1996; Landefeld et al., 2008; National Association for Continence, 1998; Resnick & Ouslander, 1990). UI studies specific to the hospital setting demonstrate that UI is present in 10%–42% of older adults (Dowd & Campbell, 1995; Fantl et al., 1996; Kresevic, 1997; Palmer et al., 1992; Schultz et al., 1997); therefore, assessment and implementation of an evidence-based protocol is essential.

IV. Parameters of Assessment
A. Document the presence or absence of UI for all patients on admission (DuBeau et al., 2010).
B. Document the presence or absence of an indwelling urinary catheter.

(continued)

C. For patients with UI, the nurse collaborates with interdisciplinary team members to:
  1. Determine whether the UI is transient, established (stress/urge/mixed/overflow/functional), or both and document (DuBeau et al., 2010; Fantl et al., 1996; Jayasekara, 2009; M. Johnson et al., 2001).
  2. Identify and document the possible etiologies of the UI (DuBeau et al., 2010; Fantl et al., 1996).

V. Nursing Care Strategies

A. General principles that apply to prevention and management of all forms of UI:
  1. Identify and treat causes of transient UI (DuBeau et al., 2010).
  2. Identify and continue successful prehospital management strategies for established UI.
  3. Develop an individualized plan of care using data obtained from the history and physical examination, and in collaboration with other team members. Implement toileting programs as needed (Ostaszkiewicz et al., 2004; Rathnayake, 2009c).
  4. Avoid medications that may contribute to UI (Newman & Wein, 2009).
  5. Avoid indwelling urinary catheters whenever possible to avoid the risk of urinary tract infection (UTI; Bouza et al., 2001; Dowd & Campbell, 1995; Gould et al., 2009; Zimakoff et al., 1996).
  6. Monitor fluid intake and maintain an appropriate hydration schedule.
  7. Limit dietary bladder irritants (Gray & Haas, 2000).
  8. Consider adding weight loss as a long-term goal in discharge planning for those with a body mass index (BMI) greater than 27 (Subak et al., 2005).
  9. Modify the environment to facilitate continence (Fantl et al., 1996; Jirovec, 2000; Palmer, 1996).
  10. Provide patients with usual undergarments in expectation of continence, if possible.
  11. Prevent skin breakdown by providing immediate cleansing after an incontinent episode and utilizing barrier ointments (Ersser et al., 2005).
  12. Pilot test absorbent products to best meet patient, staff, and institutional preferences (Dunn et al., 2002), bearing in mind adult briefs have been associated with UTIs (Zimakoff et al., 1996).
B. Strategies for specific problems:
  1. Stress UI
     a. Teach pelvic floor muscle exercises (PFMEs; DuBeau et al., 2010; B. Hodgkinson et al., 2008).
     b. Provide toileting assistance and bladder training PRN (whenever necessary; DuBeau et al., 2010).
     c. Consider referral to other team members if pharmacological or surgical therapies are warranted.
  2. Urge UI and OAB
     a. Implement bladder training (retraining; DuBeau et al., 2010; Teunissen et al., 2004).

(continued)

**Protocol 18.1: Urinary Incontinence in Older Adults
Admitted to Acute Care** *(cont.)*

    b. If patient is cognitively intact and is motivated, provide information on urge inhibition (Gray, 2005; Smith, 2000).

    c. Teach PFMEs to be used in conjunction with bladder training, and instruct in urge inhibition strategies (Flynn, Cell, & Luisi, 1994; Rathnayake, 2009a; Teunissen et al., 2004).

    d. Collaborate with prescribing team members if pharmacological therapy is warranted.

    e. Initiate referrals for those patients who do not respond to the aforementioned strategies.

3. Overflow UI

    a. Allow sufficient time for voiding.

    b. Discuss with interdisciplinary team the need for determining a post-void residual (PVR; Newman & Wein, 2009; Shinopulos, 2000). See Table 18.2.

    c. Instruct patients in double voiding and Crede's maneuver (Doughty, 2000).

    d. If catheterization is necessary, sterile intermittent catheterization is preferred over indwelling catheterization (Saint et al, 2006; Terpenning, Allada, & Kauffman, 1989; Warren, 1997).

    e. Initiate referrals to other team members for patients requiring pharmacological or surgical intervention.

4. Functional UI

    a. Provide individualized scheduled toileting, timed voiding, or prompted voiding (Eustice et al., 2000; Jirovec, 2000; Lee et al., 2009; Ostaszkiewicz et al., 2004).

    b. Provide adequate fluid intake.

    c. Refer for physical and occupational therapy PRN.

    d. Modify environment to maximize independence with continence (Fantl et al., 1996; Jirovec, 2000; Jirovec et al., 1988; Palmer, 1996).

VI. Evaluation of Expected Outcomes

A. Patients:

Will have fewer or no episodes of UI or complications associated with UI.

B. Nurses:

1. Will document assessment of continence status at admission and throughout hospital stay. If UI is identified, document and determine type of UI.

2. Will use interdisciplinary expertise and interventions to assess and manage UI during hospitalization.

3. Will include UI in discharge planning needs and refer PRN.

C. Institution:

1. Incidence and prevalence of transient UI will decrease.

2. Hospital policies will require assessment and documentation of continence status ("Assessing Care," 2007; Fung et al., 2007).

3. Will provide access to evidence-based guidelines for evaluation and management of UI.

4. Staff will receive administrative support and ongoing education regarding assessment and management of UI.

(continued)

**Protocol 18.1: Urinary Incontinence in Older Adults
Admitted to Acute Care** *(cont.)*

VII. Follow-up Monitoring of Condition
  A. Provide patient/caregiver discharge teaching regarding outpatient referral and management.
  B. Incorporate continuous quality improvement (CQI) criteria into existing program ("Assessing Care," 2007; Fung et al., 2007).
  C. Identify areas for improvement and enlist multidisciplinary assistance in devising strategies for improvement.

VIII. Relevant Practice Guidelines
  National Guideline Clearinghouse Guideline
  Synthesis.http://www.guideline.gov/syntheses/index.aspx

RESOURCES

Wound, Ostomy Continence Nurses Society
An international society providing a source of networking and research for nurses specializing in enterostomal and continence care.
http://www.wocn.org

National Association for Continence (NAFC)
A not-for-profit organization dedicated to improving the lives of individuals with incontinence.
http://www.nafc.org/

The Hartford Institute for Geriatric Nursing
This website will bring the reader to the "Try This" series to share with hospital staff.
http://www.hartfordign.org/

Society of Urologic Nurse and Associates (SUNA)
An international organization dedicated to nursing care of individuals with urologic disorders.
http://www.suna.org/

GeroNurseOnline
Geriatric Resources and tools
http://www.geronurseonline.org
Click Resources tab in Urinary Incontinence topic.

REFERENCES

Abrams, P., Cardozo, L., Fall, M., Griffiths, D., Rosier, P., Ulmsten, U., . . . Wein, A. (2003). The standardisation of terminology in lower urinary tract function: Report from the standardisation sub-committee of the International Continence Society. *Urology, 61*(1), 37–49. Evidence Level I.

Anger, J. T., Saigal, C. S., & Litwin, M. S. (2006). The prevalence of urinary incontinence among community dwelling adult women: Results from the National Health and Nutrition Examination Survey. *The Journal of Urology, 175*(2), 601–604. Evidence Level IV.

Assessing care of vulnerable elders-3 quality indicators. *Journal of the American Geriatrics Society*, *55*(Suppl 2), S464–S487. Evidence Level V.

Bayliss, V., Salter, L., & Locke, R. (2003). Pathways for continence care: An audit to assess how they are used. *British Journal of Nursing*, *12*(14), 857–863. Evidence Level IV.

Bogner, H. R., Gallo, J. J., Sammel, M. D., Ford, D. E., Armenian, H. K., & Eaton, W. W. (2002). Urinary incontinence and psychological distress in community-dwelling older adults. *Journal of the American Geriatrics Society*, *50*(3), 489–495. Evidence Level IV.

Bouza, E., San Juan, R., Muñoz, P., Voss, A., Kluytmans, J., & Co-operative Group of the European Study Group on Nosocomial Infections. (2001). A European perspective on nosocomial urinary tract infections II. Report on incidence, clinical characteristics and outcome (ESGNI-004 study). European Study Group on Nosocomial Infection. *Clinical Microbiology and Infection*, *7*(10), 532–542. Evidence Level IV.

Bradway, C. (2003). Urinary incontinence among older women. Measurement of the effect on health-related quality of life. *Journal of Gerontological Nursing*, *29*(7), 13–19. Evidence Level VI.

Bradway, C., & Hernly, S. (1998). Urinary incontinence in older adults admitted to acute care. The NICHE Faculty. *Geriatric Nursing*, *19*(2), 98–102. Evidence Level VI.

Bradway, C. W., & Yetman, G. (2002). Genitourinary problems. In V. T. Cotter & N. E. Strumpf (Eds.), *Advanced practice nursing with older adults: Clinical guidelines* (pp. 83–102). New York, NY: McGraw-Hill. Evidence Level VI.

Brandeis, G. H., Baumann, M. M., Hossain, M., Morris, J. N., & Resnick, N. M. (1997). The prevalence of potentially remediable urinary incontinence in frail older people: A study using the Minimum Data Set. *Journal of the American Geriatrics Society*, *45*(2), 179–184. Evidence Level IV.

Brittain, K. R., & Shaw, C. (2007). The social consequences of living with and dealing with incontinence—A carers perspective. *Social Science and Medicine*, *65*(6), 1274–1283. Evidence Level IV.

Brown, J. S., Sawaya, G., Thom, D. H., & Grady, D. (2000). Hysterectomy and urinary incontinence: A systematic review. *Lancet*, *356*(9229), 535–539. Evidence Level I.

Burns, P. A. (2000). Stress urinary incontinence. In D. B. Doughty (Ed.), *Urinary & fecal incontinence nursing management* (2nd ed., pp. 63–89). St. Louis, MO: Mosby. Evidence Level VI.

Bush, T. A., Castellucci, D. T., & Phillips, C. (2001). Exploring women's beliefs regarding urinary incontinence. *Urologic Nursing*, *21*(3), 211–218. Evidence Level IV.

Cassells, C., & Watt, E. (2003). The impact of incontinence on older spousal caregivers. *Journal of Advanced Nursing*, *42*(6), 607–616. Evidence Level IV.

Chiarelli, P. E., Mackenzie, L. A., & Osmotherly, P. G. (2009). Urinary incontinence is associated with an increase in falls: A systematic review. *The Australian Journal of Physiotherapy*, *55*(2), 89–95. Evidence Level I.

Choi, H., Palmer, M. H., & Park, J. (2007). Meta-analysis of pelvic floor muscle training: Randomized controlled trials in incontinent women. *Nursing Research*, *56*(4), 226–234. Evidence Level I.

Clayman, C., Thompson, V., & Forth, H. (2005). Development of a continence assessment pathway in acute care. *Nursing Times*, *101*(18), 46–48. Evidence Level IV.

Cochran, A. (2000). Don't ask, don't tell: The incontinence conspiracy. *Managed Care Quarterly*, *8*(1), 44–52. Evidence Level VI.

Coffey, A., McCarthy, G., McCormack, B., Wright, J., & Slater, P. (2007). Incontinence: Assessment, diagnosis, and management in two rehabilitation units for older people. *Worldviews on Evidence-Based Nursing*, *4*(4), 179–186. Evidence Level IV.

Colling, J., Ouslander, J., Hadley, B. J., Eisch, J., & Campbell, E. (1992). The effects of patterned urge-response toileting (PURT) on urinary incontinence among nursing home residents. *Journal of the American Geriatrics Society*, *40*(2), 135–141. Evidence Level II.

Connor, P. A., & Kooker, B. M. (1996). Nurses' knowledge, attitudes, and practices in managing urinary incontinence in the acute care setting. *Medsurg Nursing: Official Journal of the Academy of Medical-Surgical Nurses*, *5*(2), 87–92, 117. Evidence Level IV.

Cooper, G., & Watt, E. (2003). An exploration of acute care nurses' approach to assessment and management of people with urinary incontinence. *Journal of Wound, Ostomy, and Continence Nursing, 30*(6), 305–313. Evidence Level IV.

DeLancey, J. O. (1994). Structural support of the urethra as it relates to stress urinary incontinence: The hammock hypothesis. *American Journal of Obstetrics Gynecology, 170*(6), 1713–1720. Evidence Level IV.

Delancey, J. O. (2010). Why do women have stress urinary incontinence? *Neurourology and Urodynamics, 29*(Suppl 1), S13–S17. Evidence Level VI.

Ding, Y. Y., & Jayaratnam, F. J. (1994). Urinary incontinence in the hospitalised elderly—a largely reversible disorder. *Singapore Medical Journal, 35*(2), 167–170. Evidence Level VI.

Diokno, A. C., Brock, B. M., Brown, M. B., & Herzog, A. R. (1986). Prevalence of urinary incontinence and other urological symptoms in the noninstitutionalized elderly. *The Journal of Urology, 136*(5), 1022–1025. Evidence Level IV.

Doughty, D. B. (2000). Retention with overflow. In D. B. Doughty (Ed.), *Urinary & fecal incontinence nursing management* (2nd ed., pp. 159–180). St. Louis, MO: Mosby. Evidence Level VI.

Dowd, T. T. (1991). Discovering older women's experience of urinary incontinence. *Research in Nursing and Health, 14*(3), 179–186. Evidence Level IV.

Dowd, T. T., & Campbell, J. M. (1995). Urinary incontinence in an acute care setting. *Urologic Nursing, 15*(3), 82–85. Evidence Level IV.

Dowling-Castronovo, A. (2004). Urinary incontinence: An exploration of the relationship between age, COPD, and obesity. Unpublished. Evidence Level VI.

DuBeau, C. E., Kuchel, G. A., Johnson, T., II, Palmer, M. H., Wagg, A., & Fourth International Consultation on Incontinence. (2010). Incontinence in the frail elderly: Report from the 4th International Consultation on Incontinence. *Neurourology and Urodynamics, 29*(1), 165–178. Evidence Level I.

DuBeau, C. E., Simon, S. E., & Morris, J. N. (2006). The effect of urinary incontinence on quality of life in older nursing home residents. *Journal of the American Geriatrics Society, 54*(9), 1325–1333. Evidence Level IV.

Du Moulin, M. F., Hamers, J. P., Ambergen, A. W., Janssen, M. A., & Halfens, R. J. (2008). Prevalence of urinary incontinence among community-dwelling adults receiving home care. *Research in Nursing and Health, 31*(6), 604–612. Evidence Level IV.

Du Moulin, M. F., Hamers, J. P., Paulus, A., Berendsen, C., & Halfens, R. (2005). The role of the nurse in community continence care: A systematic review. *International Journal of Nursing Studies, 42*(4), 479–492. Evidence Level I.

Dunn, S., Kowanko, I., Paterson, J., & Pretty, L. (2002). Systematic review of the effectiveness of urinary continence products. *Journal of Wound, Ostomy, and Continence Nursing, 29*(3), 129–142. Evidence Level I.

Ersser, S. J., Getliffe, K., Voegeli, D., & Regan, S. (2005). A critical review of the inter-relationship between skin vulnerability and urinary incontinence and related nursing intervention. *International Journal of Nursing Studies, 42*(7), 823–835. Evidence Level I.

Eustice, S., Roe, B., & Paterson, J. (2000). Prompted voiding for the management of urinary incontinence in adults. *Cochrane Database of Systematic Reviews*, (2), CD002113. Evidence Level I.

Fader, M., Cottenden, A. M., & Getliffe, K. (2008). Absorbent products for moderate-heavy urinary and/or faecal incontinence in women and men. *Cochrane Database of Systematic Reviews*, (4), CD007408. Evidence Level I.

Fantl, A., Newman, D. K., Colling, J., DeLancey, J. O., Keeys, C., & Loughery, R. (1996). *Urinary incontinence in adults: acute and chronic management* (Report No. Publication No. 92-0047). Rockville, MD: Agency for Health Care Policy and Research. Evidence Level I.

Fink, H. A., Taylor, B. C., Tacklind, J. W., Rutks, I. R., & Wilt, T. J. (2008). Treatment interventions in nursing home residents with urinary incontinence: A systematic review of randomized trials. *Mayo Clinic Proceedings, 83*(12), 1332–1343. Evidence Level I.

Flynn, L., Cell, P., & Luisi, E. (1994). Effectiveness of pelvic muscle exercises in reducing urge incontinence among community residing elders. *Journal of Gerontological Nursing, 20*(5), 23–27. Evidence Level IV.

Fung, C. H., Spencer, B., Eslami, M., & Crandall, C. (2007). Quality indicators for the screening and care of urinary incontinence in vulnerable elders. *Journal of the American Geriatrics Society, 55*(Suppl 2), S443–S449. Evidence Level I.

Getliffe, K., Fader, M., Cottenden, A., Jamieson, K., & Green, N. (2007). Absorbent products for incontinence: 'Treatment effects' and impact on quality of life. *Journal of Clinical Nursing, 16*(10), 1936–1945. Evidence Level IV.

Gotoh, M., Matsukawa, Y., Yoshikawa, Y., Funahashi, Y., Kato, M., & Hattori, R. (2009). Impact of urinary incontinence on the psychological burden of family caregivers. *Neurourology and Urodynamics, 28*(6), 492–496. Evidence Level IV.

Gould, C. V., Umscheid, C. A., Agarwal, R. K., Kuntz, G., Pegues, D. A., & the Healthcare Infection Control Practices Advisory Committee. (2009). *Guideline for prevention of catheter-associated urinary tract infections.* Retrieved from http://www.cdc.gov/hicpac/cauti/001_cauti.html. Evidence Level I.

Gray, M. (2005). Assessment and management of urinary incontinence. *The Nurse Practitioner, 30*(7), 32–3, 36–43. Evidence Level VI.

Gray, M., Rayome, R., & Moore, K. (1995). The urethral sphincter: An update. *Urologic Nursing, 15*(2), 40–53. Evidence Level VI.

Gray, M. I. (2000). Physiology of voiding. In D. B. Doughty (Ed.), *Urinary & fecal incontinence: Nursing management* (2nd ed., pp. 1–27). St. Louis, MO: Mosby. Evidence Level V.

Gray, M. L., & Haas, J. (2000). Assessment of the patient with urinary incontinence. In D. B. Doughty (Ed.), *Urinary & fecal incontinence: Nursing management* (2nd ed.). St. Louis, MO: Mosby. Evidence Level VI.

Harmer, B., & Henderson, V. (1955). *Textbook of the principles and practice of nursing,* (5th ed.). New York, NY: MacMillan Publishing. Evidence Level VI.

Harper, C. M., & Lyles, Y. M. (1988). Physiology and complications of bed rest. *Journal American Geriatrics Society, 36*(11), 1047–1054. Evidence Level V.

Hasegawa, J., Kuzuya, M., & Iguchi, A. (2010). Urinary incontinence and behavioral symptoms are independent risk factors for recurrent and injurious falls, respectively, among residents in long-term care facilities. *Archives of Gerontology and Geriatrics, 50*(1), 77–81. Evidence Level IV.

Hay-Smith, J., Herbison, P., & Morkved, S. (2002). Physical therapies for prevention of urinary and faecal incontinence in adults. *Cochrane Database of Systematic Reviews,* (2), CD003191. Evidence Level I.

Henderson, V., & Nite, G. (1978). *Principles and practice of nursing,* (6th ed.). New York, NY: MacMillan Publishing. Evidence Level VI.

Herzog, A. R., & Fultz, N. H. (1990). Prevalence and incidence of urinary incontinence in community-dwelling populations. *Journal of the American Geriatrics Society, 38*(3), 273–281. Evidence Level V.

Hodgkinson, B., Synnott, R., Josephs, K., Leira, E., & Hegney, D. (2008). A systematic review of the effect of educational interventions for urinary and faecal incontinence by health care staff/carers/clients in the aged care, on level knowledge, frequency of incontinence episodes and hours spent on the management of incontinence episodes. *JBI Lib Syst Rev,* Publication 318. Evidence Level I.

Hodgkinson, C. P. (1965). Stress urinary incontinence in the female. *Surgery, Gynecology and Obstetrics, 120,* 595–613. Evidence Level V.

Holroyd-Leduc, J. M., Mehta, K. M., & Covinsky, K. E. (2004). Urinary incontinence and its association with death, nursing home admission, and functional decline. *Journal of the American Geriatrics Society, 52*(5), 712–718. Evidence Level I.

Holroyd-Leduc, J. M., & Straus, S. E. (2004). Management of urinary incontinence in women: Scientific review. *The Journal of the American Medical Association, 291*(8), 986–995. Evidence Level I.

Holroyd-Leduc, J. M., Tannenbaum, C., Thorpe, K. E., & Straus, S. E. (2008). What type of urinary incontinence does this woman have? *The Journal of the American Medical Association, 299*(12), 1446–1456. Evidence Level I.

Hunter, K. F., Moore, K. N., Cody, D. J., & Glazener, C. M. (2004). Conservative management for postprostatectomy urinary incontinence. *Cochrane Database Systematic Reviews,* (2), CD001843. Evidence Level I.

Jayasekara, R. (2009). Urinary incontinence: Evaluation. *JBI Database Evid Summaries,* Publication ES0610. Evidence Level I.

Jeter, K. F., & Wagner, D. B. (1990). Incontinence in the American home. A survey of 36,500 people. *Journal of the American Geriatrics Society, 38*(3), 379–383. Evidence Level IV.

Jeyaseelan, S. M., Roe, B. H., & Oldham, J. A. (2000). The use of frequency/volume charts to assess urinary incontinence. *Physical Therapy Reviews, 5*(3), 141–146. Evidence Level I.

Jirovec, M. M. (2000). Functional incontinence. In D. B. Doughty (Ed.), *Urinary and fecal incontinence nursing management,* (2nd ed., pp. 145–157). St. Louis, MO: Mosby. Evidence Level VI.

Jirovec, M. M., Brink, C. A., & Wells, T. J. (1988). Nursing assessments in the inpatient geriatric population. *The Nursing Clinics of North America, 23*(1), 219–230. Evidence Level VI.

Jirovec, M. M., Wyman, J. F., & Wells, T. J. (1998). Addressing urinary incontinence with educational continence-care competencies. *Image—The Journal of Nursing Scholarship, 30*(4), 375–378. Evidence Level VI.

Johnson, M., Bulechek, G., McCloskey-Dochterman, J., Maas, M., & Moorhead, S. (2001). *Nursing diagnoses, outcomes, and interventions: NANDA, NOC and NIC linkages.* St. Louis, MO: Mosby. Evidence Level VI.

Johnson, T. M., II, Kincade, J. E., Bernard, S. L., Busby-Whitehead, J., Hertz-Picciotto, I., & DeFriese, G. H. (1998). The association of urinary incontinence with poor self-rated health. *Journal of the American Geriatrics Society, 46*(6), 693–699. Evidence Level IV.

Kegel, A. H. (1956). Stress incontinence of urine in women; physiologic treatment. *The Journal of the International College of Surgeons, 25*(4 Part 1), 487–499. Evidence Level VI.

Kinchen, K. S., Burgio, K., Diokno, A. C., Fultz, N. H., Bump, R., & Obenchain, R. (2003). Factors associated with women's decisions to seek treatment for urinary incontinence. *Journal of Women's Health (Larchmt), 12*(7), 687–698. Evidence Level IV.

Kozier, B., Erb, G., Berman, A., & Snyder, S. (2004). *Fundamentals of nursing concepts, process, and practice* (7th ed.). Upper Saddle River, NJ: Prentice Hall. Evidence Level VI.

Kresevic, D. M. (1997). *New-onset urinary incontinence among hospitalized elders* (Doctoral dissertation, Case Western Reserve University; 1997). (UMI No. 9810934). Evidence Level IV.

Krumholz, H. M., Chen, J., Chen, Y. T., Wang, Y., & Radford, M. J. (2001). Predicting one-year mortality among elderly survivors of hospitalization for an acute myocardial infarction: Results from the Cooperative Cardiovascular Project. *Journal of the American College of Cardiology, 38*(2), 453–459. Evidence Level IV.

Landefeld, C. S., Bowers, B. J., Feld, A. D., Hartmann, K. E., Hoffman, E., Ingber, M. J., . . . Trock, B. J. (2008). National Institutes of Health state-of-the-science conference statement: Prevention of fecal and urinary incontinence in adults. *Annals of Internal Medicine, 148*(6), 449–458. Evidence Level I.

Lau, J. B. C. (2009). Urinary incontinence: Clinical assessment. *JBI Database Evid Summary,* Publication ES0599. Evidence Level I.

Lee, P. G., Cigolle, C., & Blaum, C. (2009). The co-occurrence of chronic diseases and geriatric syndromes: The health and retirement study. *Journal of the American Geriatrics Society, 57*(3), 511–516. Evidence Level IV.

Lemack, G. E., & Zimmern, P. E. (1999). Predictability of urodynamic findings based on the Urogenital Distress Inventory-6 questionnaire. *Urology, 54*(3), 461–466. Evidence Level IV.

McDowell, B. J., Engberg, S., Sereika, S., Donovan, N., Jubeck, M. E., Weber, E., & Engberg, R. (1999). Effectiveness of behavioral therapy to treat incontinence in homebound older adults. *Journal of the American Geriatrics Society, 47*(3), 309–318. Evidence Level II.

Meijer, R., Ihnenfeldt, D. S., de Groot, I. J., van Limbeek, J., Vermeulen, M., & de Haan, R. J. (2003). Prognostic factors for ambulation and activities of daily living in the subacute phase after stroke. A systematic review of the literature. *Clinical Rehabilitation, 17*(2), 119–129. Evidence Level I.

Miller, Y. D., Brown, W. J., Smith, N., & Chiarelli, P. (2003). Managing urinary incontinence across the lifespan. *International Journal of Behavioral Medicine, 10*(2), 143–161. Evidence Level IV.

Milne, J. (2000). The impact of information on health behaviors of older adults with urinary incontinence. *Clinical Nursing Research, 9*(2), 161–176. Evidence Level IV.

Mitteness, L. S. (1987a). The management of urinary incontinence by community-living elderly. *Gerontologist, 27*(2), 185–193. Evidence Level IV.

Mitteness, L. S. (1987b). So what do you expect when you're 85? Urinary incontinence in late life. In J. A. Roth & P. Conrad (Eds.), *Research in the sociology of health care* (pp. 177–219). Greenwich, CT: JAI Press. Evidence Level IV.

Morris, V., & Wagg, A. (2007). Lower urinary tract symptoms, incontinence and falls in elderly people: Time for an intervention study. *International Journal of Clinical Practice, 61*(2), 320–323. Evidence Level VI.

National Association for Continence. (1998, December). *Release of findings from consumer survey on urinary incontinence: Dissatisfaction with treatment continues to rise.* Spartansburg, SC: Author. Evidence Level IV.

Newman, D. K., & Wein, A. J. (2009). *Managing and treating urinary incontinence* (2nd ed.). Baltimore, MD: Health Professions Press. Evidence Level VI.

Nygaard, I. (2006). Urinary incontinence: Is cesarean delivery protective? *Seminars in Perinatology, 30*(5), 267–271. Evidence Level VI.

Offermans, M. P., Du Moulin, M. F., Hamers, J. P., Dassen, T., & Halfens, R. J. (2009). Prevalence of urinary incontinence and associated risk factors in nursing home residents: A systematic review. *Neurourology and Urodynamics, 28*(4), 288–294. Evidence Level I.

Ostaszkiewicz, J., Johnston, L., & Roe, B. (2004). Timed voiding for the management of urinary incontinence in adults. *Cochrane Database Systematic Reviews*, (1), CD002802. Evidence Level I.

Palese, A., Regattin, L., Venuti, F., Innocenti, A., Benaglio, C., Cunico, L., & Saiani, L. (2007). Incontinence pad use in patients admitted to medical wards: An Italian multicenter prospective cohort study. *Journal of Wound, Ostomy, Continence Nursing, 34*(6), 649–654. Evidence Level IV.

Palmer, M. H. (1988). Incontinence. The magnitude of the problem. *The Nursing Clinics of North America, 23*(1), 139–157. Evidence Level V.

Palmer, M. H. (1996). *Urinary continence: Assessment and promotion.* Gaithersburg, MD: Aspen. Evidence Level VI.

Palmer, M. H. (2004). Use of health behavior change theories to guide urinary incontinence research. *Nursing Research, 53*(6 Suppl), S49–S55. Evidence Level VI.

Palmer, M. H., Baumgarten, M., Langenberg, P., & Carson, J. L. (2002). Risk factors for hospital-acquired incontinence in elderly female hip fracture patients. *The Journals of Gerontology. Series A, Biological Sciences and Medical Sciences, 57*(10), M672–M677. Evidence Level IV.

Palmer, M. H., Bone, L. R., Fahey, M., Mamon, J., & Steinwachs, D. (1992). Detecting urinary continence in older adults during hospitalization. *Applied Nursing Research, 5*, 174–180. Evidence Level IV.

Palmer, M. H., Myers, A. H., & Fedenko, K. M. (1997). Urinary continence changes after hip-fracture repair. *Clinical Nursing Research, 6*(1), 8–21. Evidence Level IV.

Pettersen, R., Saxby, B. K., & Wyller, T. B. (2007). Poststroke urinary incontinence: One-year outcome and relationships with measures of attentiveness. *Journal of the American Geriatrics Society, 55*(10), 1571–1577. Evidence Level IV.

Rathnayake, T. (2009a). Urinary incontinence: Bladder training. *JBI Database of Evidence Summaries*, Publication ES5237. Evidence Level I.

Rathnayake, T. (2009b). Urinary incontinence: Prompted voiding. *JBI Database of Evidence Summaries*, Publication ES5396. Evidence Level I.

Rathnayake, T. (2009c). Urinary incontinence: Timed voiding. *JBI Database of Evidence Summaries*, Publication ES5330. Evidence Level I.

Rathnayake, T. (2009d). Urinary incontinence: Treatments. *JBI Database of Evidence Summaries*, Publication ES6918. Evidence Level I.

Resnick, N. M., & Ouslander, J. G. (1990). Urinary incontinence—Where do we stand and where do we go from here? *Journal of the American Geriatrics Society, 38*(3), 263–264. Evidence Level VI.

Robinson, J. P., & Shea, J. A. (2002). Development and testing of a measure of health-related quality of life for men with urinary incontinence. *Journal of the American Geriatrics Society, 50*(5), 935–945. Evidence Level IV.

Saint, S., Kaufman, S. R., Rogers, M. A., Baker, P. D., Ossenkop, K., & Lipsky, B. A. (2006). Condom versus indwelling urinary catheters: A randomized trial. *Journal of the American Geriatrics Society, 54*(7), 1055–1061. Evidence Level II.

Sampselle, C. M., Palmer, M. H., Boyington, A. R., O'Dell, K. K., & Wooldridge, L. (2004). Prevention of urinary incontinence in adults: Population-based strategies. *Nursing Research, 53*(6 Suppl), S61–S67. Evidence Level VI.

Schnelle, J. F., Cadogan, M. P., Grbic, D., Bates-Jensen, B. M., Osterwell, D., Yoshii, J., & Simmons, S. F. (2003). A standardized quality assessment system to evaluate incontinence care in the nursing home. *Journal of the American Geriatrics Society, 51*(12), 1754–1761. Evidence Level IV.

Schultz, A., Dickey, G., & Skoner, M. (1997). Self-report of incontinence in acute care. *Urologic Nursing, 17*(1), 23–28. Evidence Level IV.

Shamliyan, T., Wyman, J., Bliss, D. Z., Kane, R. L., & Wilt, T. J. (2007). Prevention of urinary and fecal incontinence in adults. *Evidence Report/Technology Assessment (Full Rep)*, (161), 1–379. Evidence Level I.

Shinopulos, N. (2000). Bedside urodynamic studies: Simple testing for urinary incontinence. *The Nurse Practitioner, 25*(6 Pt 1), 19–22. Evidence Level VI.

Shumaker, S. A., Wyman, J. F., Uebersax, J. S., McClish, D., & Fantl, J. A. (1994). Health-related quality of life measures for women with urinary incontinence: The Incontinence Impact Questionnaire and the Urogenital Distress Inventory. Continence Program in Women (CPW) Research Group. *Quality of Life Research, 3*(5), 291–306. Evidence Level IV.

Sier, H., Ouslander, J., & Orzeck, S. (1987). Urinary incontinence among geriatric patients in an acute-care hospital. *The Journal of the American Medical Association, 257*(13), 1767–1771. Evidence Level IV.

Skelly, J., & Flint, A. J. (1995). Urinary incontinence associated with dementia. *Journal of the American Geriatrics Society, 43*(3), 286–294. Evidence Level V.

Smith, D. A. (2000). Urge incontinence. In D. B. Doughty (Ed.), *Urinary & fecal incontinence: Nursing management* (2nd ed., pp. 91–104). St. Louis, MO: Mosby. Evidence Level VI.

Subak, L. L., Richter, H. E., & Hunskaar, S. (2009). Obesity and urinary incontinence: Epidemiology and clinical research update. *The Journal of Urology, 182*(6 Suppl), S2–S7. Evidence Level I.

Subak, L. L., Whitcomb, E., Shen, H., Saxton, J., Vittinghoff, E., & Brown, J. S. (2005). Weight loss: A novel and effective treatment for urinary incontinence. *The Journal of Urology, 174*(1), 190–195. Evidence Level II.

Syah, N. A. (2010). Urinary (incontinence) management. *JBI Database of Evidence Summaries*, Publication ES6985. Evidence Level I.

Tadic, S. D., Zdaniuk, B., Griffiths, D., Rosenberg, L., Schafer, W., & Resnick, N. M. (2007). Effect of biofeedback on psychological burden and symptoms in older women with urge urinary incontinence. *Journal of the American Geriatrics Society, 55*(12), 2010–2015. Evidence Level IV.

Taylor, C., Lillis, C., & LeMone, P. (2005). *Fundamental of nursing: The art and science of nursing care* (5th ed.). New York, NY: Lippincott Williams & Wilkins. Evidence Level VI.

Terpenning, M. S., Allada, R., & Kauffman, C. A. (1989). Intermittent urethral catheterization in the elderly. *Journal of the American Geriatrics Society, 37*(5), 411–416. Evidence Level IV.

Teunissen, T. A., de Jonge, A., van Weel, C., & Lagro-Janssen, A. L. (2004). Treating urinary incontinence in the elderly—conservative therapies that work: A systematic review. *The Journal of Family Practice, 53*(1), 25–30, 32. Evidence Level I.

Thomas, L. H., Barrett, J., Cross, S., French, B., Leathley, M., Sutton, C., & Watkins, C. (2005). Prevention and treatment of urinary incontinence after stroke in adults. *Cochrane Database of Systematic Reviews,* (3), CD004462. Evidence Level I.

Tsai, Y. C., & Liu, C. H. (2009). The effectiveness of pelvic floor exercises, digital vaginal palpation and interpersonal support on stress urinary incontinence: An experimental study. *International Journal of Nursing Studies, 46*(9). 1181–1186. Evidence Level II.

Uebersax, J. S., Wyman, J. F., Shumaker, S. A., McClish, D. K., & Fantl, J. A. (1995). Short forms to assess life quality and symptom distress for urinary incontinence in women: The Incontinence Impact Questionnaire and the Urogenital Distress Inventory. Continence Program for Women Research Group. *Neurourology and Urodynamics, 14*(2), 131–139. Evidence Level IV.

Vinsnes, A. G., Harkless, G. E., Haltbakk, J., Bohm, J., & Hunskaar, S. (2001). Healthcare personnel's attitudes towards patients with urinary incontinence. *Journal of Clinical Nursing, 10*(4), 455–462. Evidence Level IV.

Warren, J. W. (1997). Catheter-associated urinary tract infections. *Infectious Disease Clinics of North America, 11*(3), 609–622. Evidence Level VI.

Watson, N. M. (2004). Advancing quality of urinary incontinence evaluation and treatment in nursing homes through translational research. *Worldviews on Evidence-Based Nursing, 1*(Suppl 1), S21–S25. Evidence Level VI.

Watson, N. M., Brink, C. A., Zimmer, J. G., & Mayer, R. D. (2003). Use of the Agency for Health Care Policy and Research Urinary Incontinence Guideline in nursing homes. *Journal of the American Geriatrics Society, 51*(12), 1779–1786. Evidence Level VI.

Wilson, L., Brown, J. S., Shin, G. P., Luc, K. O., & Subak, L. L. (2001). Annual direct cost of urinary incontinence. *Obstetrics and Gynecology, 98*(3), 398–406. Evidence Level IV.

Wolf, S. L., Riolo, L., & Ouslander, J. G. (2000). Urge incontinence and the risk of falling in older women. *Journal of the American Geriatrics Society, 48*(7), 847–848. Evidence Level VI.

Wyman, J. F. (1997). The 'costs' of urinary incontinence. *European Urology, 32*(Suppl 2), 13–9. Evidence Level V.

Zimakoff, J., Stickler, D. J., Pontoppidan, B., & Larsen, S. O. (1996). Bladder management and urinary tract infections in Danish hospitals, nursing homes, and home care: A national prevalence study. *Infection Control and Hospital Epidemiology, 17*(4), 215–221. Evidence Level IV.

Catheter-Associated Urinary Tract Infection Prevention

19

*Heidi L. Wald, Regina M. Fink, Mary Beth Flynn Makic,
and Kathleen S. Oman*

EDUCATIONAL OBJECTIVES

On completion of this chapter, the reader should be able to:

1. define catheter-associated urinary tract infection (CAUTI)
2. understand the epidemiology of CAUTI
3. define indications for indwelling urinary catheters (IUC)
4. identify evidence-based strategies and interventions for the prevention of CAUTI
5. understand how to engage an interdisciplinary team in the management of CAUTIs

OVERVIEW

Health care-associated infections (HAIs) have received increasing scrutiny over the last decade and are now widely recognized as largely preventable adverse events related to medical care. CAUTIs are the single most common HAI, accounting for 34% of all HAIs (Klevens et al., 2007) and associated with significant morbidity and excess health care costs (Saint, 2000). CAUTI is disproportionately reported among older adults (Fakih et al., 2010). Although once largely overlooked as part of the price of doing business in hospitals, a significantly changed regulatory environment has emerged that will bring increased scrutiny to HAIs in general and CAUTIs in particular. Examples of this oversight include process and outcome measurement and reporting and financial incentives to improve these measures. Since 2008, the Centers for Medicare and Medicaid Services (CMS) no longer reimburses for additional costs required to treat hospital-acquired urinary tract infections (UTIs; CMS, Department of Health and Human Services [DHHS], 2007). Long-term care facilities also follow CMS regulatory guidance and their federal regulations (F-315 Tag) mandate that IUC use must be medically justified and care rendered to reduce infection risk in all residents with or without an IUC (CMS, DHHS, 2005). Enhanced public reporting and financial incentives figure prominently in the Patient Protection and Affordable Care Act of 2010;

For description of Evidence Levels cited in this chapter, see Chapter 1, Developing and Evaluating Clinical Practice Guidelines: A Systematic Approach, page 7.

HAIs are singled out for inclusion in both types of initiatives (Patient Protection and Affordable Care Act, 2010). Therefore, it is imperative that health care professional staff in various settings develop strategies and interventions to reduce IUC duration and prevent CAUTIs, thus benefitting both patient and financial outcomes.

This paradigm shift occurs as the evidence base for the prevention of CAUTI is evolving. After 25 years of stasis in the field, multiple stakeholder organizations including the Centers for Disease Control and Prevention (CDC) and several major professional societies have critically examined the literature on CAUTI prevention. Between 2008 and 2010, at least six evidence-based practice strategies, recommendations, and/or guidelines for preventing CAUTI in hospitals and long-term care have been published (Cottenden et al., 2005; Gould et al., 2009; Greene, Marx, & Oriola, 2008; Hooton et al., 2010; Joanna Briggs Institute [JBI], 2000; Lo et al., 2008; see Resources section). Prior to this proliferation of recommendations, the last evidence synthesis for CAUTI prevention in the United States occurred in 1981. In addition, in 2009, the CDC's National Healthcare Safety Network significantly revised the surveillance definition for CAUTI (CDC, National Healthcare Safety Network, 2009). In light of these rapid changes in the field, the review of policies, procedures, practices, and products is imperative for all health care facilities. In this chapter, we will review the rationale for CAUTI prevention strategies, suggest an approach to implementing a comprehensive CAUTI prevention program, and catalog the most important CAUTI prevention strategies.

BACKGROUND AND STATEMENT OF PROBLEM

Health care-associated UTIs are frequent and costly, resulting in increased morbidity and possible mortality in hospitalized older adults (Saint, 2000). There are more than 500,000 hospital-acquired UTIs in the United States annually (Gould et al., 2009; Klevens et al., 2007). At a mean cost of $589 per episode, this epidemic results in $250 million of excess health care costs each year (Tambyah, Knasinski, & Maki, 2002). Five percent of UTIs lead to bacteremias, with significantly increased mortality and costs.

The vast majority of UTIs are associated with the ubiquitous IUC, also known as a *Foley catheter* named after urologist Frederick Foley who developed the modern device. Urinary catheters are among the most widely used medical devices. Despite their utility in acutely ill patients, they have many downsides, including the CAUTI. Other complications include delirium (Inouye, 2006), local trauma, encrustation, and restriction of mobility (Saint, Lipsky, & Goold, 2002). Therefore, the benefits of managing urinary output with an IUC must be weighed against the many risks.

Unfortunately, the indiscriminate use of IUCs is widespread. IUCs are used in up to 25% of hospital admissions (Weinstein et al., 1999) and are more commonly used in the older patient (Fakih et al., 2010). Thirty percent of Medicare patients have IUCs during their hospital stay (Zhan et al., 2009) and older women are disproportionately likely to have no clear indication for catheterization (Fakih et al., 2010). Of Medicare patients undergoing elective surgery, 86% have an IUC (Wald, Ma, Bratzler, & Kramer, 2008) and nearly 50% continue to have a catheter in place beyond 48 hours postoperatively (Wald, Epstein, & Kramer, 2005). According to the Infectious Diseases Society of America (IDSA), 21%–54% of all IUCs are inappropriately placed and are not medically indicated (Hooton et al., 2010). Only 25% of attending physicians in teaching hospitals are aware that their patients have urinary catheters, and few hospitals have systematic methods for tracking which patients have catheters placed (Saint et al., 2000; Saint et al., 2008). Clearly, interventions aimed at evidence-based use of catheters are needed to prevent CAUTIs. To better understand the potential approaches to prevention of CAUTIs, an understanding of CAUTI pathogenesis is essential.

Catheter-Associated Urinary Tract Infection Pathogenesis

The urinary tract is normally a sterile body site; therefore, any positive urine culture (defined in Table 19.1) can be considered a UTI. The IDSA distinguishes between two categories of UTIs: the benign asymptomatic bacteriuria (ASB) and the clinically important symptomatic UTI. Either of these conditions can occur in the presence of an IUC (Hooton et al., 2010).

When a patient has an IUC, microorganisms can gain access to the urinary tract on either the extraluminal surface of the IUC or intraluminal surface through breaks in the catheter system (Figure 19.1). Extraluminal infection can occur early if bacteria are introduced during insertion, but more commonly, extraluminal infection occurs later (Maki & Tambyah, 2001). Once they gain access to the urinary tract, microorganisms can thrive in a "biofilm" layer on either the extraluminal or intraluminal surface of the IUC. The biofilm, made up of bacteria, host proteins, and bacterial slime, is thought to be important in the development of late CAUTIs. Because the formation of a biofilm and colonization with bacteria takes time, most CAUTI occurs after 48 hours of catheterization and increases approximately 5% per day (Schaeffer, 1986; Stamm, 1975).

The mechanisms described previously provide the rationale for evidence-based care of IUCs and highlights three potential opportunities for intervention during the use of IUCs (Figure 19.2). The first opportunity is avoidance of catheters at the time of the decision for insertion, the second is evidence-based product selection and care practices regarding IUCs (including insertion and maintenance), and the third is minimizing duration through timely removal. A fourth set of additional strategies for CAUTI prevention includes education of providers and surveillance of processes and outcomes. This set of strategies can be applied at any of the opportunities for intervention. A comprehensive program to eliminate CAUTIs includes elements of each of the aforementioned strategies.

TABLE 19.1

Definition of a Positive Urine Culture

---

1. Greater than or equal to 10^5 microorganisms/cc of urine with no more than two species of microorganisms.

OR

2. Greater than or equal to 10^3 and less than or equal to 10^5 CFU/ml with no more than two species of microorganism.

AND

A positive urinalysis:
- Positive dipstick for leukocyte esterase and/or nitrite
- Pyuria (urine specimen with = 10 WBC/mm^3 or = 3 WBC/high power field of unspun urine)
- Organisms seen on Gram stain of unspun urine.

CFU = colony forming unit; WBC = white blood cell.

FIGURE 19.1

Routes of entry of uropathogens to catheterized urinary tract.

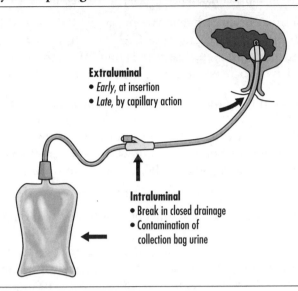

Extraluminal
- *Early*, at insertion
- *Late*, by capillary action

Intraluminal
- Break in closed drainage
- Contamination of collection bag urine

Source: Maki, D. G., & Tambyah, P. A. (2001). Engineering out the risk of infection with urinary catheters. *Emerging Infectious Diseases*, 7(2), 342–347. Retrieved from http://www.cdc.gov/ncidod/eid/vol7no2/makiG1.htm

FIGURE 19.2

Stages of catheter use and potential intervention strategies.

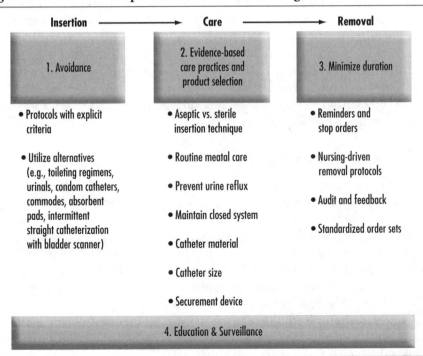

Insertion →	Care →	Removal
1. Avoidance	**2. Evidence-based care practices and product selection**	**3. Minimize duration**
• Protocols with explicit criteria	• Aseptic vs. sterile insertion technique	• Reminders and stop orders
• Utilize alternatives (e.g., toileting regimens, urinals, condom catheters, commodes, absorbent pads, intermittent straight catheterization with bladder scanner)	• Routine meatal care	• Nursing-driven removal protocols
	• Prevent urine reflux	• Audit and feedback
	• Maintain closed system	• Standardized order sets
	• Catheter material	
	• Catheter size	
	• Securement device	

4. Education & Surveillance

ASSESSMENT OF THE PROBLEM

Surveillance Definition of Catheter-Associated Urinary Tract Infection Pathogenesis

A CAUTI is a UTI that occurs while a patient has an IUC or within 48 hours of its removal. Although the clinical diagnosis of CAUTI is in the eye of the clinician, the CDC has developed explicit surveillance criteria for CAUTI for use by infection control practitioners. In brief, the patient must have the following symptoms:

1. A positive urine culture sent more than 48 hours after admission to the health care facility (Table 19.1)
2. An IUC at the time of or within 48 hours prior to the culture
3. One of the following: suprapubic tenderness, costovertebral angle pain or tenderness, or a fever higher than 38 °C without another recognized cause; or a positive blood culture with the same organism as in the urine

The CAUTI diagnosed within 48 hours of arrival to a location is attributed to the prior location.

In nonbacteremic cases, this surveillance definition requires the patient have symptoms referable to the urinary tract or a fever without another cause. ASB is of questionable clinical significance and should not be treated except in pregnant patients or those undergoing urologic surgery (Nicolle et al., 2005). For the purposes of infection control surveillance, new alterations in mental status do not meet the diagnostic criteria for CAUTI.

CAUTIs are generally reported as infections per 1,000 catheter days on a given patient care unit. More than half of all states require public reporting of hospital-acquired infections, among them, many specify reporting of CAUTIs. Such reporting of CAUTI rates is likely to increase.

Additional process measures that may be of interest include catheter days or hospital days, catheter duration per episode of catheterization (may also be referred to as *dwell time*), and proportion of catheterized or admitted patients from the emergency department (ED) or operating room (OR). Since October 2009, the Surgical Care Improvement Project collects a measure of postoperative catheter removal on postoperative Day 1 or 2 and, as of October 2010, has expanded this measure to catheter removal on catheterization Day 1 or 2 for all surgical patients (Surgical Care Improvement Project, n.d.).

Indications for Indwelling Urinary Catheters

Avoidance of unnecessary IUCs may reduce CAUTI incidence with subsequent decreases in length of stay, costs of hospitalization, and costs associated with CAUTI (Apisarnthanarak et al., 2007). Elpern et al. (2009) evaluated the inappropriate use of IUCs among inpatients and found them to be more common in female, nonambulatory, and medical ICU patients. Explicit criteria for appropriate insertion may result in significant reductions in catheter duration and CAUTI prevalence. The University of Colorado Hospital developed and disseminated an algorithm for appropriate insertion of IUCs in the ED based on guidance from the published literature (Figure 19.3).

Similar criteria can also be developed specifically for the OR and postoperative period. At the University of Colorado Hospital, a protocol for early postoperative removal was developed and disseminated (Figure 19.4).

FIGURE 19.3

Algorithm for appropriate insertions of indwelling urinary catheters.

Admission/Shift change assessment of Urine Output Management

↓

Is there a need for an indwelling urinary catheter?

Please read the following criteria for <u>appropriate use</u> of Foley catheter and check <u>your reason</u> for ordering the Foley catheter for this patient.	
☐ <u>Drainage:</u>	• Urinary obstruction (distal urinary tract) • Urinary retention (not managed with intermittent catheterization)
☐ <u>Monitoring:</u>	• Alteration in the blood pressure or volume status (unstable patient) requiring urine volume measurement. • Accurate monitoring of intake and output in a patient unable to cooperate with urine collection by other means.
☐ <u>Periprocedure:</u>	• Preoperative insertion for emergency surgery • Major trauma patients • Placement by urology for procedure or surgery
☐ <u>Therapy:</u>	• Continuous bladder irrigation • Management of urinary incontinence with **stage 3 or greater** pressure ulcerations • Comfort care for the terminally ill

↓   ↓

YES, the reason appears above.
Insert catheter

NO, the reason does not appear above. (A catheter may not be indicated for this patient.)

↓

Consider:

Re-evaluate continued need each shift.
Consider removal if indications no longer met.

1. Straight Catheterization (for Sterile specimen if needed) 2. Commode 3. Urinal 4. Bed pan 5. Incontinence Pads 6. Toileting with assistance

An IUC should not be used for routine care of patients who are incontinent, as a means to obtain urine culture or other diagnostic tests in a patient who can void, for prolonged postoperative duration without appropriate indications, or routinely in patients receiving epidural anesthesia and analgesia (see Protocol 19.1).

INTERVENTIONS AND CARE STRATEGIES

It is estimated that 20%–69% of CAUTIs are preventable (Gould et al., 2009). Specific interventions to prevent CAUTIs are summarized in the subsequent text and organized regarding the four strategies illustrated in Figure 19.2. Many of these recommendations

FIGURE 19.4

Algorithm for postoperative removal of indwelling urinary catheter placed for surgery

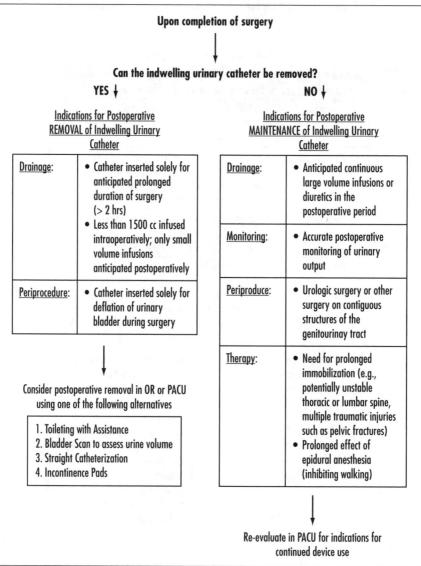

are supported by low quality evidence and expert opinion. Further study may impact these recommendations. A proposed approach to a comprehensive CAUTI intervention follows.

Strategy 1: Avoidance

To reduce the incidence of CAUTI, it is important to rethink practice systems and examine "why" behind the clinical indication for the IUC. Clearly identifying the need for the IUC can assist in the avoidance of inserting an IUC when other options for elimination are available. The use of an algorithm (Figure 19.3) to guide the insertion decision may be of assistance. To avoid catheterizations, alternative strategies for managing urine output are necessary. Completing a systems evaluation of available equipment to provide alternatives to IUC for urinary elimination is an important first step in reducing use. Developing toileting schedules incorporated with frequent nursing staff rounding is another strategy that can be used to reduce urgency and incontinence episodes.

If the patient is mobile or has limited mobility, alternatives to an IUC include the use of a bedside commode with a toileting schedule (Gray, 2010), condom catheters for male patients (Dowling-Castronovo & Bradway, 2008; Saint et al., 2006), moisture-wicking incontinence pads (BioRelief, n.d.; Cottenden et al., 2005; Medline Ultrasorb Underpad, n.d.), intermittent straight catheterization with the use of a bladder scanner to determine bladder urine volume (Hooton et al., 2010; Saint et al., 2006; Saint et al., 2009), as well as urinals and bedpans. Careful consideration of products and how and where they are stocked is essential to success. For instance, commodes need to be available in multiple sizes and need to include stable (not easy to tip) and bariatric commodes; urinals need to fit snugly on bedrails.

For less mobile male patients, the condom catheter is an effective alternative to an IUC. Research by Saint and colleagues (2006) found that the use of condom catheters for elimination were effective in reducing CAUTIs ($p = .04$). In addition, the patients in this study reported condom catheters to be more comfortable ($p = -.02$) and less painful ($p = .02$) than an IUC. The authors did not report an increase in adverse skin breakdown associated with the use of the condom catheter. Moisture-absorbing or -wicking underpads for incontinence management are a newer alternative for the acute care environment. Incontinence underpad products pull effluent moisture and urine away from the skin and can absorb up to 2 L of fluid before becoming saturated (Junkin & Selekof, 2008; Padula, Osborne, & Williams, 2008). For a full discussion of incontinence management, please refer to Chapter 18, Urinary Incontinence.

Urinary retention postsurgery or after initial IUC removal may pose clinical care challenges. To prevent IUC insertion or reinsertion, intermittent catheterization should be considered as an avoidance strategy. The bladder scanner, which utilizes ultrasound technology, is clinically beneficial in determining urinary retention, reducing unnecessary intermittent catheterizations, enhancing patient comfort, and saving costs associated with inappropriate catheterizations and possible CAUTIs (Lee, Tsay, Lou, & Dai, 2007; Palese, Buchini, Deroma, & Barbone, 2010; Sparks et al., 2004).

Strategy 2: Evidence-Based Product Selection, Insertion, and Routine Care

If an IUC is determined to be clinically indicated, selection of the right catheter, proper technique during insertion of the device, and evidence-based ongoing care management are needed to reduce infection.

Catheter material remains an area of ongoing debate. Although antimicrobial catheter materials have been shown to reduce catheter-associated bacteriuria (Johnson, Kuskowski, & Wilt, 2006), the impact of antimicrobial catheters on symptomatic CAUTIs remains unproven. Research syntheses have failed to conclusively demonstrate the effectiveness of silver-coated or antibiotic-impregnated catheters on prevention of CAUTIs for short-term catheterization of adult patients versus standard materials. There is also insufficient evidence to determine whether selection of a latex catheter, hydrogel-coated latex catheter, silicone-coated latex catheter, or all-silicone catheter influences CAUTI risk (Cottenden et al., 2005; Hooton et al., 2010; Parker et al., 2009; Patient Protection and Affordable Care Act, 2010; Schumm & Lam, 2008). The decision to use a silver-coated or antibiotic-impregnated catheter should be made with the understanding that it does not substitute for a comprehensive CAUTI prevention program.

Selecting the smallest IUC size, when possible, is an additional consideration to reduce the risk of infection (Gould et al., 2009; Greene et al., 2008; Hooton et al., 2010). The selection of a smaller catheter (e.g., less than 18 French) reduces irritation and inflammation of the urethra and reduces infection risk (Gray, 2010).

Placing an IUC is a fundamental skill for nurses; however, current evidence supporting sterile versus aseptic technique for the procedure is inconclusive (Greene et al., 2008; JBI, n.d.). Strict sterile technique involves using a sterile gown, mask, prolonged hand washing (more than 4 minutes), opening and using a sterile insertion kit, donning sterile gloves, cleansing the urethral meatus and perineal area with an antiseptic solution, and inserting the catheter using a no-touch technique (Gray, 2010). Willson and colleagues (2009) reviewed the literature and found that most clinicians employ an aseptic technique, which was most frequently defined as the use of sterile gloves, sterile barriers, perineal washing using an antiseptic cleanser, and no-touch insertion. Current recommendations suggest an IUC insertion be placed under aseptic technique with sterile equipment (Gould et al., 2009; Greene et al., 2008; Hooton et al., 2010).

Once an IUC is placed, optimal management includes care of the urethral meatus according to "routine hygiene" (e.g., daily cleansing of the meatal surface during bathing with soap and water and as needed (e.g., following a bowel movement; Gould et al., 2009; Greene et al., 2008; Hooton et al., 2010; Jeong et al., 2010; JBI, n.d.). Meatal cleansing with antiseptics, creams, lotions, or ointments has been found to irritate the meatus, possibly increasing the risk of infection (Jeong et al., 2010; Willson et al., 2009).

Securing the IUC after placement to reduce friction from movement is an important element of catheter management supported by current guidelines, researchers, and expert opinion panels (Darouiche et al., 2006; Gould et al., 2009; Hooton et al., 2010; Society of Urologic Nurses and Associates Clinical Practice Guidelines Task Force, 2006). Maintaining a closed catheter system is also supported by current guidelines (Gould et al., 2009; Greene et al., 2008; Hooton et al., 2010) to eliminate the introduction of microbes that occurs when breaking the prepackaged seals on the IUC. A systems analysis should be conducted to purchase and stock the most commonly needed IUC insertion and drainage bag kits to optimize the maintenance of a closed system. Similarly, maintaining the urine collection bag below the level of the bladder minimizes reflux into the catheter itself preventing retrograde flow of urine (Gould et al., 2009; Greene et al., 2008; Hooton et al., 2010). Establishing work flow protocols to routinely empty the drainage bag frequently and prior to transport are important in reducing urine reflux and opportunities for CAUTI.

Strategy 3: Timely Removal

Developing systems that prompt health care providers to review the need for the IUC and encourage early removal have been found to reduce IUC use and CAUTI rates

(Apisarnthanarak et al., 2007; Fernandez, Griffiths, & Murie, 2003; Loeb et al., 2008; Meddings, Rogers, Macy, & Saint, 2010). Meddings and colleagues (2010) conducted a systematic review and meta-analysis and found that urinary catheter removal reminders and stop orders appeared to reduce CAUTI rates. Implementing systems that provide physicians and nurses routine reminders to evaluate the need for the IUC were found to reduce the CAUTI rate by 56% ($p = .005$). In this study, automatic stop orders were found to reduce the rate of CAUTI by 41% ($p < .001$). Overall, urinary catheter use and mean duration of catheterization were also decreased in several studies analyzed (Meddings et al., 2010).

Other valid approaches to reducing catheter days include audit and feedback (Goetz, Kedzuf, Wagener, & Muder, 1999) and nurse-prompted reminders to recommend reevaluation of the need for the IUC and early removal (Apisarnthanarak et al., 2007; Greene et al., 2008). Some hospitals have explored nurse-driven catheter removal protocols (Wenger, 2010).

Multiple studies have examined outcomes associated with early removal of IUCs after surgery. Early removal of IUCs after uncomplicated hysterectomy decreased first ambulation time and length of hospital stay (Alessandri, Mistrangelo, Lijoi, Ferrero, & Ragni, 2006). Dunn, Shlay, and Forshner (2003) found that early removal postsurgery was not associated with adverse events in patients and subjective pain was significantly less. Keeping the IUC as long as thoracic epidural analgesia is maintained may result in a higher incidence of CAUTI and increased hospital stay. IUC removal on the morning after surgery while the thoracic epidural catheter is still in place does not lead to urinary retention, infection, or higher rates of recatheterizations (Basse, Werner, & Kehlet, 2000; Chia, Wei, Chang, & Liu, 2009; Ladak et al., 2009; Zaouter, Kaneva, & Carli, 2009).

Strategy 4: Surveillance and Education

Ensuring leadership of organizations and systems are in place to effectively evaluate and sustain practice change are essential to improving patient outcomes (Kabcenell, Nolan, Martin, & Gill, 2010; Reinertsen, Bisognano, & Pugh, 2008). In particular, surveillance is key to an effective infection control program. Metrics that are amenable to performance measurement and feedback are discussed in the Assessment of the Problem section and include process measures as well as outcomes. A 2005 survey demonstrated that only a minority of hospitals track urinary catheter use (Saint et al., 2008).

Measurement must be accompanied by provision, knowledge, and skills to front-line providers through appropriate education and training, which may be central to a multicomponent CAUTI intervention. Huang et al. (2004) found that a multifaceted educational intervention incorporating the use of algorithms, automated stop orders, and physician reminder prompts needed to be critically evaluated to effectively decrease CAUTIs in all patients. Ongoing system evaluation, nursing reeducation, practice reminders, and public reporting of unit-based CAUTI rate data are strategies to inform the health care team of current practice outcomes and effectiveness of CAUTI prevention strategies. Implementing systems that encompass the whole health care team to question the need for the IUC and, when indicated, ensuring proper care and early removal can be pivotal in reducing CAUTI rates (Wenger, 2010).

Approach to a Comprehensive Catheter-Associated Urinary Tract Infection Intervention

Evidence-based practice guidelines derived from valid, current research and other evidence sources can successfully improve patient outcomes and quality care. However, simply disseminating scientific evidence is often ineffective in changing clinical practice. Learning how to implement findings is critically important to promoting high quality and safe care (Drekonja, Kuskowski, & Johnson, 2010). To effectively facilitate the translation of best evidence into practice, processes enhancing practice change must be embraced by the health care provider (Wallin, Profetto-McGrath, & Levers, 2005). Understanding health care provider decisions, experiences, practice processes, and barriers are considered essential elements that must be explored to successfully implement practice change based on best evidence (Titler & Everett, 2006).

Developing an interdisciplinary champion team and creating a multifaceted intervention to implement evidence-based procedures for IUC insertion and maintenance must be a priority in all practice settings. The ultimate goals are to reduce routine catheter insertions, provide evidence-based catheter care, and prompt early removal when possible, thus decreasing the risk of and prevention of CAUTI.

Steps used for protocol development at the University of Colorado Hospital are highlighted in the subsequent text. Improved patient outcomes (decreased catheter days, decreased CAUTIs) and decreased costs have been realized.

Protocol Development

1. Recruit an interdisciplinary champion team to include nurses (clinical educators, OR registered nurses [RNs], ED RNs); physicians (hospitalists, infectious disease ED medical doctors [MDs], surgeons, anesthesiologists); rehabilitation therapists and transport personnel; infection control preventionists; and quality improvement, central supply, and clinical informatics representatives.
2. Examine and synthesize the evidence (search, review, critique, and hold journal clubs in various care areas to present the evidence).
3. Identify and understand product use, availability, and costs in your health care setting. Refine product use based on the best evidence and cost analysis. Examine the following:

   - Urinary catheter materials, sizes, kits, and drainage bags
   - Catheter securement device
   - Urinals and bedpan availability
   - Commodes (availability and size)
   - Bladder scanners
   - Alternatives (incontinence pads, condom catheters, etc.)

4. Identify barriers to optimal IUC care practices by surveying staff or holding focus groups throughout your health care setting.
5. Update your policy and procedures related to indwelling catheter insertion and care based on the evidence.
6. Consider breaking the project into manageable phases. Avoidance strategies may require a different approach than care or removal strategies. For instance, avoidance starts in the ED and OR, whereas removal occurs on inpatient floors.

7. Develop and use algorithms, decision aids, and factoid posters displaying evidence-based caveats.
8. Update patient and family educational materials on the importance of prompt and early removal of indwelling catheters.
9. Educate staff (including radiology, transport, rehabilitation therapy staff [PT, physical therapist; OT, occupational therapist]) focusing on policy and procedure revision, insertion indication guidelines, insertion procedures, maintenance and care, catheter bag placement, removal prompts, and bladder scanner use and procedures.
10. Work with infection control and clinical informatics staff to audit and measure outcomes. Provide feedback to staff. Potential measurable outcomes include the following:

    - CAUTIs/1,000 catheter days
    - Catheter days and hospital days
    - Postoperative catheter days and patient days
    - Proportion of catheterized and admitted patients from ED or OR

11. Continually evaluate and update practice changes.

CASE STUDY 1

Mr. T is an 84-year-old male with a history of Alzheimer's disease and incontinence presenting to your hospital with failure to thrive. The patient arrives to the medical floor with an IUC that was placed in the ED. Given the patient's incontinence and fall risk, the urinary catheter is left in place. Three days after admission while awaiting placement in a skilled nursing facility (SNF), he develops fever and delirium and is diagnosed with a UTI. This delays his transfer to the SNF.

Questions to Consider

1. Was the catheter placement medically indicated?
2. What could have been used as alternatives to indwelling catheter placement?

Discussion

Because incontinence and fall risk are not medically appropriate indications for a urethral catheter, it should have been avoided in the ED or removed as soon as the patient arrived to the floor. Alternatives to indwelling catheterization in this patient would include a bedside commode with nursing assistance, incontinence pads or diapers, or a condom catheter. Attentiveness to the appropriate medical indications for catheter use, familiarity with catheter alternatives, and recognition of the clinical and economic impacts may have prevented the infection and eased the placement of this patient.

CASE STUDY 2

Mrs. G is a 69-year-old alert female with a diagnosis of nonsmall cell lung cancer is admitted for a thoracotomy. The patient is transferred from the postanesthesia care unit (PACU) to the surgical intensive care unit (ICU) with an IUC that was placed in the OR and a thoracic epidural for pain management with morphine and bupivacaine infusion. Mrs. G is doing well 48 hours postoperatively, experiencing little pain, and is able to cough and deep breathe. She is transferred out of the ICU to the surgical floor with the urinary catheter and thoracic epidural still in place. When prompted by nursing staff to write an order for urinary catheter removal, the surgeon says he is waiting for the anesthesiology team to pull the epidural catheter before removing the urinary.

Questions to Consider

1. Was the IUC placement surgically indicated?
2. When should the IUC be removed?
3. When the IUC is removed, what can be used as alternatives?

Discussion

The IUC was probably indicated because of length of surgery (more than 2 hours) and need for accurate monitoring for intake and output. The misnomer that the IUC needs to be in place as long as the thoracic epidural remains for pain management purposes needs clarification. Multiple studies have supported IUC removal on the morning after surgery to decrease CAUTI risk (Basse et al., 2000; Chia et al., 2009; Ladak et al., 2009; Zaouter et al., 2009). Early removal does not lead to urinary retention or higher rates of recatheterization. Post-IUC removal, toileting with assistance, use of a bedpan or urinal, placement of an incontinence pad or use of a bladder scanner for post void residual volume assessment, and use of straight catheterization if indicated are alternatives.

SUMMARY

A rapidly changing evidence base and regulatory environment necessitates a renewed focus on the prevention of CAUTI, which is informed by an understanding of CAUTI pathogenesis and rational IUC use. Critical elements of a CAUTI prevention program include maximizing catheter avoidance, ensuring evidence-based practice and product use, and timely catheter removal. Additional strategies include staff education, continuing monitoring of CAUTI incidence, and catheter use. Multicomponent interventions have been used successfully in the prevention of CAUTIs.

Protocol 19.1: Prevention of Catheter-Associated Urinary Tract Infection Prevention

I. GOALS: To ensure that nurses in acute care are able to:
A. Define catheter-associated urinary tract infection (CAUTI)
B. Understand the epidemiology of CAUTI
C. Define indications for indwelling urinary catheters (IUC)
D. Identify evidence-based strategies and interventions for the prevention of CAUTI
E. Understand how to engage an interdisciplinary team in the management of CAUTIs in your setting

II. OVERVIEW
A. CAUTIs are the single most common hospital-acquired infection (HAI), accounting for 34% of all HAIs and associated with significant morbidity and excess health care costs.
B. Since 2008, the Centers for Medicare and Medicaid Services (CMS) no longer reimburse for additional costs required to treat nosocomial urinary tract infections (UTIs).
C. Between 2008 and 2010, at least six evidence-based practice strategies, recommendations, and/or guidelines for preventing CAUTI in hospitals and long-term care have been published.
D. In light of these rapid changes in the field, the review of policies, procedures, practices, and products is imperative for all health care facilities.

III. BACKGROUND AND STATEMENT OF PROBLEM
A. Introduction
1. There are more than 500,000 UTIs in the United States annually. At a mean cost of $589 per episode, this epidemic results in $250 million of excess health care costs each year.
2. Most UTIs are associated with the ubiquitous IUC, also known as a *Foley catheter*.
3. According to the Infectious Diseases Society of America, 21%–54% of all IUCs are inappropriately placed and are not medically indicated.
B. Definitions
1. *Symptomatic UTI.* A patient has at least one of the following signs or symptoms with no other recognized cause: fever (higher than 38 °C), urgency, frequency, dysuria, or suprapubic tenderness and positive urine culture (see Table 19.1).
2. *Asymptomatic bacteriuria.* A positive urine culture in a patient who does not have symptoms referable to the urinary tract; may or may not be catheter-associated.
3. *CAUTI.* A symptomatic UTI that occurs while a patient has an IUC or within 48 hours of its removal.

(continued)

**Protocol 19.1: Prevention of Catheter-Associated
Urinary Tract Infection Prevention *(cont.)***

C. Essential Elements
   1. The urinary tract is normally a sterile body site. In the presence of an IUC, microorganisms can gain access to the urinary tract on either the extraluminal surface of the IUC or intraluminal surface through breaks in the catheter system.
   2. Once bacteria gain access to the urinary tract, microorganisms can thrive in a "biofilm" layer on either the extraluminal or intraluminal surface of the IUC.
   3. Because the formation of a biofilm and colonization with bacteria takes time, most CAUTI occurs after 48 hours of catheterization and increases approximately 5% per day.
   4. The mechanisms described previously provide the rationale for evidence-based care of IUCs. Four potential opportunities for intervention include the following:
      a. Avoid the use of catheters
      b. Evidence-based care practices and product selection
      c. Timely removal
      d. Education and surveillance

IV. ASSESSMENT OF CAUTI
   A. The Centers for Disease Control and Prevention (CDC) has developed explicit surveillance criteria for CAUTI. In brief, the patient must have the following:
      1. A positive urine culture (see Table 19.1) sent more than 48 hours after admission to the health care facility
      2. An IUC at the time of or within 48 hours prior to the culture
      3. One of the following: suprapubic tenderness, costovertebral angle pain or tenderness, or a fever higher than 38 °C without another recognized cause; or a positive blood culture with the same organism as in the urine
   B. Measures
      1. Outcomes
         a. CAUTIs/1,000 catheter days
      2. Processes
         a. Catheter days and hospital days
         b. Postoperative catheter days and patient days
         c. Proportion of catheterized and admitted patients from emergency department (ED) or operating room (OR)
   C. Indications for IUCs can be operationalized using algorithms or protocols.

V. NURSING CARE STRATEGIES
Twenty percent to 69% of CAUTIs are preventable through the application of evidence-based care strategies.
   A. Catheter Avoidance
      1. Established insertion guidelines for ED and OR
      2. Alternative strategies to manage urine output available:
         a. Bedside commodes
         b. Condom catheters

(continued)

**Protocol 19.1: Prevention of Catheter-Associated
Urinary Tract Infection Prevention** *(cont.)*

    c. Moisture-wicking incontinence pads

    d. Intermittent straight catheterization

    e. Bladder scanner for monitoring and assessment

    f. Bedpans and urinals that are functional

  3. Toileting schedules and frequent nursing rounds

B. Product Selection and Routine Care

  1. Catheter material is controversial:

    a. Antimicrobial catheter materials have been shown to reduce catheter-associated bacteriuria (colonization), but impact on prevention of symptomatic CAUTIs during short-term insertions is unproven.

    b. There is insufficient evidence to determine whether selection of a latex catheter, hydrogel-coated latex catheter, silicone-coated latex catheter, or all-silicone catheter influences CAUTI risk.

  2. Select the smallest size possible (less than 18 French).

  3. Use aseptic technique and sterile product during catheter insertion.

  4. Routine urethral meatus cleansing with soap and water during bath and after bowel movement.

  5. Secure catheter to leg.

  6. Maintain a closed system at all times.

  7. Keep drainage bag below level of bladder.

  8. Empty the bag when two-third full and before transport.

C. Timely Removal

  1. Systems that prompt providers to review the need for the catheter and encourage early removal. Examples include stop orders and reminder systems: audit and feedback, nurse-prompted reminders, and nurse-driven removal protocols.

  2. Measure of removal: Surgical Care Improvement Project (SCIP), SCIP-9 measure; catheter removal on postoperative Day 1 or 2.

D. Surveillance and Education

  1. Measurement of processes and outcomes.

  2. Ongoing system evaluation, nursing reeducation, practice reminders, and public reporting of unit-based CAUTI rate data are strategies to inform the health care team of current practice outcomes and effectiveness of CAUTI prevention strategies.

VI. EVALUATION AND EXPECTED OUTCOMES

A. Plan of Care

  1. Assessment that patient meets established insertion criteria

  2. Adherence to prompts for early catheter removal

  3. Standardized catheter care guidelines followed

B. Documentation

  1. Dates of insertion and removal

  2. Type of catheter (new indwelling, chronic indwelling, reinsertion, change of device)

  3. Reason for catheter insertion

  4. Justification that catheter is still necessary

(continued)

> **Protocol 19.1: Prevention of Catheter-Associated**
> **Urinary Tract Infection Prevention** *(cont.)*
>
>   5. Post residual void after catheter removal if patient is unable to void in
>   6–8 hours; bladder volume; intervention.
> C. Catheter Utilization
>   1. Monitor unit-specific CAUTI rates.
>   2. Monitor average catheter duration (catheter days).
>   3. Monitor SCIP postoperative catheter removal on catheterization Day 1 or 2.
>   4. Trend unit-specific IUC usage.

ACKNOWLEDGMENTS

The authors would like to thank the New York University (NYU) librarians for their evidence-based search and Karis May for assistance with the formatting of this chapter.

RESOURCES

Association for Professionals in Infection Control and Epidemiology. (2008).*Guide to the elimination of catheter-associated urinary tract infections (CAUTIs): Developing and applying facility-based prevention interventions in acute and long-term care settings.*
http://www.apic.org/Content/NavigationMenu/PracticeGuidance/APICEliminationGuides/CAUTI_Guide_0609.pdf

Centers for Disease Control and Prevention. (2009). *Guideline for prevention of catheter-associated urinary tract infections, 2009.*
http://www.cdc.gov/hicpac/CAUTI/001_CAUTI.html

Gould, C. V., Umscheid, C. A., Agarwal, R. K., Kuntz, G., Pegues, D. A., & Healthcare Infection Control Practices Advisory Committee. (2009). *Guideline for prevention of catheter-associated urinary tract infections 2009.*
http://www.cdc.gov/hicpac/pdf/CAUTI/CAUTIguideline2009final.pdf

Hooton, T. M., Bradley, S. F., Cardenas, D. D., Colgan, R., Geerlings, S. E., Rice, J. C., . . . Nicolle, L. E. (2010). *Diagnosis, prevention, and treatment of catheter-associated urinary tract infection in adults: 2009 international clinical practice guideline from the Infectious Diseases Society of America.*
http://www.idsociety.org/content.aspx?id=4430#uti

International Continence Society (International Consultation on Incontinence Committee [an international group of continence researchers])
http://www.icsoffice.org

Joanna Briggs Institute
http://www.joannabriggs.edu.au/about/home.php

Society for Healthcare Epidemiology of America and the Infectious Diseases Society of America (SHEA-IDSA). (2008). *Compendium of strategies to prevent healthcare-associated infections in acute care hospitals.*
http://www.shea-online.org/about/compendium.cfm

Wound, Ostomy, and Continence Nurses Society Evidence-Based Report Card (EBRC)
http://www.wocn.org/

REFERENCES

Alessandri, F., Mistrangelo, E., Lijoi, D., Ferrero, S., & Ragni, N. (2006). A prospective, randomized trial comparing immediate versus delayed catheter removal following hysterectomy. *Acta Obstetricia Et Gynecologica Scandinavica, 85*(6), 716–720. Evidence Level II.

Apisarnthanarak, A., Rutjanawech, S., Wichansawakun, S., Ratanabunjerdkul, H., Patthranitima, P., Thongphubeth, K., . . . Fraser, V. J. (2007). Initial inappropriate urinary catheters use in a tertiary-care center: Incidence, risk factors, and outcomes. *American Journal of Infection Control, 35*(9), 594–599. Evidence Level V.

Apisarnthanarak, A., Thongphubeth, K., Sirinvaravong, S., Kitkangvan, D., Yuekyen, C., Warachan, B., . . . Fraser, V. J. (2007). Effectiveness of multifaceted hospitalwide quality improvement programs featuring an intervention to remove unnecessary urinary catheters at a tertiary care center in Thailand. *Infection Control and Hospital Epidemiology, 28*(7), 791–798. Evidence Level IV.

Basse, L., Werner, H., & Kehlet, H. (2000). Is urinary drainage necessary during continuous epidural analgesia after colonic resection? *Regional Anesthesia and Pain Medicine, 25*(5), 498–501. Evidence Level II.

BioRelief. (n.d.). *Covidien MAXICARE adult incontinence underpad*. Retrieved from http://biorelief .com/covidienkendall-maxicare-adult-underpad-super-large.html. Evidence Level VI.

Centers for Disease Control and Prevention, National Healthcare Safety Network. (2009). *Catheter-associated urinary tract infection (CAUTI) event*. Retrieved from http://www.cdc.gov/nhsn/pdfs/pscManual/7pscCAUTIcurrent.pdf/

Centers for Medicare and Medicaid Services, Department of Health and Human Services. (2005). *CMS manual system: Pub. 100-07 state operations provider certification*. Retrieved from https://www.cms.gov/transmittals/downloads/R8SOM.pdf/. Evidence Level VI.

Centers for Medicare and Medicaid Services, Department of Health and Human Services. (2007). Medicare Program; changes to the hospital inpatient prospective payment systems and fiscal year 2008 rates. *Federal Register, 72*(162), 47129–48175. Evidence Level VI.

Chia, Y. Y., Wei, R. J., Chang, H. C., & Liu, K. (2009). Optimal duration of urinary catheterization after thoracotomy in patients under postoperative patient-controlled epidural analgesia. *Acta Anaesthesiologica Taiwan: Official Journal of the Taiwan Society of Anesthesiologists, 47*(4), 173–179. Evidence Level II.

Cottenden, A., Bliss, D., Fader, M., Getliffe, K., Herrera, H., Paterson, J., . . . Wilde, M. (2005). Management with continence products. In P. Abrams, L. Cardozo, S. Khoury, & A. Wein (Eds.), *Incontinence: Basics & evaluation* (pp. 149–253). Paris, France: Health Publications Ltd. Evidence Level VI.

Darouiche, R. O., Goetz, L., Kaldis, T., Cerra-Stewart, C., AlSharif, A., & Priebe, M. (2006). Impact of StatLock securing device on symptomatic catheter-related urinary tract infection: A prospective, randomized, multicenter clinical trial. *American Journal of Infection Control, 34*(9), 555–560. Evidence Level II.

Dowling-Castronovo, A., & Bradway, C. (2008). *Nursing standard of practice protocol: Urinary incontinence (UI) in older adults admitted to acute care*. Retrieved from http://consultgerirn.org/topics/urinary_incontinence/want_to_know_more

Drekonja, D. M., Kuskowski, M. A., & Johnson, J. R. (2010). Internet survey of Foley catheter practices and knowledge among Minnesota nurses. *American Journal of Infection Control, 38*(1), 31–37. Evidence Level IV.

Dunn, T. S., Shlay, J., & Forshner, D. (2003). Are in-dwelling catheters necessary for 24 hours after hysterectomy? *American Journal of Obstetrics and Gynecology, 189*(2), 435–437. Evidence Level II.

Elpern, E. H., Killeen, K., Ketchem, A., Wiley, A., Patel, G., & Lateef, O. (2009). Reducing use of indwelling urinary catheters and associated urinary tract infections. *American Journal of Critical Care, 18*(6), 535–542. Evidence Level IV.

Fakih, M. G., Shemes, S. P., Pena, M. E., Dyc, N., Rey, J. E., Szpunar, S. M., & Saravolatz, L. D. (2010). Urinary catheters in the emergency department: Very elderly women are at high risk for unnecessary utilization. *American Journal of Infection Control, 38*(9), 683–688. Evidence Level IV.

Fernandez, R., Griffiths, R., & Murie, P. (2003). Comparison of late night and early morning removal of short-term urethral catheters. *JBI Reports, 1*(1), 1–16. Evidence Level I.

Goetz, A. M., Kedzuf, S., Wagener, M., & Muder, R. R. (1999). Feedback to nursing staff as an intervention to reduce catheter-associated urinary tract infections. *American Journal of Infection Control, 27*(5), 402–404. Evidence Level IV.

Gould, C. V., Umscheid, C. A., Agarwal, R. K., Kuntz, G., Pegues, D. A., & Healthcare Infection Control Practices Advisory Committee. (2009). *Guideline for prevention of catheter-associated urinary tract infections 2009* (pp. 1–67). Retrieved from http://www.cdc.gov/hicpac/pdf/CAUTI/ CAUTIguideline2009final.pdf/. Evidence Level VI.

Gray, M. (2010). Reducing catheter-associated urinary tract infection in the critical care unit. *AACN Advanced Critical Care, 21*(2), 247–257. Evidence Level V.

Greene, L., Marx, J., & Oriola, S. (2008). *Guide to the elimination of catheter-associated urinary tract infections (CAUTIs): Developing and applying facility-based prevention interventions in acute and long-term care settings* (pp. 1–41). Washington, DC: Association for Professionals in Infection Control and Epidemiology. Retrieved from http://www.apic.org/Content/NavigationMenu/ PracticeGuidance/APICEliminationGuides/CAUTI_Guide.pdf/

Hooton, T. M., Bradley, S. F., Cardenas, D. D., Colgan, R., Geerlings, S. E., Rice, J.C., . . . Infectious Diseases Society of America. (2010). Diagnosis, prevention, and treatment of catheter-associated urinary tract infection in adults: 2009 International Clinical Practice Guidelines from the Infectious Diseases Society of America. *Clinical Infectious Diseases, 50*(5), 625–663. Evidence Level VI.

Huang, W. C., Wann, S. R., Lin, S. L., Kunin, C. M., Kung, M. H., Lin, C, H., . . . Lin, T. W. (2004). Catheter-associated urinary tract infections in intensive care units can be reduced by prompting physicians to remove unnecessary catheters. *Infection Control and Hospital Epidemiology, 25*(11), 974–978. Evidence Level V.

Inouye, S. K. (2006). Delirium in older persons. *The New England Journal of Medicine, 354*(11), 1157–1165. Evidence Level IV.

Jeong, I., Park, S., Joeng, J., Sun Kim, D., Choi, Y. S., Lee, Y. S., & Park, Y. M. (2010). Comparison of catheter-associated urinary tract infection rates by perineal care agents in intensive care units. *Asian Nursing Research, 4*(3), 142–150. Evidence Level II.

Joanna Briggs Institute. (2000). Management of short term indwelling urethral catheter to prevent urinary tract infections. *Best Practice: Evidence Based Practice Information Sheets for Health Professionals, 4*(1), 1–6. Retrieved from http://www.joannabriggs.edu.au/pdf/BPISEng_4_1.pdf/

Johnson, J. R., Kuskowski, M. A., & Wilt, T. J. (2006). Systematic review: Antimicrobial urinary catheters to prevent catheter-associated urinary tract infections in hospitalized patients. *Annals of Internal Medicine, 144*(2), 116–126. Evidence Level I.

Junkin, J., & Selekof, J. L. (2008). Beyond "diaper rash": Incontinence-associated dermatitis: Does it have you seeing red? *Nursing, 38*(11 Suppl.), 56hn1–56hn10. Evidence Level VI.

Kabcenell, A., Nolan, T. W., Martin, L. A., & Gill, Y. (2010). *The pursuing perfection initiative: Lessons on transforming health care.* Cambridge, MA: Institute for Healthcare Improvement. Retrieved from http://www.ihi.org/IHI/Results/WhitePapers/PursuingPerfectionInitiative-WhitePaper.htm

Klevens, R. M., Edwards, J. R., Richards, C. L., Jr., Horan, T. C., Gaynes, R. P., Pollock, D. A., & Cardo, D. M. (2007). Estimating health care-associated infections and deaths in US hospitals, 2002. *Public Health Reports, 122*(2), 160–166. Evidence Level V.

Ladak, S. S., Katznelson, R., Muscat, M., Sawhney, M., Beattie, W. S., & O'Leary, G. (2009). Incidence of urinary retention in patients with thoracic patient-controlled epidural analgesia (TCPEA) undergoing thoracotomy. *Pain Management Nursing, 10*(2), 94–98. Evidence Level III.

Lee, Y. Y., Tsay, W. L., Lou, M. F., & Dai, Y. T. (2007). The effectiveness of implementing a bladder ultrasound programme in neurosurgical units. *Journal of Advanced Nursing, 57*(2), 192–200. Evidence Level IV.

Lo, E., Nicolle, L., Classen, D., Arias, K. M., Podgorny, K., Anderson, D. J., . . . Yokoe, D. S. (2008). Strategies to prevent catheter-associated urinary tract infections in acute care hospitals. *Infection Control and Hospital Epidemiology, 29*(Suppl. 1), S41–S50. Evidence Level VI.

Loeb, M., Hunt, D., O'Halloran, K., Carusone, S. C., Dafoe, N., & Walter, S. D. (2008). Stop orders to reduce inappropriate urinary catheterization in hospitalized patients: A randomized controlled trial. *Journal of General Internal Medicine, 23*(6), 816–820. Evidence Level II.

Maki, D. G., & Tambyah, P. A. (2001). Engineering out the risk of infection with urinary catheters. *Emerging Infectious Diseases, 7*(2), 342–347. Evidence Level VI.

Meddings, J., Rogers, M. A., Macy, M., & Saint, S. (2010). Systematic review and meta-analysis: Reminder systems to reduce catheter-associated urinary tract infections and urinary catheter use in hospitalized patients. *Clinical Infectious Diseases: An Official Publication of the Infectious Diseases Society of America, 51*(5), 550–560. Evidence Level I.

Medline. (n.d.). *Protection Plus disposable underpads*. Retrieved from http://www.medline.com/incontinence/underpads/ultrasorbs-ap-disposable-underpads.asp. Evidence Level VI.

Nicolle, L. E., Bradley, S., Colgan, R., Rice, J. C., Schaeffer, A., Hooton, T. M., . . . American Geriatric Society. (2005). Infectious Diseases Society of America guidelines for the diagnosis and treatment of asymptomatic bacteriuria in adults. *Clinical Infectious Disease: An official publication of the Infectious Diseases Society of America, 40*(5), 643–654. Evidence Level VI.

Padula, C. A., Osborne, E., & Williams, J. (2008). Prevention and early detection of pressure ulcers in hospitalized patients. *Journal of Wound, Ostomy, and Continence Nursing, 35*(1), 66–75. Evidence Level V.

Palese, A., Buchini, S., Deroma, L., & Barbone, F. (2010). The effectiveness of the ultrasound bladder scanner in reducing urinary tract infections: A meta-analysis. *Journal of Clinical Nursing, 19*(21–22), 2970–2979. doi: 10.1111/j.1365-2702.2010.03281.x. Evidence Level I.

Parker, D., Callan, L., Harwood, J., Thompson, D. L., Wilde, M., & Gray, M. (2009). Nursing interventions to reduce the risk of catheter-associated urinary tract infection. Part 1: Catheter selection. *Journal of Wound, Ostomy, and Continence Nursing, 36*(1), 23–34. Evidence Level V.

Patient Protection and Affordable Care Act of 2010, H.R. 3590, 111th Cong. (2010). Retrieved from http://democrats.senate.gov/reform/patient-protection-affordable-care-act-as-passed.pdf/

Reinertsen, J. L., Bisognano, M., & Pugh, M. D. (2008). *Seven leadership leverage points for organization-level improvement in health care* (2nd ed.). Cambridge, MA: Institute for Healthcare Improvement. Retrieved from http://www.ihi.org

Saint, S. (2000). Clinical and economic consequences of nosocomial catheter-related bacteriuria. *American Journal of Infection Control, 28*(1), 68–75. Evidence Level VI.

Saint, S., Kaufman, S. R., Rogers, M. A., Baker, P. D., Ossenkop, K., & Lipsky, B. A. (2006). Condom versus indwelling urinary catheters: A randomized trial. *Journal of the American Geriatrics Society, 54*(7), 1055–1061. Evidence Level II.

Saint, S., Kowalski, C. P., Kaufman, S. R., Hofer, T. P., Kauffman, C. A., Olmsted, R. N., . . . Krein, S. L. (2008). Preventing hospital-acquired urinary tract infection in the United States: A national study. *Clinical Infectious Disease: An official publication of the Infectious Diseases Society of America, 46*(2), 243–250. Evidence Level IV.

Saint, S., Lipsky, B. A., & Goold, S. D. (2002). Indwelling urinary catheters: A one-point restraint? *Annals of Internal Medicine, 137*(2), 125–127. Evidence Level VI.

Saint, S., Olmsted, R. N., Fakih, M. G., Kowalski, C. P., Watson, S. R., Sales, A. E., & Krein, S. L. (2009). Translating health care-associated urinary tract infection prevention research into practice via the bladder bundle. *Joint Commission Journal on Quality Patient Safety/Joint Commission Resources, 35*(9), 449–455. Evidence Level V.

Saint, S., Wiese, J., Amory, J. K., Bernstein, M. L., Patel, U. D., Zemencuk, J. K., . . . Hofer, T. P. (2000). Are physicians aware of which of their patients have indwelling urinary catheters? *The American Journal of Medicine, 109*(6), 476–480. Evidence Level IV.

Tambyah, P. H., Knasinski, V., & Maki, D. G. (2002). The direct costs of nosocomial catheter-associated urinary tract infection in the era of managed care. *Infection Control and Hospital Epidemiology, 23*(1), 27–31. Evidence Level IV.

Titler, M. G., & Everett, L. Q. (2006). Sustain an infrastructure to support EBP. *Nursing Management, 37*(9), 14, 16. Evidence Level VI.

Wald, H. L., Epstein, A., & Kramer, A. (2005). Extended use of indwelling urinary catheters in postoperative hip fracture patients. *Medical Care, 43*(10), 1009–1017. Evidence Level IV.

Wald, H. L., Ma, A., Bratzler, D. W., & Kramer, A. M. (2008). Indwelling urinary catheter use in the postoperative period: Analysis of the national surgical infection prevention project data. *Archives of Surgery, 143*(6), 551–557. Evidence Level VI.

Wallin, L., Profetto-McGrath, J., & Levers, M. J. (2005). Implementing nursing practice guidelines: A complex undertaking. *Journal of Wound, Ostomy, and Continence Nursing, 32*(5), 294–301. Evidence Level VI.

Weinstein, J. W., Mazon, D., Pantelick, E., Reagan-Cirincione, P., Dembry, L. M., & Hierholzer, W. J., Jr. (1999). A decade of prevalence surveys in a tertiary-care center: Trends in nosocomial infection rates, device utilization, and patient acuity. *Infection Control and Hospital Epidemiology, 20*(8), 543–548. Evidence Level IV.

Wenger, J. E. (2010). Cultivating quality: Reducing rates of catheter-associated urinary tract infection. *American Journal of Nursing, 110*(8), 40–45. Evidence Level V.

Willson, M., Wilde, M., Webb, M. L., Thompson, D., Parker, D., Harwood, J., . . . Gray, M. (2009). Nursing interventions to reduce the risk of catheter-associated urinary tract infection: Part 2: Staff education, monitoring, and care techniques. *Journal of Wound, Ostomy, and Continence Nursing, 36*(2), 137–154. Evidence Level V.

Zaouter, C., Kaneva, P., & Carli, F. (2009). Less urinary tract infection by earlier removal of bladder catheter in surgical patients receiving thoracic epidural analgesia. *Regional Anesthesia and Pain Medicine, 34*(6), 542–548. Evidence Level II.

Zhan, C., Elixhauser, A., Richards, C. L., Jr., Wang, Y., Baine, W., Pineau, M., . . . Hunt, D. (2009). Identification of hospital-acquired catheter-associated urinary tract infections from Medicare claims: Sensitivity and positive predictive value. *Medical Care, 47*(3), 364–369. Evidence Level IV.

Oral Health Care

20

Linda J. O'Connor

EDUCATIONAL OBJECTIVES

On completion of this chapter, the reader will be able to:

1. discuss the consequences of poor oral health
2. describe a thorough oral assessment in the older adult
3. describe the oral hygiene plan of care for nonintubated older adults
4. discuss nursing interventions for oral care

OVERVIEW

Poor oral health is associated with malnutrition, dehydration, brain abscesses, valvular heart disease, joint infections, cardiovascular disease, pneumonia, aspiration pneumonia, and poor glycemic control in type I and II diabetes (Abe et al., 2006; Adachi, Ishihara, Abe, & Okuda, 2007; Azarpazhooh & Leake, 2006; Bingham, Ashley, De Jong, & Swift, 2010; Coulthwaite & Verran, 2007; Ferozali, Johnson, & Cavagnaro, 2007; Kelsey & Lamster, 2008; Lockhart et al., 2009; Sato, Yoshihara, & Miyazaki, 2006; Sjögren, Nilsson, Forsell, Johansson, & Hoogstraate, 2008; Tran & Mannen, 2009; Touger-Decker & Mobley, 2007). Oral health also affects nutritional status, ability to speak, self-esteem, mental wellness, and overall well-being (Coulthwaite & Verran, 2007; Touger-Decker & Mobley, 2007; Gil-Montoya, Subirá, Ramón, & González-Moles, 2008; Kanehisa, Yoshida, Taji, Akagawa, & Nakamura, 2009; Quandt et al., 2010; Soini et al., 2006; Haumschild & Haumschild, 2009; Montero, López, Galindo, Vicente, & Bravo, 2009; Naito et al., 2010). Many oral diseases are not part of the natural aging process but side effects of medical treatment and medications.

BACKGROUND AND STATEMENT OF PROBLEM

Plaque retention is a problem in older adults who have difficulty in mechanically removing plaque caused by diminished manual dexterity, impaired vision, or chronic

For description of Evidence Levels cited in this chapter, see Chapter 1, Developing and Evaluating Clinical Practice Guidelines: A Systematic Approach, page 7.

illness (Coulthwaite & Verran, 2007; Brown, Goryakin, & Finlayson, 2009; Hakuta, Mori, Ueno, Shinada, & Kawaguchi, 2009; Ibayashi, Fujino, Pham, & Matsuda, 2008). An older adult's functional ability and cognitive status affect their ability to perform oral care and denture care. Dental plaque harbors microorganisms including *Streptococcus, Staphylococcus*, gram-positive rods, gram-negative rods, and yeasts (Coulthwaite & Verran, 2007). Dentures also have the potential to harbor *Streptococcus pneumoniae, Haemophilus influenza, Escherichia coli, Klebsiella*, and *Pseudomonas* secondary to spending time in nonhygienic environments (Coulthwaite & Verran, 2007). Dentures have been seen thrown in with patients' clothing, thrown in a washbasin or other container with bathing items, and so forth, instead of being properly cleaned and stored in a denture cup. Lack of good oral hygiene increases the risk for development of secondary infections, extended hospital stays, and significant negative health outcomes.

Multiple medications produce side effects that affect the oral cavity. Cardiac medications can cause salivary dysfunction, gingival enlargement, and lichenoid mucosal reactions. Steroid treatment can predispose a patient to oral candidiasis, and cancer treatments can cause a plethora of oral conditions such as stomatitis, salivary hypofunction, microbial infections, and xerostomia.

The mouth reflects the culmination of multiple stressors over the years and as the mouth ages, it is less able to tolerate these stressors. With an increase in chronic disease and medication usage as a person ages, the prevalence of root caries, tooth loss, oral cancers, soft tissue lesions, and periodontal problems increases significantly (Touger-Decker & Mobley, 2007; Christensen, 2007; Saunders & Friedman, 2007). Many of the oral health problems in the older adults could be avoided with routine preventive care. Many older adults believe in the myth that a decline in their oral health is a normal part of aging.

ASSESSMENT OF THE PROBLEM

Physical Assessment

The promotion of oral health through assessment and good oral hygiene is an essential of nursing care. The oral assessment is part of the nurse's head-to-toe assessment of the older adult and is done on admission and at the beginning of each shift. The nurse assesses the condition of the oral cavity, which should be pink, moist, and intact; the presence of or absence of natural teeth and/or dentures; ability to function with or without natural teeth and/or dentures; and the patient's ability to speak, chew, or swallow. Natural teeth should be intact, and dentures (partial or full) should fit comfortably and not be moving when the older adult is speaking. Any abnormal findings such as dryness, swelling, sores, ulcers, bleeding, white patches, broken or decayed teeth, halitosis, ill-fitting dentures, difficulty swallowing, signs of aspiration, and pain are documented by the nurse, and the health care team informed.

Poorly fitting dentures can cause ulcerations and candidiasis (oral fungal infection, masses, and denture stomatitis). Denture stomatitis presents as red, inflamed tissue beneath dentures, caused by fungal infections and insufficient oral hygiene. Some oral mucosal diseases that nursing may see are angular cheilitis (red and white cracked lesions in the corners of the mouth, caused by inflammation and a fungal infection), cicatricial pemphigoid (produces red, inflamed lesions on the gingival, palate, tongue, and cheek tissues), Lichen planus (most common form presents as a lacy white appearance on the tongue and/or cheeks), and Pemphigus vulgaris (red bleeding tissues result from trauma but heal without scarring). Untreated lesions can develop into large, infected regions, which require immediate medical attention. Dental professionals diagnose oral mucosal diseases, but the nurse needs to be aware of any abnormal findings and report them immediately.

The nurse also needs to assess the patient for their functional ability and manual dexterity to provide oral hygiene. The nurse needs to observe the older adult providing their oral hygiene to make sure that it is effective. The primary focus for nurses is to maintain the older adult's function so that older adults may participate in their daily care. Once the older adult provides their oral hygiene, the nurse must follow-up as appropriate to complete the oral hygiene.

Assessment Tools

The Oral Health Assessment Tool (OHAT) is an eight-category screening tool that can be used with cognitively intact or impaired older adults. The OHAT provides an organized, efficient method for nurses to document their oral assessment. The eight categories (lips, tongue, gums and tissues, saliva, natural teeth, dentures, oral cleanliness, and dental pain) are scored from 0 (*healthy*) to 2 (*unhealthy*). Total scores range from 0 to 16; the higher the score, the poorer the older adult's oral health (Chalmers, King, Spencer, Wright, & Carter, 2005). The OHAT may be implemented in any health care setting. See Resource section for access to this tool.

INTERVENTION AND CARE STRATEGIES

The gold standard for providing oral hygiene is the toothbrush. Toothbrushes should have soft nylon bristles (Pearson & Chalmers, 2004). It is the mechanical action of the toothbrush that is important for plaque removal. If the older adult has any decrease in their function or manual dexterity, the nursing staff needs to assess the older adult's ability to provide effective oral hygiene and provide assistance as needed. Foam swabs are available in numerous facilities to provide oral hygiene. Research has shown that foam swabs cannot remove plaque as well as toothbrushes (Pearson & Hutton, 2002). Foam swabs may be used for cleaning the oral mucous of an edentulous older adult.

Lemon-glycerin swabs or swab sticks are drying to the oral mucosa and cause erosion of the tooth enamel. This, combined with decreased salivary flow and an increased rate of xerostomia in the older adult, potentiates the corrosive effect of lemon-glycerin swabs (Pearson & Chalmers, 2004). Lemon-glycerin swabs or swab sticks are detrimental to the older adult and are never to be used.

Commercial mouth rinses, which contain alcohol are very trying to the oral mucosa. If an older adult is using a commercial mouth rinse with alcohol, a half-and-half mixture (commercial mouthwash and water) is recommended. Toothpaste with fluoride is currently recommended by the American Dental Association to reduce cavities and can also help to reduce periodontal disease.

The use of chlorhexidine in the geriatric patient is determined by the dentist. There are some side effects of chlorhexidine (bitter taste, change in the taste of food, mouth irritation, staining of teeth, mouth, fillings, and dentures) that may have negative outcomes for the older adult (Quagliarello et al., 2009). A good oral assessment by the nurse each shift is essential for the geriatric patient on chlorhexidine and monitoring of their nutritional intake.

Education of the nursing staff is imperative. Two of the major barriers cited by nursing staff are inadequate knowledge of how to assess and provide care and lack of appropriate supplies. Implementation of evidence-based protocols combined with ongoing educational training sessions have been demonstrated to have a positive impact on oral care being provided and on the oral health status of older adults (Touger-Decker et al., 2007; Akar & Ergül, 2008; Dharamsi, Jivani, Dean, & Wyatt, 2009; Gluhak, Arnetzl, Kirmeier, Jakse, & Arnetzl, 2010; Peltola, Vehkalahti, & Simoila, 2007; Preston, Kearns, Barber, & Gosney, 2006; Reed, Broder, Jenkins, Spivack, & Janal, 2006; Ribeiro et al., 2009; Young, Murray, & Thomson, 2008). Staff needs to be instructed on oral hygiene and the proper care of different appliances. Dentures should be brushed before placing them into a denture cup. Dentures should be removed at night, but some older adults prefer to keep their dentures in continuously. It therefore becomes even more important for the nurse to do an assessment of the oral mucosa. In the acute care and long-term care setting, the older adult may not have dental adhesive and, therefore, there is a high risk for food particles to get caught underneath of their dentures. It is important that staff remember to take the dentures out after each meal, rinse them and the patient's mouth, and place the dentures back in. Complete denture care should be given morning, night, and as needed.

Education of nursing staff, older adults, and families is imperative. Nurses need to be educated in oral assessment and nursing assistants need to be educated in observation of the oral cavity and what to report to the nurse. Both nurses and nursing assistants need to be educated in the proper techniques for providing oral hygiene and caring for oral appliances. Patients and families need to be educated in the importance of good oral health and hygiene and to dispel the oral health myths that exist about oral health and aging in general.

Education focused on the importance of good oral health and hygiene in the older adult, the myths about oral health and aging, evidence-based practice protocols, implementing these protocols, and the appropriate products for providing oral hygiene to their patients and residents must be provided to administrators. Without the proper supplies, it is impossible for the nursing staff to provide the oral hygiene care the older adult needs and to properly implement evidence-based protocols for oral health and hygiene in the older adult.

CASE STUDY

Mrs. Smith, an 84-year-old female with a history of Alzheimer's Type Dementia, was admitted for recent decreased oral intake and percutaneous endoscopic gastrostomy (PEG) placement. Mrs. Smith was alert, oriented to herself, pleasant, cooperative with care, and able to follow simple directions. She lived at home with her family and received care from a home health aide. The initial oral assessment was done on Day 2 of admission and found upper dentures and lower natural teeth, both covered with

(continued)

CASE STUDY *(continued)*

food particles. Her oral mucosa was noted to be dry. The upper dentures were difficult to remove and caused her pain. The upper denture was being "kept in place" by a collection of old food, which was found upon removal. The oral mucosa under the upper denture was covered with sores and ulcers—bleeding, infected, and very painful. The health team was notified; a dental consult was called; and an oral hygiene plan of care was implemented. Mrs. Smith's diet was changed to puree while her oral mucosa was healing and the PEG placement was put on hold. Upon inquiry, it was learned from the family that their long-time aide had just moved, and the new aide had been with them only a few months. It was during this time that they noticed the decline in Mrs. Smith's nutritional intake. The family chose to hire a new aide, and both the family and the new aide were educated on proper oral hygiene for Mrs. Smith. Once Mrs. Smith's oral mucosa had healed, the upper denture was replaced, and she was returned to her regular diet. Her oral intake returned to baseline, and a PEG was no longer required.

This case study illustrates how poor oral care often goes undetected, the importance of good oral care, the need for physical assessment by the nurse, and the need for staff and family education. This patient was being admitted for an invasive procedure secondary to poor oral health caused by poor oral care. Although the family was involved in Mrs. Smith's care (she had no contractures or skin breakdown), her lack of oral care had gone unnoticed by them. The admitting nurse documented that the patient had dentures on the admission form but did not do a physical oral assessment. The nurse caring for the patient on Day 2 had attended an oral health seminar and included the physical oral assessment in her morning rounds. She also followed up with the nursing assistants to ensure that oral care had been provided to the patient after each meal. The implementation of an oral hygiene plan of care and education of nursing staff, family, and home care staff ensured that Mrs. Smith received the oral care required for her oral mucosa to heal, her nutritional status to return to baseline, and prevented the unnecessary placement of a PEG.

SUMMARY

As previously stated, many of the oral health problems in the older adults could be avoided with routine preventive care, but many older adults believe in the myth that a decline in their oral health is a normal part of aging (Allen, O'Sullivan, & Locker, 2009; Borreani, Jones, Scambler, & Gallagher, 2010; Gagliardi, Slade, & Sanders, 2008; McKenzie-Green, Giddings, Buttle, & Tahana, 2009; Wyatt, 2009). To dispel this myth and improve the oral health of older adults, it is imperative that health care professionals provide continuing education to patients and families, advocate for oral health prevention, and provide oral care to older adults in all settings. Well-developed evidence-based oral care protocols and educational training sessions have been demonstrated to have a positive impact on the oral health status of older patients.

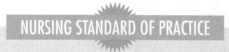

Protocol 20.1: Providing Oral Health Care to Older Adults

I. OVERVIEW: The promotion of oral health through good oral hygiene is an essential of nursing care. The registered nurse (RN) or designee provides regular oral care for functionally dependent and cognitively impaired older adults.

II. BACKGROUND:
  A. Oral hygiene is directly linked with systemic infections, cardiac disease, cerebrovascular accident, acute myocardial infarction, glucose control in diabetes, nutritional intake, comfort, ability to speak, and the patient's self-esteem and overall well-being.
  B. Definitions
    1. Oral: refers to the mouth (natural teeth, gingival and supporting tissues, hard and soft palate, mucosal lining of the mouth and throat, tongue, salivary glands, chewing muscles, upper and lower jaw, lips).
    2. Oral cavity: includes cheeks, hard and soft palate.
    3. Oral hygiene: the prevention of plaque-related disease, the destruction of plaque through the mechanical action of tooth brushing and flossing, or use of other oral hygiene aides.
    4. Edentulous: natural teeth removed.

III. PARAMETERS OF ASSESSMENT:
  A. The RN conducts an oral assessment or evaluation on admission and every shift. The nurse assesses the condition of:
    1. The oral cavity: The oral cavity should be pink, moist, and intact.
    2. The presence of or absence of natural teeth and/or dentures: Natural teeth should be intact and dentures (partial or full) should fit comfortably and not be moving when the older adult is speaking.
    3. Ability to function with or without natural teeth and/or dentures.
    4. The patient's ability to speak, chew, or swallow.
    5. Any abnormal findings such as dryness, swelling, sores, ulcers, bleeding, white patches, broken or decayed teeth, halitosis, ill-fitting dentures, difficulty swallowing, signs of aspiration, pain are documented by the nurse, and the health care team informed.
  B. Assessment Tool: The Oral Health Assessment Tool (OHAT). See Resources section for tool.

IV. NURSING CARE STRATEGIES:
  A. Oral Hygiene Plan of Care: Dependent Mouth Care of the Edentulous Patient
    1. Oral care is provided during morning care, evening care, and as needed (PRN).
    2. Wash hands and don gloves.

(continued)

Protocol 20.1: Providing Oral Health Care to Older Adults *(cont.)*

   3. Remove dentures.
   4. Brush dentures with toothbrush/toothpaste using up-and-down motion.
   5. Clean the grooved area, which fits against the gum with the toothbrush. Rinse with cool water.
   6. Brush patient's tongue.
   7. Re-insert dentures.
   8. Apply lip moisturizer.
  B. Dependent Mouth Care: Patient With Teeth or Partial Dentures
   1. Oral care is provided during morning care, evening care, and PRN.
   2. Wash hands and don gloves.
   3. Place soft toothbrush at an angle against the gum line. Gently brush teeth in an up-and-down motion with short strokes using the toothbrush.
   4. Brush patient's tongue.
   5. Apply lip moisturizer.
For partial dentures, follow procedure for full denture cleaning and insertion.
  C. Assisted or Supervised Care
   1. Oral care is provided during morning care, evening care, and PRN.
   2. Assess what patient can do and provide assistance as needed.
   3. Set up necessary items.

V. EVALUATION OF EXPECTED OUTCOMES
  A. Patient
   1. Will receive oral hygiene a minimum of once every 8 hours while in the acute care or long-term care or home setting.
   2. Patients and families will be referred to dental services for follow-up treatment.
   3. Patients and families will be educated on the importance of good oral hygiene and follow-up dental services.
  B. Professional Caregiver or RN will
   1. Conduct an assessment or evaluation of the oral cavity on admission and every shift.
   2. Notify the physician and dentist of any abnormalities present in the oral cavity.
   3. Assess what each patient can do independently.
   4. Observe aspiration precautions while providing care.
   5. Provide oral care and dental care education to patients and families.
  C. Institution
   1. Will provide access to dental services as appropriate.
   2. Will provide ongoing education to health care providers.
   3. Will provide a yearly oral health and dental care in-service to health care providers.

RESOURCES

Assessment Tools

Chalmers, J. M., King, P. L., Spencer, A. J., Wright, F. A., & Carter, K. D. (2005). The oral health assessment tool—validity and reliability. *Australian Dental Journal, 50*(3), 191–199.

Related Professional Organizations

Academy of General Dentistry
http://www.agd.org

American Dental Association
http://www.ada.org

Government Information Agencies

National Institutes on Aging
http://www.newcart.niapublications.org

National Institute of Dental and Craniofacial Research
http://www.nidcr.nih.gov

Centers for Disease Control and Prevention
http://www.cdc.gov

Regulatory or Authoritative Sites

National Institute of Dental and Craniofacial Research
http://www.nidcr.nih.gov

American Dental Association
http://www.ada.org

Continuing Education Opportunities

http://www.Hartford IGN.org

Patient and Family Resources

American Dental Association
http://www.ada.org

National Institute of Dental and Craniofacial Research
http://www.nidcr.nih.gov

REFERENCES

Abe, S., Ishihara, K., Adachi, M., Sasaki, H., Tanaka, K., & Okuda, K. (2006). Professional oral care reduces influenza infection in elderly. *Archives of Gerontology and Geriatrics, 43*(2), 157–164. Evidence Level II.

Adachi, M., Ishihara, K., Abe, S., & Okuda, K. (2007). Professional oral health care by dental hygienists reduced respiratory infections in elderly persons requiring nursing care. *International Journal of Dental Hygiene, 5*(2), 69–74. Evidence Level III.

Akar, G. C., & Ergül, S. (2008). The oral hygiene and denture status among residential home residents. *Clinical Oral Investigations, 12*(1), 61–65. Evidence Level V.

Allen, P. F., O'Sullivan, M., & Locker, D. (2009). Determining the minimally important difference for the Oral Health Impact Profile-20. *European Journal of Oral Sciences, 117*(2), 129–134. Evidence Level IV.

Azarpazhooh, A., & Leake, J. L. (2006). Systematic review of the association between respiratory diseases and oral health. *Journal of Periodontology, 77*(9), 1465–1482. Evidence Level I.

Bingham, M., Ashley, J., De Jong, M., & Swift, C. (2010). Implementing a unit-level intervention to reduce the probability of ventilator-associated pneumonia. *Nursing Research, 59*(Suppl. 1), S40–S47. Evidence Level IV.

Borreani, E., Jones, K., Scambler, S., & Gallagher, J. E. (2010). Informing the debate on oral health care for older people: A qualitative study of older people's views on oral health and oral health care. *Gerodontology, 27*(1), 11–18. Evidence Level IV.

Brown, T. T., Goryakin, Y., & Finlayson, T. L. (2009). The effect of functional limitations on the demand for dental care among adults 65 and older. *Journal of the California Dental Association, 37*(8), 549–558. Evidence Level V.

Chalmers, J. M., King, P. L., Spencer, A. J., Wright, F. A., & Carter, K. D. (2005). The oral health assessment tool—validity and reliability. *Australian Dental Journal, 50*(3), 191–199. Evidence Level III.

Christensen, G. J. (2007). Providing oral care for the aging patient. *Journal of the American Dental Association (1939), 138*(2), 239–242. Evidence Level V.

Coulthwaite, L., & Verran, J. (2007). Potential pathogenic aspects of denture plaque. *British Journal of Biomedical Science, 64*(4), 180–189. Evidence Level V.

Dharamsi, S., Jivani, K., Dean, C., & Wyatt, C. (2009). Oral care for frail elders: Knowledge, attitudes, and practices of long-term care staff. *Journal of Dental Education, 73*(5), 581–588. Evidence Level V.

Ferozali, F., Johnson, G., & Cavagnaro, A. (2007). Health benefits and reductions in bacteria from enhanced oral care. *Special Care in Dentistry, 27*(5), 168–176. Evidence Level II.

Gagliardi, D. I., Slade, G. D., & Sanders, A. E. (2008). Impact of dental care on oral health-related quality of life and treatment goals among elderly adults. *Australian Dental Journal, 53*(1), 26–33. Evidence Level V.

Gil-Montoya, J. A., Subirá, C., Ramón, J. M., & González-Moles, M. A. (2008). Oral health-related quality of life and nutritional status. *Journal of Public Health Dentistry, 68*(2), 88–93. Evidence Level IV.

Gluhak, C., Arnetzl, G. V., Kirmeier, R., Jakse, N., & Arnetzl, G. (2010). Oral status among seniors in nine nursing homes in Styria, Austria. *Gerodontology, 27*(1), 47–52. Evidence Level IV.

Hakuta, C., Mori, C., Ueno, M., Shinada, K., & Kawaguchi, Y. (2009). Evaluation of an oral function promotion programme for the independent elderly in Japan. *Gerodontology, 26*(4), 250–258. Evidence Level IV.

Haumschild, M. S., & Haumschild, R. J. (2009). The importance of oral health in long-term care. *Journal of the American Medical Directors Association, 10*(9), 667–671. Evidence Level V.

Ibayashi, H., Fujino, Y., Pham, T. M., & Matsuda, S. (2008). Intervention study of exercise program for oral function in healthy elderly people. *The Tohoku Journal of Experimental Medicine, 215*(3), 237–245. Evidence Level II.

Kanehisa, Y., Yoshida, M., Taji, T., Akagawa, Y., & Nakamura, H. (2009). Body weight and serum albumin change after prosthodontic treatment among institutionalized elderly in a long-term care geriatric hospital. *Community Dentistry and Oral Epidemiology, 37*(6), 534–538. Evidence Level IV.

Kelsey, J. L., & Lamster, I. B. (2008). Influence of musculoskeletal conditions on oral health among older adults. *American Journal of Public Health, 98*(7), 1177–1183. Evidence Level V.

Lockhart, P. B., Brennan, M. T., Thornhill, M., Michalowicz, B. S., Noll, J., Bahrani-Mougeot, F. K., & Sasser, H. C. (2009). Poor oral hygiene as a risk factor for infective endocarditis-related bacteremia. *Journal of the American Dental Association (1939), 140*(10), 1238–1244. Evidence Level II.

McKenzie-Green, B., Giddings, L. S., Buttle, L., & Tahana, K. (2009). Older peoples' perceptions of oral health: "It's just not that simple". *International Journal of Dental Hygiene, 7*(1), 31–38. Evidence Level V.

Montero, J., López, J. F., Galindo, M. P., Vicente, P., & Bravo, M. (2009). Impact of prosthodontic status on oral wellbeing: A cross-sectional cohort study. *Journal of Oral Rehabilitation*, *36*(8), 592–600. Evidence Level IV.

Naito, M., Kato, T., Fujii, W., Ozeki, M., Yokoyama, M., Hamajima, N., & Saitoh, E. (2010). Effects of dental treatment on the quality of life and activities of daily living in institutionalized elderly in Japan. *Archives of Gerontology and Geriatrics*, *50*(1), 65–68. Evidence Level V.

Pearson, A., & Chalmers, J. (2004). Oral hygiene care for adults with dementia in residential aged care facilities. *JBI Reports, 2*, 65–113. Evidence Level VI.

Pearson, L. S., & Hutton, J. L. (2002). A controlled trial to compare the ability of foam swabs and toothbrushes to remove dental plaque. *Journal of Advanced Nursing, 39*(5), 480–489. Evidence Level II.

Peltola, P., Vehkalahti, M. M., & Simoila, R. (2007). Effects of 11-month interventions on oral cleanliness among the long-term hospitalised elderly. *Gerodontology*, *24*(1), 14–21. Evidence Level II.

Preston, A. J., Kearns, A., Barber, M. W., & Gosney, M. A. (2006). The knowledge of healthcare professionals regarding elderly persons' oral care. *British Dental Journal*, *201*(5), 293–295. Evidence Level IV.

Quagliarello, V., Juthani-Mehta, M., Ginter, S., Towle, V., Allore, H., & Tinetti, M. (2009). Pilot testing of intervention protocols to prevent pneumonia in nursing home residents. *Journal of the American Geriatrics Society*, *57*(7), 1226–1231. Evidence Level II.

Quandt, S. A., Chen, H., Bell, R. A., Savoca, M. R., Anderson, A. M., Leng, X., . . . Arcury, T. A. (2010). Food avoidance and food modification practices of older rural adults: Association with oral health status and implications for service provision. *Gerontologist*, *50*(1), 100–111. Evidence Level V.

Reed, R., Broder, H. L., Jenkins, G., Spivack, E., & Janal, M. N. (2006). Oral health promotion among older persons and their care providers in a nursing home facility. *Gerodontology*, *23*(2), 73–78. Evidence Level V.

Ribeiro, D. G., Pavarina, A. C., Giampaolo, E. T., Machado, A. L., Jorge, J. H., & Garcia, P. P. (2009). Effect of oral hygiene education and motivation on removable partial denture wearers: Longitudinal study. *Gerodontology*, *26*(2), 150–156. Evidence Level II.

Sato, M., Yoshihara, A., & Miyazaki, H. (2006). Preliminary study on the effect of oral care on recovery from surgery in elderly patients. *Journal of Oral Rehabilitation*, *33*(11), 820–826. Evidence Level II.

Saunders, R., & Friedman, B. (2007). Oral health conditions of community-dwelling cognitively intact elderly persons with disabilities. *Gerodontology*, *24*(2), 67–76. Evidence Level IV.

Sjögren, P., Nilsson, E., Forsell, M., Johansson, O., & Hoogstraate, J. (2008). A systematic review of the preventive effect of oral hygiene on pneumonia and respiratory tract infection in elderly people in hospitals and nursing homes: Effect estimates and methodological quality of randomized controlled trials. *Journal of the American Geriatrics Society*, *56*(11), 2124–2130.

Soini, H., Muurinen, S., Routasalo, P., Sandelin, E., Savikko, N., Suominen, M., . . . Pitkala, K. H. (2006). Oral and nutritional status—Is the MNA a useful tool for dental clinics. *The Journal of Nutrition, Health & Aging*, *10*(6), 495–499. Evidence Level V.

Touger-Decker, R., & Mobley, C. C. (2007). Position of the American Dietetic Association: Oral health and nutrition. *Journal of the American Dietetic Association*, *107*(8), 1418–1428. Evidence Level VI.

Tran, P., & Mannen, J. (2009). Improving oral healthcare: Improving the quality of life for patients after a stroke. *Special Care in Dentistry*, *29*(5), 218–221.

Wyatt, C. C. (2009). A 5-year follow-up of older adults residing in long-term care facilities: Utilisation of a comprehensive dental programme. *Gerodontology*, *26*(4), 282–290. Evidence Level V.

Young, B. C., Murray, C. A., & Thomson, J. (2008). Care home staff knowledge of oral care compared to best practice: A west of Scotland pilot study. *British Dental Journal*, *205*(8), E15. Evidence Level V.

Managing Oral Hydration

21

Janet C. Mentes

EDUCATIONAL OBJECTIVES

On completion of this chapter, the reader should be able to:

1. describe older adults at risk for dehydration
2. identify key aspects of a hydration assessment
3. list specific interventions to promote hydration in older adults across care settings
4. identify outcomes of a hydration management program

OVERVIEW

A recent study using markers (serum sodium, osmolality, and blood urea nitrogen [BUN]/creatinine ratio) for dehydration and volume depletion from the Established Populations for Epidemiologic Studies of the Elderly (EPESE; Stookey, Pieper, & Cohen, 2005) and National Health and Nutrition Examination Survey III (NHANES III; Stookey, 2005) found that the prevalence rate for these conditions in community-dwelling older adults could range from 0.5% to 60% depending on the markers used. Another study found that 48% of older adults presenting with dehydration at an emergency room (ER) unit were from the community (Bennett, Thomas, & Riegel, 2004). Maintaining adequate fluid balance is an essential component of health across the lifespan; older adults are more vulnerable to shifts in water balance—both overhydration and dehydration—because of age-related changes and increased likelihood that an older individual has several medical conditions. Dehydration is the more frequent occurrence in older adults (Warren et al., 1994; Xiao, Barber, & Campbell, 2004). In fact, avoidable hospitalizations for dehydration in older adults have increased by 40%

For description of Evidence Levels cited in this chapter, see Chapter 1, Developing and Evaluating Clinical Practice Guidelines: A Systematic Approach, page 7.
Note. Portions of this chapter were adapted with permission from Mentes, J. C., & Kang, S. (2010). Evidence-based protocol: Hydration management. In M. G. Titler (Series Ed.), *Series on evidence-based practice for older adults.* Iowa City, IA: University of Iowa College of Nursing Gerontological Nursing Interventions Research Center, Research Translation and Dissemination Core.

from 1990 to 2000, at a cost of $1.14 billion (Xiao et al., 2004), and is one of the Agency for Healthcare Research and Quality's 13 ambulatory care-sensitive conditions.

Not only will careful attention to hydration requirements of older adults help prevent hospitalizations for dehydration but will also decrease associated conditions such as acute confusion and delirium (Foreman, 1989; Mentes & Culp, 2003; Mentes, Culp, Maas, & Rantz, 1999; O'Keeffe & Lavan, 1996; Seymour, Henschke, Cape, & Campbell, 1980); adverse drug reactions (Doucet et al., 2002); infections (Beaujean et al., 1997; Masotti et al., 2000); and increased morbidity associated with bladder cancer (Michaud et al., 1999), coronary heart disease (Chan, Knutsen, Blix, Lee, & Fraser, 2002; Rasouli, Kiasari, & Arab, 2008), stroke (Rodriguez et al., 2009), and other thromboembolytic events (Kelly et al., 2004). Further, dehydration has been associated with longer hospital stays for rehabilitation (Mukand, Cai, Zielinski, Danish, & Berman, 2003) and for readmission to the hospital (Gordon, An, Hayward, & Williams, 1998). Even in healthy community-dwelling older adults, physical performance and cognitive processing is affected by mild dehydration (Ainslie et al., 2002).

Oral hydration of older adults is particularly complex for a variety of reasons. In the following review, issues of age-related changes, risk factors, assessment measures, and nursing strategies for effective interventions for dehydration are addressed.

BACKGROUND AND STATEMENT OF PROBLEM

Water is an essential component of body composition. Intricate cellular functions such as gene expression, protein synthesis, and uptake and metabolism of nutrients are affected by hydration status. Organ systems, specifically the cardiovascular and renal systems, are particularly vulnerable to fluctuating levels of hydration (Metheny, 2000).

Older individuals are at increased risk for hydration problems stemming from several *converging age-related factors* including lack of thirst (Ainslie et al., 2002; Phillips, Bretherton, Johnston, & Gray, 1991; Phillips et al., 1984); changes in body composition, specifically loss of fluid rich muscle tissue (Bossingham, Carnell, & Campbell, 2005); increasing inability to respond efficiently to physiological stressful events where dehydration results (Farrell et al., 2008; Rolls, 1998); and renal changes including a reduced renal capacity to handle water and sodium efficiently (Macias-Nuñez, 2008). Additionally, personal, often lifetime *hydration habits*, may contribute to risk but have not been explored in relation to underhydration. As a result, older adults are often at risk for a chronic state of underhydration. Several studies (Bossingham et al., 2005; Morgan, Masterson, Fahlman, Topp, & Boardley, 2003; Raman et al., 2004) of community-dwelling older adults suggest that under normal conditions, older adults maintain adequate hydration; however, when challenged by environmental stressors—physical or emotional illness, surgery, or trauma—they are at increased risk for dehydration and rapidly become dehydrated if they are already chronically underhydrated.

DEFINITIONS

Dehydration

Dehydration is the depletion in total body water (TBW) content caused by pathologic fluid losses, diminished water intake, or a combination of both. It results in hypernatremia (more than 145 mEq/L) in the extracellular fluid compartment, which draws water from the intracellular fluids. The water loss is shared by all body fluid compartments and relatively little reduction in extracellular fluids occurs. Thus, circulation is not compromised unless the loss is very large.

Underhydration

Underhydration is a precursor condition to dehydration associated with insidious onset and poor outcomes (Mentes, 2006; Mentes & Culp, 2003). Others have referred to this condition as *mild dehydration* (Stookey et al., 2005) or *chronic dehydration* (Bennett et al., 2004).

ASSESSMENT OF THE PROBLEM

Assessment of hydration status consists of risk identification with attention to specific populations at increased risk, assessment of hydration habits, and evaluation of specific biochemical and clinical indicators.

Risk Identification

Risk for dehydration in ill or frail older adults across care settings has been more frequently studied. Although there is no outstanding risk factor for dehydration, age, gender, ethnicity, class, and number of medications taken, level of activity of daily living (ADL) dependency, presence of cognitive impairment, presence of medical conditions such as infectious processes, and a prior history of dehydration have all been associated with dehydration in older adults (Mentes & Iowa-Veterans Affairs Nursing Research Consortium [IVANRC], 2000). Therefore, although single risk factors will be discussed, it is likely that clusters of risk factors maybe more helpful in clinical settings (Leibovitz et al., 2007).

Increasing age is associated with increased likelihood of dehydration (Ciccone, Allegra, Cochrane, Cody, & Roche, 1998; Lavizzo-Mourey, Johnson, & Stolley, 1988; Warren et al., 1994). Ciccone and colleagues (1998) found that adults aged 85 years and older were three times more likely to have a diagnosis of dehydration on admission to an emergency department than adults ages 65–74 years. Older African American and Black adults have higher prevalence rates of dehydration on hospitalization than Caucasian adults (Lancaster, Smiciklas-Wright, Heller, Ahern, & Jensen, 2003; Warren et al., 1994). Female gender has been associated with risk for dehydration in nursing home residents (Lavizzo-Mourey et al., 1988); however, male hospitalized patients had an increased risk for dehydration (Warren et al., 1994) and more recently, no gender differences were detected in a large database study (Xiao et al., 2004).

In general, individuals in long-term care (LTC) settings are considered to be at increased risk, with one-third of residents experiencing a dehydration episode in a 6-month period (Mentes, 2006). However, many of the factors are also characteristic of older adult hospitalized patients as well. See Protocol 21.1 for patient-focused and staff and family issues that serve as risk factor for dehydration. The following discussion will highlight at risk groups of patients, hydration habits, and clinical parameters that indicate risk.

At-Risk Populations

Several groups of patients, based on medical diagnosis, are at increased risk. These groups include chronic mentally ill, surgical, stroke, and end-of-life patients.

Chronic Mentally Ill Patients

Special consideration should be given to chronic mentally ill older adults (e.g., individuals with schizophrenia, bipolar disorder, obsessive-compulsive disorder) because they may be at risk for hydration problems. Their antipsychotic medications may blunt their thirst response and put them at increased risk in hot weather for dehydration and heat stroke (Batscha, 1997). In addition, even small increases in their antipsychotic medications may predispose them to neuroleptic malignant syndrome (NMS), of which hyperthermia and dehydration are prominent features (Bristow & Kohen, 1996; Jacobs, 1996; Sachdev, Mason, & Hadzi-Pavlovic, 1997). In these individuals, risks for over-hydration stem from a combination of the drying side effects of prescribed psychotropic medications and the individual's compulsive behaviors that result in excessive fluid intake (Cosgray, Davidhizar, Giger, & Kreisl, 1993).

Patients With Stroke

There is increasing evidence that dehydration may play an important part in contributing to early cerebral ischemia (Rodriguez et al., 2009), and in the early recovery from stroke (Kelly et al., 2004). In fact, Kelly et al. (2004) found that dehydration in patients with stroke was hospital acquired and led to poorer outcomes for recovering patients with stroke. Dehydration, signified by increased serum osmolality, led to a 2.8- to 4.7-fold increase in the risk of hospitalized patients with stroke acquiring a venous thromboembolism (VTE). Hospitalized patients recovering from stroke should be carefully and continuously monitored for dehydration. Another sequela of stroke is dysphagia that can cause dehydration (Whelan, 2001). This appears to be related not only to the dysphagia resulting from the stroke but also the poor palatability of the thickened fluids offered to patients to prevent aspiration.

Surgical Patients

Prolonged nothing by mouth (NPO) status prior to elective surgery has been linked to increased risk of dehydration and adverse effects such as thirst, hunger, irritability, headache, hypovolemia, and hypoglycemia in surgical patients (Smith, Vallance, & Slater,1997; Yogendran, Asokumar, Cheng, & Chung, 1995). Crenshaw and Winslow (2002) have found that despite the formulation of national guidelines developed by the American Society of Anesthesiologist Task Force on Preoperative Fasting, patients were still being instructed to fast too long prior to surgery (Crenshaw & Winslow, 2002). In fact, patients may safely consume clear liquids up to 2 hours of elective surgery using general anesthesia, regional anesthesia, or sedation anesthesia.

End-of-Life Patients

Maintaining or withholding fluids at the end of life remains a controversial issue. Proponents suggest that dehydration in the terminally ill patient is not painful and lessens other noxious symptoms of terminal illness, such as excessive pulmonary secretions, nausea, edema, and pain (dehydration acts as a natural anesthetic; Fainsinger & Bruera, 1997). Some suggest additional benefit from the decreased need to stand up to use the restroom and receive bedpans or diaper changes, which could be difficult or painful for someone at the end of life.

Opponents to this position suggest that associated symptoms of dehydration such as acute confusion and delirium are stressful and reduce the quality of life for the terminally ill older adult (Bruera, Belzile, Watanabe, & Fainsinger, 1996). Most research that has been done with terminally ill patients with cancer has examined discomforts of dehydration including thirst, dry mouth, and agitated delirium. However, research has not demonstrated a link between biochemical markers of dehydration and these various symptoms in terminally ill patients (Burge, 1993; Ellershaw, Sutcliffe, & Saunders, 1995; Morita, Tei, Tsunoda, Inoue, & Chihara, 2001). It is suggested that several confounding factors influence the uncomfortable dehydration-like symptoms that accompany the end of life. These include use and dosage of opiates, type and location of cancer, hyperosmolality, stomatitis, and oral breathing (Morita et al., 2001). On the other hand, Bruera et al. (1996) have determined that small amounts of fluids delivered subcutaneously via hypodermoclysis plus opioid rotation was effective in decreasing delirium and antipsychotic use and did not cause edema in terminally ill patients. A 2-day long pilot study of parenteral hydration in terminally ill patients with cancer lead to statistically significant decreases in hallucination, myoclonus, fatigue, and sedation (Bruera et al., 2005). However, research suggests that artificial hydration does not prolong life (Bruera et al., 2005; Meier, Ahronheim, Morris, Baskin-Lyons, & Morrison, 2001; Mitchell, Kiely, & Lipsitz, 1997).

Therefore, it is recommended that maintaining or withholding fluids at the end of life be an individual decision that should be based on the etiology of illness, use of medications, presence of delirium, and family and patient preferences (Fainsinger & Bruera, 1997; Morita et al., 2001; Schmidlin, 2008). Schmidlin (2008) recommended early discussions with patients and family on their wishes as well as educating patients on the current knowledge about artificial hydration so that proper patient-centered care will be provided.

Hydration Habits

Hydration habits may indicate level of risk for dehydration in older adults. Some hydration habits may have developed over a lifetime, and others are adaptations to current health status. Four major categories of hydration habits have been identified (Mentes, 2006). The categories include those older adults who "can drink," "cannot drink," "will not drink," and older adults who are at the "end of life." For example, older adults who can drink are those who are functionally capable of accessing and consuming fluids but who may not know what is an adequate intake or may forget to drink secondary to cognitive impairment; older adults who cannot drink are those who are physically incapable of accessing or safely consuming fluids related to physical frailty or difficulty swallowing; older adults who will not drink are those who are capable of consuming fluids safely but who do not because of concerns about being able to reach the toilet with or without assistance or who relate that they have never consumed many fluids; and older adults who are terminally ill comprise the end-of-life category. Understanding hydration habits of older adults can help nurses to plan appropriate interventions to improve or ensure adequate intake (Mentes, 2006).

Indicators of Hydration Status

A priority for nursing, regardless of clinical setting, is the prevention of dehydration. Unfortunately, many of the standard tests for detection of dehydration only confirm a diagnosis of dehydration after it is too late to prevent the episode. In our fast-paced nursing environments, it is difficult to monitor the fluid intake of all our older patients. Although controversial, the use of urine color and specific gravity has been shown to be reliable indicators of hydration status (not dehydration) in older individuals in nursing homes and a Veterans Administration Medical Center with adequate renal function (Culp, Mentes, & Wakefield, 2003; Mentes, Wakefield, & Culp, 2006). Specifically, the use of urine color, as measured by a urine color chart, can be helpful in monitoring hydration status (Armstrong et al., 1994; Mentes & IVANRC, 2000). The urine color chart has eight standardized colors ranging from *pale straw* (number 1) to *greenish brown* (number 8), approximating urine-specific gravities of 1.003–1.029 (Armstrong et al., 1994). The urine color chart is most effective when an individual's average urine color is calculated over several days for an individual referent value. If the older person's urine becomes darker from his or her average color, further assessment into recent intake and health status can be conducted and fluids can be adjusted to improve hydration status before dehydration occurs. Limitations in using urine indices to estimate specific gravity include (a) certain medications and foods can discolor the urine (Mentes, Wakefield et al., 2006; Wakefield, Mentes, Diggelmann, & Culp, 2002); (b) persons must be able to give a urine specimen for a color evaluation; and (c) best results in the use of urine color as an indicator has been documented in older adults with adequate renal function (Mentes, Wakefield et al., 2006).

Bioelectrical impedance analysis (BIA) is a measurement that has been used mostly in the fitness industry to estimate body composition, including body mass index (BMI), TBW, and intracellular and extracellular water. Several nursing studies have used impedance measurements to estimate TBW and intracellular and extracellular water (Culp et al., 2003; Culp et al., 2004). Although mostly used in research, BIA is a noninvasive, reliable method to estimate body water (Ritz & Source Study, 2001). Because TBW is weight and body composition dependent, this measure is best used after a baseline value of TBW, intracellular, and extracellular fluid in liters has been documented. Then, deviations from the individual baseline can be noted.

Salivary osmolality is an emerging clinical indicator of hydration status, which is sensitive in younger healthy adults (Oliver, Laing, Wilson, Bilzon, & Walsh, 2008) and has been tested in a same sample of nursing home residents (Woods & Mentes, 2011).

Indicators of Dehydration

Dehydration is the loss of body water from intracellular and interstitial fluid compartments that is associated with hypertonicity (Mange et al., 1997). Therefore, the most reliable indicators of dehydration are elevated serum sodium, serum osmolality, and BUN/creatinine ratio (See Table 21.1). The most common clinical assessments of dehydration include the presence of dry oral mucous membranes, tongue furrows, decreased saliva, sunken eyes, decreased urine output, upper body weakness, a rapid pulse (Gross et al., 1992), and tongue dryness (Vivanti, Harvey, & Ash, 2010; Vivanti, Harvey, Ash, & Battistutta, 2008). Decreased axillary sweat production as a clinical sign of dehydration has produced contradictory results, making it an unreliable indicator of dehydration (Eaton, Bannister, Mulley, & Connolly, 1994; Gross et al., 1992). Assessment of sternal skin turgor as a sign of dehydration has been a mainstay in nursing practice; however, it is also an ambiguous indicator for dehydration in older individuals, with some researchers finding it unreliable because of age-related changes in skin elasticity

TABLE 21.1

Approximate Ranges of Laboratory Tests for Hydration Status

Test	Value Ranges for	
	Impending Dehydration	**Dehydration**
BUN/Creatinine ratio	20–24	> 25
Serum osmolality	normal 280–300 mmol/kg	> 300 mmol/kg
Serum sodium		> 150 mEq/L
Urine osmolality		> 1050 mmol/kg
Urine specific gravity	1.020–1.029	> 1.029
Urine color	dark yellow	greenish brown
Amount of urine	800–1,200 cc/day	> 800 cc/day

Note. BUN = blood urea nitrogen. Armstrong et al., 1994; Armstrong et al., 1998; Mentes, Wakefield, & Culp, 2006; Metheny, 2000; Wakefield, Mentes, Diggelmann, & Culp, 2002; Wallach, 2000

Source: Adapted with permission from Mentes, J. C., & Kang, S. (2010). Evidence-based protocol: Hydration management. In M. G. Titler (Series Ed.), *Series on evidence-based practice for older adults.* Iowa City, IA: the University of Iowa College of Nursing Gerontological Nursing Interventions Research Center, Research Translation and Dissemination Core.

(Gross et al., 1992) and others finding it reliable (Chassagne, Druesne, Capet, Ménard, & Bercoff, 2006; Vivanti et al., 2008).

INTERVENTIONS AND CARE STRATEGIES

A hydration management intervention is an individualized daily plan to promote adequate hydration based on risk factor identification that is derived from a comprehensive assessment. The intervention is divided into two phases: risk identification and hydration management.

Risk Identification

Based on the collected assessment data, a risk appraisal for hydration problems is completed using the Dehydration Risk Appraisal Checklist (Table 21.2; Mentes & Wang, 2010).

Hydration Management

Managing fluid intake for optimal fluid balance consists of (a) acute management of oral intake and (a) ongoing management of oral intake.

Acute Management of Oral Intake

Any individual who develops a fever, vomiting, diarrhea, or a nonfebrile infection should be closely monitored by implementing intake and output records and provision of additional fluids as tolerated (Wakefield et al., 2008; Weinberg et al., 1994). Individuals who are required to be NPO for diagnostic tests should be given special consideration to shorten the time that they must be NPO and should be provided with adequate amounts of fluids and food when they have completed their tests. For many procedures, a 2-hour fluid fast is recommended ("Practice Guidelines for Preoperative Fasting," 1999).

TABLE 21.2
Dehydration Risk Appraisal Checklist

The greater the number of characteristics present, the greater the risk for hydration problems. Please check all that apply.

❑ > 85 years   ❑ Female

Significant Health Conditions

❑ MMSE score < 24 (indicating cognitive impairment)   ❑ Semi-dependent in ADLs

❑ Dementia diagnosis   ❑ Repeated infections

❑ GDS score ≥ 6 (indicating depression)   ❑ History of dehydration

                                              ❑ Urinary incontinence

Medications

❑ Laxatives   ❑ Psychotropics: antipsychotics, antidepressants, anxiolytics

❑ Diuretics

Intake Behaviors

❑ BMI < 21 or > 27   ❑ Can drink independently but forgets

❑ Requires assistance to drink   ❑ Poor eater

❑ Has difficulty swallowing/chokes

Note. MMSE = mini-mental status examination; GDS = Geriatric Depression Scale; ADLs = activities of daily living; BMI = body mass index. Mentes & Wang, 2010.

Source: Reprinted with permission from Mentes, J. C., & Kang, S. (2010). Evidence-based protocol: Hydration management. In M. G. Titler (Series Ed.), *Series on Evidence-based practice for older adults.* Iowa City, IA: the University of Iowa College of Nursing Gerontological Nursing Interventions Research Center, Research Translation and Dissemination Core.

Any individual who develops unexplained weight gain, pedal edema, neck vein distension, or shortness of breath should be evaluated and closely monitored for overhydration. Fluids should be temporarily restricted and the individual's primary care provider notified. Specific attention should be focused on individuals who have renal disease or congestive heart failure (CHF); however, Holst, Strömberg, Lindholm, and Willenheimer (2008) found that a liberal fluid prescription based on body weight could be offered to patients with stable CHF. Older adults taking selective serotonin reuptake inhibitors (SSRIs) should have their serum sodium levels and their hydration status monitored carefully because they are at risk for hyponatremia and increasing fluid intake may aggravate an evolving hyponatremia (Movig, Leufkens, Lenderink, & Egberts, 1992).

Ongoing Management of Oral Intake

Ongoing management of oral intake consists of the following five components:

1. Calculate a daily fluid goal.
   All older adults should have an individualized fluid goal determined by a documented standard for daily fluid intake. There is preliminary evidence that the standard suggested by Skipper (1993)—of 100 ml/kg for first 10 kg of weight, 50 ml/kg for next 10 kg, and 15 ml/kg for the remaining kilogram—is preferred (Chidester & Spangler, 1997). Table 21.3 provides examples of daily fluid goal calculations.

TABLE 21.3
Calculating Daily Fluid Goals: Examples
70-kg (154-lb.) patient would have a fluid goal of 2,250 ml/day.
60-kg (132-lb.) patient would have a fluid goal of 2,100 ml/day.
50-kg (110-lb.) patient would have a fluid goal of 1,950 ml/day.

Because this standard reflects fluid from all sources, to calculate a standard for fluids alone, 75% of the total calculated from the formula can be used. This formula allows for at least 1,500 ml of fluid per day as a minimum, which has been shown to be well tolerated in older men aged 55–75 years (Spigt, Knottnerus, Westerterp, Olde Rikkert, & Schayck, 2006). Other standards include the following:

- 1,600 ml/m^2 of body surface per day (Gaspar, 1988; Butler & Talbot, 1944); more recently, Gaspar (1999) recommended 75% of this standard
- 30 ml/kg body weight with 1,500 ml/day minimum (Chernoff, 1994)
- 1 ml/kcal fluid for adults (National Research Council, 1989)
- 1,600 ml/day (Hodgkinson, Evans, & Wood, 2003)

2. Compare individual's current intake to the amount calculated from applying the standard to evaluate the individual's hydration status.
3. Provide fluids consistently throughout the day (Hodgkinson et al., 2003).
   a. Plan fluid intake as follows: 75%–80% delivered at meals and 20%–25% delivered during nonmeal times, such as medication times and planned nourishment times (Simmons et al., 2001).
   b. Offer a variety of fluids, keeping in mind the individual's previous intake pattern (Zembrzuski, 1997). Alcoholic beverages, which exert a diuretic effect, should not be counted toward the fluid goal. Caffeinated beverages may be counted toward the fluid goal based on individual assessment because there is evidence that in individuals who are regular users, there are no untoward effects on fluid balance and that recommendations to refrain from moderate amounts of caffeinated beverages (250–300 mg, equivalent of two to three cups of coffee or five to eight cups of tea may adversely affect fluid balance in older adults (Maughan & Griffin, 2003).
   c. Fluid with medication administrations should be standardized to a prescribed amount (e.g., at least 180 ml or 6 oz.) per administration time.
4. Plan for at-risk individuals
   For those who are at risk of underhydration because of poor intake, the following strategies can be implemented based on time, setting, and formal or informal caregiver issues:
   a. Fluid rounds mid-morning and late afternoon, where caregiver provides additional fluids (Robinson & Rosher, 2002).
   b. Provide 2- to 8-oz. glasses of fluid in morning and evening (Robinson & Rosher, 2002).
   c. "Happy hours" in the afternoon, where patients can gather together for additional fluids and socialization (Musson et al., 1990).
   d. "Tea time" in the afternoon, where patients come together for fluids, nourishment, and socialization (Mueller & Boisen, 1989).
   e. Use of modified fluid containers based on intake behaviors (e.g., ability to hold cup and swallow; Mueller & Boisen, 1989).

    f. Offer a variety of fluids and encourage ongoing intake throughout the day for those with cognitive impairment. Offer fluids that the person prefers (Simmons et al., 2001).

    g. Offer encouragement to drink, family involvement in and support, and coordination of staff communication about hydration issues (Mentes, Chang et al., 2006).

5. Fluid regulation and documentation

    a. Individuals who are cognitively intact, visually capable, and have adequate renal function can be taught how to regulate their intake through the use of a color chart to compare to the color of their urine (Armstrong et al., 1994; Armstrong et al., 1998; Mentes, Wakefield et al., 2006). For those individuals who are cognitively impaired, caregivers can be taught how to use the color chart.

    b. Frequency of documentation of fluid intake will vary from setting to setting and is dependent on an individual's condition. However, in most settings, at least one accurate intake and output recording should be documented and should include the amount of fluid consumed, intake pattern, difficulties with consumption, and a urine-specific gravity and color (Mentes & IVANRC, 2000).

    c. Accurate calculation of intake requires knowledge of the volumes of containers used to serve fluids, which should be posted in a prominent place on the care unit, because a study by Burns (1992) suggested that nurses overestimated or underestimated the volumes of common vessels.

EVALUATION

Adherence to the hydration management guideline can be monitored by the frequency of monitoring (to be determined by setting), as follows:

- Urine-specific gravity checks, preferably a morning specimen (Armstrong et al., 1994; Armstrong et al., 1998; Hodgkinson et al., 2003; Wakefield et al., 2002). A value greater than or equal to 1.020 implies an underhydrated state and requires further monitoring (Kavouras, 2002; Mentes, 2006).
- Urine color chart monitoring, preferably a morning specimen (Armstrong et al., 1994; Armstrong et al., 1998; Wakefield et al., 2002).
- 24-hour intake recording (output recording may be added; however, in settings where individuals are incontinent of urine, an intake recording should suffice; Hodgkinson et al., 2003)

Expected improved health outcomes of consistent application of a hydration management plan include the following:

- Maintenance of body hydration (Mentes & Culp, 2003; Robinson & Rosher, 2002; Simmons et al., 2001)
- Decreased infections, especially urinary tract infections (McConnell, 1984; Mentes & Culp, 2003; Robinson & Rosher, 2002)
- Improvement in urinary incontinence (Hart & Adamek, 1984; Spangler et al., 1984)
- Lowered urinary pH (Hart & Adamek, 1984)
- Decreased constipation (Robinson & Rosher, 2002)
- Decreased acute confusion (Mentes & Culp, 2003; Mentes et al., 1999)

CASE STUDY

Mrs. Chung is an 87-year-old Chinese American woman who was admitted to the hospital for observation secondary to an episode of dehydration. She has resided at Sunny Days Assisted Living Facility for the past month. Staff describes her as fiercely independent despite experiencing some declines in her health recently. Her medical diagnoses include hypertension, for which she receives a atenolol 25 mg daily and enalapril 20 mg daily; status post-mild cerebrovascular accident (CVA) with residual left-sided weakness, for which she is taking 80 mg of aspirin daily; osteoarthritis, for which she takes Tylenol extra strength twice daily; and cataracts, for which she is reluctant to have surgery. She is cognitively intact and requires only minor assistance with bathing.

Prior to hospitalization, Mrs. Chung had become more withdrawn and concerned about her health. Her family noticed that she has altered some of her daily routines. For example, she eliminated her daily tea because she finds it difficult to use the new microwave at the assisted care facility (ACF) to heat her water because of unfamiliarity. She stays in her bed much of the day, complaining that she does not have any energy. When questioned, she reluctantly admits that she has been having more problems with her long-standing urinary incontinence and she is afraid to leave her room because she is fearful that she will not be able to make it to a bathroom on time. Consequently, she has further restricted the amount of fluid that she consumes on a daily basis.

Mrs. Chung is at high risk for dehydration given that she has recently begun to restrict her fluids because of unfamiliarity with the microwave to heat her water for tea. Older adults from different cultures may wish to have their beverages served at different temperatures. Especially when ill, ethnic older adults may prefer to have warmed beverages. In addition, Mrs. Chung is "treating" her urinary incontinence by restricting her fluids, which places her at risk for dehydration and urinary tract infections. This scenario is not uncommon in older adults struggling to maintain independence. One of the major reasons for admission to a nursing home is the presence of urinary incontinence. Finally, there is some evidence that Mrs. Chung is depressed, which would also place her at risk for dehydration often secondary to decreased food and fluid intake. Additional risk factors include her age (87 years old), gender, and use of an angiotensin-converting enzyme (ACE)-inhibitor, which acts on the renin-angiotensin-aldosterone (RAA) system.

Interventions to prevent dehydration in Mrs. Chung would include evaluating her for a urinary tract infection and offering her an evaluation for her urinary incontinence that could include use of medications, if indicated; use of behavioral strategies including urge inhibition; and/or Kegel exercises. Education around the importance of maintaining adequate fluid intake to minimize urinary incontinence is indicated, which should include a discussion about the amount of daily fluids required and the provision of a graduated cup to help her ascertain appropriate amounts. Helping her simplify the use of the microwave and/or attendance at social events at the ACF where fluids are provided could be implemented. Lastly, an evaluation for depression maybe indicated if the previous interventions do not improve her mood.

SUMMARY

Dehydration in older adults is a costly yet preventable health problem. Best practices for hydration management have been identified primarily in the nursing home population. They include providing access to fluids at all times, regularly offering fluids throughout the day, assessing fluid preferences and providing the fluid of choice, and appropriate supervision of personnel who will be providing the fluids. Access to fluids means that fasting times for older adults are limited to the shortest time, fluids are available at all times, and that nursing personnel assess the ability to self-manage hydration in older individuals. Regularly offering fluids through fluid rounds, a beverage cart, or other novel means such as tea time is another principle of good hydration practices. Accommodating older peoples' preferences for type of beverage and appropriate temperature of beverage has been shown to increase fluid intake. Lastly, appropriate supervision of how much fluid per day is required and how assistance is given to older adults who are not capable of drinking themselves to ensure that required amounts are consumed is also the key in maintaining adequate hydration. The hydration practices of healthier, community-dwelling older adults are less well known and require further study.

NURSING STANDARD OF PRACTICE

Protocol 21.1: Managing Oral Hydration

I. GOAL: To minimize episodes of dehydration in older adults.

II. OVERVIEW: Maintaining adequate fluid balance is an essential component of health across the lifespan; older adults are more vulnerable to shifts in water balance, both overhydration and dehydration because of age-related changes and increased likelihood that an older individual has several medical conditions. Dehydration is the more frequently occurring problem.

III. BACKGROUND AND STATEMENT OF THE PROBLEM
  A. Definitions
    1. *Dehydration* is depletion in total body water (TBW) content caused by pathologic fluid losses, diminished water intake, or a combination of both. It results in hypernatremia (more than 145 mEq/L) in the extracellular fluid compartment, which draws water from the intracellular fluids. The water loss is shared by all body fluid compartments and relatively little reduction in extracellular fluids occurs. Thus, circulation is not compromised unless the loss is very large.
    2. *Underhydration* is a precursor condition to dehydration associated with insidious onset and poor outcomes (Mentes & Culp, 2003). Others have referred to this condition as *mild dehydration* (Stookey, 2005; Stookey et al., 2005) or *chronic dehydration* (Bennett et al., 2004).

(continued)

Protocol 21.1: Managing Oral Hydration *(cont.)*

B. Etiologic Factors Associated With Dehydration
   1. Age-related changes in body composition with resulting decrease in TBW (Bossingham et al., 2005; Lavizzo-Mourey et al., 1988; Metheny, 2000)
   2. Decreasing renal function (Lindeman, Tobin, & Shock, 1985)
   3. Lack of thirst (Farrell et al., 2008; Kenney & Chiu, 2001; Mack et al., 1994; Miescher & Fortney, 1989; Phillips et al., 1991; Phillips et al., 1984)
   4. Poor tolerance for hot weather (Josseran et al., 2009)
C. Risk Factors
   1. Patient characteristics
      a. More than 85 years of age (Ciccone et al., 1998; Gaspar, 1999; Lavizzo-Mourey et al. 1988)
      b. Female (Gaspar, 1988; Lavizzo-Mourey et al., 1988)
      c. Semi-dependent in eating (Gaspar, 1999)
      d. Functionally more independent (Gaspar, 1999; Mentes & Culp, 2003)
      e. Few fluid ingestion opportunities (Gaspar, 1988, 1999)
      f. Inadequate nutrient intake (Gaspar, 1999)
      g. Alzheimer's disease or other dementias (Albert, Nakra, Grossberg, & Caminal, 1989, 1994)
      h. Four or more chronic conditions (Lavizzo-Mourey et al., 1988)
      i. Four medications (Lavizzo-Mourey et al., 1988)
      j. Fever (Pals et al., 1995; Weinberg et al., 1994)
      k. Vomiting and diarrhea (Wakefield, Mentes, Holman, & Culp, 2008)
      l. Individuals with infections (Warren et al., 1994)
      m. Individuals who have had prior episodes of dehydration (Mentes, 2006)
      n. Diuretics: thiazide (Wakefield et al., 2008), loop and thiazide (Lancaster et al., 2003)
   2. Staff and family characteristics
      a. Inadequate staff and professional supervision (Kayser-Jones, Schell, Porter, Barbaccia, & Shaw, 1999)
      b. Depression or loneliness associated with decreased fluid intake as identified by nursing staff (Mentes, Chang, & Morris, 2006)
      c. Family or caregivers not spending time with patient (Mentes, Chang et al., 2006)

IV. PARAMETERS OF ASSESSMENT (Mentes & IVANRC, 2000).
   A. Health History
      1. Specific disease states: dementia, congestive heart failure, chronic renal disease, malnutrition, and psychiatric disorders such as depression (Albert et al., 1989; Gaspar, 1988; Warren et al., 1994)
      2. Presence of comorbidities: more than four chronic health conditions (Lavizzo-Mourey et al., 1988)
      3. Prescription drugs: number and types (Lavizzo-Mourey et al., 1988)
      4. Past history of dehydration, repeated infections (Mentes, 2006)
   B. Physical Assessments (Mentes & IVANRC, 2000)
      1. Vital signs
      2. Height and weight

(continued)

Protocol 21.1: Managing Oral Hydration *(cont.)*

    3. Body mass index (BMI; Vivanti et al., 2008)
    4. Review of systems
    5. Indicators of hydration
  C. Laboratory Tests
    1. Urine-specific gravity (Mentes, 2006; Wakefield et al., 2002)
    2. Urine color (Mentes, 2006; Wakefield et al., 2002)
    3. Blood urea nitrogen (BUN)/creatinine ratio
    4. Serum sodium
    5. Serum osmolality
    6. Salivary osmolality
  D. Individual fluid intake behaviors (Mentes, 2006)

V. NURSING CARE STRATEGIES
  A. Risk Identification (Mentes & IVANRC, 2000)
    1. Identify acute situations: vomiting, diarrhea, or febrile episodes
    2. Use a tool to evaluate risk: Dehydration Risk Appraisal Checklist
  B. Acute Hydration Management
    1. Monitor input and output (Weinberg et al., 1994)
    2. Provide additional fluids as tolerated (Weinberg et al., 1994)
    3. Minimize fasting times for diagnostic and surgical procedures ("Practice Guidelines for Preoperative Fasting," 1999)
  C. Ongoing Hydration Management
    1. Calculate a daily fluid goal (Mentes & IVANRC, 2000)
    2. Compare current intake to fluid goal (Mentes & IVANRC, 2000)
    3. Provide fluids consistently throughout the day (Ferry, 2005; Simmons, Alessi, & Schnelle, 2001)
    4. Plan for at-risk individuals
      a. Fluid rounds (Robinson & Rosher, 2002)
      b. Provide two 8-oz. glasses of fluid, one in the morning the other in the evening (Robinson & Rosher, 2002)
      c. "Happy hours" to promote increased intake (Musson et al., 1990)
      d. "Tea time" to increase fluid intake (Mueller & Boisen, 1989)
      e. Offer a variety of fluids throughout the day (Simmons et al., 2001)
    5. Fluid regulation and documentation
      a. Teach able individuals to use a urine color chart to monitor hydration status (Armstrong et al., 1994; Armstrong et al., 1998; Mentes, 2006)
      b. Document a complete intake recording including hydration habits (Mentes & IVANRC, 2000)
      c. Know volumes of fluid containers to accurately calculate fluid consumption (Burns, 1992; Hart & Adamek, 1984)

VI. EVALUATION AND EXPECTED OUTCOMES
  A. Maintenance of body hydration (Mentes & Culp, 2003; Robinson & Rosher, 2002; Simmons et al., 2001)
  B. Decreased infections, especially urinary tract infections (McConnell, 1984; Mentes & Culp, 2003; Robinson & Rosher, 2002)

(continued)

Protocol 21.1: Managing Oral Hydration *(cont.)*

C. Improvement in urinary incontinence (Spangler, Risley, & Bilyew, 1984)
D. Lowered urinary pH (Hart & Adamek, 1984)
E. Decreased constipation (Robinson & Rosher, 2002)
F. Decreased acute confusion (Mentes et al., 1999)

VII. FOLLOW-UP MONITORING OF CONDITION

A. Urine color chart monitoring in patients with better renal function (Armstrong et al., 1994; Armstrong et al., 1998; Wakefield et al., 2002)
B. Urine-specific gravity checks (Armstrong et al., 1994; Armstrong et al., 1998; Wakefield et al., 2002)
C. 24-hour intake recording (Metheny, 2000)

VIII. RELEVANT PRACTICE GUIDELINES

A. Hydration Management Evidence-Based Protocol available from the University of Iowa College of Nursing Gerontological Nursing Interventions Research Center, Research Dissemination Core. Author: Janet Mentes, revised 2010.

RESOURCES

Evidence-based website for geriatric nursing sponsored by the Hartford Institute for Geriatric Nursing
http://www.consultgerirn.org

Hydration for Health sponsored by Danone Waters
http://www.healthyhydrationcoach.com/

University of Iowa Evidence-Based Protocols
http://www.nursing.uiowa.edu/centers/gnirc/protocols.htm

REFERENCES

Ainslie, P. N., Campbell, I. T., Frayn, K. N., Humphreys, S. M., MacLaren, D. P., Reilly, T., & Westerterp, K. R. (2002). Energy balance, metabolism, hydration, and performance during strenuous hill walking: The effect of age. *Journal of Applied Physiology, 93*(2), 714–723. Evidence Level III.

Albert, S. G., Nakra, B. R., Grossberg, G. T., & Caminal, E. R. (1989). Vasopressin response to dehydration in Alzheimer's disease. *Journal of the American Geriatric Society, 37*(9), 843–847. Evidence Level III.

Albert, S. G., Nakra, B. R., Grossberg, G. T., & Caminal, E. R. (1994). Drinking behavior and vasopressin responses to hyperosmolality in Alzheimer's disease. *International Psychogeriatrics, 6*(1), 79–86. Evidence Level III.

Armstrong, L. E., Maresh, C. M., Castellani, J. W., Bergeron, M. F., Kenefick, R. W., LaGasse, K. E., & Riebe, D. (1994). Urinary indices of hydration status. *International Journal of Sport Nutrition, 4*(3), 265–279. Evidence Level IV.

Armstrong, L. E., Soto, J. A., Hacker, F. T., Jr., Casa, D. J., Kavouras, S. A., & Maresh, C. M. (1998). Urinary indices during dehydration, exercise, and rehydration. *International Journal of Sport Nutrition, 8*(4), 345–355. Evidence Level IV.

Batscha, C. L. (1997). Heat stroke. Keeping your clients cool in the summer. *Journal of Psychosocial Nursing and Mental Health Services, 35*(7), 12–17. Evidence Level V.

Beaujean, D. J., Blok, H. E., Vandenbroucke-Grauls, C. M., Weersink. A. J., Raymakers, J. A., & Verhoef, J. (1997). Surveillance of nosocomial infections in geriatric patients. *The Journal of Hospital Infection, 36*(4), 275–284. Evidence Level IV.

Bennett, J. A., Thomas, V., & Riegel, B. (2004). Unrecognized chronic dehydration in older adults: Examining prevalence rate and risk factors. *Journal of Gerontological Nursing, 30*(11), 22–28; quiz 52–23. Evidence Level IV.

Bossingham, M. J., Carnell, N. S., & Campbell, W. W. (2005). Water balance, hydration status, and fat-free mass hydration in younger and older adults. *American Journal of Clinical Nutrition, 81*(6), 1342–1350. Evidence Level II.

Bristow, M. F., & Kohen, D. (1996). Neuroleptic malignant syndrome. *British Journal of Hospital Medicine, 55*(8), 517–520. Evidence Level V.

Bruera, E., Belzile, M., Watanabe, S., & Fainsinger, R. L. (1996). Volume of hydration in terminal cancer patients. *Supportive Care in Cancer, 4*(2), 147–150. Evidence Level IV.

Bruera, E., Sala, R., Rico, M. A., Moyano, J., Centeno, C., Willey, J., & Palmer, J. L. (2005). Effects of parenteral hydration in terminally ill cancer patients: A preliminary study. *Journal of Clinical Oncology, 23*(10), 2366–2371. Evidence Level III.

Burge, F. I. (1993). Dehydration symptoms of palliative care cancer patients. *Journal of Pain Symptom Management, 8*(7), 454–464. Evidence Level IV.

Burns, D. (1992). Working up a thirst. *Nursing Times, 88*(26), 44–45. Evidence Level IV.

Butler, A. M., Talbot, N. B. (1944). Parenteral fluid therapy. *New England Journal of Medicine, 231,* 585–590. Evidence Level VI.

Chan, J., Knutsen, S. F., Blix, G. G., Lee, G. W., & Fraser, G. E. (2002). Water, other fluids, and fatal coronary heart disease: The Adventist Health Study. *American Journal of Epidemiology, 155*(9), 827–833. Evidence Level IV.

Chassagne, P., Druesne, L., Capet, C., Ménard, J. F., & Bercoff, E. (2006). Clinical presentation of hypernatremia in elderly patients: A case control study. *Journal of the American Geriatrics Society, 54*(8), 1225–1230. Evidence Level IV.

Chernoff, R. (1994). Meeting the nutritional needs of the elderly in the institutional setting. *Nutrition Reviews, 52*(4), 132–136. Evidence Level VI.

Chidester, J. C., & Spangler, A. A. (1997). Fluid intake in the institutionalized elderly. *Journal of the American Dietetic Association, 97*(1), 23–28; quiz 29–30. Evidence Level IV.

Ciccone, A., Allegra, J. R., Cochrane, D. G., Cody, R. P., & Roche, L. M. (1998). Age-related differences in diagnoses within the elderly population. *The American Journal of Emergency Medicine, 16*(1), 43–48. Evidence Level IV.

Cosgray, R., Davidhizar, R., Giger, J. N., & Kreisl, R. (1993). A program for water-intoxicated patients at a state hospital. *Clinical Nurse Specialist, 7*(2), 55–61. Evidence Level V.

Crenshaw, J. T., & Winslow, E. H. (2002). Preoperative fasting: Old habits die hard. *The American Journal of Nursing, 102*(5), 36–44; quiz 45. Evidence Level IV.

Culp, K., Mentes, J., & Wakefield, B. (2003). Hydration and acute confusion in long-term care residents. *Western Journal of Nursing Research, 25*(3), 251–266; discussion 267–273. Evidence Level IV.

Culp, K. R., Wakefield, B., Dyck, M. J., Cacchione, P. Z., DeCrane, S., & Decker, S. (2004). Bioelectrical impedance analysis and other hydration parameters as risk factors for delirium in rural nursing home residents. *The Journals of Gerontology. Series A, Biological Sciences and Medical Sciences, 59*(8), 813–817. Evidence Level II.

Doucet, J., Jego, A., Noel, D., Geffroy, C. E., Capet, C., Couffin, E., . . . Bercoff, E. (2002). Preventable and non-preventable risk factors for adverse drug events related to hospital admission in the elderly: A prospective study. *Clinical Drug Investigations, 22*(6), 385–392. Evidence Level IV.

Eaton, D., Bannister, P., Mulley, G. P., & Connolly, M. J. (1994). Axillary sweating in clinical assessment of dehydration in ill elderly patients. *British Medical Journal, 308*(6939), 1271. Evidence Level IV.

Ellershaw, J. E., Sutcliffe, J. M., & Saunders, C. M. (1995). Dehydration and the dying patient. *Journal of Pain Symptom Management, 10*(3), 192–197. Evidence Level IV.

Fainsinger, R. L., & Bruera, E. (1997). When to treat dehydration in a terminally ill patient? *Supportive Care in Cancer, 5*(3), 205–211. Evidence Level VI.

Farrell, M. J., Zamarripa, F., Shade, R., Phillips, P. A., McKinley, M., Fox, P. T., . . . Egan, G. F. (2008). Effect of aging on regional cerebral blood flow responses associated with osmotic thirst and its satiation by water drinking: A PET study. *Proceedings of the National Academy of Sciences of the United States of America, 105*(1), 382–387. Evidence Level III.

Ferry, M. (2005). Strategies for ensuring good hydration in the elderly. *Nutrition Reviews, 63*(6 Pt. 2), S22–S29. Evidence Level VI.

Foreman, M. D. (1989). Confusion in the hospitalized elderly: Incidence, onset, and associated factors. *Research in Nursing & Health, 12*(1), 21–29. Evidence Level III.

Gaspar, P. M. (1988). What determines how much patients drink? *Geriatric Nursing, 9*(4), 221–224. Evidence Level IV.

Gaspar, P. M. (1999). Water intake of nursing home residents. *Journal of Gerontological Nursing, 25*(4), 23–29. Evidence Level IV.

Gordon, J. A., An, L. C., Hayward, R. A., & Williams, B. C. (1998). Initial emergency department diagnosis and return visits: Risk versus perception. *Annals of Emergency Medicine, 32*(5), 569–573. Evidence Level IV.

Gross, C. R., Lindquist, R. D., Woolley, A. C., Granieri, R., Allard, K., & Webster, B., (1992). Clinical indicators of dehydration severity in elderly patients. *The Journal of Emergency Medicine, 10*(3), 267–274. Evidence Level IV.

Hart, M., & Adamek, C. (1984). Do increased fluids decrease urinary stone formation? *Geriatric Nursing, 5*(6), 245–248. Evidence Level III.

Hodgkinson, B., Evans, D., & Wood, J. (2003). Maintaining oral hydration in older adults: A systematic review. *International Journal of Nursing Practices, 9*(3), S19–S28. Evidence Level I.

Holst, M., Strömberg, A., Lindholm, M., & Willenheimer, R. (2008). Liberal versus restricted fluid prescription in stabilised patients with chronic heart failure: Result of a randomised cross-over study of the effects on health-related quality of life, physical capacity, thirst and morbidity. *Scandinavian Cardiovascular Journal, 42*(5), 316–322.

Jacobs, L. G. (1996). The neuroleptic malignant syndrome: Often an unrecognized geriatric problem. *Journal of the American Geriatrics Society, 44*(4), 474–475. Evidence Level V.

Josseran, L., Caillère, N., Brun-Ney, D., Rottner, J., Filleul, L., Brucker, G., & Astagneau, P. (2009). Syndromic surveillance and heat wave morbidity: A pilot study based on emergency departments in France. *BMC Medical Informatics and Decision Making, 9*, 14. Evidence Level IV.

Kavouras, S. A. (2002). Assessing hydration status. *Current Opinion in Clinical Nutrition and Metabolic Care, 5*(5), 519–524. Evidence Level IV.

Kayser-Jones, J., Schell, E. S., Porter, C., Barbaccia, J. C., & Shaw, H. (1999). Factors contributing to dehydration in nursing homes: Inadequate staffing and lack of professional supervision. *Journal of the American Geriatrics Society, 47*(10), 1187–1194. Evidence Level IV.

Kelly, J., Hunt, B. J., Lewis, R. R., Swaminathan, R., Moody, A., Seed, P. T., & Rudd, A. (2004). Dehydration and venous thromboembolism after acute stroke. *QJM: Monthly Journal of the Association of Physicians, 97*(5), 293–296. Evidence Level IV.

Kenney, W. L., & Chiu, P. (2001). Influence of age on thirst and fluid intake. *Medicine and Science in Sports and Exercise, 33*(9), 1524–1532. Evidence Level V.

Lancaster, K. J., Smiciklas-Wright, H., Heller, D. A., Ahern, F. M., & Jensen, G. (2003). Dehydration in black and white older adults using diuretics. *Annals of Epidemiology, 13*(7), 525–529. Evidence Level IV.

Lavizzo-Mourey, R., Johnson, J., & Stolley, P. (1988). Risk factors for dehydration among elderly nursing home residents. *Journal of the American Geriatrics Society, 36*(3), 213–218. Evidence Level IV.

Leibovitz, A., Baumoehl, Y., Lubart, E., Yaina, A., Platinovitz, N., & Segal, R. (2007). Dehydration among long-term care elderly patients with oropharyngeal dysphagia. *Gerontology, 53*(4), 179–183. Evidence Level IV.

Lindeman, R. D., Tobin, J., & Shock, N. W. (1985). Longitudinal studies on the rate of decline in renal function with age. *Journal of the American Geriatrics Society, 33*(4), 278–285. Evidence Level IV.

Macias-Nuñez, J. F. (2008). The normal ageing kidney–morphology and physiology. *Reviews in Clinical Gerontology, 18*, 175–197. Evidence Level V.

Mack, G. W., Weseman, C. A., Langhans, G. W., Scherzer, H., Gillen, C. M., & Nadel, E. R. (1994). Body fluid balance in dehydrated healthy older men: Thirst and renal osmoregulation. *Journal of Applied Physiology, 76*(4), 1615–1623. Evidence Level III.

Mange, K., Matsuura, D., Cizman, B., Solo, H., Ziyadeh, F. N., Goldfarb, S., & Neilson, E. G. (1997). Language guiding therapy: The case of dehydration versus volume depletion. *Annals Internal Medicine, 127*(9), 848–853. Evidence Level V.

Masotti, L., Ceccarelli, E., Cappelli, R., Barabesi, L., Guerrini, M., & Forconi, S. (2000). Length of hospitalization in elderly patients with community-acquired pneumonia. *Aging, 12*(1), 35–41. Evidence Level IV.

Maughan, R. J., & Griffin, J. (2003). Caffeine ingestion and fluid balance: A review. *Journal of Human Nutrition and Dietetics, 16*(6), 411–420. Evidence Level I.

McConnell, J. (1984). Preventing urinary tract infections. *Geriatric Nursing, 5*(8), 361–362. Evidence Level III.

Meier, D. E., Ahronheim, J. C., Morris, J., Baskin-Lyons, S., & Morrison, R. S. (2001). High short-term mortality in hospitalized patients with advanced dementia: Lack of benefit of tube feeding. *Archives of Internal Medicine, 161*(4), 594–599. Evidence Level III.

Mentes, J. C. (2006). A typology of oral hydration problems exhibited by frail nursing home residents. *Journal Gerontological Nursing, 32*(1), 13–19, quiz 20–21. Evidence Level IV.

Mentes, J. C., Chang, B. L., & Morris, J. (2006). Keeping nursing home residents hydrated. *Western Journal of Nursing Research, 28*(4), 392–406; discussion 407–418. Evidence Level IV.

Mentes, J. C., & Culp, K. (2003). Reducing hydration-linked events in nursing home residents. *Clinical Nursing Research, 12*(3), 210–225; discussion 226–228. Evidence Level III.

Mentes, J. C., Culp, K., Maas, M., & Rantz, M. (1999). Acute confusion indicators: Risk factors and prevalence using MDS data. *Research in Nursing & Health, 22*(2), 95–105. Evidence Level IV.

Mentes, J. C., & Iowa-Veterans Affairs Research Consortium. (2000). Hydration management protocol. *Journal of Gerontological Nursing, 26*(10), 6–15. Evidence Level I.

Mentes, J. C., Wakefield, B., & Culp, K. (2006). Use of a urine color chart to monitor hydration status in nursing home residents. *Biological Research for Nursing, 7*(3), 197–203. Evidence Level IV.

Mentes, J. C., & Wang, J. (2010). Measuring risk for dehydration in nursing home residents. *Research in Gerontological Nursing, 31*, 1–9. Evidence Level IV.

Metheny, N. (2000). *Fluid and electrolyte balance: Nursing considerations* (4th ed.). St. Louis, MO: Lippincott, Williams, & Wilkins. Evidence Level VI.

Michaud, D. S., Spiegelman, D., Clinton, S. K., Rimm, E. B., Curhan, G. C., Willett, W. C., & Giovannucci, E. L. (1999). Fluid intake and the risk of bladder cancer in men. *The New England Journal of Medicine, 340*(18), 1390–1397. Evidence Level IV.

Miescher, E., & Fortney, S. M. (1989). Responses to dehydration and rehydration during heat exposure in young and older men. *The American Journal of Physiology, 257*(5 Pt. 2), R1050–1056. Evidence Level III.

Mitchell, S. L., Kiely, D. K., & Lipsitz, L. A. (1997). The risk factors and impact on survival of feeding tube placement in nursing home residents with severe cognitive impairment. *Archives of Internal Medicine, 157*(3), 327–332. Evidence Level III.

Morgan, A. L., Masterson, M. M., Fahlman, M. M., Topp, R. V., & Boardley, D. (2003). Hydration status of community-dwelling seniors. *Aging Clinical and Experimental Research, 15*(4), 301–304. Evidence Level IV.

Morita, T., Tei, Y., Tsunoda, J., Inoue, S., & Chihara, S. (2001). Determinants of the sensation of thirst in terminally ill cancer patients. *Supportive Care in Cancer, 9*(3), 177–186. Evidence Level IV.

Movig, K. L., Leufkens, H., Lenderink, A., & Egberts, A. C. (1992). Serotonergic antidepressants associated with an increased risk for hyponatremia in the elderly. *European Journal of Clinical Pharmacology, 58*(2), 143–148. Evidence Level IV.

Mueller, K. D., & Boisen, A. M. (1989). Keeping your patient's water level up. *RN, 52*(7), 65–68. Evidence Level V.

Mukand, J. A., Cai, C., Zielinski, A., Danish, M., & Berman, J.. (2003). The effects of dehydration on rehabilitation outcomes of elderly orthopedic patients. *Archives of Physical Medicine and Rehabilitation, 84*(1), 58–61. Evidence Level IV.

Musson, N. D., Kincaid, J., Ryan, P., Glussman, B., Varone, L., Gamarra, N., . . . Silverman, M. (1990). Nature, nurture, nutrition: Interdisciplinary programs to address the prevention of malnutrition and dehydration. *Dysphagia, 5*(2), 96–101. Evidence Level V.

National Research Council. (1989). *Recommended dietary allowances* (10th ed.). Washington, DC: National Academy Press. Evidence Level IV.

O'Keeffe, S. T., & Lavan, J. N. (1996). Predicting delirium in elderly patients: Development and validation of a risk-stratification model. *Age and Ageing, 25*(4), 317–321. Evidence Level IV.

Oliver, S. J., Laing, S. J., Wilson, S., Bilzon, J. L., & Walsh, N. P. (2008). Saliva indices track hypohydration during 48h of fluid restriction or combined fluid and energy restriction. *Archives of Oral Biology, 53*(10), 975–980.

Pals, J. K., Weinberg, A. D., Beal, L. F., Levesque, P. G., Cunnungham, T. J., & Minaker, K. L. (1995). Clinical triggers for detection of fever and dehydration. Implications for long-term care nursing. *Journal of Gerontological Nursing, 21*(4), 13–19. Evidence Level IV.

Phillips, P. A., Bretherton, M., Johnston, C. I., & Gray, L. (1991). Reduced osmotic thirst in healthy elderly men. *The American Journal of Physiology, 261*(1 Pt. 2), R166–R171. Evidence Level III.

Phillips, P. A., Rolls, B. J., Ledingham, J. G., Forsling, M. L., Morton, J. J., Crowe, M. J., & Wollner, L. (1984). Reduced thirst after water deprivation in healthy elderly men. *The New England Journal of Medicine, 311*(12), 753–759. Evidence Level III.

Practice guidelines for preoperative fasting and the use of pharmacologic agents to reduce the risk of pulmonary aspiration: Application to health patients undergoing elective procedures: A report by the American Society of Anesthesiologist Task Force on Preoperative Fasting. (1999). *Anesthesiology, 90*(3), 896–905. Evidence Level I.

Raman, A., Schoeller, D., Subar, A. F., Troiano, R. P., Schatzkin, A., Harris, T., . . . Tylavsky, F. A. (2004). Water turnover in 458 American adults 40-79 yr of age. *American Journal of Physiology. Renal Physiology, 286*(2), F394–F401. Evidence Level IV.

Rasouli, M., Kiasari, A. M., & Arab, S. (2008). Indicators of dehydration and haemoconcentration are associated with the prevalence and severity of coronary artery disease. *Clinical and Experimental Pharmacology & Physiology, 35*(8), 889–894. Evidence Level IV.

Ritz, P., & Source Study. (2001). Bioelectrical impedance analysis estimation of water compartments in elderly diseased patients: The source study. *The Journals of Gerontology. Series A, Biological Sciences and Medical Sciences, 56*(6), M344–M348. Evidence Level IV.

Robinson, S. B., & Rosher, R. B. (2002). Can a beverage cart help improve hydration? *Geriatric Nursing, 23*(4), 208–211. Evidence Level IV.

Rodriguez, G. J., Cordina, S. M., Vazquez, G., Suri, M. F., Kirmani, J. F., Ezzeddine, M. A., & Qureshi, A. I. (2009). The hydration influence on the risk of stroke (THIRST) study. *Neurocritical Care, 10*(2), 187–194. Evidence Level IV.

Rolls, B. J. (1998). Homeostatic and non-homeostatic controls of drinking in humans. In M. J. Arnaud (Ed.), *Hydration throughout life* (pp. 19–28). Montrouge, France: John Libbey Eurotext. Evidence Level II.

Sachdev, P., Mason, C., & Hadzi-Pavlovic, D. (1997). Case-control study of neuroleptic malignant syndrome. *The American Journal of Psychiatry, 154*(8), 1156–1158. Evidence Level IV.

Schmidlin, E. (2008). Artificial hydration: The role of the nurse in addressing patient and family needs. *International Journal of Palliative Nursing, 14*(10), 485–489. Evidence Level IV.

Seymour, D. G., Henschke, P. J., Cape, R. D., & Campbell, A. J. (1980). Acute confusional states and dementia in the elderly: The role of dehydration/volume depletion, physical illness and age. *Age and Ageing, 9*(3), 137–146. Evidence Level IV.

Simmons, S. F., Alessi, C., & Schnelle, J. F. (2001). An intervention to increase fluid intake in nursing home residents: Prompting and preference compliance. *Journal of the American Geriatrics Society, 49*(7), 926–933. Evidence Level II.

Skipper, A. (1993). Monitoring and complications of enternal feeding. In *Dietitian's handbook of enteral and parenteral nutrition* (p. 298). Rockville, MD: Aspen Publishers. Evidence Level V.

Smith, A. F., Vallance, H., & Slater, R. M. (1997). Shorter preoperative fluid fasts reduce postoperative emesis. *British Medical Journal, 314*(7092), 1486. Evidence Level II.

Spangler, P. F., Risley, T. R., & Bilyew, D. D. (1984). The management of dehydration and incontinence in nonambulatory geriatric patients. *Journal of Applied Behavior Analysis, 17*(3), 397–401. Evidence Level III.

Spigt, M. G., Knottnerus, J. A., Westerterp, K. R., Olde Rikkert, M. G., & Schayck, C. P. (2006). The effects of 6 months of increased water intake on blood sodium, glomerular filtration rate, blood pressure, and quality of life in elderly (aged 55-75) men. *Journal of the American Geriatrics Society, 54*(3), 438–443. Evidence Level II.

Stookey, J. D. (2005). High prevalence of plasma hypertonicity among community-dwelling older adults: Results from NHANES III. *Journal of the American Dietetic Association, 105*(8), 1231–1239. Evidence Level IV.

Stookey, J. D., Pieper, C. F., & Cohen, H. J. (2005). Is the prevalence of dehydration among community-dwelling older adults really low? Informing current debate over the fluid recommendation for adults aged 70+years. *Public Health Nutrition, 8*(8), 1275–1285. Evidence Level IV.

Vivanti, A., Harvey, K., & Ash, S. (2010). Developing a quick and practical screen to improve the identification of poor hydration in geriatric and rehabilitative care. *Archives of Gerontology and Geriatrics, 50*(2), 156–164. Evidence Level IV.

Vivanti, A., Harvey, K., Ash, S., & Battistutta, D. (2008). Clinical assessment of dehydration in older people admitted to hospital: What are the strongest indicators? *Archives of Gerontology and Geriatrics, 47*(3), 340–355. Evidence Level IV.

Wakefield, B., Mentes, J., Diggelmann, L., & Culp, K. (2002). Monitoring hydration status in elderly veterans. *Western Journal of Nursing Research, 24*(2), 132–142. Evidence Level IV.

Wakefield, B. J., Mentes, J., Holman, J. E., & Culp, K. (2008). Risk factors and outcomes associated with hospital admission for dehydration. *Rehabilitation Nursing, 33*(6), 233–241. Evidence Level IV.

Wallach, J. (2000). *Interpretation of diagnostic tests* (7th ed., pp. 135–141). Philadelphia, PA: Lippincott, Williams & Wilkins. Evidence Level VI.

Warren, J. L., Bacon, W. E., Harris, T., McBean, A. M., Foley, D. J., & Phillips, C. (1994). The burden and outcomes associated with dehydration among US elderly, 1991. *American Journal of Public Health, 84*(8), 1265–1269. Evidence Level IV.

Weinberg, A. D., Pals, J. K., Levesque, P. G., Beal, L. F., Cunningham, T. J., & Minaker, K. L. (1994). Dehydration and death during febrile episodes in the nursing home. *Journal of the American Geriatrics Society, 42*(9), 968–971. Evidence Level IV.

Whelan, K. (2001). Inadequate fluid intakes in dysphagic acute stroke. *Clinical Nutrition, 20*(5), 423–428. Evidence Level II.

Woods, D. L., & Mentes, J. C. (2011). Spit: Saliva in nursing research, uses and methodological consideration. *Biological Research for Nursing*. Evidence Level VI.

Xiao, H., Barber, J., & Campbell, E. S. (2004). Economic burden of dehydration among hospitalized elderly patients. *American Journal of Health System Pharmacy, 61*(23), 2534–2540. Evidence Level IV.

Yogendran, S., Asokumar, B., Cheng, D. C., & Chung, F. (1995). A prospective randomized double-blinded study of the effect of intravenous fluid therapy on adverse outcomes on outpatient surgery. *Anesthesia and Analgesia, 80*(4), 682–686. Evidence Level II.

Zembrzuski, C. D. (1997). A three-dimensional approach to hydration of elders: Administration, clinical staff, and in-service education. *Geriatric Nursing, 18*(1), 20–26. Evidence Level V.

22

Nutrition

Rose Ann DiMaria-Ghalili

EDUCATIONAL OBJECTIVES

On completion of this chapter, the reader should be able to:

1. recognize factors that place the older adult at risk for malnutrition.
2. discuss methods to screen and assess nutritional status in the older adult.
3. utilize appropriate nursing interventions in the hospitalized older adult who is either at risk for malnutrition or has malnutrition.

OVERVIEW

Nutritional status is the balance of nutrient intake, physiological demands, and metabolic rate (DiMaria-Ghalili, 2002). However, older adults are at risk for poor nutrition (DiMaria-Ghalili & Amella, 2005). Furthermore, malnutrition, a recognized geriatric syndrome (Institute of Medicine [IOM], 2008), is of concern because it can often be unrecognizable and impacts morbidity, mortality, and quality of life (Chen, Schilling, & Lyder, 2001), and is a precursor for frailty in the older adult. Malnutrition in older adults is defined as "faulty or inadequate nutritional status; undernourishment characterized by insufficient dietary intake, poor appetite, muscle wasting, and weight loss" (Chen et al., 2001). In the older adult, malnutrition exists along the continuum of care (Furman, 2006). Older adults admitted to acute care settings from either the community or long-term care settings may already be malnourished or may be at risk for the development of malnutrition during hospitalization. A diagnosis of malnutrition during an acute care stay increases the cost of hospitalization estimated at US$1,726 per patient (Rowell & Jackson, 2010). Bed rest is common during hospital stay, and the associated loss of lean mass that accompanies bed rest can impact the already vulnerable nutritional status of older adults (English & Paddon-Jones, 2010). The IOM notes that although malnutrition is a problem in older adults, most health care professionals,

For description of Evidence Levels cited in this chapter, see Chapter 1, Developing and Evaluating Clinical Practice Guidelines: A Systematic Approach, page 7.

Note: This chapter is based on the geriatric nursing protocol series. See http://consultgerirn.org/topics/nFutrition_in_the_elderly/want_to_know_more

including nurses, have little training concerning the nutritional needs of older adults (IOM, 2008). Therefore, it is imperative that acute care nurses carefully assess and monitor the nutritional status of older adults to identify the risk factors of malnutrition so that appropriate interventions are instituted in a timely fashion. The focus of this nursing protocol is aimed at the discussion of nutrition in aging as it relates to risk factors, implications, and interventions for malnutrition in the older adults.

BACKGROUND AND STATEMENT OF PROBLEM

The prevalence rate of malnutrition in hospitalized older adults was 38.7% according to a recent pooled analysis of studies based on the Mini-Nutritional Assessment tool (MNA; Kaiser et al, 2010). In the same study, 47.3% of older adults were at risk for malnutrition (Kaiser et al, 2010). In addition, a 1-day international audit on nutrition in 16,455 hospitalized patients (median age, 66) found that more than half of the patients did not eat their full meal provided, and decreased food intake was associated with increased risk of dying (Hiesmayr et al., 2006). Preliminary findings from the first U.S. national nutrition day in 2009 echo these results with 40% of hospitalized patients eating half or less of their meal (NutritionDay in the US, 2011). *Marasmus, kwashiorkor, and mixed marasmus-kwashiorkor* originally described the subtypes of malnutrition associated with famine, and these terms eventually characterized disease-related malnutrition. An international guideline committee was organized to develop a consensus approach to defining adult (including older adults) malnutrition in clinical settings (Jensen et al., 2010). Inflammation is the cornerstone of the new adult disease-related malnutrition subtypes and include "starvation-related malnutrition" (without inflammation), "chronic disease-related malnutrition" (with chronic inflammation of a mild-to-moderate degree; e.g., rheumatoid arthritis), and "acute disease or injury-related malnutrition" (with acute inflammation of a severe degree; e.g., major infections or trauma; Jensen et al., 2010). Defining characteristics of this new diagnostic classification of disease-related malnutrition are under development. The new malnutrition categories underscore the impact of a loss of lean body mass and skeletal muscle associated with the catabolic nature of the inflammatory process (Jensen et al., 2010). Although *sarcopenia* is an age-related loss of muscle mass and muscle strength (Rolland, Van Kan, Gillette-Guyonnet, & Vellas, 2010), bed rest during hospitalization is also associated with a loss of lean body mass, which adversely impacts functional capacity (Rowell & Jackson, 2010).

The risk factors for malnutrition in the older adult are multifactorial and include dietary, economic, psychosocial, and physiological factors (DiMaria-Ghalili & Amella, 2005). Dietary factors include little or no appetite (Carlsson, Tidermark, Ponzer, Söderqvist, & Cederholm, 2005; Reuben, Hirsch, Zhou, & Greendale, 2005; Saletti et al., 2005), problems with eating or swallowing, eating inadequate servings of nutrients (Margetts, Thompson, Elia, & Jackson, 2003), and eating fewer than two meals a day (Saletti et al., 2005). Limited income may cause restriction in the number of meals eaten per day or dietary quality of meals eaten (Souter & Keller, 2002). Isolation is also a risk factor as older adults who live alone may lose their desire to cook because of loneliness, and appetite often decreases after the loss of a spouse (Shahar, Schultz, Shahar, & Wing, 2001). Impairment in functional status can place the older adult at risk for malnutrition (Oliveira, Fogaca, & Leandro-Merhi, 2009) since adequate functioning is needed to secure and prepare food (Sharkey, 2008). Difficulty in cooking is related to disabilities (Souter et al., 2002), and disabilities can hinder the ability to prepare or ingest food (Saletti et al., 2005). Chronic conditions can negatively influence nutritional intake as well as cognitive impairment (Kagansky et al., 2005). Psychological factors are known risk factors of malnutrition. For example, depression is related to unintentional weight loss (Morley, 2001; Thomas et al., 2002). Furthermore, poor oral health (Saletti et al., 2005) and xerostomia (dry mouth caused by decreased saliva) can impair the ability to lubricate, masticate, and swallow food (Saletti et al., 2005). Antidepressants, antihypertensives, and bronchodilators can contribute to xerostomia (DiMaria-Ghalili & Amella, 2005). Change in taste (from medications, nutrient deficiencies, or taste bud atrophy) can also alter nutritional intake (DiMaria-Ghalili & Amella, 2005).

Body composition changes in normal aging include increase in body fat, including visceral fat stores (Hughes et al., 2004) and a decrease in lean body mass (Janssen, Heymsfield, Allison, Kotler, & Ross, 2002). Furthermore, the low skeletal muscle mass associated with aging is related to functional impairment and physical disability (Janssen I, Heymsfield, & Ross, 2002).

The impact of malnutrition on the health of the hospitalized older adult is well documented. In this population, malnutrition is related to prolonged hospital stay (Pichard et al., 2004), increased risk of poor health status, recent hospitalization, and institutionalization (Margetts et al., 2003). Additionally, low MNA scores are predictors of prolonged hospital stays and mortality (Sharkey, 2008).

ASSESSMENT OF THE PROBLEM

Areas of nutrition status assessment in the hospitalized older adult should focus on identification of malnutrition and risk factors for malnutrition. The MNA (Guigoz, Lauque, & Vellas, 2002) is a comprehensive two-level tool that can be used to screen and assess the older hospitalized patient for malnutrition by evaluating the presence of risk factors for malnutrition in this age group (DiMaria-Ghalili & Guenter, 2008). The validity and reliability of the MNA for use in hospitalized older adult is well documented (Salva et al., 2004). If a patient scores less than 12 on the screen, then the assessment section should be completed in order to compute the malnutrition indicator score. The screening section of the MNA is easy to administer and is comprised of six questions. The assessment section requires measurement of midarm muscle circumference and calf circumference. Although these anthropometric measurements are relatively easy to obtain with a tape measure, nurses may first require training in these procedures prior to incorporating the MNA as part of a routine nursing assessment. Protocols should be established to identify interventions to be implemented once the screening and assessment data are obtained and should include consultation with a dietitian. See http://consultgerirn.org/resources for *Assessing Nutrition in Older Adults* (Portable document Format [PDF] file) for MNA In Nutrition topic and Resources section.

Additional assessment strategies include proper measurement of height and weight and a detailed weight history. Height should always be directly measured and never recorded via patient self-report. An alternative way to measuring standing height is knee height (Salva et al., 2004) with special calipers. An alternative to knee height measures is a demi-span measurement, half the total arm span. (For directions on estimating height based on demi-span measurement, see Appendix 2 in A Guide to Completing the Mini Nutritional Assessment at http://www.mna-elderly.com/

mna_guide.pdf). A calorie count or dietary intake analysis is a good way to quantify the type and amount of nutrients ingested during hospitalization (DiMaria-Ghalili & Amella, 2005). Laboratory indicators of nutritional status include measures of visceral proteins such as serum albumin, transferrin, and prealbumin (DiMaria-Ghalili & Amella, 2005). However, these visceral proteins are also negative acute phase reactants and are decreased during a stressed inflammatory state, limiting the ability to predict malnutrition in the acutely ill hospitalized patient. In spite of this, albumin is a strong prognostic marker for morbidity and mortality in the older hospitalized patient (Sullivan et al., 2005). As biomarkers of inflammation are translated from research to clinical practice, future nutritional assessment protocols will incorporate inflammatory markers.

INTERVENTIONS AND CARE STRATEGIES

The nursing interventions outlined in the protocol focus on enhancing or promoting nutritional intake and range in complexity from basic fundamental nursing care strategies to the administration of artificial nutrition via parenteral or enteral routes. Prior to initiating targeted nutritional interventions in the hospitalized older adult, it must first be determined if the older adult cannot eat, should not eat, or will not eat (American Society for Parenteral and Enteral Nutrition [ASPEN], 2002). Factors to consider include the gastrointestinal tract (starting with the mouth) working properly without any functional, mechanical, or physiological alterations that would limit the ability to adequately ingest, digest, and/or absorb food. Also, does the older adult have any chronic or acute health condition in which the normal intake of food is contraindicated? Or, is the older adult simply not eating, or is the appetite decreased? If the gastrointestinal tract is functional and can be used to provide nutrients then nutritional interventions should be targeted at promoting adequate oral intake.

Nursing care strategies focus on ways to increase food intake as well as ways to enhance and manage the environment to promote increased food intake. When functional or mechanical factors limit the ability to take in nutrients, nurses should obtain interdisciplinary consultations from speech therapist, occupational therapists, physical therapists, psychiatrists, and/or dietitians to collaborate on strategies that would enhance the ability of the older adult to feed themselves or to eat. Oral nutritional supplementation has been shown to improve nutritional status in malnourished hospitalized older adults (Capra et al., 2007) and should be considered in the hospitalized older adult who is malnourished or is at risk for malnutrition. When used, oral liquid nutritional supplements should be given at least 60 minutes prior to meals (Wilson et al., 2002). Specialized nutritional support should be reserved for select situations. If the provision of nutrients via the gastrointestinal tract is contraindicated, then parenteral nutrition via the central or peripheral route should be initiated (ASPEN, 2002). If the gastrointestinal tract can be utilized, then nutrients should be delivered via enteral tube feeding (ASPEN, 2002). The exact location of the tube and type of feeding tube inserted depends on the disease state, length of time tube feeding is required, and risk of aspiration. Patients started on specialized nutritional support should be routinely reassessed for the continued need for specialized nutrition support and transitioned to oral feeding when feasible. Also, advance directives, if not completed, should be addressed prior to initiating specialized nutrition support (see Chapters 28 and 29, Health Care Decision Making and Advance Directives).

CASE STUDY

Mrs. V. H. is a 75-year-old female admitted to the hospital with a myocardial infarction and is on a telemetry unit for further workup prior to coronary artery bypass grafting surgery. On admission, her standing height is 5 ft 8 in. and she weighs 140 lbs. Her BMI is 21.33. Her past medical history is significant for rheumatoid arthritis. She describes herself as generally in good health up until she was admitted to the hospital. Medications include 400 mg of ibuprofen every 6 hours, prn. Mrs. V. H. is the primary caregiver for her 80-year-old husband who has altered cognitive functioning and is bedridden after a stroke 3 years ago. She complained of being tired and lacking energy prior to admission. Her weight history is significant for a 10 lb weight loss in the past 3 months. Mrs. V. H. said she started taking oral energy drinks because she was often too tired to cook a complete dinner for herself and lacked energy and was concerned about weight loss. She reported regaining 2 lbs. after taking 3 cans of an oral nutritional supplement per day for about 4 weeks. She reported having more strength after regaining some of her weight back. Although she is married, she is isolated because she does not have any social support systems to rely on. Her only living relative is a cousin who is 70 years old and lives 60 miles away and visits twice a month. During the assessment, Mrs. V. H. continually complained of being physically exhausted from caring for her husband at home and being too tired to eat or cook a nutritious meal for herself. She is worried about how she will care for her husband upon discharge from surgery and hopes that she can recover in the same nursing home that her husband was admitted to.

Although Mrs. V. H. does not have any chronic conditions or functional limitations that may place her at risk for malnutrition, her social history is significant. As the sole caregiver for her disabled husband, she is isolated, tired, and has a decreased appetite. She reports a history of unintentional loss of 10 lbs. in 3 months. Her MNA score is 7 based on moderate loss of appetite, weight loss greater than 6.6 lbs. during the last 3 months, goes out, has suffered an acute disease, no psychological problems, and has a BMI of 21.33. Because her score is below 11, she is at risk for malnutrition, and a complete assessment level of the MNA is performed. Her total MNA assessment score is 17.5 based on an assessment score of 10.5 and a screening score of 7.0, indicating she is at risk for malnutrition. Although she is on a regular diet, she only takes in about 50% of her meals. Oral nutritional supplements are ordered twice daily between meals. Consultations obtained from the social worker, dietitian, and physical therapist.

SUMMARY

Hospitalized older adults are at risk for malnutrition. Nurses should carefully assess and monitor the nutritional status of the older hospitalized patient so that appropriate nutrition-related interventions can be implemented in a timely fashion.

Protocol 22.1: Nutrition In Aging

I. GOAL: Improvement in indicators of nutritional status in order to optimize functional status and general well being and promote positive nutritional status.

II. OVERVIEW: Older adults are at risk for malnutrition with 39% to 47% of hospitalized older adults are malnourished or at risk for malnutrition (Kaiser, 2010).

III. BACKGROUND/STATEMENT OF PROBLEM

A. Definition(s)
  1. Malnutrition: Any disorder of nutritional status, including disorders resulting from a deficiency of nutrient intake, impaired nutrient metabolism, or overnutrition.
B. Etiology and/or Epidemiology. Older adults are at risk for undernutrition because of dietary, economic, psychosocial, and physiological factors (DiMaria-Ghalili, & Amella, 2005)
  1. Dietary intake
    a. Little or no appetite (Carlsso et al., 2005; Reuben et al., 2005; Saletti et al., 2005).
    b. Problems with eating or swallowing (Margetts et al., 2003).
    c. Eating inadequate servings of nutrients (Margetts et al., 2003).
    d. Eating fewer than two meals a day (Saletti et al., 2005).
  2. Limited income may cause restriction in the number of meals eaten per day or dietary quality of meals eaten (Margetts et al., 2003).
  3. Isolation
    a. Older adults who live alone may lose desire to cook because of loneliness (Souter & Keller, 2002).
    b. Appetite of widows decreases (Souter & Keller, 2002).
    c. Difficulty cooking because of disabilities (Margetts et al., 2003).
    d. Lack of access to transportation to buy food (DiMaria-Ghalili & Amella, 2005).
  4. Chronic illness
    a. Chronic conditions can affect intake (Margetts et al., 2003).
    b. Disability can hinder ability to prepare or ingest food (Saletti et al., 2005).
    c. Depression can cause decreased appetite (Kagansky et al, 2005; Morley, 2001).
    d. Poor oral health (cavities, gum disease, and missing teeth), as is xerostomia, or dry mouth impairs ability to lubricate, masticate, and swallow food (Saletti et al., 2005).
    e. Antidepressants, antihypertensives, and bronchodilators can contribute to xerostomia (dry mouth; DiMaria-Ghalili & Amella, 2005).
  5. Physiological changes
    a. Decrease in lean body mass and redistribution of fat around internal organs lead to decreased caloric requirements (Janssen et al., 2002; Thomas et al., 2002).

(continued)

    b. Change in taste (from medications, nutrient deficiencies, or taste bud atrophy) can also alter nutritional status (DiMaria-Ghalili & Amella, 2005).

IV. PARAMETERS OF ASSESSMENT

A. General: During routine nursing assessment, any alterations in general assessment parameters that influence intake, absorption, or digestion of nutrients should be further assessed to determine if the older adult is at nutritional risk. These parameters include

    1. Subjective assessment including present history, assessment of symptoms, past medical and surgical history, and comorbidities (University of Texas School of Nursing, 2006).

    2. Social history (University of Texas School of Nursing, 2006)

    3. Drug-nutrient interactions: Drugs can modify the nutrient needs and metabolism of older people. Restrictive diets, malnutrition, changes in eating patterns, alcoholism, and chronic disease with long-term drug treatment are some of the risk factors in older adults that place them at risk for drug-nutrient interactions (National Collaborating Centre for Acute w Care, 2006).

    4. Functional limitations (Pichard et al., 2004)

    5. Psychological status (Pichard et al., 2004)

    6. Objective assessment: physical examination with emphasis on oral exam (see Chapter 20, Oral Health Care), loss of subcutaneous fat, muscle wasting, and body mass index (University of Texas School of Nursing, 2006) and dysphagia.

B. Dietary Intake: In-depth assessment of dietary intake during hospitalization may be documented with a dietary intake analysis (calorie count; DiMaria-Ghalili & Amella, 2005).

C. Risk Assessment Tool: The Mini-Nutritional Assessment (MNA) should be performed to determine if older hospitalized patient is either at risk for malnutrition or has malnutrition. The MNA determines risk based on food intake, mobility, body mass index, history of weight loss, psychological stress, or acute disease, and dementia or other psychological conditions. If score is 11 points or less, the in-depth MNA assessment should be performed (Guigoz et al., 2002). See Resources section for tool or http://consultgerirn.org/resources for Nutrition topic.

D. Anthropometry

    1. Obtain an accurate weight and height through direct measurement. Do not rely on patient recall. If patient cannot stand erect to measure height, then either a demi-span measurement or a knee-height measurement should be taken to estimate height using special knee-height calipers (Guigoz et al., 2002). Height should never be estimated or recalled due to shortening of the spine with advanced age; self-reported height may be off by as much as 2.4 cm (Guigoz et al., 2002).

    2. Weight history: A detailed weight history should be obtained along with current weight. Detailed weight history should include a history of weight loss, whether the weight loss was intentional or unintentional, and during

(continued)

Protocol 22.1: Nutrition In Aging *(cont.)*

what period. A loss of 10 lbs. over a 6-month period, whether intentional or unintentional, is a critical indicator for further assessment (Boullata, 2004; DiMaria-Ghalili & Amella, 2005).

    3. Calculate body mass index (BMI) to determine if weight for height is within normal range: 22–27. A BMI below 22 is a sign of undernutrition (Boullata, 2004).

E. Visceral proteins: Evaluate serum albumin, transferrin, and prealbumin are visceral proteins commonly used to assess and monitor nutritional status (DiMaria-Ghalili & Amella, 2005). However, keep in mind these proteins are negative acute-phase reactants, so during a stress state, the production is usually decreased. In the older hospitalized patient, albumin levels may be a better indicator of prognosis than nutritional status (Salva et al., 2004).

V. NURSING CARE STRATEGIES: (DiMaria-Ghalili & Amella, 2005)
A. Collaboration
    1. Refer to dietitian if patient is at risk for undernutrition or has undernutrition.
    2. Consult with pharmacist to review patient's medications for possible drug–nutrient interactions.
    3. Consult with a multidisciplinary team specializing in nutrition.
    4. Consult with social worker, occupational therapist, and speech therapist as appropriate.
B. Alleviate dry mouth
    1. Avoid caffeine; alcohol and tobacco; dry, bulk, spicy, salty, or highly acidic foods.
    2. If patient does not have dementia or swallowing difficulties, offer sugarless hard candy or chewing gum to stimulate saliva.
    3. Keep lips moist with petroleum jelly.
    4. Frequent sips of water.
C. Maintain adequate nutritional intake
    Daily requirements for healthy older adults include 30 kcal/kg of body weight, and 0.8 to 1 g/kg of protein per day, with no more than 30% of calories from fat. Caloric, carbohydrate, protein, and fat requirements may differ depending on degree of malnutrition and physiological stress.
D. Improve oral intake
    1. Assess each patient's ability to eat within 24 hours of admission (Jefferies, Johnson, & Ravens, 2011).
    2. Mealtime rounds to determine how much food is consumed and whether assistance is needed (Jefferies et al., 2011).
    3. Limit staff breaks to before or after patient mealtimes to ensure adequate staff available to help with meals (Jefferies et al., 2011).
    4. Encourage family members to visit at mealtimes.
    5. Ask family to bring favorite foods from home when appropriate.
    6. Ask about patient food preferences and honor them.
    7. Suggest small frequent meals with adequate nutrients to help patients regain or maintain weight (Capra, Collins, Lamb, Vanderkroft, & Wai-Chi, 2007).

(continued)

Protocol 22.1: Nutrition In Aging *(cont.)*

    8. Provide nutritious snacks (Capra et al., 2007).

    9. Help patient with mouth care and placement of dentures before food is served (Jefferies et al., 2011).

E. Provide conducive environment for meals

    1. Remove bedpans, urinals, and emesis basins from rooms before mealtime.

    2. Administer analgesics and antiemetics on a schedule that will diminish the likelihood of pain or nausea during mealtimes

    3. Serve meals to patients in a chair if they can get out of bed and remain seated.

    4. Create a more relaxed atmosphere by sitting at the patient's eye level and making eye contact during feeding.

    5. Order a late food tray or keep food warm if patients not in their rooms during mealtimes.

    6. Do not interrupt patients for round and nonurgent procedures during meal times.

F. Specialized nutritional support (American Society for Parenteral and Enteral Nutrition, 2002)

    1. Start specialized nutritional support when a patient cannot, should not, or will not eat adequately and if the benefits of nutrition outweigh the associated risks.

    2. Prior to initiation of specialized nutritional support, review the patient's advanced directives regarding the use of artificial nutrition and hydration.

G. Provide oral supplements

    1. Supplements should not replace meals but be provided between meals and not within the hour preceding a meal and at bedtime (Capra et al., 2007; Wilson, Purushothaman, & Morley, 2002).

    2. Ensure that oral supplement is at appropriate temperature (Capra et al., 2007).

    3. Ensure that oral supplement packaging is able to be opened by the patients (Capra et al., 2007).

    4. Monitor the intake of the prescribed supplement (Capra et al., 2007).

    5. Promote a sip style of supplement consumption (Capra et al., 2007).

    6. Include supplements as part of the medication protocol (Capra et al., 2007).

H. Nothing by mouth (NPO) orders

    1. Schedule older adults for test or procedures early in the day to decrease the length of time they are not allowed to eat and drink.

    2. If testing late in the day is inevitable, ask physician whether the patient can have an early breakfast.

      See American Society of Anesthesiologists (ASA) practice guideline regarding recommended length of time patients should be kept NPO for elective surgical procedures.

VI. EVALUATION/EXPECTED OUTCOMES

A. Patient

    1. The patient will experience improvement in indicators of nutritional status.

    2. The patient will improve functional status and general well-being.

(continued)

Protocol 22.1: Nutrition In Aging *(cont.)*

B. Provider
1. The provider should ensure that care provides food and fluid of adequate quantity and quality in an environment conducive to eating, with appropriate support (e.g., modified eating aids) for people who can potentially chew and swallow but are unable to feed themselves (Boullata, 2004).
2. The provider should continue to reassess patients who are malnourished or at risk for malnutrition (Boullata, 2004).
3. The provider should monitor for refeeding syndrome (Boullata, 2004).

C. Institution
1. The institution will ensure that all health care professionals who are directly involved in patient care should receive education and training on the importance of providing adequate nutrition (Boullata, 2004).

D. Quality Assurance/Quality Improvement (QA/QI)
1. Establish QA/QI measures surrounding nutritional management in aging patients.

E. Educational
1. Provider education and training includes
   a. Nutritional needs and indications for nutrition support
   b. Options for nutrition support (oral, enteral, and parenteral)
   c. Ethical and legal concepts
   d. Potential risks and benefits
   e. When and where to seek expert advice (Boullata, 2004).
2. Patient and/or caregiver education includes how to maintain or improve nutritional status as well as how to administer, when appropriate, oral liquid supplements, enteral tube feeding or parenteral nutrition

VII. FOLLOW-UP MONITORING (Boullata, 2004)

A. Monitor for gradual increase in weight over time.
1. Weigh patient weekly to monitor trends in weight.
2. Daily weights are useful for monitoring fluid status.

B. Monitor and assess for refeeding syndrome.
1. Carefully monitor and assess patients the first week of aggressive nutritional repletion.
2. Assess and correct the following electrolyte abnormalities: Hypophosphatemia, hypokalemia, hypomagnesemia, hyperglycemia, and hypoglycemia.
3. Assess fluid status with daily weights and strict intake and output.
4. Assess for congestive heart failure in patients with respiratory or cardiac difficulties.
5. Ensure caloric goals will be reached slowly more than 3–4 days to avoid refeeding syndrome when repletion of nutritional status is warranted.
6. Be aware that refeeding syndrome is not only exclusive to patients started on aggressive artificial nutrition, but may also be found in older adults with chronic comorbid medical conditions and poor nutrient intake started with aggressive nutritional repletion via oral intake.

(continued)

Protocol 22.1: Nutrition In Aging *(cont.)*

VIII: RELEVANT GUIDELINES

A. American Society of Anesthesiologists. (1999). Practice guidelines for preoperative fasting and the use of pharmacologic agents to reduce the risk of pulmonary aspiration: Application to healthy patients undergoing elective procedures: A report by the American Society of Anesthesiologist Task Force on Preoperative Fasting. *Anesthesiology, 90,* 896–905.

B. National Collaborating Centre for Acute Care. (2006). *Nutrition support in adults: Oral nutrition support, enteral tube feeding and parenteral nutrition.* London, UK: National Institute for Health and Clinical Excellence. Clinical guideline; no. 32. Electronic copies: Available in PDF from that National Institute for Health and Clinical Excellence (NICE) website.

C. American Society for Parenteral and Enteral Nutrition. (2002). Guidelines for the use of parenteral and enteral nutrition in adult and pediatric patients. *JPEN. Journal of Parenteral and Enteral Nutrition, 26,* 1SA–138SA. Note: These guidelines are undergoing revision.

D. University of Texas. (2006). *Unintentional weight loss in the elderly.* Austin, TX: Author. Note: These guidelines are located at http://www.guidelines.gov. However, the companion document with full bibliography is not in the public domain.

RESOURCES

American Dietetic Association
Position Statement: Nutrition Across the Spectrum of Aging:
http://www.eatright.org/About/Content.aspx?id=8374
Practice Paper: Individualized Nutrition Approaches for Older Adults in Health Care Communities:
http://www.eatright.org/About/Content.aspx?id=8373
Position Paper: Food and Nutrition Programs for Community-Residing Older Adults:
http://www.eatright.org/About/Content.aspx?id=6442451115

United States Department of Agriculture
Professional Development Tools: Older Adults
http://snap.nal.usda.gov/nal_display/index.php?info_center=15&tax_level=3&tax_subject=275&topic_id=1336&level3_id=5216

Regulatory/authoritative sites

American Geriatrics Society
http://www.americangeriatrics.org

American Medical Directors Association: Clinical Tools and Products
http://www.amda.com/tools/index.cfm

American Society for Parenteral and Enteral Nutrition
http://www.nutritioncare.org/

Centers for Medicare and Medicaid Services
http://www.medicare.gov/Nursing/Campaigns/NutriCareAlerts.asp

Practicing Physician Education in Geriatrics
http://www.gericareonline.net/

National Conference of Gerontological Nurse Practitioners
http://www.acnpweb.org/i4a/pages/Index.cfm?pageID=3697

National Gerontological Nursing Association
http://www.ngna.org/

National Institutes of Health
http://www.nlm.nih.gov/medlineplus/nutritionforseniors.html

The Gerontological Society of America
http://www.geron.org/

United States Department of Health and Human Services
http://www.hhs.gov/

Mini-Nutritional Assessment

Nestle Nutrition Institute
http://www.mna-elderly.com/

Nutrition in the Elderly

ConsultGeriRN website of the Hartford Institute for Geriatric Nursing
http://consultgerirn.org/resources

Knee-height Measurement

Florida International University's Long-term Care Institute Resource Materials
http://www.fiu.edu/%7Enutreldr/LTC_Institute/materials/LTC_Products.htm#7

REFERENCES

American Society for Parenteral and Enteral Nutrition. (2002). Guidelines for the use of parenteral and enteral nutrition in adult and pediatric patients. *JPEN. Journal of Parenteral and Enteral Nutrition, 26*(Suppl. 1), 1SA–138SA. Level 1.

Boullata, J. (2004). Drug-nutrient interactions. In P. Worthington, (Ed.), *Practical aspects of nutrition support. An advanced practice guide* (pp. 431–454). Philadelphia, PA: Saunders. Evidence Level VI.

Capra, S., Collins, C., Lamb, M., Vanderkroft, D., & Wai-Chi, S. (2007). Effectiveness of interventions for undernourished older inpatients in the hospital setting. *Best Practice, 11*, 1–4. Evidence Level I.

Carlsson, P., Tidermark, J., Ponzer, S., Söderqvist, A., & Cederholm, T. (2005). Food habits and appetite of elderly women at the time of a femoral neck fracture and after nutritional and anabolic support. *Journal of Human Nurtrition and Dietetics, 18*, 117–120. Evidence Level II.

Chen, C. C., Schilling, L. S., & Lyder, C. H. (2001). A concept analysis of malnutrition in the elderly. *Journal of Advance Nursing, 36*, 131–142. Evidence Level V.

DiMaria-Ghalili, R. A. (2002). Changes in nutritional status and postoperative outcomes in elderly CABG patients. *Biological Reasearch for Nursing, 4*, 73–84. Evidence Level IV.

DiMaria-Ghalili, R. A., & Amella, E. Nutrition in older adults. (2005) *The American Journal of Nursing, 105*(3), 40–50. Evidence Level V.

DiMaria-Ghalili, R. A., & Guenter, P. A. (2008). The mini nutritional assessment. *American Journal of Nursing, 108*(2), 50–59. Evidence Level V.

English, K. L., & Paddon-Jones, D. (2010). Protecting muscle mass and function in older adults during bed rest. *Current Opinion in Clinical Nutrition and Metabolic Care. 13*, 34–39. Evidence Level VI.

Furman, E. F. (2006). Undernutrition in older adults across the continuum of care: Nutritional assessment, barriers, and interventions. *Journal of Gerontological Nursing, 32*, 22–27. Evidence Level VI.

Guigoz, Y., Lauque, S., & Vellas, B. J. (2002). Identifying the elderly at risk for malnutrition. The Mini Nutritional Assessment. *Clinics in Geriatric Medicine, 18*, 737–757. Evidence Level V.

Hiesmayr, M., Schindler, K., Pernicka, E., Schuh, C., Schoeniger-Hekele, A., Bauer, P., . . . Ljungqvist, O. (2009). Decreased food intake is a risk factor for mortality in hospitalised patients: The NutritionDay survey 2006. *Clinical Nutrition, 28*, 484–491. Evidence Level IV.

Hughes, V. A., Roubenoff, R., Wood, M., Frontera, W. R., Evans, W. J., & Fiatarone Singh, M. A. (2004). Anthropometric assessment of 10-y changes in body composition in the elderly. *The American Journal of Clinical Nutrition, 80*, 475–482. Evidence Level IV.

Institute of Medicine. (2008). *Retooling for an aging America: Building the health care workforce.* Washington, DC: National Academies Press. Evidence Level VI.

Janssen, I., Heymsfield, S. B., Allison, D. B., Kotler, D. P., & Ross, R. (2002). Body mass index and waist circumference independently contribute to the prediction of nonabdominal, abdominal subcutaneous, and visceral fat. *The American Journal of Clinical Nutrition, 75*, 683–688. Evidence Level IV.

Janssen, I., Heymsfield, S. B., & Ross, R. (2002). Low relative skeletal muscle mass (sarcopenia) in older persons is associated with functional impairment and physical disability. *Journal of the American Geriatrics Society, 50*, 889–896. Evidence Level IV.

Jefferies, D., Johnson, M., & Ravens, J. (2011). Nurturing and nourishing: The nurses' role in nutritional care. *Journal of Clinical Nursing, 20*, 317–330. Evidence Level I.

Jensen, G. L., Mirtallo, J., Compher, C., Dhaliwal, R., Forbes, A., Grijalba, R. F., . . . Waitzberg, D. (2010). Adult starvation and disease-related malnutrition: A proposal for etiology-based diagnosis in the clinical practice setting from the International Consensus Guideline Committee. *JPEN. Journal of Parenteral and Enteral Nutrition, 34*, 156–159. Evidence Level VI.

Kagansky, N., Berner, Y., Koren-Morag, N., Perelman, L., Knobler, H., & Levy, S. (2005). Poor nutritional habits are predictors of poor outcome in very old hospitalized patients. *American Journal of Clinical Nutrition, 82*, 784–791. Evidence Level IV.

Kaiser, M. J., Bauer, J. M., Rämsch, C., Uter, W., Guigoz, Y., Cederholm, T., . . . Sieber, C. C. (2010). Frequency of malnutrition in older adults: A multinational perspective using the mini nutritional assessment. *Journal of the American Geriatrics Society, 58*, 1734–1738. doi:10.1111/j.1532-5415.2010.03016.x. Evidence Level 1

Margetts, B. M., Thompson, R. L., Elia, M., & Jackson, A. A. (2003). Prevalence of risk of undernutrition is associated with poor health status in older people in the UK. *European Journal of Clinical Nutrition, 57*, 69–74. Evidence Level IV.

Morley, J. E. (2001). Anorexia, sarcopenia, and aging. *Nutrition, 17*, 660–663. Evidence Level V.

National Collaborating Centre for Acute Care. (2006). Nutrition support for adults: Oral nutrition support, enteral tube feeding and parenteral nutrition. Clinical guideline; no 32 [serial on the Internet]. Retrieved from http://www.ncbi.nlm.nih.gov/books/NBK49269/

NutritionDay in the US. Retrieved from http://www.nutritiondayus.org

Oliveira, M. R., Fogaca, K. C., & Leandro-Merhi, V. A. (2009). Nutritional status and functional capacity of hospitalized elderly. *Nutrition Journal, 8*, 54. Evidence Level IV.

Pichard, C., Kyle, U. G., Morabia, A., Perrier, A., Vermeulen, B., & Unger P. (2004). Nutritional assessment: Lean body mass depletion at hospital admission is associated with an increased length of stay. *The American Journal of Clinical Nutrition, 79*, 613–618. Evidence Level IV.

Reuben, D. B., Hirsch, S. H., Zhou, K., & Greendale, G. A. (2005). The effects of megestrol acetate suspension for elderly patients with reduced appetite after hospitalization: A phase II randomized clinical trial. *Journal of the American Geriatrics Society, 53*, 970–975. Evidence Level II.

Rolland, Y., Van Kan, G. A., Gillette-Guyonnet, S., & Vellas, B. (2011). Cachexia versus sarcopenia. *Current Opinion in Clinical Nutrition and Metabolic Care, 14*, 15–21. Evidence Level VI.

Rowell, D. S., & Jackson, T. J. (2010). Additional costs of inpatient malnutrition, Victoria, Australia, 2003–2004. *European Journal of Health Economics, 12*, 353–361. Evidence Level IV.

Saletti, A., Johansson, L., Yifter-Lindgren, E., Wissing, U., Osterberg, K., & Cederholm, T. (2005). Nutritional status and a 3-year follow-up in elderly receiving support at home. Gerontology, *51*,192–198. Evidence Level IV.

Salva, A., Corman, B., Andrieu S, Salas, J., Porras, C., & Vellas, B. (2004). Minimum data set for nutritional intervention studies in the elderly IAG/ IANA task force consensus. *The Journal of Nutrition Health and Aging, 8*, 202–206. Evidence Level V.

Shahar, D. R., Schultz, R., Shahar, A., & Wing, R. R. (2001). The effect of widowhood on weight change, dietary intake, and eating behavior in the elderly population. *Journal of Aging and Health, 13*, 189–199. Evidence Level IV.

Sharkey, J. R. (2008). Diet and health outcomes in vulnerable populations. *Annals of the New York Academy of Sciences*, 1136, 210–217. Evidence Level V.

Souter, S., & Keller, C. (2002). Food choice in the rural dwelling older adult. *Southern Online Journal of Nursing Research, 3*, 1–18. Retrieved from http://www.snrs.org/members/SOJNR_articles/iss05vol03.pdf. Evidence Level IV: Non-experimental study. Level IV.

Sullivan, D. H., Roberson, P. K., & Bopp, M. M. (2005). Hypoalbuminemia 3 months after hospital discharge: Significance for long-term survival. *Journal of the American Geriatrics Society, 53*, 1222–1226. Evidence Level IV.

Thomas, D. R., Zdrowski, C. D., Wilson, M. M., Conright, K. C., Lewis, C., Tariq, S., & Morley, J. E. (2002). Malnutrition in subacute care. *The American Journal of Clinical Nutrition, 75*, 308–313. Evidence Level IV.

University of Texas School of Nursing. (2006). *Unintentional weight loss in the elderly*. Retrieved from http://www.guidelines.gov

Wilson, M. M., Purushothaman, R., & Morley, J. E. (2002). Effect of liquid dietary supplements on energy intake in the elderly. *The American Journal of Clinical Nutrition, 75*, 944–947. Evidence Level IV.

Mealtime Difficulties

23

Elaine J. Amella and Melissa B. Aselage

EDUCATIONAL OBJECTIVES

On completion of this chapter, the reader should be able to:

1. assess the older adult for critical issues related to performance at mealtimes: physical and cognitive functioning, aversion to eating, cultural/religious factors
2. modify the mealtime environment to one that promotes adequate intake and normalizes social interaction
3. educate staff and caregivers to provide individualized assistance at meals while preserving the independence and dignity of the person being assisted

OVERVIEW

Nutrition has long been recognized as a key element in promoting good health and recovery from illness across the life span; this is especially true as an individual ages. However, the process of eating and the entire ritual of meals, which together are largely culturally determined, are given little attention when nutritional problems are identified. This is especially notable in a time when interest in food and its presentation has become a national craze, with many claiming to be "foodies" and chefs raised to the status of media stars (Food Network Chef Bios, 2011). However, in institutions, restrictive diets are sometimes barely palatable, the eating environment ranges from a cluttered hospital room to a large, noisy dining room, and staff treat the meal as a task to complete rather than a process to enjoy. This chapter will address both barriers and enablers to overcoming mealtime difficulties and evidence-based strategies to support that process.

BACKGROUND AND STATEMENT OF PROBLEM

Nutrition is critical to maintaining health, and nowhere is this more important than among older adults. The ingestion of the proper balance of macronutrients and

For description of Evidence Levels cited in this chapter, see Chapter 1, Developing and Evaluating Clinical Practice Guidelines: A Systematic Approach, page 7.

micronutrients results in a pattern of eating that persists into old age and affects an individual's risk for chronic illness, especially Type 2 diabetes, heart disease, osteoarthritis, and some cancers (U.S. Centers for Disease Control and Prevention [CDC], 2009a). When older persons with multiple morbidities are hospitalized, their nutritional status is often compromised related to a complex interplay of issues from social isolation, dependence on others whether at home or in a nursing home, to depression or dementia (Arora et al., 2007). Then, as a result of these barriers to nutritional health, they are more likely to remain in hospital longer with higher rates of complications and mortality (Arora et al., 2007). Within the revised *Healthy People 2020*, determinants of health beyond individual behaviors are examined to include both the social environment, such as limitations that make it challenging for older adults to stay at home; health services–related factors such as accessibility to providers with needed expertise; and community factors such as poverty, violence, and access to healthy food (U.S. Department of Health and Human Services [USDHHS], 2011); these factors directly affect nutritional issues and disproportionately affect minorities and targeted underserved groups. A good diet in old age can be influenced by multiple factors; one study found, not surprisingly, that higher socioeconomic status, ingestion of regular fruits and vegetables since childhood, and not smoking were primary predictors (Maynard et al., 2006). Of the top 10 causes of death in the older cohort, a lifetime of good nutrition would positively improve nine causes: heart disease, cancer, stroke, chronic lower respiratory disease, Alzheimer's disease, diabetes, influenza/pneumonia, nephritic syndrome/nephritis, and septicemia, with accidents being the outlier (CDC, 2009b). However, although the examination of nutrition and maintenance of a healthy diet are primary assessment criteria, the issue of how older people choose, prepare, serve, and ingest food, or others do it for them—the phenomenon of meals—is often overlooked. *Meal* is defined as "the food served and eaten, especially at one of the customary, regular occasions for taking food during the day, as breakfast, lunch, or supper; one of these regular occasions or times for eating food" (Flexner & Hauck, 1987). Meals are custom driven and contextually based; even the time that food is eaten and what is eaten at each meal can be dictated by culture and habit.

Within a "foreign" environment such as a hospital or long-term care institution, a different culture exists—one that focuses on patient safety and quality, which has been broadly defined as preventing harm to patients and delivering quality health care (Mitchell, 2008). The overarching concern for systems outcomes may override individual needs; this has led in the long-term care environment to the "culture change" movement that focuses on quality of life as well as quality of care (Koren, 2010). Deeply embedded within this paradigm shift, which is championed by national lay and professional stakeholders, is a regard for mealtimes that reflects the comforts of home (Pioneer Network, n.d.). With a growing concern for shifting the paradigm away from solely a concern for calories consumed to a comprehensive approach to the entire phenomenon of eating, we need to explore the assessment and management of mealtimes through a new lens using a model that asks the health care provider to examine the entire context of meals for all older adults; the way that the meal assistance is rendered by caregivers, if needed, especially in the face of acute exacerbations of chronic illness and cognitive impairment; and health factors that may influence the older adult's functional and cognitive capacity to independently eat. This model—change the context, change the caregiving, change the person—has been adopted in three studies by the authors who trained caregivers in long-term care and in the community to change meals as a mechanism to promote quality of life and nutritional health (Amella & DeLegge, 2009; Amella &

Laditka, 2009; Aselage, 2011). Furthermore, the support of the routine and the familiar was shown to be critical in older persons with cognitive impairments through the work of nurse researchers who developed the Needs-Driven Dementia-Compromised Behavior framework in the late 1990s that examined dysfunctional behavior from the areas of background (personal) and proximal (environmental) factors among people with dementia (Algase et al., 1996). This work guides many interdisciplinary interventions for this compromised population today, including examination of mealtime issues (Aselage & Amella, 2010).

ASSESSMENT OF THE PROBLEM

Recommendations for assessment of nutrition among older adults vary depending on their place of residence (community, long-term care, or acute care) and their level of independence; however, a systematic review of different instruments recently supported the use of the Mini Nutritional Assessment (MNA) across sites and SCREEN II for community-dwelling older adults (Phillips, Foley, Barnard, Isenring, & Miller, 2010). However, the MNA has only one question that even indirectly deals with meals: "How many full meals does the patient eat daily?" The individual is then asked: "Do you normally eat breakfast, lunch, and dinner?" The following definition of a full meal is given: A full meal is defined as an eating occasion when the patient "sits down" to eat and consumes more than two items/dishes (Guigoz, Vellas, & Garry, 1997). An alternative assessment instrument that has been used exclusively in the community, SCREEN II, shows strong psychometrics, but does not address contextual issues beyond "eating alone" (Keller, Goy, & Kane, 2005). Assessment of the entire process of eating and mealtimes was divided into the following components by Aselage (2010) to *eating behavior* assessed by the Level of Eating Independence Scale (LEIS) and the Eating Behavior Scale (EBS); *feeding behavior* assessed by the Edinburgh Feeding in Dementia Scale (EdFED), Feeding Abilities Assessment (FAA), Self-Feeding Assessment Tool of Osborn and Marshall, the McGill Ingestive Skills Assessment (MISA), Feeding Behavior Inventory, the Feeding Traceline Technique (FTLT), Feeding Dependency Scale (FDS), and the Aversive Feeding Inventory; and *meal behavior* assessed by the Meal Assistance Screening Tool (MAST) and Structured Meal Observation. This critical appraisal of instruments determined that most are primarily used in research, most are setting specific with an emphasis on either long-term care or rehabilitation settings—few have been used in the community; are often lengthy and may not be practical in a clinical setting. Only the EdFED, which has been used across acute and long-term care settings and in the community, has strong psychometrics, and appears to be the most practical across domains (Watson, 1994b; Watson, Green, & Legg, 2001); yet, it was designed to evaluate individuals with dementia—clearly not all older persons having difficulties with meals, but in all likelihood a significant portion.

The other standardized assessment instrument worth noting is the Minimum Data Set (MDS) that, as of late 2010, underwent its third complete revision—MDS 3.0—to improve accuracy and reliability of assessment and reporting (Centers for Medicare & Medicaid Services [CMS], 2010). The MDS is administered to all residents of nursing homes in the United States receiving federal funding, and it may be a part of the assessment information that flows between agencies during transitions—nursing home to acute care. One of the foci of the MDS is determining the amount of assistance required by an individual to perform various activities, as well as health problems that may result if key factors are not addressed. The MDS dedicates only two questions in 15 sections regarding health assessment to a mealtime-like issue. In the section Preference for Customary and Routine Activities, the only relevant item is "How important is it to you to have snacks available between meals?" and in the Functional Status section, "Eating—includes eating, drinking (regardless of skill), or intake of nourishment by other means" (e.g., tube feeding, total parenteral nutrition, intravenous fluids for hydration; CMS, 2010).

As an individual ages, the likelihood of functional impairment increases. With increased frailty, loss of function follows a predictable pattern, with the ability to feed oneself the last activity of daily living (ADL) to be lost (Katz, Downs, Cash, & Grotz, 1970; Katz, Ford, Moskowitz, Jackson, & Jaffe, 1963). The most recent national data on disability showed that 19.7% of all older adults (65 years old and older) are chronically disabled, with 3.1% of those living in the community requiring assistance with five to six ADLs (Federal Interagency Forum on Age-Related Statistics, 2006). Although self-feeding must be promoted for all persons for as long as possible, techniques for promotion of independence at meals are often not used and may take too much time for caregivers resulting in increased dependence at mealtimes. Interdisciplinary researchers developed individualized nutritional interventions based on regular assessment of changing status over time; the treatment group was noted to have a declining appetite, poor posture while eating, and inadequate oral care—all amenable to alterations to the process of care with improved nutritional serological markers and depression compared to the control group (Crogan, Alvine, & Pasvogel, 2006).

Assessment is not a static event especially when an older adult experiences the downward spiral of a life-limiting cognitive or physical illness.

Different religious and cultural groups may have strict requirements for preparation and blessing of food before it can be consumed (Bermudez & Tucker, 2004). Therefore, assessment of these beliefs and preferences are vital. Individuals who follow dietary restrictions for religious or cultural reasons may not eat when rules have not been observed (Fjellström, 2004). In general, most cultures promote the washing of hands before meals; this may not be offered in institutional settings. Older adults who have serious chronic illness should be consulted regarding preferences for food and fluid intake. They should be asked about their wishes regarding treatment with artificial nutrition and hydration if not already documented in an advance directive. If the older adult loses the capacity for decision making, the proxy for health care decisions should be consulted rather than the provider assuming responsibility for the management of nutritional care.

Finally, for some older adults, social determinants of health may limit their ability to acquire and eat the foods they have preferred over a lifetime. For those individuals living at or near the poverty line, or those who live in rural or economically depressed neighborhoods, food insecurity and food deserts may be active concerns (Coates et al., 2006). In 2008, among older adults living alone, 8.8% were categorized as food insecure and 3.8% were categorized as very low food insecure, meaning they may not be eating for a whole day and this condition was present for 3 or more months (Coates et al., 2006; Seligman, Laraia, & Kushel, 2010). Inability to obtain favorite foods because one lives in an area only serviced by convenience-type stores with highly processed food (food deserts), out of fear of violence, or because of poverty may result in meals that are no longer appealing or congruent with lifelong cultural preferences. For these older adults, referral to meal programs may be vital.

INTERVENTIONS AND CARE STRATEGIES

Nutritional Health

Assessment and management of nutritional health is covered in the Nutrition chapter in this text; therefore, the reader is referred to that discussion. However, the professional nurse is reminded that nutritional health is best assessed and managed through an inter-disciplinary approach because it is a multifaceted issue. Minimally, the dietitian, provider (physician, advanced practice nurse, physician assistant), dentist, speech and language pathologist, occupational therapist, and patient/caregiver should be consulted when designing a nutritional plan of care. The social worker or case manager may be key to coordinating outside resources and should be part of discharge planning for obtaining preferred, culturally appropriate, and healthy foods. Strategies that produced better meal-time outcomes included "meal rounds" by a dietitian and food service supervisors work-ing with unit staff, which allowed for early identification of residents at risk for nutritional problems and early intervention, especially those with dysphagia and those needing assis-tance at meals (Keller, 2006). Clearly, mealtimes are an opportunity for collaboration.

Cognitive Impairments

Cognitive deficits impair the ability to eat and drink. Persons with severe cognitive impair-ments may develop refuse-like or aversive behaviors that affect their ability to be assisted at meals; this is significantly associated with mortality (Amella, 2002; Mitchell et al., 2009). In a systematic review of the literature, the only intervention that was associated with increased intake in this group was high-calorie supplements, although other nutri-tional and social interventions only showed weak association (Hanson, Ersek, Gilliam, & Carey, 2011). However, as this disease moves toward later stages, the individual's prior wishes should be respected regarding food and fluid and the focus is often placed on quality of life (Amella, 2004). Watson developed a psychometrically sound instrument, the EdFED, to measure the declining ability to consume food offered related to resis-tance (Watson & Deary, 1997). Nurses can use the principles of this instrument to deter-mine the stage of resistive eating behavior. In the earlier stages, more active behaviors are displayed (e.g., the individual pushes food away or turns his or her head away from the feeder). In later stages, passive behaviors occur, as the patient does not swallow and allows food to fall from his or her mouth. In late-stage dementia, a primitive and less forceful swallow pattern may develop. The upper airway is not well protected, making the use of bottle or syringe-type feeding not only undignified but also ineffective and unsafe.

Increasing Intake

Modifying mealtimes may result in positive nutritional outcomes—one of the most nota-ble is increasing intake of food and fluids. Interventions range from modifying a "thera-peutic" diet (including favorite foods, promoting socialization, and a team approach) to planning meals. Liberalization of diets is recommended by a major dietetic organization when intake of micronutrients (e.g., sodium) or macronutrients (e.g., fats) cannot be sup-ported and quality of life is primary, especially in those persons with life-limiting illnesses, or who have consumed minimal nutrition (Dorner, Friedrich, & Posthauer, 2010).

Equivocal results can be found regarding what activities promote greater intake at meals. Taylor and Barr (2006) reported that eating smaller more frequent meals increased intake of fluids; however, it did not increase food intake. In a randomized crossover design, researchers found that "smaller eaters" consumed more calories and protein if breakfast and lunch meals were enhanced with higher caloric food and extra protein (Castellanos, Marra, & Johnson, 2009). Additionally, in a quasi-experimental study, eating in the dining room appeared to increase total consumption of calories but did not influence intake of protein, nor did it influence weight gain (Gaskill, Isenring, Black, Hassall, & Bauer, 2009; Wright, Hickson, & Frost, 2006). Some Acute Care for the Elderly units include a dining room in their environmental modifications in order to improve the mealtime experience, increase observation of those with eating problems, and increase food intake.

Mealtimes can be a time to significantly increase social exchange, as was demonstrated through a bundled intervention including favorite foods, including chocolate; moderate exercise; and oral care. However, it was social engagement and functional ability that increased in the treatment group, with social engagement associated most with improvement (Beck, Damkjaer, & Sorbye, 2010). Furthermore, in an observational study conducted in France that promoted caregiving staff sharing meals with nursing home residents with dementia, compared to another nursing home that did not have shared meals, weight of residents in the "treatment" facility was maintained and staffs' behavior toward residents improved (Charras & Frémonteir, 2010).

Feeding Assistance and Staff Training

Within recent years, more emphasis is being placed on preparing staff in nursing homes to safely assist with meals; sadly, this has not occurred with equal vigor in acute care where older adults may be the most medically vulnerable and require knowledgeable staff to support meals. Under experimental conditions, it has been demonstrated that feeding assistance makes a critical difference for older adults with functional impairment: When nursing home residents at risk for weight loss were assisted by trained research assistants for 24 weeks, caloric intake increased and weight improved (Simmons et al., 2008). However, in the clinical world, most staff are uninformed regarding how to assist with meals and use personal beliefs and preferences to guide their delivery of meals (Lopez, Amella, Mitchell, & Strumpf, 2010). Very few elements of mealtime care are formally developed and taught: Most staff see meals as a task to be accomplished (Amella, 1999). The advent of formal paid dining assistant (DA) feeding programs in nursing homes has been supported by state survey and certification bodies to improve nutrition among residents and may include information regarding interpersonal communication in general, altering the environment and working with families. However, a careful review of an 8-hour New York State program revealed that very little time is allocated for focus on these elements (New York State Department of Health, 2007). Simmons has been working to develop and refine an interdisciplinary-informed DA training program (Simmons & Schnelle, 2006), and recently with an interdisciplinary team tested a 12-month implementation with follow-up, finding that trained DA staff were just as effective as certified nursing assistants (CNAs) at recognizing problems and assisting with meals (Bertrand et al., 2010). However this program also had a focus on safety and the task of feeding. When CNAs were trained in feeding skills, and the residents they assisted using those improved strategies were then evaluated using the EdFED, the residents receiving the new strategies had better eating behavior and were given more time to eat (Chang & Lin, 2005). In acute care, no training material could be found for direct care workers regarding the alteration of environment, personalized strategies, or methods to encourage eating.

In addition to lack of training regarding facilitation of meals and promotion of mealtime independence, mealtimes may be poorly staffed, especially in acute care settings because personnel are often taking meal breaks at the same time as patients (Crabtree, Miller, & Stange, 2005; Xia & McCutcheon, 2006). However, when hospital nurses in the United Kingdom decided to redesign meals on medical wards and address nutritional needs of patients by taking breaks at other than mealtimes, patients actually consumed more food (Dickinson, Welch, & Ager, 2008). When surveyed, CNAs and licensed nurses identified lack of time and training, as well as "working short staffed," as being related to residents not receiving enough food (Crogan, Shultz, Adams, & Massey, 2001). Mealtimes are one of the most time-consuming activities of daily living and, unfortunately, not reimbursed at the required levels. It has been reported that nursing home residents with low intake required 35–40 minutes of staff assistance despite their level of dependency (Simmons & Schnelle, 2006); the amount of time taken to support meals among acutely and critically ill older adults in hospital is not known.

Environment and Interaction

Because of the strong social and cultural components of eating, where one dines is sometimes as important as what one eats. Nurses should simply ask themselves, "Would I want to eat my next meal where this person is eating?" If the answer is no, then steps should be taken to improve the dining environment. Small changes in the dining environment may make large improvements in a patient's capacity and motivation to eat or be fed. Unfortunately in institutions, the mealtime experience is often not focused on individual needs (Sydner & Fjellström, 2005). Several patient-centered factors have been identified as critical to older adults: Each mealtime was seen as a unique process, and patients are central to the process through their actions not only at meals but also during the time surrounding meals, such as socializing while waiting (Evans, Crogan, & Shultz, 2005; Gibbs-Ward & Keller, 2005; Wikby & Fägerskiöld, 2004). External factors such as decreased noise, increased lighting, and playing of relaxing music at meals positively influenced appetite (Hicks-Moore, 2005; McDaniel, Hunt, Hackes, & Pope, 2001). Using contrasting colors (foreground/background) in tableware and tablecloth, and placing dishes in similar positions may help persons with low vision be more independent (Ellexson, 2004). Proper positioning using the appropriate, supportive chair (instead of eating in bed or sitting on the bedside) or promotes good eating posture (Rappl & Jones, 2000). Encouraging the family to eat with the patient can be beneficial; this has been shown effective in nursing homes to increase body weight and fine motor function in a randomized control trial (Altus, Engelman, & Mathews, 2002; Nijs, de Graaf, Kok, & van Staveren, 2006). Meals eaten in small groups—much like family dining—are considered an ideal method; however, this intervention had more affect on staff's perception of meals and willingness to spend time in the process of attending to meals (Kofod & Birkemose, 2004). Successful completion of the meal is dependent on who assists or feeds the patient and the interpersonal process that the person uses to interact with the patient (Altus et al., 2002; Amella, 2002). Caregivers who are able to let the patient set the tempo of the meal and allow others to make choices will be more effectual in increasing intake. These studies point to a need to patient-centered approaches that individualize mealtimes for patients and that the responsibility for ensuring this occurs rests with a sensitive and well-trained staff.

CASE STUDY

Mr. Jackson is an 82-year-old African American male who is admitted to a medical unit after a short stay in the medical intensive care unit with a diagnosis of an ischemic stroke and treatment with tissue plasminogen activator—he appears to have little residual effect, although is being closely observed because of multiple comorbidities. He has a long history of heart failure, Type 2 diabetes, and "mild" vascular dementia. His insulin has been discontinued, and he is now receiving a short-acting oral antidiabetic agent that is given at mealtimes, loop diuretic, angiotensin-converting enzyme inhibitor, and a beta-blocker. Medications can cause a decrease in appetite so Mr. Jackson needed to have a side effect profile for all drugs developed by the pharmacologist. Initially, Mr. Jackson's appetite had not improved and his blood glucose was lower than 80 mg/dl on several occasions requiring the change in antihyperglycemic. Mr. Jackson tires easily so he has been eating in the hospital bed; he is becoming more dependent in his cares and the staff is having to occasionally feed him. Within the past 48 hours, he has become incontinent and requires almost total care; his confusion is increasing and he is sometimes unaware of his surroundings. The plan was for Mr. Jackson to return to senior housing; however, his daughter now wants him to come home. Other family members are worried that he is not eating sufficiently and may need a feeding tube. They all agree that they will help the daughter with caregiving but are unable to come up with a plan that the case manager considers safe; she recommends that Mr. Jackson be discharged to a nursing home. Mr. Jackson is a member of the Seventh-Day Adventist church.

Mr. Jackson has several issues that require close monitoring, first of which are his two severe chronic illnesses—diabetes and heart failure, and superimposed delirium with dementia. All of these conditions must be medically managed before discharge can be attempted. However, these illnesses in conjunction with his change in mental status are causing him to have unmet nutritional needs that should be addressed by careful assessment and interventions.

To improve his declining intake, initially, the nurse should observe Mr. Jackson during each meal over the course of the day, noting if his capacity to eat independently or amount of assistance needed fluctuates across the day, and if he would benefit from progressive assistance. Because of the history of dementia and possible new-onset delirium, the EdFED could be used to note mealtime behaviors and see if he is amenable to environmental changes—eating out of bed, receiving cuing and prompts, provision of better lighting and use of eyeglasses, and moving him to a more stimulating environment such as the unit's dayroom. Oral care should be regularly provided. With his recently diagnosed stroke, the nurse should be especially observant of any signs of dysphagia and inability to handle dining implements. Adaptive equipment may allow him to be more independent. Consultation with the entire health care team, including the provider, speech and language pathologist, dietitian, dentist, occupational therapist, clergy, and case manager, is warranted to ensure that any unmet needs are addressed. Staff needs to be familiar with his religious preferences, such as a vegetarian diet with increased whole grain, fruits, and water instead of fruit juice.

Mr. Jackson should be allowed to rest before meals; rehabilitative therapies should be planned away from mealtimes. During mealtimes, favorite music can be played and

(continued)

CASE STUDY *(continued)*

Mr. Jackson can be assisted out of bed and supported in a therapeutic position. Family members can be encouraged to visit at mealtimes and staff should be present at meals to assist, but not rush him. Staff should also avoid performing tasks in the room while Mr. Jackson is eating—they should not distract him.

As Mr. Jackson's delirium begins to clear and with a more focused approach to his mealtime needs and improved interaction, Mr. Jackson's intake begins to improve. The family and church members bring foods he once enjoyed, and the family agrees that a stay in short-term rehab may be a better alternative to further address his medical needs and ensure needed social interaction as he recovers.

SUMMARY

In the past 5 years, a number of tailored interventions and bundled programs have been developed that have been shown to increase the caloric and fluid intake of older adults in nursing homes and hospitals. However, most evidence relies on smaller quasi-experimental or descriptive studies, some with crossover designs; most interventions are of rather short duration and few studies examine sustainability of programs (Watson & Green, 2006).

At this time, careful and regular assessment of the vulnerable older adult with multiple chronic cognitive/mental and physical illnesses is still warranted because these are the patients who are at highest risk for mealtime difficulties. A team approach to nutritional and mealtime issues is critical. Across all sites of care, attention must be paid to not just what a person eats, but how he or she eats, where he or she eats, and with whom he or she eats, because meals are powerful contributor to both health and quality of life.

NURSING STANDARD OF PRACTICE

Protocol 23.1: Assessment and Management of Mealtime Difficulties

I. GOAL: To maintain or improve nutritional intake at meals and provide a quality mealtime experience that fosters dignity and pleasure in eating, as well as respecting cultural and personal preferences, for as long as possible.

II. OVERVIEW
  Guiding Principles
    A. The adequate intake of nutrients is necessary to maintain physical and emotional health.
    B. Mealtime is not only an opportunity to ingest nutrients but also to maintain critical social aspects of life.

(continued)

Protocol 23.1: Assessment and Management of Mealtime Difficulties *(cont.)*

    C. The social components of meals will be observed, including mealtime rituals, cultural norms, and food preferences.

    D. Persons will be encouraged and assisted to self-feed for as long as possible.

    E. Persons dependent in eating will be assisted with dignity.

    F. The quality of mealtime is an indicator of quality of life and care of an individual.

III. BACKGROUND

    A. Definitions

        1. Feeding is "the process of getting the food from the plate to the mouth. It is a primitive sense without concern for social niceties" (Katz et al., 1970, p. 23).

        2. Eating is "the ability to transfer food from plate to stomach through the mouth" (Katz et al., 1970, p. 23). Eating involves the ability to recognize food, the ability to transfer food to the mouth, and the phases of swallowing.

        3. Anorexia is characterized by a refusal to maintain a minimally normal body weight and has a physiological basis in the older adults (Wilson, 2007).

        4. Dehydration is a fluid imbalance caused by too little fluid taken in or too much fluid lost or both.

        5. Dysphagia is "an abnormality in the transfer of a bolus from the mouth to the stomach" (Groher, 1997, p. 2).

        6. Apraxia is an inability to carry out voluntary muscular activities related to neuromuscular damage. As it relates to eating and feeding, it involves loss of the voluntary stages of swallowing or the manipulation of eating utensils.

        7. Agnosia is the inability to recognize familiar items when sensory cuing is limited.

    B. Etiology

    Mealtime difficulties can have multiple causes from both physiological and psychological origins. Health professionals need to consider multiple etiologies and not assume that difficulties are related only to increased confusion from a cognitive decline.

        1. Cognitive/neurological: Parkinson's disease; amyotrophic lateral sclerosis; dementia, especially Alzheimer's disease; stroke

        2. Psychological: depression

        3. Iatrogenic: lack of adaptive equipment; use of physical restraints that limit the ability to move, position, or self-feed; improper chair or table surface or discrepancy of chair to table height; use of wheelchair in lieu of table chair; use of disposable dinnerware, especially for patients with cognitive or neuromuscular impairments

IV. PARAMETERS OF ASSESSMENT

    A. Assessment of Older Adults and Caregivers

        1. Rituals used before meals (e.g., hand washing and toilet use); dressing for dinner

        2. Blessings of food or grace, if appropriate

(continued)

Protocol 23.1: Assessment and Management of Mealtime Difficulties *(cont.)*

    3. Religious rites or prohibitions observed in preparation of food or before meal begins (e.g., Muslim, Jewish, Seventh-Day Adventist; consult with pastoral counselor, if available)

    4. Cultural or special cues—family history, especially rituals surrounding meals

    5. Preferences about end-of-life decisions regarding withdrawal or administration of food and fluid in the face of incapacity, or request of designated health proxy; ethicist or social worker may facilitate process.

  B. Assessment Instruments

    1. EdFED for persons with moderate to late-stage dementia (Watson, 1994a)

    2. Katz Index of ADL for functional status (Katz et al., 1970)

    3. Food diary/meal portion method (Berrut et al., 2002)

V. NURSING INTERVENTIONS

  A. Environment

    1. Dining or patient room—encourage the older adult to eat in dining room to increase intake, personalize dining room; no treatments or other activities occurring during meals; no distractions

    2. Tableware: use of standard dinnerware (e.g., china, glasses, cup and saucer, flatware, tablecloth, napkin) versus disposable tableware and bibs

    3. Furniture: older adult seated in stable armchair; table-appropriate height versus eating in wheelchair or in bed

    4. Noise level: environmental noise from music, caregivers, and television is minimal; personal conversation between patient and caregiver is encouraged

    5. Music: pleasant, preferred by patient

    6. Light: adequate and non-glare-producing versus dark, shadowy, or glaring

    7. Contrasting background/foreground: use contrasting background and foreground colors with minimal design to aid persons with decreased vision

    8. Odor: food prepared in area adjacent to or in dining area to stimulate appetite

    9. Adaptive equipment: available, appropriate, and clean; caregivers and/or older adult knowledgeable in use; occupational therapist assists in evaluation

  B. Caregiver/Staffing

    1. Provide an adequate number of well-trained staff

    2. Deliver an individualized approach to meals including choice of food, tempo of assistance.

    3. Position of caregiver relative to elder: eye contact; seating so caregiver faces older patient in same plane

    4. Cueing: caregiver cues older adult whenever possible with words or gestures

    5. Self-feeding: encouragement to self-feed with multiple methods versus assisted feeding to minimize time

    6. Mealtime rounds: interdisciplinary team to examine multifaceted process of meal service, environment, and individual preferences

(continued)

Protocol 23.1: Assessment and Management of Mealtime Difficulties *(cont.)*

VI. EVALUATION/EXPECTED OUTCOMES
A. Individual
   1. Corrective and supportive strategies reflected in plan of care
   2. Quality-of-life issues emphasized in maintaining social aspects of dining
   3. Culture, personal preferences, and end-of-life decisions regarding nutrition respected
B. Health Care Provider
   1. System disruptions at mealtimes minimized
   2. Family and staff informed and educated to patient's special needs to promote safe and effective meals
   3. Maintenance of normal meals and adequate intake for the patient reflected in care plan
   4. Competence in diet assessment; knowledge of and sensitivity to cultural norms and preferences for mealtimes reflected in care plan
C. Institution
   1. Documentation of nutritional status and eating and feeding behavior meets expected standard
   2. Alterations in nutritional status; eating and feeding behaviors assessed and addressed in a timely manner
   3. Involvement of interdisciplinary team (geriatrician, advanced practice nurse, dietitian, speech therapist, dentist, occupational therapist, social worker, pastoral counselor, ethicist) appropriate and timely
   4. Nutritional, eating, and/or feeding problems modified to respect individual preferences and cultural norms
   5. Adequate number of well-trained staff who are committed to delivering knowledgeable and individualized care

VII. FOLLOW-UP MONITORING
A. Providers' competency to monitor eating and feeding behaviors
B. Documentation of eating and feeding behaviors
C. Documentation of care strategies, and follow-up of alterations in nutritional status and eating and feeding behaviors
D. Documentation of staffing and staff education; availability of supportive interdisciplinary team.

RESOURCES

How to Try This: The Edinburgh Feeding Evaluation in Dementia Scale: Determining How Much Help People With Dementia Need at Mealtime.
Dementia series: http://www.nursingcenter.com/prodev/ce_article.asp?tid=807225

The Mini Nutritional Assessment (MNA)
http://www.mna-elderly.com/

The Alzheimer's Association
The "Eating Well" video as part of web-based training programs, CARES: A Dementia Caregiving
   Approach.
http://www.alz.org/in_my_community_professionals.asp

REFERENCES

Algase, D. L., Beck, C., Kolanowski, A., Whall, A., Berent, S., Richards, K., & Beattie, E. (1996).
   Need-driven dementia-compromised behavior: An alternative view of disruptive behavior.
   American Journal of Alzheimer's Disease, 11(6), 10–19. Evidence Level V.

Altus, D. E., Engelman, K. K., & Mathews, R. M. (2002). Using family-style meals to increase
   participation and communication in persons with dementia. *Journal of Gerontological Nursing,
   28*(9), 47–53. Evidence Level III.

Amella, E. J. (1999). Factors influencing the proportion of food consumed by nursing home residents with dementia. *Journal of the American Geriatrics Society, 47*(7), 879–885. Evidence
   Level IV.

Amella, E. J. (2002). Resistance at mealtimes for persons with dementia. *The Journal of Nutrition,
   Heath & Aging, 6*(2), 117–122. Evidence Level IV.

Amella, E. J. (2004). Feeding and hydration issues for older adults with dementia. *The Nursing
   Clinics of North America, 39*(3), 607–623. Evidence Level V.

Amella, E. J., & DeLegge, M. (2009). Feeding in elderly with late-stage dementia: The FIELD Trial.
   NIH/NIA. Evidence Level II.

Amella, E. J., & Laditka, S. (2009). *Self-efficacy for change in a mealtime train-the-trainer program.*
   Atlanta, GA: Gerontological Society of America. Evidence Level IV.

Arora, V. M., Johnson, M., Olson, J., Podrazik, P. M., Levine, S., Dubeau, C. E., . . . Meltzer, D. O.
   (2007). Using assessing care of vulnerable elders quality indicators to measure quality of hospital care for vulnerable elders. *Journal of the American Geriatrics Society, 55*(11), 1705–1711.
   Evidence Level IV.

Aselage, M. B. (2010). Measuring mealtime difficulties: Eating, feeding and meal behaviours in older
   adults with dementia. *Journal of Clinical Nursing, 19*(5–6), 621–631. Evidence Level V.

Aselage, M. B. (2011). *A web-based dementia feeding skills training module for nursing home staff*
   (Dissertation, Medical University of South Carolina College of Nursing). Evidence Level III.

Aselage, M. B., & Amella, E. J. (2010). An evolutionary analysis of mealtime difficulties in older
   adults with dementia. *Journal of Clinical Nursing, 19*(1–2), 33–41. Evidence Level IV.

Beck, A. M., Damkjaer, K., & Sorbye, L. (2010). Physical and social functional abilities seem to
   be maintained by a multifaceted randomized controlled nutritional intervention among old
   (>65 years) Danish nursing home residents. *Archives of Gerontology and Geriatrics, 50*(3),
   351–355. Evidence Level IV.

Bermudez, O., & Tucker, K. (2004). Cultural aspects of food choices in various communities of
   elders. *Generations, 28*(3), 22–27. Evidence Level IV.

Berrut, G., Favreau, A. M., Dizo, E., Tharreau, B., Poupin, C., Gueringuili, M., . . . Ritz, P. (2002).
   Estimation of calorie and protein intake in aged patients: Validation of a method based on meal
   portions consumed. *The Journals of Gerontology. Series A, Biological Sciences and Medical Sciences,
   57*(1), M52–M56. Evidence Level III.

Bertrand, R. M., Porchak, T. L., Moore, T. J., Hurd, D. T., Shier, V., Sweetland, R., & Simmons,
   S. F. (2010). The nursing home dining assistant program: A demonstration project. *Journal of
   Gerontological Nursing, 37*(2), 34–43. Evidence Level III.

Castellanos, V. H., Marra, M. V., & Johnson, P. (2009). Enhancement of select foods at breakfast
   and lunch increases energy intakes of nursing home residents with low meal intakes. *Journal of
   the American Dietetic Association, 109*(3), 445–451. Evidence Level II.

Centers for Medicare & Medicaid Services. (2010). *Long-term care facility resident assessment instrument user's manual* (Version 3.0). Washington, DC: Services CfMaM (ed.).

Chang, C., & Lin, L. (2005). Effects of a feeding skills training programme on nursing assistants and dementia patients. *Journal of Clinical Nursing, 14*(10), 1185–1192. Evidence Level IV.

Charras, K., & Frémonteir, M. (2010). Sharing meals with institutionalized people with dementia: A natural experiment. *Journal of Gerontological Social Work, 53*(5), 436–448. Evidence Level III.

Coates, J., Frongillo, E. A., Rogers, B. L., Webb, P., Wilde, P. E., & Houser, R. (2006). Commonalities in the experience of household food insecurity across cultures: What are measures missing? *The Journal of Nutrition, 136*(5), 1438S–1448S. Evidence Level IV.

Crabtree, B. F., Miller, W. L., & Stange, K. C. (2005). Understanding practice from the ground up. *The Journal of Family Practice, 50*(10), 881–887. Evidence Level IV.

Crogan, N. L., Alvine, C., & Pasvogel, A. (2006). Improving nutrition care for nursing home residents using the INRx process. *Journal of Nutrition for the Elderly, 25*(3–4), 89–103. Evidence Level IV.

Crogan, N. L., Shultz, J. A., Adams, C. E., & Massey, L. K. (2001). Barriers to nutrition care for nursing home residents. *Journal of Gerontological Nursing, 27*(12), 25–31. Evidence Level IV.

Dickinson, A., Welch, C., & Ager, L. (2008). No longer hungry in hospital: Improving the hospital mealtime experience for older people through action research. *Journal of Clinical Nursing, 17*(11), 1492–1502. Evidence Level IV.

Dorner, B., Friedrich, E. K., & Posthauer, M. E. (2010). Position of the American Dietetic Association: Individualized nutrition approaches for older adults in health care communities. *Journal of the American Dietetic Association, 110*(10), 1549–1553. Evidence Level I.

Ellexson, M. (2004). Access to participation: Occupational therapy and low vision. *Topics in Geriatric Rehabilitation, 20*(3), 154–172. Evidence Level IV.

Evans, B. C., Crogan, N. L., & Shultz, J. A. (2005). The meaning of mealtimes: Connection to the social world of the nursing home. *Journal of Gerontological Nursing, 31*(2), 11–17. Evidence Level IV.

Federal Interagency Forum on Age-Related Statistics. (2006). *Older Americans update 2006: Key indicators of well-being. Administration on Aging, 2006.* Retrieved from http://www.agingstats .gov/agingstatsdotnet/Main_Site/Data/Data_2006.aspx

Fjellström, C. (2004). Mealtime and meal patterns from a cultural perspective. *Scandinavian Journal of Nutrition, 48*(4), 161–164. Evidence Level V.

Flexner, S., & Hauck, L. (1987). *The Random House dictionary of the English language* (2nd ed.). New York, NY: Random House.

Food Network Chef Bios. (2011, March 20). *Recipes* [Television Food Network]. Retrieved from http://www.foodnetwork.com/chefs/index.html

Gaskill, D., Isenring, E. A., Black, L. J., Hassall, S., & Bauer, J. D. (2009). Maintaining nutrition in aged care residents with a train-the-trainer intervention and Nutrition Coordinator. *The Journal of Nutrition, Health & Aging, 13*(10), 913–917. Evidence Level II.

Gibbs-Ward, A. J., & Keller, H. H. (2005). Mealtimes as active processes in long-term care facilities. *Canadian Journal of Dietetic Practice and Research, 66*(1), 5–11. Evidence Level IV.

Groher, M. E. (1997). *Dysphagia: Diagnosis and management* (3rd ed.). Boston, MA: Butterworth-Heinemann. Evidence Level V.

Guigoz, Y., Vellas, B., & Garry, P. (1997). Mini nutritional assessment: A practical assessment tool for grading the nutritional state of elderly patients. In *Facts, research and intervention in geriatrics: Nutrition in the elderly* (3rd ed., pp. 15–60). Evidence Level III.

Hanson, L. C., Ersek, M., Gilliam, R., & Carey, T. S. (2011). Oral feeding options for people with dementia: A systematic review. *Journal of the American Geriatrics Society, 59*(3), 463–472. Evidence Level I.

Hicks-Moore, S. L. (2005). Relaxing music at mealtime in nursing homes: Effect on agitated patients with dementia. *Journal of Gerontological Nursing, 31*(12), 26–32. Evidence Level III.

Katz, S., Downs, T. D., Cash, H. R., & Grotz, R. C. (1970). Progress in development of the index of ADL. *The Gerontologist, 10*(1), 20–30. Evidence Level IV.

Katz, S., Ford, A. B., Moskowitz, R. W., Jackson, B. A., & Jaffe, M. W. (1963). Studies of illness in the aged. The index of ADL: A standardized measure of biological and psychological function. *The Journal of the American Medical Association, 185*, 914–919. Evidence Level IV.

Keller, H. H. (2006). Meal programs improve nutritional risk: A longitudinal analysis of community-living seniors. *Journal of the American Dietetic Association, 106*(7), 1042–1048. Evidence Level IV.

Keller, H. H., Goy, R., & Kane, S. (2005). Validity and reliability of SCREEN II (Seniors in the community: Risk evaluation for eating and nutrition, Version II). *European Journal of Clinical Nutrition, 59*(10), 1149–1157. Evidence Level III.

Kofod, J., & Birkemose, A. (2004). Meals in nursing homes. *Scandinavian Journal of Caring Sciences, 18*(2), 128–134. Evidence Level IV.

Koren, M. J. (2010). Person-centered care for nursing home residents: The culture-change movement. *Health Affairs (Millwood), 29*(2), 312–317. Evidence Level V.

Lopez, R. P., Amella, E. J., Mitchell, S. L., & Strumpf, N. E. (2010). Nurses' perspectives on feeding decisions for nursing home residents with advanced dementia. *Journal of Clinical Nursing, 19*(5–6), 632–638. Evidence Level IV.

Maynard, M., Gunnell, D., Ness, A. R., Abraham, L., Bates, C. J., & Blane, D. (2006). What influences diet in early old age? Prospective and cross-sectional analyses of the Boyd Orr cohort. *European Journal of Public Health, 16*(3), 315–324. Evidence Level IV.

McDaniel, J. H., Hunt, A., Hackes, B., & Pope, J. F. (2001). Impact of dining room environment on nutritional intake of Alzheimer's residents: A case study. *American Journal of Alzheimer's Disease and Other Dementias, 16*(5), 297–302. Evidence Level III.

Mitchell, P. (2008). Defining patient safety and quality care. *In Patient safety and quality: An evidence-based handbook for nurses* (AHRQ Publication No. 08-0043). Rockville, MD: Agency for Healthcare Research and Quality. Evidence Level V.

Mitchell, S. L., Teno, J. M., Kiely, D. K., Shaffer, M. L., Jones, R. N., Prigerson, H. G., . . . Hamel, M. B. (2009). The clinical course of advanced dementia. *The New England Journal of Medicine, 361*(16), 1529–1538. Evidence Level IV.

New York State Department of Health. (2007). *Feeding assistant programs for nursing homes.* Services DOR, ed. Albany, NY: Author. Evidence Level V.

Nijs, K. A., de Graaf, C., Kok, F. J., & van Staveren, W. A. (2006). Effect of family style mealtimes on quality of life, physical performance, and body weight of nursing home residents: Cluster randomised controlled trial. *British Medical Journal, 332*(7551), 1180–1184. Evidence Level II.

Phillips M. B., Foley, A. L., Barnard, R., Isenring, E. A., & Miller, M. D. (2010). Nutritional screening in community-dwelling older adults: A systematic literature review. *Asia Pacific Journal of Clinical Nutrition, 19*(3), 440–449. Evidence Level I.

Pioneer Network. (n.d.). *Comparisons of nursing home cultures: Institution-directed vs. person-directed.* Retrieved from http://www.pioneernetwork.net/Providers/Comparisons

Rappl, L., & Jones, D. A. (2000). Seating evaluation: Special problems and interventions for older adults. *Topics in Geriatric Rehabilitation, 16*(2), 63–72. Evidence Level V.

Seligman, H. K., Laraia, B. A., & Kushel, M. B. (2010). Food insecurity is associated with chronic disease among low-income NHANES participants. *The Journal of Nutrition, 140*(2), 304–310. Evidence Level IV.

Simmons, S. F., Keeler, E., Zhuo, X., Hickey, K. A., Sato, H. W., & Schnelle, J. F. (2008). Prevention of unintentional weight loss in nursing home residents: A controlled trial of feeding assistance. *Journal of the American Geriatrics Society, 56*(8), 1466–1473. Evidence Level II.

Simmons, S. F., & Schnelle, J. F. (2006). Feeding assistance needs of long-stay nursing home residents and staff time to provide care. *Journal of the American Geriatrics Society, 54*(6), 919–924. Evidence Level IV.

Sydner, Y. M., & Fjellström, C. (2005). Food provision and the meal situation in elderly care—outcomes in different social contexts. *Journal of Human Nutrition and Dietetics, 18*(1), 45–52. Evidence Level IV.

Taylor, K. A., & Barr, S. I. (2006). Provision of small, frequent meals does not improve energy intake of elderly residents with dysphagia who live in an extended-care facility. *Journal of the American Dietetic Association, 106*(7), 1115–1118. Evidence Level IV.

U.S. Centers for Disease Control and Prevention. (2009a). Behavioral risk factor surveillance system survey data. *Prevention CDC* (ed.). Atlanta, GA: Author. Evidence Level V.

U.S. Centers for Disease Control and Prevention. (2009b). *Deaths and mortality*. Retrieved from http://www.cdc.gov/nchs/fastats/deaths.htm. Evidence Level V.

U.S. Department of Health and Human Services. (2011). *Healthy People 2020: Older adults*. Retrieved from http://www.healthypeople.gov/2020/topicsobjectives2020/overview.aspx?topicid=31. Evidence Level V.

Watson, R. (1994a). Measurement of feeding difficulty in patients with dementia. *Journal of Psychiatric and Mental Health Nursing, 1*(1), 45–46. Evidence Level III.

Watson, R. (1994b). Measuring of feeding difficulty in patients with dementia: Developing a scale. *Journal of Advanced Nursing, 19*(2), 257–263. Evidence Level IV.

Watson, R., & Deary, I. J. (1997). Feeding difficulty in elderly patients with dementia: Confirmatory factor analysis. *International Journal of Nursing Studies, 34*(6), 405–414. Evidence Level IV.

Watson, R., & Green, S. M. (2006). Feeding and dementia: A systematic literature review. *Journal of Advanced Nursing, 54*(1), 86–93. Evidence Level I.

Watson, R., Green, S. M., & Legg, L. (2001). The Edinburgh Feeding Evaluation in Dementia Scale #2 (EdFED #2): Convergent and discriminant validity. *Clinical Effectiveness in Nursing, 5*(1), 44–46. Evidence Level IV.

Wikby, K., & Fägerskiöld, A. (2004). The willingness to eat. *Scandinavian Journal of Caring Sciences, 18*(2), 120–127. Evidence Level IV.

Wilson, M. M. (2007). Assessment of appetite and weight loss syndromes in nursing home residents. *Missouri Medicine, 104*(1), 46–51. Evidence Level VI.

Wright, L., Hickson, M., & Frost, G. (2006). Eating together is important: Using a dining room in an acute elderly medical ward increases energy intake. *Journal of Human Nutrition and Dietetics, 19*(1), 23–26. Evidence Level III.

Xia, C., & McCutcheon, H. (2006). Mealtime in hospital—who does what? *Journal of Clinical Nursing, 15*(10), 1221–1227. Evidence Level IV.

Family Caregiving

24

Deborah C. Messecar

EDUCATIONAL OBJECTIVES

On completion of this chapter, the reader will be able to:

1. describe characteristics and factors that put family caregivers at risk for unhealthy transitions into the caregiving role
2. identify key aspects of a family caregiving preparedness assessment
3. list specific interventions to support family caregivers of older adults take on their caregiving duties
4. identify family caregiver outcomes expected from the implementation of this protocol

OVERVIEW

Family caregivers are a key link in providing safe and effective transitional care to frail older adults as they move across levels of care (e.g., acute to subacute) or across settings (e.g., hospital to home; Bauer, Fitzgerald, Haesler, & Manfrin, 2009; Coleman & Boult, 2003; Naylor, 2003). Frail older adults coping with complex chronic conditions are vulnerable to problems with care as they typically have multiple providers and move frequently between and among health care settings. Incomplete communication among providers and across health care agencies is linked to adverse outcomes and an increased risk of hospital readmission and or length of hospital stay (Bauer et al., 2009). Nurses in collaboration with family caregivers can bridge the gap between the care provided in hospital and other settings and the care needed in the community. Transitional care for frail older people can be improved if interventions address family inclusion and education, communication between health care workers and family, and interdisciplinary communication and ongoing support after the transition.

For description of Evidence Levels cited in this chapter, see Chapter 1, Developing and Evaluating Clinical Practice Guidelines: A Systematic Approach, page 7.

Helping Caregivers Take On the Caregiving Role

Helping the caregiver with the role acquisition process is a critical nursing function that facilitates good transitional care. Indicators of a healthy assumption of the caregiving role are those factors that either indicate a robust and positive role acquisition process or signal potential difficulty with assuming the caregiver role. When trying to ascertain what those indicators might be, the following questions about the caregiver role acquisition process can be posed: "What constitutes health during the role acquisition process?" "What indicates a positive state of health during this process?" and "What threats to health may occur as the process unfolds?" (Schumacher, 1995, p. 219). Because the role transition process unfolds over time, identifying process indicators that move patient and family members either in the direction of health or on the way to vulnerability and risk allow early assessment and intervention to facilitate healthy outcomes of the caregiving role acquisition (Schumacher, 2005). If unhealthy role-taking transitions can be identified, then they can either be prevented or ameliorated.

Who Is Likely to Be or Become a Caregiver?

Being a family caregiver is a widespread experience in the United States. Depending on how family caregiving is defined, national surveys estimate that anywhere from 22.4 to 52 million people provide care for a chronically ill, disabled family member or friend during any given year (National Alliance for Caregiving [NAC] & American Association for Retired Persons [AARP], 2004; Opinion Research Corporation [ORC], 2005; U.S. Department of Health and Human Services [USDHHS], 1998). Reflecting an increasing trend, 44% of all family caregivers of adults older than age 18 are men, 56% are women, and the majority is older than the age of 45 (ORC, 2005). Among the primary family caregivers of older disabled or ill adults older than age 65, the proportion of male caregivers is lower (about 32%), but this number has increased from prior years (Wolff & Kasper, 2006). Primary family caregivers are children (41.3%), spouses (38.4%), and other family or friends (20.4%; Wolff & Kasper, 2006). The most common caregiver arrangement is that of an adult female child providing care to an elderly female parent (USDHHS, 1998). Many caregivers are older and are at risk for chronic illness themselves. Nearly 45% of all primary caregivers are older than 65 years of age, with 47.4% of spousal primary caregivers being 75 years or older (Wolff & Kasper, 2006). National surveys indicate a trend in the United States of care recipients being older and more disabled, and more caregivers acting as the primary source of care (an increase from 34.9% on 1989 to 52.8% in 1999) without help from secondary caregivers (Wolff & Kasper, 2006). Family and friends now provide more than 80% of all long-term care services in the country.

Impact of Unhealthy Caregiving Transitions on Caregiver

Caregiving has documented negative consequences for the caregiver's physical and emotional health. Caregiving-related stress in a chronically ill spouse results in a 63% higher mortality rate than their noncaregiving peers (Schulz & Beach, 1999). Stress from caring for an older adult with dementia has been shown to impact the caregiver's immune system for up to 3 years after their caregiving ends (Kiecolt-Glaser et al., 2003). Spouse caregivers who provide heavy care (36 or more hours per week) are six times more likely than noncaregivers to experience symptoms of depression or anxiety; for child caregivers, the rate is twice as high (Cannuscio et al., 2002). In addition to mental health morbidity, family caregivers also experience physical health deterioration. Family caregivers have chronic conditions at more than twice the rate of noncaregivers (NAC & AARP, 2004; USDHHS, 1998). Family caregivers experiencing extreme stress have also been shown to age prematurely. It is estimated that this stress can take as much as 10 years off a family caregiver's life (Arno, 2006).

BACKGROUND AND STATEMENT OF PROBLEM

Definitions

Family Caregiving

Family caregiving is broadly defined and refers to a broad range of unpaid care provided in response to illness or functional impairment to a chronically ill or functionally impaired older family member, partner, friend, or neighbor that exceeds the support usually provided in family relationships (Arno, 2006).

Caregiving Roles

Caregiving roles can be classified into a hierarchy according to who takes on the bulk of responsibilities versus only intermittent supportive assistance. Primary caregivers tend to provide most of the everyday aspects of care, whereas secondary caregivers help out as needed to fill the gaps (Cantor & Little, 1985; Pening, 1990; Tennstedt, McKinlay, & Sullivan, 1989). Among caregivers who live with their care recipients, spouses account for the bulk of primary caregivers, whereas adult children are more likely to be secondary caregivers. The range of the family caregiving role includes protective caregiving like "keeping an eye on" an older adult who is currently independent but at risk, to full time, round-the-clock care for a severely impaired family member. Health care providers may fail to assess the full scope of the family caregiving role if they associate family caregiving only with the performance of tasks.

Caregiver Role Transition

Caregiver role acquisition is a family role transition that occurs through situated interaction as part of a role-making process (Schumacher, 2005). This is the process of taking on the caregiving role at the beginning of caregiving or when a significant change in the caregiving context occurs. Role transitions occur when a role is added to or deleted from the role set of a person—or when the behavioral expectations for an established role change significantly. Role transitions involve changes in the behavior expectations along with the acquisition of new knowledge and skills. Examples of major role transitions are becoming a new parent, getting a divorce, and changing careers. The acquisition of the family caregiving role is a specific type of role transition that occurs within families in response to the changes in health of family member who has suffered a decline in their self-care ability or health.

Indicators of Healthy Caregiver Role Transitions

The broad categories of indicators of healthy transitions include subjective well-being, role mastery, and well-being of relationships. These are the subjective, behavioral, and interpersonal parameters of health most likely to be associated with healthy role transitions (Schumacher, 2005). *Subjective well-being* is defined as "subjective responses to caregiving role transition" (Schumacher, 2005, p. 219). Subjective well-being includes any pattern of subjective reactions that arise from assuming the caregiver role within the boundary of the caregiving situation. Examples of some of the more important possible threats to subjective well-being could include role strain and depression. Role mastery is associated with accomplishment of skilled role performance and comfort with the behavior required in a new health-related care situation. Examples of threats to role mastery, which indicate a vulnerability and risk of unhealthy transitions are role insufficiency and lack of preparedness. *Well-being of relationships* refers to the quality of the relationship between the caregiver and older adult. Examples of threats to well-being of relationships are family conflict or a poor quality of relationship with the care receiver.

Family Caregiving Activities

Family caregiving activities include assistance with day-to-day activities, illness-related care, care management, and invisible aspects of care. Day-to-day activities include personal care activities (bathing, eating, dressing, mobility, transferring from bed to chair, and using the toilet) and instrumental activities of daily living (IADL; meal preparation, grocery shopping, making telephone calls, and money management; NAC & AARP, 2004; Walker, Pratt, & Eddy, 1995). Illness-related activities include managing symptoms, coping with illness behaviors, carrying out treatments, and performing medical or nursing procedures that include an array of medical technologies (Smith, 1994). Care management activities include accessing resources, communicating with and navigating the health care and social services systems, and acting as an advocate (Schumacher, Stewart, Archbold, Dodd, & Dibble, 2000). Invisible aspects of care are protective actions the caregiver takes to ensure the older adults' safety and well-being without their knowledge (Bowers, 1987).

Caregiver Assessment

Caregiver assessment refers to an ongoing iterative process of gathering information that describes a family caregiving situation and identifies the particular issues, needs, resources, and strengths of the family caregiver.

Risk Factors for Unhealthy Caregiving Transitions

Gender

Female caregivers are more likely to provide a *higher level of care* than men, which is defined as helping with at least two activities of daily living (ADL) and providing more than 40 care hours per week. Male caregivers are more likely to provide care at the lowest level, which is defined as no ADL and devoting very few hours of care per week (NAC & AARP, 2004; Pinquart & Sörensen, 2006). A number of studies have found that female caregivers are more likely than males to suffer from anxiety, depression, and other symptoms associated with emotional stress caused by caregiving (Mahoney, Regan, Katona, & Livingston, 2005; Yee & Schulz, 2000); lower levels of physical health and subjective well-being than caregiving men (Pinquart & Sörensen, 2006); and are at higher risk for adverse outcomes (Schulz, Martire, & Klinger, 2005). In the pooled analysis from the Resources for Enhancing Alzheimer's Caregiver Health (REACH) trials, females had higher initial levels of burden and depression (Gitlin et al., 2003).

Ethnicity

Rates of caregiving vary somewhat by ethnicity. Among the U.S. adult population older than age 18, 17% of White and 15% of African American families are providing informal care, whereas a slightly lower percentage of Asian Americans (14%) and Hispanic Americans (13%) are engaged in caregiving for persons older than the age of 50 (NAC & AARP, 2004). However, in another national survey, which looked only at people older than 70 years old, 44% of Latinos were found to receive informal home care compared with 34% of African Americans and 25% of non-Hispanic Whites (Weiss, González, Kabeto, & Langa, 2005). Ethnic differences are also found regarding the care recipient. Among people aged older than 70 years who require care, Whites are the most likely to receive help from their spouses; Hispanics are the most likely to receive help from their adult children; and African Americans are the most likely to receive help from a nonfamily member (National Academy on an Aging Society, 2000).

Studies show that ethnic minority caregivers provide more care (Pinquart & Sörenson, 2005) and report worse physical health than White caregivers (Dilworth-Anderson, Williams, & Gibson, 2002; Pinquart & Sörenson, 2005). African American caregivers experience less stress and depression and get more rewards related to caregiving when compared with White caregivers (Cuellar, 2002; Dilworth-Anderson et al., 2002; Gitlin et al., 2003; Haley et al., 2004; Pinquart & Sörenson, 2005). However, Hispanic and Asian American caregivers exhibit more depression than White caregivers (Gitlin et al., 2003; Pinquart & Sörenson, 2005). In addition, formal services are rarely used by ethnic minorities, which puts them at further risk for negative outcomes (Dilworth-Anderson et al., 2002; Pinquart & Sörenson, 2005). A meta-analysis of three qualitative studies examined African American, Chinese, and Latino caregiver impressions of their clinical encounters around their care receiver's diagnosis of Alzheimer's disease (Mahoney, Cloutterbuck, Neary, & Zhan, 2005). The primary issues identified in the analysis by Mahoney et al. (2005) were disrespect for concerns as noted by African American caregivers, stigmatization of persons with dementia as noted by Chinese caregivers, and fear that home care would not be supported, were among Latino caregivers. These findings indicate a need for greater culturally sensitive communications from health care providers.

Income and Educational Level

Low income is also related to being an ethnic minority and being "non-White," and the latter are risk factors for poorer health outcomes. Persons who become caregivers may be more likely to have incomes below the poverty level and be in poorer health, independent of caregiving (Vitaliano, Zhang, & Scanlan, 2003). Usually, educational level has been combined with income in most caregiving studies, so there is a lack of data on this variable. One study (Buckwalter et al., 1999) reported that caregivers who were less educated tended to report slightly more depression than those who were better educated. This is consistent with the findings from the REACH trial meta-analysis (Gitlin et al., 2003). In the meta-analysis completed by Schulz et al (2005), caregivers with low incomes and low levels of education were more at risk for adverse outcomes.

Relationship (Spouse, Nonspouse)

Past research conducted primarily among non-Hispanic White samples has shown that caregiving outcomes differ between nonspouse (who are mostly adult children) and spouse caregivers (Pinquart & Sörensen, 2004). In some literature reviews, authors noted that spousal caregivers have reported higher levels of depression than nonspouses (Gitlin, Corcoran, Winter, Boyce, & Hauck, 2001; Pruchno & Resch, 1989); intervention study found spouses reported less "upset" with the care receiver's behavior than nonspouses, who showed no decrease in "upset." In a meta-analysis of caregiving studies, spousal caregivers benefited less from existing interventions than adult children (Sörensen, Pinquart, & Duberstein, 2002).

Quality of Caregiver–Care Receiver Relationship

Disruption in the caregiver and care receiver relationship (Croog, Burleson, Sudilovsky, & Baume, 2006; Flannery, 2002) and/or a poor quality of relationship (Archbold, Stewart, Greenlick, & Harvath, 1990; Archbold, Stewart, Greenlick, & Harvath, 1992) can make caregiving seem more difficult even if the objective caregiving situation (e.g., hours devoted to caregiving, number of tasks performed) does not seem to be too demanding. Archbold et al. (1992) reported that the deleterious effects of lack of preparedness on caregiver strain faded after 9 months; however, a poor relationship with the care receiver remained strongly related to caregiver strain. Reporting a poorer quality of relationship with the care receiver was associated with a 23.5% prevalence of anxiety and 10% prevalence of depression in Mahoney and colleagues (2005) descriptive study.

Lack of Preparedness

Most caregivers are not prepared for the many responsibilities they face and receive no formal instruction in caregiving activities (NAC & AARP, 2004). According to a national opinion survey, Attitudes and Beliefs About Caregiving in the United States, 58% of respondents say they are only somewhat or not at all prepared to handle health insurance matters for an adult family member or friend, whereas 56% say they feel unprepared to assist with medications. Moreover, 64% worry about selling the home of a loved one and moving that person to another location or setting up a will or trust for that person (ORC, 2005). Stewart, Archbold, Harvath, and Nkongho, (1993) reported that although health care professionals were a caregiver's main source of information on providing physical care, the caregiver received no preparation on how to care for the patient emotionally or deal with the stresses of caregiving. Lack of preparedness can greatly increase the caregiver's perceptions of strain, especially during times of transition from hospital to home (Archbold et al., 1990; Archbold et al., 1992).

Baseline Levels of Burden and Depressive Scores

In a meta-analysis of 84 caregiving studies, Pinquart and Sörensen (2003) found that caregivers have higher levels of stress and depression as well as lower levels of subjective well-being, physical health, and self-efficacy than noncaregivers. The strongest negative effects of caregiving were observed for clinician-rated depression. Differences in perceived stress and depression between caregivers and noncaregivers were larger in spouses than in adult children (Pinquart & Sörensen, 2003). Caregivers of care receivers who have dementia (Pinquart & Sörensen, 2006) have more problems with symptom management (Butler et al., 2005; Grande, Farquhar, Barclay, & Todd, 2004) and problematic communication (Tolson, Swan, & Knussen, 2002) and have also reported increased burden, strain, and depression across studies.

Physical Health Problems

Vitaliano and colleagues' (2003) quantitative review of 23 studies from North America, Europe, and Australia examined relationships of caregiving with several health outcomes. They found that caregivers are at greater risk for health problems than are noncaregivers. These studies included 1,594 caregivers of persons with dementia and 1,478 noncaregivers who were similar in age (mean 65.6 years old) and sex ratio (65% women, 35% men). In this review, six physiological and five self-reported categories were examined that are indicators of illness risk and illness. The physiological categories included level of stress hormones, antibodies, immune counts/functioning, and cardiovascular and metabolic variables. Caregivers had a 23% higher level of stress hormones (adrenocorticotropic hormone, catecholamines, cortisol, etc.) and a 15% lower level of antibodies (Eipstein-Barr virus, herpes simplex, immunoglobulin G test) than did noncaregivers. Comorbid medical illnesses are important because many caregivers are middle aged to older adults, and they may be ill before they become caregivers. Interestingly, the relationship between caregiver status and physiological risk was stronger for men than women (Vitaliano et al., 2003).

ASSESSMENT OF THE PROBLEM

Although systematic assessment of the patient is a routine element of clinical practice, assessment of the family caregiver is rarely carried out to determine what help the caregiver may need. Effective intervention strategies for caregivers should be based on an accurate assessment of caregiver risk and strengths. According to a broad consensus of researchers and family caregiving organizations (Stewart et al., 1993), assessing the caregiver should involve addressing the following topics. These are applicable across settings (e.g., home, hospital) but may not need to be measured in every assessment. Specific topics may differ for the following:

- Initial assessments compared to reassessments (the latter focus on what has changed over time)
- New versus continuing care situations
- An acute episode prompting a change in caregiving versus an ongoing need type of setting and focus of services (Family Caregiver Alliance [FCA], 2006)

Caregiving Context

The caregiving context includes the background on the caregiver and the caregiving situation. The caregiver's relationship to the care recipient (spouse, nonspouse) is important because spouse and nonspouse caregivers have different risks and needs (Gitlin et al., 2003; Sörensen et al., 2002). The caregiver's various roles and responsibilities can either take away from or enhance their ability to provide care. For example, working caregivers may have to develop strategies to juggle family and work responsibilities, so we need to know what their employment status is (work/home/volunteer; Pinquart & Sörensen, 2006). The duration of caregiving (Sörensen et al., 2002) can give the clinician clues about how new caregiving is for the caregiver, or alert the clinician to possibility of caregiver exhaustion with the role. Questions about household status such as how many people are in the home (Pinquart & Sörensen, 2006) and the existence and involvement of extended family and social support (Pinquart &

Sörensen, 2006) can give the clinician clues about how much support the caregiver has readily available. Depending upon the type of impairment of the care receiver, the physical environment of the home, or facility where care takes place can be very important (Vitaliano et al., 2003). Determine what the caregiver's financial status is—for example, are they getting by, or are they short of funds to provide for everyday necessities (Vitaliano et al., 2003)? Ask about potential resources that the caregiver could choose to use and list these (Pinquart & Sörensen, 2006). Explore the family's cultural background (Dilworth-Anderson et al., 2002) and look for clues on how to use this as a resource.

Caregiver's Perception of Recipient's Health and Functional Status

List activities the care receiver needs help with; include both ADL and IADL (Pinquart & Sörensen, 2003; Pinquart & Sörensen, 2006). Determine if there is any cognitive impairment of the care recipient. If the answer to this question is "yes," ask if there are any behavioral problems (Gitlin et al., 2003; Sörensen et al., 2002). The presence of mobility problems can also make caregiving more difficult—assess this by simply asking if the care recipient has problems with getting around (Archbold et al., 1990; see Chapter 6, Assessment of Physical Function).

Lack of Caregiver Preparedness

Does caregiver have the skills, abilities, or knowledge to provide care recipient with needed care? To assess preparedness, use questions from the caregiving preparedness scale (see http://consultgerirn.org/resources). The Preparedness for Caregiving Scale (PCGS) was developed by Archbold and colleagues (1990, 1993). The concept of preparedness was derived from role theory, in which socialization to a role is assumed to be important for role enactment and performance. The questions prompt caregivers to rate how well prepared they think they are for caregiving in four perspectives of domain-specific preparedness: physical needs, emotional needs, resources, and stress. The clinician can interview the caregiver or ask the caregiver to complete the scale like a survey. The responses to the scale items can also be tallied and averaged for an overall score. If pressed for time, the clinician can simply ask, overall, how well prepared the caregiver thinks he or she is to care for a family member, and then follow this with more specific questions if the response indicates preparedness is low. The PCGS was evaluated in a longitudinal correlational study of family caregivers ($N = 103$) of older patients with chronic diseases (Archbold et al., 1990; Archbold et al., 1992). The scale has five Likert-type items with possible responses ranging from 1 (*not at all prepared*) to 4 (*very well prepared*). Overall scores are computed by averaging responses to the five items. Scores range from 1.00 to 4.00—the lowest score correlating with least preparedness. Archbold and colleagues (1992) reported internal reliability (Cronbach's alpha) of 0.72 at 6 weeks and 0.71 at the 9-month interview.

Quality of Family Relationships

The caregiver's perception of the quality of the relationship with the care receiver is a key predictor of the presence or lack of strain from caregiving (Archbold et al., 1990). The quality of the relationship can be assessed using the Mutuality scale (Messecar,

Parker-Walsch, & Lindauer, in press) developed by Archbold and colleagues (1990, 1992). *Mutuality* is defined as the caregiver's perceived quality of the relationship with the care receiver. Questions include "How close do you feel to him or her?"and "How much does he or she express feelings of appreciation for you and the things you do?" An overall score can be obtained by calculating the mean across all items—or the questions can be used in an open-ended interview format where the clinician then probes for more information and history about the relationship. This scale can also be completed via self-administration and then reviewed by the clinician with the caregiver (interview the caregiver apart from the care receiver). For this scale, there is no item that asks about the relationship overall; instead, the items explore several key features of the relationship such as conflict, shared positive past memories, felt positive regard, and positive reciprocity between the caregiver and care receiver. The questions open the door for the clinician to probe in a gentle way the quality of the relationship. Caregivers rate how they feel about the care recipient with possible responses ranging from 0 (*not at all*) to 4 (*a great deal*). The caregiver's mutuality score is computed by taking the average of the scores on the 15 items. Internal reliability and consistency (Cronbach's alpha) of the scale was 0.91 at both 6 weeks and 9 months from discharge from the hospital (Archbold et al., 1990).

Indicators of Problems With Quality of Care

Indicators of problems with the quality of care can include the following: evidence of an unhealthy environment, inappropriate management of finances, and demonstration of a lack of respect for older adult. The nurse's observations can be guided by The Elder Mistreatment Assessment (Fulmer, 2002), which helps the nurse identify elder abuse and neglect issues (see Elder Mistreatment Assessment instrument at http://consultgerirn.org/resources). This assessment instrument comprised seven sections that reviews signs, symptoms, and subjective complaints of elder abuse, neglect, exploitation, and abandonment (Fulmer, Paveza, Abraham, & Fairchild, 2000; Fulmer, Street, & Carr, 1984; Fulmer & Wetle, 1986). There is no "score," but the older adult should be referred to social services if there is evidence of mistreatment, a complaint by the older adult, or if there is high risk or probable abuse, neglect, exploitation, or abandonment of the older adult. Please also refer to Chapter 27, Mistreatment Detection.

Caregiver's Physical and Mental Health Status

The caregiver's perception of their own health (Pinquart & Sörensen, 2006) is one of the most reliable indicators of a physical health problem. Depression or other emotional distress (e.g., anxiety) can be assessed using the Center for Epidemiological Studies-Depression Scale (CED-S; see http://www.chcr.brown.edu/pcoc/cesdscale.pdf; Pinquart & Sörensen, 2006; Sörensen et al., 2002). The CES–D was initially designed as a screen for the community dwelling at risk for developing major depressive symptomatology. It has been used widely in intervention studies with family caregivers where it has been self-administered. The Brown University Center for Gerontology and Healthcare Research created a set of end-of-life care toolkit instruments, which are available for use on their site at no charge. For each of the 20 items, participants rate its frequency of occurrence during the past week on a 4-point scale from 0 (*rarely*) to 3 (*most of the time*).

Scores range from 0 to 60, with a higher score indicating the presence of a greater number and frequency of depressive symptoms. A score of 16 or higher has been identified as discriminatory between groups with clinically relevant and nonrelevant depressive symptoms (Fulmer et al., 2000; Radloff, 1977).

Burden or strain can be assessed using the modified Caregiver Strain Index (CSI; see http://consultgerirn.org/resources Family Caregiving; Sullivan, 2002). Pre-existing burden or strain places caregivers at greater risk and may prevent them from benefiting from interventions (Schulz & Beach, 1999; Sullivan, 2002; Vitaliano et al., 2003). The *modified CSI* is a tool that can be used to quickly identify families with potential caregiving concerns. It is a 13-question tool that measures strain related to care provision. There is at least one item for each of the following major domains: employment, financial, physical, social, and time. Positive responses to seven or more items on the index indicate a greater level of strain. Internal consistency reliability is high (Cronbach's α = 0.86) and construct validity is supported by correlations with the physical and emotional health of the caregiver and with subjective views of the caregiving situation. A positive screen (7 or more items positive) on the CSI indicates a need for more in-depth assessment to facilitate appropriate intervention.

Rewards of Caregiving

Although early family caregiving research focused almost exclusively on negative outcomes of caregiving, clearly, there are many positive aspects of providing care. Spouses can be drawn closer together by caregiving, which can act as an expression of love. Child caregivers can feel a sense of accomplishment from helping their adult parents. Caregivers should be encouraged to explore and list their perceived benefits of caregiving (Archbold et al., 1995). These can include the satisfaction of helping family member, developing new skills and competencies, and/or improved family relationships.

Self-Care Activities for Caregiver

Self-care activities can include things like setting aside time to exercise, getting time for oneself, and obtaining respite. Even if the caregiver does not use this strategy, ask them to think about strategies that would work for them. Caregivers need to be reminded that self-care is not a luxury; it is a necessity. At a minimum, caregivers need to learn how to put themselves first, manage stress, socialize, and get help.

INTERVENTIONS AND CARE STATEGIES

Definitions

Psychoeducational Interventions

Psychoeducational interventions involve a structured program geared toward providing information about the care receiver's disease process and about resources and services, and training caregivers to respond effectively to disease-related problems, such as memory and behavior problems in patients with dementia or depression and anger in patients with cancer. Use of lectures, group discussions, and written materials are always led by a trained leader. Support may be part of a psychoeducational group, but it is secondary to the educational content.

Supportive Interventions

This category subsumes both professionally led and peer-led unstructured support groups focused on building rapport among participants and creating a space in which to discuss problems, successes, and feelings regarding caregiving.

Respite or Adult Day Care

Respite care is either in-home or site-specific supervision, assistance with ADL, or skilled nursing care designed to give the caregiver time off.

Psychotherapy

This type of intervention involves a therapeutic relationship between the caregiver and a trained professional. Most psychotherapeutic interventions with caregivers follow a cognitive behavioral approach.

Interventions to Improve Care Receiver Competence

These interventions include memory clinics for patients with dementia and activity therapy programs designed to improve affect and everyday competence.

Multicomponent Interventions

Interventions in this group included various combinations of educational interventions, support, psychotherapy, and respite in Sorensen et al.'s (2002) meta-analysis. Individual studies included after the 2002 meta-analysis include nursing management and interdisciplinary care interventions and REACH II.

Overview

Past reviews of caregiver interventions, such as support groups, individual counseling, and education confirm that there is no single, easily implemented, and consistently effective method for eliminating the stresses and/or strain of being a caregiver (Knight, Lutzky, & Macofsky-Urban, 1993; Toseland & Rossiter, 1989). Sorensen and colleagues (2002) performed a more recent meta-analysis on the effects of a second generation of 78 caregiver intervention studies. The most consistent significant improvements in all outcome domains (burden, depression, well-being, ability and knowledge, care receiver symptoms) assessed in the meta-analysis resulted from psychotherapy and caregiver psychoeducational interventions aimed at improving caregiver knowledge and abilities. Multicomponent interventions, which combined features of psychotherapy and knowledge or skill building, had the largest effect on burden and in addition, were effective for improving well-being, ability, and knowledge. The effects of different types of interventions on selected indicators of unhealthy caregiver transitions from the meta-analysis and studies completed since 2002 are presented in Table 1.

Other studies of psychotherapy and psychoeducational interventions fit the same pattern of results (Akkerman & Ostwald, 2004; Burns et al., 2005; Coon, Thompson, Steffen, Sorocco, & Gallagher-Thompson, 2003; Hébert et al., 2003; Hepburn et al., 2005; Mittelman, Roth, Coon, & Haley, 2004; Mittelman, Roth, Haley, & Zarit, 2004). All of these interventions address key negative aspects of caregiving: being

TABLE 24.1

Effects of Different Types of Interventions on Indicators of Unhealthy Caregiver Transitions

Type of Intervention	Burden or Strain	Depression or Distress or Lack of Well-being	Lack of Preparedness
Psychoeducation	Significant effect (Sörensen et al., 2002)	Significant effect (Sörensen et al., 2002)	Significant effect (Sörensen et al., 2002)
Skill-building	Decreased burden—6 studies (Acton & Winter, 2002)	Decreased depression—6 studies (Acton & Winter, 2002)	Increased knowledge—9 studies (Acton & Winter, 2002)
		Significant reduction in depressive symptoms (Gallagher-Thompson et al., 2003)	14% improved reaction to CR symptoms (Hébert et al., 2003)
		Decreased bother, anxiety, depression (Mahoney et al., 2003)	
		Decreased depression (Coon et al., 2003)	
		Decreased distress (Hepburn et al., 2005)	
Supportive Interventions	Significant effect (Sörensen et al., 2002)		Significant effect (Sörensen et al., 2002)
Psychotherapy	Significant effect (Sörensen et al., 2002)	Significant effect (Sörensen et al., 2002)	Significant effect (Sörensen et al., 2002)
	Decreased objective burden	Decreased anxiety (Akkerman & Ostwald, 2004)	Some improved reaction to CR symptoms (Burns et al., 2005)
Respite	Significant effect (Sörensen et al., 2002)	Significant effect (Sörensen et al., 2002)	
		Decreased depression—3 studies (Acton & Winter, 2002)	
Focus on CR		Significant effect (Sörensen et al., 2002)	
Multicompent—added to this category:	Large significant effect (Sörensen et al., 2002)	Improved distress and depression (Bass, Clark, Looman, McCarthy, & Eckert, 2003; Callahan et al., 2006)	Significant effect (Sörensen et al., 2002)
Nursing and interdisciplinary care management—includes hospital or rehabilitation at-home and primary care	Improved carer strain (Burton & Gibbon, 2005)	Less burden (Crotty, Whitehead, Miller, & Gray 2003)	
	Decreased burden/strain—2 studies (Acton & Winter, 2002)	Less strain (Harris, Ashton, Broad, Connolly, & Richmond, 2005)	

(continued)

TABLE 24.1

Effects of Different Types of Interventions on Indicators of Unhealthy Caregiver Transitions *(continued)*

Type of Intervention	Burden or Strain	Depression or Distress or Lack of Well-being	Lack of Preparedness
	REACH interventions overall decreased burden (Gitlin et al., 2003)	More strain after intervention (Wade, 2003)	
	Decreased burden (Kalra et al., 2004)	Significant decrease in depressive symptoms (Eisdorfer et al., 2003)	
	Burden and strain were responsive to intervention (Schulz et al., 2005)	Decreased depression, distress, anxiety— 4 studies (Acton & Winter, 2002)	
		Decreased anxiety and depression (Kalra et al., 2004)	
		Decreased depression (Mittelman, Roth, Coon, et al., 2004)	
		Decreased reaction ratings (Mittelman, Roth, Haley, et al., 2004)	
		Clinically significant decreases in depression and anxiety (Schulz et al., 2005)	
		Significant effect (Sörensen et al., 2002)	
		Higher role rewards (Li et al., 2003)	
		Caregiver affect improved (Gitlin et al., 2005)	
		Well-being worse in control group (Burns et al., 2003)	
Focus on physical or emotional health of CG		Decreased psychological distress (King, Baumann, O'Sullivan, Wilcox, & Castro, 2002)	
		Decreased depression & anxiety (Waelde, Thompson, & Gallagher-Thompson, 2004)	

Note. CG = caregiver; CR = care receiver; REACH = Resources for Enhancing Alzheimer's Caregiver Health.

overwhelmed with the physical demands of care, feeling isolated, not having time for oneself, having difficulties with the care recipient's behavior, and dealing with one's own negative responses.

There are several characteristics across interventions that seem to have a moderating effect on caregiving outcomes. Focusing the caregiver training exclusively on the care receiver to alter their symptoms has almost no effect on the caregiver (Sörensen et al., 2002). In the Sorensen (2002) meta-analysis, group interventions were less effective at improving caregiver burden than individual and mixed interventions, which is consistent with Knight et al. (1993) but inconsistent with the meta-analysis performed by Yin, Zhou, and Bashford (2002). Length of an intervention appears to be important in alleviating caregiver depression and care receiver symptoms. Caregivers do less well with shorter interventions regarding depression because they lose the supportive aspects of prolonged contact with a group or a professional before they can benefit.

Characteristics of the caregiver are also associated with intervention effectiveness. Some caregivers benefit less from interventions than others do. For example, Sörensen (2002) found that spouse caregivers benefited less from interventions than did adult children. Table 2 presents caregiver characteristics associated with various indicators of unhealthy caregiver transitions. .

Interventions With Little Effect

Some intervention approaches have been consistently disappointing, showing either no significant effects or limited responses. In Lee and Cameron's (2004) update of the Cochrane database review, re-analysis of three trials of respite care found no significant effects of respite on any outcome variable. Interventions focused on medication management of the care receiver's dementing condition (Lingler, Martire, & Schulz, 2005) and/or targeted to managing problematic behavior (Livingston, Johnston, Katona, Paton, & Lyketsos, 2005) were similarly disappointing. A meta-analysis of habit training for the management of urinary incontinence interventions showed that not only were there no significant differences in incontinence between the intervention and control groups, but that caregivers found the intervention labor intensive (Ostaszkiewicz, Johnston, & Roe, 2004).

In Acton and Winter's (2002) meta-analysis of dementia, caregiving studies; small, diverse samples; lack of intervention specificity; diversity in the length, duration, and intensity of the intervention strategies; and problematic outcome measures led to nonsignificant results for many tested interventions (Cooke, McNally, Mulligan, Harrison, & Newman, 2001). They also reported that two thirds of the interventions they examined did not show any improvement in any outcome measures. Their analysis was hampered by lack of detailed description of the interventions in the studies they examined. Study limitations have also been a factor leading to disappointing results for some innovative caregiving interventions for caregivers of care receivers with other long-term, debilitating illnesses. For example, interventions designed to teach arthritis management as a couple (Martire et al., 2003), to decrease the gap between caregiver's expectations and care receiver's actual functional abilities with skill-building and nurse-coached pain management, all had disappointing results because of either small sample sizes or the complexity of the problems they were designed to address (Martin-Cook, Davis, Hynan, & Weiner, 2005; Schumacher et al., 2002). According to Price, Hermans, and Grimley Evans (2000) modification interventions for wandering have never been adequately tested because of the many flaws identified in the existing published research; outcome

TABLE 24.2

Effects of Different Types of Caregiver Characteristics on Indicators of Unhealthy Caregiver Transitions

Characteristics of Caregiving Situation	Burden	Depression or Lack of Well-being	Lack of Preparedness
CR has dementia	Less effective (Sörensen et al., 2002)	Less effective (Sörensen et al., 2002)	Less effective (Sörensen et al., 2002)
Adult child CGs	Greater improvement (Sörensen et al., 2002)	Greater improvement (Sörensen et al., 2002)	Greater improvement (Sörensen et al., 2002)
		Nonspouses did better (Gitlin et al., 2003)	
Spouse CGs	Smaller improvement (Sörensen et al., 2002)	Smaller improvement (Sörensen et al., 2002)	Smaller improvement (Sörensen et al., 2002)
		Wives with low mastery and high anxiety benefited the most (Mahoney et al., 2003)	
		Cuban husbands improved more on depressive symptoms (Eisdorfer et al., 2003)	
Older CGs	Greater improvement (Sörensen et al., 2002)	No effects (Sörensen et al., 2002)	Greater improvement (Sörensen et al., 2002)
	Higher risk for (Schulz et al., 2005)	Higher risk for (Schulz et al., 2005)	
		Greater improvement well-being (Sörensen et al., 2002)	
Female CGs	Greater improvement (Sörensen et al., 2002)	Females benefit more (Gallagher-Thompson et al., 2003)	Greater improvement (Sörensen et al., 2002)
	Better improvement (Gitlin et al., 2003)	Cuban daughters improved more on depressive symptoms (Eisdorfer et al., 2003)	
	Higher risk for (Schulz et al., 2005)	Higher risk for (Schulz et al., 2005)	
Ethnicity	Sorensen et al. (Sörensen et al., 2002)	Latinos benefit as much (Eisdorfer et al., 2003)	Sorensen et al (Sörensen et al., 2002)
		Cuban husbands and daughters improved more on depressive symptoms (Eisdorfer et al., 2003)	
		Hispanics did better (Gitlin et al., 2003)	
Lower education	Better improvement (Gitlin et al., 2003)	Better improvement (Gitlin et al., 2003)	
	Higher risk for (Schulz et al., 2005)	Higher risk for (Schulz et al., 2005)	

Note. CR = care receiver; CG = caregiver.

measurement has also been problematic. More distal outcomes, such as depression, perceived stress, caregiver strain, and self-efficacy that are less directly related to the actual intervention are less likely to change significantly (Bourgeois, Schulz, Burgio, & Beach, 2002; Burgio, Stevens, Guy, Roth, & Haley, 2003) than outcomes that are more specific to the intervention (Hebert et al., 2003).

Caregivers caring for care receivers who have conditions that worsen substantially over time (dementia, Parkinson's disease, stroke) have reported either less improvement, no improvement, or increased strain after intervention (Sörensen et al., 2002; Forster et al., 2001; Wright, Litaker, Laraia, & DeAndrade, 2001). Across many studies, Sörensen et al. (2002) reported that interventions with caregivers of dementia patients are less successful than for other caregivers. They also noted that if levels of caregiving are relatively high and cannot be reduced, as is the case for dementia caregivers, then burden and depression are less amenable to change as well. A multidisciplinary rehabilitation program for patients with Parkinson's disease resulted in no improvement in depression for caregivers after treatment (Trend, Kaye, Gage, Owen, & Wade, 2002). A meta-analysis of hospital-at-home care for patients with stroke reported no evidence from clinical trials to support a radical shift in the care of patients with acute stroke from hospital-based care (Langhorne et al., 2000). Individual studies that examined other psychoeducational and/or support and counseling interventions for stroke caregivers (albeit with relatively small samples) found no significant changes between the intervention and control groups (Clark, Rubenack, & Winsor, 2003; Gräsel, Biehler, Schimdt, & Schupp, 2005; Larson et al., 2005). Only an intensive, multicomponent skills training intervention significantly decreased burden anxiety and depression for this category of caregivers (Kalra et al., 2004). A number of family-based and symptom management interventions for patients with cancer have also found no significant intervention effects (Hudson, Aranda, & Hayman-White, 2005; Kozachik et al., 2001; Kurtz, Kurtz, Given, & Given, 2005; Northouse, Kershaw, Mood, & Schafenacker, 2005; Wells, Hepworth, Murphy, Wujcik, & Johnson, 2003). In several of these studies, there was a large dropout rate among the intervention participants because of the rapidly deteriorating condition of the care receivers.

Resources for Enhancing Alzheimer's Caregiver Health

The REACH project was designed to test promising interventions for enhancing family caregiving for persons with dementia and overcome several of the limitations of prior research (Schulz et al., 2003). More than 1,200 caregivers participated at six sites nationwide. The sample was more diverse than most caregiving studies because of the multisite design: participants were 56% White, 24% African American, and 19% Latino (Wisniewski et al., 2003). Five sites participated in this trial nationwide. The following five interventions were tested:

1. A 12-month, computer-mediated automated interactive voice response intervention designed to assist family caregivers managing care receivers with dementia (Mahoney, Tarlow, & Jones, 2003).
2. A psychoeducational (skill-building) approach modeled after community-based support groups tailored to be sensitive to ethnic groups tested (Gallagher-Thompson et al., 2003).
3. A manual-guided care-recipient–focused behavior management skill training and caregiver-focused, problem-solving training intervention tailored on cultural preferences of White and African American caregivers (Burgio et al., 2003).

4. A family therapy intervention designed to enhance communication between caregivers and other family members by identifying existing problems in communication and facilitating changes in interaction patterns (Eisdorfer et al., 2003).
5. Two primary care interventions delivered more than a period of 24 months, which included patient behavior management only and patient behavior management plus caregiver stress and coping (Burns, Nichols, Martindale-Adams, Graney, & Lummus, 2003).
6. In-home occupational therapy visits designed to help families modify the environment to reduce caregiver burden (Gitlin, Hauck, Dennis, & Winter, 2005).

When the results from the REACH interventions were pooled, overall interventions decreased burden significantly compared to the control conditions (Gitlin et al., 2003). Only the family therapy with computer technology intervention was effective for reducing depressive symptoms. Interventions were superior to control conditions on burden for women and caregivers with lower education; on depression, Hispanics, nonspouses, and caregivers with lower education had bigger responses.

REACH II followed up on REACH I, but unlike the first set of studies, which implemented a variety of interventions at six sites, REACH II implemented the same two interventions at each of five participating sites. Reach II specifically implemented a multicomponent intervention and tested new tools for assessing caregivers at risk for adverse outcomes. Intervention participants received individual risk profiles and the REACH intervention through nine in-home and three telephone sessions for more than 6 months. Caregivers receiving REACH II reported better self-rated health, sleep quality, physical health, and emotional health than for those caregivers not receiving the intervention. Findings supported using a structured, multicomponent skills training intervention that targeted caregiver self-care behaviors as one of five target areas. Overall, REACH II improved self-reported health status and decreased burden and bother in racially and ethnically diverse caregivers of people with dementia (Elliott, Burgio, & Decoster, 2010). An analysis of the findings by sociodemographic groups indicated that caregiver's age and religious coping moderated the effects of the intervention for Hispanics and Blacks. The older Hispanic and Black caregivers who received the intervention reported a decrease in caregiver burden from baseline to follow-up (Lee, Czaja, & Schulz, 2010). Findings from the REACH studies support use of multicomponent interventions tailored for specific caregiving characteristics.

Aspects of Interventions That Improve Effectiveness

A key conclusion of the REACH trial and several of the meta-analyses (Gitlin et al., 2003; Schulz et al., 2005; Sörensen et al., 2002) reviewed in this chapter was that family caregiver interventions need to be multicomponent and tailored. Multicomponent interventions have the potential to include a repertoire of various strategies that target different aspects of the caregiving experience. In focus groups conducted during a caregiving clinical trial, Farran and colleagues (2004) identified and catalogued the information and skills caregivers reported they needed to respond to their own needs or the caregiving process. This included care receiver issues such as managing difficult behaviors, worrisome symptoms, personal care problems, and caregiver concerns such as managing competing responsibilities and stressors, finding and using resources, and handling their emotional and physical responses to care (Farran et al., 2004). *Tailored interventions* are interventions that are crafted to match a specific target population, for example, spouse caregivers of patients with Alzheimer's disease and their specific caregiving issues and concerns identified through assessment (Archbold et al., 1995; Horton-Deutsch, Farran, Choi, & Fogg, 2002). Interventions that are individualized or tailored in combination with skill building demonstrated the best evidence of effectiveness (Pusey & Richards, 2001). Among the psychoeducation interventions, some of the most effective were predicated on a skills building approach (Gallagher-Thompson et al., 2003; Hepburn, Tornatore, Center, & Ostwald, 2001). Collaboration or a partnership model with the caregiver is also a key component of making the tailoring process more effective (Harvath et al., 1994). Programs that work collaboratively with care receivers and their families and are more intensive and modified to the caregiver's needs are also more successful (Brodaty, Green, & Koschera, 2003).

Nursing Care Strategies

1. *Identify content and skills needed to increase preparedness for caregiving.*
   Psychoeducational skill-building interventions include information about the care needed by the care receiver and how to provide it, as well as coaching on how to manage the caregiving role. Tasks associated with taking on the caregiving role include dealing with change, juggling competing responsibilities and stressors, providing and managing care, finding and using resources, and managing the physical and emotional responses to care (Acton & Winter, 2002; Farran, Loukissa, Perraud, & Paun, 2003; Farran et al., 2004; Gitlin et al., 2003; Sörensen et al., 2002).

2. *Form a partnership with the caregiver prior to generating strategies to address issues and concerns.*
   The goal of this partnership is blending the nurse's knowledge and expertise in health care with the caregiver's knowledge of the family member and the caregiving situation. Each party brings essential knowledge to the process of mutual negotiation between the family and the nurse. Together, they develop ideas to address the issues and concerns that are most salient for the caregiver and care receiver. One strategy that can be used in the hospital setting is to interview the caregiver using the Family Preferences Index developed by Li to assess family member's preferences to participate in care while the older adult is hospitalized (Brodaty et al., 2003; Gitlin et al., 2005; Harvath et al., 1994; Nolan, 2001).

3. *Identify the caregiving issues and concerns on which the caregiver wants to work and generate strategies.*
   Multiple strategies should be generated for each caregiving issue and concern. One of the most important findings from the review of literature on caregiving is that multicomponent interventions are superior to narrow, single-approach problem solving (Acton & Winter, 2002; Gitlin et al., 2005; Sörensen et al., 2002). Several Level II individual studies are presented in Table 1.

4. *Assist the caregiver in identifying strengths in the caregiving situation.*
   Not all outcomes from caregiving are negative, and caregiving can be rewarding for some caregivers who derive pride and satisfaction from the important role they are filling. Incorporating pleasurable activities into the daily routine or incorporating into some caregiving task something that is either fun or meaningful are ways of enhancing caregiving. Even in really difficult situations, there may be some positive benefit derived such as satisfaction in meeting an important commitment and/or recognition of personal growth (Archbold et al., 1995).

5. *Assist the caregiver in finding and using resources.*

   Navigating the health care system is one of the most difficult skills caregivers have to master (Archbold et al., 1995; Farran et al., 2004; Schumacher et al., 2002). Caregivers rarely know how to translate a need that they have into a request for help from the health care system. Learning how to speak to health care providers, how to negotiate billing, and how to request help with transportation—all of these tasks can be overwhelming. For some caregivers, Internet and other online sources of support and information can be helpful.

6. *Help caregivers identify and manage their physical and emotional responses to caregiving.*

   We know that caregiving is sometimes associated with deterioration of the caregiver's health or significant depression (Schulz et al., 2005). Generating strategies to take care of the caregiver is just as important as the strategies for caring for the care recipient.

7. *Use interdisciplinary approach when working with family caregivers.*

   Multicomponent interventions have the strongest record in terms of alleviating some of the global negative consequences of caregiving. Involving a team of other health professionals helps the nurse and family generate new ideas for strategies and brings a fresh perspective to the idea-generating process (Acton & Winter, 2002; Farran et al., 2003; Farran et al., 2004; Gitlin et al., 2003; Sorensen et al., 2002). Several Level II studies are presented in Table 1.

CASE STUDY

Alison Walsh is the oldest of two children and the only one who still lives in the same city as her widowed mother. She describes her relationship with her mother as very strained and without much love—only discipline. Her mother, who recently suffered a stroke and is considered marginal for staying home by her neurologist, is expecting that Alison will move in and take care of her. In fact, Alison's mother has virtually no resources for any other option. Alison's mother is being discharged today from the hospital. Alison says she would feel hard-pressed to take on all of the new care that her mother will require, including having to do baths and do many, if not all, of her ADL. In addition, she feels her relationship with her mother is so poor she does not understand why she should have to be the caregiver at this time when she has her own problems to deal with. Adding to her difficulties, Alison has only one other sibling to call on for help, and he lives more than 2,000 miles away in another city. Her husband has health problems as well and his care takes considerable time.

As a child caregiver, Alison is at higher risk for depression or anxiety. The goal of intervention with Alison will be to identify and address aspects of her caregiving situation amenable to modification. The possible targets for intervention will vary from one caregiver to another, and it is important that the approach be tailored. Addressing aspects of caregiving that are strong predictors of unhealthy caregiver transitions such as a lack of preparedness, stress and strain in the relationship, and overall burden can help the nurse tailor their caregiver interventions. In this case study, only three parameters of assessment (lack of preparedness, poor relationship quality, and need to find rewards of caregiving) will be addressed along with some suggested strategies for addressing the concerns indicated.

(continued)

CASE STUDY *(continued)*

First, in Alison's case, caregivers may be reluctant to raise concerns about their lack of preparedness to the nurse. They may connect lack of preparedness with being embarrassed about their own lack of understanding, or they may simply not know what it is they do not know. For example, in Alison's case, she may not realize that formal resources could be taped to provide some of the personal care that she feels unable or unwilling to perform. Exploration of her readiness to provide care will help Alison raise her concerns so that they can be fully addressed.

Second, a lack of mutuality (the positive quality of the relationship between caregiver and care recipient) is very predictive of future and sustained reported difficulty with caregiving. Alison has a difficult relationship with her mother now and a history of a poor quality relationship from childhood. This puts her at risk for experiencing more strain from caregiving. Alison is aware that her relationship with her mother is difficult, but she may not realize how much this is adding to her strain. Alison will need to think about strategies to get support and help to deal with her feelings.

Third, although in Alison's situation there might not seem to be any rewards of caregiving, it is important to ask about these anyway. There are two very important reasons for nurses exploring positive aspects of caregiving with the caregiver; caregivers want to talk about them, and these factors will be an important indicator of the quality of care provided to the care recipient. Nurses need to encourage an increase in positive affect (i.e., feelings such as gratitude, forgiveness, and the like) while at the same time working on decreasing negative feelings like depression, anxiety, and guilt.

SUMMARY

Outcomes Specific to Caregiving

The goal of the guideline is to reduce the likelihood of unhealthy transitions to the caregiving role by lowering caregiver strain, depression, and poor physical health for caregivers. Indicators of problems with this include reports of depression and/or fatigue, increased use of over-the-counter and prescription medications, increased use of health services, neglect of own health, and substance abuse. Increased focus on the caregiver system as the unit of service should increase the nurse's confidence in working with family caregivers.

Outcomes Specific to Patient

These include improvement (where possible) in patient functional status, nutrition, and hygiene. Improved symptom management for care recipients with significant chronic disease is also a desired outcome. This could include better pain management for care recipients with cancer, improved glycemic control for care recipients with diabetes, and/or diminished problematic behaviors for care recipients with dementia. The emotional well-being of the care recipient should also be an outcome of interventions to aid the caregiver. Decreased use of emergency services and increased use of formal care supports are system outcomes we might expect.

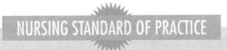

Protocol 24.1: Family Caregiving

I. GOAL: Identify viable strategies to monitor and support family caregivers.

II. OVERVIEW: Family caregivers provide more than 80% of the long-term care for older adults in this country. Caregiving can be difficult, time-consuming work added on top of job and other family responsibilities. If the caregiver suffers negative consequences from their caregiving role and these are not mitigated, increased morbidity and mortality may result for the caregiver. Not all outcomes from caregiving are negative; there are many caregivers that report rewards from caregiving.

III. BACKGROUND AND STATEMENT OF PROBLEM
  A. Definitions
    1. *Family caregiving* is broadly defined and refers to a broad range of unpaid care provided in response to illness or functional impairment to a chronically ill or functionally impaired older family member, partner, friend, or neighbor that exceeds the support usually provided in family relationships (Schumacher, Beck, & Marren, 2006).
    2. Caregiver role transitions: *Caregiver role acquisition* is a family role transition that occurs through situated interaction as part of a role-making process. This is the process of taking on the caregiving role at the beginning of caregiving or when a significant change in the caregiving context occurs. Role transitions occur when a role is added to or deleted from the role set of a person, or when the behavioral expectations for an established role change significantly (NAC & AARP, 2004).
    3. Indicators of healthy caregiver role transitions: The broad categories of indicators of healthy transitions include subjective well-being, role mastery, and well-being of relationships. These are the subjective, behavioral, and interpersonal parameters of health most likely to be associated with healthy role transitions (NAC & AARP, 2004).
    4. Family caregiving activities include assistance with day-to-day activities, illness-related care, care management, and invisible aspects of care. Day-to-day activities include personal care activities (bathing, eating, dressing, mobility, transferring from bed to chair, and using the toilet) and IADL (meal preparation, grocery shopping, making telephone calls, and money management; Walker et al., 1995). Illness-related activities include managing symptoms, coping with illness behaviors, carrying out treatments, and performing medical or nursing procedures that include an array of medical technologies (Smith, 1994). Care management activities include accessing resources, communicating with and navigating the health care and social services systems, and acting as an advocate (Schumacher et al., 2000). Invisible aspects of care are protective actions the caregiver takes to ensure the older adults' safety and well-being without their knowledge (Bowers, 1987).

(continued)

5. Caregiving roles can be classified into a hierarchy according to who takes on the bulk of responsibilities versus only intermittent supportive assistance. Primary caregivers tend to provide most of the everyday aspects of care, whereas secondary caregivers help out as needed to fill the gaps (Cantor & Little, 1985; Penning, 1990; Tennstedt et al., 1989). Among caregivers who live with their care recipients, spouses account for the bulk of primary caregivers, whereas adult children are more likely to be secondary caregivers. The range of the family caregiving role includes protective caregiving like "keeping an eye on" an older adult who is currently independent but at risk, to full-time, round-the-clock care for a severely impaired family member. Health care providers may fail to assess the full scope of the family caregiving role if they associate family caregiving only with the performance of tasks.

6. *Caregiver assessment* refers to an ongoing iterative process of gathering information that describes a family caregiving situation and identifies the particular issues, needs, resources, and strengths of the family caregiver.

B. Etiology and/or epidemiology of risk factors associated with unhealthy caregiving transitions

1. Just being a caregiver puts an individual at increased risk for higher levels of stress and depression and lower levels of subjective well-being and physical health (Pinquart & Sörensen, 2006; Vitaliano et al., 2003).

2. Female caregivers on average provide more direct care and report higher levels of burden and depression (Gitlin et al., 2003).

3. Ethnic minority caregivers provide more care, use less formal services, and report worse physical health than White caregivers (Dilworth-Anderson et al., 2002; Pinquart & Sörensen, 2006).

4. African American caregivers experience less stress and depression and get more rewards from caregiving than White (Cuellar, 2002; Dilworth-Anderson, 2002; Gitlin et al., 2003; Haley et al., 2004; Pinquart & Sörensen, 2004).

5. Hispanic and Asian American caregivers exhibit more depression (Gitlin et al., 2003; Pinquart & Sörensen, 2004).

6. Less-educated caregivers report more depression (Buckwalter et al., 1999; Gitlin et al., 2003).

7. Spouse caregivers report higher levels of depression than nonspouse caregivers (Pinquart & Sörensen, 2004; Pruchno & Resch, 1989).

8. Caregivers who have a poor quality relationship with the care recipient report more strain (Archbold et al., 1990; Croog et al., 2006; Flannery, 2002).

9. Caregivers who lack preparedness for the caregiving role also increases strain (Archbold et al., 1990; Archbold et al., 1992)

10. Caregivers of care recipients who have dementia (Pinquart & Sörensen, 2003).

IV. PARAMETERS OF ASSESSMENT

A. Caregiving context

1. Caregiver relationship to care recipient (spouse, nonspouse; Gitlin et al., Sörensen et al., 2002).

(continued)

Protocol 24.1: Family Caregiving *(cont.)*

2. Caregiver roles and responsibilities
   a. Duration of caregiving (Sörensen et al., 2002)
   b. Employment status (work/home/volunteer; Pinquart & Sörensen, 2004)
   c. Household status (number in home, etc.; Pinquart & Sörensen, 2004)
   d. Existence and involvement of extended family and social support (Pinquart & Sörensen, 2004)
3. Physical environment (home, facility; Vitaliano et al., 2003)
4. Financial status (Vitaliano et al., 2003)
5. Potential resources that caregiver could choose to use—list (Pinquart & Sörensen, 2004)
6. Family's cultural background (Dilworth-Anderson et al., 2002)

B. Caregiver's perception of health and functional status of care recipient
   1. List activities care receiver needs help with; include both ADL, and IADL (Pinquart & Sörensen, 2004).
   2. Presence of cognitive impairment—if yes, any behavioral problems (Gitlin et al., 2003; Sörensen et al., 2002)?
   3. Presence of mobility problems—assess with single question (Archbold et al., 1990).

C. Caregiver preparedness for caregiving
   1. Does caregiver have the skills, abilities, or knowledge to provide care recipient with needed care (see Preparedness for Caregiving Scale at http://consultgerirn.org/resources).

D. Quality of family relationships
   1. The caregiver's perception of the quality of the relationship with the care receiver (see Mutuality Scale; Archbold et al., 1990; Messecar et al., in press).

E. Indicators of problems with quality of care
   1. Unhealthy environment
   2. Inappropriate management of finances
   3. Lack of respect for older adult (see EAI at http://www.consultgerirn.org/resources)

F. Caregiver's physical and mental health status
   1. Self-rated health: single item—asks what is caregiver's perception of their health (Pinquart & Sölensen, 2006).
   2. Health conditions and symptoms
      a. Depression or other emotional distress (e.g., anxiety; Pinquart & Sörensen, 2003; Pinquart & Sörensen, 2006; Sörensen et al., 2002; See http://www.chcr.brown.edu/pcoc/cesdscale.pdf.)
      b. Reports of burden or strain (Schulz & Beach, 1999; Vitaliano et al., 2003; See Caregiver Stain Index at http://www.consultgerirn.org/resources—Family Caregiving topic)
   3. Rewards of caregiving
      a. List perceived benefits of caregiving (Archbold et al., 1995)
      b. Satisfaction of helping family member
      c. Developing new skills and competencies
      d. Improved family relationships
   4. Self-care activities for caregiver

(continued)

Protocol 24.1: Family Caregiving *(cont.)*

V. NURSING CARE STRATEGIES

A. Identify content and skills needed to increase preparedness for caregiving (Acton & Winter, 2002; Farran et al., 2003; Gitlin et al., 2003; Pusey & Richards, 2001; Sörensen et al., 2002).

B. Form a partnership with the caregiver prior to generating strategies to address issues and concerns (Brodaty et al., 2003; Gitlin et al., 2003; Harvath et al., 1994).

C. Invite participation in care while in the hospital using the *Family Preferences Index*, a 14-item approach to exploring caregivers' personal choices for participating in the care of hospitalized older adult family members to determine preferences to provide care (Messecar, Powers, & Nagel, 2008).

D. Identify the caregiving issues and concerns on which the caregiver wants to work and generate strategies (Acton & Winter, 2002; Gitlin et al., 2003; Sörensen et al., 2002).

E. Assist the caregiver in identifying strengths in the caregiving situation (Archbold et al., 1995).

F. Assist the caregiver in finding and using resources (Archbold et al., 1995; Farran et al., 2004; Schumacher et al., 2002). Help caregivers identify and manage their physical and emotional responses to caregiving (Schulz & Beach, 1999).

G. Use an interdisciplinary approach when working with family caregivers (Acton & Winter, 2002; Farran et al., 2003; Farran et al., 2004; Gitlin et al., 2003; Sörensen et al., 2002).

VI. EVALUATION OR EXPECTED OUTCOMES

A. Outcomes specific to caregiving transitions
   1. Lower caregiver strain
   2. Decreased depression
   3. Improved physical health
B. Outcomes specific to patient
   1. Quality of family caregiving
   2. Care recipient functional status, nutrition, hygiene, and symptom management
   3. Care recipient emotional well-being
   4. Decreased occurrence of adverse events such as increased frequency of emergent care

ACKNOWLEDGMENTS

The author wishes to gratefully acknowledge the assistance of Patricia Archbold and Barbara Stewart, the developers of the Caregiver Preparedness and Mutuality scales for their assistance in providing information and access to these valuable caregiving assessment tools. This protocol also benefited from the perspective provided by Hong Li, the developer of the Family Preference Index about the critical importance of involving family caregivers early in the hospital care process to facilitate a healthy transition into the caregiving role.

RESOURCES

CES-D
http://www.chcr.brown.edu/pcoc/cesdscale.pdf

Caregiver Strain Index
http://consultgerirn.org/uploads/File/trythis/try_this_14.pdf

Elder Assessment Instrument (EAI)
http://www.hartfordign.org/publications/trythis/issue15.pdf

Preparedness Scale
http://consultgerirn.org/uploads/File/trythis/try_this_28.pdf

REFERENCES

Acton, G. J., & Winter, M. A. (2002). Interventions for family members caring for an elder with dementia. *Annual Review of Nursing Research, 20*, 149–179. Evidence Level I.

Akkerman, R. L., & Ostwald, S. K. (2004). Reducing anxiety in Alzheimer's disease family caregivers: The effectiveness of a nine-week cognitive-behavioral intervention. *American Journal of Alzheimer's Disease and Other Dementias, 19*(2), 117–123. Evidence Level II.

Archbold, P. G., Stewart, B. J., Greenlick, M. R., & Harvath, T. A. (1990). Mutuality and preparedness as predictors of caregiver role strain. *Research in Nursing & Health, 13*(6), 375–384. Evidence Level II.

Archbold, P. G., Stewart, B. J., Greenlick, M. R., & Harvath, T. A. (1992). Clinical assessment of mutuality and preparedness in family caregivers to frail older people. In S. G. Funk, E. M. Tornquist, M. T. Champagne, & L. A. Copp (Eds.), *Key aspects of elder care* (pp. 332–337). New York, NY: Springer Publishing Company, Inc. Evidence Level II.

Archbold, P. G., Stewart, B. J., Miller, L. L., Harvath, T. A., Greenlick, M. R., Van Buren, L., . . . Schook J. E. (1995). The PREP system of nursing interventions: A pilot test with families caring for older members. Preparedness (PR), enrichment (E) and predictability (P). *Research in Nursing & Health, 18*(1), 3–16. Evidence Level II.

Arno, P. S. (2006, January). *Economic value of informal caregiving.* Presented at the Care Coordination and the Caregiving Forum, Dept. of Veterans Affairs, NIH, Bethesda, MD. Evidence Level IV.

Bass, D. M., Clark, P. A., Looman, W. J., McCarthy, C. A., & Eckert, S. (2003). The Cleveland Alzheimer's managed care demonstration: Outcomes after 12 months of implementation. *The Gerontologist, 43*(1), 73–85. Evidence Level II.

Bauer, M., Fitzgerald, L., Haesler, E., & Manfrin, M. (2009). Hospital discharge planning for frail older people and their family. Are we delivering best practice? A review of the evidence. *Journal of Clinical Nursing, 18*(18), 2539–2546.

Bourgeois, M. S., Schulz, R., Burgio, L. D., & Beach, S. (2002). Skills training for spouses of patients with Alzheimer's disease: Outcomes of an intervention study. *Journal of Clinical Geropsychology, 8*(1), 53–73. Evidence Level II.

Bowers, B. J. (1987). Intergenerational caregiving: Adult caregivers and their aging parents. *Advances in Nursing Science, 9*(2), 20–31. Evidence Level IV.

Brodaty, H., Green, A., & Koschera, A. (2003). Meta-analysis of psychosocial interventions for caregivers of people with dementia. *Journal of the American Geriatrics Society, 51*(5), 657–664. Evidence Level I.

Buckwalter, K. C., Gerdner, L., Kohout, F., Hall, G. R., Kelly, A., Richards, B., & Sime, M. (1999). A nursing intervention to decrease depression in family caregivers of persons with dementia. *Archives of Psychiatric Nursing, 13*(2), 80–88. Evidence Level II.

Burgio, L., Stevens, A., Guy, D., Roth, D. L., & Haley, W. E. (2003). Impact of two psychosocial interventions on white and African American family caregivers of individuals with dementia. *The Gerontologist*, *43*(4), 568–579. Evidence Level II.

Burns, A., Guthrie, E., Marino-Francis, F., Busby, C., Morris, J., Russell, E., . . . Byrne, J. (2005). Brief psychotherapy in Alzheimer's disease: Randomised controlled trial. *British Journal of Psychiatry*, *187*(2), 143–147. Evidence Level II.

Burns, R., Nichols, L. O., Martindale-Adams, J., Graney, M. J., & Lummus, A. (2003). Primary care interventions for dementia caregivers: 2-year outcomes from the REACH study. *The Gerontologist*, *43*(4), 547–555. Evidence Level II.

Burton, C., & Gibbon, B. (2005). Expanding the role of the stroke nurse: A pragmatic clinical trial. *Journal of Advanced Nursing*, *52*(6), 640–650. Evidence Level II.

Butler, L. D., Field, N. P., Busch, A. L., Seplaki, J. E., Hastings, T. A., & Spiegel, D. (2005). Anticipating loss and other temporal stressors predict traumatic stress symptoms among partners of metastatic/recurrent breast cancer patients. *Psycho-oncology*, *14*(6), 492–502. Evidence Level II.

Callahan, C. M., Boustani, M. A., Unverzagt, F. W., Austrom, M. G., Damush, T. M., Perkins, A. J., . . . Hendrie, H .C. (2006). Effectiveness of collaborative care for older adults with Alzheimer disease in primary care: A randomized controlled trial. *The Journal of the American Medical Association*, *295*(18), 2148–2157. Evidence Level II.

Cannuscio, C. C., Jones, C., Kawachi, I., Colditz, G. A., Berkman, L., & Rimm, E. (2002). Reverberation of family illness: A longitudinal assessment of informal caregiving and mental health status in the nurses' health study. *American Journal of Public Health*, *92*(8), 1305–1311. Evidence Level IV.

Cantor, M. H., & Little, V. (1985). Aging and social care. In R. H. Binstock & E. Shanas (Eds.), *Handbook of aging and the social sciences* (2nd ed., pp. 745–781). New York, NY: Van Nostrand Reinhold. Evidence Level V.

Clark, M. S., Rubenach, S., & Winsor, A. (2003). A randomized controlled trial of an education and counseling intervention for families after stroke. *Clinical Rehabilitation*, *17*(7), 703–712. Evidence Level II.

Coleman, E. A., & Boult, C. (2003). Improving the quality of transitional care for persons with complex care needs. *Journal of the American Geriatrics Society*, *51*(4), 556–557. Evidence Level VI.

Cooke, D. D., McNally, L., Mulligan, K. T., Harrison, M. J., & Newman, S. P. (2001). Psychosocial interventions for caregivers of people with dementia: A systematic review. *Aging & Mental Health*, *5*(2), 120–135. Evidence Level I.

Coon, D. W., Thompson, L., Steffen, A., Sorocco, K., & Gallagher-Thompson, D. (2003). Anger and depression management: Psychoeducational skill training interventions for women caregivers of a relative with dementia. *The Gerontologist*, *43*(5), 678–689. Evidence Level II.

Croog, S. H., Burleson, J. A., Sudilovsky, A., & Baume, R. M. (2006). Spouse caregivers of Alzheimer patients: Problem responses to caregiver burden. *Aging & Mental Health*, *10*(2), 87–100. Evidence Level IV.

Crotty, M., Whitehead, C., Miller, M., & Gray, S. (2003). Patient and caregiver outcomes 12 months after home-based therapy for hip fracture: A randomized controlled trial. *Archives of Physical Medicine and Rehabilitation*, *84*(8), 1237–1239. Evidence Level II.

Cuellar, N. G. (2002). A comparison of African American & Caucasian American female caregivers of rural, post-stroke, bedbound older adults. *Journal of Gerontological Nursing*, *28*(1), 36–45. Evidence Level IV.

Dilworth-Anderson, P., Williams, I. C., & Gibson, B. E. (2002). Issues of race, ethnicity, and culture in caregiving research: A 20-year review (1980–2000). *The Gerontologist*, *42*(2), 237–272. Evidence Level I.

Eisdorfer, C., Czaja, S. J., Loewenstein, D. A., Rubert, M. P., Argüelles, S., Mitrani, V. B., & Szapocznik, J. (2003). The effect of a family therapy and technology-based intervention on caregiver depression. *The Gerontologist*, *43*(4), 521–531. Evidence Level II.

Elliott, A. F., Burgio, L. D., & Decoster, J. (2010). Enhancing caregiver health: Findings from the resources for enhancing Alzheimer's caregiver health II intervention. *Journal of the American Geriatrics Society*, *58*(1), 30–37.

Family Caregiver Alliance. (2006). *Caregiver assessment: principles, guidelines and strategies for change. Report from a national consensus development conference* (Vol. I). San Francisco, CA: Author. Evidence Level VI.

Farran, C. J., Gilley, D. W., McCann, J. J., Bienias, J. L., Lindeman, D. A., & Evans, D. A. (2004). Psychosocial interventions to reduce depressive symptoms of dementia caregivers: A randomized clinical trial comparing two approaches. *Journal of Mental Health and Aging*, *10*(4), 337–350. Evidence Level II.

Farran, C. J., Loukissa, D., Perraud, S., & Paun, O. (2003). Alzheimer's disease caregiving information and skills. Part I: Care recipient issues and concerns. *Research in Nursing & Health*, *26*(5), 366–375. Evidence Level IV.

Flannery, R. B., Jr. (2002). Disrupted caring attachments: Implications for long-term care. *American Journal of Alzheimer's Disease and Other Dementias*, *17*(4), 227–231. Evidence Level VI.

Forster, A., Smith, J., Young, J., Knapp, P., House, A., & Wright, J. (2001). Information provision for stroke patients and their caregivers. *Cochrane Database of Systematic Reviews*, (3), CD001919. Evidence Level I.

Fulmer, T. (2002). *Elder abuse and neglect assessment. Try this: Best practices in nursing care to older adults*. Retrieved from: http://consultgerirn.org/resources

Fulmer, T., & Wetle, T. (1986). Elder abuse screening and intervention. *The Nurse Practitioner*, *11*(5), 33–38. Evidence Level II.

Fulmer, T., Paveza, G., Abraham, I., & Fairchild, S. (2000). Elder neglect assessment in the emergency department. *Journal of Emergency Nursing*, *26*(5), 436–443. Evidence Level II.

Fulmer, T., Street, S., & Carr, K. (1984). Abuse of the elderly: Screening and detection. *Journal of Emergency Nursing*, *10*(3), 131–140. Evidence Level II.

Gallagher-Thompson, D., Coon, D. W., Solano, N., Ambler, C., Rabinowitz, Y,, & Thompson, L. W. (2003). Changes in indices of distress among Latino and Anglo female caregivers of elderly relatives with dementia: Site-specific results from the REACH national collaborative study. *The Gerontologist*, *43*(4), 580–591. Evidence Level II.

Gitlin, L. N., Belle, S. H., Burgio, L. D., Czaja, S. J., Mahoney, D., Gallagher-Thompson, D., . . . Ory, M. G. (2003). Effect of multicomponent interventions on caregiver burden and depression: The REACH multisite initiative at 6-month follow-up. *Psychology & Aging*, *18*(3), 361–374. Evidence Level I.

Gitlin, L. N., Corcoran, M., Winter, L., Boyce, A., & Hauck, W. W. (2001). A randomized, controlled trial of a home environmental intervention: Effect on efficacy and upset in caregivers and on daily function of persons with dementia. *The Gerontologist*, *41*(1), 4–14. Evidence Level II.

Gitlin, L. N., Hauck, W. W., Dennis, M. P., & Winter, L. (2005). Maintenance of effects of the home environmental skill-building program for family caregivers and individuals with Alzheimer's disease and related disorders. *Journals of Gerontology: Series A, Biological Sciences and Medical Sciences*, *60*(3), 368–374. Evidence Level II.

Grande, G. E., Farquhar, M. C., Barclay, S. I., & Todd, C. J. (2004). Caregiver bereavement outcome: Relationship with hospice at home, satisfaction with care, and home death. *Journal of Palliative Care*, *20*(2), 69–77. Evidence Level II.

Gräsel, E., Biehler, J., Schmidt, R., & Schupp, W. (2005). Intensification of the transition between inpatient neurological rehabilitation and home care of stroke patients. Controlled clinical trial with follow-up assessment six months after discharge. *Clinical Rehabilitation*, *19*(7), 725–736. Evidence Level III.

Haley, W. E., Gitlin, L. N., Wisniewski, S. R., Mahoney, D. F., Coon, D. W., Winter, L., . . . Ory, M. (2004). Well-being, appraisal, and coping in African-American and Caucasian dementia caregivers: Findings from the REACH study. *Aging & Mental Health*, *8*(4), 316–329. Evidence Level II.

Harris, R., Ashton, T., Broad, J., Connolly, G., & Richmond, D. (2005). The effectiveness, acceptability and costs of a hospital-at-home service compared with acute hospital care: A randomized controlled trial. *Journal of Health Services Research & Policy, 10*(3), 158–166. Evidence Level II.

Harvath, T. A., Archbold, P. G., Stewart, B. J., Gadow, S., Kirschling, J. M., Miller, L., . . . Schook, J. (1994). Establishing partnerships with family caregivers: Local and cosmopolitan knowledge. *Journal of Gerontological Nursing, 20*(2), 29–35. Evidence Level V.

Hébert, R., Lévesque, L., Vézina, J., Lavoie, J. P., Ducharme, F., Gendron, C., . . . Dubois, M. F. (2003). Efficacy of a psychoeducative group program for caregivers of demented persons living at home: A randomized controlled trial. *The Journals of Gerontology. Series B: Psychological Sciences and Social Sciences, 58*(1), S58–S67. Evidence Level II.

Hepburn, K. W., Lewis, M., Narayan, S., Center, B., Tornatore, J., Bremer, K., & Kirk, L. (2005). Partners in caregiving: A psychoeducation program affecting dementia family caregivers' distress and caregiving outlook. *Clinical Gerontologist, 29*(1), 53–69. Evidence Level II.

Hepburn, K. W., Tornatore, J., Center, B., & Ostwald, S. W. (2001). Dementia family caregiver training: Affecting beliefs about caregiving and caregiver outcomes. *Journal of the American Geriatrics Society, 49*(4), 450–457. Evidence Level II.

Horton-Deutsch, S. L., Farran, C. J., Choi, E. E., & Fogg, L. (2002). The PLUS intervention: A pilot test with caregivers of depressed older adults. *Archives of Psychiatric Nursing, 16*(2), 61–71. Evidence Level III.

Hudson, P. L., Aranda, S., & Hayman-White, K. (2005). A psycho-educational intervention for family caregivers of patients receiving palliative care: A randomized controlled trial. *Journal of Pain and Symptom Management, 30*(4), 329–341. Evidence Level II.

Kalra, L., Evans, A., Perez, I., Melbourn, A., Patel, A., Knapp, M., & Donaldson, N. (2004). Training carers of stroke patients: Randomised controlled trial. *British Medical Journal, 328*(7448), 1099. Evidence Level II.

Kiecolt-Glaser, J. K., Preacher, K. J., MacCallum, R. C., Atkinson, C., Malarkey, W. B., & Glaser, R. (2003). Chronic stress and age-related increases in the proinflammatory cytokine IL-6. *Proceedings of the National Academy of Sciences of the United States of America, 100*(15), 9090–9095. Evidence Level III.

King, A. C., Baumann, K., O'Sullivan, P., Wilcox, S., & Castro, C. (2002). Effects of moderate-intensity exercise on physiological, behavioral, and emotional responses to family caregiving: A randomized controlled trial. *Journals of Gerontology. Series A: Biological Sciences and Medical Sciences, 57*(1), M26–M36. Evidence Level II.

Knight, B. G., Lutzky, S. M., & Macofsky-Urban, F. (1993). A meta-analytic review of interventions for caregiver distress: Recommendations for future research. *The Gerontologist, 33*(2), 240–248. Evidence Level I.

Kozachik, S. L., Given, C. W., Given, B. A., Pierce, S. J., Azzouz, F., Rawl, S. M., & Champion, V. L. (2001). Improving depressive symptoms among caregivers of patients with cancer: Results of a randomized clinical trial. *Oncology Nursing Forum, 28*(7), 1149–1157. Evidence Level II.

Kurtz, M. E., Kurtz, J. C., Given, C. W., & Given, B. (2005). A randomized, controlled trial of a patient/caregiver symptom control intervention: Effects on depressive symptomatology of caregivers of cancer patients. *Journal of Pain and Symptom Management, 30*(2), 112–122. Evidence Level II.

Langhorne, P., Dennis, M. S., Kalra, L., Shepperd, S., Wade, D. T., & Wolfe, C. D. (2000). Services for helping acute stroke patients avoid hospital admission. *Cochrane Database of Systematic Reviews*, (2), CD000444. Evidence Level I.

Larson, J., Franzén-Dahlin, A., Billing, E., Arbin, M., Murray, V., & Wredling, R. (2005). The impact of a nurse-led support and education programme for spouses of stroke patients: A randomized controlled trial. *Journal of Clinical Nursing, 14*(8), 995–1003. Evidence Level II.

Lee, C. C., Czaja, S. J., & Schulz, R. (2010). The moderating influence of demographic characteristics, social support, and religious coping on the effectiveness of a multicomponent psychosocial caregiver intervention in three racial ethnic groups. *Journals of Gerontology Series B: Psychological Sciences & Social Sciences, 65B*(2), 185–194.

Lee, H., & Cameron, M. (2004). Respite care for people with dementia and their carers. *Cochrane Database of Systematic Reviews*, (2), CD004396. Evidence Level I.

Li, H., Melnyk, B. M., McCann, R., Chatcheydang, J., Koulouglioti, C., Nichols, L. W., . . . Ghassemi, A. (2003). Creating avenues for relative empowerment (CARE): A pilot test of an intervention to improve outcomes of hospitalized elders and family caregivers. *Research in Nursing & Health*, *26*(4), 284–299. Evidence Level I.

Lingler, J. H., Martire, L. M., & Schulz, R. (2005). Caregiver-specific outcomes in antidementia clinical drug trials: A systematic review and meta-analysis. *Journal of the American Geriatrics Society*, *53*(6), 983–990. Evidence Level I.

Livingston, G., Johnston, K., Katona, C., Paton, J., & Lyketsos, C. G. (2005). Systematic review of psychological approaches to the management of neuropsychiatric symptoms of dementia. *The American Journal of Psychiatry*, *162*(11), 1996–2021. Evidence Level I.

Mahoney, D. F., Cloutterbuck, J., Neary, S., & Zhan L. (2005). African American, Chinese, and Latino family caregivers' impressions of the onset and diagnosis of dementia: Cross-cultural similarities and differences. *The Gerontologist*, *45*(6), 783–792. Evidence Level I.

Mahoney, D. F., Tarlow, B. J., & Jones, R. N. (2003). Effects of an automated telephone support system on caregiver burden and anxiety: Findings from the REACH for TLC intervention study. *The Gerontologist*, *43*(4), 556–567. Evidence Level II.

Mahoney, R., Regan, C., Katona, C., & Livingston, G. (2005). Anxiety and depression in family caregivers of people with Alzheimer disease: The LASER-AD study. *The American Journal of Geriatric Psychiatry*, *13*(9), 795–801.Evidence Level IV.

Martin-Cook, K., Davis, B. A., Hynan, L. S., & Weiner, M. F. (2005). A randomized, controlled study of an Alzheimer's caregiver skills training program. *American Journal of Alzheimer's Disease and Other Dementias*, *20*(4), 204–210. Evidence Level II.

Martire, L. M., Schulz, R., Keefe, F. J., Starz, T. W., Osial, T. A., Jr., Dew, M. A., & Reynolds, C. F., III. (2003). Feasibility of a dyadic intervention for management of osteoarthritis: A pilot study with older patients and their spousal caregivers. *Aging & Mental Health*, *7*(1), 53–60. Evidence Level II.

Messecar, D., Powers, B. A., & Nagel, C. L. (2008). The Family Preferences Index: Helping family members who want to participate in the care of a hospitalized older adult. *The American Journal of Nursing*, *108*(9), 52–59.

Messecar, D. C., Parker-Walsch, C., & Lindauer, A. (in press). Family caregiving. In V. Hirth (Ed.), *A case-based approach*. Burr Ridge, IL: McGraw-Hill.

Mittelman, M. S., Roth, D. L., Coon, D. W., & Haley, W. E. (2004). Sustained benefit of supportive intervention for depressive symptoms in caregivers of patients with Alzheimer's disease. *The American Journal of Psychiatry*, *161*(5), 850–856. Evidence Level II.

Mittelman, M. S., Roth, D. L., Haley, W. E., & Zarit, S. H. (2004). Effects of a caregiver intervention on negative caregiver appraisals of behavior problems in patients with Alzheimer's disease: Results of a randomized trial. *The Journals of Gerontology. Series B: Psychological Sciences and Social Sciences*, *59*(1), P27–P34. Evidence Level II.

National Academy on an Aging Society. (2000). *Caregiving: Helping the elderly with activity limitations. Challenges for the 21st century: Chronic and Disabling Conditions*, No. 7. Washington, DC: Author. Evidence Level V.

National Alliance for Caregiving & American Association for Retired Persons. (2004). *Caregiving in the U.S.* Bethesda, MD: National Alliance for Caregiving. Evidence Level IV.

Naylor, M. D. (2003). Nursing intervention research and quality of care: Influencing the future of healthcare. *Nursing Research*, *52*(6), 380–385. Evidence Level VI.

Nolan, M. (2001). Working with family carers: Towards a partnership approach. *Reviews in Clinical Gerontology*, *11*(1), 91–97. Evidence Level V.

Northouse, L., Kershaw, T., Mood, D., & Schafenacker, A. (2005). Effects of a family intervention on the quality of life of women with recurrent breast cancer and their family caregivers. *Psycho-oncology*, *14*(6), 478–491. Evidence Level II.

Opinion Research Corporation. (2005). *Attitudes and beliefs about caregiving in the U.S.: Findings of a national opinion survey.* Princeton, NJ: Author. Evidence Level IV.

Ostaszkiewicz, J., Johnston, L., & Roe, B. (2004). Habit retraining for the management of urinary incontinence in adults. *Cochrane Database of Systematic Reviews,* (2), CD002801. doi:10.1002/14651858.CD002801.pub2. Evidence Level I.

Penning, M. J. (1990). Receipt of assistance by elderly people: Hierarchical selection and task specificity. *The Gerontologist, 30,* 220–227. Evidence Level IV.

Pinquart, M., & Sörensen, S. (2003). Differences between caregivers and noncaregivers in psychological health and physical health: A meta-analysis. *Psychology and Aging, 18*(2), 250–267. Evidence Level I.

Pinquart, M., & Sörensen, S. (2004). Associations of caregiver stressors and uplifts with subjective well-being and depressive mood: A meta-analytic comparison. *Aging & Mental Health, 8*(5), 438–449. Evidence Level I.

Pinquart, M., & Sörensen, S. (2005). Ethnic differences in stressors, resources, and psychological outcomes of family caregiving: A meta-analysis. *The Gerontologist, 45*(1), 90–106. Evidence Level I.

Pinquart, M., & Sörensen, S. (2006). Gender differences in caregiver stressors, social resources, and health: An updated meta-analysis. *Journals of Gerontology. Series B: Psychological Sciences and Social Sciences, 61*(1), P33–P45. Evidence Level I.

Price, J. D., Hermans, D. G., & Grimley Evans, J. (2000). Subjective barriers to prevent wandering of cognitively impaired people. *Cochrane Database of Systematic Reviews,* (4), CD001932. doi:10.1002/14651858.CD001932. Evidence Level I.

Pruchno, R. A., & Resch, N. L. (1989). Mental health of caregiving spouses: Coping as mediator, moderator, or main effect? *Psychology and Aging, 4*(4), 454–463. Evidence Level I.

Pusey, H., & Richards, D. (2001). A systematic review of the effectiveness of psychosocial interventions for carers of people with dementia. *Aging & Mental Health, 5*(2), 107–119. Evidence Level I.

Radloff, L. (1977). The CES-D scale: A self-report depression scale for research in the general population. *Applied Psychological Measurement, 1*(3), 385–401. Evidence Level II.

Schulz, R., & Beach, S. R. (1999). Caregiving as a risk factor for mortality: The caregiver health effects study. *The Journal of the American Medical Association, 282*(23), 2215–2219. Evidence Level II.

Schulz, R., Burgio, L., Burns, R., Eisdorfer, C., Gallagher-Thompson, D., Gitlin, L. N., & Mahoney, D. F. (2003). Resources for Enhancing Alzheimer's Caregiver Health (REACH): Overview, site-specific outcomes, and future directions. *The Gerontologist, 43*(4), 514–520. Evidence Level V.

Schulz, R., Martire, L. M., & Klinger, J. N. (2005). Evidence-based caregiver interventions in geriatric psychiatry. *The Psychiatric Clinics of North America, 28*(4), 1007–1038. Evidence Level I.

Schumacher, K., Beck, C. A., & Marren, J. M. (2006). Family caregivers: Caring for older adults, working with their families. *American Journal of Nursing, 106*(8), 40–49. Evidence Level VI.

Schumacher, K. L. (1995). Family caregiver role acquisition: Role-making through situated interaction. *Scholarly Inquiry for Nursing Practice, 9*(3), 211–226.

Schumacher, K. L., Koresawa, S., West, C., Hawkins, C., Johnson, C., Wais, E., . . . Miaskowski, C. (2002). Putting cancer pain management regimens into practice at home. *Journal of Pain and Symptom Management, 23*(5), 369–382. Evidence Level IV.

Schumacher, K. L., Stewart, B. J., Archbold, P. G., Dodd, M. J., & Dibble, S. L. (2000). Family caregiving skill: Development of the concept. *Research in Nursing & Health, 23*(3), 191–203. Evidence Level IV.

Smith, C. E. (1994). A model of caregiving effectiveness for technologically dependent adults residing at home. *Advances in Nursing Science, 17*(2), 27–40. Evidence Level IV.

Sörensen, S., Pinquart, M., & Duberstein, P. (2002). How effective are interventions with caregivers? An updated meta-analysis. *The Gerontologist, 42*(3), 356–372. Evidence Level I.

Stewart, B. J., Archbold, P., Harvath, T., & Nkongho, N. (1993). Role acquisition in family caregivers of older people who have been discharged from the hospital. In S. G. Funk, E. M. Tornquist, M. T. Champagne, & R. A. Wiese (Eds.), *Key aspects of caring for the chronically ill: Hospital and home* (pp. 219–230). New York, NY: Springer Publishing Company, Inc. Evidence Level IV.

Sullivan, M. T. (2002). *Caregiver strain index (CSI). Try this: Best practices in nursing care to older adults.* Retrieved from: http://consultgerirn.org/resources

Tennstedt, S. L., McKinlay, J. B., & Sullivan, L. M. (1989). Informal care for frail elders: The role of secondary caregivers. *The Gerontologist, 29*(5), 677–683. Evidence Level IV.

Tolson, D., Swan, I., & Knussen, C. (2002). Hearing disability: A source of distress for older people and carers. *British Journal of Nursing, 11*(15), 1021–1025. Evidence Level II.

Toseland, R. W., & Rossiter, C. M. (1989). Group interventions to support family caregivers: A review and analysis. *The Gerontologist, 29*(4), 438–448. Evidence Level I.

Trend, P., Kaye, J., Gage, H., Owen, C., & Wade, D. (2002). Short-term effectiveness of intensive multidisciplinary rehabilitation for people with Parkinson's disease and their carers. *Clinical Rehabilitation, 16*(7), 717–725. Evidence Level III.

U.S. Department of Health and Human Services. (1998). *Informal Caregiving: Compassion in Action.* Washington, DC: Author. Evidence Level IV.

Vitaliano, P. P., Zhang, J., & Scanlan, J. M. (2003). Is caregiving hazardous to one's physical health? A meta-analysis. *Psychological Bulletin, 129*(6), 946–972. Evidence Level I.

Wade, D. T., Gage, H., Owen, C., Trend, P., Grossmith, C., & Kaye, J. (2003). Multidisciplinary rehabilitation for people with Parkinson's disease: A randomised controlled study. *Journal of Neurology, Neurosurgery, and Psychiatry, 74*(2), 158–162. Evidence Level II.

Waelde, L. C., Thompson, L., & Gallagher-Thompson, D. (2004). A pilot study of a yoga and meditation intervention for dementia caregiver stress. *Journal of Clinical Psychology, 60*(6), 677–687. Evidence Level III.

Walker, A., Pratt, C. C., & Eddy, L. (1995). Informal caregiving to aging family members: A critical review. *Family Relations, 44,* 404–411. Evidence Level I.

Weiss, C. O., González, H. M., Kabeto, M. U., & Langa, K. M. (2005). Differences in amount of informal care received by non-Hispanic Whites and Latinos in a nationally representative sample of older Americans. *Journal of the American Geriatric Society, 53*(1), 146–151. Evidence Level IV.

Wells, N., Hepworth, J. T., Murphy, B. A., Wujcik, D., & Johnson, R. (2003). Improving cancer pain management through patient and family education. *Journal of Pain and Symptom Management, 25*(4), 344–356. Evidence Level II.

Wisniewski, S. R., Belle, S. H., Coon, D. W., Marcus, S. M., Ory, M. G., Burgio, L. D., . . . Schulz, R. (2003). The Resources for Enhancing Alzheimer's Caregiver Health (REACH): Project design and baseline characteristics. *Psychology and Aging, 18*(3), 375–384. Evidence Level II.

Wolff, J. L., & Kasper, J. D. (2006). Caregivers of frail elders: Updating a national profile. *The Gerontologist, 46*(3), 344–356. Evidence Level I.

Wright, L. K., Litaker, M., Laraia, M. T., & DeAndrade, S. (2001). Continuum of care for Alzheimer's disease: A nurse education and counseling program. *Issues in Mental Health Nursing, 22*(3), 231–252. Evidence Level II.

Yee, J. L., & Schulz, R. (2000). Gender differences in psychiatric morbidity among family caregivers: A review and analysis. *The Gerontologist, 40*(2), 147–164. Evidence Level I.

Yin, T., Zhou, Q., & Bashford, C. (2002). Burden on family members: Caring for frail elderly: A meta-analysis of interventions. *Nursing Research, 51*(3), 199–208. Evidence Level I.

Issues Regarding Sexuality

25

Meredith Wallace Kazer

EDUCATIONAL OBJECTIVES

On completion of this chapter, the reader should be able to:

1. describe an older adult's interest in sexuality
2. identify barriers and challenges to sexual health among older adults
3. discuss normal and pathological changes of aging and their influence on sexual health
4. identify interventions that may help older adults achieve sexual health

OVERVIEW

Sexuality is an innate quality present in all human beings and is extremely important to an individual's self-identity and general well-being (Wallace, 2008). *Sexuality* is defined as "a central aspect of being human throughout life and encompasses sex, gender identities and roles, sexual orientation, eroticism, pleasure, intimacy and reproduction (World Health Organization [WHO], 2010)." *Sexual health* as a manifestation of sexuality is "a state of physical, emotional, mental and social well-being related to sexuality (WHO, 2010)." Sexual health contributes to the satisfaction of physical needs; however, it is often not as apparent that sexual contact fulfills many social, emotional, and psychological components of life as well. This is evidenced by the fact that human touch and a healthy sex life may evoke sentiments of joy, romance, affection, passion, and intimacy, whereas despondency and depression often result from an inability to express one's sexuality (Kamel & Hajjar, 2003). When this occurs, *sexual dysfunction*, defined as impairment in normal sexual functioning, may result (American Psychiatric Association [APA], 2000).

It is frequently assumed that sexual desires and the frequency of sexual encounters begin to diminish later in life. Moreover, the notion of older adults engaging in sexual activities has become taboo in today's youth-loving society (Kamel & Hajjar, 2003). Despite this stereotype, sexual identity and the need for intimacy do not disappear with

For description of Evidence Levels cited in this chapter, see Chapter 1, Developing and Evaluating Clinical Practice Guidelines: A Systematic Approach, page 7.

increasing age, and older adults do not morph into celibate, asexual beings. In a study of 3,005 U.S. older adults, current sexual activity was reported in 73% of adults aged 57–64 years, 53% of adults aged 65–74 years, and 26% of adults aged 75–84 years (Lindau et al., 2007).

BACKGROUND AND STATEMENT OF PROBLEM

Despite the persistence of sexual patterns throughout the lifespan, there is limited research and information to assist nurses to assess and intervene to promote sexual health among older adults. Lack of research literature and insufficient clinical resources are a product of the lack of societal recognition of sexuality as a continuing human need and a factor that perpetuates lack of sexual assessment and intervention among the older population. In addition to the lack of literature, there are several factors that further impact the sexual health of older adults. These factors include the presence of normal and pathological aging changes, environmental barriers to sexual health, and special problems of the older adult that interfere with sexual fulfillment, such as cognitive impairment.

Nurses' Views Toward Sexuality and Aging

Nurses' hesitancy to discuss sexuality with older adults has a significant impact on the sexual health of this population. Gott, Hinchliff, and Galena (2004) reported that general practitioners do not discuss sexual health frequently in providing primary care to older adults. Their study of 55 older men and women resulted in the finding that a major factor affecting sexual discussion between patients and their physicians included the hesitancy of discussing sexuality with a health care provider who was not the patient's age or sex. In this qualitative study, clients stated that sexuality discussions would be more comfortable and forthcoming with health care providers who matched their sex and age. Moreover, attitudes toward sexuality later in life, making jokes about sexuality, shame or embarrassment and fear, perception of sexual problems as not serious, and lack of knowledge regarding available interventions were also seen as barriers to sexual discussion between older clients and health care providers (Gott et al., 2004).

General discomfort with discussing sexuality among nurses and lack of experience in assessment and management of sexual dysfunction among older adults often prevents nurses from addressing the sexual needs of this population. Moreover, the sexuality of older adults is generally excluded from sparse gerontological curricula. Without education and experience in managing sensitive issues around sexuality, health professionals are often not comfortable discussing sexual issues with older adults. Health care providers may lessen discomfort with addressing sexual issues by increasing their knowledge on the subject and routinely introducing this dimension of health into routine assessment and management protocols.

Nurses' understanding of sexuality should be broadened beyond that of a relationship between just men and women. Many clients within various health care systems are gay or lesbian, bisexual, and transgender (GLBT) adults, and these alternative sexual preferences require respect and consideration. In a focus group study, older gay and lesbians reported extensive discrimination in accessing health care services by excluding them from program planning (Brotman, Ryan, & Cormier, 2003). Discrimination among GLBT older adults is especially seen in the development of residential services to meet the needs of older adults. In a larger study of 400,000 GLBT adults, discrimination was seen among administrators, care providers, and other residents of retirement care community (Johnson, Jackson, Arnette, & Koffman, 2005).

Normal and Pathological Aging Changes

The "sexual response cycle," or the organized pattern of physical response to sexual stimulation, changes with age in both women and men. After menopause, a loss of estrogen in women results in significant sexual changes. This deficiency frequently results in the thinning of the vaginal walls and decreased or delayed vaginal lubrication, which may lead to pain during intercourse (Lobo, 2007). Additionally, the labia atrophy, the vagina shortens, and the cervix may descend downward into the vagina and cause further pain and discomfort. Moreover, vaginal contractions are fewer and weaker during orgasm, and after sexual intercourse is completed, women return to the prearoused stage faster than they would at an earlier age. The result of these physiological age-related changes in women is the potential for significant alterations in sexual health that have traditionally received little attention from research or individual health care providers. The pain resulting from anatomical changes and vaginal dryness may result in the avoidance of sexual relationships in order to prevent painful intercourse.

Men also experience decreased hormone levels, mainly testosterone, yet this seems to have a limited impact on sexual functioning because only a minimal amount of testosterone is needed for the purposes of sex. This reduction in testosterone that has been controversially labeled *viropause* or *andropause* and male menopause generally begins between the ages of 46 and 52 years and is characterized by a gradual decrease in the amount of testosterone (Kessenich & Cichon, 2001). The loss of testosterone is not pathological and does not result in sexual dysfunction. However, men may experience fatigue, loss of muscle mass, depression, and a decline in libido. As a result of normal aging changes, older men require more direct stimulation of the penis to experience erection, which is somewhat weaker as compared to that experienced in earlier ages. As with postmenopausal women, orgasms are fewer and weaker in older men, the force and amount of ejaculation is reduced, and the refractory period after ejaculation is significantly increased (Araujo, Mohr, & McKinlay, 2004).

Bodily changes such as wrinkles and sagging skin may cause both older women and men to feel insecure about initiating a sexual encounter and maintaining emotionally secure relationships. In addition, lack of knowledge and understanding among older adults about sexuality is common because sexual education is rarely provided in formal educational systems as the older adults developed and was rarely discussed informally. Strict beliefs and values are likely to impact sexual action, freedom, and desires and may result in sexual frustration and conflict. Physical changes in the sexual response cycle that occur with increasing age do not completely explain the extensive changes in sexuality that occurs among older adults. Many individual psychosocial and cultural factors play a role in how older adults perceive themselves as sexual beings. Although sexual disorders have not been well-addressed among the older population, they have been defined and fall into four categories: hypoactive sexual desire disorder, sexual arousal disorder, orgasmic disorder, and sexual pain disorders (Walsh & Berman, 2004).

In addition to normal aging changes and pathological sexual disorders, there are a number of medical conditions that have been associated with poor sexual health and functioning in the older population (Morle & Tariq, 2003). Rosen et al. (2009) reported that the main predictors of sexual dysfunction are age, cardiovascular diseases, and diabetes. One of the most frequently occurring medical conditions among older adults includes cardiovascular disease. In a study of 2,763 postmenopausal women, the presence of coronary heart disease was associated with lack of interest, inability to relax, arousal and orgasmic disorders, and general discomfort with sex (Addis et al., 2005).

Diabetes is a large problem among older adults, affecting approximately 14.7 million individuals in the United States each year. Approximately, 40% of those with diabetes are aged 65 years or older (Centers for Disease Control and Prevention [CDC], n.d.). In a study of eight women aged 24–83 years, older women with diabetes reported lower sexual function, desire, and enjoyment than their younger counterparts (Rockliffe-Fidler & Kiemle, 2003). Moreover, in a study of 373 men aged 45–75 years with Type II diabetes, 49.8% of men reported mild or moderate degrees of erectile dysfunction (ED), and 24.8% had complete ED (Rosen et al., 2009).

The presence of depression among older adults impacts sexual health, in that depression often causes a decline in desire and ability to perform with this disease and treatment. Korfage et al. (2009) reported in a study of 3,810 men aged 57–78 years that men with ED reported significantly lower mental health than men without ED. The presence of loss and depression should be assessed among older adults and considered for the impact of these emotional and psychological factors on sexual health. (see Chapter 9, Depression in Older Adults).

Other medical conditions occurring among older adults also have the potential to impact sexual health. Older adults who have experienced strokes and subsequent aphasias reported alterations in sexual health because of communication difficulties (Lemieux, Cohen-Schneider, & Holzapfel, 2001). Additionally, Parkinson's disease (PD) that is predominantly found in an older adult has the potential to negatively impact sexual health. In a study of 444 older adults with PD, sexual limitations were reported in 73.5% of the sample as a product of difficulty in movement (Mott, Kenrick, Dixon, & Bird, 2005). Benign prostatic hypertrophy (BPH) in older men may result in altered circulation to the penis effecting erectile function and sexual arousal. Derogatis and Burnett (2008) stated that sexual dysfunction is prevalent worldwide, and its occurrence and the frequency of symptoms that impact sexual health increase directly with age for both men and women. Pathological changes of aging such as the conditions discussed are major risk factors for sexual disorders.

Medications used to treat commonly occurring medical illnesses among older adults also impact sexual function. Two of the major groups of medications include antidepressants and antihypertensives. Causative antidepressants include the commonly used selective serotonin reuptake inhibitors (SSRIs). In a study of 610 women and 412 men, 59.1% of the individuals taking SSRI antidepressant medications reported sexual dysfunction (Montejo, Llorca, Izquierdo, & Rico-Villademoros, 2001). Although the use of monoamine oxidase (MAO) inhibitors and tricyclic antidepressants has decreased in favor of the SSRIs with lower side-effect profiles, these medications also impact sexual function by reducing sexual drive and causing impotence and erectile and orgasmic disorders. Antihypertensives, angiotensin-converting enzyme (ACE) inhibitors, and alpha and beta cell blockers also result in impotence and ejaculatory disturbances among older adults (Alagiakrishnan et al., 2005). Antipsychotics, commonly used statin medications, and H2 blockers also impact the sexual health of older adults.

Special Issues Related to Older Adults and Sexuality

Cognitively impaired older adults continue to have sexual needs and desires that present a challenge to nurses. These continuing sexual needs often manifest in inappropriate sexual behavior. Sexual behaviors common to the cognitively impaired older adults may include cuddling, touching of the genitals, sexual remarks, propositioning, grabbing and groping, use of obscene language, masturbating without shame, aggression, and irritability. In a study of 41 cognitively impaired older adults, 1.8% had sexually inappropriate behavior manifesting in verbal and physical problems (Alagiakrishnan et al., 2005). In a study that used computed tomography (CT) of the head to scan 10 patients with these problematic sexual behaviors, cerebral infarction was seen in six of them, and severe disease in two others, supporting the organic basis for these symptoms (Nagaratnam & Gayagay, 2002).

Masturbation is a method in which cognitively impaired men and women may become sexually fulfilled. Nurses in long-term care facilities may assist older adults to improve sexual health by providing an environment in which the older adult may masturbate in private. Alkhalil, Tanvir, Alkhalil, and Lowenthal (2004) reported that the use of gabapentin to decrease sexual behavior problems (such as inappropriate sexual overtures and public masturbation) has demonstrated effectiveness anecdotally. Accurate assessment and documentation of the ability of cognitively impaired older adults to make competent decisions regarding sexual relationships with others while in long-term care is essential. If the resident has been determined to be incapable of decision making, then the health care staff must prevent the cognitively impaired resident from unsolicited sexual advances by a spouse, partner, or other residents.

Environmental settings may also influence sexuality among older adults. Normally, engaging in sexual intercourse occurs within the privacy of one's bedroom; however, for some older adults, extended care facilities are the substitute for what one called *home*. Residents of extended care facilities state that many of the obstacles they face regarding their sexuality include lack of opportunity, lack of available partner, poor health, feeling sexually undesirable, and guilt for having these sexual feelings. Furthermore, negative staff attitudes and beliefs regarding residents' sexual activity bar the expression of sexuality in long-term care settings (Hajjar & Kamel, 2004).

Twenty-five percent of all HIV cases are developed in adults older than the age of 50 years, underscoring the significant risk of HIV transmission in the older age group. Older adults with HIV are more likely to be diagnosed late in the disease, progress more quickly, and have a shorter survival (Martin, Fain, & Klotz, 2008). The use of antiretroviral medications among older adults may be complicated by multiple chronic comorbidities and treatments (Magalhães, Greenberg, Hansen, & Glick, 2007). Sherr et al. (2009) conducted a study of 778 patients in an HIV clinic. Of the total population, 12% were aged older than 50 years. The findings revealed that older patients reported significantly lower psychological and global burden and were more likely to take antiretrovirals than their younger cohorts. Health care providers are in a unique position to assess and manage HIV among the older population, but greater education regarding the risk for HIV in the older population is needed.

ASSESSMENT OF THE PROBLEM

A model to guide sexual assessment and intervention is available and has been well used among younger populations since the 1970s. The Permission, Limited Information, Specific Suggestion, Intensive Therapy (PLISSIT) model (Annon, 1976) begins by first seeking permission (P) to discuss sexuality with the older adult. Because many sexual disorders originate in feelings of anxiety or guilt, asking permission may put the client in control of the discussion and facilitate communication between the health care provider and client. This permission may be gained by asking general questions such as "I would like to begin to discuss your sexual health; what concerns would you like to share with me about this area of function?" Questions to guide the sexual assessment of older adults are available on many health care assessment forms. The next step of the model affords an opportunity for the nurse to share limited information (LI) with the older adult. In the case of older adults, this part of the model affords health care providers the opportunity to dispel myths of aging and sexuality and to discuss the impact of normal and pathological aging changes, as well as medications on sexual health. The next part of the model guides the nurse to provide specific suggestions (SS) to improve sexual health. In so doing, nurses may implement several of the interventions recommended for improved sexual health, such as safe sex practices, more effective management of acute and chronic diseases, removal or substitution of causative medications, environmental adaptations, or need for discussions with partners and families. The final part of the model calls for intensive therapy (IT) when needed for clients whose sexual dysfunction goes beyond the scope of nursing management. In these cases, referral to a sexual therapist is appropriate.

Sexual assessments will be most effective using open-ended questions such as "Can you tell me how you express your sexuality?" "What concerns you about your sexuality?" "How has your sexuality changed as you have aged?" "What changes have you noticed in your sexuality since you have been diagnosed or treated for disease?" "What thoughts have you had about ways in which you would like to enhance your sexual health?" The loss of relationships with significant, intimate partners is unfortunately common among older adults and often ends communication about the importance of self to the person experiencing the loss. This greatly impacts the older adult's sexual health. Asking the older adult about past and present relationships in his or her life will help to aid this assessment.

Barriers to sexual health should be assessed, including normal and pathological changes of aging, medications, and psychological problems, such as depression. Moreover, lack of knowledge and understanding about sexuality, loss of partners, and family influence on sexual practice often present substantial barriers to sexual health among older adults. Nurses should assess for presence of physiological changes through a health history, review of systems, and physical examination for the presence of normal and aging changes that impact sexual health. Older adults may view the normal changes of aging and their subsequent impact on appearance as embarrassing or indicative of illness. This may result in a negative body image and a reluctance to pursue sexual health. It is important for nurses to consider the impact of normal and pathological changes of aging on body image and assess their impact frequently.

As discussed earlier, there are a number of medical conditions that have been associated with poor sexual health and functioning including depression, cardiac disease, diabetes, stroke, and PD. Effective assessment of these illnesses using open-ended health history questions, review of systems, physical examination, and appropriate lab testing will provide necessary information for appropriate disease management and improved sexual function.

Assessing the impact of medications among older adults, especially those commonly used to treat medical illnesses such as antidepressants and antihypertensives are essential. Potential medications should be identified by reviewing the client's medication bottles and the client should be questioned about the potential impact of these medications on sexual health. If the medication is found to impact on sexual health, alternative medications should be considered. The older adult should also be questioned regarding the use of alcohol because this substance also has a potential impact on sexual response.

INTERVENTIONS AND CARE STRATEGIES

Following a thorough assessment of normal and pathological aging changes, as well as environmental factors, a number of interventions may be implemented to promote the sexual health of older adults. These interventions fall into several broad categories including (a) education regarding age-associated change in sexual function, (b) compensation for normal aging changes, (c) effective management of acute and chronic illness effecting sexual function, (d) removal of barriers associated with difficulty in fulfilling sexual needs, and (e) special interventions to promote sexual health in cognitively impaired older adults.

Client Education

The most important intervention to improving sexuality among the older population is education. It is important to remember that sexuality was likely not addressed in formal educational systems as the older adults developed and was rarely discussed informally. Older adults may possess dated values that impact sexual action, freedom, and desires and lead to both sexual frustration and conflict. Masters (1986) reported in his seminal work on the sexuality of older adults that older women were raised to believe that when menstruation ceased, they would cease to be feminine. Knowledge is essential to the successful fulfillment of sexuality for all people.

The incidence of HIV and AIDS infection is rising among older adults, with 25% of new cases resulting in adults older than the age of 50 years (Martin et al., 2008). This underscores the significant risk of HIV transmission in the older age group and the need for effective teaching regarding safe sex practices. Teaching about the use of condoms to prevent the transmission of sexually transmitted diseases is essential. In response to this rise in HIV cases and the presence of other sexually transmitted diseases, it is essential to provide older adults with safe sex information provided by the CDC.

Compensating for Normal Aging Changes

Assisting older adults to compensate for normal aging changes related to sexual dysfunction will greatly lessen the impact of these changes on sexual health. Among women, the discussion of anatomical changes in sexual anatomy will help women to anticipate these changes on sexuality. For example, the decreases in the size of the vagina and increased vaginal dryness among women may require the use of artificial water-based lubricants or topical estrogen agents. In a multicenter, double-blind, randomized, placebo-controlled study, 305 women with symptoms of vaginal atrophy were treated with a low-dose synthetic conjugated estrogen-A (SCE-A) cream twice weekly. The results revealed that the cream significantly reduced symptoms of vaginal atrophy and pain during intercourse compared to the placebo (Freedman, Kaunitz, Reape, Hait, & Shu, 2009). In men, delayed response and the increased length of time needed for erections and ejaculations are among normal changes of aging, of which older adults may not be aware. When older adults understand the impact of normal aging changes, they then understand the need to plan for more time and direct stimulation in order to become aroused.

One of the most important preventive measures older adults may undertake to reduce the impact of normal aging changes on sexual health is to continue to engage in sexual activity. Planning for more time during sexual activities; being sensitive to changes in one another's bodies; the use of aids to increase stimulation and lubrication; the exploration of foreplay, masturbation, sensual touch, and different sexual positions along with education about these common changes associated with sex and aging may help immensely. By doing so, changes in sexual response patterns are less likely to occur. Eating healthy foods, getting adequate amounts of sleep, exercising, stress-management techniques, and not smoking are also very important to sexual health.

Effective Management of Acute and Chronic Illness

Effective management of both acute and chronic illnesses that impair sexual health is also important. Interventions that improve sexual health are frameworked within the current interventions to treat disease. In other words, effective disease management using primary, secondary, and tertiary interventions will not only effectively treat the disease but also result in improved sexual health. Consequently, better glucose control among diabetics enhances circulation and may increase arousal and sexual response. Appropriate treatment of depression with medication and psychotherapy will enhance desire and sexual response. Although treatment of depression may help to improve libido and sexual dysfunctions such as orgasmic disorders, medications to treat depression often impact sexual function by lowering libido and causing orgasmic disorders. As a potential alternative to treat libido problems during antidepressant management, Seidman and Roose (2006) conducted a study of 32 depressed patients with a mean age of 52 years. The sample was randomized to receive either Enanthate (testosterone) 200 mg or sesame seed oil (placebo). Although self-reported sexual functioning improved in both groups, no significant differences were found between groups.

Oral erectile agents such as sildenafil citrate (Viagra), vardenafil HCl (Levitra), and tadalafil (Cialis) play a significant role in the treatment of sexual dysfunction that occurs with aging and are effective and well-tolerated treatments for ED in older men (Wespes et al., 2007). In men treated for prostate cancer with radical prostatectomy, the use of oral erectile agents to manage ED immediately following surgery is also gaining increased support (Miles et al., 2007). Medications used to treat diseases may result in sexual dysfunction among older adults (see http://www.netdoctor.co.uk/menshealth/feature/medicinessex.htm for a list of these medications). There are many medications that may result in decreased sexual drive and impotence as well as orgasmic and ejaculatory disorders. These medications are widely prescribed for many chronic illnesses among older adults, including psychological disorders such as depression, hypertension, elevated cholesterol, sleep disorders, and peptic ulcer diseases. Moreover, because of the hesitancy among older adults and nurses to discuss sexual problems, the effect of these medications on sexual function is often not discussed in clinical settings. This may result in either prolonged sexual dysfunction among the older adult or a noncompliance with the medication. Recognition of the continuing sexual needs of older adults among nurses is essential to beginning dialogue about sexual problems. Effective assessment will uncover medications affecting older adult's sexual function and lead to the consideration of stopping the medication in favor of alternative disease management strategies or substituting the medication causing the dysfunction with another one with less sexual effects.

Removal of Barriers to Sexual Health

One of the greatest barriers to sexual health among older adults lies within nurses' persistent beliefs that older adults are not sexual beings. Nurses should be encouraged to open lines of communication in order to effectively assess and manage the sexual health needs of aging individuals with the same consistency as other bodily systems and treat alterations in sexual health with available evidence-based strategies.

An essential intervention to promoting sexual health in this population is to educate nurses regarding the continuing sexual needs and desires persisting throughout the lifespan. Education regarding older adult sexuality as a continuing human need should be included in multidisciplinary education and staff development programs. Educational sessions may begin by discussing prevalent societal myths around older adult sexuality. Nurses should be encouraged to discuss their own feelings about sexuality and its role in the life of older adults. Moreover, the development of policies and procedures to manage sexual issues of older adult clients is important throughout environments of care.

Environmental adaptations to ensure privacy and safety among long-term care and community-dwelling residents are essential. Arrangements for privacy must be made so the dignity of older adults is protected during sexual activity. For example, nurses may assist in finding other activities for the resident's roommate so that privacy may be obtained or in securing a common room that may be used by the older adults for private visits. Call lights or telephones should be kept within reach during sexual activity and adaptive equipment such as positioning devices or trapezes may need to be obtained. Interventions such as providing rooms for privacy and offering consultations for residents regarding evaluation and treatment of their sexual problems are a few of the many ways this may be accomplished (Wallace, 2008). Roach (2004) suggested that nursing home staff and administration work to develop environments that are supportive and respectful of older resident's continuing sexual rights and promote sexual health.

Families are an integral part of the interdisciplinary team. However, for older couples, especially those in relationships with new partners, it is often difficult for families to understand that their older relative may have a sexual relationship with anyone other than the person they are accustomed to them being with. A family meeting, with a counselor if needed, is appropriate in order to help the family understand and accept the older adult's decisions about the relationship.

Special Interventions to Promote the Sexual Health of Cognitively Impaired Older Adults

Cognitively impaired older adults continue to have sexual needs and desires but may lack the capacity to make appropriate decisions regarding sexual relationships. Accurate assessment and documentation of ability to make informed decisions regarding sexual relationships must be conducted by an interdisciplinary team. If the older adult is not capable of making competent decisions, participation in sexual relationships may be considered abusive and must be prevented. On the other end of the spectrum, nurses should not attempt to prevent sexual relationships and may play an important role in promoting sexual health among older adults who are cognitively competent to make decisions regarding sexual relationships. In these cases, nurses should implement all necessary interventions to promote the sexual health of older adult clients.

Inappropriate sexual behavior such as public masturbation, disrobing, or making sexually explicit remarks to other patients or health care professionals may be a warning sign of unmet sexual needs among older adults. A full sexual assessment should be conducted using clear communication and limit setting in these situations. Following this, a plan should be developed to manage this behavior while providing the utmost respect and preserving the dignity of the client. Providing an environment in which the older adult may pursue their sexuality in private may be a simple solution to a difficult problem. Medication management for hypersexual behavior may be considered. Tricyclic antidepressants and trazodone are two medications with antilibidinal and anti-obsessive effects that may be safely used to treat hypersexual behavior (Wallace & Safer, 2009). Levitsky and Owens (1999) reported that antiandrogens, estrogens, gonadotropin-releasing hormone analogues, and serotonergic medications may be successful when other methods are ineffective.

CASE STUDY

Mrs. Jones is a highly functioning 79-year-old widow, recently admitted to a nursing home with MCI. Mrs. Jones began a friendship with Mr. Carl, who is cognitively intact and wheelchair bound. Mr. Carl is married to a woman who resides outside the facility. The nursing staff has noticed more and more intimate touches among the two residents and is concerned about Mrs. Jones's competency to make the decision to participate in this increasingly intimate relationship. Moreover, general concern about the sexual relationship within a long-term care setting prevails among the nursing staff.

The first step in this situation is to conduct a full assessment to determine Mrs. Jones's capacity to participate in this intimate relationship. The right to Mrs. Jones's autonomy is complicated by the presence of MCI and must be explored further. The question remains, does Mrs. Jones have the decisional capacity to participate in an intimate relationship?

The actual and projected outcomes of the intimate relationship would require assessment to determine what nursing actions are required regarding this relationship. If an assessment of Mrs. Jones finds that she is incapable of understanding the consequences of her relationship with Mr. Carl, then she must be protected from unsolicited sexual advances by a spouse, partner, or other residents. However, if the assessment leads nurses to believe that Mrs. Jones and Mr. Carl understand the risks and consequences of their relationship, then the right to autonomy prevails.

If clinicians determine that the older adults have the decisional capacity to consent to a sexual relationship, then a comprehensive health history, review of systems, and physical examination to determine normal and pathological changes of aging that may play a role in this sexual relationship must be conducted. Appropriate lab work for the potential presence of sexually transmitted diseases should be included. A care plan focusing the need to promote sexual health for this couple should be developed. Teaching regarding normal and pathological aging changes and the impact of these changes, as well as medications on sexual function, should be conducted. Normal changes of aging must be compensated for and diseases effecting sexual response should be treated with medications that will not impact sexual health. Safety from the transmission of sexually transmitted diseases and privacy should be provided for the residents, ensuring that their dignity is respected at all times.

SUMMARY

One of the most prevalent myths of aging is that older adults are no longer interested in sex. It is commonly believed that older adults no longer have any interest or desire to participate in sexual relationships. Because sexuality is mainly considered a young person's activity, often associated with reproduction, society does not usually associate older adults with sex. In the youth-oriented society of today, many consider sexuality among older adults to be distasteful and prefer to assume that sexuality among the older population does not exist. However, despite popular belief, sexuality continues to be important, even in the lives of older adults.

Although the sexual health of older adults has been largely ignored in the past decades, evolving images of older adults as healthy and vibrant members of society may result in a decrease in prevalence of myths of this population as nonsexual beings. Changes in the societal image of older adults as asexual celibate beings will greatly enhance removal of barriers to sexual health in the older population. Improved assessment and management of normal and pathological changes of aging and appropriate environmental adaptations and management of special issues of sexuality and aging will also result in improved sexual health in the older population. Oral erectile agents also play a substantial role in enhanced sexual health among older adults.

The fulfillment of sexual needs may be just as satisfying for older adults as it is for younger people. However, several normal and pathological changes of aging complicate sexuality among older adults. Environmental changes may create further barriers to sexual expression among older adults. Despite the many barriers to achieving sexual health among an aging population, nurses are in a critical position to understand sexual needs and capabilities in later life and assist older adults to develop compensatory strategies for improving sexual health in order to have the best possible sexual life. If these strategies and interventions are undertaken, increased awareness and acceptance of older adults' sexuality will ultimately take place, and the concept of sex in old age will no longer be such a shocking topic.

NURSING STANDARD OF PRACTICE

Protocol 25.1: Sexuality in the Older Adult

I. GOAL: To enhance the sexual health of older adults.

II. OVERVIEW: Although it is generally believed that sexual desires decrease with age, researchers have identified that sexual desires, thoughts, and actions continue throughout all decades of life. Human touch and healthy sex lives evoke sentiments of joy, romance, affection, passion, and intimacy, whereas despondency and depression often result from an inability to express one's sexuality. Health care providers play an important role in assessing and managing normal and pathological aging changes in order to improve the sexual health of older adults.

(continued)

Protocol 25.1: Sexuality in the Older Adult *(cont.)*

III. BACKGROUND AND STATEMENT OF THE PROBLEM

A. Definitions
   1. *Sexuality.* A central aspect of being human throughout life and encompasses sex, gender identities and roles, sexual orientation, eroticism, pleasure, intimacy, and reproduction (WHO, 2010).
   2. *Sexual health.* A state of physical, emotional, mental, and social well-being related to sexuality (WHO, 2010).
   3. *Sexual dysfunction.* Impairment in normal sexual functioning (APA, 2000).
B. Etiology and/or Epidemiology
   1. Despite the continuing sexual needs of older adults, many barriers prevent sexual health among older adults.
   2. Health care providers often lack knowledge and comfort in discussing sexual issues with older adults (Gott et al., 2004).
   3. The older population is more susceptible to many disabling medical conditions; a number of medical conditions are associated with poor sexual health and functioning (Morle & Tariq, 2003), including depression, cardiac disease, stroke and aphasia, Parkinson's disease (PD), and diabetes that make sexuality difficult.
   4. Medications among older adults, especially those commonly used to treat medical illnesses, also impact sexuality such as antidepressants (Montejo et al., 2001).
   5. Normal aging changes make sexual health difficult to achieve such as a higher frequency of vaginal dryness in women and erectile dysfunction (ED) in men (Kessenich & Cichon, 2001; Lobo, 2007).
   6. Environmental barriers also present barriers to sexual health among older adults (Hajjar & Kamel, 2004).

IV. ASSESSMENT

A. The Permission, Limited Information, Specific Suggestion, Intensive Therapy (PLISSIT) model (Annon, 1976) begins by first seeking permission (P) to discuss sexuality with the older adult. The next step of the model affords an opportunity for the nurse to share limited information (LI) with the older adult. What about SSIT?
B. Ask open-ended questions such as "Can you tell me how you express your sexuality?" or "What concerns you about your sexuality?" and "How has your sexuality changed as you have aged?"
C. Assess for presence of physiological changes through a health history, review of systems, and physical examination for the presence of normal and aging changes that impact sexual health.
D. Review medications among older adults, especially those commonly used to treat medical illnesses that also impact sexuality such as antidepressants and antihypertensives.
E. Assess medical conditions that have been associated with poor sexual health and functioning including depression, cardiac disease, stroke and aphasia, PD, and diabetes.

(continued)

Protocol 25.1: Sexuality in the Older Adult *(cont.)*

V. NURSING CARE STRATEGIES

A. Communication and Education
1. Discuss normal age-related physiological changes.
2. Address how the effects of medications and medical conditions may affect one's sexual function.
3. Facilitate communication with older adults and their families regarding sexual health as desired, including the following:
   a. Encourage family meetings with open discussion of issues if desired.
   b. Teach about safe sex practices.
   c. Discuss use of condoms to prevent transmission of sexually transmitted infections (STIs) and HIV.

B. Health Management
1. Perform a thorough patient assessment
2. Conduct a health history, review of systems, and physical examination
3. Effectively manage chronic illness
4. Improve glucose monitoring and control among diabetics
5. Ensure appropriate treatment of depression and screening for depression (see Chapter 9, Depression in Older Adults).
6. Discontinue and substitute medications that may result in sexual dysfunction (e.g., hypertension or depression medications).
7. Accurately assess and document older adults' ability to make informed decisions (see Chapter 28, Health Care Decision Making).
8. Participation in sexual relationships may be considered abusive if the older adult is not capable of making decisions.

C. Sexual Enhancement
1. Compensate for normal changes of aging
   a. Females:
      i. Use of artificial water-based lubricants
      ii. Use of estrogen cream (Freedman et al., 2009)
   b. Males:
      i. Recognizing the possibility for more time and direct stimulation for arousal caused by aging changes. Use of oral erectile agents for ED (Wespes et al., 2007)
2. Environmental adaptations
   a. Ensure privacy and safety among long-term care and community-dwelling residents (Wallace, 2008).

VI. EXPECTED OUTCOMES

A. Patients will:
1. Report high quality of life as measured by a standardized quality of life assessment.
2. Be provided with privacy, dignity, and respect surrounding their sexuality.
3. Receive communication and education regarding sexual health as desired.
4. Be able to pursue sexual health free of pathological and problematic sexual behaviors.

(continued)

Protocol 25.1: Sexuality in the Older Adult *(cont.)*

B. Nurses will:
   1. Include sexual health questions in their routine history and physical.
   2. Frequently reassess patients for changes in sexual health.
C. Institutions will:
   1. Include sexual health questions on intake and reassessment measures.
   2. Provide education on the ongoing sexual needs of older adults and appropriate interventions to manage these needs with dignity and respect.
   3. Provide needed privacy for individuals to maintain intimacy and sexual health (e.g., in long-term care).

VII. FOLLOW-UP MONITORING OF CONDITION

Sexual outcomes are difficult to directly assess and measure. However, with the illustrated link between sexual health and quality of life, quality of life measures such as the SF-36 Health Survey may be used to determine the effectiveness of interventions to promote sexual health. Retrieved from http://www.rand.org/health/surveys/sf36item/question.html

---

RESOURCES

American Foundation for Urological Disease, Inc.
http://www.urologyhealth.org/auafhome.asp

MedlinePlus
http://www.nlm.nih.gov/medlineplus/sexualhealthissues.html

National Institutes on Aging
http://www.nia.nih.gov/HealthInformation/Publications/sexuality.htm

Prentiss Care Networks Project
Care networks for formal and informal caregivers of older adults
http://caregiving.case.edu

World Health Organization
http://www.who.int/reproductivehealth/en/

Videos

A Rose by Any Other Name. (1976). Post Perfect Productions Backseat Bingo. Terra Nova Films

Freedom of Sexual Expression: Dementia and Resident Rights in Long-Term Care Facilities. Terra Nova Films.

The Heart Has No Wrinkles. Terra Nova Films.

REFERENCES

Addis, I. B., Ireland, C. C., Vittinghoff, E., Lin, F., Stuenkel, C. A., & Hulley, S. (2005). Sexual activity and function in postmenopausal women with heart disease. *Obstetrics and Gynecology, 106*(1), 121–127. Evidence Level II.

Alagiakrishnan, K., Lim, D., Brahim, A., Wong, A., Wood, A., Senthilselvan, A., . . . Kagan, L. (2005). Sexually inappropriate behaviour in demented elderly people. *Postgraduate Medical Journal, 81*(957), 463–466. Evidence Level IV.

Alkhalil, C., Tanvir, F., Alkhalil, B., & Lowenthal, D. T. (2004). Treatment of sexual disinhibition in dementia: Case reports and review of the literature. *American Journal of Therapeutics, 11*(3), 231–235. Evidence Level V.

American Psychiatric Association. (2000). *Diagnostic and statistical manual of mental disorders: DSM-IV-TR.* Washington, DC: Author. Evidence Level VI.

Annon, J. (1976). The PLISSIT model: A proposed conceptual scheme for behavioral treatment of sexual problems. *Journal of Sex Education Therapy, 2*(2), 1–15. Evidence Level VI.

Araujo, A. B., Mohr, B. A., & McKinlay, J. B. (2004). Changes in sexual function in middle-aged and older men: Longitudinal data from the Massachusetts male aging study. *Journal of the American Geriatrics Society, 52*(9), 1502–1509. Evidence Level IV.

Brotman, S., Ryan, B., & Cormier, R. (2003). The health and social service needs of gay and lesbian elders and their families in Canada. *The Gerontologist, 43*(2), 192–202. Evidence Level IV.

Centers for Disease Control and Prevention. (n.d.). *Diabetes data and trends.* Retrieved from http://apps.nccd.cdc.gov/DDTSTRS/default.aspx

Derogatis, L. R., & Burnett, A. L. (2008). The epidemiology of sexual dysfunctions. *The Journal of Sexual Medicine, 5*(2), 289–300. Evidence Level V.

Freedman, M., Kaunitz, A. M., Reape, K. Z., Hait, H., & Shu, H. (2009). Twice-weekly synthetic conjugated estrogens vaginal cream for the treatment of vaginal atrophy. *Menopause, 16*(4), 735–741. Evidence Level II.

Gott, M., Hinchliff, S., & Galena, E. (2004). General practitioner attitudes to discussing sexual health issues with older people. *Social Science & Medicine, 58*(11), 2093–2103. Evidence Level IV.

Hajjar, R. R., & Kamel, H. K. (2004). Sexuality in the nursing home, part 1: Attitudes and barriers to sexual expression. *Journal of the American Medical Directors Association, 5*(2 Suppl.), S42–S47. Evidence Level V.

Johnson, M. J., Jackson, N. C., Arnette, J. K., & Koffman, S. D. (2005). Gay and lesbian perceptions of discrimination in retirement care facilities. *Journal of Homosexuality, 49*(2), 83–102. Evidence Level IV.

Kamel, H. K., & Hajjar, R. R. (2003). Sexuality in the nursing home, part 2: Managing abnormal behavior-legal and ethical issues. *Journal of the American Medical Directors Association, 4*(4), 203–206. Evidence Level V.

Kessenich, C. R., & Cichon, M. J. (2001). Hormonal decline in elderly men and male menopause. *Geriatric Nursing, 22*(1), 24–27. Evidence Level V.

Korfage I. J., Pluijm, S., Roobol, M., Dohle, G. R., Schröder, F. H., & Essink-Bot, M. L. (2009). Erectile dysfunction and mental health in a general population of older men. *Journal of Sexual Medicine, 6*(2), 505–512. Evidence Level IV.

Lemieux, L., Cohen-Schneider, R., & Holzapfel, S. (2001). Aphasia and sexuality. *Sexuality and Disability, 19*(4), 253–266. Evidence Level IV.

Levitsky, A. M., & Owens, N. J. (1999). Pharmacologic treatment of hypersexuality and paraphilias in nursing home residents. *Journal of the American Geriatrics Society, 47*(2), 231–234. Evidence Level V.

Lindau, S. T., Schumm, L. P., Laumann, E. O., Levinson, W., O'Muircheartaigh, C. A., & Waite, L. J. (2007). A study of sexuality and health among older adults in the United States. *The New England Journal of Medicine, 357*(8), 762–744. Evidence Level IV.

Lobo, R. A. (2007). Menopause: Endocrinology, consequences of estrogen deficiency, effects of hormone replacement therapy, treatment regimens. In V. L. Katz, G. M. Lentz, R. A. Lobo, & D. M. Gershenson (Eds.), *Comprehensive gynecology* (5th ed.). Philadelphia, PA: Mosby Elsevier. Evidence Level VI.

Magalhães, M. G., Greenberg, B., Hansen, H., & Glick, M. (2007). Comorbidities in older patients with HIV: A retrospective study. *Journal of the American Dental Association, 138*(11), 1468–1475. Evidence Level IV.

Martin, C. P., Fain, M. J., & Klotz, S. A. (2008). The older HIV-positive adult: A critical review of the medical literature. *The American Journal of Medicine, 121*(12), 1032–1037. Evidence Level V.

Masters, W. H. (1986). Sex and aging—expectations and reality. *Hospital Practice, 21*(8), 175–198. Evidence Level VI.

Miles, C. L., Candy, B., Jones, L., Williams, R., Tookman, A., & King, M. (2007). Interventions for sexual dysfunction following treatments for cancer. *Cochrane Database of Systematic Reviews,* (4), CD005540. doi: 10.1002/14651858.CD005540.pub2. Evidence Level I.

Montejo, A. L., Llorca, G., Izquierdo, J. A., & Rico-Villademoros, F. (2001). Incidence of sexual dysfunction associated with antidepressant agents: A prospective multicenter study of 1022 outpatients. Spanish Working Group for the Study of Psychotropic-Related Sexual Dysfunction. *The Journal of Clinical Psychiatry, 62*(Suppl. 3), 10–21. Evidence Level IV.

Morle, J. E., & Tariq, S. H. (2003). Sexuality and disease. *Clinics in Geriatric Medicine, 19*(3), 563–573. Evidence Level V.

Mott, S., Kenrick, M., Dixon, M., & Bird, G. (2005). Sexual limitations in people living with Parkinson's disease. *Australasian Journal on Ageing, 24*(4), 196–201. Evidence Level IV.

Nagaratnam, N., & Gayagay, G., Jr. (2002). Hypersexuality in nursing home facilities—a descriptive study. *Archives of Gerontology and Geriatrics, 35*(3), 195–203. Evidence Level IV.

Roach, S. M. (2004). Sexual behaviour of nursing home residents: Staff perceptions and responses. *Journal of Advanced Nursing, 48*(4), 371–379. Evidence Level IV.

Rockliffe-Fidler, C., & Kiemle, G. (2003). Sexual function in diabetic women: A psychological perspective. *Sexual and Relationship Therapy, 18*(2), 143–159. Evidence Level IV.

Rosen, R. C., Wing, R. R., Schneider, S., Wadden, T. A., Foster, G. D., West, D. S., . . . Gendrano, Iii I. N. (2009). Erectile dysfunction in type 2 diabetic men: Relationship to exercise fitness and cardiovascular risk factors in the look AHEAD trial. *Journal of Sexual Medicine, 6*(5), 1414–1422. Evidence Level II.

Seidman, S. N., & Roose, S. P. (2006). The sexual effects of testosterone replacement in depressed men: Randomized, placebo-controlled clinical trial. *Journal of Sex & Marital Therapy, 32*(3), 267–273. Evidence Level II.

Sherr, L., Harding, R., Lampe, F., Johnson, M., Anderson, J., Zetler, S., . . . Edwards, S. (2009). Clinical and behavioral aspects of aging with HIV infection. *Psychology, Health & Medicine, 14*(3), 273–279. Evidence Level IV.

Wallace, M. (2008). How to try this; Sexuality assessment. *American Journal of Nursing, 108*(7), 40–48. Evidence Level V.

Wallace, M., & Safer, M. (2009). Hypersexuality among cognitively impaired older adults. *Geriatric Nursing, 30*(4), 230–237. Evidence Level V.

Walsh, K. E., & Berman, J. R. (2004). Sexual dysfunction in the older woman: An overview of the current understanding and management. *Drugs & Aging, 21*(10), 655–675. Evidence Level V.

Wespes, E., Moncada, I., Schmitt, H., Jungwirth, A., Chan, M., & Varanese, L. (2007). The influence of age on treatment outcomes in men with erectile dysfunction treated with two regimens of tadalafil: Results of the SURE study. *BJU International, 99*(1), 121–126. Evidence Level II.

World Health Organization. (2002). *Gender and human rights.* Retrieved from http://www.who.int/reproductivehealth/topics/gender_rights/sexual_health/en/. Evidence Level VI.

Substance Misuse and Alcohol Use Disorders

26

Madeline Naegle

EDUCATIONAL OBJECTIVES

On completion of this chapter, the reader should be able to:

1. describe common patterns of substance use in older adults
2. recognize common substance use disorders diagnosed in older adults
3. outline screening steps for substance use disorders in older adults
4. discuss the stepwise assessment and rationale for identifying a substance use disorder
5. analyze intervention strategies for substance use disorders in older adults
6. list potential resources on substance-related disorders for older adults and their families

OVERVIEW

Alcohol and drug use among persons aged 50 years and older is increasing as more people live longer, continue community living, and continue substance use habits established in youth and middle adulthood. Approximately 57 million persons ages 50–64 years are now living in the United States, and there are another 37.8 million persons aged 65 years and older. The projected increase in persons aged 65 years and older is expected to reach 85 million older adults by 2050 (U.S. Census Bureau, 2008). Population growth predicts greater numbers of substance-related problems in older adults, and nurses should be prepared to identify and intervene to address these issues (Han, Gfroerer, Colliver, & Penne, 2009). The estimated one third of the older population who are minority group members will also grow and because drug and alcohol use in ethnic minorities is grossly understudied, nursing interventions must be adapted in culturally competent ways and individualized to this group of older adults (Andrews, 2008; Grant et al., 2004).

BACKGROUND AND STATEMENT OF PROBLEM

Health care problems linked to substance abuse are costly to society with direct and indirect economic costs of alcohol abuse and dependence, including costs of illness and

For description of Evidence Levels cited in this chapter, see Chapter 1, Developing and Evaluating Clinical Practice Guidelines: A Systematic Approach, page 7.

crime, estimated at $184 billion in 1998. Another $143.4 billion in costs is attributed to illicit and prescription drugs (National Institute on Alcohol Abuse and Alcoholism [NIAAA], 2000). Nearly 22% of community-dwelling older adults use potentially addictive prescription medication (Simoni-Wastila & Yang, 2006), and risks of psychological and/or physical dependence associated with this phenomenon are considerable (Simoni-Wastila, Zuckerman, Singhal, Briesacher, & Hsu, 2005). This misuse of drugs in older persons costs the United States $60 billion annually, a cost that is anticipated to rise as the middle-aged population—high users of nonprescription pain relievers—grow (Wu & Blazer, 2011).

The drug most commonly misused by older adults is alcohol, followed by tobacco and psychoactive prescription drugs, with trends indicating an increase in the numbers of older individuals using marijuana (Moore et al., 2009). High personal and medical costs are linked to excessive use and abuse of alcohol, rather than moderate use. Among persons older than 60 years seen in primary care, 15% of men and 12% of women regularly drank in excess of the National Institute Alcohol Abuse and Alcoholism (NIAAA) recommended levels (i.e., one drink per day and no more than three drinks on any one occasion; Fink, Elliott, Tsia, & Beck, 2005). Heavy consumption has been shown to decrease the likelihood that older people will use preventive medical services such as glaucoma screening, vaccinations, and mammograms (Fink et al., 2005). Looking to the future, of the estimated 57 million late middle-aged persons (50–64 years old), 14% are drinking heavily, with 9% of them "at-risk" drinkers, and 23% report binge drinking (consumption of four to five drinks on an occasion; Blazer & Wu, 2009; Merrick et al., 2008).

The burden of disease derived from tobacco use continues to be heaviest among older individuals and is the leading cause of premature death in older persons (Sachs-Ericsson, Collins, Schmidt, & Zvolensky, 2011) who have smoked the longest and have the most health problems. In 2004, 18.5 million Americans older than 45 years smoked, (about 42% of all adult smokers) and in 2006, 9% of older Americans were smokers (National Center for Health Statistics [NCHS], 2007). Smoking-related deaths number 300,000 annually in this age group (Centers for Disease Control and Prevention [CDC], 2010).

As baby boomers age, their lifetime illicit drug use is anticipated to continue at the same levels, increasing the number of persons older than 55 years using illicit drugs (marijuana and cocaine; National Institute on Drug Abuse [NIDA] 2010). Using survey research and modeling methods to project trends, the number of persons aged 50 years and older who use marijuana is projected to increase from 1.0% in 1999 to at least 2.9% (3.3 million users) by 2020. Use of illicit drugs is expected to increase from 2.2% (1.6 million) to 3.1% (3.5 million) and nonmedical use of psychotherapeutic drugs is projected to increase from 1.2% to 2.4% (Colliver, Compton, Gfroerer, & Condon, 2006).

More older people in need of treatment, coupled with their reluctance to seek assistance with mental health problems (fewer than 3% of older people visit a mental health professional), suggest that nurses and health professionals caring for older adults in all settings must be knowledgeable about substance use, abuse, and dependence (Bartels et al., 2004). Psychiatric disorders often cooccur with alcohol abuse in older adults with a prevalence rate ranging from 12% to 30% (Oslin, 2005) and depression, independently and as a consequence of excessive drinking, often occurs in male smokers (Kinnunen et al., 2006).

The metabolic changes of aging are key factors in health problems related to drug or alcohol use, resulting in increased morbidity in advancing age. Older persons respond differently to alcohol because of decreased total body water, decreased rates of alcohol metabolism in the gastrointestinal tract, and increased sensitivity to alcohol combined with decreased tolerance (U.S. Department of Health and Human Services [USDHHS], 2004a). Consequently, more dramatic behavioral changes and adverse physical responses are evident at lower doses of all drugs. Social and legal problems occur more frequently and are more pronounced than in younger people, especially for older women (Center for Substance Abuse Treatment [CSAT], 1998). Because the *Diagnostic and Statistical Manual of Mental Disorders* (4th ed.; *DSM-IV*) criteria may be less applicable to older adults, these criteria must be interpreted and applied in an age-appropriate manner.

ASSESSMENT OF SUBSTANCE USE DISORDERS

Substance use and related disorders are categorized as use, misuse, abuse, and dependence. Misuse is the most common disorder in older adults because of the high number of prescription drugs used and more pronounced responses to any drugs—licit or illicit. Older people tend to "self-medicate" with alcohol and other drugs to treat physical and psychological symptoms associated with aging. Whether a problem is categorized as abuse or dependence, potential health problems are linked to the substance used; the length of time used, misuse, abuse, or dependence; and the social, legal, and health consequences for the individual. For example, persons who drink four or fewer drinks per year are considered abstinent and low-risk drinkers. For adults aged 65 years and older, one drink daily is considered moderate consumption (USDHHS, 2005). Most individuals who use and/or are dependent on alcohol, nicotine, and illicit drugs have developed drinking patterns before the age of 60. One half to two thirds of older adult alcoholics developed alcoholism or abuse patterns early in life. "Late-onset alcoholism" and patterns of prescription drug abuse, marked by increased use of alcohol or over-reliance on prescription drugs, are often linked to losses, chronic illness, psychological traumas, and common stressors of advancing age. A common example is the change from social use to risky drinking or drug misuse by people who have lost a spouse, partner, or job; are estranged from family or are facing serious illness; or any combination of situations mentioned.

Alcohol Use Disorders

The most common substance use disorders in older adults relate to alcohol consumption, including interactions of alcohol with prescription and over-the-counter (OTC) drugs (USDHHS, 2005).

At-Risk and Binge Drinking

"At-risk" drinking is a pattern that may not readily appear to cause alcohol-related problems but may cause harmful consequences to the user or others with continued use over time. Regular alcohol and tobacco use, for example, are linked to insomnia (Tibbitts, 2008), a common complaint of older persons. Negative consequences of use include accidents, health and/or mental health problems, or social and legal problems. For people older than 60 years, continuing to drink the same amounts of alcohol that did not appear to cause problems earlier in life later results in adverse consequences.

Such outcomes are determined by the individual's response to alcohol, the use of prescription drugs (alcohol interacts with at least 50% prescription drugs), and cooccurrence of other chronic medical or psychiatric disorders. Similarly, a decline in visual, auditory, or other perceptual capacities make alcohol consumption hazardous. Heavy drinking can result in ulcers, respiratory disease, stroke, and myocardial infarction, and older persons are more vulnerable to these. Most adults decrease alcohol consumption with age but significant numbers continues heavy consumption at age 60 years and older (Merrick et al., 2008).

Abuse of a substance is diagnosed when a maladaptive pattern of use, leading to impairment or distress (legal, interpersonal, emotional, or mental), is evident. These patterns include failure to fulfill role obligations and use of a drug in physically hazardous situations, all occurring over a 12-month period (modified from American Psychiatric Association [APA], 2000). Even when a person does not meet the *DSM-IV-TR* criteria for abuse or dependence, alcohol consumption at levels of more than seven drinks per week for persons older than 65 years can result in health consequences. Excessive alcohol consumption may place the older individual at risk for falls, self-neglect, and diminished cognitive capacity, and long-term alcohol use is related to the development of common medical problems such as sleep disorders, restlessness and agitation, liver function abnormalities, pneumonia, pancreatitis, gastrointestinal bleeding, and trauma as well as chronic diseases, particularly neuropsychiatric and digestive disorders, diabetes, cardiovascular disease, and pancreatic or head and neck cancer (Blow, 1998). Excess alcohol use compromises health by interfering with the absorption and utilization of prescribed drugs and nutrients.

Drug Dependence (Addiction)

Drug dependence is a maladaptive pattern of substance use that leads to impairment or distress (legal, interpersonal, emotional, or mental) occurring in a 12-month period (APA, 2000). Addiction is a chronic illness characterized by brief "slips" from sobriety and "relapses," returns to regular use of the substance. It has two components: (a) physiological dependence, induced by certain drugs, particularly alcohol, tobacco, benzodiazepines, barbiturates, amphetamines, and opioids, is evidenced in "tolerance," the need for increasing amounts of a substance to achieve the desired effect and "withdrawal," in a characteristic pattern of symptoms when use of a substance is suddenly stopped; craving accompanies withdrawal; and (b) psychological dependence, the perceived need to use the drug. Psychological dependence occurs with both abuse and dependence and is more difficult to resolve than physiologic dependence.

Illicit Drug Use

Illicit drug use is less prevalent in late adulthood than alcohol abuse or prescription drug misuse. Recent trends in the "baby boomer" generation, however, suggest that this may be changing. Marijuana use, for example, is now more prevalent among persons aged 55 years and older than among adolescents, and in 2000, more than half a million persons aged 55 years and older reported illicit drug use (Substance Abuse and Mental Health Services Administration [SAMHSA], 2001). Two recent studies, as well, indicate that among persons older than 50 years reporting illicit drug use, toxicology screens on small samples seen in urban emergency departments were positive for cocaine (63%), opiates (16%), and marijuana (14%; Rivers et al., 2004; Schlaerth, Splawn, Ong, & Smith, 2004).

Clinical observation suggests that older people are rarely asked about cocaine abuse despite strong evidence of its associated cardiovascular risks. The result is inaccurate information of the prevalence of illicit drug use among older adults (Chait, Fahmy, & Caceres, 2010).

Recovery From Drug or Alcohol Dependence

Many older persons are "in recovery" or have established long sobriety from the use of alcohol, cocaine, heroin, or other drugs. The components of recovery have been described by the Consensus Panel of the Betty Ford Institute (2007) as a lifestyle voluntarily maintained by an individual that includes sobriety, varying levels of personal health, and citizenship. Situations and life stressors may contribute to an individual's relapse to alcohol or drug use. Changes associated with aging, the numbers of losses that increase with age, and the onset of chronic illness may all become "triggers," which pose a threat to recovery and increase the risk for a return to regular, maladaptive patterns of use (relapse). On a positive note, good treatment outcomes and rates of recovery for older persons are higher than in any age group. Nurses can contribute positively by supporting the patient's attendance at self-help group meetings, continued involvement in treatment such as methadone maintenance and/or group or individual psychotherapy.

In this chapter, the term *drug* applies to OTC medications, prescription medications, nicotine, alcohol, and illicit drugs. Herbs and food supplements are also used frequently by older adults. Although knowing the chemical composition of drugs of abuse is essential to understanding their effects on mind and body, this chapter focuses primarily on drug misuse, and the effects and consequences of excessive use and use in combination, for health as well as appropriate nursing assessment and intervention strategies. Please refer to http://www.nih.nida.gov for a full listing of drugs of abuse and their chemical properties.

Psychoactive Drug Misuse and Abuse

Drug misuse, defined as use of a drug for reasons other than for which it was intended, occurs with increasing frequency with advancing age because (a) prescriptions for multiple medications and cognitive changes, ranging from early signs of dementia, can lead to medication misuse; (b) failure to discard expired medications; (c) trading medications with friends and companions; and (d) combining both nonprescription and prescription medications and alcohol. The most common resulting problems are related to (a) overdose, (b) additive effects, (c) adverse reactions to drugs used, or (d) drug interactions, especially with alcohol. Older adults are prescribed with more than 33% of all prescription drugs, and the nonmedical use of prescription drugs is increasing in persons older than 60 years (NIDA, 2007). Among older women who misuse medications and alcohol as high as 30% developed such habits after age 60 years (The National Center on Addiction and Substance Abuse [CASA] at Columbia University, 1998).

The regular use of numerous drugs for multiple medical conditions (i.e., polypharmacy) is complicated by the older adult's use of alcohol or illicit drugs (Letizia & Reinbolz, 2005). Prescription drug use or misuse contributes to falls and cognitive impairment. In persons aged 18–70 years old treated for falls, 40% of men and 8% of women tested positive for alcohol and/or benzodiazepines (9% and 3%, respectively), or both (Boyle & Davis, 2006).

Abuse of psychoactive drugs is a growing health problem for older adults and the few research findings listed as factors correlating with drug abuse are isolation, history of substance-related or mental health disorder, bereavement, chronic medical disorders, female gender, and exposure to prescription drugs with abuse potential. Use of illicit drugs by older adults is mostly limited to long-time addicts (Blow et al., 2000) and marijuana users (SAMHSA, 2000). However, substance abuse by older adults, 1 in 4 of whom receive prescriptions for psychoactive drugs with abuse potential, is becoming more common. Drugs—other than nicotine or tobacco—most commonly abused are benzodiazepines, sedative hypnotics, and opioid analgesics (Barry, Oslin, & Blow, 2001).

Smoking and Nicotine Dependence

Today's older Americans have smoked at rates among the highest of any U.S. generation (American Lung Association [ALA], 2006), resulting in many health problems and contributing to the estimated 438,000 American deaths annually caused by smoking. In 2008, more than 17 million Americans older than 45 years smoked, accounting for more than 22% of all adult smokers. By age group, the prevalence rate of smoking was 9.5% among those aged 65 years and older and 21.9% among those 45–64 years of age.

Vulnerability to the effects of smoking in an older adult varies, with men being more than twice as likely as women to die of stroke secondary to smoking (ALA, 2006). The risk of dying of a heart attack for men aged 65 years and older is twice that for women smokers and 60% higher than for nonsmoking men of the same age. Smokers also have significantly higher risks than nonsmokers for Alzheimer's disease and other types of dementia, as well as visual problems (Whitmer, Sidney, Selby, Johnston, & Yaffe, 2005).

Polysubstance Abuse

Polysubstance abuse, the misuse, abuse, or dependence of three or more drugs, is common in older adults. Prescription analgesics are frequently prescribed for chronic pain, a common complaint in older persons, and depending on the class of drug, can induce dependence. Older problem drinkers, as well, report more severe pain, greater disruption of activities caused by pain, and frequent use of alcohol to manage pain (Brennan, Schutte, & Moos, 2005). These findings underscore the importance of monitoring drinking and medication use in patients who present with complaints of pain, especially those with histories of any drug dependence, including alcohol and nicotine.

ASSESSMENT OF SUBSTANCE USE PROBLEMS

The nurse should review data collected on the most recent nursing and medical histories and findings of the most recent physical examination. When patients are using alcohol, there may be deviations in standard liver function tests (LFTs) and elevations in gamma-glutamyl transferase (GGT) and carbohydrate-deficient transferrin (CDT) levels (Godsell, Whitfield, Conigrave, Hanratty, & Saunders, 1995). Physical signs such as ecchymosis, spider angiomas, flushing, palmar erythema, or sarcopenia may be evident. The patient may have an altered level of consciousness, changes in mental status or mood, poor coordination, tremor, increased deep tendon reflexes, or a positive Romberg sign. Increased lacrimal secretions, nystagmus, and sluggish pupil reactivity may also be noted in the examination (Letizia & Reinbolz, 2005). Patients who report use of marijuana and/or other drugs should have toxicology tests to establish baseline use level. Findings can be effectively used in a motivational interview and brief interventions and/or counseling.

Nurses need to assess and document frequent changes in drug using habits and record these in substance use histories, dating from first use to the current situation. Ask if the individual ever experienced problems related to drug or alcohol use, spontaneously stopped using a drug or alcohol, or is in recovery and participating in self-help programs such as Alcoholics Anonymous or Narcotics Anonymous.

In taking the patient history, ask about a history of smoking, alcohol use, OTC medications, prescription and recreational drugs, herbal, and food and drink supplement use. Record this information using the Quantity Frequency (QF) Index (Khavari & Farber, 1978). Another helpful technique in assessing drug use is the "brown bag" technique. Ask the client to bring in a brown bag containing all of the prescribed, OTC, food supplements, and other legal or illicit drugs that he or she consumes weekly. Use these to develop the history and to open a discussion about the implications of drug use with the patient. Be sure to talk with the client about how using the drug is meaningful or helpful (i.e., relieves pain, relieves feelings of loneliness, anxiety, or comfort).

Screening, brief intervention, and referral to treatment (SBIRT) has been found to be effective with adults and older adults for smoking and alcohol use, and should be part of the nursing evaluation (Schonfeld et al., 2010). Despite federal agency guidelines supporting its use, it is rarely used with older adults. SBIRT has demonstrated efficacy and feasibility in reducing patients' alcohol consumption, decreasing dependence symptoms (Babor et al., 2007; SAMHSA, 2008), and improving general and mental health (Madras et al., 2009) following its use by nurses and nurse practitioners.

SBIRT begins with screening an individual with a valid and population-appropriate screening tool. When the patient scores positively for excess alcohol use or for smoking, a brief 3- to 5-minute advice giving or counseling session is done by the health professional. Its components are as follows:

Screening: Short, well-tested questionnaire that identifies risk (such as the Alcohol, Smoking, and Substance Involvement Screening Test [ASSIST], the Short Michigan Alcohol Screening Test—Geriatric version [SMAST-G], the Alcohol Use Disorder Identification Test [AUDIT], the Drug Abuse Screening Test [DAST], etc.)

Brief Intervention: Short, structured conversations that feature feedback and options for change

Referral: For in-depth assessment and/or diagnosis and/or treatment, if needed

Treatment: Between 1% and 10% may need some level of treatment—depending on the health care setting

The brief intervention generally consists of recommendations to stop smoking or to cut down on the amount of alcohol used. When the screening score indicates dependence on alcohol or nicotine, the nurse refers the patient to specialty treatment, providing him or her with the information needed to access a provider with expertise in this area or a specialty health care agency.

Health providers, family members, and friends may overlook substance use by older persons because no one reports the ways in which drug use is disrupting their lives, because they feel that the patient has "earned it," or patients and family do not see that use causes health problems. Health professionals may be pessimistic that older persons can change long-standing behaviors, so may not ask about drug and alcohol use.

Evidence suggests that many health professionals doubt the effectiveness of alcohol or drug treatment (Vastag, 2003). In addition, health care providers often do not recognize the association of drug use, smoking, or excessive alcohol use and health problems such as chronic obstructive pulmonary disease (COPD), stroke, or depression. Recently, dependence on alcohol and other drugs has been recognized as a chronic condition, characterized by slips and relapses, and one that responds to treatment (McLellan, Lewis, O'Brien, & Kleber, 2000). Interventions and treatment are now being matched to stages of the disease such as acute phases, exacerbations, and stages of recovery.

Screening Tools for Alcohol and Drug Use

Screening for alcohol and other drug use is equally important in the community and hospital setting. A QF Index such as the Khavari Alcohol Test (KAT) asks respondents to report their (a) usual frequency of drinking, (b) usual amount consumed per occasion, (c) maximum amount consumed on any one occasion, and (d) frequency with which one consumes the maximum amount (Allen & Wilson, 2003). The KAT consists of the four questions noted previously that are asked for each type of beverage (beer, wine, spirits, liqueurs) and can be administered in 6–8 minutes (Khavari & Farber, 1978). The amounts are then compared with NIAAA norms for persons older than 65 years, which are one drink per day for men and women and no more than three drinks per occasion. Additional questions such as (a) "Did you ever feel you had a problem related to alcohol or other drug use?" and (b) "Have you ever been treated for an alcohol or drug problem?" will yield an important additional information.

Short Michigan Alcohol Screening Test-Geriatric Version

The SMAST-G is an effective tool for screening older adults in all settings. The complete drug use history can be obtained in the comprehensive assessment. The original instrument from which this instrument was derived has a sensitivity of 93.9% and a specificity of 78.1% (Blow et al., 1992). The SMAST-G that is composed of 10 questions is quickly administered and short and has outcomes equal to the parent instrument. Each positive response counts as 1 point.

Alcohol Use Disorders Identification Test

This 10-item questionnaire has good validity in ethnically mixed groups and scores classify alcohol use as hazardous, harmful, or dependent. Administration: 2 minutes (Saunders, Aasland, Babor, de la Fuente, & Grant, 1993). The AUDIT has been found to have high specificity in adults older than 65 years (Babor, Higgins-Biddle, Saunders, & Monteiro, 2001).

Fagerström Test for Nicotine Dependence — Revised

This six-question scale provides an indicator of the severity of nicotine dependence: scores less than 4 (*low-to-moderate dependence*); 4–6 (*moderate dependence*); and 7–10 (*highly dependent on nicotine*). The questions inquire about first use early in the day, amount and frequency, inability to refrain, and smoking despite illness. This instrument has good internal consistency and reliability in culturally diverse, mixed gender samples (Pomerleau, Carton, Lutzke, Flessland, & Pomerleau, 1994).

INTERVENTIONS AND CARE STRATEGIES

Because drug and alcohol use affects physical, mental, spiritual, and emotional health, interdisciplinary collaboration is essential to providing the needed range of treatment modalities for substance use disorders and related problems. Primary care providers, psychologists, dentists, nurses, and social workers should all be equipped to detect and refer a problem, and all dimensions of health should be addressed during treatment and aftercare. The least intensive approaches to treatment for older adults should be implemented first and should be flexible, individualized, and implemented over time. Older persons are disinclined to seek or continue care with mental health or addictions specialists. Brief interventions and motivational interviewing have been found effective in producing short-term reduction in alcohol consumption for older persons and for men and women. There are some findings that motivational interviewing is more effective with smoking than brief advices (Ballesteros, González-Pinto, Querejeta, & Ariño, 2004; Wutzke, Conigrave, Saunders, & Hall, 2002). Research findings suggest that once enrolled in treatment for dependence, however, older people treated for alcohol or opioid dependence with medications such as naltrexone, methadone, or buprenorphine; and individualized, supportive, and medically based psychosocial interventions have better outcomes than younger patients (Oslin, Pettinati, & Volpicelli, 2002; Satre, Mertens, Areán, & Weisner, 2004).

Inpatient Hospitalization

Older adults who report using alcohol should be screened on admission to any care facility. A small but important percentage of them will be at risk for the development of acute alcohol withdrawal syndrome (AWS) on sudden cessation of drinking. Patients at highest risk have (a) a history of consuming large amounts of alcohol, (b) coexisting acute illness, (c) previous episodes of AWS or seizure activity, (d) a history of detoxification, and (e) intense cravings for alcohol (Letizia & Reinbolz, 2005). Symptoms of withdrawal will be intense and of greater duration than in younger persons with onset of withdrawal as early as 4–8 hours after the last drink and persisting up to 72 hours. The clinical symptoms determine the need for detoxification and are essential to medical and nursing decisions. This clinical judgment is made following a history, including history of drug and alcohol use, and physical and mental status assessments.

A 10- to 28-day period of acute care hospitalization in a mental health unit or alcohol and drug treatment center is indicated for the older person addicted to alcohol, benzodiazepines, heroin, amphetamines, or cocaine when (a) living situations and access to the drug makes abstinence unlikely, (b) there is a likelihood of severe withdrawal symptoms, (c) comorbid physical or psychiatric diagnoses such as depression and accompanying suicidal ideation or a chronic physical illness are present, (d) daily ingestion of alcohol or a sedative hypnotic has been higher than recommended doses for 4 weeks or more, and (e) mixed addiction as in alcohol and benzodiazepines or cocaine and alcohol is present. It is helpful if programs specifically designed to meet the needs of older persons are available (USDHHS, 2004a).

Ambulatory Care

Persons dependent on alcohol, tobacco, and heroin can be successfully withdrawn in community-based care through the collaboration of a medical doctor or nurse practitioner and family members and friends. Specialists in addiction should be sought as supervisors or collaborators in the process. Older persons drinking at risky levels or abusing alcohol or other drugs are generally treated in the community. Tobacco cessation protocols are now available directly to consumers as well as to primary care providers and mental health professionals.

Residential Treatment

Residential treatment is available in specialty care centers, therapeutic communities, and some long-term care facilities. Programs designed specifically for the older person are beneficial in their focus on the specific health care needs and challenges to abstinence faced by older people. These long-standing habits of use, a diminished social network, and the risks of social isolation and cost and health implications of heavy alcohol and prescription drug use make behavioral change particularly challenging.

Therapeutic Communities

Therapeutic communities provide long-term (up to 18 months) treatment and are abstinence-oriented programs. They use 12-step models of individual and group counseling, as well as participation in a social community, to address drug-related problems. For the isolated, older drug user with a history of frequent relapse, these are good treatment options.

Pharmacological Treatment

Agents for pharmacological treatment of substance abuse and dependence are more available but not all are appropriate for use with older adults. The best outcomes of pharmacological interventions occur when they are used in combination with individual and/or group counseling. Attendance at 12-step programs also supports adherence to treatment regimens.

Alcohol Abuse amd Dependence Pharmacological Treatment

There is strong evidence that naltrexone can decrease cravings and consumption in heavy drinkers. It is available in liquid form for oral use and is now available in injectable, long-acting form. It is marketed as Vivitrol or Vivitrex. These extended-release formulations of naltrexone act up to 28 days to decrease the euphoric effects of, and craving for alcohol (Bartus et al., 2003). Evidence suggests that this treatment is well tolerated by older people (Oslin et al., 2002). Contraindications for its use include renal problems, acute hepatitis, or liver failure. Some study findings stress the importance of psychosocial interventions to improve adherence to pharmacological interventions for alcohol dependence, a finding similar to those regarding smoking cessation (Mayet, Farrell, Ferri, Amato, & Davoli, 2005). Acamprosate calcium (Campral), a recent addition to prescription drug choices, has variable outcomes in reducing the craving for and consumption of alcohol. Disulfiram (Antabuse) or to deter alcohol consumption produces an elevation in vital signs and severe gastrointestinal symptoms if alcohol is ingested and is poorly tolerated by alcoholics older than 55 years. In addition, it must be taken every day if aversive effects on consumption are to occur, working with the patient's family members and support persons predicts the best outcomes with this medication.

Opioid Dependence. The use of methadone, an opioid agonist, assists the opioid-dependent person to focus on psychological and life problems. The drug buprenorphine—both an opioid antagonist and agonist—is longer acting and now available. Both are dispensed in institution-based clinic settings or by physicians specifically credentialed to prescribe and monitor buprenorphine. Evidence supports added benefit of psychosocial treatment for patient adherence to pharmacological treatment (Amato et al., 2008).

Smoking. Bupropion in doses of 75 mg with administration begun 2 weeks before the smoker intends to quit has proved a helpful adjunct to smoking cessation. Nicorette transdermal patches and nicotine gum are now available OTC and there is research support for their pharmacological contribution to smoking cessation. The best outcomes with smoking cessation are a combination of individual or group psychosocial support and the medications described previously (New York City Department of Health and Mental Hygiene, 2002).

Models of Care

Individualized care plans should be developed for older adults at risk for substance abuse or dependence in accord with the classes of drugs used and the mild, moderate, or severe nature of the disorder. Individualizing care allows flexibility for patient and nurse. Evidence is emerging, however, on models of care for older adults with complex health problems. For example, in one study, the integration of mental health into primary care increased access to mental health and substance abuse treatment for both Black and White older adult patients who are offered both enhanced specialist services and mental health services at primary care site (Ayalon, Areán, Linkins, Lynch, & Estes, 2007). Case management has also demonstrated effective outcomes with older adults with multiple social, mental health, and physical needs with problems accessing community services, including substance abuse (Hesse, Vanderplasschen, Rapp, Broekaert, & Fridell, 2007). Guidelines for all interventions should include the following:

- A nonjudgmental, health-oriented approach to substance-related problems. Drug and alcohol use and abuse are highly stigmatized in American society, particularly in minority communities, leading to denial and/or rejection by family members. Understanding addiction as a disease helps nurses and other providers adopt attitudes and approaches similar to care for other chronic illness.
- A supportive, encouraging approach to the possibilities of changing use habits. The patient or client is taught that change occurs in stages and that support and assistance are available at each stage.
- Education of patient and family on the risks associated with drug misuse. Because older persons use so many medications, the potential health consequences may be minimized in the eyes of family members and care takers.
- Assessment of substance use in relation to life style, existing chronic illnesses, nutritional patterns, sleep, exercise, sexual patterns, and recreation. Counsel the patient and/or family about the effects of substances used on these areas of the patient's life.
- Set the goal of "harm reduction" in the forms of decreased use and supervised use if abstinence is not imperative or achievable.
- Monitor substance use patterns at each encounter or visit, documenting changes and providing reinforcement of positive changes and/or movement toward treatment.

- Enhance the involvement of members of the patient's support system, including family and friends identified by the patient, community-based groups, support groups, appropriate clergy, or organizational groups such as senior centers.
- Support the development of coping mechanisms, including modifications in social, housing, and recreational environments, to minimize associations with settings and groups in which substance use and abuse are common (USDHHS, 2004a).

Counseling and Psychotherapy

Older persons tend to seek care from their primary care, medical specialist, or nurse/nurse practitioner provider even regarding assistance with mental health and substance-related problems. This practice derives from long-held beliefs that depression or anxiety indicates weakness or lack of character.

Older persons, more than others, stigmatize the excess use of alcohol or use of an illicit drug and problems with prescription drugs. Counseling done by the nurse using a brief intervention model or supportive counseling is more readily acceptable to older patients than referral to mental health or substance abuse clinics.

Optimally, short-term psychotherapy by a practitioner with education about abuse and addiction is extremely helpful. The model of cognitive behavioral therapy, in particular, has demonstrated good outcomes with excessive drinking and marijuana use (Cooney, Babor, & Litt, 2001). These approaches assist the older person to modify behavior and to deal with negative feelings and/or chronic pain that often motivate use.

Treatment Outcomes

Health care providers and older persons may feel pessimistic about the possibilities of changing their substance use behavior. Health providers often do not intervene because they believe that older people do not change. Treatment outcomes for older persons with substance use problems, however, have been shown to be as good as or better than those for younger people (USDHHS, 2004b). Good treatment outcomes, however, can be compromised by inconsistency of follow-up and limited access to aftercare for community-dwelling older adults.

CASE STUDY

Joseph and Mary P., both 71 years old, reside in a small, rural community where Mr. P. owned the only pharmacy. Retired for 5 years, Mr. P. suffers from arthritis and Mrs. P. has mitral valve insufficiency, which frequently results in cardiac symptoms that are frightening but readily managed. She has also been treated for generalized anxiety disorder for which she has been prescribed Paxil. The couple enjoys a nightly cocktail hour at which Mr. P. consumes two scotch whiskies and

(continued)

CASE STUDY *(continued)*

Mrs. P. has "wine." Recently, the visiting nurse who has been monitoring Mrs. P.'s recovery from a recent episode of congestive heart failure received a phone call from the couple's daughter who stated that on her last three evening phone calls to her parents, Mrs. P. sounded somewhat confused and her speech was slurred. When the daughter questioned Mr. P. about their drinking, he became irritable and defensive.

The visiting nurse made it a point to visit the P.'s in the early evening on her way home. She found them enjoying their cocktails and took the opportunity to conduct a drug and alcohol assessment, including making a list of all of their medications. The nurse diagnosed "drug misuse" because it appears that neither of them considered how their continued alcohol use was affecting them. She conducted a brief intervention, giving them feedback about their respective illnesses, pointed out the pros and cons of modifying their drinking such as decreasing the gastric distress Mr. P. experiences, and the benefits of limited wine intake while taking paroxetine hydrochloride (Paxil). The nurse taught them (building on autonomy and responsibility) about the relationship between physical changes and the effects of alcohol on their sleep patterns, mood, and balance. She also pointed out that both were consuming alcohol more than one daily drink and recommended that they cut down to one standard drink per day (1.5 oz of spirits, 4–5 oz wine, or 12 oz of beer). At first, they seemed unhappy about the recommendation but both committed to attempting to do so. When she visited 2 weeks later, they had begun to journal their drinking and both were recording consistent declines in the amount of alcohol consumed.

SUMMARY

Two current trends are predicted to result in an increase in the already significant number of men and women older than 55 years who experience various substance use disorders: the growing numbers of older persons in America and the continuation of tobacco, drug, and alcohol use patterns established earlier in life. Although most people decrease the amount of alcohol and kinds of drugs they use with age, anywhere from 10% to 24% of older persons do not (USDHHS, 2004a). The most common of substance use disorders is heavy drinking, especially by Caucasian men older than 65 years and living alone (USDHHS, 2004a). The frequency of heavy drinking is closely followed by smoking that causes the highest number of premature deaths among older people. The high numbers of prescription drugs used by older adults pose serious problems related to misuse and drug interactions. Health professionals are disinclined to query older adults about substance use, with the result that problems become known in the context of the diagnosis and treatment of other medical disorders. Nurses in daily contact with institutionalized and community-dwelling older adults must be skilled in screening and counseling on the use of nicotine, alcohol, prescription, illicit, and OTC drugs. Educating patient and family about health risks and referring patients to specialists and community resources are essential "best practices."

NURSING STANDARD OF PRACTICE

Protocol 26.1: Substance Misuse and Alcohol Use Disorders

I. GOAL: Implement best nursing practices to care of older persons with drug, alcohol, tobacco, or other drug misuse, abuse, or dependence.

II. OVERVIEW

A. Several factors increase the risks associated with alcohol and drug use for the older individual, continuing drug use patterns that earlier in life were commonplace, can be potentially harmful. Constitutional risk factors include changes in body composition such as decreased muscle mass, decreased organ efficiency (especially kidney and liver), and increased vulnerability of the central nervous system (CNS).

B. Alcohol use in combination with other drugs or used excessively may result in falls, impaired cognition, malnourishment, and decreased resistance to disease, interpersonal, and legal problems.

C. At-risk drinking (more than one drink per day or more than three drinks on one occasion) by older adults increases the likelihood of negative health consequences.

D. Any smoking is considered drug abuse and places the person at risk for negative health consequences: advancing age increases the likelihood of respiratory and cardiovascular illnesses.

III. BACKGROUND AND STATEMENT OF THE PROBLEM

A. Definitions (APA, 2000)

1. *Substance use disorders.* A broad category of disorders on a continuum of use or misuse of alcohol, tobacco, prescription, or illicit drugs and the abuse or dependence on these drugs.

2. *Substance abuse.* A maladaptive pattern of substance use evidenced in recurrent and significant adverse consequences related to the repeated use of substances. It is associated with repeated failure to fulfill role obligations, use in situations where use is physically hazardous, and/or when it results in legal and/or interpersonal problems.

3. *Substance dependence.* A maladaptive pattern of self-administering a drug that results in the development of tolerance, withdrawal, and compulsive drug taking behavior. Dependence is both physiological and psychological.

4. *Drug misuse.* Use of a drug for purposes other than that for which it was intended.

5. *Polysubstance-related disorder.* Misuse, abuse, or dependence on three or more drugs.

6. *Tolerance.* (a) A need for markedly increased amounts of a substance to achieve intoxication or the desired effects or (b) a markedly diminished effects with the continued use of the same amount of a substance.

7. *Withdrawal.* A characteristic group of signs and symptoms that has its onset following the sudden cessation of consumption of a drug (including alcohol and nicotine) that induces physiological dependence.

(continued)

Protocol 26.1: Substance Misuse and Alcohol Use Disorders *(cont.)*

8. *At-risk drinking.* Defined as more than one drink per day, 7 days a week or more than three drinks on any one occasion for persons 65 years and older. For older adults, at-risk drinking increases the likelihood of negative health consequences.
9. *Relapse.* Return to regular use of a substance in a maladaptive pattern.
10. *Recovery.* A lifestyle voluntarily maintained by an individual that includes sobriety, varying levels of personal health, and citizenship. Recovery is categorized as early (1–11 months), sustained (1–5 years), and beyond.

B. Etiology and/or Epidemiology: Of persons older than 50 years, 16.7% reported drinking two or more drinks per day (risky drinking) and 19.6% reported binge drinking on occasion. Among primary care patients older than 60 years, 15% of men and 12% of women regularly drank in excess of the NIAAA recommended levels (one drink per day and no more than three drinks on any one occasion).

1. The drugs used, abused, and misused most frequently by older adults are nicotine, alcohol, and prescription drugs, particularly analgesics and benzodiazepines.
2. Excessive drinking by individuals of all ethnic groups ages 65 years and older is approximately 7%, down from 12% in persons ages 55–64 years.
3. Five hundred thousand persons ages 55 years and older reported monthly use of illicit drugs in the National Household Survey on Drug Use, National Institute on Drug Abuse.
4. Approximately 11% of women older than 59 years misuse psychoactive drugs.

C. Risk Factors (USDHHS, 2004a)
1. Family history of dependence on alcohol, tobacco, prescription, or illicit drugs
2. Cooccurrence of addiction with dependency or abuse of another substance dependence (i.e., alcohol and tobacco)
3. Lifelong pattern of substance use, including heavy drinking
4. Male gender
5. Social isolation
6. Recent and multiple losses
7. Chronic pain
8. Cooccurrence with depression
9. Unmarried and/or living alone

IV. PARAMETERS OF ASSESSMENT

A. Screening for alcohol, tobacco, and other drug use is recommended for all community-dwelling and hospitalized older adults. It is essential that the nurse
1. state the purpose of questions about substances used and link them to health and safety,
2. be empathic and nonjudgmental; avoid stigmatic terms such as *alcoholic*,
3. ask the questions when the patient is alcohol- and drug-free,
4. inquire re: patient's understanding of the question (Aalto, Pekuri, & Seppä, 2003).

(continued)

Protocol 26.1: Substance Misuse and Alcohol Use Disorders *(cont.)*

B. Assessment and Screening Tools
   1. The Quantity Frequency (QF) Index (Khavari & Farber, 1978): Review all classes of drugs: alcohol, nicotine, illicit drugs, prescription drugs, OTC drugs, and vitamin supplements, for each drug used. *Record the types* of drugs, including the kinds of beverages; *Frequency*: the number of occasions on which the drug is consumed (daily, weekly, monthly); *Amount of drug consumed* on each occasion over the last 30 days. The psychological function, what the drugs does for the individual, is also important to identify. The QF Index tool should be part of the intake nursing history. The brown bag approach is also useful. Ask the patient to bring all drugs and supplements he or she uses in a brown bag to the interview.
   2. Short Michigan Alcohol Screening Test-Geriatric Version (SMAST-G): Highly valid and reliable, this is a 10-item tool that can be used in all settings. Three minutes for administration. This instrument is derived from the MAST-G with a sensitivity of 93.6% and a positive predictive value of 87.2% (Blow et al., 1992).
   3. The Alcohol Use Disorders Identification Test (AUDIT): This 10-item questionnaire has good validity in ethnically mixed groups, and scores classify alcohol use as hazardous, harmful, or dependent. Administration: 2 minutes. Sensitivity scores range from 0.74% to 0.84% and specificity around 0.90% in mixed age and ethnic groups (Allen, Litten, Fertig, & Babor, 1997). This instrument is highly effective for use with older adults (Roberts, Marshall, & MacDonald, 2005). Its derivative, the Alcohol Use Disorders Identification Test-Condensed (AUDIT-C), is composed of three questions that have proved equally valid in detecting an alcohol-related problem.
   4. Fagerström Test for Nicotine Dependence (Pomerleau et al., 1994): This six-question scale provides an indicator of the severity of nicotine dependence: scores of less than 4 (*very low*); 4–6 (*moderate*), and 7–10 (*very high*). The questions inquire about first use early in the day, amount and frequency, inability to refrain, and smoking despite illness. This instrument has good internal consistency and reliability in culturally diverse, mixed gender samples (Pomerleau et al., 1994).
C. Atypical Presentation
   Men and women older than 65 years may have substance use and dependence problems even though the signs and symptoms may be less numerous than those listed in the *Diagnostic and Statistical Manual of Mental Disorders* (4th ed., text rev.; *DSM-IV-TR*).
D. Signs of CNS Intoxication (i.e., slurred speech, drowsiness, unsteady gait, decreased reaction time, impaired judgment, disinhibition, ataxia):
   1. Assess by individual or collateral (speaking with family members) data collection, detail the consumption of amount and type of depressant medications including alcohol, sedatives, hypnotics, and opioid or synthetic opioid analgesics.

(continued)

Protocol 26.1: Substance Misuse and Alcohol Use Disorders *(cont.)*

2. Obtain a blood alcohol level. Marked intoxication 5 0.3%–0.4%, toxic effects occur at 0.4%–0.5%, coma and death at 0.5% or higher.
3. Assess vital signs and determine respiratory, cardiac, or neurological depression
4. Assess for existing medical conditions, including depression
5. Arrange for emergency room or hospitalization treatment as necessary
6. Obtain urine for toxicology, if possible
7. Assess for delirium that can be confused with intoxication and withdrawal in the older adult.

E. At-risk drinking is regular consumption of alcohol in excess of one drink per day for 7 days a week or more than three drinks on any one occasion.
   1. Assess for readiness to change behavior using stages of change model (Prochaska & DiClemente, 1992).
   2. Is drinker concerned about amount or consequences of the drinking? Has she or he contemplated cutting down?
   3. Does she or he have a plan for cutting down or stopping consumption?
   4. Has she or he previously stopped but then resumed risky drinking?
   5. Personalized feedback and education on "at-risk drinking" results in a reduction in at risk drinking among older primary care patients.

F. Treatment of acute alcohol withdrawal syndrome (guidelines are modified for other CNS depressant drugs such as barbiturates, heroin, sedative hypnotics):
   1. Assess for risk factors: (a) previous episodes of detoxification; (b) recent heavy drinking; (c) medical comorbidities including liver disease, pneumonia, and anemia; and (d) previous history of seizures or delirium (Wetterling, Weber, Depfenhart, Schneider, & Junghanns, 2006).
   2. Assess for extreme CNS stimulation and a minor withdrawal syndrome evidenced in tremors, disorientation, tachycardia, irritability, anxiety, insomnia, and moderate diaphoresis. When these signs are not detected, life-threatening situations for older adults often result. Withdrawal, occurring 24–72 hours after the last drink, can progress to seizures, hallucinosis, withdrawal delirium, extreme hypertension, and profuse diarrhea from 4 to 8 hours and for up to 72 hours following cessation of alcohol intake (delirium tremens [DTs]).
   3. Assess neurological signs, using the Clinical Institute Withdrawal Assessment for Alcohol, Revised (CIWA-Ar). This CIWA-Ar is a 10-item rating scale that delineates symptoms of gastric distress, perceptual distortions, cognitive impairment, anxiety, agitation, and headache (Sullivan, Sykora, Schneiderman, Naranjo, & Sellers, 1989).
   4. Medicate with a short-acting benzodiazepine (lorazepam or oxazepam) in doses titrated to patient's score on the CIWA-Ar, patient's age and weight; use one third to one half recommended dose (Amato, Minozzi, Vecchi, & Davoli, 2010). Continue CIWA-Ar to monitor treatment response.
   5. Provide emotional support and frequent reorientation in a cool, low stimulation setting; monitor hydration and nutritional intake. Give therapeutic dose of thiamine and multivitamins.

(continued)

Protocol 26.1: Substance Misuse and Alcohol Use Disorders *(cont.)*

G. Reported sleep disturbance, anxiety, depression, problems with attention and concentration (acute care):
1. Assess for neuropsychiatric conditions using the mental status exam, Geriatric Depression Scale, or Hamilton Anxiety Scale.
2. Obtain sleep history because drugs disrupt sleep patterns in older persons.
3. Assess intake of all drugs, including alcohol, OTC, prescription, herbal and food supplements, and nicotine. Use "brown bag" strategy.
4. If positive for alcohol use, assess for last time of use and amount used.
5. Assess for alcohol or sedative drug withdrawal as indicated.
H. Smoking cigarettes or using smokeless tobacco:
1. Assess for level of dependence using the Fagerström test (see Screening Tools for Alcohol and Drug Use section).

V. NURSING CARE STRATEGIES
A. At-risk drinking (consumption of alcohol in excess of one drink per day for 7 days a week or more than three drinks on any one occasion) or excess alcohol consumption (more than three to four drinks on frequent occasions):
1. Conduct Screening, Brief Intervention, and as indicated, Referral to Treatment: (SAMHSA, 2008)
   a. Screen using the AUDIT-C, AUDIT, or SMAST-G
   b. Feedback information to the client about current health problems or potential problems associated with the level of alcohol or other drug consumption.
   c. Stress client's responsible choice about actions in response to the information provided.
   d. Advice must be clear about reducing his or her amount of drinking or total consumption.
   e. Recommend drinking according to NIAAA levels for older adults.
   f. Provide a menu of choices to the patient or client regarding future drinking behaviors.
   g. Offer information based on scientific evidence, acknowledge the difficulty of change, and avoid confrontation. Empathy is essential to the exchange.
B. Support self-efficacy. Help client explore options for change.
1. Assist client in identifying options to solving the identified problem.
2. Review the pros and cons of behavior change options presented.
3. Help client weigh potential decisions by considering outcomes.
C. Smoking cigarettes or using smokeless tobacco
1. Apply the 5 A's Intervention (Agency for Healthcare Research and Quality [formerly the Agency for Health Care Policy and Research] Guidelines):
   a. Ask: Identify and document all tobacco use.
   b. Advise: Urge the user to quit in a strong personalized manner.
   c. Assess: Is the tobacco user willing to make a quit attempt at this time?
   d. Assist: If user is willing to attempt, refer for individual or group counseling and pharmacotherapy. Refer to telephone "quitlines" in region or state.

(continued)

Protocol 26.1: Substance Misuse and Alcohol Use Disorders *(cont.)*

    e. Arrange referrals to providers, agencies, and self-help groups. Monitor pharmacotherapy once quit date is established. The U.S. Food and Drug Administration (FDA)-approved pharmacotherapies for smoking cessation are the following:

        i. Bupropion SR (Zyban) and nicotine replacement products such as nicotine gum, nicotine inhalers, nicotine nasal spray, and nicotine patch. Nurse-initiated education about these medications is essential.

        ii. Zyban, for example, should not be combined with alcohol. Nurses working with inpatients in a case management model were found to produce outcomes in smoking cessation (Smith, Reilly, Houston Miller, DeBusk, & Taylor, 2002).

        iii. Caring, concern, and provide ongoing support

  2. Communicate caring and concern:

    a. Encourage moderate intensity exercise to reduce cravings for nicotine because 5 minutes of such exercise is associated with short-term reduction in the desire to smoke and tobacco withdrawal symptoms (Daniel, Cropley, Ussher, & West, 2004).

    b. Arrange: Schedule follow-up contact in person or by telephone within 1 week after planned quit date. Continue telephone counseling especially those using medications and nicotine patches (Boyle et al., 2005; Cooper et al., 2004).

D. Alcohol Dependence

  1. Assess patient for psychological dependence

  2. Assess patient for (a) physiological dependence and (b) "tolerance." Psychological dependence occurs with both abuse and dependence and is more difficult to resolve.

  3. Assess for need for medical detoxification (see alcohol withdrawal in Inpatient Hospitalization section)

  4. Refer patient and family to addictions or mental health nurse practitioner or physician

  5. Evaluate patient and family capacity to implement referral

  6. On successful detoxification, monitor use of medications, interpersonal therapies, and participation in self-help groups.

E. Marijuana Dependence: Little research on effective intervention for psychological dependence on marijuana is available. Some guidance can be found in smoking cessation and self-help approaches.

  1. Refer to steps for smoking cessation (see section C of Nursing Care Strategies).

  2. Refer patient to addiction specialist for counseling for psychological dependence and/or treatment with cognitive behavioral therapy.

  3. Refer to community-based self-help groups such as Narcotics Anonymous, Alcoholics Anonymous, or Al-Anon.

  4. Encourage development or expansion of patient's social support system.

(continued)

Protocol 26.1: Substance Misuse and Alcohol Use Disorders *(cont.)*

F. Heroin or Opioid Dependence
   1. Older long-term opioid users may continue use, relapse, and seek treatment. Methadone or buprenorphine are current pharmacological treatment options, effective in conjunction with self-help programs and/or psychosocial interventions
   2. Treatment with methadone, a synthetic narcotic agonist, suppresses withdrawal symptoms and drug cravings associated with opioid dependence but require daily dosing of 60 mg, minimum. It is dispensed only in state licensed clinics.
   3. Buprenorphine (Subutex or Suboxone), recently approved for use in office practice by trained physicians, is an opioid partial agonist–antagonist. Alone and in combination with naloxone (Suboxone), it can prevent withdrawal when someone ceases use of an opioid drug and then be used for long-term treatment. Naloxone is an opioid antagonist used to reverse depressant symptoms in opiate overdose and at different dosages to treat dependence (CSAT, 2010).
      a. Close collaboration with the prescriber is required because these drugs should not be abruptly terminated, used with antidepressants, and interact negatively with many prescription medications.
   4. Naltrexone, a long-acting opioid antagonist, blocks opioid effects and is most effective with those who are no longer opioid dependent but are at high risk for relapse (Srisurapanont & Jarusuraisin, 2005).
   5. Treatment of the older patient who has become addicted to Oxycontin or other opioids should be done in consultation with an addictions specialist nurse or physician.
      a. It is recommended that prescribers avoid opioids and synthetic opioids (Demerol, Dilaudid, and Oxycontin). Opioids have high potential for addiction and Demerol has been associated with delirium in older adults (CSAT, 2010).
      b. Barbiturates should be avoided for use as hypnotics and the use of benzodiazepines for anxiety should be limited to 4 months (USDHHS, 2004a).
G. Treatment and Relapse Prevention
   1. Monitor pharmacological treatment such as naltrexone as short-term treatment for alcohol dependence. The benefits of this treatment are dependent on adherence and psychosocial treatment should accompany its use (World Health Organization [WHO], 2000). Methadone or buprenorphine should be used for long-term treatment of opioid dependence.
   2. Group psychotherapy in limited studies using a cognitive behavioral approach has produced good outcomes with older adults (Payne & Marcus, 2008).
   3. Refer to community-based groups such as Alcoholics Anonymous, Narcotics Anonymous, Al-Anon groups, and encourage attendance.
   4. Educate family and patient regarding signs of risky use or relapse to heavy or alcohol-dependent behavior.

(continued)

Protocol 26.1: Substance Misuse and Alcohol Use Disorders *(cont.)*

5. Counsel patient to reduce drug use (harm reduction) and engage in relationship healing or building, community or intellectually rewarding activities, spiritual growth, and so on that increase valued nondrinking rewards.
6. Counsel in the development of coping skills:
   a. Anticipate and avoid temptation
   b. Learn cognitive strategies to avoid negative moods
   c. Make lifestyle changes to reduce stress, improve the quality of life, and increase pleasure.
   d. Learn cognitive and behavioral activities to cope with cravings and urges to use.
   e. Encourage development or expansion of patient's social support system.

VI. EVALUATION AND EXPECTED OUTCOMES

A. Patient will have:
   1. Improved physical health and function
   2. Improved quality of life, sense of well-being, and mental health
   3. More satisfying interpersonal relationships
   4. Enhanced productivity and mental alertness
   5. Decreased likelihood of falls and other accidents
B. Nurses will demonstrate:
   1. Increased accuracy in detecting patient problems related to use or misuse of substances.
   2. More evidence-based interventions resulting in better outcomes.
C. Institution will have:
   1. Increased number of referrals to ambulatory substance abuse and mental health treatment programs.
   2. Improved links with community-based organizations engaged in prevention, education, and treatment of older adults with substance-related disorders.

VII. FOLLOW-UP MONITORING OF CONDITION

A. Evaluate for increase in substance use or misuse associated with growing numbers of aging adults.
B. Increase outreach to targeted vulnerable populations.
C. Document chronic care needs of older adults diagnosed with substance-related disorders.
D. Monitor alcohol use among older adults with chronic pain.
E. Communicate findings to all members of the caregiver team.

VIII. GUIDELINES

The National Quality Forum has published "Evidence-Based Practices to Treat Substance Use Disorders." These guidelines are inclusive of primary care, the settings in which most older adults seek treatment (National Quality Forum [NQF], 2007).

RESOURCES

Important Websites

Agency for Healthcare Research and Quality (AHRQ) Guidelines
AHRQ clinical practice guidelines are available to download.
http://www.ahrq.gov

American Lung Association
http://www.ffsonline.org

American Nurses Association
http://www.ana.org

American Psychiatric Association
http://www.apa.org

American Psychiatric Nursing Association
http://www.apna.org

Centers for Disease Control and Prevention
http://www.cdc.gov/tobacco/how2quit.htm

International Nurses Society on Addictions
http://www.intnsa.org/

National Institute of Mental Health
Download patient teaching materials for panic disorders, obsessive compulsive disorder, posttraumatic stress, acute stress, and general anxiety disorders
http://www.nih.nimh.gov

National Institute on Aging
Age page: Medications: Use them safely
http://www.nia.nih.gov/healthinformation/publications/medicine.htm

National Institute on Alcohol Abuse and Alcoholism (NIAAA)
http://www.niaaa.nih.gov

National Institute on Drug Abuse (NIDA)
http://www.nida.nih.gov

New York City Department of Health and Mental Hygiene
http://www.nyc.gov/htm/doh/html

Assessment Tools

Alcohol Use Disorders Identification Test (AUDIT) Tool
Saunders, J. B., Aasland, O. G., Babor, T. F., de la Fuente, J. R., & Grant, M. (1993). Development of the Alcohol Use Disorders Identification Test (AUDIT): WHO collaborative project on early detection of persons with harmful alcohol consumption—II. *Addiction, 88*(6), 791–804. Evidence Level III.

Fagerström Test for Nicotine Dependence (FTND)
American Psychiatric Association. (2002). *Fagerström test for nicotine dependence (FTND). Revised 1991.*
American Psychiatric Association's PsychNET 2002 http://www.apa.org/videos/fagerstrom.html

FRAMES

Dyehouse, J., Howe, S., & Ball, S. (1996). *FRAMES model in the training manual for nursing using brief intervention for alcohol problems.* Rockville, MD: U.S. Department of Health and Human Services. Retrieved from Substance Abuse and Mental Health Association's (SAMSA's) pathways courses: silence hurts:

http://pathwayscourses.samhsa.gov/vawp/vawp_supps_pg20.htm

Hartford Institute for Geriatric Nursing
Substance abuse
http://consultgerirn.org/resources

Quantity Frequency Index

Khavari, K. A., & Farber, P. D. (1978). A profile instrument for the quantification and assessment of alcohol consumption. The Khavari Alcohol Test. *Journal Studies on Alcohol, 39*(9), 1525–1539.

SMAST

Naegle, M. A. (2003). *Try this: Best practices in nursing care of older adults: Alcohol use screening and assessment,* Issue # 17. A series provided by The Hartford Institute for Geriatric Nursing. Retrieved from New York University College of Nursing:

http://consultgerirn.org/uploads/File/trythis/try_this_17.pdf

Guidelines

Blow, F. C., Bartels, S. J., Brockmann, L. M., & Van Citters, A. S. (2005). *Evidence-based practices for preventing substance abuse and mental health problems in older adults.* Older Americans Substance Abuse and Mental Health Technical Assistance Center.
http://store.samhsa.gov/product/KAPT26

Michigan Quality Improvement Consortium. (2003/2005). *Screening and management of substance use disorders* (p. 1, NGC:004548).
http://www.psychiatryonline.com/pracGuide/pracGuideChapToc_5.aspx

The National Quality Forum is completing review for "Evidence-Based Practices to Treat Substance Use Disorders." These guidelines are inclusive of primary care, the settings in which most older adults seek treatment.
http://www.qualityforum.org/projects/substance_use_2009.aspx

REFERENCES

Aalto, M., Pekuri, P., & Seppä, K. (2003). Primary health care professionals' activity in intervening in patients' alcohol drinking during a 3-year brief intervention implementation project. *Drug and Alcohol Dependence, 69*(1), 9–14. Evidence Level III.

Agency for Healthcare Research and Quality. (2011). *Treating tobacco use and dependence: 2008 update.* Retrieved from http://www.ahrq.gov/path/tobbaco.htm. Evidence Level VI.

Allen, J. P., Litten, R. Z., Fertig, J. B., & Babor, T. (1997). A review of research on the Alcohol Use Disorders Identification Test (AUDIT). *Alcoholism, Clinical and Experimental Research, 21*(4), 613–619. Evidence Level III.

Allen, J. P., & Wilson, V. (Eds.). (2003). *Assessing alcohol problems: A guide for clinicians and researchers* (2nd ed., pp. 667–671). Bethesda, MD: U.S. Department of Health and Human Services. Evidence Level VI.

Amato, L., Minozzi, S., Davoli, M., Vecchi, S., Ferri, M. M., & Mayet, S. (2008). Psychosocial and pharmacological treatments versus pharmacological treatments for opioid detoxification. *Cochrane Database of Systematic Reviews,* (3), CD005031. Evidence Level I.

Amato, L., Minozzi, S., Vecchi, S., & Davoli, M. (2010). Benzodiazepines for alcohol withdrawal. *Cochrane Database of Systematic Reviews*, (3), CD005063. Evidence Level I.

American Lung Association. (2006). *Smoking among older adults*. Retrieved from http://www.lungusa .org/site/apps/s. Evidence Level IV.

American Psychiatric Association. (2000). *Diagnostic and statistical manual of mental disorders* (4th ed., Rev. ed.). Washington, DC: Author. Evidence Level VI.

Andrews, C. (2008). An exploratory study of substance abuse among Latino older adults. *Journal of Gerontological Social Work*, *51*(1–2), 87–108. Evidence Level IV.

Ayalon, L., Areán, P. A., Linkins, K., Lynch, M., & Estes, C. L. (2007). Integration of mental health services into primary care overcomes ethnic disparities in access to mental health services between black and white elderly. *The American Journal of Geriatric Psychiatry*, *15*(10), 906–912. Evidence Level IV.

Babor, T. F., Higgins-Biddle, J. C., Saunders, J. B., & Monteiro, M. G. (2001). *AUDIT: The alcohol use disorders identification test. Guidelines for use in primary care* (2nd ed.). Geneva, Switzerland: World Health Organization. Evidence Level IV.

Babor, T. F., McRee, B. G., Kassebaum, P. A., Grimaldi, P. L., Ahmed, K., & Bray, J. (2007). Screening, Brief Intervention, and Referral to Treatment (SBIRT): Toward a public health approach to the management of substance abuse. *Substance Abuse*, *28*(3), 7–30. Evidence Level III.

Ballesteros, J., González-Pinto, A., Querejeta, I., & Ariño, J. (2004). Brief interventions for hazardous drinkers delivered in primary care are equally effective in men and women. *Addictions*, *99*(1), 103–108. Evidence Level III.

Barry, K., Oslin, D., & Blow, F. (2001). *Alcohol problems in older adults: Prevention and management*. New York, NY: Guilford Press. Evidence level VI.

Bartels, S. J., Coakley, E. H., Zubritsky, C., Ware, J. H., Miles, K. M., Areán, P. A., . . . PRISM-E Investigators. (2004). Improving access to geriatric mental health services: A randomized trial comparing treatment engagement with integrated versus enhanced referral care for depression, anxiety, and at-risk alcohol use. *The American Journal of Psychiatry*, *161*(8), 1455–1462. Evidence Level III.

Bartus, R. T., Emerich, D. F., Hotz, J., Blaustein, M., Dean, R. L., Perdomo, B., & Basile, A. S. (2003). Vivitrex, an injectable, extended-release formulation of naltrexone, provides pharmokinetic and pharmacodynamic evidence of efficacy for 1 month in rats. *Neuropsychopharmacology*, *28*(11), 1973–1982.

Betty Ford Institute Consensus Panel. (2007). What is recovery? A working definition from the Betty Ford Institute. *Journal of Substance Abuse Treatment*, *33*(3), 221–228. Evidence Level VI.

Blazer, D. G., & Wu, L. T. (2009). The epidemiology of at-risk and binge drinking among middle-aged and elderly community adults: National Survey on Drug Use and Health. *The American Journal of Psychiatry*, *166*(10), 1162–1169. Evidence Level IV.

Blow, F. (1998). *Substance abuse among older adults treatment improvement protocol (TIP) Series 26*. Retrieved from http://www.ncbi.nlm.nih.gov/books/bv.fcgi?rid=hstat5.chapter.48302. Evidence Level V.

Blow, F. C., Brower, K. J., Schulenberg, J. E., Demo-Dananberg, L. M., Young, J. P., & Beresford, T. P. (1992). The Michigan Alcoholism Screening Test–Geriatric Version (MAST-G): A new elderly-specific screening instrument. *Alcoholism: Clinical and Experimental Research*, *16*(2), 372. Evidence Level III.

Blow, F. C., Walton, M. A., Barry, K. L., Coyne, J. C., Mudd, S. A., & Copeland, L. A. (2000). The relationship between alcohol problems and health functioning of older adults in primary care settings. *Journal of the American Geriatrics Society*, *48*(7), 769–774. Evidence Level III.

Boyle, A. R., & Davis, H. (2006). Early screening and assessment of alcohol and substance abuse in the elderly: Clinical implications. *Journal of Addictions Nursing*, *17*(2), 95–103. Evidence Level VI.

Boyle, R. G., Solberg, L. I., Asche, S. E., Boucher, J. L., Pronk, N. P., & Jensen, C. J. (2005). Offering telephone counseling to smokers using pharmacotherapy. *Nicotine & Tobacco Research*, *7*(Suppl. 1), S19–S27. Evidence Level III.

Brennan, P. L., Schutte, K. K., & Moos, R. H. (2005). Pain and use of alcohol to manage pain: Prevalence and 3-year outcomes among older problem and non-problem drinkers. *Addiction, 100*(6), 777–786. Evidence Level III.

Centers for Disease Control and Prevention. (2010). Annual smoking-attributable mortality, years of potential life lost, and productivity losses—United States, 1997–2001. *Morbidity and Mortality Weekly Report, 54*(25),625–628. Evidence Level V.

Center for Substance Abuse Treatment. (1998). *Substance abuse among older adults: Treatment improvement protocol (TIP) series, number 26* (DHHS Publication No. [SMA] 98-3179). Rockville, MD: Author. Evidence Level VI.

Center for Substance Abuse Treatment. (2010). *Clinical guidelines for the use of buprenorphine in the treatment of opioid addiction: A treatment improvement protocol, series 40* (DHHS Publication [SMA] 04-3939). Rockville, MD: Substance Abuse and Mental Health Services Administration. Retrieved from http://www.samhsa.gov. Evidence Level VI.

Chait, R., Fahmy, S., & Caceres, J. (2010). Cocaine abuse in older adults: An underscreened cohort. *Journal of the American Geriatrics Society, 58*(2), 391–392. Evidence Level IV.

Colliver, J. D., Compton, W. M., Gfroerer, J. C., & Condon, T. (2006). Projecting drug use among aging baby boomers in 2020. *Annals of Epidemiology, 16*(4), 257–265. Evidence Level III.

Cooney, N. L., Babor, T. F., & Litt, M. D. (2001). Matching clients to alcoholism treatment based on severity of alcohol dependence. In R. H. Longabaugh & P. W. Wirtz (Eds.). *Project MATCH hypotheses. Results and causal chain analyses.* (*NIAAA Project MATCH monograph series, 8,* pp. 134–148. Rockville, MD; NIAAA. Evidence Level III.

Cooper, T. V., DeBon, M. W., Stockton, M., Klesges, R. C., Steenbergh, T. A., Sherrill-Mittleman, D., . . . Johnson, K. C. (2004). Correlates of adherence with transdermal nicotine. *Addictive Behaviors, 29*(8), 1565–1578.

Daniel, J., Cropley, M., Ussher, M., & West, R. (2004). Acute effects of a short bout of moderate versus light intensity exercise versus inactivity on tobacco withdrawal symptoms in sedentary smokers. *Psychopharmacology, 174*(3), 320–326. Evidence Level II.

Fink, A., Elliott, M. N., Tsia, M., & Beck, J. C. (2005). An evaluation of an intervention to assist primary care physicians in screening and educating older patients who use alcohol. *Journal of the American Geriatrics Society, 53*(11), 1937–1943. Evidence Level III.

Godsell, P. A., Whitfield, J. B., Conigrave, K. M., Hanratty, S. J., & Saunders, J. B. (1995). Carbohydrate deficient transferrin levels in hazardous alcohol consumption. *Alcohol and Alcoholism, 30*(1), 61–66. Evidence Level III.

Grant, B. F., Dawson, D. A., Stinson, F. S., Chou, S. P., Dufour, M. C., & Pickering, R. P. (2004). The 12-month prevalence and trends in DSM-IV alcohol abuse and dependence: United States, 1991–1992 and 2001–2002. *Drug and Alcohol Dependence, 74*(3), 223–234. Evidence Level IV.

Han, B., Gfroerer, J. C., Colliver, J. D., & Penne, M. A. (2009). Substance use disorder among older adults in the United States in 2020. *Addiction, 104*(1), 88–96. Evidence Level VI.

Hesse, M., Vanderplasschen, W., Rapp, R. C., Broekaert, E., & Fridell, M. (2007). Case management for persons with substance use disorders. *Cochrane Database of Systematic Reviews,* (4), CD006265. Evidence Level I.

Khavari, K. A., & Farber, P. D. (1978). A profile instrument for the quantification and assessment of alcohol consumption. The Khavari Alcohol Test. *Journal of Studies on Alcohol, 39*(9), 1525–1539. Evidence Level VI.

Kinnunen, T., Haukkala, A., Korhonen, T., Quiles, Z. N., Spiro, A., III, & Garvey, A. J. (2006). Depression and smoking across 25 years of the Normative Aging Study. *International Journal of Psychiatry in Medicine, 36*(4), 413–426. Evidence Level III.

Letizia, M., & Reinbolz, M. (2005). Identifying and managing acute alcohol withdrawal in the elderly. *Geriatric Nursing, 26*(3), 176–183. Expert Level VI.

Madras, B. K., Compton, W. M., Avula, D., Stegbauer, T., Stein, J. B., & Clark, H. W. (2009). Screening, brief interventions, referral to treatment (SBIRT) for illicit drug and alcohol use at multiple healthcare sites: Comparison at intake and 6 months later. *Drug and Alcohol Dependence, 99*(1–3), 280–295. Evidence Level III.

Mayet, S., Farrell, M., Ferri, M., Amato, L., & Davoli, M. (2005). *Psychosocial treatment for opiate abuse and dependence.* The Cochrane Collaboration. Retrieved from http://www.thecochranelibrary.com. Evidence Level I.

McLellan, A. T., Lewis, D. C., O'Brien, C. P., & Kleber, H. D. (2000). Drug dependence, a chronic medical illness: Implications for treatment, insurance, and outcomes evaluation. *Journal of the American Medical Association, 284*(13), 1689–1695. Evidence Level VI.

Merrick, E. L., Horgan, C. M., Hodgkin, D., Garnick, D. W., Houghton, S. F., Panas, L., . . . Blow, F. C. (2008). Unhealthy drinking patterns in older adults: Prevalence and associated characteristics. *Journal of the American Geriatrics Society, 56*(2), 214–223. Evidence Level III.

Moore, A. A., Karno, M. P., Grella, C. E., Lin, J. C., Warda, U., Liao, D. H., & Hu, P. (2009). Alcohol, tobacco, and nonmedical drug use in older U.S. adults: Data from the 2001/02 national epidemiologic survey of alcohol and related conditions. *Journal of the American Geriatrics Society, 57*(12), 2275–2281. Evidence Level IV.

National Center for Health Statistics. (2007). Raw data from the *National Health Interview Survey.* Retrieved from http://www.cdc.gov/nchs/nhis.htm. Evidence Level III.

National Institute on Alcohol Abuse and Alcoholism. (2000). *Updating estimates of the economic costs of alcohol abuse in the United States.* Retrieved from http://pubs.niaaa.nih.gov/publications/economic-2000/index.htm. Evidence Level IV.

National Institute on Drug Abuse. (2007). *Trends in prescriptions drug abuse: Research report series.* Retrieved from http://www.http.drugabuse.gov/ResearchReports/Prescription/prescriptions5.html. Evidence Level IV.

National Institute on Drug Abuse. (2010). *Drug abuse in the 21st century: what problems lie ahead for the baby boomers?* Retrieved from http://archives/drugabuse.gov/meetings.bbsr/prevalence.html. Evidence Level V.

National Quality Forum. (2007). *National voluntary consensus standards for the treatment of substance use conditions: Evidence-based treatment practices.* Washington, DC: Author. Retrieved from http://www.qualityforum.org. Evidence Level VI.

New York City Department of Health and Mental Hygiene. (2002). Treating Nicotine Addiction. *City Health Information, 21*(6). New York, NY: New York City Department of Health and Mental Hygiene. Evidence Level III.

Oslin, D. W. (2005). Treatment of late-life depression complicated by alcohol dependence. *The American Journal of Geriatric Psychiatry, 13*(6), 491–500. Evidence Level III.

Oslin, D. W., Pettinati, H., & Volpicelli, J. R. (2002). Alcoholism treatment adherence: Older age predicts better adherence and drinking outcomes. *The American Journal of Geriatric Psychiatry, 10*(6), 740–747. Evidence Level III.

Payne, K. T., & Marcus, D. K. (2008). The efficacy of group psychotherapy for older adult clients: A meta-analysis. *Group Dynamics: Theory, Research, and Practice, 12*(4), 268–278. Evidence Level III.

Pomerleau, C. S., Carton, S. M., Lutzke, M. L., Flessland, K. A., & Pomerleau, O. F. (1994). Reliability of the Fagerstrom Tolerance Questionnaire and the Fagerstrom Test for Nicotine Dependence. *Addictive Behaviors, 19*(1), 33–39. Evidence Level V.

Prochaska, J. O., & DiClemente, C. C. (1992). Stages of change in the modification of problem behaviors. *Progress in Behavior Modification, 28*, 183–218. Evidence Level II.

Rivers, E., Shirazi, E., Aurora, T., Mullen, M., Gunnerson, K., Sheridan, B., . . . Tomlanovich, M. (2004). Cocaine use in elder patients presenting to an inner-city emergency department. *Academic Emergency Medicine, 11*(8), 874–877. Evidence Level III.

Roberts, A. M., Marshall, E. J., & MacDonald, A. J. (2005). Which screening test for alcohol consumption is best associated with "at risk" drinking in older primary care attenders? *Primary Care Mental Health, 3*(2), 131–138. Evidence Level III.

Sachs-Ericsson, N., Collins, N., Schmidt, B., & Zvolensky, M. (2011). Older adults and smoking: Characteristics, nicotine dependence and prevalence of DSM-IV 12-month disorders. *Aging & Mental Health, 15*(1), 132–141. Retrieved from http://www.informaworld.com/smpp/content. Evidence Level III.

Satre, D. D., Mertens, J. R., Areán, P. A., & Weisner, C. (2004). Five-year alcohol and drug treatment outcomes of older adults versus middle-aged and younger adults in a managed care program. *Addiction, 99*(10), 1286–1297. Evidence Level III.

Saunders, J. B., Aasland, O. G., Babor, T. F., de la Fuente, J. R., & Grant, M. (1993). Development of the Alcohol Use Disorders Identification Test (AUDIT): WHO Collaborative Project on Early Detection of Persons with Harmful Alcohol Consumption—II. *Addiction, 88*(6), 791–804. Evidence Level III.

Schlaerth, K. R., Splawn, R. G., Ong, J., & Smith, S. D. (2004). Change in the pattern of illegal drug use in an inner city population over 50: An observational study. *Journal of Addictive Diseases, 23*(2), 95–107. Evidence Level III.

Schonfeld, L., King-Kallimanis, B. L., Duchene, D. M., Etheridge, R. L., Herrera, J. R., Barry, K. L., & Lynn, N. (2010). Screening and brief intervention for substance misuse among older adults: The Florida BRITE project. *American Journal of Public Health, 100*(1), 108–114. Evidence Level IV.

Simoni-Wastila, L., & Yang, H. K. (2006). Psychoactive drug abuse in older adults. *The American Journal of Geriatric Pharmacotherapy, 4*(4), 380–392. Evidence Level IV.

Simoni-Wastila, L., Zuckerman, I. H., Singhal, P. K., Briesacher, B., & Hsu, V. D. (2005). National estimates of exposure to prescription drugs with addiction potential in community-dwelling elders. *Substance Abuse, 26*(1), 33–42. Evidence Level III.

Smith, P. M., Reilly, K. R., Houston Miller, N., DeBusk, R. F., & Taylor, C. B. (2002). Application of a nurse-managed inpatient smoking cessation program. *Nicotine & Tobbacco Research, 4*(2), 211–222. Evidence Level III.

Srisurapanont, M., & Jarusuraisin, N. (2005). Naltrexone for the treatment of alcoholism: A meta-analysis of randomized controlled trials. *The International Journal of Neuropsychopharmacology, 8*(2), 267–280. Evidence Level III.

Substance Abuse and Mental Health Services Administration. (2000). *National Household Survey on Drug Abuse, 1998, Codebook.* Rockville, MD: Office of Applied Studies, Author. Evidence Level III.

Substance Abuse and Mental Health Services Administration. (2001). *Summary of findings from the 2000 National Household Survey on Drug Abuse: Vol. 1. Summary of national findings* (NHSDA Series H-13, DHHS Publication SMA 01-3549). Rockville, MD: Office of Applied Studies, Author. Evidence Level III.

Substance Abuse and Mental Health Services Administration. (2008). *Screening, brief intervention, and referral to treatment (SBIRT): Resource manual.* Retrieved from http://www.sbirt.samhsa.gov/core_comp/index.htm2.

Sullivan, J. T., Sykora, K., Schneiderman, J., Naranjo, C. A., & Sellers, E. M. (1989). Assessment of alcohol withdrawal: The revised Clinical Institute Withdrawal Assessment for Alcohol scale (CIWA-Ar). *British Journal of Addiction, 84*(11), 1353–1357. Evidence Level III.

The National Center on Addiction and Substance Abuse at Columbia University. (1998). *Under the rug: Substance abuse and the mature woman.* New York, NY: Author. Evidence Level IV.

Tibbitts, G. M. (2008). Sleep disorders: Causes, effects, and solutions. *Primary Care, 35*(4), 817–837. Evidence Level VI.

U.S. Census Bureau. (2008). *An older and more diverse nation by midcentury.* Retrieved from http://www.census.gov/newsroom/releases/arachives/population/cb08-123.html. Evidence Level IV.

U.S. Department of Health and Human Services. (2004a). *Substance abuse among older adults: A guide for physicians.* (DHHS Publication No. SMA 00-3394). Rockville, MD: Author, Substance Abuse and Mental Health Services Administration, Center for Substance Abuse Treatment. Evidence Level VI.

U.S. Department of Health and Human Services. (2004b). *Substance abuse among older adults: A guide for social service providers.* (DHHS Publication No. SMA 00-3393). Rockville, MD: Author, Substance Abuse and Mental Health Services Administration, Center for Substance Abuse Treatment. Evidence Level VI.

U.S. Department of Health and Human Services, National Institute on Alcohol Abuse and Alcoholism. (2005). *Helping patients who drink too much: a clinician's guide.* Rockville, MD: Author. Evidence Level VI.

Vastag, B. (2003). Addiction poorly understood by clinicians: Experts say attitudes, lack of knowledge hinder treatment. *Journal of the American Medical Association, 290*(10), 1299–1303. Evidence Level III.

Wetterling, T., Weber, B., Depfenhart, M., Schneider, B., & Junghanns, K. (2006). Development of a rating scale to predict the severity of alcohol withdrawal syndrome. *Alcohol and Alcoholism, 41*(6), 611–615. Evidence Level III.

Whitmer, R. A., Sidney, S., Selby, J., Johnston, S. C., & Yaffe, K. (2005). Midlife cardiovascular risk factors and risk of dementia in late life. *Neurology, 64*(2), 277–281. Evidence Level IV.

World Health Organization. (2000). *A systematic review of opioid antagonists for alcohol dependence. Management of substance dependence: Review series.* Retrieved from http://www.who.int/entity/substance_abuse/publications/en/opioid.pdf. Evidence Level I

Wu, L. T., & Blazer, D. G. (2011). Illicit and nonmedical drug use among older adults: A review. *Journal of Aging and Health, 23*(3), 481–504. Evidence Level IV.

Wutzke, S. E., Conigrave, K. M., Saunders, J. B., & Hall, W. D. (2002). The long-term effectiveness of brief interventions for unsafe alcohol consumption: A 10-year follow-up. *Addiction, 97*(6), 665–675. Evidence Level I.

Mistreatment Detection

27

Billy Caceres and Terry Fulmer

EDUCATIONAL OBJECTIVES

On completion of this chapter, the reader should be able:

1. to educate nurses about elder mistreatment (EM)
2. to identify the factors that make older adults vulnerable for mistreatment
3. to highlight the ill effects EM may have on an older adults' overall health status
4. to provide a framework for identifying, reporting, and managing cases of EM

OVERVIEW

Most nurses in the acute care setting have likely provided care for an older adult suffering from elder mistreatment (EM) without knowing it. In a report published by the United Nations (2007), it is estimated that the number of older adults worldwide is expected to triple by the year 2050. Cases of EM are expected to become more prevalent given the expected surge of older adults. In 2000, older adults comprised 13% of the U.S. population. By 2030, it is predicted that adults older than 65 will increase to 20% of the American population (Ebersole & Touhy, 2006). With a 274% increase since 1960, adults 85 years or older, commonly referred to as the "oldest old," are the fastest growing sector of the American population (Cowen & Cowen, 2002). The oldest old are at the greatest risk for EM because of increased vulnerability and dependence on caregivers for many aspects of care. This drastic increase in older adults may only serve to exacerbate the issue of EM. Technological advances of the past century have made it possible for those with chronic diseases to live longer; however, they require greater assistance in activities of daily living (ADL) and management of care. Now, more than ever before, it is imperative for nurses to become better educated about EM and its complexities (Ploeg, Fear, Hutchison, MacMillan, & Bolan, 2009).

Nurses in the hospital setting serve an important role in recognizing EM because they are often the first health care professionals to perform a detailed medical history or

For description of Evidence Levels cited in this chapter, see Chapter 1, Developing and Evaluating Clinical Practice Guidelines: A Systematic Approach, page 7.

physical assessment. Their presence at the patient's bedside affords nurses the opportunity for direct contact with caregivers, firsthand observations of caregivers' interactions with patients, and identify red flags (Cohen, Halevi-Levin, Gagin, & Friedman, 2006). These factors place nurses in the unique and difficult role to assess, identify, and act in cases of EM more often than other members of interdisciplinary health care teams.

Nursing has had a long history in ensuring high standards of care for older adults. The identification of EM should not be the exception. In spite of this, nurses' lack of training and knowledge of the extent of EM and its presentation may hinder their ability to identify the signs of mistreatment. Abuse is often multifactorial; therefore, it is important to recognize that it is an interplay between characteristics of the abused, the perpetrator, and environmental factors (Killick & Taylor, 2009). Physical markers of abuse are often incorrectly attributed to physiological changes in the elderly rather than EM (Wiglesworth et al., 2009). Cases of EM can prove to be challenging for nurses as it is often complicated by denial on the part of the perpetrator and older adult, refusal of services by victims, as well as fears that an accusation of EM may actually worsen abuse. Serious ethical dilemmas may arise because a nurse may struggle between his or her obligation to ensure the patient's well-being and uncertainty over presence of EM (Beaulieu & Leclerc, 2006). The development of EM protocols that are grounded in evidence-based research is crucial to ensure that EM cases are properly handled by nurses and other health care professionals.

BACKGROUND AND STATEMENT OF PROBLEM

Recent data suggest that in the United States, more than 2 million older adults suffer from at least one form of EM each year (National Research Council [NRC], 2003). The National Elder Abuse Incidence Study estimated that more than 500,000 new cases of EM occurred in 1996 (National Center on Elder Abuse [NCEA], 1998). A recent study by Acierno and colleagues (2010) estimated the prevalence of EM within a 1-year period to be approximately 11%. Although 44 states and the District of Columbia have legally required mandated reporting, EM is severely underreported. There is a lack in uniformity across the United States on how cases of EM are handled. Cases of EM are managed differently state by state with varying methods of investigation and intervention (Jogerst et al., 2003). NCEA (1998) estimates that only 16% of cases of abuse are actually reported. In a systematic review, one-third of health care professionals included believe they had detected a case of EM; however, only about 50% had actually reported the case (Cooper, Selwood & Livingston, 2009). Similarly, another study found that despite 68% of emergency medical services staff surveyed stating they felt they had encountered a case of EM in the past year, only 27% had actually made a report (Jones, Walker, & Krohmer, 1995). Despite mandatory reporting on the part of health care professionals, it is believed that many are not reporting all cases of EM that they detect (Killick & Taylor, 2009).

This creates several issues in terms of obtaining an accurate sense of the scope of EM in the country and may have serious detrimental effects for the older adults suspected of being victims of EM.

Conflicting theories of causation and lack of uniform screening approaches have further complicated EM detection. Understandably, it has been difficult for nurses to adequately respond to cases of EM when they are unclear about its manifestations, causes, and detection strategies. EM researchers agree that as the population continues to age exponentially, cases of EM will reach epidemic levels.

A lack of universally accepted definitions for different types of EM has hampered efforts to ascertain what constitutes EM. In an effort to establish a clear consensus, the NRC (2003) defined *elder mistreatment* as either "intentional actions that cause harm or create serious risk of harm (whether harm is intended) to a vulnerable elder by a caregiver or other person who is in a trust relationship to the elder," or "failure by a caregiver to satisfy the elder's basic needs or to protect himself or herself from harm."

Types of Elder Mistreatment

Six types of mistreatment are generally included under the term EM. Table 27.1 describes each form of EM as well as examples of each.

The use of the term mistreatment rather than abuse further underscores a crucial feature of EM; that EM is the outcome of the actions abuse, neglect, exploitation, or abandonment. Abuse and neglect can then be further classified as intentional or unintentional. Intentional neglect might be seen as a conscious disregard for caretaking duties that are inherent for the well-being of the older adult. Unintentional neglect might occur when caregivers lack the knowledge and resources to provide quality care (Jayawardena & Liao, 2006).

TABLE 27.1

Forms of Elder Mistreatment

Type of EM	Definition	Examples
Physical abuse	The use of physical force that may result in bodily injury, physical pain, or impairment	Hitting, beating, pushing, shoving, shaking, slapping, kicking, burning, inappropriate use of drugs, and physical restraints
Sexual abuse	Any form of sexual activity or contact without consent, including with those unable to provide consent	Unwanted touching, rape, sodomy, coerced nudity, and sexually explicit photographing
Emotional/ psychological abuse	The infliction of anguish, pain, or distress through verbal or nonverbal acts	Verbal assaults, insults, threats, intimidation, humiliation, harassment, and enforced social isolation
Financial abuse/ exploitation	The illegal or improper use of an elder's funds, property, or assets	Cashing a person's checks without authorization or permission; forging a signature; misusing or stealing money or possessions; coercing or deceiving a person into signing any document; and the improper use of conservatorship, guardianship, or power of attorney
Caregiver neglect	The refusal or failure to fulfill any part of a person's obligations or duties to an older adult, including social stimulation	Refusal or failure to provide life necessities such as food, water, clothing, shelter, personal hygiene, medicine, comfort, and personal safety
Self-neglect	The behavior of an elderly person that threatens his or her own health or safety. Disregard of one's personal well-being and home environment.	Refusal or failure to provide oneself with adequate food, water, clothing, shelter, personal hygiene, medication (when indicated), and safety precautions

Source: Fulmer, T., & Greenbery, S. (n.d.). *Elder mistreatment & abuse*. Retrieved from http://consultgerirn.org/resources

Neglect, whether intentional or unintentional, is recognized as the most commonly occurring form of EM. NCEA (1998) revealed that neglect accounts for approximately half of all cases of EM reported to Adult Protective Services (APS). About 39.3% of these cases were classified as self-neglect and 21.6% attributed to caregiver neglect, including both intentional and unintentional. More than 70% of cases received by APS are attributed to cases of self-neglect with those older than 80 years thought to represent more than half of these cases (Lachs & Pillemer, 1995).

There is much debate as to whether self-neglect should be included as a type of EM. Although other forms of EM occur because of the action or inaction of an outside perpetrator, in self-neglect, the perpetrator and victim are one and the same (Anthony, Lehning, Austin, & Peck, 2009). Several international studies studying perceptions of EM identified caregiver neglect as the most common and accepted form of EM among participants (Daskalopoulos & Borrelli, 2006; Mercurio & Nyborn, 2006; Oh, Kim, Martins, & Kim, 2006; Stathopoulou, 2004; Yan & Tang, 2003). Subjects identified family members as the caregivers more likely to be perpetrators. Shockingly, neglect was seen as a "quasi-acceptable" form of abuse, whereas physical and emotional/psychological abuses were viewed as extreme and harsh.

Theories of Elder Mistreatment

The concept of vulnerability has been central to the discussion of EM. Fulmer and colleagues (2005) conducted a study of older adult patients recruited through emergency departments in two major cities. The goal was to identify factors within the older adult–caregiver relationship that may predispose some older adults to be victims of neglect over others. The theoretical framework of the study is the risk-and-vulnerability model, which posits that neglect is caused by the interaction of factors within the older adult or in his or her environment. The risk and vulnerability model adapted to EM by Frost and Willette (1994) provides an appropriate model through which to examine EM (Frost & Willette, 1994; Fulmer et al., 2005). Vulnerability is determined by characteristics within the older adult that may make him or her more likely to be victims of EM such as poor health status, impaired cognition, history of abuse, and so forth. *Risks* refer to factors in the external environment that may predispose to EM. These may include characteristics of caregivers such as health status and functional status, as well as a lack of resources and social isolation (Fulmer et al., 2005). It is the interaction between risk and vulnerability that can predispose some older adults to EM (Killick & Taylor, 2009; Paveza, Vanderweerd, & Laumann, 2008).

The risk and vulnerability model as well as other theories from the literature on family violence have been adapted from the health and social sciences literature in an effort to find probable theories for EM. However, there has been no clear consensus on one theory that explains EM (Fulmer, Guadagno, Bitondo Dyer, & Connolly, 2004). The development of assessment interventions and strategies that cross multiple theoretical frameworks is likely to be the most clinically appropriate strategy (NRC, 2003).

Theories of EM include but are not limited to the following:

1. *Situational theory:* Promotes the idea that EM is a result of caregiver strain due to the overwhelming tasks of caring for a vulnerable or frail older adult (Wolf, 2003).
2. *Psychopathology of the abuser:* Abuse is believed to stem from a perpetrator's own battle with psychological illness such as substance use, depression, and other mental disorders (Wolf, 2003).

3. *Exchange theory:* Speculates that the long-established dependencies present in the victim–perpetrator relationship are part of the "tactics and response developed in family life, which continue into adulthood" (Wolf, 2003).
4. *Social learning theory:* Attributes EM to learned behavior on the part of the perpetrator or victim from either their family life or the environment; abuse is seen as the norm (Wolf, 2003).
5. *Political economy theory:* Focuses on how older adults are often disenfranchised in society as their prior responsibilities and even their self-care are shifted on to others (Wolf, 2003).

Dementia and Elder Mistreatment

Older adults with dementia are particularly vulnerable to EM. As the population of older adults increases, it is expected that so will the number of older adults with dementia (Wiglesworth et al., 2010). It is estimated that older adults with dementia will rise from 4.5 million in 2000 to 13 million by the year 2050 (Hebert, Scherr, Bienias, Bennett, & Evans, 2003). Because of the cognitive deficits present in older adults with dementia, it is particularly difficult to screen for EM. The older adult may not be able to give a reliable history, and signs of EM may be masked or mimicked by disease (Fulmer et al., 2005). Those providing care for older adults with dementia are at particular risk for caregiver strain and burnout. Disruptive behavior such as screaming or wailing, physical aggression, or crying can be exhausting for caregivers in any setting (Lachs, Becker, Siegal, Miller, & Tinetti, 1992).

One study reported that as many as 47% of older adults with dementia were victims of some form of EM (Wiglesworth et al., 2010). The researchers used a combination of two screening instruments as well as a caregiver self-report. Similarly, in a systematic review, one-third of caregivers of older adults with dementia were willing to admit to some form of EM, whereas 5% admitted to physical abuse (Cooper, Selwood, & Livingston, 2008). In a community-based study of caregivers of older adults with dementia, 51% of caregivers admitted to verbal abuse and 16% to physical abuse. However, only 4% admitted to neglect (Cooney, Howard, & Lawlor, 2006). The ramifications of these data are sobering. If 30% will admit to EM, there is every reason to worry regarding EM in those who do not report.

Objective assessment alone cannot capture all cases of EM and, thus, a policy is needed that incorporates both objective measures as well as a discussion with both the older adult and caregiver (Cooper et al., 2008). Most caregivers are forthcoming with admission of EM and many of them ask for help in developing coping strategies and plans of care to provide better care for care recipients (Wiglesworth et al., 2010).

ASSESSMENT OF THE PROBLEM

The American Medical Association (AMA, 1992) released a set of guidelines and recommendations in 1992 on the management of EM. The AMA urged providers that all older adults should be screened for EM. Many hospitals already include EM screening as part of the admission process for all patients older than 65 years old. Assessment of EM is not an easy task. Subtle signs of EM are hard to identify and even harder to substantiate (Anthony et al., 2009). Rates of reporting on the part of health care professionals are still low due in large part to ageism in society and lack of education and training on the assessment, detection, and reporting of EM. Unsubstantiated fears exist that increasing education on assessment of EM will lead to higher rates of false positive cases and, therefore, expense and disruption in the system. However, a systematic review of 32 studies revealed that health care professionals educated about EM were not more likely to detect EM cases but were more inclined to report detected cases than those that had little or no education related to EM (Cooper et al., 2009).

The complexity and variability of most cases of EM makes it hard to describe what a typical perpetrator or a victim looks like. There is no correlation found between age, gender, race, and any association with EM (Krienert, Walsh, & Turner, 2009). Hence, it is difficult to describe who is a "typical" victim or perpetrator of EM. Some research suggests that victims of EM are more likely to be unable to provide for self-care needs on their own because of cognitive or physical deficits and have a history of depression (Giurani & Hasan, 2000). In a small scale, victims of EM had lower scores on cognitive screens using the mini-mental status exam (MMSE) and greater functional deficits as scored with the Katz Index of Independence in ADL. They also had higher rates of depression when screened with the Geriatric Depression Scale (GDS) scores (Dyer, Pavlik, Murphy, & Hyman, 2000). These studies support earlier findings from a longitudinal study on factors influencing mortality of victims of EM (Lachs, Williams, O'Brien, Pillemer, & Charlson, 1998). Others (Draper et al., 2008; Fulmer et al., 2005) have also identified a link between childhood abuse among victims and physical and sexual EM later in life. A lack of social support and social isolation increase the risk for EM in older adults (Acierno et al., 2010; Dong & Simon, 2008; Fulmer et al., 2005).

Research suggests perpetrators are more likely to be family members, report greater caregiver strain, live with the victim, have a history of mental illness and/or depression, history of substance abuse, have lived with the victim for an extended time (approximately 9.5 years), have few social supports, and have a long history of conflicts with the victim (Cowen & Cowen, 2002; Giurani & Hasan, 2000; Wiglesworth et al., 2010).

In the clinical setting while conducting an EM screen, it is recommended to separate the older adult from the caregiver and obtain a detailed history and physical assessment (Heath & Phair, 2009). Special attention should be paid to both physical and psychological signs of EM. Discrepancies between injury presentation or severity and the report of how the injury occurred as well as discrepancies between explanations from the caregiver and older adult should be paid close attention. Physically abused older adults are more likely to have significantly larger bruises and to know the cause of their bruise. Further, these abused older adults are more likely to display bruising on the face, lateral aspect of the right arm and the posterior torso (including back, chest, lumbar, and gluteal regions; Wiglesworth et al., 2009). Other possible indicators of physical abuse include bruises at various stages of healing, unexplained frequent falls, fractures, dislocations, burns, and human bite marks (Cowen & Cowen, 2002).

It is important to distinguish that signs and symptoms of EM may vary depending on the type of abuse. Table 27.2 provides strategies for assessment of each type of EM. Victims of sexual abuse are more likely to be female and exhibit "genital or urinary irritation or injury; sleep disturbance; extreme upset when changed, bathed, or examined; aggressive behaviors; depression; or intense fear reaction to an individual" (Chihowski & Hughes, 2008, p. 381). Ageist attitudes among health care professionals may limit the amount of cases of sexual abuse that are identified as older adults are rarely thought of as the usual victims of abuse (Vierthaler, 2008). Victims of financial abuse are harder to identify; however, they share similar traits such as social isolation, physical dependency, and mental disorders as victims of emotional or psychological abuse and neglect (Peisah et al., 2009).

> TABLE 27.2

Assessment of Elder Mistreatment

Type of Mistreatment	Questions Used to Assess Type of EM	Physical Assessment and Signs and Symptoms
Physical abuse	Has anyone ever tried to hurt you in any way? Have you had any recent injuries? Are you afraid of anyone? Has anyone ever touched you or tried to touch you without permission? Have you ever been tied down? Suspected evidence of physical abuse (i.e., black eye) ask: —How did that get there? —When did it occur? —Did someone do this to you? —Are there other areas on your body like this? —Has this ever occurred before?	Assess for: bruises (more commonly bilaterally to suggest grabbing), black eyes, welts, lacerations, rope marks, fractures, untreated injuries, bleeding, broken eyeglasses, use of physical restraints, sudden change in behavior. Note if a caregiver refuses an assessment of the older adult alone. Review any laboratory tests. Note any low- or high-serum prescribed drug levels. Note any reports of being physically mistreated in any way.
Emotional/ Psychological abuse	Are you afraid of anyone? Has anyone ever yelled at you or threatened you? Has anyone been insulting you and using degrading language? Do you live in a household where there is stress and/or frustration? Does anyone care for you or provide regular assistance to you? Are you cared for by anyone who abuses drugs or alcohol? Are you cared for by anyone who was abused as a child?	Assess cognition, mood, affect, and behavior. Assess for: agitation, unusual behavior, level of responsiveness, and willingness to communicate. Delirium Dementia Depression Note any reports of being verbally or emotionally mistreated.
Sexual abuse	Are you afraid of anyone? Has anyone ever touched you or tried to touch you without permission? Have you ever been tied down? Has anyone ever made you do things you did not want to do? Do you live in a household where there is stress and/or frustration? Does anyone care for you or provide regular assistance to you? Are you cared for by anyone who abuses drugs or alcohol? Are you cared for by anyone who was abused as a child?	Assess for: bruises around breasts or genital area; sexually transmitted diseases; vaginal and/or anal bleeding; or discharge, torn, stained, or bloody clothing/ undergarments. Note any reports of being sexually assaulted or raped.

(continued)

TABLE 27.2

Assessment of Elder Mistreatment *(continued)*

Type of Mistreatment	Questions Used to Assess Type of EM	Physical Assessment and Signs and Symptoms
Financial abuse/ exploitation	Who pays your bills? Do you ever go to the bank with him or her? Does this person have access to your account(s)? Does this person have power of attorney? Have you ever signed documents you did not understand? Are any of your family members exhibiting a great interest in your assets? Has anyone ever taken anything that was yours without asking? Has anyone ever talked with you before about this?	Assess for: changes in money handling or banking practice, unexplained withdrawals or transfers from patient's bank accounts, unauthorized withdrawals using the patient's bank card, addition of names on bank accounts/cards, sudden changes to any financial document/will, unpaid bills, forging of the patient's signature, appearance of previously uninvolved family members. Note any reports of financial exploitation.
Caregiver neglect	Are you alone a lot? Has anyone ever failed you when you needed help? Has anyone ever made you do things you did not want to do? Do you live in a household where there is stress and/or frustration? Does anyone care for you or provide regular assistance to you? Are you cared for by anyone who abuses drugs or alcohol? Are you cared for by anyone who was abused as a child?	Assess for: dehydration, malnutrition, untreated pressure ulcers, poor hygiene, inappropriate or inadequate clothing, unaddressed health problems, nonadherence to medication regimen, unsafe and/or unclean living conditions, animal/insect infestation, presence of lice and/or fecal/urine smell, and soiled bedding. Note any reports of feeling mistreated.
Self-neglect	How often do you bathe? Have you ever refused to take prescribed medications? Have you ever failed to provide yourself with adequate food, water, or clothing?	Assess for: dehydration, malnutrition, poor personal hygiene, unsafe living conditions, animal/insect infestation, fecal/urine smell, inappropriate clothing, nonadherence to medication regimen.

Source: Fulmer, T., & Greenbery, S. (n.d.). *Elder mistreatment & abuse*. Retrieved from http://consultgerirn.org/resources

Since the 1970s, a myriad of screening instruments have been developed to detect cases of EM, but few are appropriate for inpatient older adults. Most have had limited testing in the acute care setting and focus on in-home assessments or extensive questions that are better suited for primary care settings.

The *Elder Assessment Instrument* (EAI) developed by Fulmer and colleagues (2004) is a 41-item screening instrument that requires training on how to administer it but has been proven effective in busy hospital settings (Perel-Levin, 2008). The current EAI-R (revised in 2004) is considered more appropriate for inpatient and outpatient clinics because it relies on objective assessment by the clinician such as general appearance, assessment for dehydration, physical and psychological markers, or pressure ulcers as well as subjective information received from the patient.

The *Hwalek-Sengstock Elder Abuse Screening Test* (HS-EAST) is a 15-item instrument that relies on self-report from older adults and is documented as appropriate for detecting physical abuse, vulnerability, and high-risk situations. Some instruments focus on the caregiver, but an advantage of HS-EAST is the focus on the older adult history. It is regarded as appropriate for use in the hospital setting and can be easily administered by nurses (Fulmer et al., 2004; Perel-Levin, 2008). If a positive screen is noted, detailed physical assessment and medical history should be completed to substantiate possible abuse. Referral to experts in trauma or geriatrics, either on or off site, should take place for the best available input.

In addition to these screening instruments for EM, there are a number of other reliable and valid instruments that can aid nurses in identifying those at risk for EM. As discussed previously, victims of EM tend to have lower functional and cognitive capabilities than their counterparts. The Katz Index of Independence in ADL and/or the Lawton instrumental activities of daily living (IADL) scale may help in detecting older adults with functional deficits (Graf, 2007; Wallace, 2007). Similarly, with higher rates of depression in victims of EM, the GDS may be a useful instrument for nurses to use in the hospital setting. It is a 15-item screening instrument that is effective at distinguishing depressed older adults (Kurlowicz & Greenberg, 2007). In the literature, perpetrators of EM often report higher caregiver strain. The Modified *Caregiver Strain Index* (CSI) is a reliable and self-administered instrument that can aid in assessing caregivers that may benefit from intervention strategies to alleviate stress involved with caregiving demands (Sullivan, 2007).

The process of identifying cases of self-neglect is oftentimes even more daunting than other cases of EM. Assessing self-neglect is further complicated by a lack of standardized screening instruments or markers for detection (Dyer et al., 2006; Kelly, Dyer, Pavlik, Doody, & Jogerst, 2008; Mosqueda et al., 2008). Several researchers are currently developing screening instruments for self-neglect. However, their use in the acute care setting is limited. Most require in-depth assessments of home life and are based mostly on objective findings from the health care professional. Nevertheless, data suggests that detection of self-neglect in the hospital setting is unfortunately made easier because by the time these cases reach the hospital, they are often very severe (Mosqueda et al., 2008). Signs of self-neglect may include lack of adequate nutrition such as dehydration; changes in weight; poor hygiene and appearance such as soiled clothing, uncombed hair, debris in teeth; poor adherence to medical treatments such as unfilled prescriptions; refusing to perform dressing changes; poor glucose monitoring; and so forth (Cohen et al., 2006; Naik, Teal, Pavlik, Dyer, & McCullough, 2008). Objective measures as well as questioning of the older adult about health patterns and activities of self-care are also important factors in detecting self-neglect because it can yield important information about attitudes and opinions of the older adult.

INTERVENTIONS AND CARE STRATEGIES

Detailed screening of older adults at risk for EM is the first step in identifying cases of EM (Perel-Levin, 2008). There are various screening instruments that can help in revealing older adults and caregivers at risk for EM. Setting aside time to meet with the older patient and their caregiver separately is an important aspect of the screening process. This can highlight any inconsistencies in depictions of how injuries occur, allow the nurse to develop a closer relationship with each, as well as express his or her willingness to help each party.

Nurses should not work alone in detecting cases of EM but, instead, should include professionals from other disciplines as much as possible. According to the literature, when EM is suspected, the use of interdisciplinary teams with professionals from both the acute care and community settings is the best approach to managing such cases (Wiglesworth, Mosqueda, Burnight, Younglove, & Jeske, 2006). Institutions should develop clear guidelines for practitioners to follow when cases of EM are identified (Perel-Levin, 2008). Referral to appropriate community organizations is paramount to ensure safe discharges for suspected victims of EM. Interdisciplinary teams work best when they include team members with expertise in various disciplines including nursing, social work, law, and so forth. It is this diversity of skills that allows for innovative approaches to managing cases of EM (Jayawardena & Liao, 2006).

Educating older adults, staff, and caregivers about the nature of EM is key. It is crucial to educate older adults that have the cognitive capacity to accept or refuse interventions about patterns of EM such that abuse tends to increase in severity over time (Cowen & Cowen, 2002; Phillips, 2008). For individuals who lack the cognitive capacity to consent for interventions, it is important to report these cases to APS and develop a plan for safe discharge. Older adults should receive emergency contact information as well as community resources (Cowen & Cowen, 2002).

Interdisciplinary teams should also take into account the difficulties caregivers may experience in caring for adults with diminished functional and/or cognitive capacity and provide these caregivers with support services and interventions of their own to assist them in providing the best care they can (Lowenstein, 2009). Services should be offered not only to victims of EM but also to their suspected perpetrators. Helping caregivers gain a better understanding of proper care techniques may help alleviate cases of neglect in particular.

Because of the nature of hospital stays, most of the long-term interventions currently occur in the community setting. A systematic review of interventions for EM revealed that interventions tend to concentrate on the situational theory of abuse by focusing on education, counseling, and social support for perpetrators of EM to better cope with stressors of caregiving (Ploeg et al., 2009). However, even these community-based interventions have shown mixed results in terms of effectiveness when studying factors such as risk of recurrence of EM; levels of depression and self-esteem in older adults; and levels of caregiver strain, stress, and depression in caregivers (Ploeg et al., 2009).

In the acute care setting, patients are assumed to have the autonomy to refuse medical treatments and participate in care management as long as there are deemed to be able to give informed consent. However, what can be done if the older adult is refusing to perform activities deemed essential for their health and well-being? The answer, at the moment, is very little because there is currently no rigorously tested screening instrument to assess cognitive capacity in this population (Naik et al., 2008). Naik et al. (2008) discuss the ethical dilemma that is present when an older adult is suspected of self-neglect. If the older adult is deemed to have the cognitive capacity to make decisions about their own self-care, there is very little that health care professionals can do to intervene. Interdisciplinary health care teams are thought to be the most effective way of identifying self-neglect. Although it may seem difficult and costly to implement interdisciplinary health care teams to adequately treat this group of older adults, the costs of not connecting these individuals to proper resources can be much greater as their health conditions can go undiagnosed and untreated for longer time, therefore creating greater health care costs (Lowenstein, 2009).

There is inherent difficulty in evaluating the success of interventions implemented in acute care organizations. The nature of discharges makes it difficult to learn about outcomes in cases of EM. Not all suspected victims of EM will return to the same institution for repeat visits, and confidentiality issues can restrict information sharing among health care professionals.

CASE STUDY

Mr. Jack is an 89-year-old male admitted to a medical unit for dehydration. His 77-year-old wife is at his bedside. Upon initial assessment, the nurse notices Mr. Jack is confused, weak, and pale. He is also underweight with a body mass index (BMI) of 16. When asked about his cognitive status, Mrs. Jack reports that he was diagnosed with early dementia last year.

His vital signs are as follows: blood pressure of 88/46 mm Hg, heart rate of 123 beats per minute, respiratory rate of 26 breaths per minute, and a temperature of 101.8 °F. He is unable to verbalize a pain score; however, he does not appear to be in any pain at this moment.

Upon performing an EM assessment, the nurse gathers the following information from Mrs. Jack: Her husband has lost a total of 20 pounds in recent months and has been refusing to eat for the past week. Mrs. Jack's mobility is limited because of multiple sclerosis and their neighbor who used to accompany them to appointments has moved away. Their son, John, had to move in with them a year ago after he lost his job. Mr. Jack and his son have never had the best relationship and often argue about their living arrangements that have made them all very depressed. Also, John has stopped searching for a job and drinks alcohol often. John refuses to take Mr. Jack to see his primary care provider stating that these changes in his health are "just because he's so old."

Mr. Jack is now on intravenous hydration and is being followed by a dietitian regarding his nutrition. His vital signs and mental status have improved. Further testing reveals Mr. Jack has an esophageal tumor, which may be the cause of his discomfort.

Discussion

This may be considered a case of neglect and/or psychological abuse. Their son knows that his father's health has been deteriorating and yet refuses to obtain him proper medical attention. He also often argues with his father and may be abusing alcohol. From Mrs. Jack's report, there is no evidence of other forms of EM; however, the case should be investigated further. Although the nurse has yet to meet John, there are a number of signs to indicate that neglect or psychological/emotional abuse may be occurring in this home. As a mandated reporter, the nurse should report this case if he or she suspects any form of EM is present.

A number of risk factors are present in this family to alert the nurse to possible EM. For example, Mr. Jack has cognitive deficits because of dementia and is frail because of his present cancer diagnosis. In addition, his wife has several functional deficits because of her multiple sclerosis; she reports feeling depressed by her current situation and lacks a solid support system.

The nurse should discuss the case with Mr. Jacks' medical team as well as his social worker. The dietitian would be the good source of information for the family about Mr. Jack's nutritional needs. The nurse should collaborate with the family and interdisciplinary team to identify community services for this family.

SUMMARY

With a rapidly aging population, it is likely that cases of EM will become more prevalent. Although most research on EM has focused on EM in the community and long-term care settings, the acute care setting is a good location for the identification of those at risk for EM. EM prevalence is hard to estimate, yet most experts in the field believe it is heavily underreported because of various factors. As providers of care, it is nurses' responsibility to develop an understanding and appreciation for the complexities involved in detecting and responding to cases of EM. The recognition of markers of EM is an important step in guaranteeing that older adult patients are receiving high-quality care.

The different manifestations and types of EM often make it challenging for nurses to determine the best course of action. However, the strategies included in this chapter serve as a framework to help nurses navigate these types of situations. These strategies include best practices from the literature on EM that is applicable for acute care nurses.

Nurses serve as important advocates for older adults who may not be able to protect themselves from EM. They should encourage their institutions to develop guidelines for managing suspected cases of EM as well as establishing interdisciplinary teams to decide how to best respond in these circumstances. EM detection should be embedded within admission and nursing assessments of older adults. There is no telling how many older adults and their caregivers may benefit from a greater focus on EM. It is only through education and the use of interdisciplinary teams to respond to EM cases that nurses can ensure the safety and well-being of older adults in their care.

NURSING STANDARD OF PRACTICE

Protocol 27.1: Detection of Elder Mistreatment

I. GOAL: Identify best practices in identifying and responding to cases of EM

II. OVERVIEW: With the projected increase in the population of older adults worldwide and the rise in medical and technological advances, it is anticipated that older adults will be living longer. Therefore, it is expected that cases of EM, although currently underreported, will be on the rise. As patient advocates and providers of care, nurses serve an important function in the screening and treatment of cases of EM. However, current data shows that nurses and other health care professionals are not reporting all cases of EM they encounter either because of lack of knowledge about manifestations of EM or how reporting and investigation by state agencies functions.

III. BACKGROUND/STATEMENT OF PROBLEM
  A. Definitions
  1. *Elder mistreatment*: "Intentional actions that cause harm or create serious risk of harm (whether harm is intended) to a vulnerable elder by a caregiver or other person who is in a trust relationship to the elder," or "failure by a caregiver to satisfy the elder's basic needs or to protect himself or herself from harm (NRC, 2003)." Conflicting casual theories of EM:

(continued)

Protocol 27.1: Detection of Elder Mistreatment *(cont.)*

2. *Physical abuse:* The use of physical force that may result in bodily injury, physical pain, or impairment (NCEA, 2008).

3. *Sexual abuse:* Any form of sexual activity or contact without consent, including with those unable to provide consent (NCEA, 2008).

4. *Emotional/psychological abuse:* The infliction of anguish, pain, or distress through verbal or nonverbal acts (NCEA, 2008).

5. *Financial abuse/exploitation:* The illegal or improper use of an elder's funds, property, or assets (Naik et al., 2008).

6. *Caregiver neglect:* The refusal or failure to fulfill any part of a person's obligations or duties to an older adult, including social stimulation (NCEA, 2008).

7. *Self-neglect:* The behavior of an older adult that threatens his or her own health or safety. Disregard of one's personal well-being and home environment (NCEA, 2008).

8. *Risk-vulnerability model:* Posits that neglect is caused by the interaction of factors within the older adult and his or her environment. The risk and vulnerability model adapted to EM by Frost and Willette (1994) provides a good lens through which to examine EM. *Vulnerability* is determined by characteristics within the older adult that may make him or her more likely to be abused by caregivers such as poor health status, impaired cognition, history of abuse, and so forth. Risks refer to factors in the external environment that may contribute to EM (Frost & Willette, 1994; Fulmer et al., 2005).

9. *Psychopathology of the abuser:* Abuse is believed to stem from a perpetrator's own battle with psychological illness such as substance use, depression, and other mental disorders (Wolf, 2003).

10. *Exchange theory:* Speculates that the long-established dependencies present in the victim–perpetrator relationship are part of the "tactics and response developed in family life, which continue into adulthood" (Wolf, 2003).

11. *Social learning theory:* Attributes EM to learned behavior on the part of the perpetrator or victim from either their family life or the environment; abuse is seen as the norm (Wolf, 2003).

12. *Political economy theory:* Focuses on how older adults are often disenfranchised in society as their prior responsibilities and even their self-care are shifted on to others. [28]

B. Characteristics of Victims

1. Decreased ability to complete ADLs and more physically frail (Frost & Willette, 1994; Peisah et al., 2009; Dyer et al., 2000).

2. Cognitive deficits such as dementia (Fulmer et al., 2005; Gorbien & Eisenstein, 2005; Naik et al., 2008).

3. History of childhood trauma (Fulmer et al., 2005; Lachs et al., 1998).

4. Depression and other mental disorders, as well as an increased sense of hopelessness (Dyer et al., 2000; Fulmer et al., 2005).

5. Social isolation and lack of support systems (Draper et al., 2008; Dyer et al., 2000; Peisah et al., 2009).

6. History of substance abuse (Dyer et al., 2000; Peisah et al., 2009).

(continued)

Protocol 27.1: Detection of Elder Mistreatment *(cont.)*

C. Characteristics of Perpetrators
  1. Family member in 80% or more of cases (Cowen & Cowen, 2002).
  2. Long history of conflict with the victim (Krienert et al., 2009).
  3. Live with victim for an extended time (Wiglesworth et al., 2010).
  4. Higher rates of caregiver strain (Wiglesworth et al., 2010).
  5. History of mental illness (Wiglesworth et al., 2010).
  6. Depression and other mental disorders (Wiglesworth et al., 2010).
  7. Social isolation and lack of support systems (Wiglesworth et al., 2010).
D. Etiology and/or Epidemiology
  1. Recent data suggests that in the United States, more than 2 million older adults suffer from at least one form of EM each year (NRC, 2003).
  2. The National Elder Abuse Incidence Study estimates that more than half a million new cases of EM occurred in 1996 (NCEA, 1998).
  3. Even though 44 states and the District of Columbia have legally required mandated reporting, EM is severely underreported. There is a lack in uniformity across the United States on how cases of EM are handled (NCEA, 1998).
  4. NCEA, (1998) estimates that only 16% of cases of abuse are actually reported.
  5. The National Council on Elder Abuse revealed that neglect accounts for approximately half of all cases of EM reported to APS. About 39.3% of these cases were classified as self-neglect and 21.6% attributed to caregiver neglect, including both intentional and unintentional (NRC, 2003).
  6. Over 70% of cases received by APS are attributed to cases of self-neglect with those older than 80 years thought to represent more than half of these cases (Lachs & Pillemer, 1995).

IV. PARAMETERS OF ASSESSMENT
A. See Table 27.2.

V. NURSING CARE STRATEGIES
A. Detailed screening to assess for risk factors for EM using a combination of physical assessment, subjective information, and data gathered from screening instruments (Perel-Levin, 2008).
B. Strive to develop a trusting relationship with the older adult as well as the caregiver. Set aside time to meet with each individually (Perel-Levin, 2008).
C. The use of interdisciplinary teams with a diversity of experience, knowledge, and skills can lead to improvements in the detection and management of cases of EM. Early intervention by interdisciplinary teams can help lower risk for worsening abuse and further deficits in health status (Jayawardena & Liao, 2006; Wiglesworth et al., 2010).
D. Institutions should develop guidelines for responding to cases of EM (Perel-Levin, 2008; Wiglesworth et al., 2010).
E. Educate victims about patterns of EM such that EM tends to worsen in severity overtime (Cowen & Cowen, 2002; Phillips, 2008).
F. Provide older adults with emergency contact numbers and community resources (Cowen & Cowen, 2002).
G. Referral to appropriate regulatory agencies.

(continued)

Protocol 27.1: Detection of Elder Mistreatment *(cont.)*

VI. EVALUATION AND EXPECTED OUTCOMES

A. Reduction of harm through referrals, use of interdisciplinary interventions and/or relocation to a safer situation and environment.

B. Victims of EM express an understanding how to access appropriate services.

C. Caregivers take advantage of services such as respite care or treatment for mental illness or substance use.

D. If possible, evaluate progress in relationships between caregiver and older adult through screening instruments such as The Modified CSI and GDS.

E. Institutions establish clear and evidence-based guidelines for management of EM cases.

VII. FOLLOW-UP MONITORING OF CONDITION

A. Follow-up monitoring in the acute care setting is limited compared to the follow-up that may be performed in the community or long-term care settings.

VIII. RELEVANT PRACTICE GUIDELINES

A. American Medical Association. *Diagnostic and treatment guidelines on elder abuse and neglect.* Chicago, IL: Auhtor.

B. Aravanis, S. C., Adelman, R. D., Breckman, R., Fulmer, T. T., Holder, E., Lachs, M., . . . Sanders, A. B. (1993). Diagnostic and treatment guidelines on elder abuse and neglect. *Archives of Family Medicine, 2,* 371–388.

C. Jones, J., Dougherty, J., Schelble, D., & Cunningham, W. (1988). Emergency department protocol for the diagnosis and evaluation of geriatric abuse. *Annals of Emergency Medicine, 17*(10), 1006–1015.

D. Neale, A., Hwalek, M., Scott, R., Sengstock, M., & Stahl, C. (1991). Validation of the Hwalek-Sengstock elder abuse screening test. *Journal of Applied Gerontology, 10,* 406–418.

E. Phillips, L. R., & Rempusheski, V. F. (1985). A decision-making model for diagnosing and intervening in elder abuse and neglect. *Nursing Research, 34*(3), 134–139.

RESOURCES

Administration on Aging
http://www.aoa.gov/

Elder Mistreatment Assessment
http://consultgerirn.org/resources

Journal of Elder Abuse & Neglect
http://www.informaworld.com/smpp/title~content=t792303995~db=all

National Center on Elder Abuse
http://www.ncea.aoa.gov/ncearoot/Main_Site/index.asp

REFERENCES

Acierno, R., Hernandez, M. A., Amstadter, A. B., Resnick, H. S., Steve, K., Muzzy, W., & Kilpatrick, D. G. (2010). Prevalence and correlates of emotional, physical, sexual, and financial abuse and potential neglect in the United States: The National Elder Mistreatment Study. *American Journal of Public Health*, *100*(2), 292–297. Evidence Level IV.

American Medical Association. (1992). *Diagnostic and treatment guidelines on elder abuse and neglect.* Chicago, IL: Author.

Anthony, E. K., Lehning, A. J., Austin, M. J., & Peck, M. D. (2009). Assessing elder mistreatment: Instrument development and implications for adult protective services. *Journal of Gerontological Social Work*, *52*(8), 815–836.

Beaulieu, M., & Leclerc, N. (2006). Ethical and psychosocial issues raised by the practice in cases of mistreatment of older adults. *Journal of Gerontological Social Work*, *46*(3–4), 161–186. Evidence Level V.

Chihowski, K., & Hughes, S. (2008). Clinical issues in responding to alleged elder sexual abuse. *Journal of Elder Abuse & Neglect*, *20*(4), 377–400.

Cohen, M., Halevi-Levin, S. H., Gagin, R., & Friedman, G. (2006). Development of a screening tool for identifying elderly people at risk of abuse by their caregivers. *Journal of Aging and Health*, *18*(5), 660–685. Evidence Level IV.

Cooney, C., Howard, R., & Lawlor, B. (2006). Abuse of vulnerable people with dementia by their carers: Can we identify those most at risk? *International Journal of Geriatric Psychiatry*, *21*(6), 564–571.

Cooper, C., Selwood, A., & Livingston, G. (2008). The prevalence of elder abuse and neglect: A systematic review. *Age and Ageing*, *37*(2), 151–160. Evidence Level I.

Cooper, C., Selwood, A., & Livingston, G. (2009). Knowledge, detection, and reporting of abuse by health and social care professionals: A systematic review. *The American Journal of Geriatric Psychiatry*, *17*(10), 826–838. Evidence Level I.

Cowen, H. J., & Cowen, P. S. (2002). Elder mistreatment: Dental assessment and intervention. *Special Care in Dentistry*, *22*(1), 23–32.

Daskalopoulos, M. D., & Borrelli, S. E. (2006). Definitions of elder abuse in an Italian sample. *Journal of Elder Abuse & Neglect*, *18*(2–3), 67–85. Evidence Level IV.

Dong, X., & Simon, M. A. (2008). Is greater social support a protective factor against elder mistreatment? *Gerontology*, *54*(6), 381–388. Evidence Level IV.

Draper, B., Pfaff, J. J., Pirkis, J., Snowdon, J., Lautenschlager, N. T., Wilson, I., & Almeida, O. P. (2008). Long-term effects of childhood abuse on the quality of life and health of older people: Results from the depression and early prevention of suicide in general practice project. *Journal of the American Geriatrics Society*, *56*(2), 262–271. Evidence Level II.

Dyer, C. B., Kelly, P. A., Pavlik, V. N., Lee, J., Doody, R. S., Regev, T., . . . Smith, S. M. (2006). The making of a self-neglect severity scale. *Journal of Elder Abuse & Neglect*, *18*(4), 13–23.

Dyer, C. B., Pavlik, V. N., Murphy, K. P., & Hyman, D. J. (2000). The high prevalence of depression and dementia in elder abuse or neglect. *Journal of the American Geriatrics Society*, *48*(2), 205–208. Evidence Level IV.

Ebersole, P., & Touhy, T. A. (2006). *Geriatric nursing: Growth of a specialty* (p. 22). New York, NY: Springer Publishing Company.

Frost, M. H., & Willette, K. (1994). Risk for abuse/neglect: Documentation of assessment data and diagnoses. *Journal of Gerontological Nursing*, *20*(8), 37–45.

Fulmer, T., & Greenbery, S. (n.d.). *Elder mistreatment & abuse.* Retrieved from http://consultgerirn .org/resources

Fulmer, T., Guadagno, L., Bitondo Dyer, C., & Connolly, M. T. (2004). Progress in elder abuse screening and assessment instruments. *Journal of the American Geriatrics Society*, *52*(2), 297–304.

Fulmer, T., Paveza, G., VandeWeerd, C., Fairchild, S., Guadagno, L., Bolton-Blatt, M., & Norman, R. (2005). Dyadic vulnerability and risk profiling in elder neglect. *The Gerontologist, 45*(4), 525–534. Evidence Level IV.

Giurani, F., & Hasan, M. (2000). Abuse in elderly people: The Granny Battering revisited. *Archives of Gerontology and Geriatrics, 31*(3), 215–220. Evidence Level V.

Gorbien, M. J., & Eisenstein, A. R. (2005). Elder abuse and neglect: An overview. *Clinics in Geriatric Medicine, 21*(2), 279–292. Evidence Level V.

Graf, C. (2007). *The lawton instrumental activities of daily living scale.* Retrieved from http://consultgerirn.org/resources

Heath, H., & Phair, L. (2009). The concept of frailty and its significance in the consequences of care or neglect for older people: An analysis. *International Journal of Older People Nursing, 4*(2), 120–131. doi: 10.1111/j.1748–3743.2009.00165.x. Evidence Level V.

Hebert, L. E., Scherr, P. A., Bienias, J. L., Bennett, D. A., & Evans, D. A. (2003). Alzheimer disease in the US population: Prevalence estimates using the 2000 census. *Archives of Neurology, 60*(8), 1119–1122. Evidence Level IV.

Jayawardena, K. M., & Liao, S. (2006). Elder abuse at end of life. *Journal of Palliative Medicine, 9*(1), 127–136. Evidence Level V.

Jogerst, G. J., Daly, J. M., Brinig, M. F., Dawson, J. D. Schmuch, G. A., & Ingram, J. G. (2003). Domestic elder abuse and the law. *American Journal of Public Health, 93*(12), 2131–2136.

Jones, J. S., Walker, G., & Krohmer, J. R. (1995). To report or not to report: Emergency services response to elder abuse. *Prehospital and Disaster Medicine, 10*(2), 96–100. Evidence Level IV.

Kelly, P. A., Dyer, C. B., Pavlik, V., Doody, R., & Jogerst, G. (2008). Exploring self-neglect in older adults: Preliminary findings of the self-neglect severity scale and next steps. *Journal of the American Geriatrics Society, 56*(Suppl. 2), S253–S260.

Killick, C., & Taylor, B. J. (2009). Professional decision making on elder abuse: Systematic narrative review. *Journal of Elder Abuse & Neglect, 21*(3), 211–238. Evidence Level I.

Krienert, J. L., Walsh, J. A., & Turner, M. (2009). Elderly in America: A descriptive study of elder abuse examining National Incident-Based Reporting System (NIBRS) data, 2000–2005. *Journal of Elder Abuse & Neglect, 21*(4), 325–345. Evidence Level V.

Kurlowicz, L., & Greenberg, S. (2007). *The geriatric depression scale.* Retrieved from http://consultgerirn.org/resources

Lachs, M. S., Becker, M., Siegal, A. P., Miller, R. L., & Tinetti, M. E. (1992). Delusions and behavioral disturbances in cognitively impaired elderly persons. *Journal of the American Geriatrics Society, 40*(8), 768–773.

Lachs, M. S., & Pillemer, K. (1995). Abuse and neglect of elderly persons. *The New England Journal of Medicine, 332*(7), 437–443.

Lachs, M. S., Williams, C. S., O'Brien, S., Pillemer, K. A., & Charlson, M. E. (1998). The mortality of elder mistreatment. *Journal of the American Medical Association, 280*(5), 428–432. Evidence Level II.

Lowenstein, A. (2009). Elder abuse and neglect—"old phenomenon": New directions for research, legislation, and service developments. (2008 Roswalie S. Wolf Memorial Elder Abuse Prevention Award—International Category Lecture). *Journal of Elder Abuse & Neglect, 21*(3), 278–287. Evidence Level V.

Mercurio, A. E., & Nyborn, J. (2006). Cultural definitions of elder maltreatment in Portugal. *Journal of Elder Abuse & Neglect, 18*(2–3), 51–65. Evidence Level IV.

Mosqueda, L., Brandl, B., Otto, J., Stiegel, L., Thomas, R., & Heisler, C. (2008). Consortium for research in elder self-neglect of Texas research: Advancing the field for practitioners. *Journal of the American Geriatrics Society, 56*(Suppl. 2), S276–S280.

Naik, A. D., Teal, C. R., Pavlik, V. N., Dyer, C. B., & McCullough, L. B. (2008). Conceptual challenges and practical approaches to screening capacity for self-care and protection in vulnerable older adults. *Journal of the American Geriatrics Society, 56*(Suppl. 2), S266–S270.

National Center on Elder Abuse. (1998). *The national elder abuse incidence study: Final report.* Retrieved from http://aoa.gov/AoARoot/AoA_Programs/Elder_Rights/Elder_Abuse/docs/ABuseReport_Full.pdf

National Center on Elder Abuse. (2008). *Information about laws related to elder abuse.* Retrieved from http://www.ncea.aoa.gov/NCEAroot/Main_Site/Library/Laws/InfoAboutLaws_08_08.aspx

National Research Council. (2003). *Elder mistreatment: Abuse, neglect, and exploitation in an aging America.* Panel to Review Risk and Prevalence of Elder Abuse and Neglect. In R. J. Bonnie & R. B. Wallace (Eds.), Committee on National Statistics and Committee on Law and Justice, Division of Behavioral and Social Sciences and Education. Washington, DC: The National Academies Press.

Oh, J., Kim, H. S., Martins, D., & Kim, H. (2006). A study of elder abuse in Korea. *International Journal of Nursing Studies, 43*(2), 203–214.

Paveza, G., Vandeweerd, C., & Laumann, E. (2008). Elder self-neglect: A discussion of a social typology. *Journal of the American Geriatrics Society,* 56(Suppl. 2), S271–S275.

Peisah, C., Finkel, S., Shulman, K., Melding, P., Luxenberg, J., Heinik, J., . . . Bennett, H. (2009). The wills of older people: Risk factors for undue influence. *International Psychogeriatrics/IPA, 21*(1), 7–15. Evidence Level V.

Perel-Levin, S. (2008). *Discussing screening for elder abuse at the primary health care level.* Retrieved from World Health Organization http://www.who.int/ageing/publications/Discussing_Elder_Abuseweb.pdf

Phillips, L. R. (2008). Abuse of aging caregivers: Test of a nursing intervention. *Advances in Nursing Science, 31*(2), 164–181. Evidence Level II.

Ploeg, J., Fear, J., Hutchison, B., MacMillan, H., & Bolan, G. (2009). A systematic review of interventions for elder abuse. *Journal of Elder Abuse & Neglect, 21*(3), 187–210. Evidence Level I.

Stathopoulou, G. (2004). Greece. In K. Malley-Morrison (Ed.), *International perspectives on family violence and abuse: A cognitive ecological approach* (pp. 131–149). Mahwah, NJ: Lawrence Erlbaum Associates Publishers. Evidence Level V.

Sullivan, M. T. (2007). *The Modified Caregiver Strain Index.* Retrieved from http://consultgerirn.org/resources

United Nations. (2007). *World population prospects: The 2006 revision.* Retrieved from http://www.un.org/esa/population/publications/wpp2006/English.pdf

Vierthaler, K. (2008). Best practices for working with rape crisis centers to address elder sexual abuse. *Journal of Elder Abuse & Neglect, 20*(4), 306–322. Evidence Level V.

Wallace, M. (2007). *Katz index of independence in activities of daily living.* Retrieved from http://consultgerirn.org/resources

Wiglesworth, A., Austin, R., Corona, M., Schneider, D., Liao, S., Gibbs, L., & Mosqueda, L. (2009). Bruising as a marker of physical elder abuse. *Journal of the American Geriatrics Society, 57*(7), 1191–1196. Evidence Level IV.

Wiglesworth, A., Mosqueda, L., Burnight, K., Younglove, T., & Jeske, D. (2006). Findings from an elder abuse forensic center. *The Gerontologist, 46*(2), 277–283. Evidence Level IV.

Wiglesworth, A., Mosqueda, L., Mulnard, R., Liao, S., Gibbs, L., & Fitzgerald, W. (2010). Screening for abuse and neglect of people with dementia. *Journal of the American Geriatrics Society, 58*(3), 493–500. Evidence Level IV.

Wolf, R. (2003). Elder abuse and neglect: History and concepts. In R. J. Bonnie, & R. B. Wallace (Eds.), *Elder Mistreatment: Abuse, Neglect, and Exploitation in an Aging America. Panel to Review Risk and Prevalence of Elder Abuse and Neglect* (pp. 238–248). Committee on National Statistics and Committee on Law and Justice, Division of Behavioral and Social Sciences and Education. Washington, DC: The National Academies Press.

Yan, E., & Tang, C. S. (2003). Proclivity to elder abuse: A community study on Hong Kong Chinese. *Journal of Interpersonal Violence, 18*(9), 999–1017. Evidence Level IV.

Health Care Decision Making

28

Ethel L. Mitty and Linda Farber Post

EDUCATIONAL OBJECTIVES

On completion of this chapter, the reader should be able to:

1. define informed consent and the supporting bioethical and legal principles
2. understand the role of culture in health care decision making
3. differentiate between competence and capacity
4. understand the process of decisional capacity assessment
5. describe the nurse's role and responsibility as an advocate for the patient's voice in health care decision making

OVERVIEW

Health care is about decisions. Until the latter half of the 20th century, patients were told what health care interventions would benefit them and they rarely questioned the doctor's instructions. The rise of the rights movement in most areas of society promoted the idea that patients would benefit from robust participation in decision making affecting their health outcomes. Building on the well-established doctrine of informed consent, as well as statutory and case law, all states came to require that patient wishes and values be central to health care decisions. The result was a greater degree of clinician–patient collaboration in planning and implementing care decisions.

Although all health care activities require principled and thoughtful decision making, treatment, and diagnostic interventions—because of their benefit-burden-risk calculus—typically require specific informed consent by or on behalf of the patient. For this reason, the determination of decision-making capacity, authority, and standards becomes a most pressing clinical issue when deciding about treatment or diagnostic interventions.

For description of Evidence Levels cited in this chapter, see Chapter 1, Developing and Evaluating Clinical Practice Guidelines: A Systematic Approach, page 7.

BACKGROUND AND STATEMENT OF PROBLEM

Ethical Principles and Professional Obligations

Core ethical principles that underlie the health care decision process and give rise to clinician obligations include

- respect for autonomy: supporting and facilitating the capable patient's exercise of self-determination;
- beneficence: promoting the patient's best interest and well-being and protecting the patient from harm;
- nonmaleficence: avoiding actions likely to cause the patient harm; and
- distributive justice: allocating fairly the benefits and burdens related to health care delivery (Beauchamp & Childress, 2001).

These principles and the professional obligations they create often give rise to conflict and tension for clinicians. For example, care providers have a duty to respect patients' autonomy by honoring their decisions *and* protecting them from the harm of risky choices. Care providers are also expected to provide care to patients who need it *and* be responsible stewards of limited resources. Clinical, legal, and ethically valid decisions by or for patients invoke a careful balancing of information, principles, rights, and responsibilities in light of medical realities, cultural factors, and, increasingly, concerns about resource allocation.

Autonomy and Capacity

The well-settled right to determine what shall be done with one's own body has two equally important components: the right to consent to treatment and the right to refuse treatment. Grounded in the ethical principle of respect for persons, this right to bodily integrity is considered so fundamental that it is protected by the U.S. Constitution, state constitutions, and decisions of the U.S. Supreme Court (*Cruzan v. Director*, 1990). All persons are considered to have the potential for autonomy, expressed in the clinical setting through informed decision making. The threshold question is whether they have the *capacity* to act autonomously.

Respect for autonomy is widely considered to be the ethical principle most central to health care decision making because of its emphasis on self-governance and choices that reflect personal values. This heightened emphasis on self-determination is largely a Western phenomenon and not universally shared. Capable patients who are easily confused or with diminished or fluctuating capacity, or who are from cultures that do not consider autonomy a central value, may not be capable of or comfortable with pure autonomous decision making. Instead, they may involve trusted others in planning their care, thus exhibiting *assisted*, *supported*, or *delegated* autonomy as their preferred method of decision making. For these patients, autonomy may not be reflected in self-determined decision making about treatment, but in expressions of values and goals of care. Drawing on the assistance or support of trusted others does not diminish the integrity of the process. Voluntarily delegating decision-making authority to others is also an autonomous choice but it is one that must be explicitly confirmed, not inferred.

Diminished or fluctuating capacity is not a reason to ignore the patient's voice but is an indicator to attend more carefully to what is being communicated. The "what" and "how" of the treatment may be a decision of others to make; the "why" in the patient's voice must be heard.

Consent and Refusal

In the clinical setting, the principle of respect for autonomy is most clearly expressed in the doctrine of informed consent and refusal (Beauchamp et al., 2001). Because therapeutic and diagnostic interventions typically involve a range of benefits, burdens, and risks, express consent is almost always required before they are implemented. Consent should be a process over time rather than a single event or a signed document. Among adults with a language barrier associated with education and/or ethnicity, comprehension might be limited (Fink et al., 2010). Providing adequate time for the informed consent discussion(s) and the opportunity for "repeat back" by the patient of specific facts might improve understanding. As an expression of autonomy, the consent process can be solitary or, more likely, a collaborative process that includes consultation with clinicians, family, and trusted others.

Capable patients or surrogates acting on behalf of patients without capacity are engaged in a process, which is considered to include the following elements:

- Evidence of decisional capacity
- Disclosure of sufficient information relevant to the decision in question
- Understanding of the information provided
- Voluntariness (a patient's right to make health care choices free of any undue influence) in choosing among the options, and, based on these,
- Consent to or refusal of the intervention (Lo, 2000)

Education can improve decisional capacity to give safe, informed consent even for clinically depressed older adults (Lapid, Rummans, Pankratz, & Appelbaum, 2004). In one study, depressed patients' involvement in health care decision making not only increased the likelihood of their receiving treatment congruent with depression treatment guidelines but also showed reduced symptoms of depression over an 18-month period (Clever et al., 2006). "Framing" can be persuasive; a clinician's emphasis on the distinctions about the efficacy of a treatment and whether it would be curative or palliative can influence a patient's decision even more than information given about the disease or treatment options (Van Kleffens, van Baarsen, & van Leeuwen, 2004).

Decision-Making Authority

Treatment decisions are typically made by capable patients based on their goals and values in response to information they receive about their diagnosis, prognosis, and therapeutic options. These decisions are, thus, an expression of autonomy, reflecting the view that health care is not something that is *done to* patients; rather, it is a collaborative endeavor in which patients and clinicians contribute to the shared goal of recovery, rehabilitation, or palliation.

Readiness for decision making has a temporal, as well as a contextual, component. Older adults and their caregivers, asked in focus groups why they had or had not been involved in any advanced care planning (ACP), revealed considerable variability in their readiness for discussion of different components of the ACP process such as advance directive creation, communication with family and physicians, and consideration of their treatment goals (Fried, Bullock, Iannone, & O'Leary, 2009). Participants identified barriers and benefits to ACP and said that it was not the only way to prepare for decline in health or death. Prior experience with health care decision making for others influenced older adults' propensity to engage in ACP. Having an active role in shared decision making is associated with enhanced cancer-specific quality of life, satisfaction, and more likely use of adjuvant therapy for women with breast cancer but not for men with prostate cancer (Hack et al., 2010; Mandelblatt, Kreling, Figeuriedo, & Feng, 2006).

When patients are not capable of making decisions about their treatment, others are asked to choose for them basing their decisions as much as possible on what is known of the patients' preferences or what is considered to be in their best interest. The determination of decision-making authority is among the most critical tasks in the clinical setting. When patients lack the ability to make treatment decisions, authority to act on their behalf must be vested in others—appointed agents, family, or other surrogates. The threshold determination, then, is of the patient's decisional capacity: an assessment of an individual's ability to make decisions about health care and treatment.

Decision Aids

Decision aids assist, guide, and support a decision-making process that requires consideration of benefits, burdens, risks, and options. Studies indicate that decision aids lead to decisions that are value-based, more informed, less conflicted, and characterized by a process that is more participatory than passive compared to standard decision-making approaches (O'Connor et al., 2009). Decision aids made a difference in physician–patient discussion about the use of adjuvant therapy for women with breast cancer (Siminoff, Gordon, Silverman, Budd, & Ravdin, 2006); clarified values and options, and increased knowledge regarding breast and ovarian genetic testing counseling (Wakefield et al., 2008); and improved men's knowledge of the risks and benefits of prostate-specific antigen (PSA) testing (Watson et al., 2006). An "order effect" was discerned regarding the sequence in which information was presented in a decision aid to women with breast cancer (Ubel et al., 2010). The order of presentation of information about the risks and benefits of tamoxifen influenced their perceptions. Bias was eliminated by the simultaneous presentation of information of competing options and risks.

ASSESSMENT OF THE PROBLEM
Decision-Making Capacity

Although the terms *capacity* and *competence* are often used interchangeably, in the health care setting, their distinctions go beyond semantics. Competence is a *legal* presumption that an adult has the mental ability to negotiate various legal tasks such as entering into a contract, making a will, and standing for trial (Beauchamp & Childress, 2001). Incompetence is a judicial determination that because a person lacks this ability, she should be prevented from doing certain things (Beauchamp & Childress, 2001). Capacity is a *clinical* determination that a person has the ability to understand, make, and take responsibility for the consequences of health care decisions (Beauchamp & Childress, 2001). Because the legal system should rarely be involved in medical decisions, the patient's capacity for decision making is an assessment made by clinicians.

The importance of capacity determination resides in the presumption that adults have decisional capacity and, absent contrary evidence, treatment decisions defer to patient wishes. This deference usually extends to all decisions made by capable individuals, including those decisions that appear risky or ill advised. Capacity assessment is important because patients who lack the ability to appreciate the implications of, and accept responsibility for, their choices are vulnerable to the risks of deficient decision making. Whereas honoring the decisions of a capable patient demonstrates respect for the person, honoring the decisions of a patient without capacity is an act of abandonment. Thus, clinicians have an obligation to ensure that capable patients have the opportunity to make treatment decisions that will be implemented and incapacitated patients will be protected by having decisions made for them by others who act in their best interest.

Fulfilling this obligation requires that clinicians appreciate the characteristics of decision-making capacity, the elements of which include the ability to

- understand and process information about diagnosis, prognosis, and treatment options;
- weigh the relative benefits, burdens, and risks of the care options;
- apply a set of values to the analysis;
- arrive at a decision that is consistent over time; and
- communicate the decision (Roth, Meisel, & Lidz, 1997).

Capacity assessment depends on interaction with the patient over time rather than on specific tests. There is no gold standard instrument or "capacimeter" that assesses decisional capacity (Kapp & Mossman, 1996). The Mini-Mental Status Examination (MMSE) estimates orientation, long- and short-term memory, and mathematical and language dexterity. It is not a test of executive function (an assessment more likely to capture reasoning and recall) and is, therefore, less helpful in gauging the patient's ability to understand the implications of a decision (Allen et al., 2003). It has been suggested, however, that an MMSE score less than 19 or more than 23 might be able to distinguish those with and without capacity for decision making (Karlawish, Casarett, James, Xie, & Kim, 2005). The Assessment of Capacity for Everyday Decision-Making (ACED) is a reportedly valid and reliable instrument to assess everyday decisional capacity in those with mild-to-moderate cognitive impairment (Lai et al., 2008). Its use in facilitating assessment of health care decision-making capacity has not been reported but could be explored in future studies.

Although there is no consistent standardized definition of decisional capacity, there is sufficient evidence that safe and sufficient decision making is retained in early stage dementia (Kim, Karlawish, & Caine, 2002). Persons with mild-to-moderate dementia can make or at least participate in making treatment decisions, but impaired memory recall might be a barrier to their demonstrating their understanding of treatment options (Moye, Karel, Azar, & Gurrera, 2004). Standard assessment of appreciation of diagnostic and treatment information should focus on the patient's ability to state the importance or implications of the choice on his or her future health. Specific neuropsychological tests (e.g., MacArthur Competence Assessment Tool, Hopemont Capacity Assessment Interview) can predict decisional capacity for those with mild-to-moderate dementia, although reasoning and appreciation might differ among those with mental illness (Gurrera, Moye, Karel, Azar, & Armesto, 2006).

The standard of decision making most highly valued by a group of geriatricians, psychologists, and ethics committee members was the ability to appreciate the consequences of a decision, followed by the ability to respond "yes" or "no" to a question; the standard least supported was that the decision had to seem reasonable (Volicer & Ganzini, 2003).

Clinical Importance of Decisional Capacity

Accurate and useful capacity assessment depends on the recognition that capacity is decision-specific rather than global. For example, a person with diminished capacity may be able to decide what to have for lunch or when to shower without undue risk of harm. Evidence also suggests that adults with mild-to-moderate mental retardation are able to make and provide a rationale for their treatment decisions and evaluate the risks and benefits of treatment options (Cea & Fisher, 2003). Because most people have the ability to make some decisions and not others, respect for autonomy requires clinicians to identify the widest range of decisions each patient is capable of making. A note in the chart saying, "Patient lacks decision-making capacity" arbitrarily precludes the individual from making any decisions about anything when, in fact, the patient may only lack the ability to make complex treatment decisions. Far more helpful would be an entry that says, "Patient lacks the capacity to make decisions about participation in a drug study."

Likewise, decisional capacity may not be constant but may fluctuate, depending on the patient's clinical condition, medication, and/or time of day. Among gerontological nurses, protecting the right of older adults with diminished capacity or physical function to make those health care decisions that they can appropriately make is among their top practice concerns (Alford, 2006). It is imperative for the protection of those with mild-to-moderate dementia that their understanding and reasoning about treatments and interventions is periodically assessed (Moye, Karel, Gurrera, & Azar, 2006). Approaching patients for discussions and decisions, when they are at their most capable (e.g., during the patient's "window of lucidity"), enhances their opportunities to participate in planning their health care.

Whereas disagreement with a proposed care plan or refusal of recommended treatment does not by itself demonstrate incapacity, risky or potentially harmful decisions should be carefully scrutinized to protect vulnerable patients from the consequences of deficient decision making. Because appointing a health care agent requires a lower level of capacity than that needed to make the often complex decisions the agent will make, even patients with diminished capacity may be able to select the persons they want to speak for them (Mezey, Teresi, Ramsey, Mitty, & Bobrowitz, 2002).

Decision Making in the Absence of Capacity

The more difficult clinical scenario is decision making on behalf of patients who have lost or never had the capacity to make decisions for themselves. Two approaches have been developed in response to the needs of incapacitated patients: advance directives and surrogate decision making. Advance directives (see Chapter 29, Advance Directives) include the living will (a list of interventions the patient does or does not want in specified circumstances) and the preferred directive, the health care proxy (the appointment of a health care agent with the same decision-making authority as the patient).

It is estimated that only 19%–36% of the adult population in the United States has an advance directive. As such, the majority of health care decisions for incapacitated patients are made by surrogates. Absent explicit instructions from the patient and decisions by others are based on either substituted judgment (when the patient's wishes are known or can be inferred) or the best interest standard (when the patient did not have or articulate treatment preferences). Substituted judgment assesses what the *patient* would choose based on prior statements and patterns of decision making. The best interest standard is the *surrogate's* evaluation of the proposed intervention's benefits and burdens to the patient.

A health care surrogate may be any competent adult older than 18 years of age who, although not specifically chosen or legally appointed by a patient, assumes the responsibility for making health care decisions on behalf of a person who does not have the ability to do so. Informal surrogates are individuals, usually family or others close to the patient, who are asked by the care team to participate in making treatment decisions. Formal surrogates may be specified by state law in a hierarchy, typically in descending order of relation to the patient. Most states accord considerable latitude to surrogates, especially next of kin, in consenting to treatment. Decisions about limiting treatment are more problematic and may be significantly restricted, depending on the state in which the patient is receiving care (see Resources, American Bar Association Commission on Law & Aging for state guidelines).

Context of Health Care Decision Making

Individual treatment preferences can change as a patient's health and functional status changes (Fried et al., 2006). Previously unacceptable treatment states may become more acceptable. For example, patients already experiencing pain are less likely to refuse a treatment outcome that includes being in pain than patients who are not currently experiencing moderate-to-severe pain (Fried et al., 2006). Additionally, patients may have different treatment and comfort goals than those of their family caregivers and professional providers (Steinhauser et al., 2000).

Just as there is the right to know one's medical information, there is also a right not to be burdened with unwanted information. Older adults from cultures that traditionally shield patients from knowing about their illness may prefer to have information given to and decision making assumed by a particular family member, the family as a group, or trusted others. Although it is important to respect patient preferences and cultural traditions, a patient's waiver of the disclosure obligation must be explicitly confirmed, not presumed. Because of the implementation of Health Insurance Portability and Accountability Act of 1996 (HIPAA), many hospitals have a form for the patient to sign, designating the preferred decision maker. Another approach is to ask, "When we have information about your condition and decisions will need to be made, who would you like us to talk to? Would you like to be part of those discussions? What would make you comfortable?"

Trust in professional health care providers is a critical element in health care, certainly in decision-making situations where information is given and questions have to be answered. Various factors influence information exchange and shared decision making among providers and patients (Edwards, Davies, & Edwards, 2009). Providers are influenced by their susceptibility or responsiveness to informed patients and patients' interest in decision making, limited knowledge of patients' culture, and a tendency to stereotype patients rather than view them as individuals. Patients are influenced by their personal motivation to obtain and use information, cultural identity and expression, health literacy, and their ability to manage the possibility of receiving distressing information. Of note, a shared influence among providers and patients was sick-role expectation (Edwards et al., 2009). African American patients have been shown to be significantly more likely than White patients to report low trust, unrelated to age or socioeconomic status (Halbert, Armstrong, Gandy, & Shaker, 2006) of the U.S. health care system, and have little interest in advance directive creation and ACP (Cox et al., 2006). This is not to say, however, that Black and minority ethnic populations do not want to participate in health care decision making, including decisions at the end of life.

Quality-of-Life Considerations in Decision Making

There is almost universal acknowledgement of the patient's desire to be comfortable (i.e., relieved of pain and suffering) and to achieve a sense of completion. Attitudes about the importance of clergy, of being physically touched, and using all available technology may differ among patients, families, and caregivers. Older adults with varying degrees of functional impairment and past experiences with treatment decision making were more interested in the outcome of a serious medical event than with the curative interventions and with whether the intervention could restore or maintain their ability to participate in activities they valued (Rosenfeld, Wenger, & Kagawa-Singer, 2000). Among older adults with end-stage renal disease, the decision to begin dialysis was influenced by their family caregiving responsibilities, feeling that they had no other options, and that they currently enjoyed life and were not ready to contemplate their death (Visser et al, 2009). Those who rejected dialysis were more often male, older, and widowers in comparison to those who accepted dialysis. They imagined that they would experience a loss of autonomy and a continuing trajectory of functional loss, have difficulty getting to the dialysis center, and have to start thinking about the future—a prospect that was unappealing to them at the time. These findings speak to the contextual and temporal nature of health care decision making as has been explored by others (Fried et al., 2009).

INTERVENTIONS AND CARE STRATEGIES

Assessing the patient's orientation and understanding can provide critical information about decision-making behavior in different circumstances as well as the ability to articulate care wishes. Reporting that a patient is "disoriented to time and place" is helpful only in establishing the context in which more focused and useful assessment of decisional capacity should take place.

Documentation needs to be specific and descriptive. The entry should describe the circumstances or interaction(s) that led to the conclusion about the patient's ability to make decisions. Because capacity is decision-specific, accurate and useful statements are "Patient appears to lack the capacity to make decisions about discharge" "She is unable to describe how she will cook or get to the bathroom at home" or "Patient lacks the capacity to make decisions about surgery; he was unable to name the type of surgery, what the surgery is supposed to correct, or what is involved or to be expected during recovery."

Communicating information includes determining what the patient and/or surrogate(s) need or want to know and what they understand. Having the relevant medical facts available in lay language and avoiding jargon is essential. It is also important to consider the participants in the decision making: Who should be present? What is their relationship to the patient? What is their decisional authority? What information is necessary; at what level of detail and how will it be used? When is the information to be provided and over what period? (Popejoy, 2005) Language interpreters might be the only health care staff who recognize that surrogate decision makers and the physician or health care professionals have differing interpretations of illness, treatment, and health; disparate views about death and dying; and use language and a decision-making framework differently. An interpreter may realize that truth telling might not only be perceived as disrespectful and dangerous but able to shorten the patient's life span, as believed in certain cultures. As such, an interpreter is more than a word-for-word translator but, rather, can serve as a mediator, culture broker, patient advocate, witness, educator, and participant who interpret fact and nuance.

CASE STUDY

Mr. Peters is an 85-year-old man with advanced Alzheimer's disease who has been living in a nursing home for the past 6 months. When he stopped eating several weeks ago, he was hospitalized for percutaneous endoscopic gastrostomy (PEG) tube insertion to provide artificial nutrition and hydration. He returned to the nursing home briefly but developed uncontrolled diarrhea and apparent abdominal discomfort. Two days ago, his PEG tube fell out and he has been readmitted to the hospital for treatment of the diarrhea and possible replacement of the PEG.

Mr. Peters opens his eyes and responds to painful stimuli but does not interact and appears not to recognize family members. He is clearly incapable of participating in discussions or decisions about his care. His close family includes his son and granddaughter, who are visiting from California, and his grandson, Jason, who has been very involved for several years in providing and deciding about Mr. Peters's care.

A clinical ethics consultation has been convened, including Mr. Peters's family, his two attending physicians, the house and nursing staff who have cared for him most consistently, and the bioethicist. Discussion focuses on clarifying his condition and probable clinical course, the goals of care, and his likely care preferences.

Jason describes his grandfather as very active and fiercely independent until age 78, when his dementia began. With his wife, he had raised Jason and, when she died, he continued to raise the boy alone until Jason left for college. When the dementia worsened several years ago, Jason arranged for his grandfather and a team of 24-hour caregivers to move into an apartment next to his. That arrangement continued until Mr. Peters required care that could best be provided in a skilled nursing facility.

All three family members agree that, given Mr. Peters's personality, values, and lifetime behavior pattern, he would not have wanted to be maintained in his current condition, certainly not dependent on artificial nutrition and hydration. Nevertheless, they express concern about the ethics, legality, and clinical effect of not replacing the PEG tube, and are especially uncomfortable about whether it would be considered "starving" him to death.

According to the care team, Mr. Peters's advanced dementia is not reversible and he will continue to deteriorate mentally and physically until death. The doctors referred to the considerable literature demonstrating that, in patients with advanced dementia, artificial nutrition and hydration can cause gastrointestinal (GI) distress, including nausea, bloating, gas, and diarrhea, which appears to have happened to Mr. Peters. In the opinion of the care team, continued artificial nutrition and hydration would only contribute to the patient's suffering and prolong the dying process. The doctors also explain that, far from suffering, Mr. Peters appears more comfortable because the PEG fell out and the diarrhea has stopped. They assure the family that the patient could be admitted to the nursing home's hospice unit where he will receive comfort care, including pain and other symptom management. The bioethicist addressed the relevant ethical issues discussed in subsequent texts.

(continued)

CASE STUDY *(continued)*

Discussion

The ethics analysis of this case focuses on decision making for an incapacitated patient, promoting the patient's best interest and protecting him from harm, and forgoing life-sustaining treatment, specifically artificial nutrition and hydration, at the end of life.

Surrogate decision making on behalf of patients lacking capacity uses the following standards:

- ■ The patient's wishes as expressed directly through discussions with others or in advance directives (health care proxy appointments or living wills)
- ■ Substituted judgment (when the patient's wishes are known or can be inferred)
- ■ The best interest standard (when the patient's wishes are not known or inferable; Beauchamp & Childress, 2001).

Mr. Peters has not left any explicit instructions but, his family, knowing him very well, is able to predict with confidence what he would and would not have wanted based on his characteristic patterns of behavior and decision making. In this case, the family's substituted judgment is consistent with what was considered by the family and the care team to be in the patient's best interest—protecting him from continued artificial nutrition and hydration that would have increased his suffering without providing benefit and prolonged his dying. Framing this as *protecting* the patient from the burdens and risks of an intervention rather than *depriving* him of necessary treatment can make this decision more tolerable for distressed families.

One of the most difficult surrogate decisions is forgoing life-sustaining treatment and because providing nourishment is so intimately associated with love and nurturing, forgoing artificial nutrition and hydration is especially wrenching for families and caregivers. Clinicians, ethicists, and courts have consistently agreed that artificial nutrition and hydration is a medical treatment, the benefits, burdens, and risks of which should be assessed like those of any other intervention.

Capable patients and the appointed health care agents of incapacitated patients have a well-settled right to refuse any treatment, including those that are life-sustaining. Absent capacity or advance directives, the family's authority to make end-of-life decisions, including forgoing artificial nutrition and hydration depends on the laws of the state in which the patient is treated. Many states permit family and surrogates authorized by case or statutory law to make these decisions based on substituted judgment or their assessment of the patient's best interest in light of the patient's condition and prognosis. Other states require surrogates, even next of kin, to provide explicit evidence that the patient would have refused artificial nutrition and hydration in order to authorize withholding or withdrawing the interventions.

SUMMARY

The notion of "ownership" of one's body should apply to health care decision making even at times of crisis. Even patients with diminished or fluctuating decisional capacity should not be denied the opportunity to make the specific health care decisions they are capable of making. A vulnerable patient who lacks capacity, despite some social or conversational skills, needs to be protected from the potentially harmful effects of uninformed, poorly reasoned, and potentially risky health care decisions. It is suggested that the best way for nurses to learn older adults' informational needs, avoid paternalism, and promote their best interests is to simply ask them (Tuckett, 2006). The ethical obligations that must be assumed by health care professionals are skillfully assessing the clinical situation, the benefits, burdens and risks of the therapeutic options, the patient's capacity to make and take responsibility for the relevant decisions, and the surrogate's need for information, guidance, and support.

NURSING STANDARD OF PRACTICE

Protocol 28.1: Health Care Decision Making

I. GOALS
To ensure nurses in acute care:
  A. Understand the supporting bioethical and legal principles of informed consent.
  B. Are able to differentiate between competence and capacity.
  C. Understand the issues and processes to assess decisional capacity.
  D. Can describe the nurse's role and responsibility as an advocate for the patient's voice in health care decision making.

II. OVERVIEW
  A. Capable persons (i.e., those with decisional capacity) have a well-established right, grounded in law and Western bioethics, to determine what is done to their bodies.
  B. In any health care setting, the exercise of autonomy (self-determination) is seen in the process of informed consent to and refusal of treatment and/or care planning.
  C. Determination of decision-making capacity is a compelling clinical issue because treatment and diagnostic interventions have the potential for significant benefit, burden, and/or risk.
  D. Honoring the decisions of a capable patient demonstrates respect for the person; honoring the decisions of a patient without capacity is an act of abandonment.

III. BACKGROUND AND STATEMENT OF THE PROBLEM
  A. Introduction
    1. Core ethical principles that are the foundation of clinician obligation are the following:
      a. Respect for autonomy, beneficence, nonmaleficence, and distributive justice.
      b. Clinically, legally, and ethically valid decisions by or for patients requires a careful balancing of information, principles, rights, and responsibili-

(continued)

Protocol 28.1: Health Care Decision Making *(cont.)*

ties in light of medical realities, cultural factors and, increasingly, concerns about resource allocation.

   c. Even capable patients, including those who are older adults, easily confused or from cultures that do not consider autonomy a central value, as well as patients with diminished or fluctuating capacity, may not be capable of or comfortable with exercising purely autonomous decision making.

   d. Care professionals have an obligation to be alert to questionable or fluctuating capacity both in patients who refuse and those who consent to recommended treatment. Capable individuals may choose to make their own care decisions or they may voluntarily delegate decision-making authority to trusted others. Delegation of decisional authority must be explicitly confirmed, not inferred.

   e. The context of decision making can include cultural imperatives and taboos, perceptions of pain, suffering and quality of life and death, education and socioeconomic status, language barriers, and advance health care planning.

B. Definitions

   1. *Consent.* The informed consent process requires evidence of decisional capacity, disclosure of sufficient information, understanding of the information provided, voluntariness in choosing among the options, and, on those bases, consent to or refusal of the intervention.

   2. *Competence.* A *legal* presumption that an adult has the mental ability to negotiate various legal tasks (e.g., entering into a contract, making a will).

   3. *Incompetence.* A *judicial* determination that a person lacks the ability to negotiate legal tasks and should be prevented from doing so.

   4. *Decisional capacity.* A *clinical* determination that an individual has the ability to understand and to make and take responsibility for the consequences of health decisions. Because capacity is not global but decision-specific, patients may have the ability to make some decisions but not others. Capacity may fluctuate according to factors, including clinical condition, time of day, medications, and psychological and comfort status.

C. Essential Elements

   1. Decisional capacity reflects the ability to understand the facts, appreciate the implications, and assume responsibility for the consequences of a decision.

   2. The elements of decisional capacity: the ability to understand and process information; weigh the relative benefits, burdens, and risks of each option; apply personal values to the analysis; arrive at a consistent decision; and communicate the decision.

   3. Standards of Decision Making

      a. Prior explicit articulation: decision based on the previous expression of a capable person's wishes through oral or written comments or instructions.

      b. Substituted judgment: decision by others based on the formerly capable person's wishes that are known or can be inferred from prior behaviors or decisions.

      c. Best interests standard: decision based on what others judge to be in the best interest of an individual who never had or made known health care wishes and whose preferences cannot be inferred.

(continued)

Protocol 28.1: Health Care Decision Making *(cont.)*

IV. ASSESSMENT OF DECISIONAL CAPACITY

A. There is no gold standard instrument to assess capacity.

B. Assessment should occur over time, at different times of day, and with attention to the patient's comfort level.

C. The Mini-Mental Status Examination (MMSE) or Mini-Cog Test is not a test of capacity. Tests of executive function might better approximate the reasoning and recall needed to understand the implications of a decision.

D. Clinicians agree that the ability to understand the consequences of a decision is an important indicator of decisional capacity.

E. Safe and sufficient decision making is retained in early stage of dementia (Kim et al., 2002) and by adults with mild-to-moderate mental retardation (Cea & Fisher, 2003).

V. NURSING CARE STRATEGIES

A. Communicate with patient and family or other/surrogate decision makers to enhance their understanding of treatment options.

B. Be sensitive to racial, ethnic, religious, and cultural mores and traditions regarding end-of-life care planning, disclosure of information, and care decisions.

C. Be aware of conflict resolution support and systems available in the care-providing organization.

D. Observe, document, and report the patient's ability to
   1. articulate his or her needs and preferences,
   2. follow directions,
   3. make simple choices and decisions (e.g., "Do you prefer the TV on or off?" "Do you prefer orange juice or water?"), and
   4. communicate consistent care wishes.

E. Observe period(s) of confusion and lucidity; document the specific time(s) when the patient seems more or less "clear." Observation and documentation of the patient's mental state should occur during the day, evening, and at night.

F. Assess understanding relative to the particular decision at issue. The following probes and statements are useful in assessing the degree to which the patient has the skills necessary to make a health care decision:
   1. "Tell me in your own words what the physician explained to you."
   2. "Tell me which parts, if any, were confusing."
   3. "What do you feel you have to *gain* by agreeing to (the proposed intervention)?
   4. "Tell me what you feel you have to *lose* by agreeing to (the proposed intervention)?
   5. "Tell me what you feel you have to gain or lose by refusing (the proposed intervention)?
   6. "Tell me why this decision is important (difficult, frightening, etc.) to you."

G. Select (or construct) appropriate decision aids.

(continued)

Protocol 28.1: Health Care Decision Making *(cont.)*

H. Help the patient express what he or she understands about the clinical situation, the goals of care, their expectation of the outcomes of the diagnostic, or treatment interventions.

I. Help the patient identify who should participate in diagnostic and treatment discussions and decisions.

VI. EVALUATION AND EXPECTED OUTCOME(S)

A. The number of referrals to the ethics committee or ethics consultant in situations of decision-making conflict between any of the involved parties.

B. The use of interpreters in communication of, or decision-making about, diagnostic and/or treatment interventions.

C. Plan of care: instructions regarding frequency of observation to ascertain the patient's lucid periods, if any.

D. Documentation
   1. Is the process of the capacity assessment described?
   2. Is the assessment specific to the decision at issue?
   3. Is the informed consent and refusal interaction described?
   4. Are the specifics of the patient's degree or spheres of orientation described?
   5. Is the patient's language used to describe the diagnostic or treatment intervention under consideration recorded? Is the patient's demeanor during this discussion recorded?
   6. Are the patient's questions and the clinician(s) answers recorded?
   7. Are appropriate mental status descriptors used consistently?

RESOURCES

American Bar Association (ABA)
http://www.americanbar.org

American Bar Association Commission on Law & Aging, Legislative Updates
See link for chart that summarizes the wide variation on how states allocate decisional authority in the absence of patient capacity to make health care decisions, *as well as legislative updates and other relevant information.*
http://www.americanbar.org/groups/law_aging.html

American Society of Bioethics and Humanities
http://www.asbh.org

The Hastings Center
http://www.thehastingscenter.org

Health Insurance Portability and Accountability Act of 1996 (HIPAA)
http://www.hhs.gov/ocr/privacy/

The Office for Civil Rights (OCR) enforces the HIPAA Privacy Rule
http://www.hhs.gov/ocr/privacy/hipaa/understanding/summary/index.html

REFERENCES

Alford, D. M. (2006). Legal issues in gerontological nursing—part 2: Responsible parties and guardianships. *Journal of Gerontological Nursing, 32*(2), 15–18. Evidence Level VI.

Allen, R. S., DeLaine, S. R., Chaplin, W. F., Marson, D. C., Bourgeois, M. S., Dijkstra, K., & Burgio, L. D. (2003). Advance care planning in nursing homes: Correlates of capacity and possession of advance directives. *The Gerontologist, 43*(3), 309–317. Evidence Level IV.

Beauchamp, T. L., & Childress, J. F. (2001) *Principles of biomedical ethics* (5th ed.). New York, NY: Oxford University Press. Evidence Level VI.

Cea, C. D., & Fisher, C. B. (2003). Healthcare decision-making by adults with mental retardation. *Mental Retardation, 41*(2), 78–87. Evidence Level IV.

Clever, S. L., Ford, D. E., Rubenstein, L. V., Rost, K. M., Meredith, L. S., Sherbourne, C. D., . . . Cooper, L. A. (2006). Primary care patients' involvement in decision-making is associated with improvement in depression. *Medical Care, 44*(5), 398–405. Evidence Level IV.

Cox, C. L., Cole, E., Reynolds, T., Wandrag, M., Breckenridge, S., & Dingle, M. (2006). Implications of cultural diversity in do not attempt resuscitation (DNAR) decision-making. *Journal of Multicultural Nursing and Health, 12*(1), 20–28. Evidence Level I.

Cruzan v. Director, Missouri Department of Health, 497 U.S. 261 (1990)

Edwards, M., Davies, M., & Edwards, A. (2009). What are the external influences on information exchange and shared decision-making in healthcare consultations: A meta-synthesis of the literature. *Patient Education and Counseling, 75*(1), 37–52. Evidence Level I.

Fink, A. S., Prochazka, A. V., Henderson, W. G., Bartenfeld, D., Nyirenda, C., Webb, A., . . . Parmelee, P. (2010). Predictors of comprehension during surgical informed consent. *Journal of the American College of Surgeons, 210*(6), 919–926. Evidence Level II.

Fried, T. R., Bullock, K., Iannone, L., & O'Leary, J. R. (2009). Understanding advance care planning as a process of health behavior change. *Journal of the American Geriatrics Society, 57*(9), 1547–1555. Evidence Level IV.

Fried, T. R., Byers, A. L., Gallo, W. T., Van Ness, P. H., Towle, V. R., O'Leary, J. R., & Dubin, J. A. (2006) Prospective study of health status preferences and changes in preferences over time in adults. *Archives of Internal Medicin, 166*(8), 890–895. Evidence Level IV.

Gurrera, R. J., Moye, J., Karel, M. J., Azar, A. R., & Armesto, J. C. (2006). Cognitive performance predicts treatment decisional abilities in mild to moderate dementia. *Neurology, 66*(9), 1367–1372. Evidence Level IV.

Hack, T. F., Pickles, T., Ruether, J. D., Weir, L., Bultz, B. D., Mackey, J., & Degner, L. F. (2010). Predictors of distress and quality of life in patients undergoing cancer therapy: Impact of treatment type and decisional role. *Psycho-Oncology, 19*(6), 606–616. Evidence Level II.

Halbert, C. H., Armstrong, K., Gandy, O. H., Jr., & Shaker, L. (2006). Racial differences in trust in health care providers. *Archives of Internal Medicine, 166*(8), 896–901. Evidence Level IV.

Kapp, M. B., & Mossman, D. (1996). Measuring decisional capacity: Cautions on the construction of a "capacimeter." *Psychology, Public Policy, and Law, 2*(1), 73–95. Evidence Level VI.

Karlawish, J. H., Casarett, D. J., James, B. D., Xie, S. X., & Kim, S. Y. (2005). The ability of persons with Alzheimer disease (AD) to make a decision about taking an AD treatment. *Neurology, 64*(9), 1514–1519. Evidence Level IV.

Kim, S. Y., Karlawish, J. H., & Caine, E. D. (2002). Current state of research on decision-making competence of cognitively impaired elderly persons. *The American Journal of Geriatric Psychiatry: Official Journal of the American Association for Geriatric Psychiatry, 10*(2), 151–165. Evidence Level V.

Lai, J. M., Gill, T. M., Cooney, L. M., Bradley, E. H., Hawkins, K. A., & Karlawish, J. H. (2008). Everyday decision-making ability in older persons with cognitive impairment. *The American Journal of Geriatric Psychiatry: Official Journal of the American Association for Geriatric Psychiatry, 16*(8), 693–696. Evidence Level IV.

Lapid, M. I., Rummans, T. A., Pankratz, V. S., & Appelbaum, P. S. (2004). Decisional capacity of depressed elderly to consent to electroconvulsive therapy. *Journal of Geriatric Psychiatry and Neurology, 17*(1), 42–46. Evidence Level II.

Lo, B. (2000). *Resolving ethical dilemmas: A guide for clinicians* (2nd ed.). Philadelphia, PA: Lippincott Williams & Wilkins. Evidence Level VI.

Mandelblatt, J., Kreling, B., Figeuriedo, M., & Feng, S. (2006). What is the impact of shared decision making on treatment and outcomes for older women with breast cancer? *Journal of Clinical Oncology: Official Journal of the American Society of Clinical Oncology, 24*(30), 4908–4913. Evidence Level IV.

Mezey, M., Teresi, J., Ramsey, G., Mitty, E., & Bobrowitz, T. (2002). Determining a resident's capacity to execute a health care proxy. Voices of decision in nursing homes: Respecting residents' preferences for end-of-life care. New York, NY: United Hospital Fund. Evidence Level IV.

Moye, J., Karel, M. J., Azar, A. R., & Gurrera, R. J. (2004). Capacity to consent to treatment: Empirical comparison of three instruments in older adults with and without dementia. *The Gerontologist, 44*(2), 166–175. Evidence Level IV.

Moye, J., Karel, M. J., Gurrera, R. J., & Azar, A. R. (2006). Neuropsychological predictors of decision-making capacity over 9 months in mild-to-moderate dementia. *Journal of General Internal Medicine, 21*(1), 78–83. Evidence Level IV.

O'Connor, A. M., Stacey, D., Entwistle, V., Llewellyn-Thomas, D., Rovner, D., Holmes-Rovner, M., . . . Jones, J. (2004). *Decision aids for people facing health treatment or screening decisions.* Chichester, United Kingdom: John Wiley & Sons. Evidence Level I.

Popejoy, L. (2005). Health-related decision-making by older adults and their families: How clinicians can help. *Journal of Gerontological Nursing, 31*(9), 12–18. Evidence Level V.

Rosenfeld, K. E., Wenger, N. S., & Kagawa-Singer, M. (2000). End-of-life decision making: A qualitative study of elderly individuals. *Journal General Internal Medicine, 15*(9), 620–625. Evidence Level IV.

Roth, L. H., Meisel, A., & Lidz, C. W. (1997). Tests of competency to consent to treatment. *The American Journal of Psychiatry, 134*(3), 279–284. Evidence Level VI.

Siminoff, L. A., Gordon, N. H., Silverman, P., Budd, T., & Ravdin, P. M. (2006). A decision aid to assist in adjuvant therapy choices for breast cancer. *Psycho-Oncology, 15*(11), 1001–1013. Evidence Level II. Steinhauser, K. E., Christakis, N. A., Clipp, E. C., McNeilly, M., McIntyre, L., & Tulsky, J. A. (2000). Factors considered important at the end of life by patients, family, physicians, and other care providers. *Journal of the American Medical Association, 284*(19), 2476–2482. Evidence Level IV.

Tuckett, A. G. (2006). On paternalism, autonomy and best interests: Telling the (competent) aged-care resident what they want to know. *International Journal of Nursing Practice, 12*(3), 166–173. Evidence Level V.

Ubel, P. A., Smith, D. M., Zikmund-Fisher, B. J., Derry, H. A., McClure, J., Stark, A., . . . Fagerlin, A. (2010). Testing whether decision aids introduce cognitive biases: Results of a randomized trial. *Patient Education and Counseling, 80*(2), 158–163. Evidence Level II.

Van Kleffens, T., van Baarsen, B., & van Leeuwen, E. (2004). The medical practice of patient autonomy and cancer treatment refusals: A patients' and physicians' perspective. *Social Science and Medicine, 8*(11), 2325–2336. Evidence Level IV.

Visser, A., Dijkstra, G. J., Kuiper, D., de Jong, P. E., Franssen, C. F., Gansevoort, R. T., . . . Reijneveld, S. A. (2009). Accepting or declining dialysis: Considerations taken into account by elderly patients with end-stage renal disease. *Journal of Nephrology, 22*(6), 794–799. Evidence Level IV.

Volicer, L., & Ganzini, L. (2003). Health professionals' views on standards for decision-making capacity regarding refusal of medical treatment in mild Alzheimer's disease. *Journal of the American Geriatrics Society, 51*(5), 1270–1274. Evidence Level IV.

Wakefield, C. E., Meiser, B., Homewood, J., Taylor, A., Gleeson, M., Williams, R., . . . Australian GENetic testing Decision Aid Collaborative Group. (2008). A randomized trial of a breast/ovarian cancer genetic testing decision aid used as a communication aid during genetic counseling. *Psycho-Oncology, 17*(8),844–854. Evidence Level II.

Watson, E., Hewitson, P., Brett, J., Bukach, C., Evans, R., Edwards, A., . . . Austoker, J. (2006). Informed decision making and prostate specific antigen (PSA) testing for prostate cancer: A randomised controlled trial exploring the impact of a brief patient decision aid on men's knowledge, attitudes and intention to be tested. *Patient Education and Counseling, 63*(3), 367–379. Evidence Level II.

Advance Directives

29

Ethel L. Mitty

EDUCATIONAL OBJECTIVES

On completion of this chapter, the reader should be able to:

1. differentiate between a durable power of attorney for health care and a living will
2. describe assessment parameters to ensure that older adults receive advance directive information
3. identify strategies to ensure good communication about advance directives among patients, families, and health care professionals
4. guide a discussion of the benefits and burdens of various treatment options to assist proxy treatment decision making
5. describe measurable outcomes to be expected from implementation of this practice protocol

OVERVIEW

One of the most difficult situations health care professionals face is treatment decision making for those who can no longer communicate their treatment preferences. Decision-making capacity of older adults may be diminished, fluctuating, or lapsed. The justification for advance care planning (ACP) is that a person with capacity can prospectively state their wishes, values, and treatment preferences so that their authentic voice will be heard when their capacity and/or ability to communicate has lapsed. Approximately 30% of older adults do not have a relative, friend, or guardian who can make health care decisions for them. The right to *not* complete an advance directive (AD) must also be respected. Patients should be informed (and in some cases, reassured) that neither providers nor the facility will abandon them or provide substandard care if they elect not to formulate an AD.

For description of Evidence Levels cited in this chapter, see Chapter 1, Developing and Evaluating Clinical Practice Guidelines: A Systematic Approach, page 7.

BACKGROUND AND STATEMENT OF PROBLEM

The *Patient Self-Determination Act* (PSDA, 1992), enacted in 1991, is the federal statutory codification of an individual's right to conduct health planning and decision making in advance. Predicated on the Western philosophic tradition of individual freedom and choice, and that self-determination is a moral right, the U.S. Supreme Court articulated the requirement of "clear and convincing evidence" that an incompetent patient would not want a specific treatment. Because few oral statements could meet this standard, written ADs were promulgated as constituting clear and convincing evidence.

ADs are value neutral and can be used to request as well as refuse treatment(s). They provide guidance for health care professionals and families. Importantly, ADs provide immunity from civil and criminal liability for health care professionals and families when an AD is followed in good faith. State statutes generally outline the conditions under which an AD is legally valid and when it should be followed (see ADs by State link in Resources section).

Quality-of-life concerns, the influence of the family, and pragmaticism influence most adults' decisions to create an AD (Crisp, 2007). Older adults who create ADs feel that their physicians know their wishes and do not feel that the AD would be a constraint on their care. Those who do not create an AD want their families to make decisions for them and apparently fail to see the flexibility that having an AD provides (Beck, Brown, Boles, & Barrett, 2002). Among participants of the original Framingham Heart Study, almost 70% discussed their end-of-life (EOL) care preferences and ADs with someone but not necessarily with a physician or health care provider. More than half had a health care proxy (HCP) or a living will (LW); slightly under half had both. Most respondents wanted comfort care at the end of life but few wanted to forego life-sustaining treatment (LST) interventions (e.g., ventilator, feeding tube) and would endure a burdensome health status (e.g., intense pain, confusion, forgetfulness) to prolong life, rather than die (McCarthy et al., 2008).

Hospice patients who talk with their surrogate decision makers (i.e., proxy) about their treatment wishes for their last week(s) of life have a higher rate of agreement with their surrogate's understanding of their treatment wishes than patients who do not have these discussions (Engelberg, Patrick, & Curtis, 2005).

Although family surrogate decision making is more accurate than primary physicians regarding older patients' preferences for LST in hypothetical scenarios, having an AD does not necessarily improve congruence between patients' wishes and decisions made by others (Coppola, Ditto, Danks, & Smucker, 2001). Substitute decision makers are not necessarily making treatment choices or decisions that represent the patient's preferences (Ditto et al., 2001; Mitchell, Berkowitz, Lawson, & Lipsitz, 2000). The evidence, to date, is inconclusive with regard to patient–surrogate information sharing and decision making. Whereas a small study found that communication between patients and their proxies improved the accuracy of proxies representations of patient preferences (Barrio-Cantalejo et al., 2009), a meta-analysis of surrogate decision making found no improvement in accuracy of representing patient preferences as a result of prior discussion between patient and proxy (Shalowitz, Garrett-Mayer, & Wendler, 2006). However, lack of concordance between a patient's stated wishes and physician orders cannot simply be viewed as a denial of a patient's rights; physicians might be relying on additional information to guide their treatment decisions (Hardin & Yusufaly, 2004).

TYPES OF ADVANCE DIRECTIVES

Treating a patient without their explicit permission is *battery*. In most states, unless the patient has severely limited the proxy's decision-making scope, the proxy's decision has the same weight and power as the patient speaking on his or her own behalf. A proxy's power is no greater or less than the capable patient himself or herself. Vague or ambiguous language in an AD (e.g., refusal of "heroic measures") deprives the proxy as well as providers the guidance needed to honor the patient's wishes. There are two types of ADs: DPAHC (also called HCP) and LW.

Durable Power of Attorney for Health Care

The DPAHC allows an individual to appoint a relative, friend, or trusted other—called a *health care proxy*, *agent*, *attorney-in-fact*, or *surrogate*—to make health care decisions if the individual loses the ability to make decisions or communicate his or her wishes. (An alternate agent should also be appointed.) A key presumption of HCP appointment is that the patient and proxy have discussed the patient's treatment wishes. Older adults with a DPHAC and an LW are less likely to die in a hospital or receive all care possible in comparison to those without a DPAHC (Silveira, Kim, & Langa, 2010). (Some states require the proxy's signature on the AD as an attempt to assure that the proxy is aware of his or her appointment and has accepted decision-making responsibilities as the patient's voice in care planning decision making.) Whereas an LW is in effect at the end of life, the DPAHC springs into effect at any time that the patient has a temporary (or permanent) absence of decisional capacity, as might be associated with trauma, illness, or mental impairment (dementia, stroke, delirium). A proxy has the legal authority to interpret the patient's wishes based on the medical circumstances of the situation and is not restricted to only deciding if LST can be withdrawn or withheld. Thus, the proxy can make decisions as the need arises, and such decisions can respond directly to the situation at hand rather than being restricted only to circumstances that were thought of previously.

"Family consent laws" designate the order in which persons can make decisions for an incapacitated patient who did not appoint a proxy; a spouse is usually first, then adult children, parents, and distant relatives. Decisions of family members acting in this capacity are restricted in various ways by many states including the requirement that the patient must be terminal or in a persistent vegetative state, comatose, and so forth. Disputes between family members who bear the same relationship to the patient (e.g., two children) are not uncommon and often very difficult to resolve. A proxy's decision legally supersedes a decision made by a family member or nonproxy concerned party. This is not to say, however, that a proxy's decision is always easy and conflict-free or that the burden is light.

Living Will

For adults who have no one to appoint as their proxy, completing an LW that outlines their wishes is preferable to not providing any information at all about their care preferences. An LW is also helpful for those with a DPAHC who want to provide their proxy some guidance about their treatment preferences and EOL care wishes, including artificial nutrition and hydration (ANH), ventilator support, and pain management.

An LW is a prospective declaration that provides specific instructions to health care providers about particular kinds of health care treatments or interventions that an individual would or would not want in specific clinical circumstances, usually at the end of life. All but three states (New York, Massachusetts, and Michigan) have detailed statutes recognizing LWs. However, the usefulness of LWs is limited to those clinical circumstances that were thought of before the person became incapable of making or communicating decisions. If a situation occurs that the LW does not address, providers and families may not know how to proceed and still respect the patient's wishes. Hence, it is recommended that individuals also appoint a proxy—a trusted other who knows their values and wishes. When an individual completes both the LW and DPAHC, the proxy or agent might not be obligated (in some states) to follow the wishes outlined in the LW; the LW serves as a guide. When presented with the opportunity to complete a "traditional" LW that limited LST in terminal illness and a "modified" LW with three treatment options (i.e., limiting LST in critical illness; providing LST on a trial basis; refusing LST and/or ANH in advanced dementia), almost 90% of hospitalized general medical patients preferred the modified LW and a number of subjects subsequently chose to create one (Abbo, Sobotka, & Meltzer, 2008).

Some states have a combined directive that includes elements of the LW and the DPAHC. A section on organ donation ("anatomical gift") has been added to the AD document of some states that allows the individual to indicate if they wish to donate an organ(s). However, in New York State, for example, the proxy cannot effect this wish unless the proxy is also the identified decision maker for *organ donation*, a distinct statutory authority separate from an HCP's rights and responsibilities.

"Instructional or medical directives" have been suggested to compensate for the deficiencies of LWs. They address specific clinical situations and interventions. Individuals must decide prospectively which interventions they would want in the face of four scenarios: coma with virtually no chance of recovery; coma with a small chance of recovery but restored to an impaired physical and mental state; advanced dementia and a terminal illness; and advanced dementia. Among the interventions are cardiopulmonary resuscitation (CPR), ANH, dialysis, invasive diagnostic tests, antibiotics, and blood transfusion. The instructional/medical directive does not, however, address the patient's desired goals of care, willingness to allow a short-term intervention, or treatment choices associated with stage of chronic illness or exacerbation.

Two other AD documents further the goals of ACP and are accepted in many states: the physician order for life-sustaining treatment (POLST) and the Five Wishes document. *POLST* originated in Oregon in 1995 and is a state-endorsed protocol to honor an individual's wish to die in a setting of his or her choice without unwanted life-supporting interventions. It contains four separate categories of physician's orders that are based on patient–physician discussion: comfort measures, antibiotics, parenteral feeding, and CPR. Nursing home residents with POLST forms are more likely to have documented restricted LST preferences as well as be less likely to be hospitalized if their POLST indicated comfort measures only. There is no evidence of differences in symptom assessment or management among residents with and without POLST forms (Hickman et al., 2010). The POLST has greater specificity and accuracy in communicating EOL preferences in comparison to traditional ads (Bomba & Vermilyea, 2006).

The *Five Wishes document* meets the legal requirements of ADs in almost all states and is available in 26 languages. It combines the HCP, LW, instructional directions, and proxy designation. Open-ended statements guide the individual to express their thoughts and wishes about how they want to be physically and emotionally supported, the medical treatments they want and do not want, and the funeral arrangements and eulogy they would like. The "values statements" embedded in the Five Wishes AD generally do not explore or express the patient's understanding of the benefits and burdens of various treatments, thereby making it difficult to act on the patient's wishes and preferences (Lo & Steinbrook, 2004).

Location of death (e.g., home or hospice rather than in acute care), less likelihood of being on a respirator or having a feeding tube, fewer concerns with family/significant other being informed about what to expect, and good physician communication are associated with ADs and quality EOL care (Bakitas et al., 2008; Detering, Hancock, Reade, & Silvester, 2010; Teno, Grunier, Schwartz, Nanda, & Wetle, 2007). Patients facing the need for EOL care for advanced illness, randomized to an advanced illness coordinated care program, experienced increased satisfaction with care and communication, completed more ADs, and their surrogates reported fewer support problems than patients receiving usual care (Engelhardt et al., 2006). As with another study (Teno et al., 2007), there was no difference in survival rates between the two groups. However, unmet needs were for adequate pain management and emotional support for patient and family (Teno et al., 2007).

Factors important to older patients with regard to their medical decision making and ADs include their religious beliefs, dignity, physical comfort, dependency, and finances (Hawkins, Ditto, Danks, & Smucker, 2005). Few patients want to document their specific medical treatment preferences; they highly value verbal communication. Spouse surrogates are less likely than child surrogates to believe that recording wishes in advance is necessary. Most patients gave their surrogate leeway in decision making. The spouse surrogate was more likely than the child surrogate to feel that financial issues were important. Patients had more confidence in their child surrogate understanding their wishes than their spouse surrogate understanding. The effect of a recent hospitalization on a reduced desire to receive LSTs (e.g., CPR, ANH) was noted during an interview conducted just after recovery but returned to normal several months after hospitalization. These results challenge assumptions about the stability of treatment preferences and the temporal context during which treatment decisions are made (Ditto, Jacobson, Smucker, Danks, & Fagerlin, 2006; Hawkins et al., 2005).

Research Advance Directive

The notion of a research advance directive (RAD) has been suggested (National Bioethics Advisory Commission, 1998). The conduct of research with participants suffering from a dementing illness is daunting with regard to obtaining informed consent. An RAD must be executed while the individual still retains decisional capacity and must contain a fairly detailed description of the person's understanding of the research intention and possible risks, benefits, and burdens. The proxy decision maker must make a determination whether the person's intention to participate in research is congruent with the proposed research. A study involving patients with moderate dementia and their family proxies sought to learn whether the patients wanted to retain decision making about their participation in research in the future or allow their proxy to make the decision. Although many, but not all, patients granted future decision making about research participation to their proxies, it was also clear that proxies did not always want to make research participation decisions (Stocking et al., 2006).

Psychiatric Advance Directive

Psychiatric advance directives (PAD) are presumably written by individuals with decisional competence. Given the opportunity to meet with a trained facilitator, adults with psychotic disorders sufficiently increased their competence to make treatment decisions within their PADs (Elbogen et al., 2007). Psychiatric outpatients want assistance to create a PAD. Of these, most are female, non-White, have limited personal autonomy, a history of self-harm or arrest, and a felt pressure to take medications (Swanson, Swartz, Ferron, Elbogen, & Van Dorn, 2006). Completion of a PAD is associated with patients with good insight and their need to keep their outpatient mental health treatment appointment (Swanson et al., 2006).

Patient identification in their PAD of their preferred psychiatric medications predicted not only that it was likely to be prescribed but that medication adherence persisted over time (Wilder, Elbogen, Moser, Swanson, & Swartz, 2010). Among mental health professionals (i.e., psychiatrists, psychologists, social workers), most agree that PADs would be helpful for patients with severe mental illness. However, their positive attitude is supported by their knowledge that their respective state laws do not require them to follow a directive that contained a patient's refusal of appropriate mental health treatment (Elbogen et al., 2006).

Oral Advance Directive

Although the courts prefer written ADs, oral advance directives are respected, especially in emergency situations, and can be persuasive in a judicial decision to withhold an LST. Some states permit a patient to orally designate a proxy in discussion with their physician, rather than execute a written AD (Lo & Steinbrook, 2004). In determining the validity of an oral AD, the court seeks information about whether the statement was made on serious or solemn occasions, consistently repeated, made by a mature person who understood the underlying issues, was consistent with the values demonstrated in other aspects of the patient's life (including the patient's religion), made before the need for the treatment decision, and specifically addressed the actual condition of the patient (Lo & Steinbrook, 2004). What might seem like an occasional comment made by a patient (whether in a practitioner's office or at the bedside) should be recorded for just such an occasion when "clear and convincing evidence" is required. It has been argued that oral instructions explicated during conversation with one's physician can be taken to signify the patient's genuine intent on having his or her instructions followed.

Do Not Resuscitate Orders

Consent to CPR is presumed unless a physician writes a do-not-resuscitate (DNR) order. Respecting (or not) a patient's resuscitation wishes is a frequent cause of moral distress for nurses. It has been suggested that CPR should not be instituted when it will not offer a medical benefit or when death is inevitable and expected. All states have a Natural Death Act that recognizes the right of competent patients, in their written AD, to refuse LSTs. Patients have a right to refuse CPR after they have been informed of the risks and benefits involved and may, in fact, request a DNR order. If the physician is unwilling to write a DNR order to comply with the patient's request, the physician has a duty to notify the patient or family and assist the patient to obtain another physician.

It is important that otherwise healthy hospitalized older adults who may benefit from CPR should not be denied this life-saving intervention.

For patients on a palliative home care program, their interest and willingness to have a DNR order is associated with sleep and incontinence problems, acceptance of their situation and nearness to death, and their wish to die at home. Once again, the temporal nature of AD care preferences has to be factored in (Brink, Smith, & Kitson, 2008).

Artificial Nutrition and Hydration

ANH poses ethical, legal, and cultural challenges. The U.S. Supreme Court, in 1990 (before the PSDA), established that competent patients have a "constitutionally protected liberty" to refuse unwanted medical treatment. The court further established that ANH is no different than other forms of medical treatment. Many ethicists and legal scholars hold that there is no legal difference between forgoing and discontinuing ANH. The legal evidence and procedures required to forgo or discontinue ANH vary by state. Several states hold that proxies cannot make decisions about withholding unless the patient specifically directs, in the AD, that the proxy can make this decision on his or her behalf. (The DPAHC document contains a statement and box to check, if the patient wishes, that states: "My proxy knows my wishes." Nothing has to be written regarding precisely what those wishes are.) The LW statutes in some states regard ANH as a medical treatment, whereas other states consider ANH a comfort measure (Gillick, 2006). Nurses need to be aware of their state law in this regard and, also, the extent to which patients (and proxies) are correctly informed about the clinical benefits and burdens of ANH at the end of life and the caring/comfort treatment alternatives. Whether or not to institute ANH or to withdraw it once started has the moral equivalence, for many people, of "killing" the patient.

ASSESSMENT OF THE PROBLEM

A primary consideration in approaching a patient about AD creation is the person's capacity to not only make decisions about his or her health care but also to accept responsibility for the consequences of the decision. "Competence" and "capacity" are not the same, yet they are frequently used synonymously and interchangeably (see Chapter 28, Health Care Decision Making). The law presumes competency unless shown otherwise; only the court can rule that an individual is incompetent. Capacity is a clinical determination and is not determined solely by a medical or psychiatric diagnosis or test. Inability to make financial decisions or communicate verbally does not preclude the ability to communicate important information about one's treatment preferences. The determination that a patient lacks capacity is often made based on a *mental status assessment test*—an inappropriate measure of decisional capacity. Thus, there is a grave risk that individuals with communication disorders or those with mild dementia might not have the opportunity to appoint an HCP or to execute an LW.

Decisional Capacity to Create an Advance Directive

The steps in determining whether a patient has sufficient decisional capacity to create an AD are similar to the basic elements of a valid consent and are based on observation of a specific set of abilities. These steps include (a) the patient appreciates and understands that he or she has the right to make a choice; (b) the patient understands the medical situation, prognosis, risks, benefits, and consequences of treatment consent (or refusal); (c) the patient can communicate the decision; and (d) the patient's decision is stable and consistent over a period (Roth, Meisel, & Lidz, 1977).

Decision-making capacity is not an all-or-none, "on-off" switch. Not all health decisions require the same level of decision-making capacity. Rather, capacity should be viewed as "task specific." An individual may be able to perform some tasks adequately and may have the ability to make some decisions, but is unable to perform all tasks or make all decisions. The notion of "decision-specific capacity" assumes that an individual has or lacks capacity for a particular decision at a particular time and under a particular set of circumstances (Meisel, 2002). Most older adults have sufficient cognitive capability to make some, but not all, decisions. An individual might have the requisite capacity or understanding that they can choose someone to make health care decisions for them when they no longer have the capacity to make treatment choices. The determination of decisional capacity becomes more exacting in relationship to the complexity and risk associated with the health care decision (Midwest Bioethics Center, 1996).

Appreciation of the consequences of an option or decision is a key component of capacity determination. There is no gold standard or "capacimeter" to assess. The *mini-mental status examination* (MMSE) is a cognitive screen; it was not designed for, nor is it applicable to, capacity determination (Mezey, Teresi, Ramsey, Mitty, & Bobrowitz, 2002). Bioethicists, legal scholars, and clinicians generally agree that a lower level of capacity is needed to create a DPAHC in comparison to an LW (Mezey et al., 2002). Objective assessment of capacity can avoid two types of mistakes. First, mistakenly preventing persons who ought to be considered capacitated from directing the course of their treatment and, second, failing to protect incapacitated persons from the harmful effects of their decisions. Failure to take language barriers and hearing and visual deficits into account can result in the erroneous conclusion that a person lacks the capacity to execute an AD. Residents with dementia who are White and have some higher education are likely to have an AD that is primarily used to restrict, not request, many forms of aggressive LST care at the end of life. Pain management and comfort care are routinely requested, however (Triplett et al., 2008).

Benefit–Burden Assessment

A benefit–burden analysis considers the intended and unintended consequences of a particular treatment, estimates the likelihood that the intended benefit will occur, and weighs the importance of the benefit and burden to the patient. Patients are not necessarily consistent in their treatment preferences, especially if the chance to avoid death or the degree of burden is unclear. Many patients are in variable stages of readiness for ACP that includes creation of an AD and communication with their families and physicians about their treatment goals. Prior experience with health care treatment decision making can influence a patient's perceptions of his or her readiness (Fried, Bullock, Iannone, & O'Leary, 2009; Fried, O'Leary, Van Ness, & Fraenkel, 2007). The proxy can be helped to infer how the patient would evaluate the benefits and burdens based on knowledge of the patient's values, preferences, and past behavior. The nurse can ask the proxy, "If [the patient] could join this discussion, what would he say?" "Faced with similar situations in the past, how did he decide?" Higher congruence between patient and proxy regarding patients' EOL care preferences is associated with a nurse-led discussion intervention: patients were more knowledgeable about LSTs, less willing to receive LSTs for a new serious medical event, and less willing to live in a state of poor health (Schwartz et al., 2002).

The rationale for withholding or withdrawing a treatment is to eliminate a burdensome intervention/treatment that is not producing the desired result. In those situations where the proxy has scant knowledge about the patient for whom he or she must make health care decisions (or there is no AD, proxy appointment, or person who speaks for the patient), a decision is made on what would be in the patient's best interest. Known as the "reasonable person" or "best interest" standard, the decision relies on the notion of what an average person in the patient's particular situation would consider beneficial or burdensome. Questions that could move the process along would ask, "What does [this patient] have to gain or lose as a result of this treatment?" In what ways will [this patient] be better or worse off as a result of this treatment—or not having this treatment?"

CULTURAL PERSPECTIVES ON ADVANCE CARE PLANNING

The notion of ACP and written directives is not universally acceptable. In some cultures, for the close-knit family, an AD is intrusive, irrelevant, and a refusal if not a legal denial of care. Many in the Black and ethnic minority populations do not view the DPAHC as relevant, nor do they regard a DNR order as a summative value statement (Cox et al., 2006). Disinterest in creating an AD because of a present-day, rather than a future, orientation and an unwillingness to write, speak, or plan for one's death are pervasive cultural influences on a decision not to create an AD. As well, deference to physician decision making, the family's role in protecting the patient from the burdens of life and death decision making, and spiritual obligations or beliefs can exert a powerful influence on the decision.

Studies indicate different LST preferences and decision-making contexts among racial and ethnic groups (Cox et al., 2006). Overall, Asian and Hispanic patients prefer family-centered decision making in contrast to White and African American patients' preference for patient-directed decision making (Kwak & Haley, 2005). As many have shown, White patients are more interested in and likely to discuss treatment preferences, execute an LW, refuse certain LST, and appoint an HCP decision maker than Black or Hispanic patients (Hopp & Duffy, 2000). AD completion is more concentrated among White patients with higher education and income levels than among Black and Hispanic patients with low income levels and less than a high school education (Mezey, Leitman, Mitty, Bottrell, & Ramsey, 2000). Latino patients in comparison to White patients are less likely to complete an AD or communicate their preferences even though there are no differences between groups with regard to AD preferences (Froman & Owen, 2005).

In contrast, African American patients are more likely to want LSTs to prolong life. Some Black patients believe that having an AD is a legal way to deny access to treatment and care, and tend to distrust the health care system more than Mexican Americans and European Americans (Perkins, Geppert, Gonzales, Cortez, & Hazuda, 2002). Among African American patients, spirituality and beliefs that are in conflict with palliative care goals, views of suffering and death and dying, and mistrust of the health care system negatively influence their creation of an AD (Bullock, 2006; Gerst & Burr, 2008; Johnson, Kuchibhatla, & Tulsky, 2008). An intervention study using same-race peer mentors to discuss ACP with dialysis patients demonstrated a significant positive effect on Black patients but not on White patients. Positive outcomes included increased comfort in discussion, completion of ADs, and improved feelings of well-being (Perry et al., 2005).

Cultural assimilation as well as cultural diversity make even a simplistic assumption about why people do and do not create an AD extremely hazardous. When patients and health care professionals are from different ethnic backgrounds, the value systems that form the basis for AD decision making may conflict, often leading to distinct ethical and interpersonal tensions. Older Japanese American patients in the United States prefer to make their own decisions about withholding LST, whereas older Japanese patients residing in Japan defer decision making to their physicians and families (Matsui, Braun, & Karel, 2008). Subtle themes pertain to elder Japanese patients with regard to their feelings about being a burden to others, the family obligation to support the dying person, and the overall usefulness of an AD as a means to reduce conflict, yet not be intrusive (Bito et al., 2007). High religiosity, a strong family decision-making history, and a belief that the family should support the patient's wishes are negatively correlated with AD creation among many cultural groups in the United States, such as patients who are Greek (Makridou, Efklides, Economidis, & Peonidis, 2006), Bosnian (Searight & Gafford, 2005), Asian Indian (Doorenbos & Nies, 2003), and Malaysian (Htut, Shahrul, & Poi, 2007). Predictors of AD completion for multiethnic urban seniors include what investigators called *modifiable factors*, such as an established relationship with a primary care physician and their doctor's willingness to start the discussion, being knowledgeable about ACP, recognition of the family role in decision making, and prior experience with decision making about mechanical ventilation (Morrison & Meier, 2004).

NURSES' ROLES IN ADVANCE DIRECTIVES

All adult patients, regardless of their gender, religion, socioeconomic status, diagnosis, or prognosis should be approached with information about and encouraged to discuss ACP and ADs. These conversations occur over time; they are not interviews, per se. Discussion is always patient centered, not proxy or provider centered. Nurses can have a major role in checking their patients' knowledge about EOL treatment options and the benefits, burdens, and consequences of each option. Correct information/knowledge about the difference between euthanasia and assisted suicide, treatment refusal, and treatment withdrawal is associated with being college educated, being White, and having prior experience as a proxy for another (Silveira, DiPiero, Gerrity, & Feudtner, 2000). Oncology nurses are knowledgeable about ADs but less so about the PSDA and their respective state laws. They lack confidence in their knowledge and ability to assist patients to create an AD (Jezewski et al., 2005). Interestingly, they view their role as one of advocacy, especially for adequate pain management (even though it may hasten death).

Patients say that they complete ADs to ease their family's financial and emotional burden and to ease decision making. They want to discuss EOL care and LWs, but they expect providers to initiate these discussions. Community-dwelling older patients attending a general medical clinic were more likely to create an AD when they received AD information by mail in advance of their appointment, and their physician received a reminder to discuss ADs, in comparison to patients whose physicians only received a reminder to document ADs (Heiman, Bates, Fairchild, Shaykevich & Lehmann, 2004). Discussions of EOL care and ADs are a statistically significant predictor of patient satisfaction with their primary care physician (Tierney et al., 2001). Attitude, skills, and knowledge about ACP among medical residents caring for hospitalized older adults revealed that they had incomplete and often erroneous understanding of patients' decision-making process, all of which influenced their willingness to have such a discussion (Gorman, Ahern, Wiseman, & Skrobik, 2005). Training in ACP for medical residents not only improved their knowledge in and comfort with discussion of Ads, but also positively influenced patient interest in creating an AD (Alderman, Nair, & Fox, 2008). Case managers vary in their level of ACP knowledge and skills, reaction to family involvement and patient receptivity, and in supporting their clients in creating an AD (Black & Fauske, 2007). Directives that address hospitalization and ED treatment are the most useful for physicians yet are not always available, especially in emergency departments (Cohen-Mansfield & Lipson, 2008; Weinick, Wilcox, Park, Griffey, & Weissman, 2008).

A pervasive myth among patients, and one influenced by a history of abuse and denial of health care, is that an AD means "do not treat" or, conversely, means being kept alive against their wishes, with all manner of tubes and technology. Some patients believe, erroneously, that a lawyer is needed to execute an AD and that each state has its own specific AD document that must be used. It is partially correct that in the absence of an AD "surrogate decision maker," a family member is most often the designated decision maker. This reflects custom as well as recognition of the pivotal role of the family in important decisions as well as the fact that a family member is most likely to be aware of the patient's values, wishes, and preferences. The reality in many cases is that families disagree or might be ignorant of the patient's wishes. Nurses are in a position to identify pending family conflict and act to mitigate the drastic effects of poor or delayed treatment decisions.

The language of ADs can be confounding, especially for those with limited literacy. Randomized to a standard AD (12th-grade reading level) form and one which was modified to address literacy needs (i.e., 5th-grade reading level; graphics), most English- and Spanish-speaking patients preferred the modified form, which resulted in higher AD creation among them (Sudore et al., 2007). Most community-dwelling older adults know about treatment purposes but least about outcomes (Porensky & Carpenter, 2008). Phrases such as "improvement" or "vegetable" were idiosyncratically interpreted.

INTERVENTIONS AND CARE STRATEGIES

One way for a nurse to begin the discussion about ACP is by helping the patient and/or proxy explore and express what quality of life means for the patient, the importance of preservation of life, and how the patient's illness (and death) will affect others (emotionally, financially, etc.). Some patients might want to focus on the quality of their living, whereas others focus on the quality of their dying. Some patients might want to talk about from whom and where they will receive care at the end of life. Some may abhor their coming dependence on others; others may not like or want it, but will accept it. Still others might opt for hospice care out of the home to distance their dependency on family caregivers. Patients (and proxies) might need or want to talk about what they each fear most and what will be important when dying.

Communication About Advance Care Planning

Under state law and Joint Commission standards, patients have the right to have a qualified interpreter translate and transmit discussion between themselves and their health care professional. The interpreter may be the only person who recognizes that patients and their families have a totally different "take" than the health care team on words like "health" and "illness," on what a treatment is supposed to do, and on what dying is and what it is not. If "telling bad news" is prohibited (e.g., Navajo, Greece, Korea, Horn of Africa nations), then it might be difficult to discuss EOL planning. It should not be assumed that facility, family, or other interpreters are neutral and will simply "translate" words. An interpreter is communicating fact and nuance, explanation and rationale, and might influence a treatment decision by virtue of attempting a 1:1 word translation or a clumsy approximation of two distinct languages. In the presence of conflict about a treatment decision, or an unexpected decision, it may be in the patient's best interest to bring in another interpreter and repeat the exchange of information and questions.

CASE STUDY

Mrs. R. is an 88-year-old female, widowed for 22 years, and with no next of kin who lived alone prior to her admission to the nursing home 2 years ago, at which time she consented to a DNR order. She has severe chronic obstructive pulmonary disease (COPD), chronic renal failure (blood urea nitrogen of 58), dementia mild/mod (MMSE score of 20/30), is mildly depressed (by Geriatric Depression Scale score), and is below her initial body weight (−22 lbs). Mrs. R. now requires another person for all personal care; she bruises easily. Her prognosis is poor; goals of care are symptom management with comfort/palliative care. She has had multiple hospitalizations for pneumonia; the latest was 10 weeks ago after which she had further weight loss and developed a Grade II pressure ulcer on her right hip. She is receiving the standard medications for COPD, antianxiety medication, a short-acting sleeping medication, and appetite stimulants. Recent discussion about her quality of life by the interdisciplinary team noted that she no longer attends parties, Sabbath candle lighting, or discussions, all of which she used to enjoy. Mrs. R. seemed unable to make health care decisions as of 6 months ago; her decisional capacity appears to fluctuate in relation to her oxygen saturation.

Five years ago, Mrs. R. created an LW that stipulated "aggressive comfort care, including ventilator support." There are no verbal statements documented that might indicate Mrs. R.'s feelings about being hospitalized if she has another COPD exacerbation, which is to be expected given the trajectory of this disease.

Two days ago, Mrs. R. began to have stertorous breathing, a nonproductive cough, and episodes of diaphoresis. She appears exhausted; her solid food intake is minimal, and she gets very dyspneic when taking small sips of fluid. A chest x-ray was equivocal and is to be repeated today. At present, her vital signs are as follows: tem-

(continued)

CASE STUDY *(continued)*

perature, 100.8; pulse oximeter, 82%; pulse and blood pressure are within normal limits. The nursing home has the resources to provide oxygen and IV fluids including antibiotics.

Discussion

The difficulty of this case is an LW instruction written before the disease trajectory had reached a terminal state, and that now might not be in Mrs. R.'s best interests; aggressive intervention might be more burdensome than beneficial. Whose voice will articulate the benefits and burdens of hospitalization or remaining in the nursing home for palliative/terminal care? The nurse assistants feel she should be hospitalized; their advocacy is based on 2 years of knowing her and feelings of great affection for her. The clinical professional staff argue from prognostications about the likely outcome of an aggressive intervention (e.g., ventilator support) and probable multiple skin breakdowns if she is hospitalized. The standard of "substituted judgment" that a proxy uses when deciding on behalf of a patient whose wishes and preferences are known is not available to us. One could ask, "What would Mrs. R. choose if she could join the discussion?" The "best interest" standard of decision making asks what we think would promote Mrs. R.'s well-being. Can we bring her back to baseline (the status at which staff knew and loved her)? At this point, the benefit–burden assessment becomes a critical part of the discussion.

Conflict between the professional and paraprofessional staff has to be addressed. For the nurses, administering morphine to provide respiratory comfort might well hasten Mrs. R.'s death. Are we prolonging life or prolonging death? Are we treating resident or institutional anxiety? What is quality of life? Is it a complex personal phenomenon and judgment? A medical determination? To what extent can the facility provide a reasonable quality of life, a degree of comfort and safety, that might meet Mrs. R.'s interests at this time—different from that which the staff previously enjoyed with her? What are the legal and ethical implications of departing from Mrs. R.'s AD? What are the implications of morphine administration and of the principle of double (i.e., unintended) effect?

After discussion with an ethics consultant at an interdisciplinary meeting that included the nurse assistants involved in her care, a consensus decision was made not to hospitalize Mrs. R. The decision was guided by the clinical facts, Mrs. R.'s prior wishes (for "aggressive comfort care"), the likely trajectory of COPD, fact gathering, values discussion, and reflection about Mrs. R.'s condition after each hospitalization. Mechanical ventilation was likely to be more of a burden than a benefit at this point in her illness; Mrs. R. could be made comfortable with judicious use of medication and intensive nursing care. This case teaches us that ACP is not a static one-time event. Whether a person's wishes and preferences are stated through an AD document or verbally, they must be periodically reviewed upon a person's change of condition, lifestyle, proxy, heart, and mind. The ability to reach consensus through mediation that addressed each person's concerns, but kept the discussion resident centered, was key to arriving at a medically and ethically appropriate decision that focused on the goals of care.

SUMMARY

Discussions about care at the EOL should occur over time. Having such discussions shortly after hospitalization for an acute event can blur the goals of ACP, focusing more on resuscitation preferences than on the long range goals of care and treatment (Happ et al., 2002). Notions of quality of life, confusion about what it looks and feels like, and how to measure this complex phenomenon influence EOL care preference interventions. Rather than discussing the technology of LST and EOL care, nurses can help recenter the discussion on the patient's wishes and preferences. It may be wiser and more humane to discuss with patients, families, and proxies the acceptable state of health, desired functionality, and the "valued life activities" that patients want. Construing quality of life in this manner might be more meaningful and helpful.

An environment conducive to meaningful discussions about ADs and EOL care requires an appropriate time and location. An emergency admission is not an appropriate time. Distribution without discussion, commonly done in hospital admission offices at the time of an elective admission, is not an appropriate time either. (Nursing homes tend to wait 2 weeks before discussing ADs with a new admission.). Many studies report that the most effective interventions for patient creation of an AD is oral information provided over several interactive sessions (Bravo, Dubois, & Wagneur, 2008; Tamayo-Velázquez et al., 2010) and the opportunity to ask questions (Jezewski, Meeker, Sessana, & Finnell, 2007). Passive use of print material and lack of opportunity to receive assistance in creating an AD does not elicit AD creation (Ramsaroop, Reid, & Adelman, 2007). It is unlikely that education and information about ADs will completely counteract the natural discomfort associated with discussing death and dying; this is generally as true for patients and families as it is for care providers. Awareness of the patient and family's spiritual and cultural "surround" as well as the provider's moral biases about LST can give rise to sensitive and realistic discussion.

NURSING STANDARD OF PRACTICE

Protocol 29.1: Advance Directives

I. GUIDING PRINCIPLES
   A. All people have the right to decide what will be done with their bodies.
   B. All individuals are presumed to have decision-making capacity until deemed otherwise.
   C. All patients who can participate in a conversation, either verbally or through alternate means of communication, should be approached to discuss and record their treatment preferences and wishes.
   D. Health care professionals can improve EOL care for older adult patients by encouraging the use of ADs.

(continued)

Protocol 29.1: Advance Directives *(cont.)*

II. BACKGROUND
A. Education About Advance Directives
   1. Patients uniformly state that they want more information about ADs.
   2. Patients want nurses (and physicians) to approach them about ADs.
   3. It is estimated that 19% to 36% of Americans have completed an AD.
B. Advance Directives
   1. Allow individual to provide directions about the kind of medical care they do or do not want if they become unable to make or communicate their decisions;
   2. Provide guidance for health care professionals, families, and substitute decision makers about health care decision making that reflect the person's wishes; and
   3. Provide immunity for health care professionals, families, and appointed proxies from civil and criminal liability when health care professionals follow the AD in good faith.
C. Two Types of Advance Directives: DPAHC (also called HCP) and LW.
   1. A *durable power of attorney* allows an individual to appoint someone, called HCP, agent, or surrogate, to make health care decisions for him or her should he or she lose the ability to make decisions or communicate his or her wishes.
   2. A *living will* provides specific instructions to health care providers about particular kinds of health care treatment an individual would or would not want to prolong life. LWs are often used to declare a wish to refuse, limit, or withhold LST.
D. Instructional or Medical Directive: intended to compensate for the weaknesses of LWs. This kind of directive identifies specific interventions that are acceptable to a patient in specific clinical situations (e.g., POLST).
E. Oral Advance Directives (Verbal Directives): allowed in some states if there is clear and convincing evidence of the patient's wishes. Clear and convincing evidence can include evidence that the patient made the statement consistently and seriously, over time, specifically addressed the actual condition of the patient, and was consistent with the values seen in other areas of the patient's life. Legal rules surrounding oral advance directives vary by state.

III. ASSESSMENT PARAMETERS
A. All adult patients regardless of age (with the exception of patients with persistent vegetative state, severe dementia, or coma) should be asked if they have an LW or if they have designated a proxy.
B. All patients regardless of age, gender, religion, socioeconomic status, diagnosis, or prognosis should be approached to discuss ADs and ACP.
C. Discussions about ADs should be conducted in the patient's preferred language to enable information transfer and questions and answers.
D. Discussions should be conducted with sensitivity to the patient's stage of wellness and illness, that is, to their temporal as well as physical status.
E. Patients who have been determined to lack capacity to make other decisions may still have the capacity to designate a proxy or make some health care decisions. Decision-making capacity should be determined for each individual based on whether the patient has the ability to make the specific decision in question.

(continued)

F. If an LW has been completed or proxy has been designated:
   1. The document should be readily available on the patient's current chart.
   2. The attending physician should know that the directive exists and has a copy.
   3. The designated HCP should have a copy of the document.
   4. The directive should be reviewed periodically by the patient, attending physician/nurse, and the proxy to determine if it reflects the patient's current wishes and preferences.

IV. CARE STRATEGIES

A. Nurses should assist patients and families trying to deal with EOL care issues.
B. Patients may be willing to discuss their health situation and mortality with a nurse or clergyman rather than with a family member and should be supported in doing so.
C. Patients should be assisted in talking with their family/proxy about their treatment and care wishes.
D. Patients should be assessed for their ability to cope with the information provided.
E. Nurses must be mindful of and sensitive to the fact that race, culture, ethnicity, and religion can influence the health care decision-making process. The fact that patients from non-Western cultures may not subscribe to Western notions of autonomy does not mean that these patients do not want to talk about their treatment wishes, or that they would not have conversations with their families about their treatment preferences.
F. Patient's must be respected for their decision to not complete an AD and reassured that they will not be abandoned or receive substandard care if they do not elect to formulate an AD.
G. Nurses should be aware of the institution's mechanism for resolving conflicts between family members and the patient or proxy or between the patient/family and care providers and assist the parties in using this resource.
H. Nurses should be aware of which professional in their agency/institution is responsible for checking with the patient that copies of the AD have been given to their primary health care provider(s), to their proxy, *and* that the patient is carrying a wallet-size card with AD and contact information.

V. EVALUATION OF EXPECTED OUTCOMES

To determine whether implementation of this protocol influenced the type as well as the number of ADs created, changes should be measurable and should contribute to the facility's ongoing quality improvement program. Look at:

A. As documented in the record
   1. Whether patients are asked about ACP and directives
   2. Whether patients do or do not have an AD
B. Of those patients with an AD, the percentage of ADs included in patient charts;
C. The use of interpreters to assist staff discussion of ADs with patients for whom English is not their primary language;
D. The number of ADs completed in association with admission to, or receipt of services from, the agency/institution;
E. The number of nurse referrals to the ethics committee of patient or staff situations regarding ADs.

RESOURCES

American Nurses Association (ANA)
www.nursingworld.org

- Code for Nurses with Interpretive Statements
- Position statements on assisted suicide and active euthanasia, do-not-resuscitate, comfort and relief, patient self-determination act
- Selected bibliographies on ethical issues such as EOL decisions, foregoing, nursing ethics committees, and assisted suicide and euthanasia

The American Society for Bioethics and Humanities
www.asbh.org

- International Journal of Nursing Ethics

Caring Connections
A program of the National Hospice and Palliative Care Organization (NHPCO)
Includes Partnership for Caring, Inc. (formerly, Choice in Dying)
http://www.caringinfo.org

- Questions and Answers: Advance directives and EOL decisions, medical treatments and your advance directives, artificial nutrition and hydration and EOL decision making, do-not-resuscitate orders and EOL decisions
- Video: Who's Death Is It, Anyway? (PBS special)

Aging With Dignity
Five Wishes
www.agingwithdignity.org/five-wishes.php

Washington State Medical Association
Physician's Orders for Life-Sustaining Treatment (POLST)
http://www.wsma.org/patient_resources/polst.cfm

American Association of Colleges of Nursing
End-of-Life Nursing Education Consortium (ELNEC)
www.aacn.nche.edu/elnec/curriculum.htm

Physician Education Research Center
End of Life/Palliative Education Resource Center (EPERC)
www.eperc.mcw.edu/EPERC/FastFactsandConcepts

Advance Directives, by State
http://www.noah-health.org/en/rights/endoflife/adforms.html
http://www.caringinfo/stateaddownload

REFERENCES

Abbo, E. D., Sobotka, S., & Meltzer, D. O. (2008). Patient preferences in instructional advance directives. *Journal of Palliative Medicine*, *11*(4), 555–562. Evidence Level IV.

Alderman, J. S., Nair, B., & Fox, M. D. (2008). Residency training in advance care planning: Can it be done in the outpatient clinic? *The American Journal of Hospice & Palliative Care*, *25*(3), 190–194. Evidence Level IV.

Bakitas, M., Ahles, T. A., Skalla, K., Brokaw, F. C., Byock, I., Hanscom, B., . . . Hegel, M. T. (2008). Proxy perspectives regarding end-of-life care for persons with cancer. *Cancer, 112*(8), 1854–1861. Evidence Level IV.

Barrio-Cantalejo, I. M., Molina-Ruiz, A., Simón-Lorda, P., Cámara-Medina, C., Toral López, I., del Mar Rodríguez del Aguila, M., & Bailon-Gómez, R. M. (2009). Advance directives and proxies' predictions about patients' treatment preferences. *Nursing Ethics, 16*(1), 93–109. Evidence Level II.

Beck, A., Brown, J., Boles, M., & Barrett, P. (2002). Completion of advance directives by older health maintenance organization members: The role of attitudes and beliefs regarding life-sustaining treatment. *Journal of the American Geriatrics Society, 50*(2), 300–306. Evidence Level II.

Bito, S., Matsumura, S., Singer, M. K., Meredith, L. S., Fukuhara, S., & Wenger, N. S. (2007). Acculturation and end-of-life decision making: Comparison of Japanese and Japanese-American focus groups. *Bioethics, 21*(5), 251–262. Evidence Level IV.

Black, K., & Fauske, J. (2007). Exploring influences on community-based case managers' advance care planning practices: Facilitators or barriers? *Home Health Care Services Quarterly, 26*(2), 41–58. Evidence Level IV.

Bomba, P. A., & Vermilyea, D. (2006). Integrating POLST into palliative care guidelines: A paradigm shift in advance care planning in oncology. *Journal of the National Comprehensive Cancer Network, 4*(8), 819–829. Evidence Level V.

Bravo, G., Dubois, M. F., & Wagneur, B. (2008). Assessing the effectiveness of interventions to promote advance directives among older adults: A systematic review and multi-level analysis. *Social Science and Medicine, 67*(7), 1122–1132. Evidence Level I.

Brink, P., Smith, T. F., & Kitson, M. (2008). Determinants of do-not-resuscitate orders in palliative home care. *Journal of Palliative Medicine, 11*(2), 226–232. Evidence Level IV.

Bullock, K. (2006). Promoting advance directives among African Americans: A faith-based model. *Journal of Palliative Medicine, 9*(1), 183–195. Evidence Level IV.

Cohen-Mansfield, J., & Lipson, S. (2008). Which advance directive matters? An analysis of end-of-life decisions made in nursing homes. *Research on Aging, 30*(1), 74–92. Evidence Level IV.

Coppola, K. M., Ditto, P., Danks, J. H., & Smucker, W. D. (2001). Accuracy of primary care and hospital-based physicians' predictions of elderly outpatients' treatment preferences with and without advance directives. *Archives of Internal Medicine, 161*(3), 431–440. Evidence Level II.

Cox, C. L., Cole, E., Reynolds, T., Wandrag, M., Breckenridge, S., & Dingle, M. (2006). Implications of cultural diversity in do not attempt resuscitation (DNAR) decision-making. *Journal of Multicultural Nursing & Health, 12*(1), 20–28. Evidence Level V.

Crisp, D. H. (2007). Healthy older adults' execution of advance directives: A qualitative study of decision making. *Journal of Nursing Law, 11*(4), 180–190. Evidence Level IV.

Detering, K. M., Hancock, A. D., Reade, M. C., & Silvester, W. (2010). The impact of advance care planning on end of life care in elderly patients: Randomised controlled trial. *British Medical Journal, 340*, c1345.doi: 10.1136/bmj.c1345. Evidence Level II.

Ditto, P. H., Danks, J. H., Smucker, W. D., Bookwala, J., Coppola, K. M., Dresser, R., . . . Zyzanski, S. (2001). Advance directives as acts of communication: A randomized controlled trial. *Archives of Internal Medicine, 161*(3), 421–430. Evidence Level II.

Ditto, P. H., Jacobson, J. A., Smucker, W. D., Danks, J. H., & Fagerlin, A. (2006). Context changes choices: A prospective study of the effects of hospitalization on life-sustaining treatment preferences. *Medical Decision Making, 26*(4), 313–322. Evidence Level IV.

Doorenbos, A. Z., & Nies, M. A. (2003). The use of advance directives in a population of Asian Indian Hindus. *Journal of Transcultural Nursing, 14*(1), 17–24. Evidence Level IV.

Elbogen, E. B., Swanson, J. W., Appelbaum, P. S., Swartz, M. S., Ferron, J., Van Dorn, R. A., & Wagner, H. R. (2007). Competence to complete psychiatric advance directives: Effects of facilitated decision making. *Law and Human Behavior, 31*(3), 275–289. Evidence Level II.

Elbogen, E. B., Swartz, M. S., Van Dorn, R., Swanson, J. W., Kim, M., & Scheyett, A. (2006). Clinical decision making and views about psychiatric advance directives. *Psychiatric Services, 57*(3), 350–355. Evidence Level IV.

Engelberg, R. A., Patrick, D. L., & Curtis, J. R. (2005). Correspondence between patients' preferences and surrogates' understandings for dying and death. *Journal of Pain and Symptom Management*, *30*(6), 498–509. Evidence Level III.

Engelhardt, J. B., McClive-Reed, K. P., Toseland, R. W., Smith, T. L., Larson, D. G., & Tobin, D. R. (2006). Effects of a program for coordinated care of advanced illness on patients, surrogates, and healthcare costs: A randomized trial. *American Journal of Managed Care*, *12*(2), 93–100. Evidence Level II.

Fried, T. R., Bullock, K., Iannone, L., & O'Leary, J. R. (2009). Understanding advance care planning as a process of health behavior change. *Journal of the American Geriatrics Society*, *57*(9), 1547–1555. Evidence Level IV.

Fried, T. R., O'Leary, J., Van Ness, P., & Fraenkel, L. (2007). Inconsistency over time in the preferences of older persons with advanced illness for life-sustaining treatment. *Journal of the American Geriatrics Society*, *55*(7), 1007–1014. Evidence Level IV.

Froman, R. D., & Owen, S. V. (2005). Randomized study of stability and change in patients' advance directives. *Research in Nursing & Health*, *28*(5), 398–407. Evidence Level II.

Gerst, K., & Burr, J. A. (2008). Planning for end-of-life care: Black-White differences in the completion of advance directives. *Research on Aging*, *30*(4), 428–449. Evidence Level IV.

Gillick, M. R. (2006). The use of advance care planning to guide decisions about artificial nutrition and hydration. *Nutrition in Clinical Practice*, *21*(2), 126–133. Evidence Level V.

Gorman, T. E., Ahern, S. P., Wiseman, J., & Skrobik, Y. (2005). Residents' end-of-life decision making with adult hospitalized patients: A review of the literature. *Academic Medicine: Journal of the Association of American Medical Colleges*, *80*(7), 622–633. Evidence Level V.

Happ, M. B., Capezuti, E., Strumpf, N. E., Wagner, L., Cunningham, S., Evans, L., & Maislin, G. (2002). Advance care planning and end-of-life care for hospitalized nursing home residents. *Journal of the American Geriatrics Society*, *50*(5), 829–835. Evidence Level IV.

Hardin, S. B., & Yusufaly, Y. A. (2004). Difficult end-of-life treatment decisions: Do other actors trump advance directives? *Archives of Internal Medicine*, *164*(14), 1531–1533. Evidence Level II.

Hawkins, N. A., Ditto, P. H., Danks, J. H., & Smucker, W. D. (2005). Micromanaging death: Process, preferences, values, and goals in end-of-life medical decision making. *The Gerontologist*, *45*(1), 107–117. Evidence Level IV.

Heiman, H., Bates, D. W., Fairchild, D., Shaykevich, S., & Lehmann, L. S. (2004). Improving completion of advance directives in the primary care setting: A randomized controlled trial. *The American Journal of Medicine*, *117*(5), 318–324. Evidence Level II.

Hickman, S. E., Nelson, C. A., Perrin, N. A., Moss, A. H., Hammes, B. J., & Tolle, S. W. (2010). A comparison of method to communicate treatment preferences in nursing facilities: Traditional practice versus the physician orders for life-sustaining treatment program. *Journal of the American Geriatrics Society*, *58*(7), 1241–1248. Evidence Level IV.

Hopp, F. P., & Duffy, S. A. (2000). Racial variations in end-of-life care. *Journal of the American Geriatrics Society*, *48*(6), 658–663. Evidence Level IV.

Htut, Y., Shahrul, K., & Poi, P. J. (2007). The views of older Malaysians on advanced directive and advanced care planning: A qualitative study. *Asia-Pacific Journal of Public Health*, *19*(3), 58–67. Evidence Level IV.

Jezewski, M. A., Brown, J., Wu, Y. W., Meeker, M. A., Feng, J. Y., & Bu, X. (2005). Oncology nurses' knowledge, attitudes, and experiences regarding advance directives. *Oncology Nursing Forum*, *32*(2), 319–327. Evidence Level IV.

Jezewski, M. A., Meeker, M. A., Sessanna, L., & Finnell, D. S. (2007). The effectiveness of interventions to increase advance directive completion rates. *Journal of Aging and Health*, *19*(3), 519–536. Evidence Level I.

Johnson, K. S., Kuchibhatla, M., & Tulsky, J. A. (2008). What explains racial differences in the use of advance directives and attitudes toward hospice care? *Journal of the American Geriatrics Society*, *56*(10), 1953–1958. Evidence Level IV.

Kwak, J., & Haley, W. E. (2005). Current research findings on end-of-life decision making among racially or ethnically diverse groups. *The Gerontologist*, *45*(5), 634–641. Evidence Level V.

Lo, B., & Steinbrook, R. (2004). Resuscitating advance directives. *Archives of Internal Medicine*, *164*(14), 1501–1506. Evidence Level V.

Makridou, S., Efklides, A., Economidis, D., & Peonidis, F. (2006). Advance directives: A study in Greek adults. *Hellenic Journal of Psychology*, *3*(3), 227–258. Evidence Level IV.

Matsui, M., Braun, K. L., & Karel, H. (2008). Comparison of end-of-life preferences between Japanese elders in the United States and Japan. *Journal of Transcultural Nursing*, *19*(2), 167–174. Evidence Level IV.

McCarthy, E. P., Pencina, M. J., Kelly-Hayes, M., Evans, J. C., Oberacker, E. J., D'Agostino, R. B., Sr, . . . Murabito, J. M. (2008). Advance care planning and health care preferences of community-dwelling elders: The Framingham Heart Study. *The Journals of Gerontology, Series A, Biological Sciences and Medical Sciences*, *63*(9), 951–959. Evidence Level IV.

Meisel, A. (2002). *The right to die* (Vols. 1–2). New York, NY: Aspen Law & Business. Evidence Level VI.

Mezey, M. D., Leitman, R., Mitty, E. L., Bottrell, M. M., & Ramsey, G. C. (2000). Why hospital patients do and do not execute an advance directive. *Nursing Outlook*, *48*(4), 165–171. Evidence Level IV.

Mezey, M., Teresi, J., Ramsey, G., Mitty, E., & Bobrowitz, T. (2002). *Determining a resident's capacity to execute a health care proxy. Voices of decision in nursing homes: Respecting residents' preferences for end-of-life care*. New York, NY: United Hospital Fund of New York. Evidence Level IV.

Midwest Bioethics Center. (1996). *Ethics Committee Consortium: Guidelines for the determination of decisional incapacity*. Kansas City, MO: Author. Evidence Level VI.

Mitchell, S. L., Berkowitz, R. E., Lawson, F. M., & Lipsitz, L. A. (2000). A cross-national survey of tube-feeding decisions in cognitively impaired older persons. *Journal of the American Geriatrics Society*, *48*(4), 391–397. Evidence Level IV.

Morrison, R. S., & Meier, D. E. (2004). High rates of advance care planning in New York City's elderly population. *Archives of Internal Medicine*, *164*(22), 2421–2426. Evidence Level IV.

National Bioethics Advisory Commission. (1998). *Research involving persons with mental disorders that may affect decision making capacity* (Vol 1). Rockville, MD: Author.

Patient Self-Determination Act, Pub. L. No. 101-508, 42 U.S.C.A.1395cc(f) (1992).

Perkins, H. S., Geppert, C. M., Gonzales, A., Cortez, J. D., & Hazuda, H. P. (2002). Cross-cultural similarities and differences in attitudes about advance care planning. *Journal of General Internal Medicine*, *17*(1), 48–57. Evidence Level IV.

Perry, E., Swartz, J., Brown, S., Smith, D., Kelly, G., & Swartz, R. (2005). Peer mentoring: A culturally sensitive approach to end-of-life planning for long-term dialysis patients. *American Journal of Kidney Diseases*, *46*(1), 111–119. Evidence Level II.

Porensky, E. K., & Carpenter, B. D. (2008). Knowledge and perceptions in advance care planning. *Journal of Aging and Health*, *20*(1), 89–106. Evidence Level IV.

Ramsaroop, S. D., Reid, M. C., & Adelman, R. D. (2007). Completing an advance directive in the primary care setting: What do we need for success? *Journal of the American Geriatrics Society*, *55*(2), 277–283. Evidence Level V.

Roth, L. H., Meisel, A., & Lidz, C. W. (1977). Tests of competency to consent to treatment. *American Journal of Psychiatry*, *134*(3), 279–284.

Schwartz, C. E., Wheeler, H. B., Hammes, B., Basque, N., Edmunds, J., Reed, G., . . . Yanko, J. (2002). Early intervention in planning end-of-life care with ambulatory geriatric patients: Results of a pilot trial. *Archives of Internal Medicine*, *162*(14), 1611–1618. Evidence Level II.

Searight, H. R., & Gafford, J. (2005). "It's like playing with your destiny": Bosnian immigrants' views of advance directives and end-of-life decision-making. *Journal of Immigrant Health*, *7*(3), 195–203. Evidence Level IV.

Shalowitz, D. I., Garrett-Mayer, E., & Wendler, D. (2006). The accuracy of surrogate decision makers: A systematic review. *Archives of Internal Medicine, 166*(5), 493–497. Evidence Level I.

Silveira, M. J., DiPiero, A., Gerrity, M. S., & Feudtner, C. (2000). Patients' knowledge of options at the end of life: Ignorance in the face of death. *Journal of the American Medical Association, 284*(19), 2483–2488. Evidence Level IV.

Silveira, M. J., Kim, S. Y., & Langa, K. M. (2010). Advance directives and outcomes of surrogate decision making before death. *The New England Journal of Medicine, 362*(13), 1211–1218. Evidence Level IV.

Stocking, C. B., Hougham, G. W., Danner, D. D., Patterson, M. B., Whitehouse, P. J., & Sachs, G. A. (2006). Speaking of research advance directives: Planning for future research participation. *Neurology, 66*(9), 1361–1366. Evidence Level IV.

Sudore, R. L., Landefeld, C. S., Barnes, D. E., Lindquist, K., Williams, B. A., Brody, R., & Schillinger, D. (2007). An advance directive redesigned to meet the literacy level of most adults: A randomized trial. *Patient Education and Counseling, 69*(1–3), 165–195. Evidence Level II.

Swanson, J., Swartz, M., Ferron, J., Elbogen, E., & Van Dorn, R. (2006). Psychiatric advance directives among public mental health consumers in five U.S. cities: Prevalence, demand, and correlates. *Journal of the American Academy of Psychiatry and the Law, 34*(1), 43–57. Evidence Level IV.

Tamayo-Velázquez, M. I., Simón-Lorda, P., Villegas-Portero, R., Higueras-Callejón, C., García-Gutiérrez, J. F., Martínez-Pecino, F., & Barrio-Cantalejo, I. M. (2010). Interventions to promote the use of advance directives: An overview of systematic reviews. *Patient Education and Counseling, 80*(1), 10–20. Evidence Level I.

Teno, J. M., Gruneir, A., Schwartz, Z., Nanda, A., & Wetle, T. (2007). Association between advance directives and quality of end-of-life care: A national study. *Journal of the American Geriatrics Society, 55*(2), 189–194. Evidence Level IV.

Tierney, W. M., Dexter, P. R., Gramelspacher, G. P., Perkins, A. J., Zhou, X. H., & Wolinsky, F. D. (2001). The effect of discussion about advance directives on patients' satisfaction with primary care. *Journal of General Internal Medicine, 16*(1), 32–40. Evidence Level II.

Triplett, P., Black, B. S., Phillips, H., Richardson Fahrendorf, S., Schwartz, J., Angelino, A. F., . . . Rabins, P. V. (2008). Content of advance directives for individuals with advanced dementia. *Journal of Aging and Health, 20*(5), 583–596. Evidence Level IV.

Weinick, R. M., Wilcox, S. R., Park, E. R., Griffey, R. T., & Weissman, J. S. (2008). Use of advance directives for nursing home residents in the emergency department. *The American Journal of Hospice & Palliative Care, 25*(3), 179–183. Evidence Level IV.

Wilder, C. M., Elbogen, E. B., Moser, L. L., Swanson, J. W., & Swartz, M. S. (2010). Medication preferences and adherence among individuals with severe mental illness and psychiatric advance directives. *Psychiatric Services, 61*(4): 380–385. Evidence Level II.

Comprehensive Assessment and Management of the Critically Ill

30

Michele C. Balas, Colleen M. Casey, and Mary Beth Happ

EDUCATIONAL OBJECTIVES

On completion of this chapter, the reader should be able to:

1. identify factors that influence an older adult's ability to survive and rehabilitate from a catastrophic illness
2. list examples of atypical presentation of illness in critically ill older adults
3. describe geriatric-specific assessment and physical examination of critically ill older adults
4. identify nursing interventions that decrease critically ill older adults' risk for adverse medical outcomes

OVERVIEW

More than half (55.8%) of all intensive care unit (ICU) days are incurred by patients older than the age of 65, and this number is expected to increase to unprecedented levels over the next 10 years as the population ages (Angus et al., 2000). For example, it is projected that by the year 2020, more than 350,000 older adults will annually require acute mechanical ventilation for more than 4 days (Zilberberg, de Wit, Pirone, & Shorr, 2008). Although older adults are an extremely heterogeneous group, they share some age-related characteristics and are susceptible to various geriatric syndromes and diseases that may influence ICU treatments and outcomes (Milbrandt, Eldadah, Nayfield, Hadley, & Angus, 2010; Pisani, 2009).

Ideally, the goals of providing nursing care to the critically ill older adult include restoring physiologic stability, preventing complications, maintaining comfort and

For description of Evidence Levels cited in this chapter, see Chapter 1, Developing and Evaluating Clinical Practice Guidelines: A Systematic Approach, page 7.

Note: This chapter has been adapted from the American Association of Colleges of Nursing, "Preparing Nursing Students to Care for Older Adults: Enhancing Gerontology in Senior-Level Undergraduate Courses" curriculum module. Assessment and Management of Older Adults with Complex Illness in the Critical Care Unit, prepared by Michele C. Balas, Colleen M. Casey, and Mary Beth Happ.

safety, and preserving or preventing decline in preillness functional ability and quality of life (QOL). There is evidence, however, suggesting that many critically ill older adults are at risk for poor outcomes. Once hospitalized for a life-threatening illness, older adults suffer from high ICU, hospital, and long-term crude mortality rates and are at risk for deterioration in functional ability, cognitive impairment, and postdischarge institutional care (de Rooij, Abu-Hanna, Levi, & de Jonge, 2005; Esteban et al., 2004; Ford, Thomas, Cook, Whitley, & Peden, 2007; Hennessy, Juzwishin, Yergens, Noseworthy, & Doig, 2005; Hopkins & Jackson, 2006; Kaarlola, Tallgren, & Pettilä, 2006; Marik, 2006; Wunsch et al., 2010). Older age is also one of the factors that may lead to physician bias in refusing ICU admission (Joynt et al., 2001; Mick & Ackerman, 2004); the decision to withhold mechanical ventilation, surgery, or dialysis (Hamel et al., 1999); and an increased frequency of do-not-resuscitate orders (Hakim et al., 1996). Despite these findings, most critically ill older adults demonstrate resiliency, report being satisfied with their QOL postdischarge, and, if needed, would reaccept ICU care and mechanical ventilation (Guentner et al., 2006; Hennessy et al., 2005; Kleinpell & Ferrans, 2002).

BACKGROUND AND STATEMENT OF PROBLEM

Chronologic age *alone* is not an acceptable or accurate predictor of poor outcomes after critical illness (Milbrandt et al., 2010; Nagappan & Parkin, 2003). Factors influencing an older adult's ability to survive a critical illness include severity of illness, nature and extent of comorbidities, diagnosis, the need for mechanical ventilation, complications, preadmission of cognitive and functional status, malnutrition, and patient preference (de Rooij et al., 2005; Marik, 2006; Wunsch et al., 2010). Other less well investigated variables include senescence, vasoactive drug use, ageism, decreased social support, and the critical care environment (Ford et al., 2007; Mick & Ackerman, 2004; Tullmann & Dracup, 2000). The onset of new geriatric syndromes for an older hospitalized adult such as urinary incontinence, infection, delirium, or falls are also harbingers of undesirable events that can often be prevented with appropriate and timely ICU nursing interventions (for more information, visit http://www.geronurseonline.org). This chapter presents strategies and rationale for comprehensive assessment of critically ill older adults to guide optimal care management.

ASSESSMENT OF PROBLEM AND NURSING CARE STRATEGIES

Assessment of Baseline Health Status

Comprehensive assessment of a critically ill older adult's preadmission health status, functional and cognitive ability, and social support systems helps the nurse identify risk factors that make the older adult susceptible to cascade iatrogenesis (Creditor, 1993), the development of life-threatening conditions, and frequently encountered geriatric syndromes.

Preexisting Cognitive Impairment

Several anatomic and physiologic changes occur in the aged central nervous system (see Table 30.1; Miller, 2009). The additive effect of chronic illness (e.g., diabetes, hypertension, or coronary artery disease [CAD]) coupled with common aging changes and acute

TABLE 30.1

Age-Associated Changes by Body System in the Older ICU Patient

System	Age-Associated Changes
Respiratory	Decrease in chest wall compliance, rib mobility, lung size and elasticity, ventilatory response to hypoxia and hypercapnia, strength of respiratory muscles, PaO_2 level, mucociliary clearance, total lung capacity (minimal), forced vital capacity, forced inspiratory and expiratory volume, peak and maximal expiratory flow rate, tidal volume (slight), diffusing capacity, and maximal inspiratory and expiratory pressure Increases in residual volume, closing volume, A/A gradient, ventilation/perfusion (VQ) imbalance, and chest wall stiffness Physical assessment findings: possible kyphosis and an increased anteroposterior diameter of the chest upon auscultation, a few bibasilar crackles that clear with deep breathing and coughing
Gastrointestinal	Decrease in number of mucus-secreting cells, mucosal prostaglandin concentrations, bicarbonate secretion, transit time of feces, pepsin and acid secretion, gastric emptying, and thinning of smooth muscle in gastric mucosa; decrease in the number and velocity of peristaltic contractions in esophagus, enteric nervous system neurons, capacity to repair gastric mucosa, calcium absorption, lean muscle mass and strength, daily energy expenditure, intracellular water, number of hepatocytes, and overall weight and size of liver (compensatory increase in cell size and proliferation of bile ducts), hepatic blood flow, and metabolism of and sensitivity to drugs Increase in body fat, changes to interstitial tissue (predisposing to soft tissue injury and increasing the time and course for mobilization of extracellular water)
Genitourinary	Increase in proportion of sclerotic nephrons or glomeruli, functional unit hypertrophy, afferent and efferent arteriole atrophy, collagen in the bladder, benign prostatic hypertrophy (men), hypertrophy of bladder muscle, thickening of the bladder Decline in number of functioning nephrons, glomerular filtration rate, renal tubular cell function and number, renal blood flow, and creatinine clearance; ability to conserve sodium and excrete hydrogen ions; ability to excrete salt and water loads, ammonia, and certain drugs in the activity of the renin-angiotensin system and end-organ responsiveness to antidiuretic hormone, tone of sphincters, and alterations in estrogen cause further changes in urethral sphincter of women
Skin	Decrease in surface area between dermis and epidermis, subcutaneous and connective tissue, number of eccrine and sebaceous glands, sebum amount, vascular supply to dermis, epidermal turnover, skin turgor, moisture content, and dermal thickness Physical assessment findings: thin, fragile, wrinkled, loose, or transparent, dry, flaky, rough, and often itchy skin
Neurologic	Decrease in size of brain/brain weight, number of neurons and dendrites, length of dendrite spines, cerebral blood flow, neurotransmitters or their binding sites, in dopaminergic function, visual acuity and depth perception (secondary to anatomic and functional changes to the auditory and vestibular apparatus) and proprioception, balance and postural control, and tactile and vibratory sensation Increase in liposuscins, neuritic plaques, neurofibrillary bodies, ventricle size, and sulci widening Physical assessment findings: decreased papillary response to penlight, decrease in near and peripheral vision, loss of visual acuity to dim light, evidence of muscle wasting and atrophy, presentation of a benign essential tumor, slower and less agile movement as compared to younger adults, diminished peripheral reflexes, and a decreased vibratory sense in the feet and ankles

(continued)

TABLE 30.1

Age-Associated Changes by Body System in the Older ICU Patient *(continued)*

System	Age-Associated Changes
Cardiovascular	Decrease in number of myocytes and pacemaker cells, ventricular compliance, rate of relaxation, baroreceptor sensitivity, vein elasticity, compliance of arteries, response of myocardium to catecholamine stimulation, resting heart rate, heart rate with stress, and cardiac reserve
	Increase in myocardial collagen content, amyloid deposits, myocardial irritability, stiffening of the outflow tract and great vessels (causing resistance to vascular emptying), ventricular hypertrophy (slight), pulse wave velocity, time required to complete the cycle of diastolic filling and systolic emptying, vein dilation, and valvular stiffening
	Physical assessment findings: Upon auscultation, many healthy older adults display a fourth heart sound (S_4), an aortic systolic murmur, higher systolic blood pressure with a widening pulse pressure, and a slower resting heart rate.
Immune/ hematopoietic	Change in T-cell populations, products, and response to stimuli; defects in B-cell function; mix of immunoglobulins change (i.e., IgM decreases, IgG and IgA increase) and decline in neutrophil function

Note. ICU = intensive care unit; IgG = immunoglobulin G; IgA = immunoglobulin A; IgM = immunoglobulin M.
Source: Based on Bickley & Szilagyi (2008); Marik, Vasu, Hirani, & Pachinburavan (2010); Menaker & Scalea (2010); Miller (2009); Pisani (2009); Rosenthal & Kavic (2004); and Urden, Stacy, & Lough (2002).

pathology may, however, place older adults at higher risk for some commonly encountered ICU syndromes such as delirium (McNicoll et al., 2003; Pisani, Murphy, Van Ness, Araujo, & Inouye, 2007). High rates of preexisting cognitive impairment (31%–42%) are reported in older adults admitted to both medical and surgical ICUs (Balas et al., 2007; Pisani, Redlich, McNicoll, Ely, & Inouye, 2003). Unfortunately, this cognitive impairment is often unrecognized by both the older adults family and health care providers (Balas et al., 2007; Pisani et al., 2003). Relatives or other caregivers should be asked for baseline information about memory, executive function (problem solving, planning, organization of information), and overall functional ability in daily living prior to the critical care admission (Kane, Ouslander, & Abrass, 2004; see Chapter 8, Assessing Cognitive Function). Because knowledge of an older adult's preadmission cognitive status may also assist in treatment decisions, ICU clinicians should consider familiarizing themselves with dementia screening tools such as the Informant Questionnaire on Cognitive Decline in the Elderly (IQCODE) that were specifically designed for proxy administration (Jorm, 1994).

Psychosocial Factors

Critical illness often renders older adults physically unable to effectively communicate with the health care team. The inability to communicate may stem from multiple factors including physiologic instability, tracheal intubation, and/or sedative and narcotic use (Happ, 2000, 2001). Family members, or significant others, are therefore a crucial source for obtaining important preadmission information such as the older adult's past medical and surgical history, drug and alcohol use, nutritional status, home environment, infectious disease exposure, medication use, religious preference, and social support systems. Further, the lack of presence of family or a significant other threatens the nurse's ability to obtain accurate data about the person, which is often needed to make urgent, important care management and end-of-life discussions. (See Chapters 28, Health Care Decision Making, and Chapter 29, Advance Directives).

Functional Ability

Although most older adults report having at least one chronic condition, they remain relatively independent (Administration on Aging, 2009). Assessing preadmission functional status is essential when caring for critically ill older adults because many studies have found it to be an important prognostic indicator in this population (Marik, 2006; Mick & Ackerman, 2004; Tullmann & Dracup, 2000). Both the Katz Index of Independence in Activities of Daily Living (KATZ ADLs; Katz, Ford, Moskowitz, Jackson, & Jaffe, 1963) and the Functional Independence Measure (FIM; Kidd et al., 1995) have been recommended for use with an older population (Kresevic & Mezey, 2003; see Chapter 6, Assessment of Physical Function). Upon admission to the ICU, nurses should also investigate whether the older adult uses glasses, hearing aids, or other devices to perform their ADLs. Having these assistive devices available to the older adult while they are in the ICU is important to enhance communication and rehabilitation.

Assessment and Interventions During ICU Stay

Although a full discussion of the physiologic changes that accompany common aging is beyond the scope of this chapter, in the following sections we hope to provide readers with (a) an overview of the major age-related changes to organ systems and description of how these changes often manifest on physical exam (Table 30.1); (b) a discussion of atypical presentations of some common ICU diagnoses; and (c) a description of interventions that may decrease the risk of untoward medical events for critically ill older adults (also see Protocol 30.1). Common nursing interventions that benefit multiple organ systems will only be discussed in the first section in which the intervention is introduced. These interventions include encouraging early, frequent mobilization or ambulation; obtaining timely and appropriate consults (e.g., physical, occupational, speech, respiratory, nutritional therapy); providing proper oral hygiene and adequate pain control; securing and ensuring the proper functioning of tubes or catheters; maintaining normothermia; deep vein thrombosis prophylaxis; and reviewing and assessing medication appropriateness. The importance of these interventions and vigilance to these elements of nursing care cannot be overstated.

Respiratory System

Because of a decrease in respiratory reserve with aging (Table 30.1; Pisani, 2009), an older ICU patient's respiratory status can become the most tenuous component of his or her recovery. Common pulmonary changes in aging elevate an older adult's risk for aspiration, atelectasis, pneumonia, and acute lung injury (Menaker & Scalea, 2010; Nagappan & Parkin, 2003; Pisani, 2009; Rosenthal & Kavic, 2004; Urden, Stacy, & Lough, 2002). These risks are further heightened in older adults who undergo thoracic or abdominal surgery; sustain rib fractures or chest injury; receive narcotics or sedatives; have tubes that bypass the oropharyngeal airway; or who are weak, deconditioned, dehydrated, and have poor oral hygiene (Menaker & Scalea, 2010; Nagappan & Parkin, 2003; Rosenthal, 2004; Rosenthal & Kavic, 2004; Urden et al., 2002). Preexisting pulmonary disease and manipulations of the abdominal and thoracic cavities may further lead to unreliability of traditional values associated with central venous pressure (CVP) and pulmonary artery occlusion pressures (PAOPs; Rosenthal & Kavic, 2004). Consequently, it is important to discuss with the ICU team any unusual preexisting or acute influences on these hemodynamic parameters so that accurate trends can be monitored.

Caring for the older adult who requires mechanical ventilation is particularly challenging. Although debate exists about whether age influences outcome in this population, evidence suggests that chronic ventilatory dependency disproportionately affects older patients, whether as a complication of a critical illness or as a result of a chronic respiratory system limitation (Esteban et al., 2004; Kleinhenz & Lewis, 2000; Zilberberg et al., 2008). Patients who require 4 or more days of mechanical ventilation are more likely to die in the hospital, or if they survive, to spend a considerable amount of time in an extended care facility upon discharge, experience an increased risk of hospital readmission, suffer from continued morbidity, and experience a decreased QOL (Chelluri et al., 2004; Daly et al., 2009; Douglas, Daly, Brennan, Gordon, & Uthis, 2001; Douglas, Daly, Gordon, & Brennan, 2002; Douglas, Daly, Kelley, O'Toole, & Montenegro, 2007; Douglas, Daly, O'Toole, Kelley, & Montenegro, 2009; Oeyen, Vandijck, Benoit, Annemans, & Decruyenaere, 2010). These patients and their family members often experience symptoms of depression and posttraumatic stress disorder following discharge from the ICU (Douglas, Daly, Kelley, O'Toole, & Montenegro, 2005; Douglas, Daly, O'Toole, & Hickman, 2010; Griffiths, Fortune, Barber, & Young, 2007; Jubran et al., 2010). These potential consequences should be included as part of a discussion of treatment options and postdischarge follow-up with older adults and their families.

The aforementioned findings also highlight the need for the ICU team to aggressively pursue means of early ventilator liberation. A protocol that paired spontaneous awakening trials (SATs) with spontaneous breathing trials (SBTs) was recently found to improve mechanically ventilated patients' outcomes (Girard et al., 2008). In this study, patients treated with both SATs and SBTs spent more days breathing without assistance, were discharged from intensive care and the hospital earlier, and, at any instant during the year after enrollment, were less likely to die than were patients in the control group (Girard et al., 2008). It has also been suggested that even more benefit may be accrued by adding SATs and SBTs to protocols of early mobilization of mechanically ventilated patients (Bailey, Miller, & Clemmer, 2009; King, Render, Ely, & Watson, 2010; Morris et al., 2008). Finally, recent advances in techniques and applications of noninvasive ventilation provide an exceedingly useful means of managing respiratory compromise, thus potentially avoiding mechanical ventilation, in the older adult population (Muir, Lamia, Molano, & Cuvelier, 2010).

Older patients with preexisting obstructive or restrictive lung disease who are mechanically ventilated either in the ICU or in long-term care facilities are also at increased risk for ventilator-assisted pneumonia (VAP; Buczko, 2010). To minimize this complication, nurses should aggressively exercise standard VAP precautions, including elevating the head of the bed to at least 30 degrees, providing frequent oral care, maintaining adequate cuff pressures, using continuous subglottic suctioning, avoiding the routine changing of ventilator circuit tubing, assessing the need for stress ulcer and deep venous thrombosis (DVT) prophylaxis, turning the patient as tolerated, providing optimal hygiene, and advocating for weaning trials as early as possible (American Association of Critical Care Nurses [AACN], 2004; American Thoracic Society [ATS] & Infectious Diseases Society of America [IDSA], 2005; Dezfulian et al., 2005; Institute for Healthcare Improvement [IHI] & 5 Million Lives Campaign, 2008; Krein et al., 2008). Several studies have also reported that early tracheostomy may be of benefit in decreasing VAP in older critically ill patients (Menaker & Scalea, 2010).

Nurses should consider that older adults with common respiratory pathology often do not present with symptoms traditionally considered "hallmarks of infection"—fever, chills, and other constitutional symptoms. In fact, the typical signs of pneumonia—fever, cough, and sputum production—can be absent in older adult, with only 33%–60% of older patients presenting with a fever (Bellmann-Weiler & Weiss, 2009). Instead, older patients with either sepsis or pneumonia can often present with acute confusion, tachypnea, and tachycardia (Girard & Ely, 2007). This vague symptomatology can delay diagnosis, and importantly antibiotic administration, leading to poorer outcomes (Iregui, Ward, Sherman, Fraser, & Kollef, 2002).

Cardiovascular System

Because so many older adults live with hypertension, peripheral vascular disease, or CAD, individual responses to treatment can dramatically differ depending on the severity of their illness and any preexisting comorbidities. Even the "disease-free" older adult may experience a decrease in their ability to respond to stressful situations because of many changes that accompany cardiovascular aging (see Table 30.1; Pisani, 2009).

Cardiovascular-associated aging changes ultimately render the myocardium less compliant and responsive to catecholamine stimulation, can cause ventricular hypertrophy, and predispose the older adult to the development of several different types of arrhythmias (Nagappan & Parkin, 2003; Rosenthal & Kavic, 2004; Urden et al., 2002). During times of stress, an older adult achieves an increase in cardiac output by increasing diastolic filling rather than increasing heart rate (Nagappan & Parkin, 2003; Rosenthal & Kavic, 2004; Urden et al., 2002). The practical implication of this finding is that older adults often require higher filling pressures (i.e., CVPs in the 8–10 cm range, PAOPs in the 14–18 cm range) to maintain adequate stroke volume and may be especially sensitive to hypovolemia (Rosenthal & Kavic, 2004). However, overhydration of the older adult should also be avoided because it can lead to systolic failure, poor organ perfusion, and hypoxemia with subsequent diastolic dysfunction (Rosenthal & Kavic, 2004). Careful monitoring of hemodynamic and fluid status is therefore essential to optimize the older patient's cardiac status.

Cardiac complications are among the highest causes of mortality in the elderly surgical patient (Menaker & Scalea, 2010). Although many of the randomized controlled trials of beta-blocker therapy are small, the weight of evidence, in aggregate, suggests that the use of preoperative beta-adrenergic blockade decreases the incidence of postoperative cardiac complications and death in patients considered high risk (Fleisher et al., 2007). High cardiovascular risk includes older adults with unstable coronary syndromes, decompensated heart failure, significant arrhythmias, previous myocardial infarction, and even patients with diabetes mellitus and renal insufficiency (Fleisher et al., 2007). Certain other drugs commonly used in the ICU setting to treat cardiac conditions may prove to be either not as effective (e.g., isoproterenol and dobutamine) or more effective (e.g., afterload reducers) in the older adult population (Rosenthal & Kavic, 2004).

Symptoms of a myocardial infarction and congestive heart failure may be blunted in critically ill older adults (Menaker & Scalea, 2010; Pisani, 2009), requiring the need to monitor for nonspecific and atypical presentations in this patient population, including shortness of breath, acute confusion, or syncope (Miller, 2009). Worsening clinical status or difficulty weaning from mechanical ventilation should prompt the ICU team to investigate the possibility of myocardial ischemia in this population (Pisani, 2009).

Neurologic System

The central and peripheral nervous system changes that accompany aging may partially explain why older adults often present to emergency departments or the ICU with acute neurologic symptoms. These acute neurologic changes may represent an atypical presentation of an acute illness, including alterations caused by infection, an imbalance of electrolytes, or drug toxicity. A thorough physical examination, with follow-up testing, must be conducted to accurately diagnose the etiology of an older adult's neurologic changes as well as a thorough review of medication use.

Age-related changes to the neurologic system, when coupled with acute pathology and the ICU environment, may increase a critically ill older adult's risk for cognitive dysfunction, falls, restraint use, oversedation, alterations in body temperature, and anorexia. Most importantly, these changes also elevate the risk of delirium that occurs in up to 70% of older adults admitted to an ICU (Balas et al., 2007; Kresevic & Mezey, 2003; Peterson et al., 2006) and is associated with increased morbidity, mortality, length of hospital stay, and poor functional outcomes (Balas et al., 2007; Balas, Happ, Yang, Chelluri, & Richmond, 2009; Ely et al., 2001). Pain, sleep deprivation, visual impairment, illness severity, prior cognitive impairment, dehydration, comorbidities, laboratory abnormalities, multiple medications, chemical withdrawal syndromes, infections, fever, windowless units, and ICU length of stay may place the critically ill older adult at risk for delirium (Morandi, Jackson, & Ely, 2009). Although management of delirium in hospitalized patients is discussed more fully in Chapter 11, clinicians must be particularly aware of the interconnectedness of delirium, mechanical ventilation, and immobility in the critical care environment. Nurse-led interdisciplinary, multicomponent strategies such as the awakening and breathing coordination, delirium monitoring/management, and early mobility (ABCDE) bundle proposed by Vasilevskis et al. (2010) have the potential to decrease delirium rates and subsequent poor outcomes in the older adult population.

In addition to the physical barriers to speech imposed by mechanical ventilation, older adult patients are at greater risk for impaired communication than their younger counterparts because of preexisting vision, hearing, and cognitive or language impairments (Bartlett, Blais, Tamblyn, Clermont, & MacGibbon, 2008; Happ & Paull, 2008; Patak et al., 2009). Accurate interpretation of patient messages, including pain and symptom descriptions, may be difficult and frustrating for patients and care providers. Partnering with speech-language pathologists on tools and techniques to facilitate patient comprehension and communication can improve this process (Bartlett et al., 2008; Happ & Paull, 2008).

Achieving adequate pain control for critically ill older adults is of utmost importance, both related to and independent of its relationship to delirium; however, the nurse also needs to avoid oversedation and undertreatment of pain in this population because both are associated with multiple negative outcomes, including distress, delirium, sleep disturbances, and impaired mobility (Graf & Puntillo, 2003; Rosenthal & Kavic, 2004). Several tools exist to assess a critically ill patient's level of sedation and delirium status. The Richmond Agitation and Sedation Scale (RASS; Ely et al., 2001; Sessler et al., 2002) and the Confusion Assessment Method-ICU (CAM-ICU; Ely et al., 2001) are two of the most common tools in the critical care setting (see Resources section for additional information on these tools and Practice Protocol for interventions to reduce delirium).

Gastrointestinal System

Common age-related changes to the gastrointestinal (GI) system can predispose older ICU patients to complications during their ICU stay, ranging from altered presentation of illness to issues of medication effectiveness (Table 30.1). Older adults also experience changes in their body composition (i.e., decrease in lean body mass) and energy use that can potentiate the effect of medications on these GI system changes.

Ironically, although many conditions affecting the GI system are more common in older adults (e.g., constipation, undernutrition and malnutrition, gastritis), their presence is not fully explained by the aging processes (Rosenthal & Kavic, 2004). When assessing the GI function of a critically ill older adult, it is important for the nurse to realize that age may blunt the manifestations of acute abdominal disease. For example, pain may be less severe, fever may be less pronounced or absent, and signs of peritoneal inflammation, such as muscle guarding and rebound tenderness, may be diminished or even absent (Bickley & Szilagyi, 2008). Because of changes in the secretion of gastric enzymes, the stomach wall of older adults can be more susceptible to acid injury, especially in the face of critical illness. The practice of routine stress ulcer prophylaxis in the critically ill patient, part of the VAP bundle and common in many ICUs, however, has more recently been challenged as a potential contributor to pneumonia with more narrow indications that has been assumed, even in mechanically ventilated patients (Herzig, Howell, Ngo, & Marcantonio, 2009; Logan, Sumukadas, & Witham, 2010; Marik, Vasu, Hirani, & Pachinburavan, 2010).

Delayed gastric emptying may predispose older adults to abdominal distension, nausea, vomiting, aspiration, and constipation. This delayed motility is especially true in the postoperative period when many older adults are immobile and receiving narcotics. Many older adults take multiple medications, which along with age-related changes such as altered thresholds for taste and smell, a hypersensitive hypothalamic satiety center, and oropharyngeal atrophy, can inhibit their intake of solids and liquids (Rosenthal & Kavic, 2004). This baseline GI functionality, in combination with their critical illness, must be proactively addressed. The nurse needs to be alert for ill-fitting dentures, swallowing difficulties, silent aspiration, and the possibility of decreased saliva production (caused by either salivary dysfunction or the use of drugs such as sympathomimetics). These alterations can lead to insufficient mastication and can combine with other risk factors that put the older ICU patient at risk for aspiration. Aspiration should be considered a life-threatening situation requiring immediate nursing intervention.

Older adults facing stress from illness, injury, or infection are also at high risk for protein–calorie malnutrition, as evidenced by low serum albumin and prealbumin levels, a decline in hepatic function, decreased muscle mass and strength, and dysfunction in those tissues with high cell turnover (Nagappan & Parkin, 2003; Rosenthal & Kavic, 2004). These changes lead to a breakdown in barrier function, increased susceptibility to infection, delayed wound healing, fluid shifts, deconditioning, and further impairment in absorption of essential nutrients (Rosenthal, 2004). Thus, early enteral or parental nutritional support is crucial while taking advance directives into consideration.

Reductions with age in the activity of the drug-metabolizing enzyme system and blood flow through the liver influence the liver's capacity to metabolize various drugs (Kane et al., 2004; Urden et al., 2002). Splanchnic blood flow is further compromised in states of shock or even mild hypotension. These changes may predispose older adults to adverse drug reactions (Urden et al., 2002). For example, drugs such as warfarin that work directly on hepatocytes may reach their therapeutic effect at lower doses

(Rosenthal & Kavic, 2004). Common pharmacologic agents used in the critical care setting and their common side effects often experienced by the gerontologic patient are given in Table 30.2 (see Chapter 17, Reducing Adverse Drug Events).

Finally, many older adults have diabetes and even those older adults without preexisting diabetes may experience elevated blood glucose levels as a result of medications and a stress response to critical illness. Therefore, glycemic control in the older ICU patient may be more difficult because of a declining glucose tolerance associated with aging. Although initial studies indicated tight control of blood sugar, with blood glucose levels 80–110 mg/dL, optimized recovery, and outcomes (Humbert, Gallagher, Gabbay, & Dellasega, 2008; Van den Berghe et al., 2001), more recent study has revealed that this tight control actually increases mortality (Van den Berghe, Bouillon, & Mesotten, 2009).

TABLE 30.2

High-Risk Medications Commonly Used in Older ICU Patients

Drug	Severity Rating[†]	Potential Adverse Effects
*Amiodarone (Cordarone)	High	May provoke torsades de pointes and QT interval problems. Lack of efficacy in older adults.
*Clonidine (Catapres)	Low	Orthostatic hypotension, CNS adverse effects
*Diazepam (Valium)	High	Increased sensitivity to benzodiazepines; long half-life in older patients (can be several days); prolonged sedation; increasing risk of falls and fractures; short- and intermediate-acting benzodiazepines preferred
Digoxin (Lanoxin)	Low	Decreased renal clearance may lead to increased risk of toxic effects; dose should not exceed >0.125 mg/day except when treating atrial arrhythmias
*Diphenhydramine (Benadryl)	High	Strong anticholinergic effects, confusion, oversedation; can also cause dry mouth and urinary retention; aggravates benign prostatic hypertrophy and glaucoma; use smallest possible dose
*Ketorolac (Toradol)	High	Peptic ulceration, GI bleeding, perforation; GI effects can be asymptomatic
*Meperidine (Demerol)	High	Active metabolite accumulation may cause CNS toxicity, tremor, confusion, irritability; other narcotics preferred
*Promethazine (Phenergan)	High	Highly anticholinergic; confusion, oversedation; can also cause dry mouth, urinary retention; aggravates benign prostatic hypertrophy and glaucoma
Propofol (Diprivan)	Unrated	Lipophilic drug; decreased clearance in older adults related to increased total body fat
Cimetidine (Tagamet) and Ranitidine (Zantac)	Low	CNS effects, confusion

[†]Severity Rating—Adverse effects of medications rated as high or low severity based on the probability of event occurring and significance of the outcome (Beers, 1997; Bonk et al., 2006)

*Identified in Bonk et al. (2006) as seven most commonly prescribed Beers medications used in older hospitalized patients.

CNS = central nervous system; GI = gastrointestinal.

Source: Adapted from Bonk, Krown, Matuszewski, & Oinonen (2006);
and Fick, Cooper, Wade, Waller, Maclean, & Beers (2003).

Genitourinary System

Preservation of the older adult's preadmission renal status is one of the goals of ICU care. Common age-related changes in the genitourinary (GU) system decrease the older adult's ability to excrete ammonia and drugs, diminish their capacity to regulate fluid and acid–base balance, and often impair their ability to properly empty their bladder (Nagappan & Parkin, 2003; Rosenthal & Kavic, 2004; Urden et al., 2002). The coupling of these common age-related changes with conditions commonly seen in the ICU environment such as hypovolemia, shock, sepsis, and polypharmacy render the older adult at increased risk for acute renal failure, metabolic acidosis, and adverse drug events (Yilmaz & Erdem, 2010). The increased prevalence in the older population of asymptomatic bacteriuria also exacerbates an older ICU patient's infection risk related to Foley catheter use (Richards, 2004).

The nurse must take into consideration an older patient's baseline cardiovascular status relative to their renal function. If an older patient was typically hypertensive prior to hospitalization, for example, this patient's renal vasculature may be accustomed to a higher-than-normal pressure to perfuse the kidneys. Furthermore, common indicators of dehydration, such as skin turgor, should be considered an unreliable sign in an older adult, related to their loss of subcutaneous tissue (Sheehy, Perry, & Cromwell, 1999). Although the Cockcroft–Gault formula (see Chapter 17, Reducing Adverse Drug Events) has been derived to estimate creatinine clearance in the healthy aged, care must be taken when applying this formula to critically ill older patients or to those patients on medications that directly affect renal function (Rosenthal & Kavic, 2004). Finally, the nurse should be especially cognizant of medications known to contribute to renal failure including aminoglycosides, certain antibiotics, and contrast dyes, and closely monitor laboratory results as warranted (Urden et al., 2002).

Immune and Hematopoietic System

The changes that occur in the aged immune and hematological system mainly involve altered T- and B-cell functioning and a decrease in hematopoietic reserve (Nagappan & Parkin, 2003; Rosenthal & Kavic, 2004; Urden et al., 2002; see Table 30.1). The consequences of these changes include an increased susceptibility to infection, increases in autoantibodies and monoclonal immunoglobulins, and tumorigenesis (Rosenthal & Kavic, 2004). These common aging changes coupled with the stress, malnutrition, and number of invasive procedures seen in the critical care environment may heighten the older adult's risk for a nosocomial infection. Furthermore, because an older adult's ability to mount a febrile response to infection diminishes with age (related to a decline in hypothalamic function), the older patient may even be septic without the warning of a fever (Urden et al., 2002) and instead may exhibit only a decline in mental status. Close assessment of other nonfebrile signs of infection (i.e., restlessness, agitation, delirium, hypotension, and tachycardia) is essential and warranted.

Although recent research suggests that giving blood more liberally to patients may be associated with worse patient outcomes, these findings may not necessarily apply to the older adult population for several reasons: (a) the chronic anemia often seen in aging, (b) the exclusion of many older adults from previous clinical trials, (c) research findings that suggest higher transfusion triggers in older patients with acute myocardial infarction actually decrease mortality, and (d) the association of low hemoglobin levels with increased incidence of delirium, functional decline, and decreased mobility (Rosenthal & Kavic, 2004).

Skin and Wounds

Older adults are at high risk for skin breakdown in the ICU setting because of loss of elastic, subcutaneous, and connective tissues; a decrease in sweat gland activity; and a decrease in capillary arterioles supplying the skin with age (Bickley & Szilagyi, 2008; Urden et al., 2002; see Table 30.1). Because the skin changes that occur in older adults can cause difficulty with thermoregulation, can heighten the risk for skin breakdown and IV infiltrations, may delay wound healing, and make hydration assessment difficult, the nurse should make every effort to prevent heat loss, carefully monitor hydration status, and conduct thorough skin assessments (Bickley & Szilagy, 2008; Urden et al., 2002; see Chapter 16, Preventing Pressure Ulcers and Skin Tears).

CASE STUDY

Ned Saunders is a 71-year-old man who fell off a ladder while stringing holiday lights and suffered serious complications, including adult respiratory distress syndrome (ARDS), after laminectomy. He required a second back surgery (revision of the laminectomy) during the same hospital stay and developed a *Clostridium difficile* (*C. difficile*) infection and nutritional problems secondary to the severe diarrhea. Infection with antibiotic-resistant organisms necessitated the use of isolation protocol. Tracheostomy placement occurred on the 17th ICU day and progressive weaning trials began.

Preadmission

Mr. Saunders was a former smoker and his past medical history included mild chronic obstructive pulmonary disease and hypertension. His medications prior to admission were albuterol inhaler, two puffs every 6 hours, and hydrochlorothiazide 50 mg for blood pressure. He smoked a half pack per day for 30 years. A retired school teacher, Mr. Saunders was slightly overweight but active around the house and enjoyed an active social life, especially dancing with his wife at local dance halls. He was a "social drinker," as reported by his wife, having three to four glasses of wine per week. Mr. Saunders was completely independent in all ADLs before this hospitalization. Mini-Mental State Examination (MMSE) score on admission before surgery was 29. CAM-ICU (for delirium) on admission to the ICU was positive for delirium.

Psychosocial

Mr. Saunders was unable to focus attention for more than 5 seconds at a time and was intermittently agitated during the early stages of ICU stay. Delirium was treated with around-the-clock dosages of IV haloperidol. He also received fentanyl patch for pain and lorazepam (dose and frequency taken) as needed for anxiety and sedation. Efforts were made to minimize and taper the use of the benzodiazepine (lorazepam) in an attempt to clear the delirium.

Anxiety and communication difficulties were identified by nurses as problems possibly influencing his "mental state" during ventilator weaning. Communication

(continued)

CASE STUDY *(continued)*

was inhibited by respiratory tract intubation, cognition problems, and lack of dentures and eyeglasses. Because his thinking was unclear, nurses used visual cues in the form of written words, gestures, and pictures to augment their messages to Mr. Saunders. They cued him to use a simple communication board and asked yes/no questions by categories (e.g., family, your body, comfort needs) whenever possible. After the tracheostomy procedure was completed, his wife was advised to bring in his dentures to improve lip reading. He began using a tracheostomy speaking valve after 5.5 weeks of hospitalization.

The patient's wife was his sole support. They had no children or close relatives. A reserved woman, she remained positive when at the patient's bedside. Nurses coached her to use touch and encouragement at the bedside. Mrs. Saunders asked the therapists to teach her range-of-motion exercises and she performed these during afternoon visits. She provided calm and distracting talk during weaning trials, reading get-well cards from friends.

Cardiac

Mr. Saunders remained in a sinus tachycardia through most of the hospitalization with occasional premature ventricular contractions. His hemoglobin and hematocrit dropped to 10 mg/dL and 36 percent respectively during the hospitalization with no identified source of bleeding. He received one unit of packed red blood cells and diuretics before weaning trials were resumed.

Respiratory

Mr. Saunders progressed from dependence on mechanical ventilation in assist control mode (FiO_2 = 40%, continuous positive airway pressure [CPAP] = 5 cmH$_2$O, PS [pressure support] = 10 cmH$_2$O) to tracheostomy mask oxygen at 50% FiO_2 over a 10-day period.

Gastrointestinal

Nutritional balance was particularly challenging with Mr. Saunders because of the impaired absorption of nutrients during *C. difficile* infection. Nutrition or dietitian consult should be obtained. The infection was treated with IV vancomycin. A jejunostomy tube was placed for continuous tube feeding and caloric requirements adjusted frequently with careful attention to albumin levels. Vancomycin drug levels must also be monitored.

Skin

Meticulous attention to wound healing at the back surgery site and fit of "turtle shell" to prevent friction or skin tears.

(continued)

CASE STUDY *(continued)*

Rehabilitation

Mr. Saunders received early physical therapy, beginning as passive range during the most critical phase of his illness and progressing to active range of motion and chair sitting. His mobility was limited by the protective "turtle shell" appliance required for healing of his spine during any out-of-bed activity. A daily chair-sitting period was arranged, requiring coordination between physical therapy and nursing. The team initiated speech and swallowing rehabilitation (i.e., speech and swallowing evaluation) beginning with lollipops to reestablish swallowing.

Discharge Planning

Mr. Saunders's progress was slow and his respiratory status was still tenuous at the end of his ICU stay. He required significant physical rehabilitation following his critical illness. A long-term acute care hospital (LTACH) was the best choice for continued care and rehabilitation. As Mr. Saunders's respiratory status and speaking ability improved, his anxiety diminished. Because Mr. Saunders had multiple risk factors for delirium, the exact cause of the delirium was unknown at discharge. Attention to normalizing the fluid and electrolyte balance, reestablishing and maintaining normal sleep–wake cycles, and gradually withdrawing the use of benzodiazepines continued as care was transferred to the LTACH. His mental status improved as evidenced by less frequent periods of inattention and confusion. Short-term memory problems persisted and required frequent cueing and reminders from staff and his wife.

SUMMARY

Nurses in the acute care setting must recognize and respond to the many factors that influence a critically ill older adult's ability to survive and rehabilitate from a catastrophic illness. In order to identify some of these risk factors, it is essential that the nurse perform a comprehensive assessment of each older adult's preadmission health status, functional and cognitive ability, and social support systems. It is equally important that the nurse understand the implications of common aging changes, comorbidities, and acute pathology that interacts with and heightens the risk of adverse and often preventable medical outcomes. The application of evidence-based interventions aimed at restoring physiologic stability, preventing complications, maintaining comfort and safety, and preserving preillness functional ability and QOL are crucial components of caring for this extremely vulnerable population.

NURSING STANDARD OF PRACTICE

Protocol 30.1: Comprehensive Assessment and Management of the Critically Ill

I. GOAL: To restore physiologic stability, prevent complications, maintain comfort and safety, and preserve preillness functional ability and quality of life (QOL) in older adults admitted to critical care units.

II. OVERVIEW: Caring for an older adult who is experiencing a serious or life-threatening illness often poses significant challenges for critical care nurses. Although older adults are an extremely heterogeneous group, they share some age-related characteristics that leave them susceptible to various geriatric syndromes and diseases. This vulnerability may influence both their ICU utilization rates and outcomes. Critical care nurses caring for this population must not only recognize the importance of performing ongoing, comprehensive physical, functional, and psychosocial assessments tailored to the older ICU patient, but also must be able to identify and implement evidence-based interventions designed to improve the care of this extremely vulnerable population.

III. BACKGROUND
  A. Definition
       Critically ill older adult. A person, age 65 or older, who is currently experiencing, or at risk for, some form of physiologic instability or alteration warranting urgent or emergent, advanced, nursing/medical interventions and monitoring.
  B. Etiology and Epidemiology
      1. More than one half (55.8%) of all ICU days are incurred by patients older than the age of 65 (Angus et al., 2000).
      2. Older adults are living longer, are more racially and ethnically diverse, often have multiple chronic conditions, and more than one quarter report difficulty performing one or more ADLs. These factors may affect both the course and outcome of critical illness.
      3. Once hospitalized for a life-threatening illness, older adults often:
          a. Experience high ICU, hospital, and long-term crude mortality rates and are at risk for deterioration in functional ability and postdischarge institutional care (de Rooij et al., 2005; Esteban et al., 2004; Ford et al., 2007; Hennessy et al., 2005; Hopkins & Jackson, 2006; Kaarlola et al., 2006; Marik, 2006; Wunsch et al., 2010)
          b. Older age is also a factor that may lead to:
              i.   Physician bias in refusing ICU admission (Joynt et al., 2001; Mick & Ackerman, 2004)
              ii. The decision to withhold mechanical ventilation, surgery, or dialysis (Hamel et al., 1999)
              iii. An increased likelihood of an established resuscitation directive (Hakim et al., 1996)
          c. Most critically ill older adults
              i.   Demonstrate resiliency
              ii. Report being satisfied with their QOL postdischarge

(continued)

**Protocol 30.1: Comprehensive Assessment and Management
of the Critically Ill *(cont.)***

    iii. Would reaccept ICU care and mechanical ventilation if needed (Guentner et al., 2006; Hennessy et al., 2005; Kleinpell & Ferrans, 2002)

  d. Chronologic age *alone* is not an acceptable or accurate predictor of poor outcomes after critical illness (Nagappan & Parkin, 2003; Milbrandt et al., 2010).

  e. Factors that may influence an older adult's ability to survive a catastrophic illness include the following:

    i. Severity of illness

    ii. Nature and extent of comorbidities

    iii. Diagnosis, reason for/duration of mechanical ventilation

    iv. Complications

    v. Others

      a) Prehospitalization functional ability

      b) Vasoactive drug use

      c) Preexisting cognitive impairment

      d) Senescence

      e) Ageism

      f) Decreased social support

      g) Critical care environment (de Rooij et al., 2005; Ford et al., 2007; Marik, 2006; Mick & Ackerman, 2004; Tullmann & Dracup, 2000; Wunsch et al., 2010)

IV. PARAMETERS OF ASSESSMENT

  A. Preadmission: Comprehensive assessment of a critically ill older adult's preadmission health status, cognitive and functional ability, and social support systems helps identify risk factors for cascade iatrogenesis, the development of life-threatening conditions, and frequently encountered geriatric syndromes. Factors that the nurse needs to consider when performing the admission assessment include the following:

  1. Preexisting cognitive impairment: Many older adults admitted to ICUs suffer from high rates of unrecognized, preexisting cognitive impairment (Balas et al., 2007; Pisani et al., 2003).

    a. Knowledge of preadmission cognitive ability could aid practitioners in:

      i. Assessing decision-making capacity, informed consent issues, and evaluation of mental status changes throughout hospitalization (Pisani, Inouye, McNicoll, & Redlich, 2003)

      ii. Making anesthetic and analgesic choices

      iii. Considering one-to-one care options

      iv. Weaning from mechanical ventilation

      v. Assessing fall risk

      vi. Planning for discharge from the ICU

    b. Upon admission to the ICU, the nurse should ask relatives or other caregivers for baseline information about the older adult's:

      i. Memory, executive function (e.g., fine motor coordination, planning, organization of information), and overall cognitive ability (Kane et al., 2004)

(continued)

**Protocol 30.1: Comprehensive Assessment and Management
of the Critically Ill** *(cont.)*

     ii. Behavior on a typical day; how the patient interacts with others; their responsiveness to stimuli; how able they are to communicate (reading level, writing, and speech); and their memory, orientation, and perceptual patterns prior to their illness (Milisen, DeGeest, Abraham, & Delooz, 2001)

     iii. Medication history to assess for potential withdrawal syndromes (Broyles, Colbert, Tate, Swigart, & Happ, 2008)

c. Psychosocial factors: Critical illness can render older adults unable to effectively communicate with the health care team, often related to physiologic instability, technology that leaves them voiceless, and sedative and narcotic use (Happ, 2000, 2001). Family members are therefore often a crucial source for obtaining important preadmission information. Upon ICU admission, the nurse needs to determine the following:

     i. What is the older adult's past medical, surgical, and psychiatric history? What medications was the older adult taking before coming to the ICU? Does the older adult regularly use illicit drugs, tobacco, or alcohol? Do they have a history of falls, physical abuse, or confusion?

     ii. What is the older adult's marital status? Who is the patient's significant other? Will this person be the one responsible to make decisions for the older adult if they are unable to do so? Does the older adult have an advanced directive for health care? Is the older adult a primary caregiver to an aging spouse, child, grandchild, or other person?

     iii. How would the older adult describe his or her ethnicity? Do they practice a particular religion or have spiritual needs that should be addressed? What was their QOL like before becoming ill?

d. Preadmission functional ability and nutritional status: Limited preadmission functional ability and poor nutritional status are associated with many negative outcomes for critically ill older adults (Marik, 2006; Mick & Ackerman, 2004; Tullmann & Dracup, 2000). Therefore, the nurse should assess the following:

     i. Did the older adult suffer any limitations in the ability to perform their ADLs preadmission? If so, what were these limitations?

     ii. Does the older adult use any assistive devices to perform his or her ADLs? If so, what type?

     iii. Where did the patient live prior to admission? Did he or she live alone or with others? What was the older adult's physical environment like (house, apartment, stairs, multiple levels, etc.)?

     iv. What was the older adult's nutritional status like preadmission? Does he or she have enough money to buy food? Does he or she need assistance with making meals and obtaining food? Does he or she have any particular food restrictions or preferences? Where he or she using supplements and vitamins on a regular basis? Does he or she have any signs of malnutrition, including recent weight loss or gain, muscle wasting, hair loss, or skin breakdown?

(continued)

**Protocol 30.1: Comprehensive Assessment and Management
of the Critically Ill *(cont.)***

B. During ICU stay: There are many anatomic and physiologic changes that occur with aging (see Table 30.1). The interaction of these changes with the acute pathology of a critical illness, comorbidities, and the ICU environment leads not only to atypical presentation of some of the most commonly encountered ICU diagnoses, but may also elevate the older adult's risk for complications. The older adult must be systematically assessed for the following:

1. Comorbidities and common ICU diagnoses
   a. Respiratory: chronic obstructive pulmonary disease, pneumonia, acute respiratory failure, adult respiratory distress syndrome, and rib fractures/ flail chest
   b. Cardiovascular: acute myocardial infarction, coronary artery disease, peripheral vascular disease, hypertension, coronary artery bypass grafting, valve replacements, abdominal aortic aneurysm, dysrhythmias
   c. Neurologic: cerebral vascular accident, dementia, aneurysms, Alzheimer's disease, Parkinson's disease, closed head injury, transient ischemic attacks
   d. Gastrointestinal (GI): biliary tract disease, peptic ulcer disease, GI cancers, liver failure, inflammatory bowel disease, pancreatitis, diarrhea, constipation, and aspiration
   e. Genitourinary (GU): renal cell cancer, chronic renal failure, acute renal failure, urosepsis, and incontinence
   f. Immune/hematopoietic: sepsis, anemia, neutropenia, and thrombocytopenia
   g. Skin: necrotizing fasciitis, pressure ulcers
2. Acute pathology: thoracic or abdominal surgery, hypovolemia, hypervolemia, hypothermia/hyperthermia, electrolyte abnormalities, hypoxia, arrhythmias, infection, hypotension/hypertension, delirium, ischemia, bowel obstruction, ileus, blood loss, sepsis, disrupted skin integrity, multisystem organ failure
3. ICU/environmental factors: deconditioning, poor oral hygiene, sleep deprivation, pain, immobility, nutritional status, mechanical ventilation, hemodynamic monitoring devices, polypharmacy, high-risk medications (e.g., narcotics, sedatives, hypnotics, nephrotoxins, vasopressors), lack of assistive devices (e.g., glasses, hearing aids, dentures), noise, tubes that bypass the oropharyngeal airway, poorly regulated glucose control, Foley catheter use, stress, invasive procedures, shear/friction, intravenous catheters
4. Atypical presentation: Commonly seen in older adults experiencing the following: myocardial infarction, acute abdomen, infection, and hypoxia

V. NURSING CARE STRATEGIES

A. Preadmission: Based on their preadmission assessment findings, the nurse should consider the following:
1. Obtaining appropriate consults (i.e., nutrition, physical/ occupational/ speech therapist)
2. Implementing safety precautions
3. Using pressure-relieving devices
4. Organizing family meetings
5. Providing the older adult with a consistent primary nurse

(continued)

Protocol 30.1: Comprehensive Assessment and Management of the Critically Ill *(cont.)*

B. During ICU: Nursing interventions that may benefit:
   1. Multiple organ systems:
      a. Encouraging early, frequent mobilization/ambulation
      b. Providing proper oral hygiene
      c. Ensuring adequate pain control
      d. Reviewing/assessing medication appropriateness
      e. Avoiding polypharmacy/high-risk medications (see Table 30.2)
      f. Securing and ensuring the proper functioning of tubes/catheters
      g. Actively taking measures to maintain normothermia
      h. Closely monitoring fluid volume status.
   2. Respiratory
      a. Encourage and assist with coughing, deep breathing, incentive spirometer use; use alternative device when appropriate (e.g., positive expiratory pressure [PEP])
      b. Assess for signs of swallowing dysfunction and aspiration
      c. Closely monitor pulse oximetry and arterial blood gas results
      d. Consider the use of specialty beds
      e. Advocate for early weaning trials and extubation as soon as possible
      f. Exercise standard VAP precautions (AACN, 2004; ATS & IDSA, 2005; Dezfulian et al., 2005; IHI & 5 Million Lives Campaign, 2008; Krein et al., 2008):
         i. Keep the head of the bed elevated to more than 30 degrees.
         ii. Provide frequent oral care.
         iii. Maintain adequate cuff pressures.
         iv. Use continuous subglottic suctioning devices.
         v. Do not routinely change ventilator circuit tubing.
         vi. Assess the need for stress ulcer and deep venous thrombosis (DVT) prophylaxis.
         vii. Turn the patient as tolerated.
         viii. Maintain general hygiene practices.
   3. Cardiovascular
      a. Carefully monitor the older adult's hemodynamic and electrolyte status.
      b. Closely monitor the older adult's ECG with an awareness of many conduction abnormalities seen in aging. Consult with physician regarding prophylaxis when appropriate.
      c. Advocate for the removal of invasive devices as soon as the patient's condition warrants. The least restrictive device may include long-term access.
      d. Recognize that both preexisting pulmonary disease and manipulations of the abdominal and thoracic cavities may lead to unreliability of traditional values associated with central venous pressures (CVPs) and pulmonary artery occlusion pressures (PAOPs; Rosenthal & Kavic, 2004).
      e. Because of age-related changes to the cardiovascular system, the nurse should acknowledge (Rosenthal & Kavic, 2004):
         i. Older adults often require higher filling pressures (i.e., CVPs in the 8–10 cm range, PAOPs in the 14–18 cm range) to

(continued)

Protocol 30.1: Comprehensive Assessment and Management of the Critically Ill *(cont.)*

maintain adequate stroke volume and may be especially sensitive to hypovolemia.

　ii. Overhydration of the older adult should also be avoided because it can lead to systolic failure, poor organ perfusion, and hypoxemia with subsequent diastolic dysfunction.

　iii. Certain drugs commonly used in the ICU setting may prove to be either not as effective (e.g., isoproterenol and dobutamine) or more effective (e.g., afterload reducers).

4. Neurologic/pain
   a. Closely monitor the older adult's neurologic and mental status.
   b. Screen for delirium and sedation level at least once per shift.
   c. Implement the following interventions to reduce delirium:
   　i. Promote sleep, mobilize as early as possible, review medications that can lead to delirium, treat dehydration, reduce noise or provide "white noise," close doors/drapes to allow privacy, provide comfortable room temperature, encourage family and friends to visit, allow the older adult to assume their preferred sleeping positions, discontinue any unnecessary lines or tubes, and avoid the use of physical restraints, using least restraint for minimum time only when absolutely necessary.
   　ii. Maximize the older adult's ability to communicate his or her needs effectively and interpret his or her environment.
   　　a) Promote the older adult wearing glasses, hearing aids, and other appropriate assistive devices.
   　　b) Face the patients when speaking to them, get their attention before talking, speak clearly and loud enough for them to understand, allow them enough time (pause time) to respond to questions, provide them with a consistent provider (i.e., a primary nurse), use visual clues to remind them of the date and time, and provide written or visual input for a message (Garett, Happ, Costello, & Fried-Oken, 2007).
   　　c) Provide the older adult with alternate means of communication (e.g., providing him or her with a pen and paper, using nonverbal gestures, and/or using specially designed boards with alphabet letters, words, or pictures; Garett et al., 2007; Happ et al., 2010).
   　　d) Provide translators/interpreters as needed.
   d. Provide adequate pain control while avoiding oversedation or undersedation. For a full discussion, see Chapter 14, Pain Management.

5. Gastrointestinal
   a. Monitor for signs of GI bleeding and delayed gastric emptying and motility.
   　i. Encourage adequate hydration, assess for signs of fecal impaction, and implement a bowel regimen.
   　ii. Avoid use of rectal tubes.
   b. Advocate for stress ulcer prophylaxis.

(continued)

**Protocol 30.1: Comprehensive Assessment and Management
of the Critically Ill** *(cont.)*

  c. Provide dentures as soon as possible.

  d. Implement aspiration precautions.

    i. Keep the head of the bed elevated to a high Fowler's position, frequently suction copious oral secretions, bedside evaluate swallowing ability by a speech therapist, assess phonation and gag reflex, monitor for tachypnea.

  e. Advocate for early enteral/parenteral nutrition.

  f. Ensure tight glucose control.

 6. Genitourinary

  a. Assess any GU tubes to ensure patency and adequate urinary output. If the older adult should experience an acute decrease in urinary output, consider using bladder scanner (if available), rather than automatic straight catheterization, to check for distension.

  b. Advocate for early removal of Foley catheters. Use other less invasive devices/methods to facilitate urine collection (i.e., external or condom catheters, offering the bedpan on a scheduled basis, and keeping the nurse's call bell/signal within the older adult's reach).

  c. Monitor blood levels of nephrotoxic medications as ordered.

 7. Immune/hematopoietic

  a. Ensure that the older adult is ordered appropriate DVT prophylaxis (i.e., heparin, sequential compression devices)

  b. Monitor laboratory results, assess for signs of anemia relative to patient's baseline

  c. Recognize early signs of infection—restlessness, agitation, delirium, hypotension, tachycardia—because older adults are less likely to develop fever as a first response to infection.

  d. Meticulously maintain infection control/prevention protocols.

 8. Skin

  a. Conduct thorough skin assessment.

  b. Vigilantly monitor room temperature, make every effort to prevent heat loss, and carefully use and monitor rewarming devices.

  c. Use methods known to reduce the friction and shear that often occurs with repositioning in bed.

  d. In severely compromised patients, the use of specialty beds may be appropriate.

  e. Techniques such as frequent turning, pressure-relieving devices, early nutritional support, as well as frequent ambulation may not only protect an older adult's skin, but also promote the health of their cardiovascular, respiratory, and GI systems.

  f. Closely monitor IV sites, frequently check for infiltrations and use of nonrestrictive dressings and paper tape.

VI. EVALUATION/EXPECTED OUTCOMES

 A. Patient

  1. Hemodynamic stability will be restored.

  2. Complications will be avoided/minimized.

(continued)

> **Protocol 30.1: Comprehensive Assessment and Management
> of the Critically Ill** *(cont.)*

  3. Preadmission functional ability will be maintained/optimized.
  4. Pain/anxiety will be minimized.
  5. Communication with the health care team will be improved.
 B. Provider
  1. Employ consistent and accurate documentation of assessment relevant to the older ICU patient.
  2. Provide consistent, accurate, and timely care in response to deviations identified through ongoing monitoring and assessment of the older ICU patient.
  3. Provide patient/caregiver with information and teaching related to his or her illness and regarding transfer of care and/or discharge.
 C. Institution: includes quality assurance/quality assessment (QA/QI)
  1. Evaluate staff competence in the assessment of older critically ill patients.
  2. Utilize unit-specific, hospital-specific, and national standards of care to evaluate existing practice.
  3. Identify areas for improvement and work collaboratively across disciplines to develop strategies for improving critical care to older adults.

VII. RELEVANT PRACTICE GUIDELINES

Clinical practice guidelines for the sustained use of sedatives and analgesics in the critically ill adult. Task Force of the American College of Critical Care Medicine (ACCM) of the Society of Critical Care Medicine (SCCM), American Society of Health-System Pharmacists (ASHP), and American College of Chest Physicians ACC/AHA 2006 guideline update on perioperative cardiovascular evaluation for noncardiac surgery: Focused update on perioperative beta-blocker therapy: A report of the American College of Cardiology/American Heart Association Task Force on Practice Guidelines. Developed in collaboration with the American Society of Echocardiography, American Society of Nuclear Cardiology, Heart Rhythm Society, Society of Cardiovascular Anesthesiologists, Society for Cardiovascular Angiography and Interventions, and Society for Vascular Medicine and Biology.

ACKNOWLEDGMENTS

The authors would like to acknowledge the continual support and commitment to improving nursing care of older adults provided by the John A. Hartford Foundation. Case study provided by the "Study of Ventilator Weaning: Care and Communication Processes" database using composite patient information and pseudonyms (R01-NR007973).

RESOURCES

The Richmond Agitation and Sedation Scale (RASS) and The Confusion Assessment Method-ICU (CAM-ICU)
http://www.icudelirium.org/delirium/training-pages/CAM-ICU%20trainingman.2005.pdf

Training manual includes information for administering both the RASS and the CAM-ICU.
Copyright © 2002, E. Wesley Ely and Vanderbilt University
http://geronurseonline.org

Hartford Institute for Geriatric Nursing
http://www.consultgerirn.org/resources

Topics relevant to this chapter include the following:

- Brief Evaluation of Executive Dysfunction: An Essential Refinement in the Assessment of Cognitive Impairment
- Decision Making and Dementia
- Recognition of Dementia in the Hospitalized Older Adult
- Beers' Criteria for Potentially Inappropriate Medication Use in the Elderly Assessing Pain in Older Adults
- KATZ Index of Independence in ADL

REFERENCES

Administration on Aging. (2009). *A profile of older Americans: 2009*. Retrieved from http://www.aoa.gov/AoARoot/Aging_Statistics/Profile/2009/docs/2009profile_508.pdf. Evidence Level IV.

American Association of Critical Care Nurses. (2004). *Ventilator-associated pneumonia*. Retrieved from http://www.aacn.org/AACN/practiceAlert.nsf/Files/VAPi. Evidence Level I.

American Thoracic Society, & Infectious Diseases Society of America. (2005). Guidelines for the management of adults with hospital-acquired, ventilator-associated, and healthcare-associated pneumonia. *American Journal of Respiratory and Critical Care Medicine, 171*(4), 388–416. Evidence Level I.

Angus, D. C., Kelley, M. A., Schmitz, R. J., White, A., Popovich, J., Jr., & Committee on Manpower for Pulmonary and Critical Care Societies. (2000). Caring for the critically ill patient. Current and projected workforce requirements for care of the critically ill and patients with pulmonary disease: Can we meet the requirements of an aging population? *Journal of the American Medical Association, 284*(21), 2762–2770. Evidence Level IV.

Bailey, P. P., Miller, R. R., III, & Clemmer, T. P. (2009). Culture of early mobility in mechanically ventilated patients. *Critical Care Medicine, 37*(10 Suppl.), S429–S435. Evidence Level VI.

Balas, M. C., Deutschman, C. S., Sullivan-Marx, E. M., Strumpf, N. E., Alston, R. P., & Richmond, T. S. (2007). Delirium in older patients in surgical intensive care units. *Journal of Nursing Scholarship, 39*(2), 147–154. Evidence Level IV.

Balas, M. C., Happ, M. B., Yang, W., Chelluri, L., & Richmond, T. (2009). Outcomes associated with delirium in older patients in surgical ICUs. *Chest, 135*(1), 18–25. Evidence Level IV.

Bartlett, G., Blais, R., Tamblyn, R., Clermont, R. J., & MacGibbon, B. (2008). Impact of patient communication problems on the risk of preventable adverse events in acute care settings. *Canadian Medical Association Journal, 178*(12), 1555–1562. Evidence Level IV.

Bellmann-Weiler, R., & Weiss, G. (2009). Pitfalls in the diagnosis and therapy of infections in elderly patients—a mini-review. *Gerontology, 55*(3), 241–249. Evidence Level VI.

Bickley, L. S., & Szilagyi, P. G. (2008). *Bates' guide to physical examination and history taking* (10th ed.). Philadelphia, PA: Lipincott Willlams & Wilkins. Evidence Level VI.

Bonk, M. E., Krown, H., Matuszewski, K., & Oinonen, M. (2006). Potentially inappropriate medications in hospitalized senior patients. *American Journal of Health System Pharmacists, 63*(12), 1161–1165. Evidence Level IV.

Broyles, L. M., Colbert, A. M., Tate, J. A., Swigart, V. A., & Happ, M. B. (2008). Clinicians' evaluation and management of mental health, substance abuse, and chronic pain conditions in the intensive care unit. *Critical Care Medicine, 36*(1), 87–93. Evidence Level IV.

Buczko, W. (2010). Ventilator-associated pneumonia among elderly Medicare beneficiaries in long-term care hospitals. *Health Care Financing Review, 31*(1), 1–10. Evidence Level IV.

Chelluri, L., Im, K. A., Belle, S. H., Schulz, R., Rotondi, A. J., Donahoe, M. P., . . . Pinsky, M. R. (2004). Long-term mortality and quality of life after prolonged mechanical ventilation. *Critical Care Medicine, 32*(1), 61–69. Evidence Level IV.

Creditor, M. C. (1993). Hazards of hospitalization of the elderly. *Annals of Internal Medicine, 118*(3), 219–223. Evidence Level VI.

Daly, B. J., Douglas, S. L., Gordon, N. H., Kelley, C. G., O'Toole, E., Montenegro, H., & Higgins, P. (2009). Composite outcomes of chronically critically ill patients 4 months after hospital discharge. *American Journal of Critical Care, 18*(5), 456–464. Evidence Level IV.

de Rooij, S. E., Abu-Hanna, A., Levi, M., & de Jonge, E. (2005). Factors that predict outcome of intensive care treatment in very elderly patients: A review. *Critical Care, 9*(4), R307–R314. Evidence Level V.

Dezfulian, C., Shojania, K., Collard, H. R., Kim, H. M., Matthay, M. A., & Saint, S. (2005). Subglottic secretion drainage for preventing ventilator-associated pneumonia: A meta-analysis. *The American Journal of Medicine, 118*(1), 11–18. Evidence Level I.

Douglas, S. L., Daly, B. J., Brennan, P. F., Gordon, N. H., & Uthis, P. (2001). Hospital readmission among long-term ventilator patients. *Chest, 120*(4), 1278–1286. Evidence Level IV.

Douglas, S. L., Daly, B. J., Gordon, N., & Brennan, P. F. (2002). Survival and quality of life: Short-term versus long-term ventilator patients. *Critical Care Medicine, 30*(12), 2655–2662. Evidence Level IV.

Douglas, S. L., Daly, B. J., Kelley, C. G., O'Toole, E., & Montenegro, H. (2005). Impact of a disease management program upon caregivers of chronically critically ill patients. *Chest, 128*(6), 3925–3936. Evidence Level II.

Douglas, S. L., Daly, B. J., Kelley, C. G., O'Toole, E., & Montenegro, H. (2007). Chronically critically ill patients: Health-related quality of life and resource use after a disease management intervention. *American Journal of Critical Care, 16*(5), 447–457. Evidence Level II.

Douglas, S. L., Daly, B. J., O'Toole, E., & Hickman, R. L., Jr. (2010). Depression among white and nonwhite caregivers of the chronically critically ill. *Journal of Critical Care, 25*(2), 364.e11–364.e19. Evidence Level IV.

Douglas, S. L., Daly, B. J., O'Toole, E. E., Kelley, C. G., & Montenegro, H. (2009). Age differences in survival outcomes and resource use for chronically critically ill patients. *Journal of Critical Care, 24*(2), 302–310. Evidence Level IV.

Ely, E. W., Inouye, S. K., Bernard, G. R., Gordon, S., Francis, J., May, L., . . . Dittus, R. (2001). Delirium in mechanically ventilated patients: Validity and reliability of the confusion assessment method for the intensive care unit (CAM-ICU). *The Journal of the American Medical Association, 286*(21), 2703–2710. Evidence Level IV.

Esteban, A., Anzueto, A., Frutos-Vivar, F., Alía, I., Ely, E. W., Brochard, L, . . . Mechanical Ventilation International Study Group. (2004). Outcome of older patients receiving mechanical ventilation. *Intensive Care Medicine, 30*(4), 639–646. Evidence Level IV.

Fick, D. M., Cooper, J. W., Wade, W. E., Waller, J. L., Maclean, J. R., & Beers, M. H. (2003). Updating the Beers criteria for potentially inappropriate medication use in older adults: Results of a US consensus panel of experts. *Archives of Internal Medicine, 163*(22), 2716–2724. Evidence Level I.

Fleisher, L. A., Beckman, J. A., Brown, K. A., Calkins, H., Chaikof, E. L., Fleischmann, K. E., . . . Society for Vascular Medicine and Biology. (2007). ACC/AHA 2006 guideline update on perioperative cardiovascular evaluation for noncardiac surgery: Focused update on perioperative beta-blocker therapy—a report of the American College of Cardiology/American Heart Association Task Force on Practice Guidelines (Writing Committee to update the 2002 guidelines on perioperative cardiovascular evaluation for Noncardiac Surgery). *Anesthesia and Analgesia, 104*(1), 15–26. Evidence Level I.

Ford P. N., Thomas, I., Cook, T. M., Whitley, E., & Peden, C. J. (2007). Determinants of outcome in critically ill octogenarians after surgery: An observational study. *British Journal of Anaesthesia, 99*(6), 824–829. Evidence Level IV.

Garett, K. L., Happ, M. B., Costello, J., & Fried-Oken, M. (2007). AAC in intensive care units. In D. R. Beukelman, K. L. Garrett, & K. M. Yorkston (Eds.), *Augmentative communication strategies for adults with acute or chronic medical conditions*. Baltimore, MD: Brookes Publishing. Evidence Level VI.

Girard, T. D., & Ely, E. W. (2007). Bacteremia and sepsis in older adults. *Clinics in Geriatric Medicine, 23*(3), 633–647. Evidence Level VI.

Girard, T. D., Kress, J. P., Fuchs, B. D., Thomason, J. W., Schweickert, W. D., Pun, B. T., . . . Ely E. W. (2008). Efficacy and safety of a paired sedation and ventilator weaning protocol for mechanically ventilated patients in intensive care (Awakening and Breathing Controlled trial): A randomised controlled trial. *Lancet, 371*(9607), 126–134. Evidence Level II.

Graf, C., & Puntillo, K. (2003). Pain in the older adult in the intensive care unit. *Critical Care Clinics, 19*(4), 749–770. Evidence Level VI.

Griffiths, J., Fortune, G., Barber, V., & Young, J. D. (2007). The prevalence of post traumatic stress disorder in survivors of ICU treatment: A systematic review. *Intensive Care Medicine, 33*(9), 1506–1518. Evidence Level V.

Guentner, K., Hoffman, L. A., Happ, M. B., Kim, Y., Dabbs, A. D., Mendelsohn, A. B., & Chelluri, L. (2006). Preferences for mechanical ventilation among survivors of prolonged mechanical ventilation and tracheostomy. *The American Journal of Critical Care, 15*(1), 65–77. Evidence Level IV.

Hakim, R. B., Teno, J. M., Harrell, F. E., Jr., Knaus, W. A., Wenger, N., Phillips, R. S., . . . Lynn, J. (1996). Factors associated with do-not-resuscitate orders: Patients' preferences, prognoses, and physicians' judgments. SUPPORT Investigators. Study to Understand Prognoses and Preferences for Outcomes and Risks of Treatment. *Annals of Internal Medicine, 125*(4), 284–293. Evidence Level III.

Hamel, M. B., Teno, J. M., Goldman, L., Lynn, J., Davis, R. B., Galanos, A. N., . . . Phillips, R. S. (1999). Patient age and decisions to withhold life-sustaining treatments from seriously ill, hospitalized adults. SUPPORT Investigators. Study to Understand Prognoses and Preferences for Outcomes and Risks of Treatment. *Annals of Internal Medicine, 130*(2), 116–125. Evidence Level III.

Happ, M. B. (2000). Interpretation of nonvocal behavior and the meaning of voicelessness in critical care. *Social Science & Medicine, 50*(9), 1247–1255. Evidence Level IV.

Happ, M. B. (2001). Communicating with mechanically ventilated patients: State of the science. *AACN Clinical Issues, 12*(2), 247–258. Evidence Level IV.

Happ, M. B., Baumann, B. M., Sawicki, J., Tate, J. A., George, E. L., & Barnato, A. E. (2010). SPEACS-2: Intensive care unit "communication rounds" with speech language pathology. *Geriatric Nursing, 31*(3), 170–177. Evidence Level III.

Happ, M. B., & Paull, B. (2008). Silence is not golden. *Geriatric Nursing, 29*(3), 166–168. Evidence Level VI.

Hennessy, D., Juzwishin, K., Yergens, D., Noseworthy, T., & Doig, C. (2005). Outcomes of elderly survivors of intensive care: A review of the literature. *Chest, 127*(5), 1764–1774. Evidence Level V.

Herzig, S. J., Howell, M. D., Ngo, L. H., & Marcantonio, E. R. (2009). Acid-suppressive medication use and the risk for hospital-acquired pneumonia. *Journal of American Medical Association, 301*(20), 2120–2128. Evidence Level IV.

Hopkins, R. O., & Jackson, J. C. (2006). Long-term neurocognitive function after critical illness. *Chest, 130*(3), 869–878. Evidence Level VI.

Humbert, J., Gallagher, K., Gabbay, R., & Dellasega, C. (2008). Intensive insulin therapy in the critically ill geriatric patient. *Critical Care Nursing Quarterly, 31*(1), 14–18. Evidence Level VI.

Institute for Healthcare Improvement, & 5 Million Lives Campaign. (2008). *Getting started kit: Prevent ventilator associated pneumonia*. Retrieved from http://www.ihi.org. Evidence Level VI.

Iregui, M., Ward, S., Sherman, G., Fraser, V. J., & Kollef, M. H. (2002). Clinical importance of delays in the initiation of appropriate antibiotic treatment for ventilator-associated pneumonia. *Chest, 122*(1), 262–268. Evidence Level IV.

Jorm, A. F. (1994). A short form of the Informant Questionnaire on Cognitive Decline in the Elderly (IQCODE): Development and cross-validation. *Psychological Medicine, 24*(1), 145–153. Evidence Level IV.

Joynt, G. M., Gomersall, C. D., Tan, P., Lee, A., Cheng, C. A., & Wong, E. L. (2001). Prospective evaluation of patients refused admission to an intensive care unit: Triage, futility and outcome. *Intensive Care Medicine, 27*(9), 1459–1465. Evidence Level IV.

Jubran, A., Lawm, G., Duffner, L. A., Collins, E. G., Lanuza, D. M., Hoffman, L. A., & Tobin, M. J. (2010). Post-traumatic stress disorder after weaning from prolonged mechanical ventilation. *Intensive Care Medicine, 36*(12), 2030–2037. Evidence Level IV.

Kaarlola, A., Tallgren, M., & Pettilä, V. (2006). Long-term survival, quality of life, and quality-adjusted life-years among critically ill elderly patients. *Critical Care Medicine, 34*(8), 2120–2126. Evidence Level IV.

Kane, R. L., Ouslander, J. G., & Abrass, I. B. (2004). *Essentials of clinical geriatrics* (5th ed.). New York, NY: McGraw-Hill. Evidence Level VI.

Katz, S., Ford, A. B., Moskowitz, R. W., Jackson, B. A., & Jaffe, M. W. (1963). Studies of illness in the aged. The index of ADL: A standardized measure of biological and psychosocial function. *The Journal of the American Medical Association, 185*, 914–919. Evidence Level IV.

Kidd, D., Stewart, G., Baldry, J., Johnson, J., Rossiter, D., Petruckevitch, A., & Thompson, A. J. (1995). The Functional Independence Measure: A comparative validity and reliability study. *Disability and Rehabilitation, 17*(1), 10–14. Evidence Level III.

King, M. S., Render, M. L., Ely, E. W., & Watson, P. L. (2010). Liberation and animation: Strategies to minimize brain dysfunction in critically ill patients. *Seminars in Respiratory and Critical Care Medicine, 31*(1), 87–96. Evidence Level IV.

Kleinhenz, M. E., & Lewis, C. Y. (2000). Chronic ventilator dependence in elderly patients. *Clinics in Geriatric Medicine, 16*(4), 735–756. Evidence Level VI.

Kleinpell, R. M., & Ferrans, C. E. (2002). Quality of life of elderly patients after treatment in the ICU. *Research in Nursing & Health, 25*(3), 212–221. Evidence Level IV.

Krein, S. L., Kowalski, C. P., Damschroder, L., Forman, J., Kaufman, S. R., & Saint, S. (2008). Preventing ventilator-associated pneumonia in the United States: A multicenter mixed-methods study. *Infection Control and Hospital Epidemiology, 29*(10), 933–940. Evidence Level IV.

Kresevic, D. M., & Mezey, M. (2003). Assessment of function. In M. D. Mezey, T. Fulmer, & I. Abrahams (Eds.), *Geriatric nursing protocols for best practice* (2nd ed., pp. 31–46). New York, NY: Springer Publishing. Evidence Level VI.

Logan, I. C., Sumukadas, D., & Witham, M. D. (2010). Gastric acid suppressants—too much of a good thing? *Age and Ageing, 39*(4), 410–411. Evidence Level VI.

Marik, P. E. (2006). Management of the critically ill geriatric patient. *Critical Care Medicine, 34*(9 Suppl.), S176–S182. Evidence Level VI.

Marik, P. E., Vasu, T., Hirani, A., & Pachinburavan, M. (2010). Stress ulcer prophylaxis in the new millennium: A systematic review and meta-analysis. *Critical Care Medicine, 38*(11), 2222–2228. Evidence Level I.

McNicoll, L., Pisani, M. A., Zhang, Y., Ely, E. W., Siegel, M. D., & Inouye, S. K. (2003). Delirium in the intensive care unit: Occurrence and clinical course in older patients. *Journal of the American Geriatrics Society, 51*(5), 591–598. Evidence Level IV.

Menaker, J., & Scalea, T. M. (2010). Geriatric care in the surgical intensive care unit. *Critical Care Medicine, 38*(9 Suppl.), S452–S459. Evidence Level VI.

Mick, D. J., & Ackerman, M. H. (2004). Critical care nursing for older adults: Pathophysiological and functional considerations. *The Nursing Clinics of North America, 39*(3), 473–493. Evidence Level VI.

Milbrandt, E. B., Eldadah, B., Nayfield, S., Hadley, E., & Angus, D. C. (2010). Toward an integrated research agenda for critical illness in aging. *American Journal of Respiratory and Critical Care Medicine, 182*(8), 995–1003. Evidence Level VI.

Milisen, K., DeGeest, S., Abraham, I. L., & Delooz, H. H. (2001). Delirium. In T. T. Fulmet, M. D. Foreman, & M. Walker (Eds.), *Critical care nursing of the elderly* (2nd ed., pp. 41–52). New York, NY: Springer Publishing. Evidence Level VI.

Miller, C. A. (2009). *Nursing for wellness in older adults* (5th ed.). Philadelphia, PA: Lippincott Willams & Wilkins. Evidence Level VI.

Morandi, A., Jackson, J. C., & Ely, E. W. (2009). Delirium in the intensive care unit. *International Review of Psychiatry*, *21*(1), 43–58. Evidence Level VI.

Morris, P. E., Goad, A., Thompson, C., Taylor, K., Harry, B., Passmore, L., . . . Haponik, E . (2008). Early intensive care unit mobility therapy in the treatment of acute respiratory failure. *Critical Care Medicine*, *36*(8), 2238–2243. Evidence Level IV.

Muir, J. F., Lamia, B., Molano, C., & Cuvelier, A. (2010). Respiratory failure in the elderly patient. *Seminars in Respiratory and Critical Care Medicine*, *31*(5), 634–646. Evidence Level VI.

Nagappan, R., & Parkin, G. (2003). Geriatric critical care. *Critical Care Clinics*, *19*(2), 253–270. Evidence Level VI.

Oeyen, S. G., Vandijck, D. M., Benoit, D. D., Annemans, L., & Decruyenaere, J. M. (2010). Quality of life after intensive care: A systematic review of the literature. *Critical Care Medicine*, *38*(12), 2386–2400. Evidence Level V.

Patak, L., Wilson-Stronks, A., Costello, J., Kleinpell, R. M., Henneman, E. A., Person, C., & Happ, M. B. (2009). Improving patient-provider communication: A call to action. *The Journal of Nursing Administration*, *39*(9), 372–376. Evidence Level VI.

Peterson, J. F, Pun, B. T., Dittus, R. S., Thomason, J. W., Jackson, J. C., Shintani, A. K., & Ely, E. W. (2006). Delirium and its motoric subtypes: A study of 614 critically ill patients. *Journal of the American Geriatrics Society*, *54*(3), 479–484. Evidence Level IV.

Pisani, M. A. (2009). Considerations in caring for the critically ill older patient. *Journal of Intensive Care Medicine*, *24*(2), 83–95. Evidence Level VI.

Pisani, M. A., Inouye, S. K., McNicoll, L., & Redlich, C. A. (2003). Screening for preexisting cognitive impairment in older intensive care unit patients: Use of proxy assessment. *Journal of the American Geriatrics Society*, *51*(5), 689–693. Evidence Level IV.

Pisani, M. A., Murphy, T. E., Van Ness, P. H., Araujo, K. L., & Inouye, S. K. (2007). Characteristics associated with delirium in older patients in a medical intensive care unit. *Archives of Internal Medicine*, *167*(15), 1629–1634. Evidence Level VI.

Pisani, M. A., Redlich, C., McNicoll, L., Ely, E. W., & Inouye, S. K. (2003). Underrecognition of preexisting cognitive impairment by physicians in older ICU patients. *Chest*, *124*(6), 2267–2274. Evidence Level IV.

Richards, C. L. (2004). Urinary tract infections in the frail elderly: Issues for diagnosis, treatment and prevention. *International Urology and Nephrology*, *36*(3), 457–463. Evidence Level VI.

Rosenthal, R. A. (2004). Nutritional concerns in the older surgical patient. *Journal of the American College of Surgeon*, *199*(5), 785–791. Evidence Level VI.

Rosenthal, R. A., & Kavic, S. M. (2004). Assessment and management of the geriatric patient. *Crititical Care Medicine*, *32*(4 Suppl.), S92–S105. Evidence Level VI.

Sessler, C. N., Gosnell, M. S., Grap, M. J., Brophy, G. M., O'Neal, P. V., Keane, K. A., . . . Elswick, R. K. (2002). The Richmond Agitation-Sedation Scale: Validity and reliability in adult intensive care unit patients. *American Journal of Respiratory and Critical Care Medicine*, *166*(10), 1338–1344. Evidence Level I.

Sheehy, C. M., Perry, P. A., & Cromwell, S. L. (1999). Dehydration: Biological considerations, age-related changes, and risk factors in older adults. *Biological Research for Nursing*, *1*(1), 30–37. Evidence Level V.

Tullmann, D. F., & Dracup, K. (2000). Creating a healing environment for elders. *AACN Clinical Issues*, *11*(1), 34–50. Evidence Level VI.

Urden, L. D., Stacy, K. M., & Lough, M. E. (2002). Gerontological alterations and management. In L. D. Urden, K. M. Stacy, M. E. Lough, & L. A. Thelan (Eds.), *Thelan's critical care nursing: Diagnosis and management* (4th ed., pp. 199–220). St. Louis, MO: Mosby. Evidence Level VI.

Van den Berghe, G., Bouillon, R., & Mesotten, D. (2009). Glucose control in critically ill patients. *The New England Journal of Medicine, 361*(1), 89–92. Evidence Level II.

Van den Berghe, G., Wouters, P., Weekers, F., Verwaest, C., Bruyninckx, F., Schetz, M., . . . Bouillon, R. (2001). Intensive insulin therapy in the critically ill patients. *The New England Journal of Medicine, 345*(19), 1359–1367. Evidence Level II.

Vasilevskis, E. E., Ely, E. W., Speroff, T., Pun, B. T., Boehm, L., & Dittus, R. S. (2010). Reducing iatrogenic risks: ICU-acquired delirium and weakness—crossing the quality chasm. *Chest, 138*(5), 1224–1233. Evidence Level VI.

Wunsch, H., Guerra, C., Barnato, A. E., Angus, D. C., Li, G., & Linde-Zwirble, W. (2010). Three-year outcomes for Medicare beneficiaries who survive intensive care. *The Journal of the American Medical Association, 303*(9), 849–856. Evidence Level IV.

Yilmaz, R., & Erdem, Y. (2010). Acute kidney injury in the elderly population. *International Urology and Nephrology, 42*(1), 259–271. Evidence Level VI.

Zilberberg, M. D., de Wit, M., Pirone, J. R., & Shorr, A. F. (2008). Growth in adult prolonged acute mechanical ventilation: Implications for healthcare delivery. *Critical Care Medicine, 36*(5), 1451–1455. Evidence Level IV.

Fluid Overload: Identifying and Managing Heart Failure Patients At Risk for Hospital Readmission

31

Judith E. Schipper, Jessica Coviello, and
Deborah A. Chyun

EDUCATIONAL OBJECTIVES

On completion of this chapter, the reader will be able to:

1. describe the older adult with heart failure who is at risk for hospital re-admission
2. conduct a comprehensive cardiac history
3. identify three physical findings that may be associated with fluid overload in the older adult patient with heart failure
4. name three key symptoms associated with fluid overload in the older adult patient with heart failure
5. define cardiovascular stability in relation to the five key indicators
6. plan monitoring strategies to reduce fluid overload in the older adult with heart failure.

OVERVIEW

Heart failure (HF) is the most common cause of hospital admission in the older adult (Funk & Krumholz, 1996; Krumholz, Wang, et al., 1997). Hospitalizations for HF account for approximately 50% of all cardiovascular hospital admissions (Krumholz, Wang, et al., 1997; Lloyd-Jones et al., 2010) The evidenced-based literature demonstrates that as many as half of these admissions are readmissions and are preventable (Lloyd-Jones, et al., 2004; Rich et al., 1995; Ross et al., 2008). Early identification of patients at risk for rehospitalization during the hospital stay provides opportunity for interventions to impact the readmission rate. The epidemic growth in HF prevalence is commensurate with an aging population and has stimulated a focus of research to identify those patients at high risk for hospitalization and readmission. Symptoms

For description of Evidence Levels cited in this chapter, see Chapter 1, Developing and Evaluating Clinical Practice Guidelines: A Systematic Approach, page 7.

Note: This chapter was adapted from the American Association of Colleges of Nursing Preparing Nursing Students to Care for Older Adults: Enhancing Gerontology in Senior-Level Undergraduate Courses curriculum module, *Assessment and Management of Hypertension and Heart Failure,* prepared by Deborah A. Chyun and Jessica Coviello.

of HF compel patients to seek medical aid; however, evidence to date has shown HF patients postpone seeking medical assistance 12 hours to 14 days before recognition of these changes as harmful to bodily functioning (Koenig, 1998; Rich MW & Kitman DW, 2005). The delay causes further deterioration in cardiac status requiring acute hospitalization. This chapter presents the complex nature and pathophysiology of HF symptoms, with nursing management strategies to reduce hospital re-admission rates. A detailed protocol for nursing practice of the aging population is presented highlighting the nursing assessment and management of HF.

BACKGROUND AND STATEMENT OF PROBLEM

HF is a public health problem affecting an estimated 5.8 million Americans yearly (Lloyd-Jones et al., 2010; Thom et al., 2006). Cardiovascular disease (CVD), which includes hypertension (HTN) and HF, valvular heart disease and arrhythmias, along with the atherosclerotic disease that causes coronary heart disease (Hay et al., 1993), stroke, and peripheral vascular disease (PVD), is the major contributor to mortality and comorbidity in older adults. CVD accounts for 40% of all deaths in those aged 75 to 85 years, and 48% of all deaths in those 85 years and older (Lloyd-Jones et al., 2010; Thom et al., 2006). Acute or chronic HF is the leading cause of hospital admission in patients older than 65 years of age with readmission rates to acute care facilities averaging 17.2% nationally in 1996 now increased to 23.6% in 2010 (Funk & Krumholz, 1996; Lloyd-Jones et al., 2010). Risk of readmission has been shown to be four times higher in older adults aged 80 years and older, higher in ethnicities other than Whites, and higher with lower economic status (Giamouzis et al., 2011).

The prevalence of HF increases with age, and more than 75% of those affected are older than 65 years of age. Development of HF is higher with male sex, lower level of education, low levels of physical activity, cigarette smoking, overweight, diabetes mellitus (DM), HTN, valvular heart disease, left ventricular hypertrophy (LVH) and atherosclerosis of the coronaries or CHD. HTN is a precursor in 75% of individuals diagnosed with HF (Thom et al., 2006). Both the incidence and prevalence of HF continues to increase as the population ages.

Risk Factors for Developing Heart Failure in Older Adults

The primary clinical risk factors for developing HF are advancing age, male sex, HTN, myocardial infarction (MI), DM, valvular heart disease, and obesity. HTN is the most common cause of HF in patients without CHD, accounting for 24% of the cases of HF (Ho et al., 1993). HTN is also extremely common in type 2 DM, as it occurs in 40% to 60% of older adults with type 2 DM (Hypertension in Diabetes Study Group, 1993). Women with DM are at extremely high-risk for developing HF (Levy, Larson, Vasan, Kannel, & Ho, 1996). Individuals with HTN and DM often develop HF with preserved systolic function or so-called diastolic HF rather than systolic dysfunction (Piccini, Klein, Gheorghiade, & Bonow, 2004).

Other related clinical risk factors of HF include smoking, dyslipidemia of genetic and dietary etiology; sleep disordered breathing, chronic kidney disease, albuminuria, sedentary lifestyle, low socioeconomic status, and psychological stress. Toxic substances such as chemotherapeutic agents (anthracyclines, cyclophosphamide, 5-FU, trastuzumab), illicit drugs (amphetamines, cocaine), medications (nonsteroidal anti-inflammatory drugs [NSAIDs], thiazolidinediones [TZDs], alcohol) can precipitate HF (Schocken et al., 2008).

DM is a CVD equivalent and, as such, is an important contributor to HF. Women and those individuals treated with insulin are at the greatest risk. In a sample of older Medicare patients with type 2 DM, 22% had a diagnosis of HF, and this prevalence increased with advancing age (Bertoni et al., 2004). In addition, the presence of type 2 DM is associated with higher HF-related morbidity and mortality. After MI or coronary revascularization procedures, individuals with type 2 DM also have a high morbidity and mortality, which is largely caused by the development of HF. An earlier analysis of outcomes in Medicare patients 1 year after a MI revealed that 11% of patients without DM had HF, whereas 17% of patients with DM on oral agents and 25% of those treated with insulin were admitted for HF (Chyun, Vaccarino, Murillo, Young, & Krumholz, 2002).

The initial diagnosis of HF is most often an acute index event requiring hospitalization. Patients at risk for re-admission after initial diagnosis of HF include the following (Bertoni et al., 2004; Chyun et al., 2002; Lewis et al., 2003):

- Age 70 years and older, and even more so for age 80 years and older
- Newly diagnosed HF with hospitalization (Krumholz, Parent, et al., 1997)
- Low systolic blood pressure (SBP; Pocock et al., 2006)
- Increased heart rate (Stefenelli, Bergler-Klein, Globits, Pacher, & Glogar, 1992; Triposkiadis et al., 2009) or arrhythmia atrial fibrillation (Koitabashi et al., 2005)
- Hospitalizations for any reason in the last 5 years (Kossovsky et al., 2000)
- Social isolation (Faris, Purcell, Henein, & Coats, 2002)
- HF related to acute MI or uncontrolled HTN
- History of alcohol abuse (Evangelista, Doering, & Dracup, 2000)
- HF with acute infection
- HF with an exacerbation of a comorbidity; anemia with hemoglobin of less than 12 (Young et al., 2008), kidney disease (Metra et al., 2008), COPD (Braunstein et al., 2003; Mascarenhas, Lourenço, Lopes, Azevedo, & Bettencourt, 2008), and sleep apnea (Kasai et al., 2008)
- History of depression or anxiety (Faris et al, 2002; Rumsfeld et al., 2003)
- Nonadherence to diet, fluid intake, or medications

Pathophysiology of Heart Failure

Understanding the pathophysiology of HF provides insight into the rationale for treatment. Defined, *heart failure* is the inability of the heart to pump blood sufficient to metabolic needs of the body or cannot do so without greatly elevated filling pressures (Miller & Piña, 2009). The inability of the left ventricle to eject blood sufficiently represents systolic HF and is diagnosed with a measurement of ejection fraction (EF) less than 50%. Diastolic dysfunction and failure are the result of inadequate filling of the left ventricle. Diastolic HF is also more descriptively named HF with preserved systolic function because the EF is essentially normal: approximately 60%. The symptoms of HF are directly related to impairment in the filling and ejecting of the blood in the left ventricle (Owan et al., 2006).

All of the risk factors and disease entities listed previously can cause direct damage to the myocardium, as in MI and toxic exposure, or subject it to increased level of wall stress, as in HTN or valvular lesions. Such insult initiates compensatory actions by the heart that are mediated by the neurohormones of the sympathetic nervous system (SNS) and the renin angiotension aldosterone system (RAAS), which are active both systemically and directly in the myocardium. Rather than offering benefit, the SNS (epinephrine and norepinephrine) and RAAS (angiotensin II vasopressin, aldosterone) hormones promote cardiac remodeling and hypertrophy, causing dilatation of the ventricle and buildup of fibrous tissue that weakens the cardiomyocytes. These changes occur during compensated (asymptomatic) as well as decompensated (symptomatic) failure. The overexpression of neurohormones causes salt and water retention and vasoconstriction, which in turn produce increased hemodynamic stress on the left ventricle. These factors are cyclical unless treated. Untreated, there is further disruption of left ventricle architecture and performance (Miller & Piña, 2009).

Because this process begins without symptoms, for patients at risk, it is essential to identify factors that are a hazard to cardiovascular health and initiate treatment before significant damage to the myocardium occurs. The American College of Cardiology/ American Heart Association Task Force (ACC/AHA) developed guidelines to classify HF in 4 stages (2005):

Stage A is considered a pre-HF stage or an "at-risk" stage. It includes patients with HTN, atherosclerotic disease, DM, obesity, metabolic syndrome, those using cardiotoxic substances, or those with a family history of cardiomyopathy

Stage B includes asymptomatic individuals with previous MI, LVH, decreased EF, and asymptomatic valvular disease

Stage C includes individuals with known heart disease and symptoms—shortness of breath, fatigue, and reduced exercise tolerance—or those who are now asymptomatic after effective treatment for their heart disease,

Stage D includes individuals with refractory HF requiring the use of specialized interventions and includes patients with marked symptoms at rest despite maximal medical therapy.

Atherosclerosis and ischemia in CHD is the most common etiology of HF in the United States, followed closely by HTN alone and valvular disease, although thyroid dysfunction and excessive alcohol intake may also lead to HF. In the absence of known CVD, systolic function of the heart remains relatively unchanged in older adults, as does exercise tolerance. Diastolic dysfunction, however, is predominately a disease of the elderly and may be present even in the absence of HTN or hypertrophic cardiomyopathy, which are also known to contribute to diastolic failure (Bhatia et al., 2006; Olsson et al., 2006; Yancy, Lopatin, Stevenson, De Marco, & Fonarow, 2006). The archetypical patient presenting with diastolic HF is 70 to 80 years of age, female, obese, diabetic, and often has atrial fibrillation (Coats, 2001). Diastolic dysfunction is characterized by an exaggerated heart rate (HR) with activity, which is often one of the first clinical findings. The severity of symptoms varies among patients and may not correlate to left ventricular ejection fraction (LVEF; Brucks et al., 2005).

HTN, CHD, and hypertrophic cardiomyopathy are all abnormalities that are exacerbated by tachycardia underscoring the importance of avoiding a high heart rate in all older individuals. Diastolic abnormalities caused by HTN, aortic stenosis or CHD may precipitate HF. Patients with either systolic or diastolic HF are at risk for fluid overload. Although discussed as two separate entities, many older adults have components of both systolic and diastolic dysfunction.(Gheorghiade et al., 2010)

ASSESSMENT OF THE PROBLEM

For older adults diagnosed with HF, the health history and physical assessment is directed at monitoring symptoms and assessing cardiovascular function. For the nurse assessing and managing the patient with HF, it is important to note that the recognition of fluid overload is not always straightforward. Unlike the classic picture of HF observed in younger adults, the symptoms of fluid overload can be subtle and elusive in older adults (Coviello, 2004). Once symptoms become pronounced in the older adult, the nurse has a challenging task to resolve the HF, especially if it is of a long-standing duration (Giamouzis et al., 2011). Monitoring parameters must be established where the patient and nurse actively identify subtle changes and seek intervention as early as possible (Grady et al., 2000).

The Health History

HF has both symptomatic and nonsymptomatic phase. When symptoms occur, they are related to intravascular and interstitial fluid overload and inadequate tissue perfusion. Symptoms become evident with exertion and in severe HF, even at rest. The New York Heart Association functional capacity is another important method for classifying the HF patient according to how much activity patients are able to do without symptoms (see Table 31.1). Classifying patients in this way offers evidence of the extent of volume overload and activity limitation caused by symptoms, which then leads the nurse to realize a level of disease. Patients, with proper treatment, can improve their functional status and classification from a NYHA Class III to II or even I; however, they do not reclaim earlier stages. For example, a Stage C patient does not return to Stage B.

Both patients and providers frequently attribute symptoms of fluid overload to aging. When symptoms occur during exertion, senior patients may simply decrease their activities to prevent symptoms, yet when asked, they report activity from a memory of months earlier. Because of inaccurate reporting of activity, HF in older adults is often difficult to recognize and, therefore, goes untreated. Thus, the nurse should routinely ask questions related to activity-limiting dyspnea. A key indicator in establishing a baseline for functional capacity is to ask the patient what their maximal asymptomatic activity is now, what it was 6 months ago, and what it was 1 year ago. Other important questions include "How far can you walk without getting short of breath"? "What is the activity that commonly produces shortness of breath"? "Do you experience shortness of

TABLE 31.1	
New York Heart Association Functional Capacity Classification	
Class I	No limitation of physical activity. Ordinary physical activity does not cause undue fatigue, palpitation, dyspnea, or angina.
Class II	Slight limitation of physical activity. Ordinary physical activity results in fatigue, palpitation, dyspnea, or angina.
Class III	Marked limitation of physical activity. Comfortable at rest, but less than ordinary of physical activity results in fatigue, palpitation, dyspnea, or angina.
Class IV	Unable to carry on any physical activity without discomfort. Symptoms present at rest. With any physical activity, symptoms increase.

Source: Adapted from: American Heart Association. (1994). Revisions to classification of functional capacity and objective assessment of patients with disease of the heart. *Circulation, 90,* 644–645.

breath when simply sitting?" "Do you wake at night feeling short of breath?" Repeating these questions in subsequent interviews will help monitor changes in activity associated with treatment or with suspected fluid gain. Is the patient physically capable of performing activities of daily living?

HF is a pathophysiological process in which left ventricular dysfunction occurs independently from symptom development (Brucks et al., 2005). Symptom expression is dependent upon compensatory mechanisms and the length of time HF has been present. Patients with acute HF, as seen with MI, may be more symptomatic because their compensatory mechanisms have not fully developed. In comparison, the patient with long-standing HF may have severe dysfunction but may not become symptomatic at all until they eat a high-sodium meal and develop fluid overload rapidly, oftentimes overnight. In this case, compensatory mechanisms are now exhausted and as a result, fail. The window of opportunity to successfully intervene is narrow, as is the margin of error. Treatment for fluid overload in this case must be swift and brisk but gentle enough to maintain BP (Grady, et al, 2000). Nurses need to be aware of the importance of both early recognition and early intervention in the patient with fluid overload. A few hours delay in providing treatment can mean the difference between successful management at home or need for hospital admission with variable outcomes.

Knowledge of the past medical history will help to anticipate problems related to other conditions because their presence may complicate assessment and management of HF. Cardiac risk factors; levels of physical activity; and control of lipids, HTN, obesity, DM, and smoking need to be determined. Older adult responses to HF medications and treatment are variable. In addition, other drugs commonly used in this age group, such as nonsteroidal anti-inflammatory agents, can actually exacerbate fluid overload by increasing sodium retention. Previous questions related to cardiovascular functional capacity may have already provided some information, but additional information on musculoskeletal and neurological function is important.

Assessment of additional symptoms is also important. *Orthopnea* is the most sensitive and specific symptom of elevated filling pressures, and it tends to reliably parallel filling pressures in patients with this symptom (Ankler et al., 2003; Stevenson & Perloff, 1989). Nocturnal or exertional cough is often a dyspnea equivalent and should not be confused with the cough from an angiotensin-converting enzyme (ACE) inhibitor, which is not associated with activity or position. Individual patients generally exhibit reproducible patterns of fluid overload. These should be documented, be made available to all on the care team, and be used in patient education and subsequent monitoring. Questions related to symptoms and function should be part not only of the initial assessment, but also of subsequent visits as a means of surveillance (Stevenson & Perloff, 1989).

The clinical presentation of HF may include a variety of symptoms reflective of pulmonary congestion and decreased cardiac output. The questions related to health history are important to include and/or observe during the health encounter. Although the presence of any one symptom is sufficient to warrant consideration of HF when they occur with other physical findings, orthopnea, paroxysmal nocturnal dyspnea, and progressive dyspnea on exertion are virtually diagnostic of fluid overload.

The presence of other comorbidities among older adults, such as DM, renal dysfunction, and liver disease, along with systemic physiological changes associated with aging, further complicate the assessment and management of HF in the older adult. Comorbidities should also be carefully assessed by reviewing laboratory data. DM may necessitate monitoring of blood glucose since wide variations in glucose can affect ischemic threshold. Renal and liver disease may affect pharmacodynamics of drugs used to treat HF. Anemia, a common medical condition in older adults, affects oxygenation, activity tolerance, and subsequent fluid balance (Young et al., 2008). The presence of chronic obstructive pulmonary disease (COPD), as well as other comorbidites, may necessitate special precautions when assessing and managing oxygen therapy and beta-blockers.

Since over use of salt in the diet may precipitate fluid overload, a comprehensive dietary history is absolutely essential. The nurse should include specific questions about what the patient eats at meal and who prepares those meals. Additionally, does the patient use the salt shaker or salt substitutes at the table or in cooking? A review of foods high in sodium on a printed list often reveals foods the patient is eating but previously did not admit to. For instance, important dietary questions related to use of canned products or deli meats, which contain higher amounts of sodium should be included. A list of the sodium and the potassium content of a variety of foods, including fruits and vegetables, can be helpful in providing the information necessary for the patient to make appropriate daily choices. Because assessment of nutritional status is critical to elicit accurate fluid and sodium intake, it is prudent in the acute care setting for the older adult to have a dietary consultation. Additionally, since cachexia is a harbinger of a downward spiral in patients with HF, questions need to be included on the health history related to appetite and weight loss (Evangelista et al., 2000; Lavie, Osman, Milani, & Mehra, 2003).

Current prescription and over-the-counter medication taking should be assessed, along with any alternative therapies. Many older adult who are eligible for aspirin, beta-blockers, and ACE inhibitors do not receive these medications despite the important role that these agents have in reducing CHD-related morbidity and mortality (Anker et al., 2003; Colucci et al., 1996; Colucci et al., 2007; Packer, Bristow, et al., 1996; Packer, 1998; Schocken et al., 2008).

Included in the health history should be questions related to medication adherence and the patient's decision to either take or not to take medications (Grady et al., 2000; Riegel et al., 2009). Understanding a patient's rationale to selectively not take certain medications at certain times will help reveal ways for the nurse to intervene. Patients may wish to adjust their diuretic dose so that they can function socially during the day. This is not an adherence issue but a sound decision based on the patient's rationale as to how to fit the medication regimen into their lifestyle. The interview can reveal if "nonadherence" has such a rationale. If a cause is not found, other issues need to be explored such as cost, number of medications, and/or the frequency of the doses. Ways to simplify the drug regimen should be explored.

Psychosocial factors, personal beliefs and behaviors, along with cultural and environmental influences, all contribute to management of chronic disease. The importance of depression and social support has been well documented in the older adult; therefore, all of these factors need to be assessed (Davos et al., 2003; Faris et al., 2002). The nursing assessment in individuals with HF should identify the individual's response to treatment, which can then be used to assist the individual in subsequent management of symptoms and the underlying condition, health promotion and disease prevention activities, and chronic disease management. Awareness of the patient's own perception of why they sought medical care and a detailed analysis of the symptoms will assist in assessing the individual's or caregiver's ability to identify symptoms, their knowledge regarding their condition, its prognosis, and general health beliefs, along with their prior ability to manage this or other medical conditions.

The Physical Assessment of the Older Adult With Fluid Overload

Physical assessment of the patient with suspected fluid overload includes inspection; palpation; and auscultation of the peripheral vasculature, heart, lungs, abdomen, and extremities. Orientation, functional limitations, and mental clarity are observed during examination of vital signs, which include height and weight and waist circumference.

A patient's height and baseline weight are important indicators of both nutritional and fluid status. The importance of daily weights should be emphasized in the hospital setting and, each day with each weight, a reinforcement of the need to not only continue this practice at home, but to record the daily weight in a log as well. Weights should subsequently be taken by the patient daily, typically the first thing in the morning upon arising, before breakfast, and with no clothes or wearing light clothing to avoid false fluctuations (Grady et al., 2000; Riegel et al., 2009; Riegel, Naylor, Stewart, McMurray, & Rich, 2004). This provides the best baseline for consistency. Hospitalized patients with HF have a weight measurement each day. With each daily weight, give reinforcement again of the importance and also the significance of weight gain and actions to take with 3 to 5-lb weight gain. A 2-lb. weight gain overnight or a 3-lb weight gain in a week is an indication that medical management must change. Measurement of a senior's waist circumference is also important to determine at baseline, since many times, this is the location for fluid accumulation (Grady et al., 2000). Once height and weight are measured, a body mass index (BMI) should be calculated. Research has shown that higher BMIs (25–30 kg/m^2) are associated with longer survival (Horwich et al., 2001; Lavie et al., 2003; Pickering et al., 2005; Pickering et al, 2008).

A thorough evaluation of the blood pressure (BP) should be performed. A variety of environmental factors can influence BP determination; therefore, the room should be of a comfortable temperature, the patient as relaxed as possible, and a 5-minute rest before taking the first reading. Clothing that covers the area where the cuff will be placed should be removed, and the individual should be seated comfortably, with legs uncrossed, with the back and arm supported; the middle of the cuff on the upper arm should be at a level of the right atrium (Sansevero, 1997). The initial BP reading should be taken in both arms. Proper cuff size is critical to obtaining an accurate measurement. Obese individuals with large arm circumference need to have the appropriate cuff size for accuracy. Conversely, thin, cachectic patients will also have inaccurate reading with a standard cuff. The bladder length should be 80% of the arm circumference and width at least 40%. The midline of the bladder should be placed above the brachial artery, 2 to 3 cm above the antecubital fossa, where the artery should have first been palpated. When using the auscultatory method, which remains the "gold standard" for BP measurement, palpating the radial pulse first while inflating the cuff will identify the point at which the pulse disappears. For the subsequent auscultatory measurement, the cuff should then be inflated to at least 30 mmHg above this point. The rate of deflation is also extremely important with a rate of 2 to 3 mmHg/second recommended. The first and last audible sounds are the SBP and diastolic BP (DBP) respectively. Two readings, taken 5 minutes apart should be averaged and if there is greater than 5 mm Hg difference, additional readings should be obtained (Pickering et al., 2005; Pickering et al., 2008; Sansevero, 2007).

Pseudohypertension is a rare phenomenon resulting from noncompressibility of thickened arteries and will result in the recording of falsely high BP when indirect methods are used. A high BP over time without any indication of end-organ damage, and treatment of the BP creates symptoms of hypotension such as dizziness, confusion, and decreased urine output points to this diagnosis. This tendency for peripheral arteries to become rigid with aging may result in a need to increase cuff pressure in order to compress the artery. If suspected, an intra-arterial reading has been suggested to avoid overmedication with antihypertensives; however, this is an extreme measure and is rarely done. Most providers, who treat HTN in the elderly, consider 160/90 as a hypertensive BP and will treat gently with appropriate antihypertensives and pull back on treatment if symptoms of hypotension or orthostasis occur. Isolated systolic HTN is also common in the older adult and is defined by a SBP greater than 140 and a DBP of less than 90 mm Hg. Care must be taken not to overtreat in this population, especially if aortic stenosis or other valvular disease is present. Older adults are also more likely to exhibit white-coat HTN, where the BP may be elevated over 140/90 mm Hg in the presence of a health care worker and an actual reading at home is usually 135/85 mm Hg. Therefore, assessment of the BP not only requires careful attention to technique but also consideration of the physiological abnormalities associated with aging. Home BP monitoring has been suggested as a means for patients to partner with their providers to provide care. For those patients who are unable for whatever reason, 24-hour ambulatory BP monitoring is available to more accurately assess BP fluctuations during the day (Arzt et al., 2006).

In addition, the standing BP should be assessed because older adults have a tendency for postural hypotension. Orthostatic hypotension is diagnosed when the SBP falls by at least 20 mm Hg or the DBP by 10 mm Hg within 3 minutes. The presence of orthostatic hypotension may also reveal early dehydration in a patient who is usually otherwise stable (Arzt & Bradley, 2006). Because dehydration is the second most common admission for the older adult with HF, with falling following closely behind, standing BPs should be part of the routine assessment. In addition, patients should be assessed for dehydration whenever a condition exists where fluid loss could occur. This includes not only with vomiting or diarrhea but also with diaphoresis caused by extremes in temperature and humidity.

Inspection is the first step of the physical assessment. General inspection of the periphery includes the following:

- Observing color of the skin and mucous membranes.
- Inspecting the patient's nails, including nail beds, and the angle between the base of the nail and the skin of the cuticle (normally less than 160 degrees). An angle of 180 degrees is called *clubbing*; the distal phalanx appears rounded. Clubbing is associated with chronic hemoglobin desaturation.
- If cachexic, check dependent areas for decubiti.
- Hair on distal extremities—adequate arterial perfusion.

Palpation of the extremities occurs following inspection of the skin color for temperature and turgor as well as the color of the nail beds. Capillary refill of the nail should be assessed by compressing the nail for 2 to 3 seconds and then releasing. Note the time elapsed until the original color returns. Normally, the nail bed is pink; capillary refill occurs within 2 to 3 seconds. A pale or cyanotic nail with delayed capillary refill may indicate decreased peripheral perfusion. The peripheral pulses should be palpated bilaterally, including radial, femoral, pedal, and posterior tibial pulse. Note pulse rate, rhythm, and symmetry.

Respiratory rate and effort should be assessed prior to auscultation of the lungs. If possible, oxygen saturation during rest and activity should be recorded. Patients whose oxygen level desaturates during activity to 86% or lower may require oxygen support at home. In addition, surveillance of oxygen saturation during sleep may be required if the patient or family reports difficulty with sleep at night. It is not uncommon to see sleep apnea in patients with HF (Bennett & Sauvé, 2003; Cormican & Williams, 2004; Kaneko, Hajek, Zivanovic, Raboud, Bradley, 2003; Lanfranchi & Somers, 2003; Maisel, 2001a; Mansfield et al., 2003). Use the diaphragm of the stethoscope to assess the lungs. Listen in all the lobes for diminished sounds, crackles, wheezes, or rhonchi. Lung sounds are an important part of the assessment, particularly in patients with a history of HF.

The cardiovascular assessment begins by locating the apex and apical pulse by feeling for the point of maximal impulse (PMI). In systolic HF, the PMI is displaced laterally and indicates the heart is dilated. Assessment of apical pulse rate and regularity, with attention to fullness and amplitude, also are important. Heart sounds should be ascertained with both the diaphragm and the bell of the stethoscope. Note the presence of S1 and S2 and of extra sounds, S3 gallop, S4, murmurs, clicks, or rubs. If extra heart sounds are present, also examine the carotid arteries by listening on both sides of the neck with the bell. Bruits sound like murmurs, so it is important to differentiate between the two. Some aortic murmurs will radiate into the neck and may even be audible when auscultating the lungs posteriorly. Always listen to the heart before listening for extra sounds in the neck. In addition, the carotids should not be palpated bilaterally because this can lead to dysrhythmias and decreased blood flow to the brain

Jugular veins are assessed best with the patient in semi-Fowler's position but if the patient is severely dyspneic, Fowler's position may be necessary. With the patient's head in straight alignment, observe the jugular neck veins for the presence of jugular venous distention (JVD). Turning the head slightly to the left and shining a penlight angularly on the vein allows for easier visualization of JVD and *a* and v waves, particularly in obese patients. The jugular venous pulse waves will vary with respiration and decrease during inspiration. The jugular vein is compressible and varies with the angle of the neck. In the absence of pathology, venous distention is not present. *Jugular venous distention* is the most sensitive sign of elevated filling pressures and is present with fluid overload, cor pulmonale, or high venous pressure (Stevenson, et al. 1989).

The abdomen should then be examined. First, auscultate for bowel sounds in a distended abdomen to assess for other pathology-causing distention. Next, palpate to determine if the abdomen is soft and nontender. A protuberant abdomen with bulging flanks suggests the possibility of ascites. Because ascitic fluid characteristically sinks with gravity while gas-filled loops of bowel float to the top, percussion gives a dull note in dependent areas of the abdomen. Look for such a pattern by percussing outward in several directions from the central area of tympany. Map the area between tympany and dullness. To palpate the liver, place your hand behind the patient, parallel to and supporting the right 11th and 12th ribs and adjacent soft tissues below. Remind the patient to relax. By pressing your left hand forward, the patient's liver may be felt more easily by the other hand. Patients who are sensitive to palpation can rest their hand on your palpating hand. Note any tenderness. If at all palpable, the edge of the liver is soft, sharp, and regular. The liver can be enlarged in HF because of congestion. To further assess for volume excess, place the patient in semi-Fowler's position at the highest level at which the jugular neck pulsations remain visible. Firmly apply pressure with the palmar surface of the hand over the right upper quadrant of the patient's abdomen for 1 minute.

A 1-cm rise in the jugular distention called *hepatojugular reflux* confirms the presence of fluid overload. Hepatojugular reflux may be associated with or without tenderness. Patients may also complain of a feeling of fullness.

The presence of *peripheral edema*, a symptom that can be related to fluid overload from cardiac renal disease or PVD, should be evaluated. Edema can also occur in response to medications such as calcium channel blockers. Dependent parts of the body such as the feet, the ankles, and the sacrum are the most likely locations to find edema. The presence and location of edema and whether it is pitting or nonpitting should be assessed. Depress an edematous area over a bony prominence for 5 to 15 seconds, then release. Grading scale for edema is as follows:

$0 =$ *no pitting*
$1+ =$ *trace*
$2+ =$ *moderate*, disappears in 10 to 45 seconds
$3+ =$ *deep*, disappears in 1 to 2 minutes
$4+ =$ *very deep*, disappears in 3 to 5 minutes

The neurological assessment cannot be overlooked because changes in heart rate and rhythm, a decrease in cardiac output, and side effects of cardiac medications may cause significant changes in mental status. The nurse can observe and assess the patient's mood, thought processes, thought content, abnormal perceptions, insight, judgment, memory, and retention throughout the exam from intake of history and throughout treatment. Because depression is common among both the older adult and the chronically ill, signs of depression should be assessed (Koenig, 1998; Maisel, 2001b). Examples of signs of depression include feelings of hopelessness and sadness (also see Chapter 9, Depression). The time, the day, and the year as well as orientation to place should be included. Memory of hospitalization, teaching that occurred while hospitalized; subsequent events postdischarge can be addressed depending on whether the patient is hospitalized or being seen as an outpatient (Grady et al., 2000; Wang, FitzGerald, Schulzer, Mak, & Ayas, 2005).

To summarize, the physical examination findings consistent with HF include the following:

- JVD
- Basilar crackles, bronchospasm and wheezing
- Displaced apical impulse
- Presence of S3 or S4; heart murmur
- Elevated heart rate and BP
- Hepatomegaly/splenomegaly
- Hepatojugular reflux
- Elevated heart rate and BP
- Temperature of extremities, warm versus cool

Laboratory and Diagnostic Studies

The initial laboratory evaluation of patients presenting with symptoms of HF should include complete blood count, serum electrolytes including calcium and magnesium, blood urea nitrogen, serum creatinine, fasting blood glucose, glycosylated hemoglobin A1c (HbA1c), lipid profile, liver function tests, thyroid stimulating hormone, and urinalysis. B-type natriuretic peptide (BNP) is useful in the evaluation of symptomatic patients presenting in the urgent care setting in whom the clinical diagnosis of HF is uncertain (Cygankiewicz et al., 2009; Huang et al., 2007; Hunt et al., 2005). A baseline BNP in the patient with a confirmed diagnosis of HF in the compensated state can provide a comparison measurement when both the presence of fluid overload is suspected. A BNP level below 100 indicates a very low probability of HF; however, a level between 100 to 400 pg/mL should raise suspicion of HF. Levels greater than 400 pg/mL have a 95% probability of HF and congestion caused by volume overload (Cygankiewicz et al., 2009; Hunt et al., 2005) and response to therapy. Electrolyte abnormalities are common in the older adult, particularly in individuals on chronic diuretic therapy. Of critical importance is the serum potassium whose level should not drop below 3.8 mmol/l. Renal function, as well as electrolyte levels, should remain current and repeated whenever a patient has to increase diuretic therapy for longer than 3 days because of fluid overload. Anemia is frequently observed and may contribute to hypoxia, myocardial ischemia, and fluid overload.

The index episode or first acute HF is most often ischemic in etiology. Cardiac enzymes assist in determining the presence of acute MI when an acute fluid overload event occurs (Bertoni et al., 2004; Chyun et al., 2002; Lewis et al., 2003). Older adults may have a MI in the total absence of symptoms or with atypical symptoms. All of these factors make a review of diagnostic tests results very important.

A 12-lead electrocardiogram (ECG) and chest x-ray (PA and lateral) should be performed initially in all patients presenting with symptoms of HF. A baseline ECG is vital so that ST and T waves; axis changes; prolongation in PR, QRS, and QT intervals can be assessed for indication of ongoing ischemia and response to medications. A new onset arrhythmia heralded by an episode of fluid overload is not uncommon. The excess volume in HF can cause a stretch of the atrium, which, in turn, can precipitate atrial fibrillation, a common arrhythmia in patients with chronic HF. Two-dimensional echocardiography with Doppler should be performed during the initial evaluation to assess LVEF, LV size, wall thickness, and valve function. Radionucleotide ventriculography (MUGA scan) can be performed to assess ventricular volumes, LVEF, and myocardial perfusion abnormalities although the current advanced technology of echocardiography makes the radionucleotide method of MUGA unnecessary. Cardiac catheterization should be performed on patients presenting with symptoms of HF who have angina or significant ischemia or who have known, suspected, or at high-risk for CHD, unless the patient is not eligible for revascularization of any kind.

Halter monitoring may be considered in patients presenting with HF who have a history of MI and/or syncope and are being considered for an electrophysiology study to document an inducible ventricular tachycardia. In addition, other candidates for electrophysiology include those with an LVEF of 30% or less with a QRS complex duration that exceeds 120 ms. Patients who meet this criteria may receive biventricular pacemaker in combination with an automatic implantable defibrillator in order to prevent sudden death from ventricular arrhythmia (Prystowsky & Nisam, 2000), as well as improve cardiac output (Bonds et al., 2010; Chobanian et al., 2003; Glant & Raz, 2010).

INTERVENTIONS AND CARE STRATEGIES

Initial goals in the acute management of HF are to alleviate symptoms and improve oxygenation, improve circulation, and correct the underlying causes of the HF. Longer term goals are to improve exercise tolerance and functional capacity, and through treatment improve ventricular function thereby reducing admission and readmission rates and decreasing morbidity and mortality. The management of HF follows standard ACC/ AHA Task Force expert consensus recommendations, including intensive treatment of co-existent HTN, CHD, and renal disease (Chobanian et al., 2003). Importantly, optimal treatment of HTN is critical to both the prevention and treatment of HF. Although the level at which medication should be started is still debated (Lee, Lindquist, Segal, & Covinsky, 2006), the goal BP should be 130/80 mm Hg (Baruch et al., 2004).

There are key prognostic indicators of 4-year mortality for older adults diagnosed with HF. Patients with renal dysfunction, pulmonary disease, a BMI of less than 25 kg/m², diabetes, HTN, and cancer, as well as those who continue to smoke have a greater risk of mortality. Those with a functional deficit in activities of daily living (ADLs; difficulty bathing, managing finances, walking several blocks, or pushing or pulling heavy objects) combined with one or more of the earlier mentioned factors are at greater risk not only for mortality but additionally the need for hospitalization. A chart review and history during hospitalization should then include not only the standard accepted cardiac risk factors but also the key indicators as listed previously. Detecting these additional prognostic indicators can aid in developing interventions that can affect quality of life and survival (Carson, Tognoni, & Cohn, 2003). Goals for therapy should include reaching goals for fasting blood sugar and HbA1c, BP, cholesterol, and HF therapy through the use of evidenced based standards of care.

In *Stage A*, HF, HTN, and lipid disorders are treated with lifestyle modification and medication as indicated to achieve guideline recommended goals for BP and cholesterol. Smoking cessation assistance, in the form of counseling and medication, is offered at every interaction with a patient that smokes. A goal of increasing activity or exercise should be mutually established with patients. For some, this may be as little as standing and sitting during television commercials, whereas for others, it may mean a walk before or after dinner or more for others. The control of metabolic syndrome is achieved through lifestyle modification. *Alcohol* is a simple sugar, and in excess contributes to the development of insulin resistance and diabetes, increasing cardiovascular risk. Illicit drug use must be identified, treatment offered and encouraged. Both ACE inhibitors and angiotension-receptor blockers (ARBs; Maggioni et al., 2005) treat HTN and HF but, importantly, have been shown to prevent cardiovascular events, cerebrovascular events, and progression of renal disease. Their use is especially important in patients with vascular disease or in those with DM.

In *Stage B*, these same cited measures are used with ACE inhibitors, ARBs, and beta-blockers used in certain patients. All ACE inhibitors are indicated in HF; however, there are only two ARBs with evidence strong enough to be indicated in HF. Valsartan and candesartan, both ARBs, obtained recognition for benefit in HF in their respective studies (Cohn, 1999; Cohn & Tognoni, 2001; Ostergren, 2006; Packer, 1998; Packer, Bristow, et al., 1996; Packer, Colucci, et al., 1996; Shah, Desai, & Givertz, 2010). In *Stage C*, dietary sodium restriction is added to this regimen, and as a symptomatic stage, diuretics are needed to be added to treat the fluid retention that causes symptoms, along with ACE inhibitors or ARB and beta-blockers. Carvedilol and metoprolol, in extended release form, are the two drugs in the beta-blocker category that are indicated in the treatment of HF (Barrella & Della Monica, 1998; Carmody & Anderson, 2007; Colucci et al., 1996; Colluci et al., 2007; Goldstein & Hjalmarson, 1999; Hjalmarson et al., 2000; Hjalmarson & Fagerberg, 2000; Naylor et al., 1994).

In certain patients, aldosterone antagonists, ARBs, and/or digitalis are used and are effective (Baruch et al., 2004; Carson et al., 2003; Cohn & Tognoni, 2001; Maggioni et al., 2005). Hydralazine in combination with isordil or other nitrates are beneficial in the African American population (Rich & Nease, 1999). Most of the *Stage C* patients qualify for a biventricular pacemaker and/or implantable defibrillators to treat life-threatening arrhythmias. In *Stage D*, patients under the age of 70 without significant comorbidities may be offered options such as cardiac transplant or left ventricular assist device (LVAD, VAD). A trial of inotrope therapy, such as milrinone or dobutamine, may serve as a temporary boost to end-stage patients and may lead to treatment as palliative therapy, offering patients at end of life an improved quality and ability to be with their family. Palliative care offers the end-stage patient comfort that affords the patient a quality of life in an environment where the patient can be at ease rather than the frequent and recurrent hospital visits on an emergent basis. While the LVAD first was designed as a bridge to transplant, VADs are now offered as a bridge to decision about transplant. Additionally, the LVAD as destination therapy is a palliative measure, again offering the patient a quality of life their heart is able to give. Hospice care is also offered to the end-stage HF patient who is not a candidate for any further therapy. The nurse has an important role in assisting the individual and their caregivers in understanding the disease process and treatment options, including end-of-life care (Coviello, Hricz-Borges, & Masulli, 2002).

Open and honest discussion regarding the chronic, progressive nature of HF must begin early in the disease process since the natural history of HF involves declining physical as well as psychological functioning. Although depression is commonly seen in the older adult, as well as individuals with CVD, there are few studies that have addressed this important problem in older adult with HF (Faris et al., 2002). In a study of patients at Duke University over the age of 60, Koenig found 107 patients of 342 depressed patients had HF, with 36.5 % having a major depression and 25.5% having a minor depression (Koenig, 1998). Because pharmacotherapy and behavioral interventions have demonstrated effectiveness, all older individuals should be screened for depression and treated appropriately. Early discussions related to the goals of care and advanced directives with frequent revisiting of patient understanding of the disease course and patient preferences as the illness progresses ensures patient and care partner participation in decision making. A multidisciplinary team including a spiritual and/or a psychological representative should be developed to offer support for all involved: the patient, family, and all involved in the care of the patient.

The benefits of the multidisciplinary team to provide care to HF patients have been discussed for the last several years. In most cases, this has been related to the use of the team approach to help keep patients stable in order to prevent hospital re-admissions (Naylor, 2006; Naylor et al., 2004; Naylor & Keating, 2008). Comprehensive transitional care interventions have been shown not only to reduce costs and cardiac outcomes, but also have a beneficial effect on hospitalization for comorbid conditions (Chriss et al., 2004; Coviello et al., 2002; Dickson et al., 2008; Naylor et al., 2009; Riegel et al., 2004). In the case of the patient in end-stage HF, a multidisciplinary team either for inpatient or outpatient management can provide cost-effective service providing patients with their last wishes in the environment that they choose (Grady et al., 2000; Riegel et al., 2006).

Once the initial history and physical assessment have been completed, an individualized care plan to monitor and treat fluid overload should be implemented. The care plan should include teaching that begins early in the hospital stay while the patient's memory of a decompensated state is fresh. The teaching of principles of HF self-care relies on the patient ability to learn to recognize the beginnings of decompensation. Techniques to prevent a congested state and manage self-care to maintain euvolemia, are crucial to begin as early as possible (Cavallari et al., 2004; Lancaster, Smiciklas-Wright, Heller, Ahern, & Jensen, 2003; Riegel et al., 2009; Taylor et al., 2004). A 3-lb weight gain in 1 to 2 days or a 5-lb weight gain in the course of the week is reason to alter diuretic dosage for up to 3 days. If the patient returns to baseline weight before the 3-day period, they may reduce their dose back to standard daily dose (Grady et al., 2000). Patients can be taught how to regulate their diuretic doses based on their symptoms and weight. The nurse and patient can construct a self-care algorithm that gives them a sound "recipe" to follow if fluid overload occurs. The important factor here is early recognition and swift, brief action. Clear guidelines as to when to contact caregivers, if they are not living with the patient, should also be provided. Consideration should be given to the patient's baseline functional capacity, as well as renal function. Diuretics are used in both systolic and diastolic HF to relieve congestive symptoms by promoting the excretion of sodium and water and by decreasing cardiac filling pressures, thereby decreasing preload. They should be used effectively but cautiously in the elderly with diastolic dysfunction, where maintaining an adequate cardiac output is heavily preload dependent in order to avoid syncope, falls, or confusion.

A double dose of oral diuretics for up to 3 days is usually well tolerated in both systolic as well as diastolic HF. When diuretics are used, serum potassium levels should be monitored because of an increased risk of hypokalemia with loop diuretics and of hyperkalemia with potassium-sparing agents especially if renal impairment exists. Patients should be forewarned about signs of hypokalemia such as profound weakness. Loop diuretics may be useful for patients who are volume sensitive or who have a tendency to retain fluid because of renal impairment. Aldosterone antagonists, as potassium sparing diuretics, abate some degree of hypokalemia, resulting from loop diuretics; however, serum potassium levels should be monitored. In some patients, ACE inhibitors can cause hyperkalemia and in combination with aldosterone inhibitors this may be exacerbated. Recent evidence suggests that many individuals, particularly African Americans, may still require potassium supplementation (Gonseth, Guallar-Castillón, Banegas, & Rodríguez-Artalejo, 2002). In addition, dehydration is an important problem in older adults taking diuretics and appears to be an even greater concern in African Americans (McKelvie et al., 2002), making assessment of hydration status an important nursing concern (Arzt & Bradley, 2006).

Use of diuretic agents increases the risk for sudden loss of urinary control (urinary incontinence) in older adults, a very common, potentially reversible geriatric syndrome (http://consultgerirn.org/resources and select "Try This Urinary Incontinence Assessment"). Practice with an older adult population requires frequent monitoring and detection of symptoms related to the onset of urinary incontinence, which is often signaled by symptoms of urinary frequency, urgency, or nocturia. These symptoms may actually be present in the older adult from other coexisting comorbidities. Nocturia is particularly evident in patients with heart disease because the supine position increases vascular return and precipitates frequent rising at night to urinate. Nighttime falls in the older adult most often occur when the patient wakes to travel to the bathroom. Pre-existing comorbidities such as visual impairment or osteoarthritis of the hip and or knees, as well as prostate hypertrophy in men, make safety strategies a priority in urgent bathroom requirements. Overall, management considerations for the older adult with heart disease and a new development of urinary incontinence or falls include re-evaluation of medication regimen, activity considerations, and the use of additional adaptive aides to assist in avoidance of preventable events. Use of a nighttime bedpan, urinal, or commode with frequent toileting rounds and reduction of nighttime fluids all are possible and worthwhile solutions. Furosemide, as the most commonly used diuretic, has a half-life of 6 hours. Inpatients who are a falling risk, timing the completion of diuresis before bedtime can decrease nocturia.

Beta-blockers are useful in the management of diastolic HF because of their inhibition of the SNS and resultant negative chronotropic effect, which decreases heart rate and increases time for diastolic filling. Beta-blockers are beneficial in the treatment of systolic HF (Cohn, 1999; Colucci et al., 1996; Colucci et al., 2007; Goldstein & Hjalmarson, 1999; Hjalmarson & Fagerberg, 2000; Packer, 1998; Packer, Bristow, et al., 1996; Packer, Colucci, et al., 1996; Ostergren, 2006; Shah et al., 2010) and are initiated in a euvolemic state after symptoms have resolved. These agents should be initiated at low doses and titrated up to optimal tolerated dose. Use of beta-blockers in combination with ACE inhibitors has demonstrated both an improvement in LVEF and functional capacity once optimized. Although beta-blockers may potentially worsen insulin resistance, mask hypoglycemia or aggravate orthostatic hypotension in older individuals with DM, these agents have been shown to contribute to improved outcomes. Therefore, careful monitoring for adverse effects is required with beta-blocker treatment to realize the beneficial effects of this important medication.

Digoxin increases contractility and decreases heart rate. It is not routinely indicated; however, it may be useful in those patients with persistent symptoms despite diuretic and ACE inhibitor therapy and in those patients who also have atrial fibrillation. Blood levels of digoxin should be monitored for toxicity and interactions with other medications such as amiodarone, verapamil, and vasodilators. Quinidine is no longer indicated or used therapeutically. The narrow therapeutic range for potassium is extremely important to monitor to prevent hypokalemia, which can precipitate arrhythmias in older adult patients with HF who are predisposed to both atrial and ventricular arrhythmias. Other medications that have a positive inotropic effect are dopamine and dobutamine. Both of these drugs can improve contractility and subsequent cardiac output; however, they also increase myocardial oxygen demand. *Milrinone* is a phosphodiesterase inhibitor that has been shown to be beneficial in the management of the hospitalized patient with HF, providing a positive inotropic effect, as well as a vasodilation (see Chapter 17, Adverse Drug Events, for potential sequelae to several CV medications).

Vasodilators are also useful in the treatment of systolic and diastolic failure through reduction in preload. As with diuretics, they should be used cautiously in those with diastolic HF. Hydralazine and isosorbide reduce both preload and afterload, relieving symptoms and improving exercise tolerance. This combination is commonly used when patients do not tolerate ACE therapy. African Americans, in particular, had reduction in morbidity and mortality with hydralazine/nitrate combination (Piepoli, Davos, Francis, & Coats, 2004). Morphine sulfate, often used in an emergent situation, also has a peripheral vasodilating effect and is useful with pulmonary edema or in patients with breathlessness at end of life.

With appropriate titration of these medications, an improvement in both left ventricular function and functional capacity can be achieved. Medications to treat HTN and lipid abnormalities may not be well tolerated, and the potential for side effects and drug interactions is increased in the setting of polypharmacy. Both anti-hypertensive agents as well as lipid-lowering agents should be used in the lowest doses possible to bring about the desired goal for treatment.

Patients and caregivers need to understand the warning signs of HF and recurrent MI such as chest pain, pressure, shortness of breath, indigestion, nausea, dizziness, palpitations, confusion, weakness, and weight gain. A clear plan for obtaining immediate medical attention should be developed. This is especially important if the older person lives alone; some type of "medical alert" system may be needed. Telemonitoring may be an option for some patients to consider. Understanding and ability to follow the medication regimen is paramount. A thorough assessment of the patient and their caregivers is therefore vital. The older individual may be on multiple medications and the schedule may be confusing. The need to maintain cardiac medications must be stressed and the risk of the patient abruptly discontinuing beta-blocker, nitrates, and anti-arrhythmics must be assessed. All medications should be reviewed with the patient and their caregivers, stressing desired effects, common side effects, and possible interactions with over-the-counter medications (http://consultgerirn.org/resources and select Geriatric Topics "Medication"). The nurse should also review what to do if medications are accidentally omitted or become too costly to maintain. Long-term management of HF requires a multidisciplinary team approach (Lloyd-Jones, et al., 2004) and disease management programs have been effective in reducing re-admission rates (Exercise-based rehabilitation for heart failure [database on the Internet], 2006). Furthermore, even though many of these individuals are debilitated, exercise training has been shown to improve functional ability (Masoudi et al., 2005; Nesto et al., 2004; Pharmacotherapy of hypertension in the elderly [database on the Internet], 2006). Referral to inpatient cardiac rehabilitation is an important stepping-stone to reconditioning patients so they can better function at home when discharged.

Optimization of the medication for HF, coupled with activity progression can enhance the patient's capacity for ADLs and quality of life. An active patient may notice early signs of fluid overload when unable to accomplish standard activities done the previous week. Therefore, questions related to activity tolerance can provide insight for the nurse who monitors the patient. The patient with gradual fluid gain will first notice a change in their level of fatigue, which will translate into a change in their daily routine. Previous experience with fluid overload will also reveal to the nurse the patient's own unique signs and symptoms because not every patient has the same indicators. It is not only important to assess these factors directly with the patient during the interview but to also reinforce that these symptoms are important for the patient to monitor as well (Grady et al., 2000). In addition to changes in weight, deviation from the baseline functional ability is an early clue, even before peripheral edema or lung congestion is present.

The prevention and treatment of HF in patients with DM requires optimal management of co-existent HTN, CHD, and left ventricular dysfunction. Additionally, control of hyperglycemia is an important issue because the presence of HF affects the choice of medications used to treat type 2 DM. Although insulin and insulin secretagogues are considered safe for use in individuals with HF, TZDs are contraindicated, and metformin should be used only cautiously with careful monitoring of renal function (Hope-Ross, Buchanan, Archer, & Allen, 1990). Decreased clearance of metformin in individuals with HF caused by hypoperfusion or renal insufficiency can lead to potentially dangerous lactic acidosis. TZDs are associated with fluid retention, pedal edema, and weight gain, particularly when used in conjunction with insulin, and contribute to HF (Yusuf et al.,

2000). Careful clinical assessment and ongoing monitoring should be implemented in the presence of known structural heart disease or a prior history of HF.

Adequate control of BP is also essential in the management of HF. Treatment of older persons with HTN has been shown to reduce CVD morbidity and mortality (Di Bari et al., 2004). An important nursing consideration is to monitor for adverse effects of medications used to manage HF, as well as HTN, along with patient and caregiver education. ACE inhibitors are important in the management of systolic HF and may also be helpful in diastolic failure. In the Heart Outcomes Prevention Evaluation Study (Wing et al., 2003), ACE inhibitors prevented cardiac events in high-risk patients without HF or known low EFs (Brenner et al., 2001). In addition, ACE inhibitors have a renal protective benefit that is extremely important in preventing the development or worsening of HF, especially in patients with DM. Recent evidence suggests that use of ACE inhibitors is associated with a larger lower extremity muscle mass, which may have benefit in wasting syndromes and prevention of disability (Riegel, Lee, Dickson, & Carlson, 2009) and that they are particularly efficacious in older adults (Bonow et al., 2006). ARBs are also used widely for the prevention and treatment of HF, particularly when patients are unable to use ACE inhibitors because of the development of cough (Bonow et al., 2006). Renal function and hyperkalemia should be assessed when using both classes of agents, especially in the presence of underlying renal dysfunction.

CASE STUDY

CTG is a 72-year-old woman with a history of diet-controlled glucose intolerance and HF with normal renal function. She is seen in the geriatric clinic with a 3-day history of poor appetite, nausea, and occasional vomiting. She complains of a constant feeling of fullness. She was last hospitalized 3 months ago because of fluid overload related to newly diagnosed HF. Her diuretic was increased 6 weeks ago for mild ankle swelling. She denies recent lower extremity swelling, orthopnea, or paroxysmal nocturnal dyspnea. Her blood sugars have been well controlled in the 90–130 range without hypoglycemic episodes. She denies fever, chills, cough, or urinary symptoms. She says she never misses her medications. Up until 5 days ago, she was able to walk 30 minutes a day without difficulty. She had noticed a gradual increase in fatigue over the last 10 days and found herself too tired to attend several social and church events in the evening. When asked what her daily weights have been, she confessed that since she had been feeling so good she had abandoned this as a daily practice. Concerned, however, about her recent symptoms, she weighed herself this morning and found that she had gained 6 pounds since she last weighed herself 2 weeks ago. Although she has been compliant to her medications for HF which include the following:

Coreg 6.25 mg twice a day
Altace 5 mg daily
Aldactone 12.5 mg daily
Lasix 20 mg daily
Imdur 15 mg daily

(continued)

CASE STUDY *(continued)*

She has not taken a double dose of Lasix with the additional weight gain as shown in her self-care action plan. She had been unaware of that weight gain because she had not been weighing herself. In addition, she had attended two social events 2 weekends ago that included eating out. Her self-care action plan had shown that she should increase her diuretic for 1 day following eating out the day before.

On physical examination, her BP is 132/86 with a heart rate of 88 bpm. She is afebrile. She has fine crackles in the lower bases bilaterally. There is 1l edema. Heart sounds demonstrate S1, S2, and S3. Her apical impulse is displaced to the left. There is jugular neck vein distention. Her abdominal girth has increased 2 inches since her last visit.

Lasix was increased to 40mg for a maximum of 3 days. If at any point during the 3 days her weight returned to baseline, she was instructed to return to her usual dose of Lasix. She was advised of the importance of daily weights in order to maintain her baseline weight. She was referred back to her self-care action plan for changes in diuretic depending upon her daily weight and the maintenance of her low-sodium diet in light of her social schedule. She will return to the clinic in 1 week.

Discussion

This patient exemplifies the need for educational reinforcement in a newly diagnosed patient with HF, who is just learning how to incorporate a self-care action plan. Like many patients who have had to take antibiotics in the past, compliance can wane when the patient feels well. Assessment of self care knowledge and ability should be ongoing throughout the hospital stay, but is critical at the time of discharge in order to provide appropriate focus in outpatient care and support. The use of a tool to quantify knowledge and ability of self-care such as the Self-Care in Heart Failure Index is useful to identify patients who have continued needs for assistance after discharge (Riegel, Lee, Dickson, & Carlson, 2009). It is important to make contact with a newly diagnosed patient with HF fairly frequently in order to address questions that might influence the self-care decision making of the patient.

SUMMARY

Hospital admissions can be reduced in older adults with HF

1. When care is spent in identifying the patients' own unique signs and symptoms of fluid overload.
2. By creating monitoring parameters for the nurse in the form of the history and the physical assessment.
3. By creating monitoring parameters for the patient in the form of a self-care algorithm with clear guidelines for self-care action.
4. By achieving goals for clinical stability.

NURSING STANDARD OF PRACTICE

Protocol 31.1: Heart Failure: Early Recognition, and Treatment of the Patient At Risk for Hospital Readmission

I. GOAL: To reduce the incidence of hospital readmission of older adult patients with heart failure (HF).

II. OVERVIEW

A. HF is the most common cause of hospitalization of adults over the age of 65 (Krumholz et al., 1997; Funk & Krumholz, 1996) and is the cause of functional impairment and ultimate morbidity and mortality as well as significant hospital costs (Lloyd-Jones et al., 2010; Thom et al., 2006).

B. Hospitalization can be prevented by identifying the high-risk HF patients, early recognition of sign and symptoms of decompensation, and timely initiation or regulation of medical therapy (Lloyd-Jones et al., 2004; Rich et al., 1995; Ross et al., 2008).

C. Recognition of risk factors and routine monitoring for potential HF decompensation should be part of comprehensive nursing care of older adults (Lloyd-Jones et al., 2004; Rich et al., 1995; Ross et al., 2008).

III. BACKGROUND AND STATEMENT OF PROBLEM

A. Definition

HF is the inability of the heart to pump blood sufficient to metabolic needs of the body or cannot do so without greatly elevated filling pressures (Miller & Pina, 2009). Acute HF can develop swiftly or over the preceding weeks as the primary initial event. Acute decompensated HF is the result of chronic HF (Brucks et al., 2005).

B. Etiology and Epidemiology

1. *Prevalence and incidence:* There are over 5.8 million individuals with HF in the United States and approximately half a million new cases every year (Lloyd-Jones et al., 2010; Thom et al., 2006).

2. *Etiology:* Deficiency in myocardial pump function as a result of nonischemic progressive cardiomyopathy or more prevalent ischemic causes such as coronary heart disease and MI with a resulting development of signs and symptoms such as edema, dyspnea, and orthopnea (Bertoni et al., 2004; Chyun et al., 2002; Lewis et al, 2003).

3. *Risk factors: Predisposing* age (70 years old and older), severity of illness, comorbidities such as HTN, coronary artery disease, diabetes, valvular heart disease, and obesity. Additionally, cognitive impairment, depression, sensory impairment, fluid and electrolyte disturbances, and polypharmacy also impose an increased risk (Ho et al., 1993; Hypertension in Diabetes Study Group, 1993; Levy et al., 1996; Piccini et al., 2004). *Precipitating*: High-sodium diet, excess fluid intake, sleep disordered breathing, chronic kidney disease, anemia, cardiotoxims such as chemotherapeutic agents, NSAIDS, illicit drugs, or alcohol (Schocken et al., 2008). *Environmental factors*: low socioeconomic status, psychological stress (Schocken et al., 2008).

(continued)

**Protocol 31.1: Heart Failure: Early Recognition, and Treatment
of the Patient At Risk for Hospital Readmission *(cont.)***

4. *Outcomes:* HF has a downward trajectory that through preventative measures can be delayed; however, not without considerable impact on quality of life (Grady et al., 2000).

IV. PARAMETERS OF ASSESSMENT

A. Assess at initial encounter and every shift
   1. *Baseline:* Health history NYHA classification of functional status and stage of HF, cognitive and psychosocial support systems (Brucks et al., 2005)
   2. *Symptoms:* dyspnea, orthopnea, cough, edema; Vital signs: BP, HR, RR (Pickering et al., 2005; Pickering et al., 2008; Sansevero, 1997). Physical assessment with signs: rales or "crackles"; peripheral edema, ascites, or pulmonary vascular congestion of chest x-ray (Stevenson & Perloff, 1989)
   3. *Medications review* – Optimal medical regimen according to ACC/AHA/HFSA guideline unless contraindicated (Brenner et al., 2001; Riegel et al., 2009; Wing et al., 2003)
   4. *Electrocardiogram/telemetry review:* Heart rate, rhythm, QRS duration, QT interval (Bertoni et al., 2004; Chyun et al., 2002; Chyun et al., 2003)
   5. Review echocardiography, cardiac angiogram, muga scan, cardiac CT or MRI for left ventricle and valve function: left ventricular ejection fraction (LVEF; Bertoni et al., 2004; Chyun et al., 2002; Lewis et al., 2003)
   6. Laboratory value review (Cygankiewicz et al., 2009; Huang et al., 2007; Hunt et al., 2005)
      Metabolic evaluation: Electrolytes (hyponatremia, hypokalemia), thyroid function, liver function, kidney function
      Hematology: Evaluation for anemia: Hemoglobin, hematocrit, iron, iron-binding capacity, and B12 folic acid
      Evaluation for infection (fever, WBCs with differential, cultures)
   7. *Impaired mobility/deconditioned status:* physical therapy or structured cardiac rehabilitation inpatient or outpatient
B. Sensory impairment—vision, hearing—limitations in ability for self-care (Davos et al., 2003; Faris et al., 2002)
C. Signs and symptoms—assess for changes in mental status every shift (Davos et al., 2003; Faris et al., 2002)

V. NURSING CARE STRATEGIES

A. Obtain HF/cardiology and geriatric consultation (Rich et al., 1995; Naylor, 2006; Naylor & Keating, 2008; Naylor et al., 2004).
B. Eliminate or minimize risk factors
   1. Administer medications according to guidelines and patient assessment (Brenner et al., 2001; Riegel et al., 2009; Wing et al., 2003)
   2. Avoid continuous intravenous infusion especially of saline (Cavallari et al., 2004; Lancaster et al., 2003; Riegel et al., 2009; Taylor et al., 2004).
   3. Maintain euvolemia once fluid overload is treated. Prevent/promptly treat fluid overload, dehydration, and electrolyte disturbances. Maximize oxygen delivery (supplemental oxygen, blood, and BP support as needed (Cavallari, et al., 2004; Lancaster, et al., 2003; Riegel et al., 2009; Taylor, et al., 2004).

(continued)

Protocol 31.1: Heart Failure: Early Recognition, and Treatment of the Patient At Risk for Hospital Readmission *(cont.)*

4. Ensure daily weights accurately charted (Grady et al., 2000; Riegel et al., 2004; Riegel et al., 2009).
5. Provide adequate nutrition with a 2-g sodium diet (see Chapter 22, Nutrition).
6. Provide adequate pain control (see Chapter 14, Pain Management).
7. Use sensory aids as appropriate.
8. Regulate bowel/bladder function.

D. Provide self-care education with maintenance and management strategies (Masoudi et al., 2005; Nesto et al., 2004; Pharmacotherapy for Hypertension in the Elderly, 2006)
   1. Activity recommendation as appropriate to functional status. Assess for safety in ambulation hourly rounds with encouragement to toilet.
   2. Facilitate rest with schedule of diuretic medications for limited nocturia.
   3. Maximize mobility: limit use of urinary catheters.
   4. Communicate clearly; provide explanations.
   5. Emphasize purpose and importance of daily weights.
   6. Dietician referral for educational needs re-sodium.

E. Identify care partners. Reassure and educate
   1. Foster care support of family/friends
   2. Assess willingness and ability of care partner to assist with self-care: dietary needs of sodium restriction, daily weight logging, symptom recognition, and medical follow-up.

VI. EVALUATION/EXPECTED OUTCOMES

A. Patient
   1. Absence of symptoms of congestion
   2. Hemodynamic status remains stable (prior to acute decompensation)
   3. Functional status returned to baseline (prior to acute decompensation)
   4. Improved adherence to medical and self-care regimen
   5. Discharged to same destination as prehospitalization

B. Health Care Provider
   1. Regular use of self-care heart failure index screening tool
   2. Increased detection of symptoms before acute decompensation
   3. Implementation of appropriate interventions to prevent/treat volume overload
   4. Improved nurse awareness of patient/caregiver self-care confidence and ability
   5. Increased management using guideline-directed therapy

C. Institution
   1. Staff education and interprofessional care planning
   2. Implementation of HF specific treatments
   3. Decreased overall cost
   4. Decreased preventable readmission and length of hospital stay
   5. Decreased morbidity and mortality
   6. Increased referrals and consultation to above-specified specialists
   7. Improved satisfaction of patients, families, and nursing staff

(continued)

**Protocol 31.1: Heart Failure: Early Recognition, and Treatment
of the Patient At Risk for Hospital Readmission *(cont.)***

VII. FOLLOW-UP MONITORING OF CONDITION

A. Decreased frequency of readmission as a measure of quality care
B. Incidence of decompensated HF to decrease
C. Patient days with symptoms of congestion to decrease
D. Staff competence in prevention, recognition, and treatment of HF
E. Documentation of a variety of interventions for HF

Na^+ = sodium; BUN/Cr = blood urea nitrogen/creatinine ratio; BP = blood pressure;
HR=heart rate; RR respiratory rate; Hgb/Hct = hemoglobin and hematocrit;
SpO_2 = pulse oxygen saturation; WBCs = white blood cells; URI = upper respiratory infection;
UTI = urinary tract infection; ROM = range of motion

RESOURCES

American Association of Heart Failure Nurses
http://aahfn.org/

Heart Failure Society of America
http://www.hfsa.org

REFERENCES

American Heart Association. (1994). Revisions to classification of functional capacity and objective assessment of patients with disease of the heart. *Circulation, 90,* 644–645.

Anker, S. D., Negassa, A., Coats, A. J., Afzal, R., Poole-Wilson, P. A., Cohn, J. N., & Yusuf, S. (2003). Prognostic importance of weight loss in chronic heart failure and the effect of treatment with angiotension-converting-enzyme inhibitors: An observational study. *Lancet, 361*(9363), 1077–1083. Evidence Level III.

Arzt, M., & Bradley, T. D. (2006). Treatment of sleep apnea in heart failure. *American Journal of Respiratory and Critical Care Medicine, 173*(12), 1300–1308. Evidence Level V.

Arzt, M., Young, T., Finn, L., Skatrud, J. B., Ryan, C. M., Newton, G. E., . . . Bradley, T. D. (2006). Sleepiness and sleep in patients with both systolic heart failure and obstructive sleep apnea. *Archives of Internal Medicine, 166*(16), 1716–1722. Evidence Level III.

Barrella, P., & Della Monica, E. (1998). Managing congestive heart failure at home. *AACN Clinical Issues, 9*(3), 377–388. Evidence Level VI.

Baruch, L., Glazer, R. D., Aknay, N., Vanhaecke, J., Heywood, J. T., Anand, I., . . . Cohn, J. N. (2004). Morbidity, mortality, physiologic and functional parameters in elderly and non-elderly patients in the Valsartan Heart Failure Trial (Val-HeFT). *American Heart Journal, 148*(6), 951–957. Evidence Level I.

Bennett, S. J., & Sauvé, M. J. (2003). Cognitive deficits in patients with heart failure: A review of the literature. *Journal of Cardiovascular Nursing, 18*(3), 219–242. Evidence Level VI.

Bertoni, A. G., Hundley, W. G., Massing, M. W., Bonds, D. E., Burke, G. L., & Goff, D. C., Jr. (2004).Heart failure prevalence, incidence, and mortality in the elderly with diabetes. *Diabetes Care, 27,* 699–703. Level IV.

Bhatia, R. S., Tu, J. V., Lee, D. S., Austin, P. C., Fang, J., Haouzi, A., . . . Liu, P. P. (2006). Outcome of heart failure with preserved ejection fraction in a population-based study. *The New England Journal of Medicine, 355*(3), 260–269. Evidence Level III.

Bonds, D. E., Miller, M. E., Bergenstal, R. M., Buse, J. B., Byington, R. P., Cutler J. A., . . . Sweeney, M. E. (2010). The association between symptomatic, severe hypoglycaemia and mortality in type 2 diabetes: Retrospective epidemiological analysis of the ACCORD study. British Medical Journal, *340*, b4909. doi: 10.1136/bmj.b4909. Evidence Level II.

Bonow, R. O., Carabello, B. A., Chatterjee, K., de Leon, A. C. Jr, Faxon, D. P., Freed, M. D., . . . Riegel, B. (2006). ACC/AHA 2006 guidelines for the management of patients with valvular heart disease. *Circulation, 114*(5), e84–e131. Evidence Level I.

Braunstein, J. B., Anderson, G. F., Gerstenblith, G., Weller, W., Niefeld, M., Herbert, R., & Wu, A. W. (2003). Noncardiac comorbidity increases preventable hospitalizations and mortality among Medicare beneficiaries with chronic heart failure. *Journal of the American* College *of Cardiology, 42*(7), 1226–1233. Evidence Level IV.

Brenner, B. M., Cooper, M. E., de Zeeuw, D., Keane, W. F., Mitch, W. E., Parving, H. H., Shahinfar, S. (2001). Effects of losartan on renal and cardiovascular outcomes in patients with type 2 diabetes and nephropathy. *The New England Journal of Medicine, 345*(12), 861–869. Evidence Level I.

Brucks, S., Little, W. C., Chao, T., Kitzman, D. W., Wesley-Farrington, D., Gandhi, S., & Shihazabi, Z, K. (2005). Contribution of left ventricular diastolic dysfunction to heart failure regardless of ejection fraction. *The American Journal of Cardiology, 95*(5), 603–606. Evidence Level II.

Carmody, M. S., & Anderson, J. R. (2007). BiDil (isosorbide dinitrate and hydralazine): A new fixed-dose combination of two older medications for the treatment of heart failure in black patients. *Cardiology Review, 15*(1), 46–53. Evidence Level I.

Carson, P., Tognoni, G., & Cohn, J. N. (2003). Effect of Valsartan on hospitalization: Results from Val-HeFT. *Journal of Cardiac Failure, 9*(3), 164–171. Evidence Level II.

Cavallari, L. H., Fashingbauer, L. A., Beitelshees, A. L., Groo, V. L., Southworth, M. R., Viana, M. A., . . . Dunlap, S. H. (2004). Racial differences in patients' potassium concentrations during spironolactone therapy for heart failure. *Pharmacotherapy, 24*(6), 750–756. Evidence Level III.

Chobanian, A. V., Bakris, G. L., Black, H. R., Cushman, W. C., Green, L. A., Izzo, J. L., Jr., . . . Rocella, E. J. (2003). The seventh report of the Joint National Committee on Prevention, Detection, Evaluation, and Treatment of High Blood Pressure. *Journal of the American Medical Association, 289*, 1560–1572. Evidence Level VI.

Chriss, P. M., Sheposh, J., Carlson, B., & Riegel, B. (2004). Predictors of successful heart failure self-care maintenance in the first three months after hospitalization. *Heart Lung, 33*(6), 345–353. Evidence level III.

Chyun, D., Vaccarino, V., Murillo, J., Young, L. H., & Krumholz, H. M. (2002). Mortality, heart failure and recurrent myocardial infarction in the elderly with diabetes. *American Journal of Critical Care, 11*, 504–19. Evidence Level II.

Coats, A. J. (2001). Heart failure: What causes the symptoms of heart failure? *Heart, 86*(5), 574–578. Evidence Level V.

Cohn, J. N. (1999). Improving outcomes in congestive heart failure: Val-HeFT. Valsartan in Heart Failure Trial. *Cardiology, 91*(Suppl. 1), 19–22. Evidence Level II.

Cohn, J. N., & Tognoni, G. (2001). A randomized trial of the angiotensin-receptor blocker valsartan in chronic heart failure. *The New England Journal of Medicine, 345*(23), 1667–1675. Evidence Level I.

Colucci, W. S., Kolias, T. J., Adams, K. F., Armstrong, W. F., Ghali, J. K., Gottlieb, S. S., . . . Sugg, J. E. (2007). Metoprolol reverses left ventricular remodeling in patients with asymptomatic systolic dysfunction: The REversal of VEntricular Remodeling with Toprol-XL (REVERT) trial. *Circulation, 116*(1), 49–56. Evidence Level II.

Colucci, W. S., Packer, M., Bristow, M. R., Gilbert, E. M., Cohn, J. N., Fowler, M. B., . . . Lukas, M. A. (1996). Carvedilol inhibits clinical progression in patients with mild symptoms of heart failure. US Carvedilol Heart Failure Study Group. *Circulation, 94*(11), 2800–2806. Evidence Level II.

Cormican, L. J., & Williams, A. (2005). Sleep disordered breathing and its treatment in congestive heart failure. *Heart, 91*(10), 1265–1270. Evidence Level V.

Coviello, J. S. (2004). Cardiac assessment 101: A new look at the guidelines for cardiac homecare patients. *Home Healthcare Nurse, 22*(2),116–123. Evidence Level VI.

Coviello, J. S., Hricz-Borges, L., & Masulli, P. S. (2002). Accomplishing quality of life in end-stage heart failure: A hospice multidisciplinary approach. *Home Healthcare Nurse, 20*(3), 195–198. Evidence Level VI.

Cygankiewicz, I., Gillespie, J., Zareba, W., Brown, M. W., Goldenberg, I., Klein, H., . . . Moss, A. J. (2009). Predictors of long-term mortality in Multicenter Automatic Defibrillator Implantation Trial II (MADIT II) patients with implantable cardioverter-defibrillators. *Heart Rhythm, 6*(4), 468–473. Evidence Level II.

Davos, C. H., Doehner, W., Rauchhaus, M., Cicoira, M., Francis, D. P., Coats, A. J., . . . Anker, S. D. (2003). Body mass and survival in patients with chronic heart failure without cachexia: The importance of obesity. *Journal of Cardiac Failure, 9*(1), 29–35. Evidence Level IV.

Di Bari, M., van de Poll-Franse, L. V., Onder, G., Kritchevsky, S. B., Newman, A., Harris T. B., . . . Pahor, M. (2004). Antihypertensive medications and differences in muscle mass in older persons: The Health, Aging and Body Composition Study. *Journal of the American Geriatrics Society, 52*(6), 961–966. Evidence Level IV

Dickson, V. V., Deatrick, J. A., & Riegel, B. (2008). A typology of heart failure self-care management in non-elders. *European Journal of Cardiovascular Nursing, 7*(3),171–81. Evidence Level IV.

Evangelista, L. S., Doering, L. V., & Dracup, K. (2000). Usefulness of a history of tobacco and alcohol use in predicting multiple heart failure readmissions among veterans. *The American Journal of Cardiology, 86*(12),1339–1342. Evidence Level III.

Exercise-based rehabilitation for heart failure [database on the Internet]2006.QM

Faris, R., Purcell, H., Henein, M. Y., & Coats, A. J. (2002). Clinical depression is common and significantly associated with reduced survival in patients with non-ischaemic heart failure. *European Journal of Heart Failure, 4*(4), 541–551. Evidence Level III.

Funk, M., & Krumholz, H. M. (1996). Epidemiologic and economic impact of advanced heart failure. *Journal of Cardiovascular Nursing, 10*(2), 1–10. Evidence Level V.

Gheorghiade, M., Follath, F., Ponikowski, P., Barsuk, J. H., Blair, J. E., Cleland, J. G., . . . Filippatos, G. (2010). Assessing and grading congestion in acute heart failure: A scientific statement from the acute heart failure committee of the heart failure association of the European Society of Cardiology and endorsed by the European Society of Intensive Care Medicine. *European Journal of Heart Failure, 12*(5), 423–433. Evidence Level VI.

Giamouzis, G., Kalogeropoulos, A., Georgiopoulou, V., Laskar, S., Smith, A. L., Dunbar, S., . . . Butler, J. (2011). Hospitalization epidemic in patients with heart failure: Risk factors, risk prediction, knowledge gaps, and future directions. *Journal of Cardiac Failure, 17*(1), 54–75. Evidence Level V.

Glandt, M., & Raz, I. (2010). Pharmacotherapy: ACCORD blood pressure and ACCORD lipid: How low can we go? *Natural Reviews, Endocrinology, 6*(9), 483–484. Evidence Level II.

Goldstein, S., & Hjalmarson, A.. (1999). The mortality effect of metoprolol CR/XL in patients with heart failure: Results of the MERIT-HF trial. *Clinical Cardiology, 22*(Suppl. 5), 30–5. Evidence Level V.

Gonseth, J., Guallar-Castillón, P., Banegas, J. R., & Rodríguez-Artalejo, F. (2004). The effectiveness of disease managament programmes in reducing hospitla re-admission in older persons with heart failure: A systematic review and meta-analysis of published reports. *European Heart Journal, 25*(18),1570–1595. Evidence Level I.

Grady, K. L., Dracup, K., Kennedy, G., Moser, D. K., Piano, M., Stevenson, L. W., & Young, J. B. (2000). Team management of patients with heart failure: A statement for healthcare professionals from The Cardiovascular Nursing Council of the American Heart Association. *Circulation, 102*(19), 2443–2456 Evidence Level VI

Hay, P., Sachdev, P., Cumming, S., Smith, J. S., Lee, T., Kitchener, P., & Matheson, J. (1993). Treatment of obsessive-compulsive disorder by psychosurgery. *Acta Psychiatrica Scandinavica*, *87*(3), 197–207. Evidence Level III,

Hjalmarson, A., & Fagerberg, B. (2000). MERIT-HF mortality and morbidity data. *Basic Research in Cardiology*, *95*(Suppl. 1), 198–103. Evidence Level V.

Hjalmarson, A., Goldstein, S., Fagerberg, B., Wedel, H., Waagstein, F., Kjekshus, J., . . . Deedwania, P. (2000). Effects of controlled-release metoprolol on total mortality, hospitalizations, and well-being in patients with heart failure: The Metoprolol CR/XL Randomized Intervention Trial in congestive heart failure (MERIT-HF). MERIT-HF study group. *Journal of the American Medical Association*, *283*(10), 1295–1302 . Level I.

Ho, K. K., Pinsky, J. L., Kannel, W. B., & Levy, D. (1993). The epidemiology of heart failure: The Framingham study. *Journal of the American College of Cardiology*, *22*(4 Suppl. A), 6A–13A. Level V.

Hope-Ross, M., Buchanan, T. A., Archer, D. B., & Allen, J. A. (1990). Autonomic function in Holmes Adie syndrome. *Eye (Lond)*, *4*(Pt. 4), 607–612. Evidence Level V.

Horwich, T. B., Fonarow, G. C., Hamilton, M. A., MacLellan, W. R., Woo, M. A., & Tillisch, J. H. (2001). The relationship between obesity and mortality in patients with heart failure. *Journal of the American College of Cardiology*, *38*(3), 789–795. Evidence Level IV.

Huang, D. T., Sesselberg, H. W., McNitt, S., Noyes, K., Andrews, M. L., Hall, W. J., . . . Moss, A. J. (2007). Improved survival associated with prophylactic implantable defibrillators in elderly patients with prior myocardial infarction and depressed ventricular function: A MADIT-II substudy. *Journal of Cardiovascular Electrophysiology*, *18*(8), 833–888. Evidence Level II.

Hunt, S. A., Abraham, W. T., Chin, M. H., Feldman, A. M., Francis, G. S., Ganiats, T. G., . . . Riegel, B. (2005). ACC/AHA 2005 Guideline update for the diagnosis and management of chronic heart failure in the adult. *Circulation*, *112*(12), e154–e235. Evidence Level I.

Hypertension in Diabetes Study Group. (1993). HDS: 1: Prevalence of hypertension in newly presenting type 2 diabetic patients and the association with risk factors for cardiovascular disease and diabetic complications. *Journal of Hypertension*, *11*, 309–17. Evidence Level III.

Kaneko, Y., Hajek, V. E., Zivanovic, V., Raboud, J., & Bradley, T. D. (2003). Relationship of sleep apnea to functional capacity and length of hospitalization following stroke. *Sleep*, *26*(3), 293–297. Evidence Level II.

Kasai, T., Narui, K., Dohi, T., Yanagisawa, N., Ishiwata, S., Ohno, M., . . . Momomura, S. (2008). Prognosis of patients with heart failure and obstructive sleep apnea treated with continuous positive airway pressure. Chest, *133*(3),690–696. Evidence Level II.

Koenig, H. G. (1998). Depression in hospitalized older patients with congestive heart failure. General Hospital Psychiatry, *20*(1), 29–43. Evidence Level III.

Koitabashi, T., Inomata, T., Niwano, S., Nishii, M., Takeuchi, I., Nakano, H., . . Izumi, T. (2005). Paroxysmal atrial fibrillation coincident with cardiac decompensation is a predictor of poor prognosis in chronic heart failure. *Circulation Journal*, *69*(7), 823–830. Evidence Level III.

Kossovsky, M. P., Sarasin, F. P., Perneger, T. V., Chopard, P., Sigaud, P., & Gaspoz, J. (2000). Unplanned readmissions of patients with congestive heart failure: Do they reflect in-hospital quality of care or patient characteristics? *The American Journal of Medicine*, *109*(5), 386–390. Evidence Level III.

Krumholz, H. M., Parent, E. M., Tu, N., Vaccarino, V., Wang, Y., Radford, M. J., & Hennen, J. (1997). Readmission after hospitalization for congestive heart failure amoung Medicare beneficiaries. *Archives of Internal Medicine*, *157*(1), 99–104. Evidence Level IV.

Krumholz, H. M., Wang, Y., Parent, E. M., Mockalis, J., Petrillo, M., & Radford, M. J. (1997). Quality of care for elderly patients hospitalized with heart failure. *Archives of Internal Medicine*, *157*(19), 2242–2247. Evidence Level II.

Lancaster, K. J., Smiciklas-Wright, H., Heller, D. A., Ahern, F. M., & Jensen, G. (2003). Dehydration in black and white older adults using diuretics. *Annals of Epidemiology*, *13*(7), 525–529. Evidence Level IV.

Lanfranchi, P. A., & Somers, V. K. (2003). Sleep-disordered breathing in heart failure: Characteristics and implications. *Respiratory Physiology* & *Neurobiology*, *136*(2–3), 153–165. Evidence Level VI.

Lavie, C. J., Osman, A. F., Milani, R. V., & Mehra, M. R. (2003). Body composition and prognosis in chronic systolic heart failure: The obesity paradox. *American Journal of Cardilology, 91*(7), 891–894. Evidence Level IV.

Lee, S. J., Lindquist, K., Segal, M. R., & Covinsky, K. E. (2006). Development and validation of a prognostic index for 4-year mortality in older adults. *Journal of the American Medical Association, 295*(7), 801–808. Evidence Level III.

Levy, D., Larson, M. G., Vasan, R. S., Kannel, W. B., & Ho, K. K. (1996). The progression from hypertension to congestive heart failure. *Journal of the American Medical Association, 275*(20), 1557–1562. Evidence Level II.

Lewis, E. F., Moye, L. A., Rouleau, J. L., Sacks, F. M., Arnold, J. M., Warnica, J. W., . . . Pfeffer, M. A. (2003). Predictors of late development of heart failure in stable survivors of myocardial infarction: The CARE study. *Journal of the American College of Cardiology, 42*(8), 1446–1453. Evidence Level II.

Lloyd-Jones, D., Adams, R. J., Brown, T. M., Carnethon, M., Dai, S., De Simone . . . American Heart Association Statistics Committee and Stroke Statistics Subcommittee. (2004). Comprehensive discharge planning with post discharge support for older persons with congestive heart failure. *Journal of the American Medical Association, 291*(11),1358–1367. Evidence Level I.

Lloyd-Jones, D., Adams, R. J., Brown, T. M., Carnethon, M., Dai, S., De Simone G., . . . Wylie-Rosett, J. (2010). Heart disease and stroke statistics—2010 update: A report from the American Heart Association. *Circulation, 121*(7), e46–e215. Evidence Level IV.

Maggioni, A. P., Latini, R., Carson, P. E., Singh, S. N., Barlera, S., Glazer, R., . . . Cohn, J. N. (2005). Valsartan reduces the incidence of atrial fibrillation in patients with heart failure: Results from the Valsartan Heart Failure Trial (Val-HeFT). *American Heart Journal, 149*(3), 548–557. Evidence Level II.

Maisel, A. S. (2001a). B-type natriuretic peptide (BNP) levels: Diagnostic and therapeutic potential. *Reviews in Cardiovascular Medicine, 2*(Suppl. 2), S13–S18. Evidence Level VI.

Maisel, A. S. (2001b). B-type natriuretic peptide in the diagnosis and management of congestive heart failure. *Cardiology Clinics, 19*(4), 557–571. Evidence Level VI.

Mansfield, D. R., Solin, P., Roebuck, T., Bergin, P., Kaye, D. M., & Naughton, M. T. (2003). The effect of successful heart transplant treatment of heart failure on central sleep apnea. *Chest, 124*(5),1675–1681. Evidence Level III.

Mascarenhas, J., Lourenço, P., Lopes, R., Azevedo, A., & Bettencourt, P. (2008). Chronic obstructive pulmonary disease in heart failure. Prevalence, therapeutic and prognostic implications. *American Heart Journal, 155*(3), 521–525. Evidence Level IV.

Masoudi, F. A., Inzucchi, S. E., Wang, Y., Havranek, E. P., Foody, J. M., & Krumholz, H. M. (2005). Thiazolidinediones, metformin, and outcomes in older patients with diabetes and heart failure: An observational study. *Circulation, 111*, 583–590. Evidence Level II.

McKelvie, R. S., Teo, K. K., Roberts, R., McCartney, N., Humen, D., Montague, T. . . Yusuf, S. (2002). Effects of exercise training in patients with heart failure: The exercise rehabilitation trial (EXERT). *American Heart Journal, 144*(1), 23–30. Evidence Level II.

Metra, M., Nodari, S., Parrinello, G., Bordonali, T., Bugatti, S., Danesi, R., . . . Dei Cas, L. (2008). Worsening renal function in patients hospitalized for acute heart failure: Clinical implications and prognostic significance. *European Journal of Heart Failure, 10*(2), 188–195. Evidence Level III.

Miller, A. B., & Piña, I. L. (2009). Understanding heart failure with preserved ejection fraction: Clinical importance and future outlook. Congestive Heart Failure, *15*(4), 186–192. Evidence Level V.

Naylor, M., Brooten, D., Jones, R., Lavizzo-Mourey, R., Mezey, M., & Pauly, M. (1994) Comprehensive discharge planning for the hospitalized elderly. A randomized clinical trial. *Annals of Internal Medicine, 120*(12), 999–1006. Evidence Level II.

Naylor, M., & Keating, S. A. (2008). Transitional care. *American Journal of Nursing, 108*(9 Suppl.), 58–63.

Naylor, M. D. (2006). Transitional care: A critical dimension of the home healthcare quality agenda. *Journal for Healthcare Quality, 28*(1), 48–54. Evidence Level VI.

Naylor, M. D., Feldman, P. H., Keating, S., Koren, M. J., Kurtzman, E. T., Maccoy., . . . Krakauer, R. (2009). Translating research into practice: Transitional care for older adults. *Journal of Evaluation in Clinical Practice, 15*(6),1164–1170. Evidence Level VI.

Naylor, C. J., Griffiths, R. D., & Fernandez, R. S. (2004). Does a multidisciplinary total parenteral nutrition team improve patient outcomes? A systematic review. *Journal of Parenteral and Enteral Nutrition, 28*(4), 251–258. Evidence Level I

Nesto, R. W., Bell, D., Bonow, R. O., Fonseca, V., Grundy, S. M., Horton, E. S., . . . Kahn, R. (2004). Thiazolidinedione use, fluid retention, and congestive heart failure: A consensus statement from the American Heart Association and American Diabetes Association. *Diabetes Care, 27*, 256–263. Evidence Level V.

Olsson, L. G., Swedberg, K., Ducharme, A., Granger, C. B., Michelson, E. L., McMurray, J. J., . . . Pfeffer, M. A. (2006). Atrial fibrillation and risk of clinical events in chronic heart failure with and without left ventricular systolic dysfunction: Results from the candesartan in heart failure—Assessment of Reduction in Mortality and Morbidity (CHARM) program. *Journal of the American College of Cardiology, 47*(10), 1997–2004. Evidence Level I.

Ostergren, J. B. (2006). Angiotensin receptor blockade with candesartan in heart failure: Findings from the Candesartan in Heart failure—assessment of reduction in mortality and morbidity (CHARM) programme. *Journal of Hypertension, 24*(1), S3–S7. Evidence Level II.

Owan, T. E., Hodge, D. O., Herges, R. M., Jacobsen, S. J., Roger, V. L., & Redfield, M. M. (2006). Trends in prevalence and outcome of heart failure with preserved ejection fraction. *The New England Journal of Medicine, 355*(3), 251–259. Evidence Level II.

Packer, M. (1998). Beta-blockade in heart failure. Basic concepts and clinical results. *American Journal of Hypertension, 11*(1 Pt 2), 23S–37S. Evidence Level V.

Packer, M., Bristow, M. R., Cohn, J. N., Colucci, W. S., Fowler, M. .B., Gilbert, E. M., & Shusterman, N. H. (1996). The effect of carvedilol on morbidity and mortality in patients with chronic heart failure. U.S. Carvedilol Heart Failure Study Group.. *The New England Journal of Medicine, 334*(21), 1349–1355. Evidence Level I.

Packer, M., Colucci, W. S., Sackner-Bernstein, J. D., Liang, C. S., Goldscher, D. A., Freeman, I., . . . Shusterman, N. H. (1996). Double-blind, placebo-controlled study of the effects of carvedilol in patients with moderate to severe heart failure. The PRECISE trial. Prospective randomized evaluation of carvedilol on symptoms and exercise. *Circulation, 94*(11), 2793–2799. Evidence Level I.

Pharmacotherapy for hypertension in the elderly [database on the Internet]. (2006). Evidence Level V.

Piccini, J. P., Klein, L., Gheorghiade, M., & Bonow, R. O. (2004). New insights into diastolic heart failure: Role of diabetes mellitus. *American Journal of Medicine, 116*(Suppl. 5A), 64S–75S. Evidence Level V.

Pickering, T. G., Hall, J. E., Appel, L. J., Falkner, B. E., Graves, J., Hill, M. N., . . . Roccella, E. J. (2005) Recommendations for blood pressure measurements in humans and experimental animals: Part 1: Blood pressure measurement in humans: A statement for professionals from the Subcommittee of Professional and Public Education of the American Heart Association Council on High Blood Pressure Research. *Circulation, 111*, 697–716. Evidence Level VI.

Pickering, T. G., Miller, N. H., Ogedegbe, G., Krakoff, L. R., Artinian, N. T., & Goff, D. (2008). Call to action on use and reimbursement for home blood pressure monitoring: Executive summary: A joint scientific statement from the American Heart Association, American Society of Hypertension, and Preventive Cardiovascular Nurses Association. *Hypertension, 52*(1), 1–9. Evidence Level VI.

Piepoli, M. F., Davos, C., Francis, D. P., & Coats, A. J. (2004). Exercise training meta-analysis of trials in patients with chronic heart failure (ExTraMATCH). *British Medical Journal, 328*(7433), 189. Evidence Level II

Pocock, S. J., Wang, D., Pfeffer, M. A., Yusuf, S., McMurray, J. J., . . .Granger, C. B. (2006). Predictors of mortality and morbidity in patients with chronic heart failure. *European Heart Journal, 27*(1), 65–75. Evidence Level IV.

Prystowsky, E. N., & Nisam, S. (2000). Prophylactic implantable cardioverter defibrillator trials: MUSTT, MADIT, and beyond. Multicenter Unsustained Tachycardia Trial. Multicenter Automatic Defibrillator Implantation Trial. *American Journal of Cardiology. 86*(11),1214–1215. Evidence Level I.

Rich, M. W., Beckham, V., Wittenberg, C., Leven, C. L., Freedland, K. E., & Carney, R. M. (1995). A multidisciplinary intervention to prevent the readmission of elderly patients with congestive heart failure. *The New England Journal of Medicine, 333*(18), 1190–1195. Evidence Level II.

Rich, M. W., & Kitman, D. W. (2005). Third pivotal research in cardiology in the elderly (PRICE-III) symposium: Heart failure in the elderly: Mechanisms and management. *American Journal of Geriatric Cardiology, 14*(5), 250–261. Evidence Level V.

Rich, M. W., & Nease, R. F. (1999). Cost-effectiveness analysis in clinical practice: The case of heart failure. *Archives of Internal Medicine, 159*(15), 1690–1700. Evidence Level IV.

Riegel, B., Dickson, V. V., Hoke, L., McMahon, J. P., Reis, B. F., & Sayers, S. (2006). A motivational counseling approach to improving heart failure self-care: Mechanisms of effectiveness. *Journal of Cardiovascular Nursing, 21*(3), 232–241. Evidence Level II.

Riegel, B., Lee, C. S., Dickson, V. V., & Carlson, B. (2009). An update on the self-care of heart failure index. *Journal of Cardiovascular Nursing, 24*(6), 485–497. Evidence Level II.

Riegel, B., Moser, D. K., Anker, S. D., Appel, L. J., Dunbar, S. B., Grady, K. L., . . . Whellan, D. J. (2009). State of the science: Promoting self-care in persons with heart failure: A scientific statement from the American Heart Association. *Circulation, 120*(12), 1141–1163. Evidence Level VI.

Riegel, B., Naylor, M., Stewart, S., McMurray, J. J., & Rich, M. W. (2004). Interventions to prevent readmission for congestive heart failure. *Journal of the American Medical Association, 291*(23), 2816.

Ross, J. S., Mulvey, G. K., Stauffer, B., Patolla, V., Bernheim, S. M.., Keenan, P. S., & Krumholz, H. M. (2008). Statistical models and patient predictors of readmission for heart failure: A systematic review. *Archives of Internal Medicine, 168*(13), 1371–1386. Evidence Level I.

Rumsfeld, J. S., Havranek, E., Masoudi, F. A., Peterson, E. D., Jones, P., Tooley, J. F., . . . Spertus, J. A. (2003). Depressive symptoms are the strongest predictors of short-term declines in health status in patients with heart failure. *Journal of the American College of Cardiology, 42*(10), 1811–1817. Evidence Level III.

Sansevero, A. C. (1997). Dehydration in the elderly: Strategies for prevention and management. *Nurse Practitioner, 22*(4), 41–42, 51–67, 63–66. Evidence Level VI.

Schocken, D. D., Benjamin, E. J., Fonarow, G. C., Krumholz, H. M., Levy, D., Mensah, G. A., . . . Hong, Y. (2008). Prevention of heart failure: A scientific statement from the American Heart Association Councils on Epidemiology and Prevention, Clinical Cardiology, Cardiovascular Nursing, and High Blood Pressure Research; Quality of Care and Outcomes Research Interdisciplinary Working Group; and Functional Genomics and Translational Biology Interdisciplinary Working Group. Circulation, *117*(19), 2544–2565. Evidence Level VI.

Shah, R. V., Desai, A. S., & Givertz, M. M. (2010). The effect of renin-angiotensin system inhibitors on mortality and heart failure hospitalization in patients with heart failure and preserved ejection fraction: A systematic review and meta-analysis. *Journal of Cardiac Failure, 16*(3), 260–267. Evidence Level I.

Stefenelli, T., Bergler-Klein, J., Globits, S., Pacher, R., & Glogar, D. (1992). Heart rate behavior at different stages of congestive heart failure. *European Heart Journal, 13*(7), 902–907. Evidence Level III.

Stevenson, L. W., & Perloff, J. K. (1989). The limited reliability of physical signs for estimating hemodynamics in chronic heart failure. *Journal of the American Medical Association, 261*(6), 884–888. Evidence Level II.

Taylor, A. L., Ziesche, S., Yancy, C., Carson, P., D'Agostino, R., Jr, Ferdinand, K., . . . Cohn, J. N. (2004). Combination of isosorbide dinitrate and hydralazine in blacks with heart failure. *The New England Journal of Medicine, 351*, 2049–2057. Evidence Level II.

Thom, T., Haase, N., Rosamond, W., Howard, V. J., Rumsfeld, J., Manolio, T., . . . Wolf, P. (2006). Heart disease and stroke statistics—2006 update: A report from the American Heart Association Statistics Committee and Stroke Statistics Subcommittee. *Circulation, 113*(6), e85–e151. Available from http://circ.ahajournals.org. Evidence Level IV.

Triposkiadis, F., Karayannis, G., Giamouzis, G., Skoularigis, J., Louridas, G., & Butler, J. (2009). The sympathetic nervous system in the heart failure physiology, pathophysiology, and clinical implications. *Journal of the American College of Cardiology, 54*(19),1747–1762. Evidence Level I.

Wang, C. S., FitzGerald, J. M., Schulzer, M., Mak, E., & Ayas, N. T. (2005). Does this dyspneic patient in the emergency department have congestive heart failure? *Journal of the American Medical Association, 294*(15), 1944–1956. Evidence Level V.

Wing, L. M., Reid, C. M., Ryan, P., Beilin, L. J., Brown, M. A., Jennings, G. L., . . . West, M. J. (2003). A comparison of outcomes with angiotensin-converting—enzyme inhibitors and diuretics for hypertension in the elderly. *The New England Journal of Medicine, 348*(7), 583–592. Evidence Level II.

Yancy, C. W., Lopatin, M., Stevenson, L. W., De Marco, T., & Fonarow, G. C. (2006). Clinical presentation, management, and in-hospital outcomes of patients admitted with acute decompensated heart failure with preserved systolic function: A report from the Acute Decompensated Heart Failure National Registry (ADHERE) database. *Journal of the American College of Cardiology, 47*(1), 76–84. Evidence Level I.

Young, J. B., Abraham, W. T., Albert, N. M., Gattis Stough, W., Gheorghiade, M., Greenberg, B. H., . . . Fonarow, G. C. (2008). Relation of low hemoglobin and anemia to morbidity and mortality in patients hospitalized with heart failure (insight from the OPTIMIZE-HF registry). *The American Journal of Cardiology, 101*(2),223–230. Evidence Level II.

Yusuf, S., Sleight P., Pogue, J., Bosch, J., Davies, R., & Dagenais, G. (2000). Effects of an angiotensin-converting enzyme inhibitor, ramipril, on cardiovascular events in high-risk patients. The Heart Outcomes Prevention Evaluation Study Investigators. *The New England Journal of Medicine, 342*,145–153. Evidence Level I.

Cancer Assessment and Intervention Strategies

32

Janine Overcash

EDUCATIONAL OBJECTIVES

On completion of this chapter, the reader should be able to:

1. recognize the incidence and prevalence of U.S. statistics on malignancy in the older adult
2. identify three common malignancies in the older adult
3. recognize three common comorbidities in the older adult with cancer
4. identify three common cancer-related emergencies in the older adult
5. identify three assessment instruments useful in the assessment of the older person
6. identify three important elements of a health history specific to the older patient with cancer
7. identify three important elements of a physical examination specific to the older patient with cancer
8. define clinical parameters of frailty of an older adult with cancer

OVERVIEW

The probability of developing a malignancy increases with age. In the years between 1975 and 2007, the National Cancer Institute (NCI) Surveillance, Epidemiology, and End Results (SEER) Program found that the mean age of a cancer diagnosis is 66 years old (NCI, 2010). According to the Centers for Disease Control and Prevention (CDC), the number of people aged 65 years and older are expected to increase from 12.4% in 2000 to 19.6% in 2030 (National Center for Health Statistics, 2006). Older people diagnosed with cancer are often resilient; however, they are also faced with issues associated with diminished identity, suffering, and social isolation (Hughes, Closs, & Clark, 2009) especially when hospitalized. Acute care nurses must appreciate that cancer is common in older adult patients and be aware of potential health limitations and emergencies associated with the diagnosis and treatment of malignancy.

For description of Evidence Levels cited in this chapter, see Chapter 1, Developing and Evaluating Clinical Practice Guidelines: A Systematic Approach, page 7.

This chapter will present assessment strategies and instruments that can be used in an acute care setting and detail potential medical emergencies associated with cancer disease process and treatment.

ASSESSMENT OF THE OLDER HOSPITALIZED PATIENT
Comorbid Conditions

A diagnosis of cancer may be only one of several comorbidities and it is important to understand how the malignant and nonmalignant conditions affect the older adult's health. An acute health crisis may be the result of the culmination of several comorbidities interacting with the cancer diagnosis and treatment (Reiner & Lacasse, 2006). Older adults with cancer, those with multiple comorbidities (Koroukian, 2009), and those who are hospitalized more than 120 days are likely to die in the hospital (Kozyrskyi, Black, Chateau, & Steinbach, 2005). Additionally, the timing of diagnosis of comorbid conditions between 6 and 18 months prior to a diagnosis of cancer have been associated with lower survival (Shack, Rachet, Williams, Northover, & Coleman, 2010). The more severe the comorbidity, the less opportunity of survival at 1 year and 5 years after a diagnosis of cancer (Iversen, Nørgaard, Jacobsen, Laurberg, & Sørensen, 2009). For patients who are diagnosed with the comorbid condition of diabetes, there is a twofold risk of recurrence or development of a new breast cancer as compared to people who do not have diabetes (Patterson et al., 2010). Existence, management, and severity of comorbid conditions are a principle aspect of the acute nursing assessment. Unmanaged or uncontrolled comorbid conditions have the potential to modify cancer treatment plans and outcomes.

Comprehensive Geriatric Assessment

The comprehensive geriatric assessment (CGA) can predict completion of chemotherapy and pending mortality in older patients diagnosed with cancer (Aaldriks et al., 2010). The CGA is a 2-year prognostic predictor of mortality (Pilotto et al., 2007) in gastrointestinal patients and has been used to determine the comorbid condition severity and extent of geriatric conditions (Koroukian, 2009). The American Geriatrics Society (2008) recommendations suggests that CGA is an important component of care for older persons who have or are at risk for functional limitations. Older patients receiving acute care can benefit from the CGA by revealing health concerns and creating a baseline for care management strategies (Mion, Odegard, Resnick, & Segal-Galan, 2006).

CGA used in oncology has been found to influence cancer treatment decisions in terms of dosing, delaying treatment, and other health considerations (Chaibi et al., 2010). No one definition of a CGA exists. A CGA can be developed to include screening instruments necessary to meet the needs of a particular older patient population (Panel on Prevention of Falls in Older Persons, American Geriatrics Society, & British Geriatrics Society, 2011). The instruments that commonly make up the CGA and that guide screening practices in many health care domains are all found on http://www.consultgerirn.org and other chapters in this text. Whereas a CGA may be relevant to primary care settings, understanding such issues as medication history and polypharmacy, caregiver situation, and emotional condition are also important to an acute assessment.

A CGA can include various laboratory tests as well, in addition to self-report and performance evaluations. Laboratory data such as C-reactive protein can predict morbidity or mortality and help identify individual risk factors (Chundadze et al., 2010; Pal, Katheria, & Hurria, 2010). Serum 25(OH)D will assess vitamin D levels to determine if falls or muscle weakness can be a risk factor (Dhesi et al., 2004). Serum albumin levels at 3.3 mg/dl at admission, serum creatinine levels at 1.3 mg/dl or higher, history of heart failure, immobility, and advanced age are all predictors of inpatient mortality (Silva, Jerussalmy, Farfel, Curiati, & Jacob-Filho, 2009). Other mortality risk factors in older hospitalized patients are red blood cell and platelet transfusions that increase the opportunity for venous and arterial thrombotic events (Khorana et al., 2008). Another predictor of inpatient mortality while hospitalized is being uninsured or underinsured (Allareddy & Konety, 2006). It is important to consider inpatient risk factors for mortality and conduct assessments to anticipate potential problems before they become a crisis.

Assessment for the existence of a caregiver that will be available in the home following discharge is another important element of the CGA. For many older patients with cancer, lack of a caregiver can be a problem and can impact health and medical treatment. Older patients who are married tend to take advantage of preventative health care services compared to those older persons who live with an adult child who often do not receive preventative health services (Lau & Kirby, 2009).

Assessment of the older patient should occur upon admission to the hospital and prior to discharge to understand trends in health and functional and behavioral ability. Discharge planning should include interventions based on the CGA findings and communication is vital with outpatient providers to continue to address the limitations that may affect the health, quality of life, and independence of the older person with cancer.

Developing a Comprehensive Geriatric Assessment for Hospitalized Patients

The following are instruments that can identify functional, physical, emotional, medication history, and cognitive impairment in the acute care patient and are generally included in a CGA (see related chapters):

A. Assess for emotional distress
 1. The Geriatric Depression Scale (GDS; Yesavage et al., 1982–1983)
 2. The SF-12 Tool (Ware, Kosinski, & Keller, 1996). The SF-12 is a general health-related quality-of-life instrument that is widely used in research and clinical assessment. Two summary scores are the culmination of the measures from the mental health aspect and the physical health domain. The SF-12 is simple to administer and provides the clinician with a measure of emotional and physical health.
B. Assessment for cognitive limitations
 1. The Mini-Cog test is used in the assessment of cognition (Borson, Scanlan, Brush, Vitaliano, & Dokmak, 2000; Borson, Scanlan, Chen, & Ganguli, 2003). The instrument is comprised of the clock drawing test and recall.
 2. Assess the number and indications of medications. Look for medications with the same indications and potential harmful interactions and consider any difficulty with cancer treatment agents. For more information on polypharmacy screening, visit http://www.consultgerirn.org and select "Try This: Beers' Criteria for Potentially Inappropriate Medication Use in the Elderly."

C. Assess for geriatric syndromes such as urinary incontinence, falls, or depression (for more information, visit http://www.consultgerirn.org/resources and select "Try This: Urinary Incontinence Assessment in Older Adults," "Fall Risk Assessment," or "The Geriatric Depression Scale").

D. Assess functional status and potential for falls

1. Ask the patient if a fall had been experienced within the last year.

   a. The physical performance test battery (Simmonds, 2002) has age-related norms and is a valid and reliable tool used with patients with cancer.

   b. The 6-minute walk that assesses the speed and ability to ambulate for the entire time (Enright et al., 2003).

   c. The Timed Up and Go test help considers rising from a chair, walking 3 m, and returning to the chair in a sitting position (Podsiadlo & Richardson, 1991).

   d. Assessment of physical status can take place on observation of gait (Tinetti, 1986) using the Gait Assessment Scale (Tinetti, Mendes de Leon, Doucette, & Baker, 1994).

   e. Berg Balance Scale (BBS) is a 14-item scale developed for use in a clinical setting (Berg, Wood-Dauphinee, Williams, & Maki, 1992). The BBS can be helpful in predicting falls and functional status problems.

E. Assess the ability to perform self-care activities

1. Activities of Daily Living (ADL) Scale (Katz, Downs, Cash, & Grotz, 1970)

2. Instrumental Activities of Daily Living (IADL) Scale (Lawton & Brody, 1969)

Health History

The subjective information obtained from the older adult is a critical factor in the development of the plan of care. Respect and confidence are not only prudent but standard practice for the acute care nurse and can set the stage for a productive health-centered dialogue. The nurse should assess the reason(s) for seeking care (chief complaint) and include the family and support person(s). The following are issues that should be considered when conducting a health history of the older adult with cancer:

A. Assess history of present illness regarding cancer diagnosis, cancer stage at diagnosis, cancer stage currently, and cancer treatment (surgical, chemotherapy, radiation therapy, hormonal therapy).

B. Assess past medical history as related to a diagnosis of cancer (include dates of diagnosis and treatments and regular oncological assessment continue).

C. Assess family medical history of malignancy and ages on diagnosis (some families have strong familial histories of malignancy and perhaps younger generations should consider genetic counseling).

D. Assess regular cancer screening examinations.

E. Assess for common geriatric syndromes (issues such as incontinence or falls that have many motivating factors).

Physical Examination

Conducting a physical examination of an older adult must orchestrate an understanding of normative aging changes and knowledge of pathology likely for an older adult. The physical examination is also an opportunity to teach about the importance of self-examination (breast and skin exams) and provide relevant health information. When older adults perceive the physical examination as informative and understandable, they are more likely to be more satisfied with their health care encounter (Foxall, Barron, & Houfek, 2003).

Physical examination provides objective information to the nurse that is synergistic to self report measures. Self-report measures are instruments such as the IADL assessment (Lawton & Brody, 1969) and ADL (Katz et al., 1970) that focus on tasks vital to independent living. It has been shown that self-report instruments tend to overestimate abilities (Kuriansky, Gurland, & Fleiss, 1976; Naeim & Reuben, 2001), and objective assessments such as observing gait or balance may produce more realistic data.

Functional status, and not chronological age, is an important indicator of cancer treatment tolerance (Balducci & Yates, 2000; Garman & Cohen, 2002). Changes in functional status may help determine cancer treatment tolerance or disease progression (Chen et al., 2003; Given, Given, Azzouz, & Stommel, 2001; Reiner & Lacasse, 2006). Assessment of physical function and recognition of patients with physical deficiency can also identify those patients who have an increased risk of hospitalization (Wyrwich & Wolinsky, 2000). It is important to conduct a functional assessment at regular intervals while the patient is receiving acute care to look at trends throughout the cancer treatment process. Patients may show functional compromise during periods following cancer therapy and become more functionally apt when not receiving treatment.

Physical examination and functional status assessment can help reveal a clinical presentation of frailty. Fried et al. (2001) suggests that *frail* can, in part, be defined as follows:

1. Older than age 85
2. Dependent in one or more ADLs
3. The presence of one or more geriatric syndromes

Older adults who are considered frail are more likely to receive palliative cancer treatment as compared to those not considered frail and receive curative therapy (Balducci & Yates, 2000).

A complete head-to-toe assessment including the general elements of subjective and objective physical exam, accompanied with the CGA assessment instruments and performance evaluations, provide the infrastructure to develop a reasonable treatment plan. Assessment of the older adult with cancer is a vital, dynamic component of care for the interdisciplinary health care team.

MEDICAL EMERGENCIES ASSOCIATED WITH CANCER AND CANCER TREATMENT

A diagnosis of cancer can lead to medical emergencies such as electrolyte imbalances, unstable fractures, and neutropenia leading to infection. It is important to obtain cancer-related history and physical information concerning the type of treatment and the exact diagnosis with metastasis (spread of the malignancy from the original site). It is also important for the acute care nurse to know the cycle of chemotherapy administration for a particular patient. Often, chemotherapy such as doxorubicin and cyclophamide are given four times, 3 weeks apart. As the chemotherapy proceeds, various issues such as nausea and vomiting, low white cell counts (neutropenia), and mouth sores may occur and be present upon acute evaluation. The following are considered oncological emergencies and require acute care.

Hypercalcemia

Hypercalcemia is a reasonably common complication associated with multiple myeloma, breast, and lung cancers. The most common cause of hypercalcemia is malignancy (Fisken, Heath, Somers, & Bold, 1981) and generally found in 3%–5% of emergency admission patients (Lee et al., 2006). Nonmalignant causes are hyperparathyroidism and renal failure. When hyperthyroidism is associated with hyperparathyroidism and malignancy, survival is much greater as compared to hypercalcemia caused by malignancy alone (Hutchesson, Bundred, & Ratcliffe, 1995). It is important to measure parathyroid hormone in patients with hypercalcemia in order to predict time of survival (Hutchesson et al., 1995).

Hypercalcemia is defined as calcium concentration of more than 10.2 mg/dl (Lee et al., 2006). Signs and symptoms of hypercalcemia are often not evident in patients with mild or moderate hypercalcemia (calcium levels of 10.3–14.0 mg/dl). Gastrointestinal discomfort, changes in level of consciousness, and general nonspecific discomfort can be experienced in cases of moderate hypercalcemia. Other signs and symptoms are lethargy, confusion, anorexia, nausea, constipation, polyuria, and polydipsia (Halfdanarson, Hogan, & Moynihan, 2006).

Treatment of hypercalcemia depends on the severity. Thiazide diuretics should be discontinued. Hydration must be maintained to diminish risk of exacerbation of hypercalcemia. Severe hypercalcemia should be considered a medical emergency. Intravenous normal saline and loop diuretics should be implemented but will only last as long as the treatments are infusing. Bisphosphonates can help reduce bone reabsorption resulting in reduced serum calcium levels (Budayr et al., 1989). Calcitonin also can be administered subcutaneous or intramuscularly and can also reduce calcium levels (Halfdanarson et al., 2006).

Tumor Lysis Syndrome

Tumor lysis syndrome (TLS) is caused when a tumor breaks down and intercellular ions, nucleic acids, proteins and their metabolites release into the extracellular space (Del Toro, Morris, & Cairo, 2005). The syndrome develops when chemotherapy or radiation therapy causes hyperkalemia, hyperuricemia, and hyperphosphatemia, which can enhance the risk for renal failure and reduced cardiac function (Cantril & Haylock, 2004). As chemotherapy agents become more effective, the risks increase for TLS. Agents including cisplatin, etoposide, flurarabine, intrathecal methotrexate, paclitaxel, rituximab, radiation therapy, interferon alpha, corticosteroids and tamoxifen can cause TLS (Davidson et al., 2004; Lin, Lucas, & Byrd, 2003).

Hyperphosphatemia and hypocalcemia can occur about 24–48 hours following the first chemotherapy administration. Signs and symptoms such as muscle cramps, anxiety, depression, confusion, hallucinations, cardiac arrhythmia, and seizures can result (Cantril & Haylock, 2004). Untreated TLS can lead to renal failure (Davidson et al., 2004).

Hyperkalemia is created by a release of potassium from the debilitation of the tumor cells. High serum potassium levels can cause severe arrhythmias and sudden death (Cairo & Bishop, 2004).

Hyperuricemia (uric acid more than 10 mg/dl) can result in acute obstruction uropathy and cause hematuria, flank pain, hypertension, edema, lethargy, and restlessness (Cairo & Bishop, 2004; Cantril & Haylock, 2004). Hydration, administration of allopurinol, and diuresis are generally the first-line treatment (Cantril & Haylock, 2004). Treatment with rasburicase has been found to be effective in the treatment and prevention of hyperuricemia and TLS (Annemans et al., 2003).

The signs and symptoms associated with TLS include decreased urine output, seizures, and arrhythmias. Electrolytes must be assessed to determine presence of hyperkalemia, hyperuricemia, and hyperphosphatemia. Electrocardiograms should be obtained to assess arrhythmia.

Spinal Cord Compression

Spinal cord compression is not uncommon and can occur when metastasis spreads to the vertebral bodies and invades the spinal cord. The area of the spinal column in the thoracic area is the most common location and must be recognized immediately to prevent critical, irreversible damage (Halfdanarson et al., 2006). Spinal cord compression can lead to paraplegia and long-term neurological deficits (Hirschfeld, Beutler, Seigle, & Manz, 1988).

Signs and symptoms are numbness and tingling in the extremities, upper thorax, and back pain (Lowey, 2006). Pain can radiate or localize and may seem chronic, which may disguise the emergent spinal cord compression and delay critical treatment. Bowel and bladder dysfunction can also result.

Diagnosis is often made with magnetic resonance imaging (MRI) and computed tomography (CT) and sometimes plain radiographic films of the affected area. Treatment is often initiated with glucocorticoids followed by either radiation therapy and/or surgery. Surgery has been debated but many agree that it is reasonable in conjunction with radiation therapy and sometimes chemotherapy (McLain & Bell, 1998; Schmidt, Klimo, & Vrionis, 2005). Nurses have the ability to recognize the signs and symptoms of this debilitating and often lethal oncological emergency (Bucholtz, 1999).

Neutropenic Fever

Neutropenic fever is an oncological medical emergency that is caused by the diminishment of neutrophils by various chemotherapeutic agents. Neutropenia is considered present when the neutrophil count is less than 1.0×10^9/L and severe neutropenia is neutrophil counts less than 0.5×10^9/L (Halfdanarson et al., 2006).

Generally, fever is the presenting sign; however, skin rashes and mucositis may also be present. For some patients, neutropenic fever can occur after the first cycle of chemotherapy and patients who have undergone aggressive surgery with bowel resections are at enhanced risk (Sharma, Rezai, Driscoll, Odunsi, & Lele, 2006).

An instrument has been developed to help screen for the likelihood of neutropenia and the identification of patients who are likely to benefit from prophylaxis granulocyte colony-stimulating factors (G-CSFs; Donohue, 2006). G-CSF works to elevate white blood cell counts necessary in fighting infection. A great amount of nursing literature exists on the definition, prevention, and management of neutropenic fever. Prevention of neutropenia and neutropenic fever should be proactive in the administration of G-CSFs in patients who are considered at high risk for neutropenia (Krol et al., 2006). An older cancer patient receiving myelotoxic chemotherapy (cyclophosphamide, doxorubicin, vincristine, and prednisolone) is considered high risk and should receive prophylactic G-CSF administration (Repetto et al., 2003).

CASE STUDY

A 76-year-old White woman presents to the emergency department with delirium and trauma to her left hip. The patient's daughter reports that the patient fell in the bathroom several hours earlier. She has a diagnosis of breast cancer and is currently undergoing chemotherapy and has received four cycles of Adriamycin and cyclophosphamide. She also has a history of osteoarthritis, hypertension, and gastric reflux disease. Presenting signs and symptoms are delirium, cracked mucus membranes, low blood pressure (BP) at 88/42, and tachycardia.

Situations such as dehydration are not uncommon in an older person undergoing chemotherapy. Patients may have vomiting or diarrhea and become dehydrated as a result. Seniors have less functional reserve and are, therefore, more likely to suffer from complications of cancer treatment (Balducci, 2006). Older adults require careful examination and intervention in order to maintain and enhance health and independence.

1. In this clinical scenario, which geriatric syndromes are present?
   Answer: Falls, delirium, pain associated with trauma, functional status limitations, and ambulatory difficulty
   Rationale: This patient has multiple geriatric syndromes and is at risk for further deconditioning. It is important to recognize the geriatric syndromes present and anticipate any additional injuries. Ensure caregiver support and help facilitate a plan for care while at home.
2. In this clinical scenario, which oncological emergency is this patient at greatest risk to develop?
   Rationale: Based on the signs and symptoms of dehydration, hypercalcemia is of concern. Hydrate to prevent hypercalcemia and to reduce signs and symptoms of dementia. Falls are also of concern because the risk of future falls is associated with prior falls. Dehydration in an older adult patient with cancer can be associated with many problematic health and functional limitations.

SUMMARY

Acute care of the older patient requires nurses' health assessment skills to be proactive in detecting and addressing limitations that can result from a cancer diagnosis and treatment. Nonmalignant comorbidities and geriatric syndromes play a role in the diagnosis and treatment of cancer and should be assimilated into the critical thinking involved in developing the nursing plan of care. Careful health assessment and evaluation are critical to the acute care nurse in understanding the disease progress, treatment tolerance, and the presence of oncological emergencies. Nurses working in acute settings must be acquainted with principles of geriatric care that should be applied to patients with any type of diagnosis and not limited to malignancy. Understanding normative aging changes versus pathology can help facilitate a specialized plan of care with enhanced health and independence as the intended patient outcomes.

RESOURCES

The National Comprehensive Cancer Network offers clinical practice guidelines, including senior adult oncology.
http://www.nccn.org/professionals/physician_gls/default.asp

The American Geriatric Society offers clinical guidelines in using the CGA in the older person.
http://www.americangeriatrics.org

The Oncology Nursing Society offers recommendations for practice of the oncology patient.
http://www.ons.org

REFERENCES

Aaldriks, A. A., Maartense, E., le Cessie, S., Giltay, E. J., Verlaan, H. A., van der Geest, L. G., . . . Nortier, J. W. (2010). Predictive value of geriatric assessment for patients older than 70 years, treated with chemotherapy. *Critical Reviews in Oncology/Hematology*. Evidence Level I.

Allareddy, V., & Konety, B. R. (2006). Characteristics of patients and predictors of in-hospital mortality after hospitalization for head and neck cancers. *Cancer*, *106*(11), 2382–2388. Evidence Level IV.

American Gericatrics Society. (2008). Comprehensive geriatric assessment position statement. Retrieved from Annals of Long Term Care website: http://www.annalsoflongtermcare.com/article/5473

Annemans, L., Moeremans, K., Lamotte, M., Garcia Conde, J., van den Berg, H., Myint, H., . . . Uyttebroeck, A. (2003). Pan-European multicentre economic evaluation of recombinant urate oxidase (rasburicase) in prevention and treatment of hyperuricaemia and tumour lysis syndrome in haematological cancer patients. *Supportive Care in Cancer*, *11*(4), 249–257. Evidence Level I.

Balducci, L. (2006). Management of cancer in the elderly. *Oncology (Williston Park, NY)*, *20*(2), 135–143; discussion 144, 146, 151–152. Evidence Level V.

Balducci, L., & Yates, J. (2000). General guidelines for the management of older patients with cancer. *Oncology (Williston Park, NY)*, *14*(11A), 221–227. Evidence Level V.

Berg, K. O., Wood-Dauphinee, S. L., Williams, J. I., & Maki, B. (1992). Measuring balance in the elderly: Validation of an instrument. *Canadian Journal of Public Health*, *83*(Suppl. 2), S7–S11. Evidence Level V.

Borson, S., Scanlan, J., Brush, M., Vitaliano, P., & Dokmak, A. (2000). The mini-cog: A cognitive "vital signs" measure for dementia screening in multi-lingual elderly. *International Journal of Geriatric Psychiatry*, *15*(11), 1021–1027. Evidence Level IV.

Borson, S., Scanlan, J. M., Chen, P., & Ganguli, M. (2003). The Mini-Cog as a screen for dementia: Validation in a population-based sample. *Journal of the American Geriatrics Society*, *51*(10), 1451–1454. Evidence Level IV.

Bucholtz, J. D. (1999). Metastatic epidural spinal cord compression. *Seminars in Oncology Nursing*, *15*(3), 150–159. Evidence Level II.

Budayr, A. A., Nissenson, R. A., Klein, R. F., Pun, K. K., Clark, O. H., Diep, D., . . . Strewler, G. J. (1989). Increased serum levels of a parathyroid hormone-like protein in malignancy-associated hypercalcemia. *Annals of Internal Medicine*, *111*(10), 807–812. Evidence Level I.

Cairo, M. S., & Bishop, M. (2004). Tumour lysis syndrome: New therapeutic strategies and classification. *British Journal of Haematology*, *127*(1), 3–11. Evidence Level V.

Cantril, C. A., & Haylock, P. J. (2004). Emergency. Tumor lysis syndrome. *The American Journal of Nursing*, *104*(4), 49–52. Evidence Level V.

Chaïbi, P., Magné, N., Breton, S., Chebib, A., Watson, S., Duron, J. J., . . . Spano, J. P. (2010). Influence of geriatric consultation with comprehensive geriatric assessment on final therapeutic decision in elderly cancer patients. *Critical Reviews in Oncology/Hematology*. Evidence Level VI.

Chen, H., Cantor, A., Meyer, J., Beth Corcoran, M., Grendys, E., Cavanaugh, D., . . . Extermann, M. (2003). Can older cancer patients tolerate chemotherapy? A prospective pilot study. *Cancer, 97*(4), 1107–1114. Evidence Level IV.

Chundadze, T., Steinvil, A., Finn, T., Saranga, H., Guzner-Gur, H., Berliner, S., . . . Paran, Y. (2010). Significantly elevated C-reactive protein serum levels are associated with very high 30-day mortality rates in hospitalized medical patients. *Clinical Biochemistry, 43*(13–14), 1060–1063. Evidence Level III.

Davidson, M. B., Thakkar, S., Hix, J. K., Bhandarkar, N. D., Wong, A., & Schreiber, M. J. (2004). Pathophysiology, clinical consequences, and treatment of tumor lysis syndrome. *The American Journal of Medicine, 116*(8), 546–554. Evidence Level V.

Del Toro, G., Morris, E., & Cairo, M. S. (2005). Tumor lysis syndrome: Pathophysiology, definition, and alternative treatment approaches. *Clinical Advances in Hematology & Oncology, 3*(1), 54–6. Evidence Level IV.

Dhesi, J. K., Jackson, S. H., Bearne, L. M., Moniz, C., Hurley, M. V., Swift, C. G., & Allain, T. J. (2004). Vitamin D supplementation improves neuromuscular function in older people who fall. *Age and Ageing, 33*(6), 589–595. Evidence Level III.

Donohue, R. (2006). Development and implementation of a risk assessment tool for chemotherapy-induced neutropenia. *Oncology Nursing Forum, 33*(2), 347–352. Evidence Level III.

Enright, P. L., McBurnie, M. A., Bittner, V., Tracy, R. P., McNamara, R., Arnold, A., . . . Cardiovascular Health Study. (2003). The 6-min walk test: A quick measure of functional status in elderly adults. *Chest, 123*(2), 387–398. Evidence Level II.

Fisken, R. A., Heath, D. A., Somers, S., & Bold, A. M. (1981). Hypercalcaemia in hospital patients. Clinical and diagnostic aspects. *Lancet, 1*(8213), 202–207. Evidence Level IV.

Foxall, M. J., Barron, C. R., & Houfek, J. (2003). Women's satisfaction with breast and gynecological cancer screening. *Women & Health, 38*(1), 21–36. Evidence Level IV.

Fried, L. P., Tangen, C. M., Walston, J., Newman, A. B., Hirsch, C., Gottdiener, J., . . . Cardiovascular Health Study Collaborative Research Group. (2001). Frailty in older adults: Evidence for a phenotype. *The Journals of Gerontology. Series A, Biological Sciences and Medical Sciences, 56*(3), M146–M156. Evidence Level II.

Garman, K. S., & Cohen, H. J. (2002). Functional status and the elderly cancer patient. *Critical Reviews in Oncology/Hematology, 43*(3), 191–208. Evidence Level III.

Given, B., Given, C., Azzouz, F., & Stommel, M. (2001). Physical functioning of elderly cancer patients prior to diagnosis and following initial treatment. *Nursing Research, 50*(4), 222–232. Evidence Level II.

Halfdanarson, T. R., Hogan, W. J., & Moynihan, T. J. (2006). Oncologic emergencies: Diagnosis and treatment. *Mayo Clinic Proceedings. Mayo Clinic, 81*(6), 835–848. Evidence Level II

Hirschfeld, A., Beutler, W., Seigle, J., & Manz, H. (1988). Spinal epidural compression secondary to osteoblastic metastatic vertebral expansion. *Neurosurgery, 23*(5), 662–665. Evidence Level IV.

Hughes, N., Closs, S. J., & Clark, D. (2009). Experiencing cancer in old age: A qualitative systematic review. *Qualitative Health Research, 19*(8), 1139–1153. Evidence Level I.

Hutchesson, A. C., Bundred, N. J., & Ratcliffe, W. A. (1995). Survival in hypercalcaemic patients with cancer and co-existing primary hyperparathyroidism. *Postgraduate Medical Journal, 71*(831), 28–31. Evidence Level III.

Iversen, L. H., Nørgaard, M., Jacobsen, J., Laurberg, S., & Sørensen, H. T. (2009). The impact of comorbidity on survival of Danish colorectal cancer patients from 1995 to 2006—a population-based cohort study. *Diseases of the Colon and Rectum, 52*(1), 71–78. Evidence Level I.

Katz, S., Downs, T. D., Cash, H. R., & Grotz, R. C. (1970). Progress in development of the index of ADL. *The Gerontologist, 10*(1), 20–30. Evidence Level V.

Khorana, A. A., Francis, C. W., Blumberg, N., Culakova, E., Refaai, M. A., & Lyman, G. H. (2008). Blood transfusions, thrombosis, and mortality in hospitalized patients with cancer. *Archives of Internal Medicine, 168*(21), 2377–2381. Evidence Level IV.

Koroukian, S. M. (2009). Assessment and interpretation of comorbidity burden in older adults with cancer. *Journal of the American Geriatrics Society, 57*(Suppl. 2), S275–S278. Evidence Level IV.

Kozyrskyi, A. L., Black, C., Chateau, D., & Steinbach, C. (2005). Discharge outcomes in seniors hospitalized for more than 30 days. *Canadian Journal on Aging, 24*(Suppl. 1), 107–119. Evidence Level II.

Krol, J., Paepke, S., Jacobs, V. R., Paepke, D., Euler, U., Kiechle, M., & Harbeck, N. (2006). G-CSF in the prevention of febrile neutropenia in chemotherapy in breast cancer patients. *Onkologie, 29*(4), 171–178. Evidence Level IV.

Kuriansky, J. B., Gurland, B. J., & Fleiss, J. L. (1976). The assessment of self-care capacity in geriatric psychiatric patients by objective and subjective methods. *Journal of Clinical Psychology, 32*(1), 95–102. Evidence Level IV.

Lau, D. T., & Kirby, J. B. (2009). Living arrangement and colorectal cancer screening: Updated USPSTF guidelines. *American Journal of Public Health, 99*(10), 1733–1734. Evidence Level V.

Lawton, M. P., & Brody, E. M. (1969). Assessment of older people: Self-maintaining and instrumental activities of daily living. *The Gerontologist, 9*(3), 179–186. Evidence Level II.

Lee, C. T., Yang, C. C., Lam, K. K., Kung, C. T., Tsai, C. J., & Chen, H. C. (2006). Hypercalcemia in the emergency department. *The American Journal of the Medical Sciences, 331*(3), 119–123. Evidence Level II.

Lin, T. S., Lucas, M. S., & Byrd, J. C. (2003). Rituximab in B-cell chronic lymphocytic leukemia. *Seminars in Oncology, 30*(4), 483–492. Evidence Level II.

Lowey, S. E. (2006). Spinal cord compression: An oncologic emergency associated with metastatic cancer: Evaluation and management for the home health clinician. *Home Healthcare Nurse, 24*(7), 439–446. Evidence Level IV.

McLain, R. F., & Bell, G. R. (1998). Newer management options in patients with spinal metastasis. *Cleveland Clinic Journal of Medicine, 65*(7), 359–366. Evidence Level IV.

Mion, L., Odegard, P. S., Resnick, B., & Segal-Galan, F. (2006). Interdisciplinary care for older adults with complex needs: American Geriatrics Society position statement. *Journal of the American Geriatrics Society, 54*(5), 849–852. Evidence Level V.

Naeim, A., & Reuben, D. (2001). Geriatric syndromes and assessment in older cancer patients. *Oncology (Williston Park, NY), 15*(12), 1567–1577, 1580; discussion 1581, 1586, 1591. Evidence Level V.

National Cancer Institute. (2010). *SEER cancer statistics review, 1975–2007.* Retrived from http://seer.cancer.gov/csr/1975_2007/index.html

National Center for Health Statistics. (2006). *Trends in health and aging.* U.S. Department of Health and Human Services, Centers for Disease Control and Prevention. Atlanta, Georgia.

Pal, S. K., Katheria, V., & Hurria, A. (2010). Evaluating the older patient with cancer: Understanding frailty and the geriatric assessment. *CA: A Cancer Journal for Clinicians, 60*(2), 120–132. Evidence Level V.

Panel on Prevention of Falls in Older Persons, & American Geriatrics Society and British Geriatrics Society. (2011). Summary of the updated American Geriatrics Society/British Geriatrics Society clinical practice guideline for prevention of falls in older persons. *Journal of the American Geriatrics Society, 59*(1), 148–157. Evidence Level V.

Patterson, R. E., Flatt, S. W., Saquib, N., Rock, C. L., Caan, B. J., Parker, B. A., . . . Pierce, J. P. (2010). Medical comorbidities predict mortality in women with a history of early stage breast cancer. *Breast Cancer Research and Treatment, 122*(3), 859–865. Evidence Level I.

Pilotto, A., Ferrucci, L., Scarcelli, C., Niro, V., Di Mario, F., Seripa, D., . . . Franceschi, M. (2007). Usefulness of the comprehensive geriatric assessment in older patients with upper gastrointestinal bleeding: A two-year follow-up study. *Digestive Diseases, 25*(2), 124–128.

Podsiadlo, D., & Richardson, S. (1991). The timed "Up & Go": a test of basic functional mobility for frail elderly persons. *Journal of the American Geriatrics Society, 39*(2), 142–148. Evidence Level II.

Reiner, A., & Lacasse, C. (2006). Symptom correlates in the gero-oncology population. *Seminars in Oncology Nursing, 22*(1), 20–30. Evidence Level II.

Repetto, L., Biganzoli, L., Koehne, C. H., Luebbe, A. S., Soubeyran, P., Tjan-Heijnen, V. C., & Aapro, M. S. (2003). EORTC Cancer in the Elderly Task Force guidelines for the use of colony-stimulating factors in elderly patients with cancer. *European Journal of Cancer*, *39*(16), 2264–2272. Evidence Level I.

Schmidt, M. H., Klimo, P., Jr., & Vrionis, F. D. (2005). Metastatic spinal cord compression. *Journal of the National Comprehensive Cancer Network*, *3*(5), 711–719. Evidence Level IV.

Shack, L. G., Rachet, B., Williams, E. M., Northover, J. M., & Coleman, M. P. (2010). Does the timing of comorbidity affect colorectal cancer survival? A population based study. *Postgraduate Medical Journal*, *86*(1012), 73–78. Evidence Level I.

Sharma, S., Rezai, K., Driscoll, D., Odunsi, K., & Lele, S. (2006). Characterization of neutropenic fever in patients receiving first-line adjuvant chemotherapy for epithelial ovarian cancer. *Gynecologic Oncology*, *103*(1), 181–185. Evidence Level II.

Silva, T. J., Jerussalmy, C. S., Farfel, J. M., Curiati, J. A., & Jacob-Filho, W. (2009). Predictors of in-hospital mortality among older patients. *Clinics (São Paulo, Brazil)*, *64*(7), 613–618. Evidence Level IV.

Simmonds, M. J. (2002). Physical function in patients with cancer: Psychometric characteristics and clinical usefulness of a physical performance test battery. *Journal of Pain and Symptom Management*, *24*(4), 404–414. Evidence Level II.

Tinetti, M. E. (1986). Performance-oriented assessment of mobility problems in elderly patients. *Journal of the American Geriatrics Society*, *34*(2), 119–126. Evidence Level II.

Tinetti, M. E., Mendes de Leon, C. F., Doucette, J. T., & Baker, D. I. (1994). Fear of falling and fall-related efficacy in relationship to functioning among community-living elders. *Journal of Gerontology*, *49*(3), M140–M147. Evidence Level II.

Ware, J., Jr., Kosinski, M., & Keller, S. D. (1996). A 12-Item Short-Form Health Survey: Construction of scales and preliminary tests of reliability and validity. *Medical Care*, *34*(3), 220–233. Evidence Level II.

Wyrwich, K. W., & Wolinsky, F. D. (2000). Physical activity, disability, and the risk of hospitalization for breast cancer among older women. *The Journals of Gerontology. Series A, Biological Sciences and Medical Sciences*, *55*(7), M418–M421. Evidence Level IV.

Yesavage, J. A., Brink, T. L., Rose, T. L., Lum, O., Huang, V., Adey, M., & Leirer, V. O. (1982–1983). Development and validation of a geriatric depression screening scale: A preliminary report. *Journal of Psychiatric Research*, *17*(1), 37–49. Evidence Level II.

Acute Care Models

33

Elizabeth Capezuti, Marie Boltz, and Cynthia J. Nigolian

EDUCATIONAL OBJECTIVES

On completion of this chapter, the reader should be able to:

1. identify the objectives common to all geriatric acute care models
2. describe the various types of models employed in North American hospitals
3. understand the evidence to support implementation of geriatric acute care models

OVERVIEW

Advances in geriatric science, coupled with the increasing older adult patient population, have led to the development of several geriatric models of care across all health care settings. Acute care models addressing the unique needs of older hospitalized patients began with the comprehensive geriatric assessment (CGA) programs first developed in the 1970s (Rubenstein, 2008).

Geriatric acute care models aim to facilitate improved overall outcomes by promoting a rehabilitative approach while preventing adverse events that occur more commonly in older patients. Also known as *geriatric syndromes*, these are clinical conditions in older persons that do not fit into discrete disease categories (Rubenstein, 2008) and include functional decline, pressure ulcers, fall-related injury, undernutrition or malnutrition, urinary tract infection, and delirium (see Chapter 12, Iatrogenesis). These syndromes or complications contribute to prolonged hospital stays as well as increased likelihood for rehospitalization, institutionalization, emergency department usage, and postacute rehabilitation therapy services. These complications rarely occur alone; the interrelationships among these various syndromes during hospitalization is well documented (Inouye, Studenski, Tinetti, & Kuchel, 2007; Rubenstein, 2008).

Acute care models attend to the age-specific vulnerabilities (i.e., frailty, comorbidities, cognitive impairment) of older hospitalized patients. These models also address the

For description of Evidence Levels cited in this chapter, see Chapter 1, Developing and Evaluating Clinical Practice Guidelines: A Systematic Approach, page 7.

role of institutional factors that determine staff practices and the physical environment that can contribute to iatrogenic complications. Thus, the overall goals of acute geriatric models of care are (a) prevention of complications that occur more commonly in older adults and (b) address hospital factors that contribute to complications (Capezuti, Boltz, & Kim, in press). This chapter provides an overview of care delivery issues that are addressed by acute models of care for older adults and a description of the most commonly employed hospital models.

GERIATRIC ACUTE CARE MODEL OBJECTIVES

There are several geriatric acute care models, each with their own approach to prevent complications and address institutional/staff practices that can contribute to complications. All of these models, however, share a common set of general objectives (Hickman, Newton, Halcomb, Chang, & Davidson, 2007; Hickman, Rolley, & Davidson, 2010). The six general objectives of geriatric acute care models are discussed herein.

Educate Health Care Providers in Core Geriatric Principles

Many health care providers have not received in their basic or continuing education the core geriatric care principles such as recognition of age-specific factors that increase the risk of complications (Berman et al., 2005; Wald, Huddleston, & Kramer, 2006). All acute care models require a coordinator with advanced geriatric education; however, successful implementation depends on direct care staff with the knowledge and competencies to deliver evidence-based care to older patients. Thus, the coordinator or a clinician with geriatric specialization will facilitate staff learning via individual patient consultation, in-service group education, unit rounds, journal clubs, web-based discussion groups, conferences, and other internal institutional educational venues (Fletcher, Hawkes, Williams-Rosenthal, Mariscal, & Cox, 2007; Smyth, Dubin, Restrepo, Nueva-Espana, & Capezuti, 2001).

Target Risk Factors for Complications

The ideal method to prevent complications is by timely screening of potential geriatric syndromes, early identification, and subsequent reduction of risk factors. Some of the models focus on a particular syndrome; however, because of the interrelationship of shared risk factors, reduction of one complication will affect the prevention of other geriatric syndromes. To properly identify risk factors, standardized assessment tools known to be valid and reliable for older adults is recommended. The Hartford Institute for Geriatric Nursing website includes the "Try This" and "How To Try This" series of assessment instruments (ConsultGeriRN, n.d.). At the institutional level, incorporating these risk assessments into routine everyday practice requires hospital policies, procedures, and protocols that will promote usage such as embedding these tools within the health care record.

Incorporate Patient or Family Choices and Treatment Goals

Informed patient's choices are essential whether they are decisions about activity level and medication use to more complex issues such as advance directives.

Family members of patients who can no longer participate in decision making must often deal with the complicated balance between quality-of-life considerations and potential length of life. The decision to employ life-sustaining treatments consistent with patients' preferences is typically and unfortunately only considered when the patient is hospitalized (Somogyi-Zalud, Zhong, Hamel, & Lynn, 2002). For this reason, many geriatric models work collaboratively or in conjunction with palliative care programs.

Employ Evidence-Based Interventions

The high proportion of complications in older hospitalized patients is partly attributed to the lack of evidence-based geriatric care practices. There is tremendous variability in the adoption of geriatric protocols (Neuman, Speck, Karlawish, Schwartz, & Shea, 2010). Issues with overuse or inappropriate medications (e.g., overuse of psychoactive drugs), unnecessary restraints, inadequate detection of cognitive or affective changes (e.g., delirium, depression), and poor pain control are examples of hospital factors that can lead to adverse outcomes. Thus, geriatric acute care models promote the use of standardized evidence-based protocols described in this book.

Promote Interdisciplinary Communication

The detection of management of geriatric syndromes are not limited to medical intervention but require other disciplines such as nursing, pharmacy, social work, and physical and occupational therapy to address the complex interaction of medical, functional, psychological, and social issues leading to these complications. Most importantly, it is the communication of the various disciplines' input that is facilitated by geriatric care models that is essential.

Emphasize Proactive Discharge Planning

Older hospitalized patients are more likely to experience delays in discharge, greater emergency service use hospital readmission, and rehabilitation in an institution or at home (Coleman, Min, Chomiak, & Kramer, 2004). Hospital readmission for older patients is most likely associated with medical errors in medication continuity (Coleman, Smith, Raha, & Min, 2005; Foust, Naylor, Boling, & Cappuzzo, 2005), diagnostic workup, or test follow-up (Forster, Murff, Peterson, Gandhi, & Bates, 2003). Geriatric acute care models address the posthospital care environment and the care transition following hospital discharge by promoting coordination among health care providers, facilitating medication reconciliation, preparing patients and their caregivers to carry out discharge instructions, and making appropriate home care referrals (Bowles, Naylor, & Foust, 2002; Flacker, Park, & Sims, 2007; Moore, McGinn, & Halm, 2007). Two of the six models consider the care transition as the primary focus of their programs.

ACUTE CARE MODEL TYPES

Although there are several types of geriatric acute care models that are used in U.S. hospitals, all address both common health problems and care delivery issues. Most consider all geriatric syndromes, whereas others target specific ones such as delirium. The models are implemented in various degrees from a hospital-wide to unit-based approach or some focus on specific processes of hospitalization such as discharge planning.

Geriatric Consultation Service

The consultants in a geriatric service may include a geriatrician, a geropsychiatrist, a geriatric clinical nurse specialist, or an interdisciplinary team of geriatric health care providers to conduct a CGA or evaluate a specific condition (older adult mistreatment), symptom (wandering), or situation (adequacy of spouse to care for patient at home). Some hospitals will require that all patients who are screened at high risk for geriatric-related complications or are admitted from a homebound program or a nursing home will receive a geriatric consult (Agostini, Baker, Inouye, & Bogardus, 2001), whereas most are requested by another primary service for an individual patient. These consultation services have been associated with reduced length of stay (Harari, Martin, Buttery, O'Neill, & Hopper, 2007); however, it is difficult to evaluate any consultation service because their recommendations may not be followed or the hospital may not have the resources or staff to adequately implement the recommendations (Allen et al., 1986).

Acute Care for the Elderly Units

These discrete geriatric units provide CGA delivered by a multidisciplinary team with a focus on the rehabilitative needs of older patients. Team rounds and patient-centered team conferences are considered essential. The core team includes a geriatrician, clinical nurse specialist, social worker, as well as specialists from other disciplines providing consultation—occupational and physical therapy, nutrition, pharmacy, audiology, and psychology. Geriatric evaluation and management (GEM) units developed in the U.S. Department of Veterans Affairs (VA) system have documented significant reductions in functional decline and suboptimal medication use as well as return to home postdischarge and, more recently, decreased rate of nursing home placement among hospitalized veterans on GEM units compared to general medical units (Phibbs et al., 2006). There have been mixed outcomes in nonveteran populations with some demonstrating improved drug prescribing (Spinewine et al., 2007) and reduced mortality (Saltvedt, Mo, Fayers, Kaasa, & Sletvold, 2002), whereas others showing no differences in clinical outcomes compared to usual medical units (Kircher et al., 2007).

Since the 1990s, acute care for the elderly (ACE) units have been implemented in non-VA hospitals. An interdisciplinary team consisting of staff with geriatric expertise work collaboratively using strategies such as team rounds and family conferences. Most ACE units have made physical environment adaptations to address age-related changes (e.g., flooring to reduce glare), support orientation (writeboards indicating staff names, discharge goals), and promote staff observation (e.g., alarmed exit doors, communal space for meals). Led by geriatricians and/or geriatric advanced practice nurses (GAPNs), the interdisciplinary team facilitates care coordination and identification of modifiable risk factors for geriatric syndromes and prevents avoidable discharge delay.

Compared with other medical units, patients hospitalized on ACE units demonstrate reduced incidence of delirium (Bo et al., 2009) and have maintained prehospital or improved functional status at discharge of patients and fewer were discharged to nursing homes without increases in hospital or postdischarge costs (Landefeld, Palmer, Kresevic, Fortinsky, & Kowal, 1995). These positive outcomes are attributed to processes of care more likely found in ACE units: less restraint use, early mobilization, fewer days to discharge planning, and less use of high-risk medications (Counsell et al., 2000). Recently, more hospitals are using ACE units for those at highest risk for age-related complications, with ACE staff providing consultation to export ACE principles throughout the health system. This mobile-ACE approach facilitates reaching a greater number of hospitalized older adults.

Nurses Improving Care for Healthsystem Elders

A national program aimed at system improvement to achieve positive outcomes for hospitalized older adults, Nurses Improving Care for Healthsystem Elders (NICHE) seeks to improve the quality of care provided to older patients and improve nurse competence by "modifying the nurse practice environment with the infusion of geriatric-specific: (a) core values into the mission statement of the institution; (b) special equipment, supplies, and other resources; and (c) protocols and techniques that promote interdisciplinary collaboration" (Boltz et al., 2008b, p. 283). NICHE includes several approaches that promote dissemination of evidence-based geriatric best practices into hospital care. The system-level approach of NICHE provides a structure for nurses to collaborate with other disciplines and to actively participate in or coordinate other geriatric acute care models. A NICHE coordinator acts in a leadership role by facilitating, teaching, and mentoring others and changing systems of care (Fletcher, Hawkes, Williams-Rosenthal, Mariscal, & Cox, 2007). In some hospitals, a GAPN functions in this role as well as providing direct clinical consultation for evaluating and managing patients. The geriatric resource nurse (GRN) model is foundational to NICHE; it is an educational intervention whereby the NICHE coordinator or the GAPN prepares staff nurses as the clinical resource person on geriatric issues to other nurses on their unit (Lee, Fletcher, Westley, & Fankhauser, 2004). The GRN model provides staff nurses, via education and role modeling (e.g., nursing bedside rounds) by a geriatric APN or NICHE coordinator, with content focusing on care management for geriatric syndromes (Lopez et al., 2002; Mezey, Quinlan, Fairchild, & Vezina, 2006). Application of evidence-based practice at the bedside is facilitated by organizational strategies such as incorporation of institution-wide clinical protocols provided in this book.

The GRN model fosters professional development and enhanced work satisfaction for nurses who feel that they have institutional support to provide quality care. These supports include geriatric-specific resources (continuing education, equipment, and specialty services), interdisciplinary collaboration, as well as patient, family, and nurse involvement in treatment-related decision making. Evaluation in NICHE hospitals have reported improved clinical outcomes, rate of compliance with geriatric institutional protocols, cost-related outcomes, and improved nurse knowledge (Pfaff, 2002; Swauger & Tomlin, 2002; Turner, Lee, Fletcher, Hudson, & Barton, 2001). The GRN model is associated with positive outcomes such as reduced delirium in a NICHE orthopedic unit (Guthrie, Schumacher, & Edinger, 2006) and reduced complications among hospitalized older adults with dementia (Allen & Close, 2010). In studies aggregating results from several NICHE hospitals, NICHE implementation is associated with improved processes of care (Fulmer et al., 2002; Mezey et al., 2004) as well as higher nurse perceived quality of care (Boltz et al., 2008a).

NICHE also promotes implementation of ACE model. The ACE model within NICHE emphasizes nurse-driven protocols and geriatric continuing education of all nursing staff. Similar to other ACE units, study of a NICHE-ACE unit found lower fall and pressure ulcer rates and lower length of stay when compared to overall hospital rates (LaReau & Raphelson, 2005).

The Hospital Elder Life Program

The Hospital Elder Life Program (HELP) is an intervention program using clinicians (geriatric specialists of various disciplines) working together as an interdisciplinary team with trained volunteers that target risk factors for delirium (mental orientation, therapeutic activities, early mobilization, vision and hearing adaptations, hydration and feeding assistance, and sleep enhancement). Protocols based on several well-designed clinical trials are employed to reduce incidence of new delirium and, among those who did develop delirium, reduce total number of episodes and days with delirium, functional decline, costs of hospital services, and use of long-term nursing home services (Inouye, Baker, Fugal, Bradley, & for the HELP Dissemination Project, 2006; Inouye, Bogardus, Baker, Leo-Summers, & Cooney, 2000; Inouye et al., 1999). The program depends on well-trained and supervised volunteers in patient care interventions (Bradley, Webster, Schlesinger, Baker, & Inouye, 2006b) that are coordinated by Elder Life Specialists. The Elder Life Nurse Specialist typically has advanced geriatric nursing education and will supervise the implementation of nursing-related assessments and tracking of delirium risk factor protocol adherence.

Transitional Care Models

Transitional care models aim to specifically address the needs of older adult patients with complex medical and social needs and their caregivers to navigate the health care system across settings. Two models with demonstrated positive outcomes include the advanced practice nurse (APN) transitional care model (Naylor & Keating, 2008) and the care transitions coaching or care transitions intervention (Coleman, Parry, Chalmers, & Min, 2006; Coleman et al., 2004). (These are described in more detail in Chapter 34, Transitional Care.)

Combination and Specialty Geriatric Acute Care Models

In some hospitals, a combination of geriatric models is implemented such as a geriatric consultation team and transitional care (Arbaje et al., 2010) or inpatient geriatric assessment and intensive home care (Buurman, Parlevliet, van Deelen, de Haan, & de Rooij, 2010). In others, a core geriatric interdisciplinary team provides direct consultation as well as screens patients for other related services such as palliative care, rehabilitative services, or pain management programs. Some hospitals have developed dual-function units such as merging an ACE unit with a palliative care (Gelfman, Meier, & Morrison, 2008; Tomasovic;aa, 2005), stroke (Allen et al., 2003), or oncology (Flood, Brown, Carroll, & Locher, 2011) unit as well as incorporating a "delirium room" within an ACE unit (Flaherty et al., 2003) or a geriatric assessment unit within an emergency department (Pareja et al., 2009).

Others have developed programs that incorporate geriatric comanagement with other specialties such as rehabilitation, orthopedics, trauma, and oncology (Allen et al., 2003; Gelfman et al., 2008; Kammerlander et al., 2010). These programs have demonstrated increased detection of and reduced incidence of delirium, as well as reduced length of stay, readmission rates, morbidity, and mortality (Flaherty et al., 2003; Flood et al., 2011; Milisen et al., 2001; Pareja et al., 2009). Programs promoting collaboration between hospitalists and geriatric consultation team have resulted in lower length of hospital stay (Sennour, Counsell, Jones, & Weiner, 2009), although preliminary evidence suggests that hospitalists leading transitional care teams (Better Outcomes for Older Adults through Safer Transitions [BOOST]) can prevent postdischarge complications and readmissions within 30 days and increases the patients' confidence in self-management (Dedhia et al., 2009). Administered by the Society of Hospital Medicine, the BOOST program provides technical support to optimize the hospital discharge process and diminish discontinuity and fragmentation of care (Williams & Coleman, 2009).

New Model Approaches

The availability of geriatric clinicians is essential to implementing any model; however, there is a significant shortage of fellowship-trained geriatricians, geriatric psychiatrists, master's prepared geriatric nurse specialists, as well as specialists in other disciplines (Committee on the Future Health Care Workforce for Older Americans, 2008). This is especially true for hospitals located in rural areas as well as small hospitals without the financial capacity to employ geriatric specialists (Jayadevappa, Bloom, Raziano, & Lavizzo-Mourey, 2003). Some hospitals are working with other hospitals in their health system or in their region to create learning collaboratives or "knowledge networks" by using web-based and other long-distance communication strategies. Thus, a geriatrician (Malone et al., 2010) or a GAPN (Capezuti, 2010) can participate in "virtual" rounds with staff in another location (Friedman, Mendelson, Kates, & McCann, 2008; Pallawala & Lun, 2001) to foster communication; that is, the e-geriatrician or e-APN has access to a system-wide electronic health record such as the ACE Tracker and the TeleGeriatric system (Pallawala & Lun, 2001) or similar web-based assessment tool (Gray & Wootton, 2008). In this way, collaboration and mentoring of professional colleagues is facilitated while enhancing the care provided to older adults.

SUMMARY

Despite differences in approaches or foci, all models share common goals. The model employed in a hospital or health system is based on the unique needs of that hospital's patient population, the resources available (geriatric clinicians, bed size, volunteers, etc.), and especially the senior administrator's commitment to geriatric programming. Because there is currently no direct reimbursement for many components of these models, administrators are motivated by the model's alignment to the institution's strategic plan or mission, consumer or community satisfaction, and costs savings (such reduced costly and nonreimbursable complications; Adunsky et al., 2005; Boult et al., 2009; Bradley, Webster, Schlesinger, Baker, & Inouye, 2006a; Hart, Frank, Hoffman, Dickey, & Kristjansson, 2006; Kammerlander et al., 2010; Siu, Spragens, Inouye, Morrison, & Leff, 2009). Although all of the models have demonstrated positive outcomes, only a small number (approximately 500) have been implemented in U.S. acute care facilities. Most are located in academic or teaching hospitals. Expansion to more than 3,000 hospitals that serve a high proportion of older adults may depend on advancing the unique contributions of each within an integrated model that will enhance the hospital experience of the older patient (Capezuti & Brush, 2009; Marcantonio, Flacker, Wright, & Resnick, 2001).

REFERENCES

Adunsky, A., Arad, M., Levi, R., Blankstein, A., Zeilig, G., & Mizrachi, E. (2005). Five-year experience with the 'Sheba' model of comprehensive orthogeriatric care for elderly hip fracture patients. *Disability and Rehabilitation, 27*(18–19), 1123–1127. Evidence Level IV.

Agostini, J. V., Baker, D. I., Inouye, S. K., & Bogardus, S. T. (2001). *Multidisciplinary geriatric consultation services. Agency for Healthcare Research and Quality Evidence Report 43: Making health care safer: A critical analysis of patient safety practices* (AHRQ Publication No. 01-E058). U.S. Department of Health and Human Services. Evidence Level V.

Allen, C. M., Becker, P. M., McVey, L. J., Saltz, C., Feussner, J. R., & Cohen, H. J. (1986). A randomized, controlled clinical trial of a geriatric consultation team. Compliance with recommendations. *The Journal of the American Medical Association, 255*(19), 2617–2621. Evidence Level II.

Allen, J., & Close, J. (2010). The NICHE geriatric resource nurse model: Improving the care of older adults with Alzheimer's disease and other dementias. *Geriatric Nursing, 31*(2), 128–132. Evidence Level V.

Allen, K. R., Hazelett, S. E., Palmer, R. R., Jarjoura, D. G., Wickstrom, G. C., Weinhardt, J. A., . . . Counsell, S. R. (2003). Developing a stroke unit using the acute care for elders intervention and model of care. *Journal of the American Geriatrics Society, 51*(11), 1660–1667. Evidence Level V.

Arbaje, A. I., Maron, D. D., Yu, Q., Wendel, V. I., Tanner, E., Boult, C., . . . Durso, S. C. (2010). The geriatric floating interdisciplinary transition team. *Journal of the American Geriatrics Society, 58*(2), 364–370. Evidence Level III.

Berman, A., Mezey, M., Kobayashi, M., Fulmer, T., Stanley, J., Thornlow, D., & Rosenfeld, P. (2005). Gerontological nursing content in baccalaureate nursing programs: Comparison of findings from 1997 and 2003. *Journal of Professional Nursing, 21*(5), 268–275. Evidence Level V.

Bo, M., Martini, B., Ruatta, C., Massaia, M., Ricauda, N. A., Varetto, A., . . . Torta, R. (2009). Geriatric ward hospitalization reduced incidence delirium among older medical inpatients. *The American Journal of Geriatric Psychiatry, 17*(9), 760–768. Evidence Level IV.

Boltz, M., Capezuti, E., Bowar-Ferres, S., Norman, R., Secic, M., Kim, H., . . . Fulmer, T. (2008a). Changes in the geriatric care environment associated with NICHE (Nurses Improving Care for HealthSystem Elders). *Geriatric Nursing, 29*(3), 176–185. Evidence Level IV.

Boltz, M., Capezuti, E., Bowar-Ferres, S., Norman, R., Secic, M., Kim, H., . . . Fulmer, T. (2008b). Hospital nurses' perception of the geriatric nurse practice environment. *Journal of Nursing Scholarship, 40*(3), 282–289. Evidence Level IV.

Boult, C., Green, A. F., Boult, L. B., Pacala, J. T., Snyder, C., & Leff, B. (2009). Successful models of comprehensive care for older adults with chronic conditions: Evidence for the Institute of Medicine's "retooling for an aging America" report. *Journal of the American Geriatrics Society, 57*(12), 2328–2337. Evidence Level I.

Bowles, K. H., Naylor, M. D., & Foust, J. B. (2002). Patient characteristics at hospital discharge and a comparison of home care referral decisions. *Journal of the American Geriatrics Society, 50*(2), 336–342. Evidence Level IV.

Bradley, E. H., Webster, T. R., Schlesinger, M., Baker, D., & Inouye, S. K. (2006a). Patterns of diffusion of evidence-based clinical programmes: A case study of the Hospital Elder Life Program. *Quality & Safety in Health Care, 15*(5), 334–338. Evidence Level V.

Bradley, E. H., Webster, T. R., Schlesinger, M., Baker, D., & Inouye, S. K. (2006b). The roles of senior management in improving hospital experiences for frail older adults. *Journal of Healthcare Management, 51*(5), 323–336. Evidence Level IV.

Buurman, B. M., Parlevliet, J. L., van Deelen, B. A., de Haan, R. J., & de Rooij, S. E. (2010). A randomised clinical trial on a comprehensive geriatric assessment and intensive home follow-up after hospital discharge: The Transitional Care Bridge. *BMC Health Services Research, 10*, 296. Evidence Level II.

Capezuti, E. (2010). An electronic geriatric specialist workforce: Is it a viable option? *Geriatric Nursing, 31*(3), 220–222. Evidence Level V.

Capezuti, E., Boltz, M., & Kim, H. (in press). Geriatric models of care. In R. A. Rosenthal et al. (Eds.), *Principles and practice of geriatric surgery*. New York, NY: Springer Publishing. Evidence Level VI.

Capezuti, E., & Brush, B. L. (2009). Implementing geriatric care models: What are we waiting for? *Geriatric Nursing, 30*(3), 204–206. Evidence Level V.

Coleman, E. A., Min, S. J., Chomiak, A., & Kramer, A. M. (2004). Posthospital care transitions: Patterns, complications, and risk identification. *Health Services Research, 39*(5), 1449–1465. Evidence Level IV.

Coleman, E. A., Parry, C., Chalmers, S., & Min, S. J. (2006). The care transitions intervention: Results of a randomized controlled trial. *Archives of Internal Medicine, 166*(17), 1822–1828. Evidence Level II.

Coleman, E. A., Smith, J. D., Frank, J. C., Min, S. J., Parry, C., & Kramer, A. M. (2004). Preparing patients and caregivers to participate in care delivered across settings: The Care Transitions Intervention. *Journal of the American Geriatrics Society, 52*(11), 1817–1825. Evidence Level III.

Coleman, E. A., Smith, J. D., Raha, D., & Min, S. J. (2005). Posthospital medication discrepancies: Prevalence and contributing factors. *Archives of Internal Medicine, 165*(16), 1842–1847. Evidence Level IV.

Committee on the Future Health Care Workforce for Older Americans. (2008). *Retooling for an aging America: Building the health care workforce*. Washington, DC: National Academies Press. Evidence Level VI.

ConsultGeriRN.org. (n.d.). Retrieved from http://consultgerirn.org/resources

Counsell, S. R., Holder, C. M., Liebenauer, L. L., Palmer, R. M., Fortinsky, R. H., Kresevic, D. M., . . . Landefeld, C. S. (2000). Effects of a multicomponent intervention on functional outcomes and processes of care in hospitalized older patients: A randomized controlled trial of Acute Care for Elders (ACE) in a community hospital. *Journal of the American Geriatrics Society, 48*(12), 1572–1581. Evidence Level II.

Dedhia, P., Kravet, S., Bulger, J., Hinson, T., Sridharan, A., Kolodner, K., . . . Howell, E. (2009). A quality improvement intervention to facilitate the transition of older adults from three hospitals back to their homes. *Journal of the American Geriatrics Society, 57*(9), 1540–1546. Evidence Level V.

Flacker, J., Park, W., & Sims, A. (2007). Hospital discharge information and older patients: Do they get what they need? *Journal of Hospital Medicine, 2*(5), 291–296. Evidence Level IV.

Flaherty, J. H., Tariq, S. H., Raghavan, S., Bakshi, S., Moinuddin, A., & Morley, J. E. (2003). A model for managing delirious older inpatients. *Journal of the American Geriatrics Society, 51*(7), 1031–1035. Evidence Level V.

Fletcher, K., Hawkes, P., Williams-Rosenthal, S., Mariscal, C. S., & Cox, B. A. (2007). Using nurse practitioners to implement best practice care for the elderly during hospitalization: The NICHE journey at the University of Virginia Medical Center. *Critical Care Nursing Clinics of North America, 19*(3), 321–337. Evidence Level V.

Flood, K. L., Brown, C. J., Carroll, M. B., & Locher, J. L. (2011). Nutritional processes of care for older adults admitted to an oncology-acute care for elders unit. *Critical Reviews in Oncology/Hematology, 78*(1), 73–78. Evidence Level IV.

Forster, A. J., Murff, H. J., Peterson, J. F., Gandhi, T. K., & Bates, D. W. (2003). The incidence and severity of adverse events affecting patients after discharge from the hospital. *Annals of Internal Medicine, 138*(3), 161–167. Evidence Level IV.

Foust, J. B., Naylor, M. D., Boling, P. A., & Cappuzzo, K. A. (2005). Opportunities for improving post-hospital home medication management among older adults. *Home Health Care Services Quarterly, 24*(1–2), 101–122. Evidence Level V.

Friedman, S. M., Mendelson, D. A., Kates, S. L., & McCann, R. M. (2008). Geriatric co-management of proximal femur fractures: Total quality management and protocol-driven care result in better outcomes for a frail patient population. *Journal of the American Geriatrics Society, 56*(7), 1349–1356. Evidence Level V.

Fulmer, T., Mezey, M., Bottrell, M., Abraham, I., Sazant, J., Grossman, S., & Grisham, E. (2002). Nurses Improving Care for Healthsystem Elders (NICHE): Using outcomes and benchmarks for evidenced-based practice. *Geriatric Nursing, 23*(3), 121–127. Evidence Level IV.

Gelfman, L. P., Meier, D. M., & Morrison, R. S. (2008). Does palliative care improve quality? A survey of bereaved family members. *Journal of Pain and Symptom Manage, 36*(1), 22–28. Evidence Level IV.

Gray, L., & Wootton, R. (2008). Comprehensive geriatric assessment 'online.' *Australasian Journal on Ageing, 27*(4), 205–208. Evidence Level V.

Guthrie, P. F., Schumacher, S., & Edinger, G. (2006). A NICHE delirium prevention project for hospitalized elders. In N. M. Silverstein & K. Maslow (Eds.), *Improving hospital care for persons with dementia* (pp. 139–157). New York, NY: Springer Publishing. Evidence Level V.

Harari, D., Martin, F. C., Buttery, A., O'Neill, S., & Hopper, A. (2007). The older persons' assessment and liaison team 'OPAL': Evaluation of comprehensive geriatric assessment in acute medical inpatients. *Age and Ageing, 36*(6), 670–675. Evidence Level III.

Hart, B., Frank, C., Hoffman, J., Dickey, D., & Kristjansson, J. (2006). Senior friendly health services. *Perspectives, 30*(1), 18–21. Evidence Level V.

Hickman, L., Newton, P., Halcomb, E. J., Chang, E., & Davidson P. (2007). Best practice interventions to improve the management of older people in acute care settings: A literature review. *Journal of Advanced Nursing, 60*(2), 113–126. Evidence Level V.

Hickman, L. D., Rolley, J. X., & Davidson, P. M. (2010). Can principles of the Chronic Care Model be used to improve care of the older person in the acute care sector? *Collegian, 17*(2), 63–69. Evidence Level V.

Inouye, S. K., Baker, D. I., Fugal, P., Bradley, E. H., & for the HELP Dissemination Project. (2006). Dissemination of the hospital elder life program: Implementation, adaptation, and successes. *Journal of the American Geriatrics Society, 54*(10), 1492–1499. Evidence Level IV.

Inouye, S. K., Bogardus, S. T., Jr., Baker, D. I., Leo-Summers, L., & Cooney, L. M., Jr. (2000). The Hospital Elder Life Program: A model of care to prevent cognitive and functional decline in older hospitalized patients. Hospital Elder Life Program. *Journal of the American Geriatrics Society, 48*(12), 1697–1706. Evidence Level IV.

Inouye, S. K., Bogardus, S. T., Jr., Charpentier, P. A., Leo-Summers, L., Acampora, D., Holford, T. R., & Cooney, L. M., Jr. (1999). A multicomponent intervention to prevent delirium in hospitalized older patients. *The New England Journal of Medicine, 1340*(9), 669–676. Evidence Level II.

Inouye, S. K., Studenski, S., Tinetti, M. E., & Kuchel, G. A. (2007). Geriatric syndromes: Clinical, research, and policy implications of a core geriatric concept. *Journal of the American Geriatrics Society, 55*(5), 780–791. Evidence Level VI.

Jayadevappa, R., Bloom, B. S., Raziano, D. B., & Lavizzo-Mourey, R. (2003). Dissemination and characteristics of acute care for elders (ACE) units in the United States. *International Journal of Technology Assessment in Health Care, 19*(1), 220–227. Evidence Level V.

Kammerlander, C., Roth, T., Friedman, S. M., Suhm, N., Luger, T. J., Kammerlander-Knauer, U., . . . Blauth M. (2010). Ortho-geriatric service—a literature review comparing different models. *Osteoporosis International, 21*(Suppl. 4), S637–S646. Evidence Level V.

Kircher, T. T., Wormstall, H., Müller, P. H., Schwärzler, F., Buchkremer, G., Wild, K., . . . Meisner, C. (2007). A randomised trial of a geriatric evaluation and management consultation services in frail hospitalised patients. *Age and Ageing, 36*(1), 36–42. Evidence Level II.

Landefeld, C. S., Palmer, R. M., Kresevic, D. M., Fortinsky, R. H., & Kowal, J. (1995). A randomized trial of care in a hospital medical unit especially designed to improve the functional outcomes of acutely ill older patients. *The New England Journal of Medicine, 332*(20), 1338–1344. Evidence Level II.

LaReau, R., & Raphelson, M. (2005). The treatment of the hospitalized elderly patient in a specialized acute care of the elderly unit: A southwest Michigan perspective. *Southwest Michigan Medical Journal, 2*(3), 21–27. Evidence Level V.

Lee, V., Fletcher, K., Westley, C., & Fankhauser, K. A. (2004). Competent to care: Strategies to assist staff in caring for elders. *Medsurg Nursing, 13*(5), 281–288. Evidence Level V.

Lopez, M., Delmore, B., Ake, J. M., Kim, Y. R., Golden, P., Bier, J., . . . Fulmer, T. (2002). Implementing a geriatric resource nurse model. *The Journal of Nursing Administration, 32*(11), 577–585. Evidence Level V.

Malone, M. L., Vollbrecht, M., Stephenson, J., Burke, L., Pagel, P., & Goodwin, J. S. (2010). Acute Care for Elders (ACE) tracker and e-Geriatrician: Methods to disseminate ACE concepts to hospitals with no geriatricians on staff. *Journal of the American Geriatrics Society, 58*(1), 161–167. Evidence Level IV.

Marcantonio, E. R., Flacker, J. M., Wright, R. J., & Resnick, N. M. (2001). Reducing delirium after hip fracture: A randomized trial. *Journal of the American Geriatrics Society, 49*(5), 516–522. Evidence Level II.

Mezey, M., Kobayashi, M., Grossman, S., Firpo, A., Fulmer, T., & Mitty, E. (2004). Nurses Improving Care to Health System Elders (NICHE): Implementation of best practice models. *The Journal of Nursing Administration, 34*(10), 451–457. Evidence Level V.

Mezey, M., Quinlan, E., Fairchild, S., & Vezina, M. (2006). Geriatric competencies for RNs in hospitals. *Journal for Nurses in Staff Development, 22*(1), 2–10. Evidence Level IV.

Milisen, K., Foreman, M. D., Abraham, I. L., De Geest, S., Godderis, J., Vandermeulen, E., . . . Broos, P. L. (2001). A nurse-led interdisciplinary intervention program for delirium in elderly hip-fracture patients. *Journal of the American Geriatrics Society, 49*(5), 523–532. Evidence Level III.

Moore, C., McGinn, T., & Halm, E. (2007). Tying up loose ends: Discharging patients with unresolved medical issues. *Archives of Internal Medicine, 167*(12), 1305–1311. Evidence Level IV.

Naylor, M., & Keating, S. A. (2008). Transitional care. *The American Journal of Nursing, 108*(Suppl. 9), 58–63. Evidence Level V.

Neuman, M. D., Speck, R. M., Karlawish, J. H., Schwartz, J. S., & Shea, J. A. (2010). Hospital protocols for the inpatient care of older adults: Results from a statewide survey. *Journal of the American Geriatrics Society, 58*(10), 1959–1964. doi:10.1111/j.1532-5415.2010.03056.x. Evidence Level IV.

Pallawala, P. M., & Lun, K. C. (2001). EMR-based TeleGeriatric system. *Studies in Health Technology and Informatics, 84*(Pt. 1), 849–853. Evidence Level V.

Pareja, T., Hornillos, M., Rodríguez, M., Martínez, T., Madrigal, M., Mauleón, C., & Alvarez, B. (2009). Unidad de observación de urgencias para pacientes geriátricos: Beneficios clínicos y asistenciales [Medical short stay unit for geriatric patients in the emergency department: Clinical and healthcare benefits]. *Revista Española De Geriatría y Gerontología, 44*(4), 175–179. Evidence Level IV.

Pfaff, J. (2002). The Geriatric Resource Nurse Model: A culture change. *Geriatric Nursing, 23*(3), 140–144. Evidence Level V.

Phibbs, C. S., Holty, J. E., Goldstein, M. K., Garber, A. M., Wang, Y., Feussner, J. R., & Cohen, H. J. (2006). The effect of geriatrics evaluation and management on nursing home use and health care costs: Results from a randomized trial. *Medical Care, 44*(1), 91–95. Evidence Level II.

Rubenstein, L. Z. (2008). Geriatric assessment programs. In E. A. Capezuti, E. L. Siegler, & M. D. Mezey (Eds.), *The encyclopedia of elder care: The comprehensive resource on geriatric and social care* (2nd ed., pp. 346–349). New York, NY: Springer Publishing. Evidence Level VI.

Saltvedt, I., Mo, E. S., Fayers, P., Kaasa, S., & Sletvold, O. (2002). Reduced mortality in treating acutely sick, frail older patients in a geriatric evaluation and management unit. A prospective randomized trial. *Journal of the American Geriatrics Society, 50*(5), 792–798. Evidence Level II.

Sennour, Y., Counsell, S. R., Jones, J., & Weiner, M. (2009). Development and implementation of a proactive geriatrics consultation model in collaboration with hospitalists. *Journal of the American Geriatrics Society, 57*(11), 2139–2145. Evidence Level V.

Siu, A. L., Spragens, L. H., Inouye, S. K., Morrison, R. S., & Leff, B. (2009). The ironic business case for chronic care in the acute care setting. *Health Affairs, 28*(1), 113–125. Evidence Level V.

Smyth, C., Dubin, S., Restrepo, A., Nueva-Espana, H., & Capezuti, E. (2001). Creating order out of chaos: Models of GNP practice with hospitalized older adults. *Clinical Excellence for Nurse Practitioners, 5*(2), 88–95. Evidence Level V.

Somogyi-Zalud, E., Zhong, Z., Hamel, M. B., & Lynn, J. (2002). The use of life-sustaining treatments in hospitalized persons aged 80 and older. *Journal of the American Geriatrics Society, 50*(5), 930–934. Evidence Level IV.

Spinewine, A., Swine, C., Dhillon, S., Lambert, P., Nachega, J. B., Wilmotte, L., & Tulkens, P. M. (2007). Effect of a collaborative approach on the quality of prescribing for geriatric inpatients: A randomized, controlled trial. *Journal of the American Geriatrics Society, 55*(5), 658–665. Evidence Level II.

Swauger, K., & Tomlin, C. (2002). Best care for the elderly at Forsyth Medical Center. *Geriatric Nursing, 23*(3), 145–150. Evidence Level V.

Tomasovic;aa, N. (2005). Geriatric-palliative care units model for improvement of elderly care. *Collegium Antropologicum, 29*(1), 277–282. Evidence Level V.

Turner, J. T., Lee, V., Fletcher, K., Hudson, K., & Barton, D. (2001). Measuring quality of care with an inpatient elderly population: The geriatric resource nurse model. *Journal of Gerontological Nursing, 27*(3), 8–18. Evidence Level V.

Wald, H., Huddleston, J., & Kramer, A. (2006). Is there a geriatrician in the house? Geriatric care approaches in hospitalist programs. *Journal of Hospital Medicine, 1*(1), 29–35. Evidence Level IV.

Willams, M. V., & Coleman, E. (2009). BOOSTing the hospital discharge. *Journal of Hospital Medicine, 4*(4), 209–210. Evidence Level V.

Transitional Care

34

Fidelindo Lim, Janice Foust, and Janet Van Cleave

EDUCATIONAL OBJECTIVES

On completion of this chapter, the reader will have gained knowledge on the challenges and opportunities associated with transitional care and should be able to:

1. describe various transitional care models
2. identify potential for nurse-led and advanced practice nurses (APN)-led transitional care
3. identify essential elements of successful transitional care

OVERVIEW

Persons with continuous complex care needs frequently require care in multiple settings. The American Geriatrics Society (2003) defines *transitional care* as "a set of actions designed to ensure the coordination and continuity of health care as patients transfer between different locations or different levels of care within the same location." (p. 556). Representative locations include (but are not limited to) hospitals, subacute and post-acute nursing facilities, the patient's home, primary and specialty care offices, and long-term care facilities (Coleman & Boult, 2003). During transitions between settings, this population is particularly vulnerable to experiencing poor care quality and problems of care fragmentation. For example, among Medicare patients, 20% were hospitalized within 30 days and 34% were rehospitalized within 60 days (Jencks, Williams, & Coleman, 2009). Despite how common these transitions have become, the challenges of improving care transitions have historically received little attention from policy makers, clinicians, and quality improvement entities (Coleman, 2003), until recently. With hospital readmission now heralded as a quality indicator, there is more incentive to correct transition-related problems. The enactment of the Patient Protection and Affordable Care Act (PPACA) in 2010 (see relevant practice guidelines in this chapter) will help formalize and implement transitional care services with federal funding.

For description of Evidence Levels cited in this chapter, see Chapter 1, Developing and Evaluating Clinical Practice Guidelines: A Systematic Approach, page 7.

Many factors contribute to gaps in care during critical transitions. Poor communication, incomplete transfer of information, inadequate education of older adults and their family caregivers, limited access to essential services, and the absence of a single-point person to ensure continuity of care all contribute transition-associated problems (Naylor, 2002; Naylor & Keating, 2008). The practice of nursing is closely tied to health illness transitions in a person's lifetime. The quality of the outcomes during these transitional events is largely determined by the degree of care coordination among health care environments and proactive involvement of the patient and their families in the process, wherein a nurse plays a pivotal role. Success in implementing evidence-based transition care strategies will help curtail preventable rehospitalizations and save health care dollars.

This chapter reviews issues associated with transitional care mainly from the acute care setting and presents evidence-based transitional care models (TCMs) as well as strategies to enhance outcome performance. The authors searched the CINAHL, Cochrane databases of systematic Reviews, Medline/PubMed, PsycINFO and Evidence-Based Resources from the Joanna Briggs Institute using combinations of the following terms: research, ages 65 years or older, care transitions, case management, critical pathways, continuity of patient care, patient transfer, patient discharge, discharge planning and discharge education, and readmission and transfer. The articles search are rated by level of evidence according to Stetler and colleagues' (1998) and Melnyk and Fineout-Overholt's (2005) Level of Evidence guidelines. The search period was 2000 to 2010.

BACKGROUND AND STATEMENT OF PROBLEM

In 2004, older adults represent 50% of hospital days; 60% of all ambulatory adult primary care visits; 70% of all home care visits; and 85% of residents in nursing homes (National Center for Healthcare Statistics, 2004). Of the 1.5 million current residents in U.S. Nursing Homes, nearly one half (48.2%) were admitted from a hospital or health care facility other than a nursing home or assisted-living-type facility (Centers for Disease Control and Prevention [CDC], 2009). In 2007, older adults aged 65 years and older accounted for just 13% of the U.S. population, but 37% of the hospital discharges (CDC, 2007). Therefore, the likelihood of older adults being in a state of transition between care environments is very high.

Transitions are considered high-stress events for patients, their families, and care providers alike. Evidence suggests that transitions are particularly vulnerable to breakdowns in care and, thus, there is a need for transitional care services (Naylor & Keating, 2008). Two especially problematic areas are medication discrepancies and poor post-hospital follow-up with primary care providers. Forster, Murff, Peterson, Gandhi, & Bates (2003) found that nearly 20% of recently discharged medical patients experienced an adverse event during the first several weeks at home. Of these, 66% involved medications and were the most common type of adverse event (Forster et al., 2003). Corbett, Setter, Daratha, Neumiller, & Wood, (2010) found in a study on home medication discrepancies that the problems were astoundingly widespread, with 94% of the participants having at least one discrepancy. The average number of medication discrepancies identified was 3.3 per patient during hospital to home transition (Corbett et al., 2010). Another major area of breakdown is patient follow-up visits after discharge. For example, one study reported that among Medicare patients rehospitalized within

30 days, up to 50% did not have documentation of physician follow-up visits postdischarge (Coleman, 2003). Patients and their caregivers are often unprepared for transitions and are overwhelmed by discharge information. Poor preparation of the patient and their informal caregivers for their next level of care interface, be it the home or another facility, compromises overall patient safety. Follow-up visits after discharges provide opportunities to reinforce discharge education and monitor for changes in conditions. The lack of incentives and accountability make these transfers particularly susceptible to medical errors (Nurses Improving Care for Healthsystem Elders [NICHE], 2010).

The 2001 Institute of Medicine (IOM) landmark report *Crossing the Quality Chasm: A New Health System for the 21st Century*, pointed out that the health care delivery system is poorly organized to meet the challenges at hand. The delivery of care is often overly complex and uncoordinated, requiring steps and patient "hand offs" that slowdown care and decrease rather than improve safety (IOM, 2001). Increasingly, patients are being discharged home or to other health care environments with both complex and complicated treatment plans with limited; timely follow-through by professionals, causing undue stress to the patient and their informal caregivers once they leave the hospital. Levine, Halper, Peist, & Gould (2010) has described informal caregivers' essential role and called for more proactive involvement of them as partners during transitions, especially when they could be the major source of continuity for the patient. The stress of caregiving is likely to be exacerbated during episodes of acute illness (Naylor & Keating, 2008), readmissions and transfers to various health care environments.

Health care disparity and lack or inadequate access to transition care resources will be more pronounced in the disenfranchised segment of older adults, namely those who are living alone, undomiciled, suffering from mental illness, victims of elder abuse and neglect, the uninsured, and those lacking in legal status.

ASSESSMENT OF THE PROBLEM

The lack of sustained transition care programs outside of funded randomized controlled trials (RCTs) is largely caused by the almost nonexistent third-party reimbursement of transition care services, although its necessity have been well described in the literature (Naylor & Keating, 2008). However, this pattern is about to be rectified with the enactment of Public Law 111–148, known as the PPACA. This groundbreaking legislation offers significant provisions and funding for creating community-based transition care services starting from 2011 to 2015 (PPACA, 2010).

Coleman, Smith, et al. (2004) identified four major content areas that patients and caregivers who recently underwent posthospital care transitions expressed as most essential and most needed: medication self-management, a patient-centered health record, primary care and specialist follow-up, and knowledge of "red-flags" warning symptoms or signs indicative of a worsening condition. Similarly, Miller, Piacentine, & Weiss (2008) identified posthospital difficulties faced by adults during the first 3 weeks at home. Among those patients who had difficulty coping, pain was the most frequent stressor, followed by managing complications and recovery challenges. These recently discharged patients also described relying on family or friends for emotional support, and were concerned about being a burden.

A study that compared the referral decisions of hospital clinicians with those of nurses with expertise in discharge planning and transitional care, found that transitional care nurses (TCNs) judged that 96 of 99 of the control group patients discharged without home care had unmet discharge needs that may have benefited from a postdischarge referral (Bowles, Naylor, & Foust, 2002). In investigating patient perceptions of the quality-of-discharge instruction by assessing inpatients' ratings of care and service in the United States between 1997 and 2001 ($n = 4,901,178$), Clark and colleagues (2005) found that patient satisfaction with discharge instructions decreased significantly each year ($p < 0.001$). They point out that patients gave lower ratings to the quality-of-discharge instruction than to the overall quality of their hospital stay, and that U.S. hospitals (in general) are not meeting The Joint Commission (TJC) standards for patient education and discharge.

In a Sentinel Event Alert publication in January, 2006, TJC reported that from September 2004 to July 2005, the United States Pharmacopeia (USP) received 2,022 reports of medication reconciliation errors. Of those reports, 66% occurred during the patient's transition or transfer to another level of care, 22% occurred during the patient's admission to the facility, and 12% occurred at the time of discharge (Cumbler, Carter, & Kutner, 2008). The report added that of those medication errors causing death or major injury, about 63%, at least part, are related to breakdown in communication.

The most common example of communication breakdown is when systems of care fail to ensure that the essential elements of the patient's care plan that were developed in one setting are communicated to the next team of clinicians (e.g., preparation for the goals of care delivered in the next setting, arrangements for follow-up appointments and laboratory testing, and reviewing the current medication regimen; Coleman, 2003). Language and health literacy issues and cultural differences exacerbate the communication breakdowns encountered in health care transition (Naylor & Keating, 2008). For example, a review of literature noted direct communication between hospital and community physicians was relatively rare (3%–20%), and available discharge summaries at the first primary care visit were low (12%–34%; Kripalani et al., 2007). Additionally, discharge summaries did not always have essential information (e.g., medications, diagnostic results) when available.

INTERVENTIONS AND CARE STRATEGIES

Various TCMs have been described in the literature, and several RCTs have tested interventions. Key outcome variables from these RCTs include rehospitalization rate, cost reduction, patient satisfaction, and quality of care. Specific features of the two well-known evidence-based models are summarized in Table 34.1.

The Two Leading Examples of Transition Care Interventions:

The Advanced Practice Nurses Transitional Care Model (Naylor & Keating, 2008; Naylor et al., 2004; Naylor et al., 2009)

The TCM developed at the University of Pennsylvania provides a comprehensive in-hospital planning and home follow-up for chronically ill, high-risk older adults hospitalized for common medical and surgical conditions (Naylor & Keating, 2008).

TABLE 34.1

Transition Care—Strategies for Implementation

Model	Transition Interface	Target Population	Implementation	Primary Provider	Duration of Follow-Up
Transitional Care Model (TCM; Jencks et al., 2009; Naylor, 2002; Naylor & Sochalski, 2010; Naylor et al., 2009; Naylor et al., 2004)	Hospital to home Home to hospital	65 years or older, high-risk, cognitively intact older adults with a variety of medical and surgical conditions (e.g., CHF and comorbidities)	Initial APN visit within 24 hours of hospital admission. APN visits at least daily the index hospitalization. APN home visits (one within 24 hours of discharge), weekly visits during the first month (with one of these visits coinciding with the initial follow-up visit to the patient's physician). Bimonthly visits during the second and third months. Additional APN visits based on patients' needs and APN telephone availability 7 days per week. If a patient was re-hospitalized for any reason during the intervention period, the APN resumed daily hospital visits to facilitate the transition from hospital to home. Use of care management strategies foundational to the quality-cost model of APN transitional care model, including identification of patients' and caregivers' goals, individualized and collaborative plan of care. Implementation of an evidence-based protocol, guided by national heart failure guidelines.	APN in a "manager coordinator" role	From admission to 3 months postdischarge
Care Transitions Intervention (Coleman, 2003; Coleman, Smith, et al., 2004; Coleman et al., 2006; Coleman, Min, et al., 2004)	Hospital to home and hospital to skilled nursing facility	65 years or older with at least 1 of the following diagnoses: stroke, congestive heart failure, coronary artery disease, cardiac arrhythmias, COPD, diabetes mellitus, spinal stenosis, hip fracture, peripheral vascular disease, deep venous thrombosis, and pulmonary embolism.	The transition coach first met with the patient in the hospital before discharge Arrange a home visit, ideally within 48 to 72 hours after hospital discharge. For those patients transferred to a skilled nursing facility, the transition coach telephoned or visited at least weekly). The home visit involved the transition coach, the patient, and the caregiver. The primary goal of the home visit is to reconcile all of the patient's medication regimens (e.g., pre-hospitalization and posthospitalization medications).	APN "transition coach" in a supportive role	From admission to 28 days postdischarge

Transition coach imparted skills on how to effectively communicate care needs during subsequent encounters with health care professionals.

The patient and transition coach rehearsed or role-played effective communication strategies. The transition coach reviewed with the patient any red flags that indicated a condition was worsening and provided education about the initial steps to take to manage the red flags and when to contact the appropriate health care professional.

Following the home visit, the transition coach maintained continuity with the patient and caregiver by telephoning three times during a 28-day posthospitalization discharge period. The first telephone call generally focused on determining whether the patient had received appropriate services (e.g., whether new medications had been obtained or durable medical equipment had been delivered). In the two subsequent telephone calls, the transition coach reviewed the patient's progress toward goals established during the home visit, discussed any encounters that took place with other health care professionals, reinforced the importance of maintaining and sharing the personal health record and supported the patient's role in chronic illness self-management.

The heart of the model is the TCN, who follows patients from the hospital into their homes and provides services designed to streamline plans of care, interrupt patterns of frequent acute hospital and emergency department (ED) use, and prevent health status decline. Although the TCM is nurse led, it is a multidisciplinary model that includes doctors, other nurses, social workers, discharge planners, pharmacists, and other members of the health care team, all of whom implement tested protocols uniquely focused on increasing the ability of patients and their caregivers to manage their care (Naylor et al., 2009).

This model involves APNs who assume a primary role in managing patients and coordinating the transition from hospital to home and vice-versa. APNs implement a comprehensive discharge planning and home follow-up protocol. When compared with the control group, members of the intervention group had improved physical function, quality of life, and satisfaction with care. People in the intervention group had fewer rehospitalizations during the year after discharge, resulting in a mean savings in total health care costs of $5,000 per patient (Naylor & Keating, 2008). An RCT using the TCM for older adults hospitalized with heart failure showed increase in the length of time between hospital discharge and readmission or death, reduced total number of rehospitalizations and decreased health care costs (Naylor et al., 2004; NICHE, 2010).

The Care Transitions Intervention Model (Coleman, Parry, Chalmers, & Min, 2006)

Coleman and colleagues (2006) developed this model through the Division of Health Care Policy and Research at the University of Colorado Health Sciences Center in Denver.

This model involves a specialized nurse or "transition coach," who teaches patients self-management skills and ensures their needs are met during transition. The transition coach helps the patient self-manage medications, maintain patient-centered health records, complete follow-up care with their primary physician, and learn how to recognize and respond to red flags that indicate their condition is worsening. Providing patients with support and tools to participate in their transition care using this model has been shown to reduce hospital readmissions and associated costs (Coleman et al., 2006; NICHE, 2010). An RCT found that patients who received this intervention had lower all cause rehospitalization rates through 90 and 180 days after discharge compared with control patients. At 6 months, mean hospital costs were approximately $500 less for patients in the intervention group compared with controls (Coleman et al., 2006; Naylor & Keating, 2008)

Other transition models that have been described in the literature include the following:

Community-based transitions—hospital at home and day hospital models (Naylor & Keating, 2008).

Transitions within settings—acute care for elders (ACE) and professional–patient partnership model (Naylor, & Keating, 2008).

Hospital-to-home transition—geriatric floating interdisciplinary transition team (Geri-FITT) model (Arbaje et al., 2010) and chronic care model (2011)

Multi-setting transitions—Florida's Medicare Quality Improvement Organization (FMQAI; 2010). It is one of Medicare's Quality Improvement Organization (QIOs).

Naylor and Sochalski (2010) describes the core features of transitional care, which can be used as a guide for program planning and implementation to include the following:

A. A comprehensive assessment of an individual's health goals and preferences; physical, emotional, cognitive, and functional capacities and needs; and social and environmental considerations.
B. Implementation of an evidence-based plan of transitional care.
C. Transition care that is initiated at hospital admission but extends beyond discharge through home visit and telephone follow-up.
D. Mechanisms to gather and appropriately share information across sites of care.
E. Engagement of patients and family caregivers in planning and executing the plan of care.
F. Coordinated services during and following the hospitalization by a health care professional with special preparation in the care of chronically ill people, preferably a master's-prepared nurse.

Whichever model is adopted by the institution and stakeholders, staff training is of vital importance. Competency in cross-site collaboration is critical to the management of patients with complex acute and chronic illnesses; however, very few clinicians have any formal training in this area (Coleman, 2003).

Starting January 1, 2011 the government has established support of community-based transition programs under the PPACA, section 3025. This 5-year program comes with a 500 million dollar funding with the primary aim in implementing improved care transition services to high-risk Medicare beneficiaries. By "high risk," the law aims to dedicate transition care services to patients with multiple chronic conditions or other risk factors associated with a hospital readmission or substandard transition into posthospitalization care. Target populations are those diagnosed with cognitive impairment, depression, and a history of multiple readmissions (PPACA, 2010). To qualify for funding, the transition care program proposal must meet the following criteria (PPACA, 2010):

A. Initiates care transition services for a high-risk Medicare beneficiary not later than 24 hours prior to discharge.
B. Arranges timely postdischarge follow-up services to provide the beneficiary and the primary caregiver with information regarding responding to symptoms that may indicate additional health problems or a deteriorating condition.
C. Provides the high-risk Medicare beneficiary and the primary caregiver with assistance to ensure productive and timely interactions between patients and post-acute and outpatient providers.
D. Assesses and actively engages with the high-risk Medicare beneficiary and the primary caregiver through the provision of self-management support and relevant information that is specific to the beneficiary's condition.
E. Conducts comprehensive medication review and management, including, if appropriate, counseling and self-management support.
F. Provide services to medically underserved populations, small communities, and rural areas.

These criteria reflect the findings from the RCTs implementing Naylor's TCM (Naylor & Keating, 2008; Naylor et al., 2004) and the Care Transitions Intervention model by Coleman (Coleman, Smith, et al., 2004). The adaptation of these best practice models into legislation is a fine example of research translated into practice.

CASE STUDY

Lin Kwon Ying is a 70-year-old widow who lives alone in an apartment in Chinatown. He was mostly independent up until 5 months ago when he started to develop shortness of breath, increasing fatigue, and cough. He has had three admissions for congestive heart failure (CHF) exacerbation. His medical–surgical history includes hypertension (HTN), arthritis, peptic ulcer disease, and GI bleeding. He is back in the hospital for another CHF exacerbation, a small left pleural effusion, and a left leg deep venous thrombosis. Although cognitively intact, Mr. Ying does not speak English and his family is very much involved in his care. A relative is present during most of the day and evening while he is in the hospital. Most of his relatives have poor English proficiency. Mr. Ying is scheduled for discharge home the next day after being in the hospital for 6 days. His current medications have been satisfactorily reconciled, with the addition of enoxaparin (low-molecular–weight heparin) injection for 7 days and to check with his primary care provider for possible oral anticoagulation. He is to continue taking prehospitalization medications such as metoprolol, esomeprazole, multivitamins, and furosemide. The family reports that Mr. Ying uses Chinese liniment to ease his joint pains. He is described by his family as an obedient patient who will do whatever his doctor recommends although he has received little advice or "teachings" during his previous CHF admissions. He cannot recall being informed what lifestyle changes are required of him.

Factors such as Mr. Ying's rehospitalization, a diagnosis of CHF, language barrier, family involvement, being cognitively intact, and a complex plan of care (e.g., self-injection of enoxaparin) indicate that he is an ideal candidate to receive dedicated transitional care services. If transition care service were available in the current institution, he would have been referred for a consult upon his admission. An assessment would have been made by an advanced practice TCN or "coach," preferably in the presence of the informal caregiver and a staff translator. From this transition care evaluation, a multidisciplinary plan of care with emphasis applying best practices, on family involvement and patient teaching by the staff nurses would be drawn up. The handoff report would mention Mr. Ying's status as a transition care patient and a disease-specific clinical pathway (in his case CHF) would be implemented and followed through during rounds and discharge planning.

To satisfy TJC standards, all his medication should have been reconciled within 24 hours of his admission and the record placed in a prominent location in his chart. The challenge is to create a medication reconciliation record written in Mr. Ying's own language (Mandarin) that he can take with him upon discharge.

At the bedside level, the nurses (mostly bilingual Chinese) provided random or "ambush" teachings when they saw Mr. Ying consuming Chinese food brought from home that they considered high in sodium. No dedicated patient teachings were delivered and no printed materials in the patient's language were provided. How best to standardized patient teachings in acute care transitions is an ongoing challenge. Staff often reports not having the time to teach the patient and their family. Patient education must be held as an essential and independent nursing intervention. The facility must provide adequate training, not only for the licensed independent practitioners (nurses, NPs, MDs, and social workers), but also of the auxiliary staff

(continued)

CASE STUDY *(continued)*

such as patient-care technicians and other staff members with direct patient contact. Repetition and reinforcement with use of traditional printed media can easily be achieved. Numerous online patient teaching materials are now available. The institution could translate these materials into various languages based on local needs. In Mr. Ying's case, his ability to self-inject enoxaparin should be assessed, reinforced, and documented. During handoff, the nurse would include the patient's teaching needs and the follow-up needed, focusing on health promotion content, follow-up appointments, telephone numbers to call for questions, or report changes in condition.

Depending on the TCM applied, Mr. Ying would receive a home visit from the APN transition care coordinator or "coach" within 24 hours postdischarge with an individualized and explicit plan of care; including following up on medications, availability of equipment, and self-report of any "red-flag" signs for CHF exacerbation or pulmonary embolism. On his first visit to his primary care provider, he would be accompanied by his transition care coordinator/coach. In this visit and in future encounters with health care providers, Mr. Ying would be encouraged and provided with the skills necessary for self-advocacy and self-management of his condition. Success would depend on various factors such as patient readiness, literacy, and longitudinal follow-up. From the evidence-based models mentioned in this chapter, follow-up varies from Day 1 of hospitalization to up to 3 months postdischarge. Patient follow-up must also address patients' and informal caregivers' satisfaction with the care received. Additionally, the postacute TCN could also coordinate referrals to relevant, local community organizations to provide greater continuity and longer term support.

SUMMARY

High-quality transitional care is especially important for older adults with multiple chronic conditions and complex therapeutic regimens, as well as for their family caregivers (Naylor & Keating, 2008). Nurses must recognize their critical role in safe transitions. Breakdown in communication is often cited as one of the major cause of poor quality transitions that may lead to untimely rehospitalization, injury, and poor patient satisfaction. Clinicians and institutions must actively collaborate and communicate to ensure an appropriate exchange of information, coordination of care across health care settings among multiple providers (IOM, 2001). The current evidence indicates that hospital discharge planning for frail older people can be improved if interventions address family inclusion and education, communication between health care workers and family, interdisciplinary communication, and ongoing support after discharge (Bauer, Fitzgerald, Haesler, & Manfrin, 2009). In addition, evidence supports the need for close follow-up posthospitalization including home visits, telephone calls, and timely primary care provider visits. This provides opportunities to reinforce previous patient and family education, especially medications, and monitoring of condition changes (Naylor et al., 2004; Coleman et al., 2006; Rich et al., 1995).

As more and more evidence on the value of transitional programs in improving health outcomes emerge, we hope to see sustainable adaptation of best practice models in transition care as nurse-sensitive quality indicator of health care delivery. With the full implementation and evaluation of the PPACA community-based transition program legislation, we can expect to gain the benefits of evidence-based transition care interventions for the ever-growing older adult population.

NURSING STANDARD OF PRACTICE

Protocol 34.1: Transitional Care

I. GOAL
A. Nurses will assume a proactive role in transitional care across health care settings.
B. Nurses will identify barriers to successful transitions and offer sustainable solutions.
C. Increase coordination of care during transitions across health care settings amongst all members of the health care system, including the family and informal caregivers.

II. OVERVIEW
A. Evidence that both quality and patient safety are jeopardized for patients undergoing transitions across care settings continues to expand (Coleman, Mahoney, & Parry, 2005).
B. Care transitions are clinically dangerous times, particularly for older adults with complex health problems (Corbett et al., 2010).
C. Problems encountered with poor transition process can lead to unplanned readmission and ED visits (Jacob & Poletick, 2008).
D. Transitions are particularly vulnerable to breakdowns in care and, thus, have the greatest need for transitional care services (Naylor & Keating, 2008; Coleman et al., 2006).
E. Family caregivers play a major—and perhaps the most important—role in supporting older adults during hospitalization and especially after discharge (Naylor & Keating, 2008).

III. BACKGROUND AND STATEMENT OF PROBLEM
A. Definition
   Transitional care: The American Geriatrics Society (2003) defines transitional care as "a set of actions designed to ensure the coordination and continuity of health care as patients transfer between different locations or different levels of care within the same location. Representative locations include (but are not limited to) hospitals, subacute and postacute nursing facilities, the patient's home, primary and specialty care offices, and long-term care facilities. Transitional care, which encompasses both the sending and the receiving aspects of the transfer, is based on a comprehensive plan of care and includes logistical arrangements, education of the patient and family, and coordination among the health professionals involved in the transition." (Coleman & Boult, 2003)

(continued)

Protocol 34.1: Transitional Care *(cont.)*

Transitional care encompasses a broad range of services and environments designed to promote the safe and timely passage of patients between levels of health care and across care settings (Naylor & Keating, 2008).

B. Etiology and/or Epidemiology

1. Situations likely to result in failed transitions include poor social support, discharge during times when ancillary services are unavailable, uncertain medication reconciliation, depression, and patients' cognitive limitations (Cumbler et al., 2008).

2. Medication errors related to medication reconciliation typically occur at the "interfaces of care"—when a patient is admitted to, transferred within, or discharged from a health care facility (Sentinel Event Alert, 2006).

3. Hospital discharge practices are placing an increasing burden of care on the family caregiver (Bauer et al., 2009).

4. RCTs of transitional care interventions has been shown to reduce hospital readmissions and health care costs (Arbaje et al., 2010; Coleman et al., 2006; Naylor et al., 2004).

5. APN interventions in transition care has consistently resulted in improved patient outcomes and reduced health care costs (Naylor, 2002).

IV. PARAMETERS OF ASSESSMENT

A. Patient population who are most likely to benefit from transition care interventions are those who are diagnosed with one or more of the following diseases: CHF, chronic obstructive pulmonary disease, coronary artery disease, diabetes, stroke, medical and surgical back conditions (predominantly spinal stenosis), hip fracture, peripheral vascular disease, cardiac arrhythmias, deep venous thrombosis, and pulmonary embolism (Coleman, Min, Chomiak, & Kramer, 2004).

B. Upon admission to an acute care setting, starting at the ED; patient evaluation must include referral of vulnerable older adults for transitional care services.

C. Compliance with TJC standards in medication reconciliation will be used as one of the quality indicators and predictor in overall patient safety.

V. NURSING CARE STRATEGIES

A. General guidelines that may be adapted in implementing transition care strategies based on the TMC are as follows (Bowles et al., 2002):

1. The TCN as the primary coordinator of care to assure consistency of provider across the entire episode of care.

2. In-hospital assessment, preparation, and development of an evidence-based plan of care.

3. Regular home visits by the TCN with available, ongoing telephone support (7 days per week) through an average of 2 months postdischarge.

4. Continuity of medical care between hospital and primary care physicians facilitated by the TCN, accompanying patients to first follow-up visits.

5. Coordinate a timely appointment with patient's primary care provider.

6. Comprehensive, holistic focus on each patient's needs including the reason for the primary hospitalization as well as other complicating or coexisting events.

(continued)

Protocol 34.1: Transitional Care *(cont.)*

7. Active engagement of patients and their family and informal caregivers including education and support.

8. Emphasis on early identification and response to health care risks and symptoms to achieve longer term positive outcomes and avoid adverse and untoward events that lead to readmissions.

9. Multidisciplinary approach that includes the patient, family, informal and formal caregivers, and health care providers as part of a team.

10. Physician–nurse collaboration across episodes of acute care.

11. Communication to, between, and among the patient, family and informal caregivers, and health care providers.

B. Successful and safe transitions demands active patient and informal caregiver involvement. To improve patient advocacy and safety, the nurse can:

1. Promote the "Speak Up" initiative by the TJC in 2002. The brochure "Planning Your Follow Up Care" lists patient-centered and safety-focused questions to be asked by the patients from their health care provider before they are discharged from the hospital (Joint Commission on Accreditation of Health Care Organization, 2002).

2. Encourage family involvement and direct them to the "Next Steps in Care" website (see resources).

3. Provide the patient a complete and updated medication reconciliation record. The record should include medications the patient was taking prior to admission, medications prescribed during hospitalization, and medications to be continued upon discharge (Sentinel Event Alert, 2006).

4. Implement evidence-based interventions to reduce transition-related medication discrepancies (Corbett et al., 2010). Encourage the patient to carry their medication list (e.g., a copy of recent medication reconciliation from a recent hospital admission) and to share the list with any providers of care, including primary care and specialist physicians, nurses, pharmacists and other caregivers (Sentinel Event Alert, 2006).

Critical Elements of Successful Transitions

A. Team approach and preferably nurse led (APN or specialized nurse; Coleman et al., 2006; Naylor & Keating, 2008)

B. Active and early family involvement across transitions (Almborg, Ulander, Thulin, & Berg, 2009; Bauer et al., 2009; Naylor & Keating, 2008)

C. Proactive patient roles and self-advocacy (Coleman et al., 2006)

D. High-quality and individualized patient and family discharge instructions (Clark et al., 2005)

E. Apply interventions for improving comprehension among patients with low health literacy and impaired cognitive function (Chugh, Williams, Grigsby, & Coleman, 2009), such as the National Patient Safety Foundation's "Ask Me 3" campaign available at: http://www.npsf.org/askme3/

F. Patient and informal caregiver empowerment through education

G. Commence interventions well before discharge (Bauer et al., 2009)

(continued)

Protocol 34.1: Transitional Care *(cont.)*

Coleman identified elements of effective and successful transitions as follows (Coleman, 2003):

A. Communication between the sending and receiving clinicians regarding a common plan of care
B. A summary of care provided by the sending institution (to the next care interface providers)
C. The patient's goals and preferences (including advance directives)
D. An updated list of problems, baseline physical and cognitive functional status, medications, and allergies
E. Contact information for the patient's caregiver(s) and primary care practitioner
F. Preparation of the patient and caregiver for what to expect at the next site of care
G. Reconciliation of the patient's medication prescribed before the initial transfer with the current regimen
H. A follow-up plan for how outstanding tests and follow-up appointments will be completed
I. An explicit discussion with the patient and caregiver regarding warning symptoms or signs to monitor that may indicate that the condition has worsened and the name and phone number of who to contact if this occurs.

Barriers to Successful Transitions

Coleman identified barriers to effective care transitions at three levels: the delivery system, the clinician, and the patient (Coleman, 2003).

A. The Delivery System Barriers
1. The lack of formal relationships between care settings represents a barrier to cross-site communication and collaboration.
2. Lack of financial incentives promoting transitional care and accountability in fee-for-service Medicare. Although such incentives exist in Medicare managed care, most plans do not fully address care integration.
3. The different financing and contractual relationships that facilities have with various pharmaceutical companies impede effective transitions. As patients are transferred across settings, each facility has incentives to prescribe or substitute medications according to its own medication formulary. This constant changing of medications creates confusion for the patient, caregiver, and receiving clinicians.
4. Neither fee-for-service nor managed care Medicare has implemented quality or performance indicators designed to assess the effectiveness of transitional care.
5. The lack of information systems designed to facilitate the timely transfer of essential information.
B. The Clinician Barriers
1. The growing reliance on designated institution-based physicians (i.e., "hospitalists") and productivity pressures have made it difficult for primary care physicians to follow their patients when they require hospitalization or short-term rehabilitation.

(continued)

Protocol 34.1: Transitional Care *(cont.)*

   2. Nursing staff shortages have forced an increasing number of acute hospitals to divert patients to other facilities where a completely new set of clinicians, who often do not have timely access to the patients' prior medical records, manages them. Skilled nursing facility (SNF) staff are also overwhelmed and do not have the time or initiative to request necessary information.
   3. Clinicians do not verbally communicate patient information to one another across care settings.
C. The Patient Barriers
   1. Lack of advocacy or outcry from patients for improving transitional care until they or a family member is confronted with the problem firsthand.
   2. Older patients and their caregivers often are not well prepared or equipped to optimize the care they will receive in the next setting.
   3. They may have unrealistic expectations about the content or duration of the next phase of care and may not feel empowered to express their preferences or provide input for their care plan.
   4. Patients may not feel comfortable expressing their concern that the primary factor that led to their disease exacerbation was not adequately addressed.

Evaluation/Expected Outcomes

Clinician outcomes
   A. Increase nurse involvement in leading transition care teams.
   B. Enhance staff training of transitional care by a multidisciplinary team.
   C. Include patient's transitional care needs during in-hospital "hand off".
   D. Improve medication reconciliation throughout all transition interfaces.

Patient outcomes
   A. Improve patient satisfaction, increase involvement with their care during hospitalization and transitions of care across health care settings.
   B. Increase feeling of empowerment in making health care decision.
   C. Reduce rehospitalization and ED visits because of primary disease and comorbidities.

Informal caregiver outcomes
   A. Improve informal caregiver satisfaction and exercise proactive roles during transitions across health care settings.
   B. Increase informal caregiver participation in all transitions interface.

Institutional outcomes
   A. Adopt evidence-based TCMs and provide logistic support.
   B. Provide orientation and on-going education on transitional care strategies.
   C. Introduce transitional care content into nursing core curriculum both in baccalaureate and graduate levels.

VI. FOLLOW-UP MONITORING

   A. Institute comprehensive and multidisciplinary transition care planning as soon as the patient is admitted and sustained throughout hospitalization.

(continued)

Protocol 34.1: Transitional Care *(cont.)*

B. Identify transition care team members and perform periodic role re-assessment, including roles of informal caregivers.

C. Incorporate continuous quality improvement criteria into transition care programs such as monitoring for rehospitalization of targeted older adult, quality of discharge instruction, and medication reconciliation.

D. Develop ongoing transitional care educational programs for both formal and informal caregivers, using high-tech and traditional media.

E. Provide orientation and ongoing education on procedures for reconciling medications to all health care providers, including ongoing monitoring (Sentinel Event Alert, 2006).

F. Periodic "debriefing" of high-risk discharges as quality improvement strategy.

G. Improve recognition of condition changes or adverse events caused by medications.

H. Increase patient and caregivers' knowledge concerning action steps if condition worsens including who to contact and 24-hour contact information.

VII. RELEVANT PRACTICE GUIDELINES

A. Ongoing chart and medical records review of patients being considered for discharge or awaiting transition should reflect the quality indicators (QI) outlined in the Assessing Care of Vulnerable Elders (ACOVE) under the Continuity and Coordination of Care QI heading (Assessing Care of Vulnerable Elders-3 Quality Indicators, 2007).

B. TJC National Patient Safety Goals (NPSG, effective July 2011) related to transitions of care include the following:

NPSG.03.06.01—Maintain and communicate accurate patient medication information. The elements of performance (EP) include the following: (TJC, 2010)

1. Obtain information on the medications the patient is currently taking when he or she is admitted to the hospital or is seen in an outpatient setting. This information is documented in a list or other format that is useful to those who manage medications.

   Note 1: Current medications include those taken at scheduled times and those taken on an as-needed basis.

   Note 2: It is often difficult to obtain complete information on current medications from a patient. A good faith effort to obtain this information from the patient and/or other sources will be considered as meeting the intent of the EP.

2. Define the types of medication information to be collected in non–24-hour settings and different patient circumstances.

   Note 1: Examples of non–24-hour settings include the ED, primary care, outpatient radiology, ambulatory surgery, and diagnostic settings.

   Note 2: Examples of medication information that may be collected include name, dose, route, frequency, and purpose.

3. Compare the medication information the patient brought to the hospital with the medications ordered for the patient by the hospital to identify and resolve discrepancies.

   Note: Discrepancies include omissions, duplications, contraindications, unclear information, and changes. A qualified individual, identified by the hospital, does the comparison.

(continued)

Protocol 34.1: Transitional Care *(cont.)*

4. Provide the patient (or family as needed) with written information on the medications the patient should be taking when he or she is discharged from the hospital or at the end of an outpatient encounter (e.g., name, dose, route, frequency, purpose).

   Note: When the only additional medications prescribed are for a short duration, the medication information the hospital provides may include only those medications.

5. Explain the importance of managing medication information to the patient when he or she is discharged from the hospital or at the end of an outpatient encounter.

   Note: Examples include instructing the patient to give a list to his or her primary care physician; to update the information when medications are discontinued, doses are changed, or new medications (including over-the-counter products) are added; and to carry medication information at all times in the event of emergency situations.

Standard PC.04.02.01 (Provision of Care; U.S. Department of Health and Human Services Agency for Healthcare Research and Quality, 2011).

When a [patient] is discharged or transferred, the [organization] gives information about the care, treatment, and services provided to the [patient] to other service providers who will provide the [patient] with care, treatment, or services.

At the time of the patient's discharge or transfer, the hospital informs other service providers who will provide care, treatment, or services to the patient about the following:

1. The reason for the patient's discharge or transfer
2. The patient's physical and psychosocial status
3. A summary of care, treatment, and services it provided to the patient
4. The patient's progress toward goals
5. A list of community resources or referrals made or provided to the patient

C. Project Better Outcomes for Older Adults through Safe Transitions (BOOST)–www.hospitalmedicine.org/BOOST - provides a "toolkit" for quality improvement based on best practices, provides technical support to hospitals implementing the toolkit, and provides mentoring to promote long-term sustainability of transitional care programs (Chugh et al., 2009).

D. Position Statement of The American Geriatrics Society Health Care Systems Committee on Improving the Quality of Transitional Care for Persons with complex care needs must be considered in developing practice guidelines (Coleman et al., 2003)

E. The National Transitions of Care Coalition (NTOCC) developed the guidebook *Improving on Transitions of Care: How to Implement and Evaluate a Plan* (http://www.ntocc.org/Portals/0/ImplementationPlan.pdf). This book is intended for institutions ready to make changes in the processes their facilities use to send and receive patients. It includes an educational component about transitions of care, implementation manual, and evaluation methodology that

(continued)

Protocol 34.1: Transitional Care *(cont.)*

relates to nursing home to emergency department (ED)/hospital and vice-versa. This implementation and evaluation plan aims to empower institutions to take the first step at measuring their own performance in transitions of care and identify areas for improvement (National Transitions of Care Coalition, 2008). Guidelines on hospital to home and ED to home transitions are also available from the NTOCC website:

http://www.ntocc.org/Portals/0/ImplementationPlan_HospitalToHome.pdf
http://www.ntocc.org/Portals/0/ImplementationPlan_EDToHome.pdf

F. The PPACA addresses community-based transition program under section 3026 of the law. The law provides incentive for hospital to establish and cultivate partnerships with community-based organizations to implement evidence-based transition care intervention. Proposals and programs must meet the criteria stipulated in the law (see Intervention/Care Strategies above). This criteria will lend itself to evaluation of relevant practice guidelines (Patient Protection and Affordable Care Act, 2010).

ACKNOWLEDGMENT

With gratitude to Nigel Morgan and Malvina Kluger for their assistance in reviewing the manuscript.

RESOURCES

Administration on Aging
http://www.aoa.gov/

The American Geriatrics Society Transitional Care Information Page
http://www.healthinaging.org/public_education/pef/transitional_care.php

The Care Transitions Program: Eric Coleman. MD
http://www.caretransitions.org

Centers for Medicare and Medicaid Services
Value Project: Transitional Care Weekly Learning Sessions
http://www.cfmc.org/value/co/index.htm

Centers for Medicare and Medicaid Services: Patient Discharge Checklist
http://www.medicare.gov/Publications/Pubs/pdf/11376.pdf

Institute for Healthcare Improvement (IHI)
Provides educational resources on transitional care and medication reconciliation including samples of a reconciliation tracking tool and a medication reconciliation flow sheet.
http://www.ihi.org/ihi

The Joint Commission: "Speak Up" Initiative: Planning Your Follow-Up Care
http://www.jointcommission.org/PatientSafety/SpeakUp/speak_up_recovery.htm

Meals on Wheels Association of America
http://www.mowaa.org/

National Cancer Institute Transitional Care Planning
http://www.cancer.gov/cancertopics/pdq/supportivecare/transitionalcare/patient

National Transitions of Care Coalition: Transition Care Advocacy Group
http://www.ntocc.org/

The Next Steps in Care: Family Caregivers and Health Professionals Working Together. United Hospital Fund.
http://www.nextstepincare.org/

NICHE –Transitional Care Models
http://www.nicheprogram.org/niche_encyclopedia-geriatric_models_of_care-transitional_models

Partnership for Clear Health Communication and National Patient Safety Foundation "Ask Me 3" campaign
http://www.npsf.org/askme3/

Promising Practices: APN Transitional Care
http://promisingpractices.fightchronicdisease.org/programs/detail/apn_transitionalcare_model

Robert Wood Johnson Foundation's (RWJF) Speaking Together Toolkit
This toolkit provides advice to hospitals on improving the quality and accessibility of their language services for limited English proficient populations.
http://www.rwjf.org/qualityequality/product.jsp?id=29653

Transition Care Model: Mary Naylor, PhD, R.N
http://www.nursing.upenn.edu/research/ncth/Pages/default.aspx

Visiting Nurse Associations of America
http://vnaa.org/vnaa/siteshelltemplates/homepage_navigate.htm

REFERENCES

Almborg, A. H., Ulander, K., Thulin, A., & Berg, S. (2009). Discharge planning of stroke patients: The relatives' perceptions of participation. *Journal of Clinical Nursing, 18*(6), 857–865. Evidence Level IV.

Arbaje, A. I., Maron, D. D., Yu, Q., Wendel, V. I., Tanner, E., Boult, C., . . . Durso, S. C. (2010). The geriatric floating interdisciplinary transition team. *Journal of the American Geriatrics Society, 58*(2), 364–370. Evidence Level V.

Assessing care of vulnerable elders-3 quality indicators. (2007). *Journal of the American Geriatrics Society, 55*(Suppl. 2), S464-S487.

Bauer, M., Fitzgerald, L., Haesler, E., & Manfrin, M. (2009). Hospital discharge planning for frail older people and their family: Are we delivering best practice? A review of the evidence. *Journal of Clinical Nursing, 18*(18), 2539–2546. Evidence Level V

Bowles, K. H., Naylor, M. D., & Foust, J. B. (2002). Patient characteristics at hospital discharge and a comparison of home care referral decisions. *Journal of the American Geriatrics Society, 50*(2), 336–342. Evidence Level III.

Centers for Disease Control and Prevention. (2007). *National health statistics reports. Number 29. National hospital discharge survey: 2007 summary.* Retrieved from http://www.cdc.gov/nchs/data/nhsr/nhsr029.pdf

Centers for Disease Control and Prevention. (2009). National Nursing Home Survey: 2004 overview. *Vital and Health Statistics,* Series 13, No. 167. Retrieved from http://www.cdc.gov/nchs/data/series/sr_13/sr13_167.pdf

The Chronic Care Model. (2011). *Improving Chronic Illness Care.* Retrieved from http://www.improvingchroniccare.org/index.php?p=The_Chronic_Care_Model&s=212.

Chugh, A., Williams, M. V., Grigsby, J., & Coleman, E. A. (2009). Better Transitions: Improving comprehension of discharge instructions. *Frontiers of Health Services Management, 25*(3),11–32. Evidence Level V.

Clark, P. A., Drain, M., Gesell, S. B., Mylod, D. M., Kaldenberg, D. O., & Hamilton, J. (2005). Patient perceptions of quality in discharge instruction. *Patient Education and Counseling, 59*(1). 56–68. Evidence Level IV.

Coleman, E. A. (2003). Falling through the cracks: Challenges and opportunities for improving transitional care for persons with continuous complex care needs. *Journal of the American Geriatrics Society, 51*(4), 549–555. Evidence Level V.

Coleman, E. A., & Boult, C. (2003). Improving the quality of transitional care for persons with complex care needs. *Journal of the American Geriatrics Society, 51*(4), 556–557. Level VI

Coleman, E. A., Mahoney, E., & Parry, C. (2005). Assessing the quality of preparation for post-hospital care from the patient's perspective: The care transitions measure. *Medical Care, 43*(3), 246–255. Evidence Level.

Coleman, E. A., Min, S. J., Chomiak, A., & Kramer, A. M. (2004). Posthospital care transitions: Patterns, complications, and risk identification. *Health Services Research, 39*(5), 1449–1465. Evidence Level V.

Coleman, E. A., Parry, C., Chalmers, S., & Min, S. J. (2006). The care transitions intervention: Results of a randomized controlled trial. *Archives of Internal Medicine, 166*(17), 1822–1828. Evidence Level II.

Coleman, E. A., Smith, J. D., Frank, J. C., Min, S. J., Parry, C., & Kramer, A. M. (2004). Preparing patients and caregivers to participate in care delivered across settings: The care transitions intervention. *Journal of the American Geriatrics Society, 52*(11), 1817–25. Evidence Level III.

Corbett, C. F., Setter, S. M., Daratha, K. B., Neumiller, J. J., & Wood, L. D. (2010). Nurse identified hospital to home medication discrepancies: Implications for improving transitional care. *Geriatric Nursing, 3*(31), 188–196. Evidence Level IV.

Cumbler, E., Carter, J., & Kutner, J. (2008). Failure at the transition of care: Challenges in the discharge of the vulnerable elderly patient. *Journal of Hospital Medicine, 3*(4), 349–352. Evidence Level V.

Florida's Medicare Quality Improvement Organization. (2010). Retrieved from http://www.fmqai.com/default.aspx

Forster, A. J., Murff, H. J., Peterson, J. F., Gandhi, T. K., & Bates, D. W. (2003). The incidence and severity of adverse events affecting patients after discharge from the hospital. *Annals of Internal Medicine, 138*(3), 161–167. Evidence Level IV.

Institute of Medicine. (2001). *Crossing the quality chasm: a new health system for the 21st century.* Washington, DC: National Academy Press. Evidence Level I.

Jacob, L., & Poletick, E. B. (2008). Systematic review: Predictors of successful transition to community-based care for adults with chronic care needs. *Care Management Journals, 9*(4), 154–165. Evidence Level I.

Jencks, S. F., Williams, M. V., & Coleman, E. A. (2009). Rehospitalizations among patients in the Medicare fee-for-service program. *The New England Journal of Medicine, 360*(14), 1418–1428. Evidence Level V

Joint Commission on Accreditation of Health Care Organization. (2002). *Speak up: planning your follow-up care.* Retrieved from http://www.jointcommission.org/PatientSafety/SpeakUp/speak_up_recovery.htm. Evidence Level VI.

Kripalani, S., LeFevre, F., Phillips, C. O., Williams. M. V., Basaviah, P., & Baker, D. W (2007). Deficits in communication and information transfer between hospital-based and primary care physicians: Implications for patient safety and continuity of care. *The Journal of the American Medical Association. 297*(8), 831–841. Evidence Level IV.

Levine, C., Halper, D., Peist, A., & Gould, D. A. (2010). Bridging troubled waters: Family caregivers, transitions, and long-term care. *Health Affairs (Project Hope), 29*(1), 116–124. Evidence Level VI.

Melnyk, B. M., & Fineout-Overholt, E. (2005). Evidence-based practice in healthcare. Philadelphia, PA: Lippincott Williams & Wilkins. Evidence Level I.

Miller, J. F., Piacentine, L. B., & Weiss, M. (2008). Coping difficulties after hospitalization. *Clinical Nursing Research, 17*(4), 278–296. Evidence Level IV.

National Center for Healthcare Statistics. (2004). Retrieved from http://www.cdc.gov/nchs/

National Transitions of Care Coalition. (2008). *Improving on transitions of care: how to implement and evaluate a plan.* Retrieved from http://www.ntocc.org/Portals/0/ImplementationPlan.pdf.

Naylor, M. D. (2002). Transitional care of older adults. *Annual Review of Nursing Research, 20,* 127–147. Evidence Level I.

Naylor, M. D., Brooten, D. A., Campbell, R. L., Maislin, G., McCauley, K. M., & Schwartz, J. S. (2004). Transitional care of older adults hospitalized with heart failure: A randomized, controlled trial. *Journal of the American Geriatrics Society, 52*(5), 675–684. Evidence Level II.

Naylor, M. D., Feldman, P. H., Keating, S., Koren, M. J., Kurtzman, E. T., Maccoy, M. C., & Krakauer, R. (2009). Translating research into practice: Transitional care for older adults. *Journal of Evaluation in Clinical Practice, 15*(6),1164–1170. Evidence Level IV.

Naylor, M. D., & Keating, S. A. (2008). Transitional care. *The American Journal of Nursing, 108*(9 Suppl), 58–63; quiz 63. Evidence Level V.

Naylor, M. D., & Sochalski, J. A. (2010). *Scaling up: Bringing the transitional care model into the mainstream.* The Commonwealth Fund. Retrieved from http://www.commonwealthfund.org/Content/Publications/IssueBriefs/2010/Nov/Scaling-Up-Transitional-Care.aspx. Evidence Level V: Overview.

Nurses Improving Care for Healthsystem Elders. (2010). Retrieved from http://www.nicheprogram.org/niche_encyclopedia-geriatric_models_of_care-transitional models. Evidence Level VI: Expert Opinion.

Patient Protection and Affordable Care Act. (2010). Retrieved from http://docs.house.gov/energycommerce/ppacacon.pdf

Rich, M. W., Beckham, V., Wittenberg, C., Leven, C. L., Freedland, K. E., & Carney, R. M. (1995). A multidisciplinary intervention to prevent the readmission of elderly patients with congestive heart failure. *The New England Journal of Medicine, 333*(18), 1190–1195. Evidence Level II.

Sentinel Event Alert. (2006). *Issue 35: Using medication reconciliation to prevent errors.* Joint Commission. Retrieved from http://www.jointcommission.org/assets/1/18/SEA_35.PDF. Evidence Level: Quality Measures.

Stetler, C. B., Morsi, D., Rucki, S., Broughton, S., Corrigan, B., Fitzgerald, J., . . . Sheridan, E. A. (1998). Utilization-focused integrative reviews in a nursing service. *Applied Nursing Research, 11*(4), 195–206. Evidence Level I.

The Joint Commission. (2010). *National patient safety goal on reconciling medication information.* Retrieved from http://www.jointcommission.org/assets/1/6/Communications_NPSG_Med_Rec_HAP_20101115[1].pdf

U.S. Department of Health and Human Services, Agency for Healthcare Research and Quality. (2011). *Care transitions measure summary.* Retrieved from http://www.qualitymeasures.ahrq.gov/content.aspx?id=15178

Index